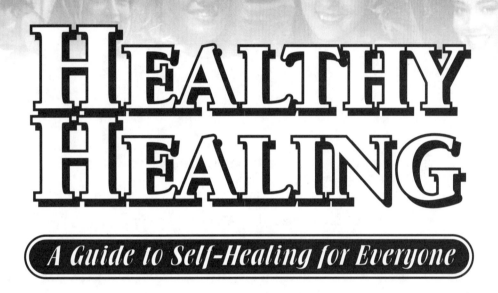

ALL NEW TENTH EDITION
UPDATED & EXPANDED

HEALTHY HEALING

A Guide to Self-Healing for Everyone

Linda Rector Page, N.D., Ph.D.

This reference is to be used for educational information.
It is not a claim for cure or mitigation of disease, but rather an adjunctive approach,
supplying individual nutritional needs
that otherwise might be lacking
in today's lifestyle.

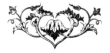

FIRST EDITION, JUNE 1985. COPYRIGHT REQ. NOV. 1985.
SECOND EDITION, JANUARY 1986.
THIRD EDITION, REVISED, SEPTEMBER 1986.
FOURTH EDITION, REVISED/UPDATED, MAY 1987.
FIFTH EDITION, NOVEMBER 1987.
SIXTH EDITION, REVISED/UPDATED, JUNE 1988.
SEVENTH EDITION, REVISED/UPDATE, JAN. 1989, SEPT. 1989, MARCH 1990.
EIGHTH EDITION, REVISED/UPDATED/EXPANDED, JULY, 1990.
NINTH EDITION, REVISED/UPDATED/EXPANDED, SEPT., 1992 AND 1994.
TENTH EDITION, REVISED/UPDATED/EXPANDED, JAN., 1997.

About the Author....

$\mathcal{L}$inda Rector-Page has been working in the fields of nutrition and herbal medicine both professionally and as a personal lifestyle choice, since the early seventies. She is a certified Doctor of Naturopathy and Ph.D., with extensive experience in formulating and testing herbal combinations. She received a Doctorate of Naturopathy from the Clayton College of Natural Healing in 1988, and a Ph.D. in Nutritional Therapy from the American Holistic College of Nutrition in 1989. She is a member of both the American and California Naturopathic Medical Associations. Linda has recently become an adjunct professor at the Clayton College, where she participates in an advisory capacity for the school's Master Herbalist programs.

Linda opened and operated the "Rainbow Kitchen," a natural foods restaurant, then became a working partner in The Country Store Natural Foods store. She has written four successful books and a Library Series of specialty books in the nutritional healing field. Today, she lectures around the country and in the media on a wide range of natural healing topics.

Linda is the founder, developer and formulator of Crystal Star Herbal Nutrition, a manufacturer of over 250 premier herbal compounds. A major, cutting edge influence in the herbal medicine field, Crystal Star Herbal Nutrition products are carried by over twenty-five hundred natural food stores in the U.S. and around the world.

Broad, continuous research in all aspects of the alternative healing world, from manufacturers, to natural food stores, to consumers, has been the cornerstone of success for her reference work HEALTHY HEALING now in its tenth edition. Feedback from all these sources provides up-to-the-minute contact with the needs, desires and results being encountered by people taking more responsibility for their own health. Much of the lifestyle information and empirical observation detailed in her books comes from this direct experience - knowledge that is then translated into Crystal Star Herbal Nutrition products, and recorded in every HEALTHY HEALING edition.

COOKING FOR HEALTHY HEALING, now in its second revised edition, is a companion to HEALTHY HEALING. It draws on both the recipes from the Rainbow Kitchen and the more defined, lifestyle diets that she has developed from healing results since then. The book contains thirty-three separate diet programs, and over 900 healthy recipes. Every recipe has been taste-tested and time-tested as a part of each recommended diet, so that the suggested healing program can be easily maintained with optimum nutrition.

In HOW TO BE YOUR OWN HERBAL PHARMACIST, Linda addresses the rising appeal of herbs and herbal healing in America. Many people are interested in clearly understanding herbal formulation knowledge for personal use. This book is designed for those wishing to take more definitive responsibility for their health through individually developed herbal combinations.

Linda's newest work is a party reference book called PARTY LIGHTS, written with restaurateur and noted chef Doug Vanderberg. PARTY LIGHTS takes healthy cooking one step further by adding in the fun to a good diet. More than sixty party themes are completely planned in this book, all with healthy party foods, earthwise decorations, professional garnishing tips, festive napkin folding, games and activities.

Dedication

The tenth edition of Healthy Healing is dedicated to the profound wonders of healing herbs.
I believe that herbs are an eye of the needle through which we can look to glimpse
the miracle of creation...because herbs help us care for each other.
They grow eyes on our hearts.

HERBS ARE WITHOUT A DOUBT...UNIVERSAL.
THEY DO NOT DISCRIMINATE,
BUT EMBRACE HUMANS OF ALL SORTS AND ANIMALS OF ALL KINDS, WITH THEIR BENEFITS.
WHILE IT SEEMS, ON A DAY-TO-DAY BASIS, THAT WE ARE HOPELESSLY DIVIDED,
IN THE END WE ARE ALL ONE.
OUR HOPES AND DREAMS ARE THE SAME.

THE HIGHEST CALLING OF THE HEALER
IS TO RALLY THE MIND AND BODY AGAINST THE DISEASE.

Even one miracle cure can show the value of a therapy
with the body's own healing powers.
When the evidence is good enough to affect the behavior of researchers,
why pretend it is too preliminary for consumers?
If a therapy is natural, non-invasive and does no harm,
consumers should be able to act upon it as a valid choice.

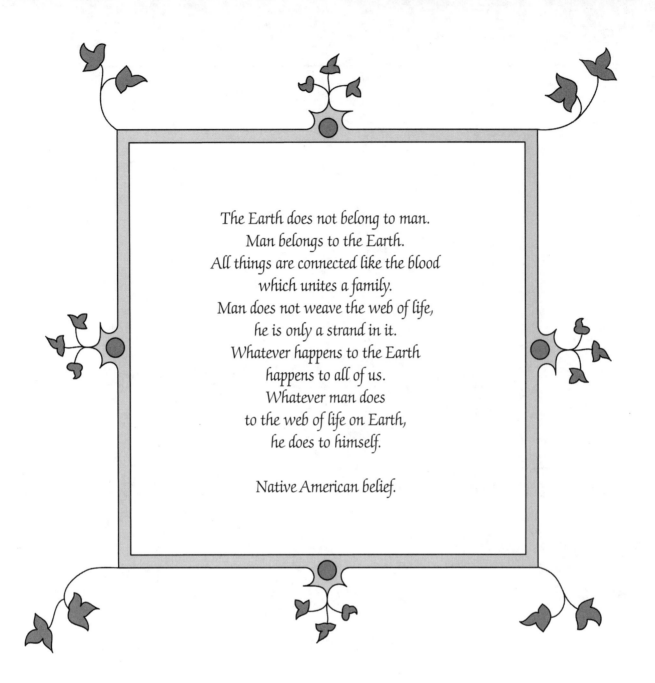

The Earth does not belong to man.
Man belongs to the Earth.
All things are connected like the blood
which unites a family.
Man does not weave the web of life,
he is only a strand in it.
Whatever happens to the Earth
happens to all of us.
Whatever man does
to the web of life on Earth,
he does to himself.

Native American belief.

Visit HEALTHY HEALING PUBLICATIONS on the web for the latest, updated information on natural healing techniques, herbal remedies, the appearance and seminar schedule for Dr. Linda Rector Page, and more.

www.healthyhealing.com

Dr. Page is the editor of a new national newsletter that you can receive every month in your home. She'll keep you up to date on your health choices with the latest alternative health information - in depth - on subjects and choices everybody needs to know for optimum, personal well-being.

Call 1-800-289-9222 for more information and a free brochure.

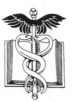

OTHER BOOKS BY

Linda Rector Page, N.D., Ph.D.

Cooking For Healthy Healing

How To Be Your Own Herbal Pharmacist

Party Lights
(with Doug Vanderberg)

AND

The Healthy Healing Library
Book Series

About the Cover

The "Faces of the World" cover for the tenth edition reminds us
that natural healing is eternal and universal.

Natural healing helps us grow in maturity
because to use it we must take a measure of responsibility for our health.
It increases our wisdom because it shows us how to work with great diversity.
It brings us together because it helps us care for each other.

Natural healing represents timeless knowledge.
It is for everyone.

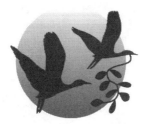

NEITHER DRUGS NOR HERBS NOR VITAMINS ARE A CURE FOR ANYTHING.
THE BODY HEALS ITSELF.
THE HUMAN BODY IS INCREDIBLY INTELLIGENT.
IT USUALLY RESPONDS TO INTELLIGENT THERAPIES.
THE HEALING PROFESSIONAL CAN HELP THIS PROCESS
BY OFFERING INTELLIGENT THERAPIES.

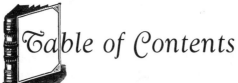

Table of Contents

Section One

Section Two

Section Three

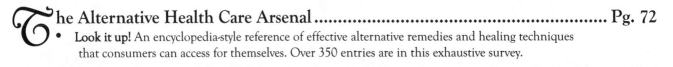

How to Use this Book....

This book is a reference for people who are interested in a more personal kind of healing and preventive health care. I call it "Lifestyle Therapy." For long-lasting health, your body must do its own work. The natural healing recommendations described here help rebalance specific areas of the body so that it can function normally. They work *with* body functions, not outside them. They are free of harmful side effects and do not traumatize the system.

There are four remedy categories:
- DIET & SUPERFOOD THERAPY
- HERBAL THERAPY
- SUPPLEMENTS
- LIFESTYLE SUPPORT THERAPY (INCLUDING BODYWORK AND RELAXATION TECHNIQUES)

Each person is an individual, so there are many effective recommendations to choose from in each category. Each person can put together the best healing program for him-or-her self.

The bold print suggestions are those we have found to be the most helpful for the most people. These highlighted recommendations can many times be considered complete programs in themselves, and can often be used effectively together. All given doses are daily amounts unless otherwise specified.

- **Where a remedy has proven especially effective for women, a female symbol ♀ appears by the recommendation.**
- **Where a remedy has proven especially effective for men, a male symbol ♂ appears by the recommendation.**
- **Where a remedy has also proven effective for children, a small child's face ☺ appears by the recommendation.**

While no one will use everything in any one category, or even use every category, diet must be considered a primary, long-term healing tool. The diets I recommend are "real people" diets, used by people with specific health conditions who have related their experiences to us. We find that over the years, diseases change - through mutation, environment, or treatment, for instance - and a person's immune response to them changes. HEALTHY HEALING's diet programs are continually modified to meet new and changing needs.

The "foot" and "hand" diagrams on the ailment pages show the reflexology pressure points for each body area, so that you can use reflexology therapy when it is indicated. In some cases, the points are very tiny, particularly for the glands. They take practice to pinpoint. The best sign that you have reached the right spot is that it will be very tender, denoting crystalline deposits or congestion in the corresponding body part. There is often a feeling of immediate relief in the area as the waste deposit breaks up for removal by the body.

You can have every confidence that the recommended remedies have been used by thousands of people in some cases, and found to be effective. As I develop and work with the healing programs over the years, they are constantly updated with new information.

Every edition of HEALTHY HEALING offers you the latest knowledge from a wide network of natural healing professionals - nutritional consultants, holistic practitioners, naturopaths, nurses, world health studies and traditional physicians, both in America and around the world with whom we work.

But the most important information is the empirical evidence from the people who have tried the natural healing methods for themselves, experienced real improvement in their health, and wish to share their measure of success with others.

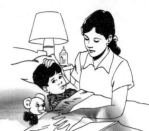

Section One

A CLEAR LOOK AT YOUR HEALTH CARE OPTIONS TODAY

Without question, Americans want to take more responsibility for their own health care. But what are the real options you have to choose from? How can you judge the pros and cons of conventional and alternative healing systems? Can they work together?

What's the difference between drugs and herbal medicines? Can you use them together? Can chemical drugs and herbal remedies complement each other? Can you wean yourself off drugs with herbal medicines?

This chapter offers a clear review of the alternative healing systems available today, with a brief analysis of how you can best use each of them.

Here are the topics we'll consider:
- Naturopathy
- Homeopathy
- Chiropractic
- Massage Therapy
- Reflexology
- Acupuncture and Acupressure
- Biofeedback
- Guided Imagery and Hypnotherapy
- Enzyme Therapy
- Overheating Therapy
- Aromatherapy

and also
- Natural Healing Pre-Op and Post-Op Techniques

for optimal healing after surgery or serious illness.

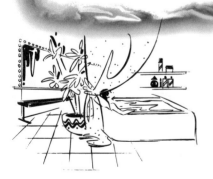

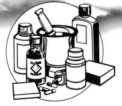

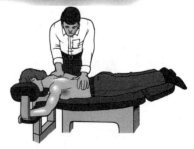

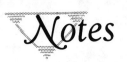

Notes

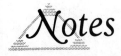

Notes

Your Health Care Choices Today

Personal health empowerment and traditional healing knowledge in western industrial populations has dropped away over the years, as medical advances and "letting the doctor do it" have become a way of life in modern society. Our culture has allowed the entire health care industry to become so powerful and so disproportionately lucrative that it is now in the business of illness rather than health. In one disconcerting example, a cancer physician, returning from an extended vacation, found an empty waiting room. His colleague had been treating his patients nutritionally. The physician wailed, "This is terrible. It took me years to build a long-term, regular patient clientele!"

Thoughtful people everywhere are realizing that our doctors receive no reward for health, only for treating illness, and conventional medicine can only go so far before expense outweighs the value of the treatment. Drug and medical costs, even basic medical insurance payments, have escalated beyond the reach of most families. And, we are realizing that the doctor can't always "do it."

The turn of the twentieth century finds many people using more natural, less drug-oriented therapies, sometimes as an alternative to conventional medicine, sometimes in a team approach along with it. As orthodox medicine becomes more invasive, and less in touch with the person who is ill, informed people are becoming more willing to take a measure of responsibility for their own health.

Health is a lifestyle process. It is based in wellness care, instead of just illness treatment. The best news is that natural remedies work - often far better than current medical prescriptions for many health conditions.

ALLOPATHIC, OR ORTHODOX, MEDICINE PUTS ITS EMPHASIS ON CRISIS INTERVENTION. IT IS ABOUT DOING BATTLE WITH A DISEASE OR AN IMMINENT THREAT TO LIFE. MANY MODERN MEDICAL TECHNIQUES WERE DEVELOPED DURING WAR TIME, FOR EMERGENCY CARE. THEY ARE AT THEIR BEST IN THIS "HEROIC MODE," BRINGING UP THE BIG GUNS OF SURGERY AND DRUGS TO SEARCH OUT AND DESTROY DANGEROUS ORGANISMS. IT IS THE KIND OF TREATMENT NECESSARY FOR ACUTE DISEASE, ACCIDENTS, EMERGENCIES AND WARTIME LIFE-SAVING.

Allopathic medicine is less successful in treating chronic illness. Respected studies show that most illnesses don't just drop out of the sky and hit us over the head. Diseases such as arthritis, osteoporosis, lower back pain, high blood pressure, coronary-artery disease, ulcers and hormone imbalances are related to aging and lifestyle. In these instances the big guns and emergency measures are usually not applicable. They tend to overkill, and don't allow the body to use its own immune response.

Most illness is self-limiting. The human body is a beautifully designed healing system that can meet the majority of its problems without outside intervention. Even when outside help is required, healing can be enhanced if the patient can be kept free of emotional devastation, depression and panic. Emotional trauma impairs immune function by decreasing the body's interleukins, vital immune defense substances. Panic constricts blood vessels, putting additional burden on the heart. Depression intensifies existing diseases, and opens the door to others. There is a direct connection between one's mental state and the ability of the immune system to do its job.

But medical schools do not teach disease prevention, or proper diet and exercise as a part of health. Although many alternative techniques are widely accepted in Europe, American physicians downplay the interaction of mind and body, saying that a patient's state of mind does not matter to bacteria or a virus. Objective measures of health are emphasized - the number of white blood cells, blood pressure readings, etc., instead of how the patient feels.

For all its brilliant achievements, modern medicine is still only pathology oriented. Doctors see the disease, not the person, and are only trained to use drugs, surgery, and the latest laboratory technologies. To paraphrase Abraham Maslow: "If all you're trained to use is a hammer, the whole world looks like a nail."

This approach does not sit well with the informed public today, who want more control over their health problems, and intend to be a part of the decision making process for their health needs.

Conventional medicine teaches that pain means sickness, treating it as a powerful enemy, and assaulting the symptoms with prescription medicines that either mask it or drive it underground - a practice that usually means it will resurface later with increased intensity.

Alternative healers recognize that pain is also the body's way of informing us that we are doing something wrong, not necessarily that something *is* wrong. Pain can tell us that we are smoking too much, eating too much, or eating the wrong things. It can notify us when there is too much emotional congestion in our lives, or too much daily stress. Pain can be a friend with useful information about our health, so that we can effectively address the cause of a problem.

We are constantly pressured by the medical community to have exhaustive tests, to be screened for cholesterol, high blood pressure, breast lumps, and cancer cells. If there is acute pain or other symptoms that indicate the need for a doctor, obvious common sense dictates that a doctor should be called, or emergency medical steps taken. But mammography, pap smears, and many other tests are not prevention, simply early detection.

Many physicians have a financial interest in ordering an array of tests, in performing surgeries, and in prescribing certain medications; many times, the pressure for testing is driven by these issues rather than for information. The fear of malpractice lawsuits also causes doctors to be overly zealous in ordering tests. Yet medical tests can be hazardous to your health. Faulty diagnoses and inaccurate readings are common in poorly trained, rushed labs. The more tests a person undergoes, the greater the odds of being told, often incorrectly, that something is wrong. Mental anxiety is brought on by needless testing, medication, or treatment, and a brusque or rushed doctor. You can literally worry yourself sick when there is nothing particularly wrong.

NOT EVERY PROBLEM REQUIRES COSTLY, MAJOR MEDICAL ATTENTION. A SENSIBLE LIFESTYLE, WITH GOOD HEALTHY FOOD, REGULAR MODERATE EXERCISE AND RESTFUL SLEEP IS STILL THE BEST MEDICINE FOR MANY HEALTH CONDITIONS. THE PRINCIPLES OF NATURE GOVERNING HEALTH AND ILLNESS ARE AGELESS; THEY APPLY EQUALLY EVERYWHERE AT ALL TIMES. THERE IS NO DOWN TIME WITH THE LAWS OF NATURE, AND THEY DO NOT PLAY FAVORITES.

We need to be re-educated about our health - to be less intimidated by doctors and disease. I believe that the greatest ally of alternative medicine will be science itself - not the restricted view of science that assumes its basic concepts are complete, but the open-ended science that sets preconceived notions aside. Today's consumers are not only more aware of alternative health care choices, and more confident in their own healing strength, but also want to do something for themselves to get better. The time has clearly come for a partnership between health care professionals and patients, so that the healing resources from both sides can be optimally employed.

No prescription is more valuable than knowledge. This book is a ready reference for the alternative health care choices open to those wishing to take more responsibility for their own well-being. The recommended suggestions are backed up by extensive research into therapies for each specific ailment, and by contributing health care professionals and nutritional consultants from around the country, with many years of eyewitness and hands-on experience in natural healing results.

> "When health is absent,
> Wisdom cannot reveal itself,
> Art cannot become manifest,
> Strength cannot be exerted.
> Wealth is useless,
> and Reason is powerless."
> Herophiles, 300B.C.

The Pros & Cons of Orthodox & Alternative Medicine
How Do They Compare?

The paradigm shift in medicine at the beginning of this century constituted enormous reform for health care and medical education. The ability to isolate microbes that cause infectious disease, and to create treatments that would kill those microbes without killing the patient, meant tremendous acceptance for the practice of allopathic medicine, characterizing it as both heroic and scientific. But the pendulum swung too far as the sledge hammers of drugs and surgery were driven more by profit than by healing. *Today, another paradigm shift in health care is in the making, from emphasis on disease treatment to emphasis on disease prevention.*

Chronic diseases, like cancer and arthritis are the scourge of modern times. Drug and laboratory advances, the cornerstones of allopathic medicine, are less effective in treating chronic diseases. Health care systems must provide more protective, less invasive, more readily accepted treatments for chronic disorders. Conventional medicine is devoted to eliminating uncertainty about the validity, effectiveness, and safety of its science and techniques, an emphasis that has resulted in an authoritarian, heavily regulated approach to its action and thinking. Many defend these rigid values and regulations because they have brought about a health care system that is arguably the most technologically advanced in the world. Yet, even with the broad medical arsenal available to doctors, they can only cure about one-fourth of the illnesses presented to them. *A recent report by the U.S. Office of Technology Assessment shows only 10 to 20% of standard medical procedures are effective!*

As disease prevention becomes the watchword of wellness, medical strategies must change to avoid expensive, invasive modalities. Today's medicine depends on surgical procedures, lab tests, high-tech intervention equipment, a warehouse of antibiotics, and powerful biochemicals. These are hit-or-miss more often than we are willing to admit. They are frequently ineffective, and generally ignore the person in favor of the illness and its symptoms. Many have serious side effects and sometimes make the patient worse. Alternative medicine methods are less expensive, effective and much safer.

Yet, some aspects of orthodox medicine are very valuable. Many naturopathic physicians believe that building bridges with conventional medicine has tangible benefits, and a broad range of healing methods makes sense. Medical diagnostic tools can monitor a disorder; some drugs can reduce crippling symptoms, often dramatically at first; some of the new drugs can retard progression of a disease.

I feel we need both types of medicine. **Clearly, orthodox medicine has saved many lives. Just as clearly, alternative medicine has prevented much illness.** Our bodies are so complicated........with an incredibly complex immune system, thousands of enzymes, delicate fluid balance, and interlocking circulatory pathways - just a few things that our healing system has to take into account. Multiply those things by the uniqueness of each person, and you can see why we need a wealth of choices for our health.

If there is no one "right" path, then multi-disciplinary health care is a better way. A team approach can take the best tools from each. A new study by the New England Journal of Medicine shows that American health care consumers are doing just that.

One in three are using some form of complementary or alternative medicine today.

Nor are doctors as resistant to alternative practices as they used to be. Some doctors now recognize that mental and spiritual factors influence disease, that drugs and surgery are frequently over used, and that human touch is vital in the doctor/patient relationship.

An increasing number of MDs are even including holistic treatments, adopting some of the practices of natural medicine, in order to offer their patients the best of both worlds. In the field of mental health, for instance, traditional doctors admit that alternative approaches are more effective, less expensive, and safer than conventional drug treatment.

Alternative medicine is really all about choices, something Americans consider to be a fundamental right. The realm of alternative medical practice is huge, because there isn't a "one-size-fits-all" for health care. Every person is an individual, and different therapies work for different people.

Alternative health care emphasizes prevention over crisis intervention, seeking to improve health rather than simply extend life through heroic means. Holistic practitioners as a whole, believe that healing originates within the human body from innate vitality, and not from medicines or machines. In general, they believe that toxins in the body cause disease; removing toxins through the use of natural remedies helps the body regain health.

Lifestyle therapy is more subtle than drugs or surgery-based health care. One should expect the therapeutic effects of natural medicines to be slower but more permanent - a normal result of the body taking the time to do it right. *The natural healing rule of thumb is one month of healing for every year you have had the problem.*

HERE ARE THE CORE PRINCIPLES THAT DISTINGUISH ALTERNATIVE MEDICINE FROM ORTHODOX MEDICINE.

1 *It is important to know the cause of the disease,* not just recognize the symptoms. Understanding the cause means the patient can eliminate it. When people seek alternative care, they're asking, "Why do I have this problem? I'm tired of having the doctor just treat the symptoms."

2 *The person is more important than the disease.* Alternative treatments are highly individualized. Ten people going to an alternative doctor for a headache may leave with ten different remedies. Practitioners of conventional medicine often see only the similarities and treat everyone the same.

3 *Lifestyle is significant.* Alternative practitioners look beyond the physical symptoms and take into account a patient's mental, emotional, and even spiritual life as inseparable from physical health.

4 *The body can heal itself.* Alternative medicine practitioners view symptoms such as fever or inflammation, as signs that the body is mounting an immune response to heal itself. Instead of trying to eliminate symptoms, lifestyle therapy treatments work to enhance natural defenses and healing vitality.

5 *Preventive medicine is the best medicine.* Alternative caregivers teach that daily habits create the conditions for health or disease. Alternative practitioners believe that removing disease-causing conditions will prevent disease.

6 *The cure and the preventive are often the same.* Most alternative medicine practitioners teach that just as avoiding the causative agents will **prevent** an illness, removing them will **cure** the illness. For instance, if obesity is the condition, then the cure, a restricted diet, is the same as the preventive.

7 *Alternative practitioners are also teachers who can empower you to help yourself.* Many adopt the position of coach rather than doctor to give patients the power of their own healing systems.

"HEALTHY HEALING" takes empowerment into account by offering a wealth of lifestyle choices for health problems...things you can do for yourself to improve almost every health condition. Even if the condition is serious, and even if you are under traditional medical care, there are always significant things you can do to help your body's healing process. Healing is both a physical process and an accomplishment of the spirit. It takes place in the physical world, and also in the universe of the soul. I have seen this to be undeniably true over the last 20 years, in case after case, regardless of the problem or its duration.

"HEALTHY HEALING" details the results of both empirical evidence and clinical studies to offer you tried and true choices......choices that are non-invasive, health supporting, body balancing and disease preventing, as well as healing.

Good information is the key. I find that most people have a lot of common sense and intuitive knowledge about themselves and their health problems. With access to solid information, people invariably make good choices for their health.

Naturopathy

aturopathy is the fastest growing of all the alternative healing disciplines. Until very recently, because the allopathic medical world did not recognize or accredit Naturopathy, those trained in naturo pathic methods were either denied a clinical practice under American medical laws, or forced into a strictly educative posture as a way of discrediting naturopathic techniques.

As more people become disillusioned with conventional health care, naturopathy is seen as having respect for all ways of healing, and as combining the best of both orthodox and alternative medicine. The appeal of naturopathic physicians is that while many have an educational background similar to that of a conventional M.D., modern naturopathic medicine incorporates extensive training in other disciplines. The medical establishment is more willing to accept clinical naturopaths than other alternative practitioners because of their rigorous schooling, which includes herbal therapy, homeopathy, hydrotherapy, massage therapy, chiropractic, behavioral, and Oriental and Ayurvedic medicine.

Naturopathic students are trained in therapeutic nutrition, and psychological counseling, subjects not required in traditional medical schools. They may even work in conventional hospitals. As physicians, they can provide diagnostic and therapeutic services, including physical exams, lab testing and X-rays. Many can deliver babies, usually in a home setting. Others specialize in pediatrics, gynecology or geriatrics. The current scope of clinical Naturopathy covers the full practice of medicine excluding major surgery, and the prescribing of most drugs. Minor surgery, such as the removal of a mole or wart, is allowed.

Naturopaths are, for the most part, primary care and general practice family physicians. They have enormous scope. Since they specialize in non-invasive, gentle lifestyle therapy, they can offer almost unlimited recommendations. Instead of prescribing a standard treatment for a common health complaint, a naturopathic physician can offer an individual approach.

Conventional doctors, because their drug and surgical treatments can be so dangerous or full of side effects, have few choices, and are bound by what has been officially approved or authorized.

NATUROPATHIC MEDICINE MAY BE APPLIED IN ANY HEALTH CARE SITUATION, BUT ITS STRONGEST SUCCESSES ARE IN THE TREATMENT OF CHRONIC AND DEGENERATIVE DISEASE. NATUROPATHIC MEDICINE IS NOT RECOMMENDED FOR SEVERE, ACUTE TRAUMA, SUCH AS A SERIOUS AUTOMOBILE ACCIDENT, A CHILDBIRTH EMERGENCY, OR ORTHOPEDIC PROBLEMS REQUIRING CORRECTIVE SURGERY, ALTHOUGH IT CAN CONTRIBUTE TO MUCH FASTER RECOVERY IN THESE CASES.

Naturopaths fall into two groups. Those who are trained medically have extensive hands-on coursework in anatomy, physiology, biochemistry, pathology, neurosciences, histology, immunology, pharmacology, epidemiology, public health and other conventional disciplines as well as various natural therapies.

Non-medically trained naturopaths use the naturopathy degree as an accreditation to teach, to write and to access research. One of the core beliefs of naturopathy is education - the passing on of knowledge to empower the patient.

Although all naturopaths emphasize therapeutic choices based on individual interest and experience, they maintain a consistent philosophy. All are trained in the basic tools of natural therapeutics, and all work with diet and nutrition while specializing in one or more other therapeutic methods.

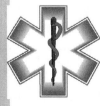

Naturopathic medicine sees disease as a manifestation of the natural causes by which the body heals itself, and seeks to stimulate its vital healing forces. If the cause of the imbalance is not removed, the responses will continue either at a lower level of intensity or intermittently to become chronic disease. Fever and inflammation are good examples of the way the body deals with an imbalance that is hindering healthy function.

NATUROPATHY IS FOUNDED ON FIVE THERAPEUTIC PRINCIPLES.

A typical visit to a Naturopath generally incorporates these beliefs.

[1] ***The healing power of nature.*** The belief that the body has considerable power to heal itself, and that the role of the physician or healer is to facilitate and enhance this process, preferably with the aid of natural, non-toxic, non-invasive therapies. Above all, the physician or healer must do no harm.

[2] ***The person is viewed and diagnosed as a whole.*** The Naturopath must work to understand the patient's complex interaction of physical, mental, emotional, spiritual and social factors. Understanding the patient as an individual is essential when searching for causative factors.

[3] ***The goal is to identify and treat the cause of the problem.*** Naturopathic medicine does not simply suppress symptoms, but seeks the underlying causes of a disease, especially as manifested in the four major elimination systems: the lungs, kidneys, bowels, and skin. A naturopath views symptoms as expressions of the body's attempt to heal. The causes of a disease spring from the physical, mental, emotional and spiritual levels. Healing a chronic disease requires the removal of the underlying cause.

Some illnesses are the result of spiritual disharmony, experienced as a feeling of deep unease or inadequate strength of will necessary to support the healing process. For lasting good health, this disharmony must be overcome. Naturopathic physicians can play an important role in guiding patients to discover the appropriate action in these cases.

In acute cases such as ear infections, inflammation or fever, the naturopath addresses associated pain, infection and inflammation as well as the relationship of the acute condition to the underlying causes, such as diet, life stresses, and occupational hazards.

- Homeopathy and acupuncture are frequently used to stimulate recovery.
- Herbal medicines are frequently used as tonics and nutritive agents to strengthen weak systems.
- Dietary supplements and glandular extracts may also be used to overcome nutritional deficiencies.
- Hydrotherapy and various types of physical therapy may be required.
- Relaxation techniques are often suggested to alleviate emotional stresses, and to allow the digestive system to function in an environment required for proper digestion.

[4] ***The physician is a healing teacher.*** A naturopath should be foremost a teacher, educating, empowering and motivating the patient to assume more personal responsibility for their own wellness by adopt- ing a healthy attitude, lifestyle and diet. After identifying the conditions that cause the illness, a naturopathic physician discusses with the patient the most appropriate methods for creating a return to health.

[5] ***Prevention is the best cure.*** Prevention of disease is best accomplished through dietary and lifestyle habits which support health.

> Care more than others think is wise.
> Risk more than others think is safe.
> Dream more than others think is
>   practical.
> Expect more than others think is
>   possible.

Homeopathy

Homeopathy is a kinder, gentler medical philosophy that recognizes disease as an energy imbalance, a disturbance of the body's "vital force." Its techniques are based on the premise that the body is a self healing entity, and that symptoms are the expression of the body attempting to restore its balance. Homeopathic remedies are formulated to stimulate and increase this curative ability. Each remedy has a number of symptoms that make it unique, just as each person has traits that make him or her unique. Homeopathic physicians are trained to match the patient's symptoms with the precise remedy, which is mild and non-toxic. Even the highest potencies do not create the side effects of allopathic drugs. The remedies themselves neither cover up nor destroy disease, but stimulate the body's own healing action to rid itself of the problem.

Homeopathic medicine is based on three prescription principles:

1. The **LAW OF SIMILARS**: expressed as "like curing like." From the tiny amount of the active principle in the remedy, the body learns to recognize the hostile microbe in a process similar to DNA recognition. The LAW OF SIMILARS is the reason that a little is better than a lot, and why such great precision is needed.

2. The **MINIMUM DOSE PRINCIPLE**: the dilution of the "like" substance to a correct strength for the individual (strong enough to stimulate the body's vital force without overpowering it). Dilutions, usually in alcohol, are shaken or succussed, a certain number of times (3, 6, or 12 times in commercial use) to potentiate therapeutic power through the vibratory effect. Each successive dilution decreases the actual amount of the substance in the remedy. In the strongest dilutions, there is virtually none of the substance remaining, yet potentiation is the highest for healing effect.

3. The **SINGLE REMEDY PRINCIPLE**: where only one remedy is administered at a time.

❦

Although homeopathic treatments are specific to the individual patient in private practice, we have found two things to be true about the remedies available in most stores today:

THEY WORK ON THE ANTIDOTE PRINCIPLE. MORE IS NOT BETTER FOR A HOMEOPATHIC REMEDY. SMALL AMOUNTS OVER A PERIOD OF TIME ARE MORE EFFECTIVE. FREQUENCY OF DOSAGE IS DETERMINED BY INDIVIDUAL REACTION TIME, INCREASING AS THE FIRST IMPROVEMENTS ARE NOTED. WHEN SUBSTANTIAL IMPROVEMENT IS EVIDENT, INDICATING THAT THE BODY'S OWN HEALING FORCES ARE STIMULATED AND HAVE COME INTO PLAY, THE REMEDY SHOULD BE DISCONTINUED.

THEY WORK ON THE TRIGGER PRINCIPLE. A GOOD WAY TO START A HEALING PROGRAM IS WITH A HOMEOPATHIC MEDICINE. THE BODY'S ELECTRICAL ACTIVITY, STIMULATED BY THE REMEDY, CAN MEAN MUCH MORE RAPID RESPONSE TO OTHER, SUCCEEDING THERAPIES.

Homeopathic medicine differs from conventional medicine in two significant ways:

1. Conventional medicines usually mask or reduce the symptoms of a disease without addressing the underlying problem. Homeopathic remedies act as catalysts to the body's immune system to wipe out the root cause.

2. Although both medicinal systems use weak doses of a disease-causing agent to stimulate the body's defenses against that illness, homeopathy uses plants, herbs and earth minerals for this stimulation, whereas conventional medicine uses viruses or chemicals.

The recent worldwide rise in popularity for homeopathy is due to its effectiveness in treating epidemic diseases, such as HIV-positive and other life-threatening viral conditions. Many tests are showing that homeopathy not only treats the acute infective stages, but also helps reduce the intake of antibiotics and other drugs that cause side effects, which further weakens an already deficient immune system.

In significant 1991 tests, Internal Medicine World Magazine reported six HIV-infected patients who became HIV-negative after homeopathic treatment. Following this and other reports, success with AIDS has been widely experienced by homeopaths as follows:

> PREVENTION - generating resistance to the virus and subsequent infection.
> SUPPORT DURING ACUTE ILLNESSES - reducing the length and severity of the infection.
> RESTORATION OF HEALTH - revitalizing the body so that overall health does not deteriorate.

HOW TO TAKE HOMEOPATHIC REMEDIES

For maximum effectiveness, take $1/2$ dropperful under the tongue at a time, and hold for 30 seconds before swallowing; or dissolve the tiny homeopathic lactose tablets under the tongue. These remedies are designed to enter the bloodstream directly through the mouth's mucous membranes. For best absorption, do not eat, drink or smoke for 10 minutes before or after taking. Do not use with chemical medicines, caffeine, cayenne, mint or alcohol; they overpower homeopathy's subtle stimulus.

Store homeopathic remedies at room temperature out of heat and sunlight, and away from perfumes, camphor, liniments and paints.

The basic rule for dosage is to repeat the medicines as needed.

Occasionally, aggravation of symptoms may be noted at first as the body restructures and begins to rebuild its defenses, in much the same way as a healing crisis occurs with other natural cleansing therapies. This effect usually passes in a short period of time.

Healing can be quite long lasting. The right homeopathic remedy can restore health on all levels.

HERE ARE THE MOST POPULAR HOMEOPATHIC REMEDIES AND HOW TO USE THEM:

- **APIS** - macerated bee tincture. Relieves stinging, burning and rapid swelling after bee sting or insect bites. Recommended for sunburn and other minor burns, skin irritations, hives, early stages of boils, and frostbite. Helps relieve joint pain, eye inflammation and fevers. Apis is effective against pain that is improved by cold and made worse by pressure.

- **ARNICA** - often the first medicine given after an injury or a fall, to counter bruising, swelling, and local tenderness. Excellent for pain relief and rapid healing, particular from sports injuries, such as sprains, strains, stiffness or bruises. Unlike herbal preparations of Arnica, homeopathically diluted Arnica tablets are safe for internal consumption to relieve contusions, calm someone who has had a great shock, and dispel the distress that accompanies accidents and injuries. Used before and after surgery and childbirth to prevent bruising and speed recovery. Apply externally only to unbroken skin.

- **ACONITE** - for children's earaches. Helps the body deal with the trauma of sudden fright or shock.

- **ARSENICUM ALBUM** - for food poisoning accompanied by diarrhea. For allergic symptoms such as a runny nose; for asthma and colds.

- **BELLADONNA** - for rapid relief from sudden fever, sunstroke or swelling. Used to treat sudden onset conditions characterized by redness, throbbing pain, and heat, including certain types of cold, high fever, earache and sore throat. Recommended for a person who has a flushed face, hot and dry skin, and dilated pupils. A remedy for teething, colds and flu, earache, fever, headache, menstrual problems, sinusitis, and sore throat.

- **BRYONIA** - for certain types of flu, fevers, coughs and colds that come on slowly. For some headaches, indigestion, muscle aches and pains. Helpful for irritability and aggravation by motion. Also for swelling, inflammation and redness of arthritis when symptoms are worse with movement and better with cold applications.
- **CALENDULA** - promotes healing of minor cuts and scrapes, cools sunburns, and relieves skin irritations.
- **CANTHARIS** - for treating bladder infections and genito-urinary tract problems, especially where there is burning and urgency to urinate. Also good for skin burns.
- **CAPSICUM** - a digestive aid, and stimulant. Apply topically to stop minor bleeding, joint pain and bruises.
- **CHAMOMILLA** - to calm fussy children during teething pains, colic and fever. Good for childhood cold symptoms of runny nose, tight cough, stringy diarrhea and earache. Treats childhood and adult restlessness, insomnia, toothache and joint pains. Recommended for those who are frequently irascible, stubborn and inconsolable.
- **EUPHRASIA** - used as both an external and internal treatment for eye injuries especially when there is profuse watering, burning pain, and swelling. Also used for abrasions, stuffy headache, and mucus in the throat.
- **GELSEMIUM** - to energize people with chronic lethargy. To overcome dizziness from colds or flu.
- **HYPERICUM** - used topically and internally to relieve pain and trauma related to nerves and the central nervous system. For an injury that causes the type of shooting pain that ascends the length of a nerve, and for wounds to an area with many nerve endings, like the ends of the fingers and toes. Accelerates healing of jagged cuts and relieves the pain from dental surgery, toothaches, and tailbone injuries. Effective for depression and insomnia, A powerful anti-inflammatory for ulcers and nerve damage; also for cuts scrapes, mild burns and sunburn.
- **IGNATIA** - a female remedy to relax emotional tension. Effective during times of great grief or loss.
- **LACHESIS** - for PMS symptoms that improve once menstrual flow begins. For menopausal hot flashes, irritability and bloating.
- **LEDUM** - for bruises. Use after Arnica treatment to fade a bruise after it becomes black and blue.
- **LYCOPODIUM** - a mood booster that often increases personal confidence. Favored by estheticians to soothe irritated complexions and as an antiseptic.
- **MAGNESIUM PHOS** - for abdominal cramping, spasmodic back pain and menstrual cramps.
- **NATRUM MURIATICUM** - for the water retention experienced during PMS.
- **NUX VOMICA** - used principally to treat headache, nausea and vomiting, when due to overeating or drinking. A prime remedy for hangover, recovering alcoholics and drug addiction. Beneficial for gastrointestinal tract problems, such as abdominal bloating, peptic ulcer, heartburn, flatulence, constipation and motion sickness.
- **OSCILLOCOCCINUM** - a premiere remedy for flu.
- **PASSIFLORA** - a prime remedy for insomnia and nervousness.
- **PODOPHYLLUM** - helps diarrhea, especially for children.
- **PULSATILLA** - for childhood asthma, allergies and earaches, when the child is tearful and passive. For colds characterized by a profusely running nose and coughing. For certain eye and ear ailments, skin eruptions, allergies, fainting episodes, and gastric upsets, particularly when the patient is sensitive and prone to crying. A common ingredient in homeopathic combination remedies for colds and flu, sinusitis, indigestion and insomnia.
- **RHUS TOX** - a poison ivy derivative, dilutions are taken to alleviate poison ivy and other red, swollen skin rashes, hives, and burns, as well as joint stiffness. A sports medicine for pain and swelling that affects muscles, ligaments, and tendons from sprains and overexertion. A "rusty gate" remedy, for the person who feels stiff and sore at first but better after movement. For stiffness in the joints when the pain is worse with cold, damp weather. A common ingredient in homeopathic combination remedies for back pain, strains and sprains and skin conditions.
- **SEPIA** - effective in treating herpes, eczema, hair loss and PMS.
- **SULPHUR** - commonly taken for certain chronic, as opposed to acute, conditions, skin problems, and during the early stages of the flu. May also be used to treat sore throats, allergies, and earaches.
- **THUJA** - effective for treating warts and moles, and for sinusitis.
- **VALERIAN** - soothes nerves and eases muscle tension. Used as a sedative and for insomnia.

Homeopathic Cell Salts

Mineral, or tissue salts in the body can be used as healing agents for specific health problems. Homeo-pathic doctor, William Schuessler, discoverer of the twelve cell salts, and the Biochemic System of Medicine, felt that all forms of illness were associated with imbalances of one or more of the indispensable mineral salts. In addition, his research indicates that homeopathically prepared minerals help to maintain mineral balance in the body, and are used by the body as core, building nutrients at the cellular level.

CELL SALTS ARE BASED ON HOMEOPATHIC REMEDIES AND MAY BE USED IN HEALING PROGRAMS THAT INCORPORATE OTHER HOMEOPATHIC TREATMENT. AS WITH OTHER HOMEOPATHIC REMEDIES, MINERAL SALTS ARE USED TO STIMULATE CORRESPONDING BODY CELL SALTS TOWARD NORMAL METABOLIC ACTIVITY AND HEALTH RESTORATION. THEY RE-TUNE THE BODY TO RETURN IT TO A HEALTHY BALANCE. ONLY VERY SMALL AMOUNTS ARE NEEDED TO PROPERLY NOURISH THE CELLS.

THE TWELVE CELL SALTS

Many of today's cell salts are extracted from organic plant sources. These medicines are available both in tinctures and as tiny lactose-based tablets that are easily dissolved under the tongue.

❖ **CALCAREA FLUOR** - *calcium fluoride* - contained in the elastic fibers of the skin, blood vessels, connective tissue, bones and teeth. Used in the treatment of dilated or weakened blood vessels, such as those found in hemorrhoids, varicose veins, hardened arteries and glands.

❖ **CALCAREA PHOS** - *calcium phosphate* - abundant in all tissues. Strengthens bones, and helps build new blood cells. Deficiency results in anemia, emaciation and weakness, slow growth and poor digestion.

❖ **CALCAREA SULPH** - *calcium sulphate* - found in bile; promotes continual blood cleansing. When deficient, toxic build-up occurs in the form of skin disorders, respiratory clog, boils and ulcerations, and slow healing.

❖ **FERRUM PHOS** - *iron phosphate* - helps form red corpuscles to oxygenate the bloodstream. Treats congestive colds and flu, and skin inflammation. A good remedy for the first stages of infections.

❖ **KALI MUR** - *potassium chloride* - deficiency results in coating of the tongue, gland swelling, skin scaling, and excess mucous discharge. Used after FERRUM PHOS for inflammatory arthritic and rheumatic conditions.

❖ **KALI PHOS** - *potassium phosphate* - found in all fluids and tissues. Deficiency is characterized by intense body odor. Used to treat mental problems such as depression, irritability, neuralgia, dizziness, headaches, and nervous stomach.

❖ **KALI SULPH** - *potassium sulphate* - an oxygen-carrier for the skin. Deficiency causes a deposit on the tongue, and slimy nasal, eye, ear and mouth secretions.

❖ **MAGNESIA PHOS** - *magnesium phosphate* - an infrastructure constituent. Deficiency impairs muscle and nerve fibers, causing cramps, spasms and neuralgia pain, usually accompanied by prostration and profuse sweating.

❖ **NATRUM MUR** - *sodium chloride* - found throughout the body. Regulates moisture within the cells. Deficiency causes fatigue, chills, craving for salt, bloating, profuse secretions from the skin, eyes and mucous membranes, excessive salivation, and watery stools.

❖ **NATRUM PHOS** - *sodium phosphate* - regulates the body's acid/alkaline balance. Catalyzes lactic acid and fat emulsion. Imbalance is indicated by a coated tongue, itchy skin, sour stomach, low appetite, diarrhea and flatulence.

❖ **NATRUM SULPH** - *sodium sulphate* - an imbalance produces edema in the tissues, dry skin with watery eruptions, poor bile and pancreas activity, headaches, and gouty symptoms.

❖ **SILICEA** - *silica* - essential to the health of bones, joints, skin, and glands. Deficiency produces catarrh in the respiratory system, pus discharges from the skin, slow wound healing, and offensive body odor. Very successful in treating boils, pimples and abscesses, for hair and nail health, blood cleansing, and rebuilding the body after illness or injury.

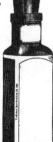

Chiropractic

Overwhelming evidence has changed the medical community's attitude toward chiropractic as a method for both healing and normalizing the nervous system. With almost 15 million patients annually, and 35,000 licensed practitioners, chiropractic therapy is now America's second largest health-care system.

Meaning "done with the hands," chiropractic therapy uses physical manipulation of the spine to relieve pain and return energy to the body. The central belief of chiropractic is that proper alignment of the spinal column is essential for health, because the spinal column acts as a switchboard for the nervous system. Its practitioners feel that the nervous system holds the key to the body's healing potential because it coordinates and controls the functions of all other body systems.

Today's chiropractors incorporate such techniques as physical therapy, nutritional counseling and muscle rehabilitation into their practices. Many have also branched out into treatment of PMS, candida albicans yeast overgrowth, chronic fatigue syndrome, insomnia and asthma, because of the relationship of these problems to nerve obstruction. Some chiropractors encourage their patients to use them as primary-care physicians, because ailments such as respiratory conditions, digestive troubles and circulatory problems respond well to chiropractic care.

While the most common complaint for chiropractic treatment is still lower back pain, chiropractic adjustment can be helpful in preventing wear and tear on joints and ligaments by maintaining their proper positioning. It can help decrease scar tissue formation after serious injury, and help prevent later stiffness of the affected joints. Chiropractic is also successful in treating menstrual difficulties, and new evidence shows that chiropractic adjustment combined with proper nutrition can improve, and in some cases reverse, arthritis and osteoarthritis.

Most chiropractors today are no longer "back crackers," but instead use a hand-held activator that delivers a controlled, light, fast thrust to the problem area. The thrust is so quick that it accelerates ahead of the body's tightening-up resistance to the adjustment. A chiropractor locates the fixated area of the spine, makes the quick adjustment, and corrects the subluxation. Other problems aggravated by the fixation usually begin to heal immediately. The gentleness of this method makes adjustments far safer and more comfortable for the patient.

THE SPINAL COLUMN AND THE NERVOUS SYSTEM WORK TOGETHER TO AFFECT YOUR HEALTH:

The spinal column is made up of twenty-four bones called vertebrae that surround and protect the spinal cord. Between each vertebra, pairs of spinal nerves extend to every part of the body, including muscles, bones, organs and glands. Each vertebra affects its neighbor and one portion of the spine may affect or damage other areas of the body.

The nervous system is comprised of three overlapping systems: the central nervous system, the autonomic nervous system and the peripheral nervous system. Health relies upon the balance and equilibrium of these three interrelated nerve systems, which can be disrupted by misalignment, stress or illness. Almost every nerve in the body runs through the spine, and stress-caused constriction tends to accumulate in the lower back, neck and shoulders. Chiropractic adjustments therefore, can address many seemingly unrelated dysfunctions, both physical and subconscious.

Misalignments in the spine, known as subluxations, cause nerve interference, and result in both pain and reduced immune response. A subluxation can have a direct effect on organ function. When subluxations occur, the electrical impulse flow from the brain to the nerve structures is interrupted, interfering with the normal function. By adjusting spinal joints to remove subluxations, normal nerve function can be restored. While subluxations may not be the sole cause of a given disease, they are still a major predisposing factor to it because they prevent the nervous system from working optimally.

Massage Therapy

Massage therapy has been a healing method for thousands of years. The ancient Romans and Greeks used it regularly to treat a variety of medical conditions. Since its re-discovery as a New Age relaxation technique, today's massage therapy has joined the alternative medicine techniques of chiropractic and reflexology as a viable health discipline. Within the past decade, overwhelming scientific evidence has accumulated to support the claim that massage therapy is effective for many health problems.

The Physicians Guide to Therapeutic Massage states that massage therapy benefits conditions such as muscle spasms and pain, spinal curvatures, body soreness, headaches, whiplash, temporo-mandibular joint syndrome (TMJ), tension-related respiratory disorders like bronchial asthma, and emphysema. It can help reduce swelling, correct posture, improve body motion, and through lymphatic massage, facilitate the elimination of toxins from the body.

Massage therapy can be used as an adjunct treatment for cardiovascular disorders, neurological and gynecological problems; it is often effective in place of drugs for these problems.

Massage therapists also treat PMS, chronic fatigue syndrome, candida albicans, gastro-intestinal conditions, epilepsy, psoriasis and skin problems, as well as traditional spinal/nerve problems. Most use a holistic approach, recommending diet correction, nutritional supplements, and enzyme therapy in a personally developed program for their patients.

Massage therapy is particularly helpful for pain control, stimulating the production of endorphins, the body's natural pain relievers. It stimulates the body's immune response and natural healing powers.

MODERN RESEARCH INDICATES THAT MASSAGE THERAPY:

- calms the nervous system and promotes muscle relaxation.
- promotes recovery from fatigue and pain after hard exercise.
- helps break up scar tissue and adhesions which develop as a result of injury.
- can relieve certain types of pain, especially back pain.
- effectively treats chronic inflammatory conditions by increasing limbic circulation.
- helps reduce inflammation and swelling from fractures or injuries.
- improves blood circulation throughout the entire circulatory system.
- promotes mucous and fluid drainage from the lungs by percussion and vibration techniques.
- can increase peristaltic action in the intestines to promote fecal elimination.

THERE ARE MANY TECHNIQUES OF THERAPEUTIC MASSAGE. THE CHOICE IS LIMITED ONLY BY PERSONAL PREFERENCE AND DESIRED RESULTS. FOR LASTING BENEFITS, USE MASSAGE THERAPY AS PART OF A PROGRAM THAT INCLUDES DIET IMPROVEMENT AND EXERCISE.

HERE ARE THE MOST POPULAR MASSAGE THERAPY METHODS:

Alexander technique - This system strives to improve posture by properly positioning the head and neck. A favorite of actors and singers, the Alexander technique works to expand the chest cavity, improve breathing and body movement. The sessions involve guided body movement as well as table-work massage techniques.

Feldenkrais - This system believes that to change the way we act, we must change the way we move. Through simple body manipulations and exercises, Feldenkrais practitioners help patients change unbalanced muscle patterns and the thought and feeling patterns associated with them.

Polarity therapy - Besides the muscles, glands and nerves, the human body has a magnetic field that directs these systems and maintains energy balance. A polarity practitioner works to access the magnetic current and its movement patterns to release energy blocks.

Reflexology - Under this system, the feet and hands are seen as the end points of energy zones and associated organs and glands throughout the body. The points are manipulated to open blocked energy pathways. Since the feet serve as reflexes for the entire body, foot reflexology is most often used. Reflexology is best used in conjunction with other massage techniques.

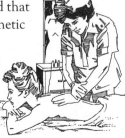

Rolfing - Rolfers attempt to realign the body with gravity by deeply manipulating the connective tissue that contains the muscles and links them to the bones.

Swedish massage - This system uses kneading, stroking, friction, tapping and sometimes body shaking to stimulate or relax. The techniques help muscles, joints, nerves and the endocrine system, and when used *before* an athletic workout, can prevent soreness, relieve swelling and tension and improve muscular performance. By stimulating the body's circulation, it can speed rehabilitation from injury.

MASSAGE THERAPY IS A WONDERFUL HEALTH TOOL. *I am continually amazed myself at how good I feel after a massage treatment. Certainly use it when you are ill, but let its benefits improve your everyday life, too.*

- Massage calms your nervous system and relaxes your muscles.
- It wipes away fatigue and re-energizes you
- It breaks up scar tissue and reduces fibrosis and adhesions from injuries
- It soothes many types of pain.
- It relieves chronic inflammation by stimulating lymphatic circulation (great for arthritis sufferers).
- It improves blood flow to all your organs, including your heart and brain.
- It increases blood flow throughout your body, helping it to work more efficiently.
- It strengthens the digestive system, which aids in the elimination of toxins from your body.
- It stimulates the release of brain chemicals that lift your mood and stimulate your immune system.
- Massage actually helps prevent future health problems, like heart disease!

As wonderful as massage therapy is, there are some health conditions where massage is not a good idea.

- Don't massage a person with high fever, cancer, tuberculosis or other infections or malignant conditions which might be further spread throughout the body.
- Don't massage the abdomen of a person with high blood pressure or ulcers.
- Don't massage the legs of a person with varicose veins, diabetes, phlebitis or blood vessel problems.
- Massage no closer than six inches on either side of bruises, cysts, skin breaks or broken bones.
- Massage people with swollen limbs gently, only above the swelling and towards the heart.

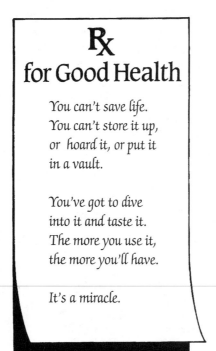

Rx
for Good Health

*You can't save life.
You can't store it up,
or hoard it, or put it
in a vault.*

*You've got to dive
into it and taste it.
The more you use it,
the more you'll have.*

It's a miracle.

Reflexology

Reflexology is an ancient natural science based on the belief that each part of the body is interconnected through the nerve system to specific points on the feet and hands. A history of foot massage spans time and place from the Physician's Tomb in Egypt of 2300 B.C. to the Physicians Temple in Nara, Japan, of 700 A.D. The ancient Egyptians are believed to have actually developed hand and foot reflexology, with specific pressure points corresponding to parts of the body.

Today reflexology is often known as zone therapy, and is an important part of massage therapy treatment. We know that stress is involved in over 80% of all illness. And we know the first step in healing is relaxation. Reflexology helps the body to heal itself through relaxation. Its goal is to clear the pathways of energy flow throughout the body, to return body balance, and increase immune response. It does this by stimulating the lymphatic system to eliminate wastes adequately, and the blood to circulate easily. By bringing needed nutrients to poorly functioning areas, reflexology treatments can make the organs, the lymph system and the nervous system stronger and healthier.

THE SCIENCE OF REFLEXOLOGY BELIEVES THAT ALL BODY PARTS HAVE ENERGY AND SHARE INFORMATION. PRESSURE TO A PARTICULAR MERIDIAN POINT BRINGS ABOUT BETTER FUNCTION IN ALL PARTS OF THAT MERIDIAN ZONE, NO MATTER HOW REMOTE THE POINT IS FROM THE BODY PART IN NEED OF HEALING. THUS, REFLEXOLOGY CAN ALSO BE USED FOR A MEASURE OF SELF-DIAGNOSIS AND TREATMENT.

The nervous system is very like an electrical system, and contact can be made through the feet and hands with each of the electro-mechanical zones in the body to the nerve endings. The nerve endings are called reflex points, and ten reflexology zone meridians have been extensively mapped by reflexologists connecting all the organs and glands, and culminating in the hands and feet. (SEE ILLUSTRATION IN ACUPUNCTURE SECTION.)

The term "reflex" refers to the fact that these points are reflexive, automatic stimulus responses, like a knee-jerk reaction. Today, reflexology treatments are used for pain relief, and for faster recovery from injuries or illness without surgery or heavy medication. Reflexology can also be part of a good health maintenance program. You don't have to be sick to appreciate the benefits. Many people simply enjoy the tension release a session gives.

Fifteen pounds of applied force can send a surge of energy to the corresponding body area, removing obstructive crystals, restoring circulation, and clearing congestion. The nerve reflex point on the foot for any afflicted area will be tender or sore indicating crystalline deposits brought about by poor capillary circulation of fluids. The amount of soreness on the foot point can also indicate the size of the crystalline deposit, and the amount of time it has been accumulating.

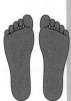

Reflexologists look at the feet as a mini-map of the entire body, with the big toes serving as the head, the balls of the feet representing the shoulders, and the narrowing the waist area. Any illness, injury or tension in the body produces tenderness in the corresponding foot zone. Reflexologists rely on an inchworm-like massage motion of the thumb to produce light or deep pressure on each zone, concentrating on the tender spots, which often feel like little grains of salt under the skin.

For your own individual use in this book, it is helpful to picture the hands and feet as the body's control panels. The "foot" and "hand" diagrams on the specific ailment pages graphically show the pressure points for each area, so that you can use reflexology when indicated. In some cases, the points are very tiny, particularly for the glands. They will take practice to pinpoint.

The best rule for knowing when you have reached the right spot is that it will probably be very tender, denoting crystalline deposits or congestion in the corresponding organ. However, there is often an immediate feeling of relief in the area as waste deposits break up for removal by the body.

HERE ARE SOME EASY REFLEXOLOGY TECHNIQUES YOU CAN USE:

Pressing on the sore point three times for 10 seconds each time is effective. The pressure treatment may be applied for twenty to thirty minute sessions at a time, about twice a week. Sessions more often than this will not give Nature the chance to use the stimulation or do its necessary repair work. Most people notice frequent and easy bowel movements in the first twenty-four hours after zone therapy as the body throws off released wastes.

Finger-Walking: Your thumb acts as a brace as the fingers move, bending at the first joint and applying steady pressure.

Thumb-Walking: Let the fingers grasp, while thumb tip exerts pressure. The thumb bends only at the first joint.

Pinch-Grip: The flats of the thumb and finger grasp and exert pressure on an area.

Multiple Finger Grip: Let the palm act as a brace while the tips of all four fingers make contact.

Direct-Grip: The flat of the thumb remains stationary and exerts pressure; the heel of the hand is the moving force.

HERE ARE SOME REFLEXOLOGY TECHNIQUES TO INCREASE ENERGY AND RELIEVE BOTH MIND AND BODY STRESS.

*   Use finger walking technique to walk across each toe. Cover nails and base of toe.

*   Grasp toe between fingers and thumb. Using the pinch-grip, bring fingers and thumb together. The corner of the thumb exerts pressure on top of the toe. Then using pinch-grip, exert pressure on webbing between toes.

*   Separate the big toe and second toe, exposing trough. Place finger at base of toe. Use finger walking technique to walk down side of trough to inside of foot. Switch hands to work outside of foot.

*   Place finger in the trough between first and second toes on top of foot. Use multiple-finger grip on inside of the trough. Reposition and work another part of the trough. Work on each trough. Switch hands. Use multiple-finger grip on side of trough toward outside of foot.

*   Place tips of fingers on the ledge formed across base of toes. Grasp foot, and wrap fingers around to provide leverage. Use multiple-finger grip, with fingers in downward direction.

*   Place thumb on the bottom of the foot, with fingers resting on top of the foot. Use thumb-walking technique to work webbing between toes, as far into trough as padding on ball of foot will allow. Don't work into soft skin between toes.

*   For direct-grip method, grasp the foot with the holding hand. Place flat of thumb of other hand on bottom of foot in area to be worked. With holding hand, rotate foot against stationary thumb of working hand.

*   Grasp the foot. Rest thumb of working hand on inside edge of the foot for leverage. Place finger on outside edge of the foot. Use finger-walking technique to walk around outside edge of foot.

Complete health and awakening are really the same thing.

Acupuncture & Acupressure

Acupuncture and acupressure are ancient systems of natural healing from the Orient, now gaining respect in the western world. The central belief of Traditional Chinese Medicine is that the body must be in balance to function at its peak. Acupuncture is based on this belief.

Traditional Oriental medicine believes that all emotional and physical energy, known as chi, flows through the body along specific bioelectric and chemical pathways called meridians, or "energy pathways." When chi energy is flowing smoothly, the body is in perfect balance. If chi energy flow is slowed down or blocked, by factors like injury, poor diet, stress or climate, then physical or emotional illness often results.

The meridian points are connected to specific organs and body functions. The pathways regulate and coordinate the body's well-being by distributing Chi energy throughout it. Acupuncture and acupressure are a painless, non-toxic therapy for redirecting and restoring Chi energy flow. Most patients feel relaxed during acupuncture treatment, but response is highly individualized, relaxing some, energizing others.

Acupuncture uses hair thin needles and/or electrodes to direct and rechannel body energy. Western science believes that acupuncture needling stimulates certain nerve cells to release chemicals found in the spine, muscles and brain. These chemicals help relieve pain by releasing endorphins, the body's pain-relieving substances. They also stimulate the release of other chemicals and hormones that normalize body processes. Acupuncture is used in the U.S. mainly for pain relief, but is valuable in the treatment of environmentally-induced illnesses caused by radiation poisoning or air pollution, and useful in carpal tunnel syndrome, and withdrawal complications from smoking, alcoholism, and other addictions.

Chinese medicine sees acupuncture as stimulating the release of blocked chi energy, which then flows throughout the body allowing it to begin healing itself. Because the body meridians are interconnected with the internal organs, Chinese practitioners use acupuncture to treat everything from immune disorders, like chronic fatigue syndrome, to allergies and asthma. Acupuncture is also extremely effective in treating rheumatoid conditions, bringing relief to 80% of those who suffer from arthritis.

The World Health Organization cites 104 different conditions that acupuncture can treat, including, migraines, sinusitis, the common cold, tonsillitis, eye inflammation, myopia, duodenal ulcer and other gastrointestinal disorders, neuralgia, Meniere's disease, tennis elbow, paralysis from stroke, speech aphasia and sciatica.

Acupuncturists specialize in treating people, not symptoms. They look for lifestyle patterns that affect health, and place great emphasis on balance and harmony with the patient's environment for the best results from their treatments. They see noticeable immune response reduction when there are excesses in the patient's life, from daily stress to emotional upsets, even the weather. When the patient's underlying imbalance is corrected, not only does the main complaint improve, but secondary complaints are also treated. Depending on the patient's needs, Chinese herbs, vitamin suppplements, therapeutic exercises, and changes in diet and lifestyle are part of the complete healing process.

Modern acupuncture also uses several adjunct treatments: moxibustion, a form of heat therapy in which certain herbs, like Chinese wormwood are burned near acupuncture points to radiate through the skin and influence the meridian below; cupping, a circulation stimulating technique, in which heated glass cups are placed over acupuncture points to draw blood to the area; and massage therapy.

The nature of the problem determines the number of acupuncture treatments a patient will require. Someone suffering acute pain in a specific area may need only a few months of treatments; someone with a chronic diseases usually requires a longer-term treatment program.

𝒜cupressure uses the same principles and meridian points as acupuncture, but works through finger pressure, and massage and stroking rather than needles to effect stimulation. Fourteen major meridians or channels of energy, run through your body. (See diagram below.) Each meridian is named for the organ or function connected to its energy flow. Stimulating these points manually can release blocked energy. Acupressure is also effective for general preventative care. Acupressure and massage therapy are frequently combined in a healing stimulation session.

For optimum benefits, two acupressure points may be simultaneously stimulated at the same time, one with each hand, while the part of the body in between is stretched to effect maximum energy flow between the points. Or, one can duplicate the pressure on both sides of the body. Immediately after finding and massaging the point on one side, repeat the technique on the opposite side. In most cases the points only need to be triggered about 15 seconds apiece to get prompt relief.

THE PRIMARY ADVANTAGE OF ACUPRESSURE IS THAT IT IS A SELF-ACCESS THERAPY. IN FACT, THE CHINESE CONSIDER ACUPRESSURE A PERSONAL FIRST AID METHOD. ALMOST EVERY TECHNIQUE CAN EASILY BE DONE AT HOME AS NEEDED, TO RELIEVE PAIN, AND OPEN UP BODY CLEANSING AND HEALING CHANNELS.

YOU CAN USE SOME OF THE MOST EFFECTIVE ACUPRESSURE POINTS YOURSELF:

Acupressure is a two-step process. **Step one** is finding the right pressure point. They are tiny - only about the size of a pin-head - so this may be more difficult than it seems. If you can't find the exact spot on your body at first, poke around a bit~acupressure points are generally more tender than the surrounding area. **Step two** is massaging the point properly. Use the tip of your index finger, your middle finger, or both side by side. In some spots, it may be easier to use your thumb. The point should be stimulated as deeply as can be managed - in a digging kind of massage. A few seconds of pressure, repeated several times, will often be enough. You should push until you feel some discomfort.

BODY   ZONES

There are certain "acupressure reactions" that generally accompany proper stimulation. Within about 30 seconds of "triggering" an effective point, you should feel a sensation of warmth, clamminess and/or a slight flush of perspiration forming across the brow or shoulders, along with a perceptible, light-headed feeling. This type of reaction is a good indication that you have found the right point, and relief should be felt. If you don't get prompt, satisfactory relief after triggering a point, it usually means one of several things:
1. You didn't find the right point for your symptom. Try another point.
2. You didn't find the point. Make sure you feel the twinge when you probe and press.
3. The point may not have been stimulated properly. Did you use the tip of your thumb or finger? Did you stimulate both sides of your body for enough time?

ACUPRESSURE TECHNIQUES FOR COMMON HEALTH PROBLEMS:
- For a sore back, press on the points on either side of the lower spine, just around the corner from the bottom-most rib. Press both sides simultaneously.
- Give a lift to an aching back with a little pressure just beneath the tip of the tailbone.
- For low back pain, press hard in the center of the depression at the sides of your buttocks. Press both sides simultaneously.
- A finger press right between the eyes can bring headache relief.
- For menstrual pain, press two finger widths below your belly button. Start therapy several days before your period is due and continue for several days after.
- For menstrual congestion, press three finger widths under each kneecap, at the side of your leg.
- Press a point just above the breastbone for nagging hiccups.
- To relieve nocturnal leg cramps, apply strong pressure to the points behind the knee, in the center of the calf, and where the Achilles tendon joins the calf muscle.

- To treat insomnia, press a point below the little finger at the first crease of the wrist.
- Also for insomnia, press two points, right at the natural hairline on either side of the spine.
- To quiet a cough, press the points just below the collarbone. The same pressure points are also helpful in easing an asthmatic cough.
- For a sore throat, press the center of your forehead about midway between the eyebrows and the natural hairline. Massage the point until the acupressure reaction occurs.
- For temporary relief of toothache, press right above the corner of the jaw on the affected side.
- For more athletic energy, press the nape of the neck, hard and quickly, just before the event.
- For lower abdomen problems, such as bowel disorders or indigestion, run your thumb up the inner, rear edge of the shin bone directly in line with your ankle bone toward the knee. At about 3" up, you'll feel the unmistakable tingling that announces the point.

- **To relieve neck tension,** place your right hand with the palm facing the floor, then bend it back slightly so that a crease appears at your wrist. Remember where this crease is, and measure the width of two left thumbs (about two inches) back from the crease towards your elbow. Press very deeply with the middle finger in the small hollow between your two arm bones. Duplicate the process on your left forearm.
- **To relieve tension in the neck and shoulders,** press about 2 inches down from your elbow toward your hand, on the hairy side of your upper forearm. Probe deeply in the muscle until you feel a very tender spot. It will be quite tender with even moderate pressure, since it's a judo disabling point.
- **To relieve a headache,** place your right hand with the palm facing the floor. Squeeze your thumb tightly against your pointer finger so a fleshy mound pops up on the back of the right hand between them. Place the bent knuckle of the left index finger on top of the mound. Keeping the knuckle in place, relax the right hand and press deeply in that area until you feel the tender point. The more it hurts, the better it is likely to be for your headache.
- **Acupressure can be a dieting tool.** Locate the cleft between the bottom of the nose and top of the upper lip. Pinch it when you're hungry, and within moments your hunger will be gone.

Because both acupuncture and acupressure are free of toxins and additive side effects, they have become alternatives for people who used to live on Motrin, Advil and other pain pills that harm the liver. Western medicine is just beginning to realize the valuable role of acupressure and acupuncture in disease prevention care, the way these techniques are used in the Orient. Both methods are also effective for animals, and are often recommended for hip dysplasia and arthritis in large animals.

As with other natural therapies, the aim is to regulate, balance and normalize so the body can function normally. Surgery and drugs may often be avoided, and there are sometimes spectacular results. In addition, traditional western doctors are finding that acupuncture and acupressure work well in conjunction with conventional medicine. Both acupuncture and acupressure can positively influence the course of a therapeutic program, and should be considered as a means of mobilizing a person's own healing energy and balance.

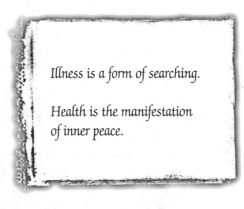

Illness is a form of searching.

Health is the manifestation of inner peace.

Biofeedback

Biofeedback uses electronic devices to give auditory, verbal, and visual information back to the body about how it is working, It is perhaps the most accepted by the mainstream medical community of all alternative healing techniques - probably because it uses expensive, high-tech equipment. Before the advent of the biofeedback machine, conventional medicine held that an individual had no control over heart rate, body temperature, brain activity, or blood pressure. When biofeedback experiments proved, in the 1960's, that people *could* voluntarily affect these functions, a great deal of research began into how it might be employed for human health.

Here's how biofeedback works. The patient is wired with sensors, and by giving auditory and/or visual signals to his body, learns to control what are usually subconscious responses, such as circulation to the hands and feet, tension in the jaw, or heartbeat rate. Biofeedback computers then provide a rapid, detailed analysis of the target activities within the body. Biofeedback practitioners interpret changes in the computer readings which help the patient learn to stabilize erratic and unhealthy biological functions. A normal, healthy reading includes fairly warm skin, low sweat gland activity, and a slow, even heart rate.

Today, biofeedback is being used by all kinds of health professionals - physicians, psychologists, social workers and nurses. It is seen as a useful medical tool for controlling health problems like asthma, chronic fatigue, epilepsy, drug addiction and chronic pain. It is a successful specific in the treatment of migraines, cold extremities, and psoriasis, a skin disease that has a psychological foundation.

Biofeedback is used in relaxation therapy to help overcome insomnia and anxiety. Sleep disorders, hyperactivity and other behavior problems in children, dysfunctions stemming from inadequate control over muscles, bladder incontinence, back pain, temporo-mandibular joint syndrome (TMJ), and even loss of control due to brain or nerve damage, all show improvement under biofeedback training.

Biofeedback also helps problems such as heart malfunction, stress-related intestinal disorders like ulcers and irritable bowel syndrome, hiatal hernia, ringing in the ears (Meniere's syndrome), facial tics, and cerebral palsy.

THE EFFECTS OF BIOFEEDBACK CAN BE MEASURED BY:
1. monitoring skin temperature influenced by blood flow beneath the skin;
2. monitoring galvanic skin response, the electrical conductivity of the skin;
3. observing muscle tension with an electro-myogram;
4. tracking heart rate with an electro-cardiogram;
5. using an electroencephalogram to monitor brain wave activity.

One of the most common vital signs monitored by biofeedback to affect health is muscle tension, because this can be used to treat tension headaches, muscle pain, incontinence and partial paralysis. Another is skin temperature, which can be used to treat Reynaud's syndrome, migraines, hypertension and anxiety.

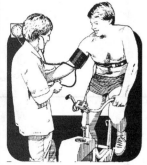

Other signs are perspiration, which is used to treat anxiety and body odor; pulse, which is used to treat hypertension, stress and arrhythmia; and breathing rate, which is used to treat asthma, hyperventilation and anxiety.

Biofeedback is seldom used by itself, but is instead combined with other relaxation techniques and lifestyle changes. Biofeedback doesn't work for everyone. Its success stories are from people who are willing to make lifestyle improvements.

Guided Imagery

Guided imagery uses the mind/body connection to help give people more control over their health. It is a communication technique for accessing the network between mind and body as a source of power in the healing process.

Imagery is the normal way the nervous system finds, stores, and processes information. In essence, it is a flow of thoughts that we can see, hear, feel, smell, or taste in our imagination. It has its roots in the ancient Greek understanding of how the mind influences the subconscious, and has been employed under many different names, throughout the history of medicine, to speed healing by reducing stress and calming the mind.

Imagery is used in modern times to encourage athletes and performers to better performance, minimizing discomfort from all kinds of acute injuries, including sprains, strains, and broken bones. In healing, it is successful in overcoming chronic pain and persistent infections, and in shrinking tumor growths. Even serious, degenerative illness such as cancer has responded to guided imagery, with patients showing heightened immune activity as they imagine cancer cells being gobbled up by immune antibodies.

Imagery can be a healing factor in dealing with either a simple tension headache or a life-threatening disease. It is a proven method for helping people tolerate medical procedures and treatments, for reducing side effects, and for supporting a less painful, faster recuperation. Experts claim that imagery can help both physical and psychological disorders, from high blood pressure and acne, to diabetes, cancer and addictions.

Imagery is often used for relief of neck tension and back pain, allergies, asthma, benign arrhythmias, stress-related gastrointestinal symptoms like chronic abdominal pain and spastic colon, urinary complaints, and reproductive irregularities including premenstrual syndrome, irregular menstruation, dysmenorrhea, and even excessive uterine bleeding. It can also accelerate healing from the symptoms of the common cold, flus, and infections.

IMAGERY CAN BE AN EFFECTIVE TOOL IN CLARIFYING ATTITUDES, EMOTIONS, BEHAVIORS, AND LIFESTYLE PATTERNS THAT PRODUCE ILLNESS. IT CAN ALSO AFFECT THE MENTAL AND EMOTIONAL PART OF ILLNESS RECOVERY, BY HELPING PEOPLE FIND MEANING IN THEIR HEALTH PROBLEMS AS THEY LEARN TO COPE WITH AN ILLNESS. BY DIRECTLY ACCESSING EMOTIONS, IMAGERY CAN HELP THE INDIVIDUAL UNDERSTAND THE HEALING NEEDS THAT MAY BE REPRESENTED BY AN ILLNESS AND CAN HELP DEVELOP WAYS TO MEET THOSE NEEDS IN ORDER TO CHOOSE WELLNESS.

We know that stress is an emotional response to life's situations, and that an emotional reaction to a stressful situation manifests itself in one's physical health. If a person responds to a loss with a prolonged state of depression, the body, too, will fall into a prolonged state of depression, manifested as illness. However, if the person is able to integrate the loss into a broader meaning of life, the feelings of loss, grief and depression will be relatively temporary. We experience a more wholesome view of life when we feel ourselves in control - as participants in life rather than as victims of undesirable circumstances.

The school of imagery believes that the body will be in a better position to cope with disease-causing factors if it is not under stress. If stress levels are high, immune response is reduced, so learning to relax is fundamental to self-healing. Today, guided imagery in one form or another is a part of almost every relaxation and stress-reduction technique. For many people, imagery is the easiest way to learn to relax, and its active nature makes it more satisfying than other methods of relaxation.

Scientifically, imagery works like a computer to program directions into the hypothalamus that a patient wants for his body. This happens almost instantaneously, traveling from the brain through the nervous system, to the endocrine system through the hypothalamus-pituitary-adrenal axis, and then through the vagus nerve for both psychological and physical accord.

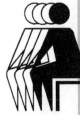

Everything that is registered in our minds is registered in our bodies. Messages you send your body through imagery, for example, are immediately translated through the parasympathetic nervous system into neurotransmitters, that direct the immune system to work better against abnormal cells, or the hormone system to rebalance and stop creating abnormal cells.

Deepak Chopra M.D., a well-known expert on the mind-body connection, explains that "the mind is in every cell of the body. Every thought we think causes a release of neuropeptides that are transmitted to all the cells in the body." Thoughts of love cause the release of interleukin and interferon, which help to heal the body. Anxious thoughts cause the release of cortisone and adrenaline, which suppress the immune system. Peaceful, calming thoughts release chemicals in the body similar to valium, which help the body to relax.

THERE ARE TWO TYPES OF GUIDED IMAGERY TECHNIQUES - RECEPTIVE IMAGERY AND ACTIVE IMAGERY:

- **Receptive imagery** involves entering a relaxed state, then focusing on the area of the body with the ailment. You envision an embodiment of the illness - perhaps a mischievous demon- and ask it why it is causing the trouble. Your unconscious can provide a great deal of information about what your body needs.

- **Active imagery** involves envisioning an illness being cured. This may mean anything from imagining your immune system attacking a tumor, to picturing arm pain as a ball that rolls down your arm and out of your body.

Guided imagery therapists use a near-trance condition, induced through spoken suggestion to affect healing. Patients are asked to envision themselves in a tranquil place like a quiet woods or a mountain lake, then directed to describe what they see, hear, smell, or feel, in order to reach a deeper state of relaxation. This technique is called *sensory recruitment* because it calls on areas of the brain that control each different sense.

When relaxation has been reached, patients are asked to visualize their immune system as an energy force battling for their health. Their immune responses are analyzed in great detail. They are then asked to join forces with the immune system, by mentally envisioning the illness and then imagining their antibodies and white cells overcoming it.

Not everyone is capable of working with guided imagery treatment. An active imagination is a must, because the vividness of the image plays a role in the treatment's effectiveness. Successful subjects are those who can understand its value in relation to their problems, and who do not mentally fight it.

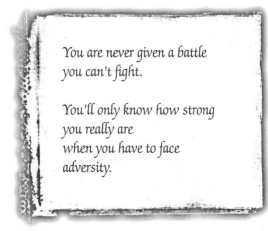

You are never given a battle you can't fight.

You'll only know how strong you really are when you have to face adversity.

Hypnotherapy

The power of suggestion has always played a major role in healing. Hypnosis is an artificially induced mental state that heightens receptivity to suggestion. Hypnotherapy uses both suggestion and trance to access the deepest levels of the mind in order to effect positive changes in a person's behavior. It maximizes the mind's contribution to healing by producing a multilevel relaxation state - a state which allows enhanced focus to increase tolerance to adverse stimuli, ease anxiety, and enhance affirmative imagery.

Physiologically, hypnosis stimulates the limbic system, the region of the brain linked to emotion and involuntary responses, like adrenal spurts and blood pressure. Habitual patterns of thought and reaction are temporarily suspended during hypnosis, rendering the brain capable of responding to healthy suggestions. The physiological shift can actually be observed during a hypnotic state, as can greater control of autonomic nervous system functions that are normally beyond one's ability to control. Stress and blood pressure reduction are common occurrences.

RESEARCH DEMONSTRATES THAT BODY CHEMISTRY ACTUALLY CHANGES DURING A HYPNOTIC TRANCE. IN ONE EXPERIMENT, A YOUNG GIRL WAS UNABLE TO HOLD HER HAND IN A BUCKET OF ICE WATER FOR MORE THAN THIRTY SECONDS. BLOOD LEVELS OF CORTISOL IN HER BODY WERE HIGH, INDICATING SHE WAS IN SEVERE STRESS. UNDER HYPNOSIS, SHE WAS ABLE TO KEEP THE SAME HAND IN ICE WATER FOR THIRTY MINUTES. THERE WAS NO RISE IN BLOOD CORTISOL LEVELS.

Hypnotherapy has therapeutic applications for both psychological and physical disorders.

A skilled hypnotherapist can effect profound changes in respiration and relaxation to create enhanced well-being. Today, hypnotherapy techniques are becoming widely used to help you quit smoking, lose weight, or get a good night's sleep. Professional sports trainers use it to boost athletic performances. It is also a method for treating medical conditions, like facial neuralgia, sciatica, arthritis, whiplash, menstrual pain and tennis elbow. Migraines, ulcers, respiratory conditions, tension headaches, and even warts respond to hypnotherapy.

New applications show that hypnotherapy can help people tolerate the discomfort of medical procedures. Some patients have even undergone surgery without anesthesia using hypnosis. Dentists regularly use hypnosis for root-canal patients who cannot tolerate anesthesia.

Hypnotherapy is also useful in surgical operations where regular anesthesia isn't a good option, in cases like hysterectomies, hernias, breast biopsies, hemorrhoidectomies and cesarian sections. A recent study shows that burn victims heal considerably faster with less pain and fewer complications if they are hypnotized shortly after they are injured.

Scientists are now examining a new aspect of hypnotherapy: its effect on the immune system. Recent research shows that hypnotherapy can be used to train your immune system to fight disease.

Hypnotherapy works best as a partnership between doctor and patient. Surprisingly, while most people do not think that they can be hypnotized, 90% of the general population *can* achieve a trance, and another 30% have a high enough susceptibility to enter a state that is receptive to treatment.

THREE CONDITIONS ARE ESSENTIAL FOR SUCCESSFUL HYPNOTHERAPY:
- A comfortable environment, free of distraction, so the patient can reach the deepest possible level.
- Trustful rapport between the hypnotist and the patient.
- A willingness and desire by the subject to be hypnotized. People who benefit most from hypnotherapy understand that hypnosis is not a surrender of personal control, but instead, an advanced form of relaxation.

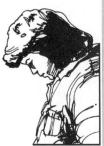

Overheating Therapy

Overheating therapy, or hyperthermia, is once again becoming known for the valuable healing tool that it is. Its known use dates from ancient Greek physicians, who raised body temperature as an immune defense mechanism against infection. It was also used in the elaborate bath complexes of the Romans, and the sweat lodges of the American Indians and Scandinavians. Herbs, minerals, healing clays and especially sea plants, are used in overheating therapy for body detoxification.

Increased body temperature speeds up metabolism, inhibits the growth of infective organisms, and literally burns or sweats harmful substances out. Even slight temperature increases lead to considerable reduction in virus replication. Overheating therapy is used successfully against pathogenic bacteria and viruses, including infectious flus, cancer, arthritis, leukemia and most recently, against the HIV virus.

Despite skepticism by conventional medicine, drastic diseases like AIDS that have no drug related cure mean that other methods must be tried. CNN HEALTH recently showed a blood-overheating procedure for an AIDS patient in the treatment of Kaposi's sarcoma, the cancer that produces the severe skin lesions in HIV-infected patients. The sores vanished in about four months, along with other symptoms. Since then, other AIDS sufferers with sarcoma have undergone hyperthermia with the same success. In some cases, the blood has even tested negative for the HIV virus. Since only blood hyperthermia has been tried for AIDS, the virus may still be in the bone and resurface, but the reduction of symptoms is obvious.

Our bodies use overheating therapy as an immune system response mechanism in the form of a fever, to help kill infective organisms. When exposed to heat, blood vessels in the skin dilate to allow more blood to flow to the surface, activating the sweat glands, which then pour the water onto the skin's surface. As the water evaporates from the skin, it draws both heat and toxins from the body, becoming a natural detoxification treatment as well as a cooling system. Today, many health care professionals believe that a non-life-threatening fever should be allowed to do its healing work.

Even though the natural work of the kidneys takes out many toxic accumulations, therapeutic internal cleansing by regular sweating can be an important part of health maintenance. German scientists recently tested marathon runners logging 20 miles a day. Analyzing their sweat, they found it contained heavy metals like cadmium, lead and nickel. They concluded that sweating excretes potential cancer-causing elements, and that regular profuse sweating could help maintain good health.

Overheating therapy also aids in weight loss. A dry sauna places great demand on the body in terms of burning calories, which, of course assists in fat loss. Sweat glands must work harder to produce sweat in a dry sauna, requiring more energy and burning more calories. The energy required for these processes is derived from the conversion of fat and carbohydrates to calories. ***To lose weight, take a daily sauna!***

SWEATING BY OVERHEATING THE BODY IN A DRY SAUNA PRODUCES THE FOLLOWING EFFECTS:

- Speeds up metabolic processes to inhibit the growth of pathogenic bacteria and viruses.
- Creates a fever reaction that kills potentially dangerous viruses and bacteria, and increases the number of leukocytes in the blood to strengthen the immune system.
- Provides a deep, prolonged, therapeutic sweat that will flush out toxins and heavy metals.
- Accelerates cardiovascular action, making the heart pump harder and dropping diastolic blood pressure.
- Stimulates vasodilatation of peripheral vessels to relieve pain and speed healing of sprains, strains, bursitis, peripheral vascular diseases, arthritis and muscle pain.
- Promotes relaxation and a feeling of well-being.

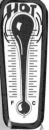

NOTE: Simple overheating therapy may be practiced in the home, via either a dry sauna or an overheating bath. See bodywork techniques for successful cleansing, page 178, for method and technique of a therapeutic bath.

Enzymes & Enzyme Therapy
What They Are ⚘ How They Work ⚘ Why You Need Them

Modern science is trumpeting the amazing powers of its new discovery, enzyme therapy; yet both enzymes and enzyme therapy have been known for thousands of years. Ancient Chinese medicine knew of the energetic powers of enzymes in its search for the harmony of life. We know that the Egyptians, the Greeks and the Arabs felt that an unseen force existed which changed grape juice into wine, dough into bread, and malt into beer.

Enzymes exist in all living things. They make life possible. No substances in our bodies are more important than enzymes. Without them we could not breathe, digest food, or move a muscle. No vitamin, mineral, or hormone can do its job without enzymes. They act as catalysts for every activity, and are involved in *every* bio-chemical process. Every second of our lives, more than 2,700 different types of enzymes are performing a complicated interlocking network of activities which no computer could even begin to imitate, sometimes at breathtaking speed.

Enzyme activity and integration works in milliseconds, with 100% productivity. In fact, digestive enzymes in human beings are stronger than any of the body's other enzymes, and more concentrated than any other enzyme combination found in nature. A very good thing, since our processed, overcooked, nutrient-poor diets demand a great deal of enzymatic work!

Enzyme activity is incredibly specialized. There is a special enzyme for each biochemical reaction in the body, and the reaction is so specific that it cannot take place without the presence of its particular enzyme. There is even an enzyme, *cathepsin*, which is stored in our systems for our death, to break down cells and tissue for the body's return to the earth's organic matrix. Yet, enzyme activity is truly holistic, too. Most enzymes act together as co-enzymes, or as co-factors with vitamins, minerals and other food elements for optimum body efficiency.

THERE ARE THREE CATEGORIES OF ENZYMES:
1. Metabolic enzymes, which run the body processes, repair damage and decay, and heal disease.
2. Digestive enzymes, which assimilate carbohydrates, proteins and fats into the body.
3. Fresh plant enzymes, which start food digestion, and aid human digestive enzymes. The best food sources of enzymes for humans are bananas, mangos, sprouts, papayas, avocados and pineapples.

THERE ARE THREE INTERESTING FACTS ABOUT FOOD ENZYMES:
• All food, whether plant or animal, has enzymes that serve it in life. When eaten, these become the property of the eater, are now *its* food enzymes, and begin immediately to work for the eater's digestive benefit, helping in its own breakdown for the good of the eater.

• **All foods in their natural state contain the enzymes required to digest them.** Animal organisms even have the proteolytic enzyme, cathepsin, which comes into play after death, becoming the prime factor for autolysis.

• Only enzymes found in whole, unprocessed foods give the body what it needs to work properly, to replace and rebuild cells. Humans cannot independently assimilate food; our bodies must have the help of the food itself.

Enzymes are the body's delivery system. Most nutrient deficiencies result from the body's inability to absorb them, not from the lack of the nutrients themselves. While science has not been able to manufacture enzymes synthetically, many have been isolated, and can be used by man to support enzyme deficiencies. Hydrochloric acid and bile activity are essential parts of good digestion. HCl sterilizes and acidifies foods in the stomach, working with pepsin and water to make chyme. The chyme is then neutralized by highly alkaline juices from the pancreas and the intestine, and by bile from the liver and gall bladder. Bile also works with lipase to emulsify fats and convert them to beneficial fatty acids. Supplementing digestive enzymes and acids such as HCl and bile, help insure assimilation and maximize utilization of core nutrients for health and healing. If you can't make them, take them.

SIGNIFICANT DIGESTIVE ENZYMES:

Note: Digestive enzymes are categorized by the function they perform, plus the ending "ase". For example, *lactase* breaks down milk sugar into glucose and galactose.

- **Pancreatin**, a proteolytic digestive secreted by the pancreas, contains essential enzymes essential for the digestion of protein, carbohydrates and fat. The pancreas releases about $1^1/_2$ **quarts** of pancreatic juice into the small intestine every day. Pancreatin therapy use has centered on degenerative disease.
- **Papain and chymopapain**, proteolytic food enzymes from papaya, are vegetable pepsins for digestion of proteins. Papain also contains substances that break down starch and work on fat, so it is a prime meat tenderizer.

  Papain therapy helps:

  Loosen necrotic, encrusted waste material from the intestinal walls.

  Treat phlogistic edemas, inflammatory processes and accelerates wound healing.

  Relieve bites and stings when tablets are mixed into a paste with water.

- **Bromelain**, a proteolytic, anti-inflammatory food enzyme from pineapple, aids digestion of fats. When combined with papain (above), the two together break down protein into amino acids.

  Bromelain therapy helps improve:

  All stress-related conditions, especially pre-op preparation and post-op trauma.

  Inflammatory conditions and diseases like arthritis, hemorrhoids, thrombophlebitis.

  Gastrointestinal diseases like ileitis, diverticulitis, gastritis, colitis and ulcers.

  The cleansing of coronary arteries, preventing narrowing and clogging.

  Mouth and gum swelling from dental surgery

- **SOD (Superoxide Dismutase)**, a copper/zinc-containing enzyme found in all body cells, protects the cells and fights to destroy free radicals. Some diseases related to a free-radical problem are arthritis, allergies, cancer, heart problems, leukemia, lupus and premature aging.

  SOD therapy works with Bromelain therapy for the following conditions:

  Reduces the inflammation of arthritis. Reduces risk of cancer and other degenerative diseases.

  Aids in the healing of wounds. Alleviates symptoms related to radiation sickness.

  Greatly aids damaged heart, kidney, intestines, pancreas, and skin tissue.

  Reduces the number and severity of abnormal heart arrhythmias.

  Slows down the aging process through cell protection.

- **Lactase,** the enzyme which digests the milk sugars, is plentiful in children and decreases with age. Almost 65% of adults have some deficiency in lactase.
- **Catalase** works with SOD to reduce free radical production for immune health.
- **Amylase** digests sugars and starches.
- **Cellulase** digests cellulose, the fibrous component of most vegetable matter.
- **Trypsin and Chymotrypsin,** proteolytic enzymes that help convert chyme, (see papain).
- **Diastase and Mycozyme** are potent vegetable starch digestants.
- **Lipase**, along with bile, digests fats and oils, converting them to heat and energy.
- **Pepsin,** breaks down proteins into peptides, can digest 3500 times its weight in proteins.
- **Protease,** with pepsin and HCl, breaks up proteins into amino acids.
- **Rennin** helps digest cow's milk products.

About Co-enzyme Q10

CO-ENZYME Q_{10} is a biochemical enzyme activator found in every body cell, and a vital enzyme catalyst for cell energy. All live foods contain a form of Coenzyme Q_1 to Q_{10}. CoQ_{10} therapy has a long history of effectiveness in boosting immunity, increasing cardiac strength, reversing high blood pressure, promoting natural weight loss, inhibiting aging, and overcoming periodontal disease. Other specific enzyme therapy treatments are for congestive heart failure, angina, ischemic heart disease, cardiomyopathy, mitral valve prolapse, diabetes, cancer tumors and candida albicans. CoQ_{10} can alleviate toxic effects of drugs commonly used to treat cancer and hypertension.

The body's ability to assimilate food source CoQ_{10} declines with age. One to three months may be necessary to saturate deficient tissues with supplementation.

HERBS ARE AN EXCELLENT CHOICE FOR ENZYME THERAPY BECAUSE THEY CARRY THEIR OWN PLANT ENZYMES ALONG WITH THEIR MEDICINAL PROPERTIES. SOME OF THE MOST ACTIVE YOU CAN USE FOR YOURSELF:

- **Ginger** contains plant enzymes that break down proteins. It inhibits inflammation, tones the heart, stimulates liver function, and helps the conversion of cholesterol into bile acids.
- **Milk Thistle** contains silymarin, a biochemical, which concentrates in the liver, the bile, and the intestines.
- **Nettles** drive toxins and metabolic waste products out of the body by stimulating the kidneys to excrete more water. An extract of nettles inhibits the enzyme activity that contributes to an enlarged prostate (BPH).
- **Licorice** contains glycyrrhizin, a biochemical that suppresses the main enzyme responsible for inactivating progesterone, aldosterone and cortisol in humans, for a balancing effect on estrogen metabolism.
- **Aloe Vera** has proteolytic enzymes that slough off dead skin cells, and opens pores. An enzyme called carboxpeptidase in aloe hydrolyzes inflammatory mediators responsible for burn wound healing and pain relief.
- **Green Tea and Black Tea** selectively change the ratio of two specific metabolic enzymes in the liver, helping the body to moderate toxic elements, and makes it easier for them to be excreted.
- **Oregon grape root** contains the alkaloid berberine which stimulates the secretion of bile, and has shown antibiotic action against E. coli, Streptococcus, cholera and flu viruses.
- **Hawthorn** has PCOs, and other flavonoids that help prevent collagen destruction by inhibiting free radical damage, and the synthesis of histamines, prostaglandins, and leukotrienes, compounds that promote inflammation.
- **Dandelion** enhances the flow of bile which helps break down fats.
- **Cayenne** triggers the flow of saliva and stomach secretions needed to break down food.
- **Catnip** provides enzyme therapy for indigestion or heartburn.

MAXIMIZE YOUR DAILY ENZYME BENEFITS:

Enzyme protection and enzyme therapy are dramatically affected by the use of a microwave because it destroys enzymes. Enzymes are also destroyed by substances like tobacco, alcohol, caffeine, fluorides, chlorine in drinking water, air pollution, chemical additives and many medicines. Enzymes are extremely sensitive to heat. Even low degrees of heat can destroy food enzymes and greatly reduce digestive ability. Heat above 120° F. completely destroys them. Eating fresh foods not only requires much less digestive work from the body, the foods can provide more of their own enzymes to work with yours.

Nearly 80% of the calories consumed by Americans today come from processed foods. There are well over 6,000 synthetic chemicals which are "legally" added to food. And that number doesn't include pesticide and herbicide residues, which appear in the majority of commercial food at measurable levels. It is no wonder that pancreatic disease is common today. **Enzymes are a major pancreatic protector.**

HOW DOES ENZYME THERAPY WORK? HOW CAN WE USE IT FOR OURSELVES?

Enzyme therapy uses metabolic enzymes to stimulate immune response. Metabolic enzymes are involved in every process in the body, but the link between *enzymes and immunity* comes from lymphocytes, or white blood cells. Immune organs, like the thymus and lymph nodes, keep a constant level of white blood cells circulating through the body to attack foreign invader cells. When toxins and foreign substances invade the body, white blood cells attack them, and break them up or digest them by secreting enzymes on their surfaces. Certain diseases, such as cancer, leukemia, anemia, and heart disease can even be diagnosed by measuring the amount of various enzymes in the blood and body fluids.

Enzyme therapy helps conquer ailments like heart disease, malignancies, skin problems, low and high blood sugar, stomach and colon pain, eye diseases and headaches. Proteolytic enzymes serve as anti-inflammatory agents for sports injuries, respiratory problems, degenerative diseases, and healing from surgery. Other enzymes clean wounds, dissolve blood clots, and control allergic reactions to drugs.

Enzymes therapy is effective against sprains and strains; enzymes curb inflammation by breaking up debris in the injured area and allow the vessels to unclog, leading to a decrease in swelling, a reduction in pain and more rapid repair of the injured area. One of the most important functions of enzymes is to neutralize toxins in the body. Antioxidant co-enzymes, such as glutathione peroxidase, and superoxide dismutase, (SOD), scavenge and neutralize cell-damaging free radicals by turning them into stable oxygen and H_2O_2, and then into oxygen and water.

High quality enzymes from your health food store are therapeutically active for enzyme healing. Most types are now able to state on the bottle their specific area of activity.

Aromatherapy
What It Is ℞ How To Use It

Aromatherapy, a branch of herbal medicine that uses essential plant oils to produce physical and emotional effects in the body, is both an ancient art and science. Aromatherapy works on different levels to accelerate healing, especially restoring energy and body balance through the nervous system. Aromatherapy oils have deep subconscious effects on emotions, triggering memory, and altering attitudes. Depending on the oils chosen, they may either calm and relax, or stimulate and energize. On the spiritual plane, aromatherapy elevates and soothes the spirit to restore harmony between mind and body.

Records of aromatherapy date back thousands of years. Every ancient civilization used some form of aromatherapy to improve health and daily life. Egyptians burned scented oils 5,000 years ago, and also embalmed their corpses with resin and essence compounds. Hippocrates, the father of modern Western medicine, successfully fought a plague in Athens 2,000 years ago using aromatic fumigations throughout the city.

In the middle ages, people burned pine oil in the streets during disease epidemics, and rubbed their bodies with oil of garlic, a powerful antibacterial agent. Aromatic frankincense was as precious as gold in the ancient world. Its vapor was believed to elevate the spirit, linking the human psyche with higher energies. In 1981, German scientists investigated the "mind-altering" effects of frankincense, and found that its vapor produced a powerful consciousness-expanding, psychoactive reaction in the brain.

As modern lifestyles become more chaotic and medical costs keep rising, many people are re-discovering aromatherapy as a natural, self-help technique to restore harmony between mind and body. Aromatherapy is widely practiced in Europe as a healing technique today, because it helps restore the natural balance of the body instead of merely suppressing the symptoms of an ailment. In England, for instance, it is used in hospitals with diffusers, which pump the relaxing aroma of lavender through the wards to help boost patient morale. Lavender relaxes stress, so it is felt that patients are able to heal faster. At night, patients are given a choice of a tranquilizer drug or an aromatherapy oil massage.

Essential oils, 75 to 100 times more concentrated than dried herbs and flowers, are the heart of aromatherapy. During the life of the plant, essential oils deliver messages through the plant structure to regulate its functions, trigger immune response to environmental stress, protect it from harm and attract insects for pollination and propagation. In essence, aromatherapy oils act in plants much like hormones do in humans. They are some of the most potent of all herbal medicines.

Essential oils affect people first through the sense of smell. Smell is the most rapid of all the senses because its information is directly relayed to the hypothalamus. Motivation, moods and creativity all begin in the hypothalamus, so odors affect all of these processes. Scents are intimately intertwined with our emotions, feelings, and memories.

A familiar scent can instantly flood your head with a field of flowers, or paint pictures of your past on the movie screen of your mind.

Scents also influence the endocrine system responsible for hormone levels, metabolism, insulin production, stress levels, sex drive, body temperature and appetite. The volatile molecules of essential oils work through hormone-like chemicals to produce their sensations. Certain oils can enhance your emotional equilibrium merely by inhaling them. (The smelling salts of Victorian days were used for more than just reviving a fainting lady.)

Aromatherapy oils aren't really oils, but distilled condensations, formed by rushing steam through plant material. The resulting fluids are volatile, non-oily essences with molecules so small they can penetrate the skin. Aromatherapy essences are highly active, and may be taken in by inhalation, steams, infusers, or applied topically in massages, compresses or baths.

USING AROMATHERAPY OILS

Essential oils are highly concentrated and should only be used in 1 to 5 drop doses.

Skin Care

Your skin is your body's largest organ, both for ingestion and elimination. It is a major part of the immune system, too, protecting against the elements, and preventing harmful chemicals or too much water from entering the body. Stress, emotions, poor nutrition, and pollution all take a heavy toll on skin.

Essential oils are especially effective for skin, acting as transporters to carry therapeutic benefits to skin layers. Aromatherapy helps improve your skin's condition by stimulating circulation. It encourages cell growth through phytohormone activity and cell regeneration to create a fresher, more vibrant complexion. Stress-reducing benefits also keep skin looking clear and calm. Floral waters are the easiest way to use essential oils on the skin. Waters have the healing properties of the oil itself, and are well-suited to sensitive skin. Make floral waters in a spray bottle if possible, for convenience. Simply blend 5 to 10 drops of the essential oil into 4 oz. distilled water, and use as needed. Essential oils may also be added to body lotions and moisturizers. However, since the oils are volatile, you cannot make up the preparation in advance. Pour some lotion into your hand; add 3 drops of oil and apply to skin.

- *Oils for general skin care - chamomile, geranium, lavender, lemon, ylang ylang.*
- *Oils for dry, or aging skin - rose, carrot seed, rosemary, jasmine, red sage, sandlewood.*
- *Oils for oily skin - lavender, eucalyptus, geranium, ylang ylang, basil, camphor, lemon.*
- *Oils for sensitive skin - chamomile, neroli, rose.*
- *Oils for wrinkled skin - lemon, fennel, palmarosa, carrot seed, myrrh.*
- *Oils to promote the growth of healthy skin cells - lavender, rose*

Facial Oil for Dry to Normal Skin: in a base of $\frac{1}{4}$ ounce Jojoba or vitamin E oil, add 2 drops geranium oil, 1 drop frankincense oil, and 1 drop myrrh oil. Massage several drops into your skin twice daily.

Facial Oil for Normal to Oily Skin: in a base of $\frac{1}{4}$ ounce Jojoba or vitamin E oil, add 3 drops lavender oil and 1 drop ylang-ylang oil.

Aromatherapy Facial Steam Cleanse: add 3 drops lemongrass oil and 1 drop eucalyptus oil to a bowl of steaming water. Put your face 6 to 10 inches above the water, and tent a towel over your head.

Aromatherapy Skin Wash: in a base of 4 ounces of liquid soap, add 5 drops peppermint oil, 1 drop eucalyptus oil, 1 drop chamomile oil, and 2 drops sage oil to revitalize troubled skin.

Hair Care

The easiest way to use the aromatherapy oils for your hair is to mix 12 to 15 drops of oils into an 8-oz. bottle of your favorite shampoo or conditioner.
Note: Some essential oils may strip peroxide-based hair coloring. Do a sample test area if you are concerned.

- *Oils for dry hair - cedarwood, lavender*
- *Oils for oily hair - lemongrass, rosemary*
- *Oils for dandruff - rosemary, cedarwood*
- *Oils to reduce hair loss - cedarwood, lavender, rosemary, sage, juniper.*

Essential Brushing Oil: to balance, shine, and scent hair and scalp; add equal amounts rosemary and lavender oil to a small perfume bottle; shake out 2 drops on a brush and run several times through hair.

Aromatherapy Scalp Rub For Scalp Diseases: to 2-oz. sweet almond oil, add 2 drops rosemary oil, 2 drops sage oil and 2 drops cedarwood oil to relieve scalp distress.

Oral Hygiene
Follow directions exactly when using aromatherapy oils in the mouth.

- *For fresh breath and better digestion - use 1 drop peppermint oil on the tongue; or blend five drops peppermint oil with 1 oz. of cider vinegar and 3 oz. water, and use as a regular mouthwash.*
- *For toothache - blend 20 drops clove oil with 1-oz. brandy and apply with a cotton swab.*
- *For gum problems - Put 3 or 4 drops of sage or tea tree oil on a cotton swab and apply to gums.*

Mental, Emotional & Spiritual Health
Use in a massage oil, in a diffuser, in an aromatic bath, or inhale the aromas from the bottle.

- *Oils for refreshment and invigoration - sage, lemon, lime, pine, eucalyptus, vervain.*
- *Oils to calm nervous tension and emotional stress - sage, pine, geranium, rosemary, pennyroyal.*
- *Oils for pleasant dreams and insomnia - anise, chamomile, ylang ylang.*
- *Oils for libido - ylang-ylang, patchouli, sandalwood, cinnamon.*
- *Oils for stimulating intellect and memory - rosemary, petitgrain.*
- *Oils for serenity and calmness - lavender, pine, chamomile, orange.*
- *Oils for positive motivation - peppermint, lemon, eucalyptus.*

Stress Reduction & Relaxation
Reducing stress is an aromatherapy specialty. Essential oils appear to influence hormones that regulate body metabolism and insulin production. Chronic stress lowers immunity, elevates blood pressure, and raises cholesterol levels; Stress depletes all your body's energies, and its nutrient supplies. Signs of stress include anger, anxiety, depression, paranoia, hostility, lethargy, and mental fatigue.

Stress-Soothing Massage Oil - to 2 ounces sweet almond oil, add 4 drops bergamot oil, 4 drops chamomile oil, 4 drops lavender oil, 4 drops sandalwood oil, 3 drops marjoram oil, 2 drops elemi oil and 2 drops frankincense oil.

Stress-Buster Diffuser Oil - in a small glass bottle, combine 15 drops lavender oil, 10 drops sage oil, 10 drops elemi oil, 10 drops geranium oil, 8 drops bergamot oil, 8 drops orange oil, 8 drops rosewood oil, 6 drops ylang ylang oil and 5 drops coriander oil. Add a few drops to your diffuser or lamp bowl as necessary to reduce tension.

One of the best ways to use aromatherapy is in a therapeutic bath. Aromatherapy baths can help control stress, alleviate tension and minimize muscular aches and pains. Swish oils in warm bath water and soak.

Winter Bath: to help ward off colds and stimulate circulation, use 3 drops juniper oil, 2 drops pepper oil and 5 drops lavender oil.

Summer Bath: to cool your skin, refresh and invigorate, use 3 drops peppermint oil, 4 drops bergamot oil and 2 drops basil oil.

Morning Bath: to start the day with an invigorating tonic, use 5 drops rosemary oil, 5 drops juniper oil and 2 drops peppermint oil.

Evening Bath: for better quality sleep, use 2 drops chamomile, 5 drops lavender, 2 drops orange blossom oil.

Aphrodisiac Bath: helps put you in the mood for love, use 2 drops ylang-ylang oil, 8 drops sandalwood oil and 2 drops Jasmine oil.

Lemon Detox Bath: to freshen and cleanse the body, use the juice from 1 lemon, 5 drops lemon oil and 2 drops geranium oil.

Relaxing Mineral Bath Salts: add 1 cup Dead Sea salts, 1 cup Epsom salts, $\frac{1}{2}$ cup sea salt and $\frac{1}{4}$ baking soda to a tub; swish in 3 drops lavender oil, 2 drops chamomile oil, 2 drops marjoram oil and 1 drop ylang-ylang oil.

Aromatherapy For Energy & Stimulation

Some essential oils have a direct effect on the central nervous system. Peppermint energizes while easing headaches. Ginger and fennel stimulate circulation. Rose influences hormonal activity. Lavender and geranium can either stimulate or sedate, according to the individual's physiological needs.

Rosemary Fatigue-Fighting Bath: Use 4 drops rosemary oil, 2 drops orange oil, 1 drop thyme oil.

Energizing Body Oil: mix, then massage into skin in the morning, 2 ounces sweet almond oil, 6 drops lavender oil, 4 drops rosemary oil, 3 drops geranium oil, 3 drops lemon oil, 2 drops coriander oil, 2 drops patchouli oil

Energy Inhalant Oil: in a small glass bottle, combine 8 drops rosemary oil, 6 drops elemi oil, 4 drops peppermint oil, 3 drops basil oil, 1 drop ginger oil. Inhale directly from the bottle for an energy boost.

Energy Boosting Diffuser Blend: in a small glass bottle, combine 15 drops rosemary oil, 12 drops pine oil, 10 drops lavender oil, 10 drops lemon oil, 2 drops peppermint oil. Add a few drops to your diffuser or lamp bowl.

Aromatherapy Oils For Healing:

Blend just before using for best results.

- **Body cleansing and rejuvenation** - massage skin with a blend of 15 drops geranium, 35 drops neroli and 1-oz. vegetable oil, to promote cell regeneration, rid the body of toxins and relieve tension.
- **Antiseptic oils** - lemon, clove, eucalyptus, pine, cinnamon, rosemary, thyme, tea tree. *Note:* These are excellent in a diffuser to keep harmful bacteria count down. Effective for upper respiratory infections, colds and flu. Use approx. 30 to 50 drops oils, and let diffuser run for 30 minutes twice a day.
- **Skin abrasions** - apply one drop of sage or lavender oil to speed healing. If used for first aid to cuts or bruises, put a few drops on a cotton swab and apply to area.
- **Sore throat and cough** - oils such as eucalyptus and tea tree may be applied topically to the throat. Cypress may be taken as a "tea," at a dose of 1 drop to a cup of hot water every hour.
- **Chest congestion** - make a vapor rub, using 50 drops eucalyptus, 15 drops peppermint, and 10 drops wintergreen to 1 oz. vegetable oil. Rub into chest for relief.
- **Allergy and asthma relief** - add a few drops of eucalyptus, lavender, sage, peppermint or wintergreen oil to a pot of boiling water or a vaporizer.
- **Bladder problems** - make a bladder "tea", using 2 drops of lavender, juniper, thyme oil in a cup of hot water.
- **Indigestion** - take 1 to 2 drops with meals of either rosemary, peppermint or lemon oil.
- **Intestinal or bowel irritation** - use a "tea" with 1 drop geranium oil to a cup of hot water.
- **Sunburn** - use 1 part tea tree oil to 1 part aloe vera gel and apply.
- **Headache** - apply 1 drop of lavender, peppermint or rosemary oil to back of the neck and temples.
- **Analgesic rub for sore joints and muscles** - use 20 drops each of clove, eucalyptus, tea tree, and wintergreen oils in 1 oz. vegetable oil. Rub into affected area, or add 1/4 oz. to a bath.

THERE'S A WIDE RANGE OF THERAPEUTIC OILS FOR YOU TO CHOOSE FROM. HERE ARE SOME OF THE EASIEST TO USE:

- *Bergamot* - eases digestion, relaxes nervous system.
- *Chamomile* - stimulates the mind, memory and respiratory system; helps overcome exhaustion.
- *Clove* - rejuvenates, soothes irritability and allays temper.
- *Eucalyptus* - loosens mucous, treats asthma and bronchitis.
- *Geranium* - stimulates the psyche, acts as an antidepressant, averts tension.
- *Jasmine* - is uplifting and soothing; known for its erogenous quality.
- *Lavender* - induces sleep, alleviates stress, reduces depression and nervous tension.
- *Lemongrass* - helps sedate the nervous system, soothes headaches, stimulates thyroid.
- *Patchouli* - a nerve sedative and antidepressant.
- *Peppermint* - cools a fever, decongests sinuses, soothes headaches and calms the mind.
- *Pine* - antiseptic for respiratory tract, soothes mental stress and relieves anxiety.
- *Rosemary* - encourages intuition and enhances memory.
- *Sage* - a cleansing and detox oil; also for mental strain and exhaustion.
- *Tangerine* - soothes psyche, calms, eases nervous tension.
- *Vanilla* - calming and soothing with aphrodisiac qualities.

The aromatherapy formulas in this section have been exerpted from many sources, both ancient and modern. See resource listing for details.

NOTE: *A DROP OF THE FOLLOWING IS PARTICULARLY EFFECTIVE FOR TREATING A BLEMISH THAT IS JUST ERUPTING. PUT ON A COTTON SWAB AND APPLIED DIRECTLY.*

- **Oils for inflamed skin** - chamomile, lavender, neroli, rosewood, geranium, cedarwood.
- **Oils for acne** - eucalyptus, juniper, lavender, cajeput, palmarosa, tea tree.
- **Oils for eczema or psoriasis** - cedarwood, patchouli, lavender, chamomile.

HERE'S THE WAY TO USE AROMATHERAPY OILS FOR THE BEST RESULTS:

Aromatherapy oils are customarily used by adding a few drops to a massage oil or facial care product, or using a diffuser or lamp, or in a steam inhaler to ease respiratory distress. When inhaled into the lungs, molecules of essential oils attach to oxygen molecules, enter the blood stream and journey throughout the body with therapeutic activity. Oils evaporate easily and completely. They don't leave marks on your clothing or towels.

- Use only pure essential oils. Never substitute synthetics.
- Buy your essential oils from reliable sources that guarantee the purity of their oils.
- Always dilute essential oils in a carrier oil, such as almond, apricot, canola or jojoba oil, before applying them. Essential oils are highly concentrated - sometimes as much as 100 times stronger than the fresh or dried plant. Even one drop of pure essential oil applied directly to your skin may cause irritation.
- Uncap the bottle for a few seconds only. Drop oils into the palm of your hand or a clean container for blending. Keep bottles tightly capped and away from sunlight and heat when not in use.
- Follow the directions for aromatherapy blends carefully. Never add more than the recommended number of drops. When using essential oils on infants or children, dilute them.
- Use glass containers for all blends of essential oils. Oils can damage plastic containers.
- Do not shake essential oils. Just gently roll the bottle between your hands for a few minutes.
- Trust your nose. If you dislike the smell of a certain oil, don't use it.
- Inhale essential oils for short periods only; run a diffuser for only five to ten minutes at a time.
- If you experience any irritation, sensitivity, or reaction, discontinue use of the suspect oil.
- Never take essential oils internally, except as directed by a professional of medical aromatherapy.
- The essential oils and aromatherapy blends discussed in this book are safe for most people to use.

As always, people with certain medical conditions should be cautious. Some essential oils can trigger asthma attacks or epileptic seizures in susceptible people. Some can elevate or depress blood pressure. Consult a health care professional before using aromatherapy if you have any of these conditions. Essential oils can also counteract or diminish the effectiveness of homeopathic remedies. If you are using any homeopathic preparations, check with a homeopathic physician.

"Here first she bathes, and round
    her body pours
Soft oils of fragrance and ambrosial
showers,
The winds, perfumed, the balmy
    gale conveys.
Through heaven, through earth, and
    all the aerial ways."

_____ Homer

Optimal Healing After Surgery
Pre-Op & Post-Op Techniques
Strengthening Your Body For Surgery ❖ Accelerating Healing
Cleaning Out Drug Residues ❖ Getting Over The Side Effects

Orthodox medicine is at its best in a heroic role. It is crisis intervention technology that can stabilize an emergency condition, or arrest a life-threatening disease long enough to give the body an opportunity to fight and a chance to heal itself. But surgery and major medical treatments are always traumatic on the body. You can do much to strengthen your system, alleviate body stress, and increase your chances of rapid recovery and healing.

Starting 2 to 3 weeks before your scheduled surgery:

Strengthen your immune system and supply your body with healing nutrients. Include daily:
- A high vegetable protein diet. *You must have protein to heal.* Eat brown rice and other whole grains.
- Vitamin C 3000mg with bioflavonoids and rutin for tissue integrity.
- B Complex 100mg with pantothenic acid 500mg for adrenal strength.
- A multivitamin/mineral with anti-oxidants, beta-carotene, zinc, calcium and magnesium for tissue repair.
- Take a full spectrum, pre-digested amino acid compound drink, about 1000mg daily.
- OPCs, pycnogenol or grape seed, 50mg 2x daily, as powerful antioxidants.
- Garlic capsules, 4-6 daily, a natural antibiotic that enhances immune function.

Strengthen your ability to heal. Include daily:
- Bromelain 750mg twice daily (with Quercetin 250mg. if you expect inflammation).
- CoQ_{10}, 60mg 2x daily and/or germanium 150mg. capsules, 2x daily - free radical destroyers
- Sun CHLORELLA 15 tablets, 1 packet of powder, or Crystal Star ENERGY GREEN™ drink.
- Centella asiatica capsules 2 caps 2x daily for nerve tissue strength.
- Crystal Star GINSENG SIX SUPER™ tea, 2x daily.
- Vitamin K for blood clotting. Food sources: leafy greens and blackstrap molasses, alfalfa sprouts.
- Take a potassium juice (page 167), potassium supplement liquid, and/or a protein drink daily.

Note 1: because the medical community uses information and testing results from synthetic, rather than naturally-occurring vitamin E sources, such as wheat germ and soy, many doctors insist that no vitamin E be taken four weeks prior to surgery in an effort to curb powdered ginger to relieve nausea and vomiting. post-operative bleeding. We have not found this to be the case with natural vitamin E, but suggest that you consult your physician if you are in doubt.

Note 2: prior to surgery, take 1gm. powdered ginger helps relieve nausea and vomiting

Herbal combinations can contribute a great deal to the success of surgical procedures offering nurturing, normalizing nutrients to support the healing process.

Here are some system-healing-specific areas that herbs can help:
- Cardiovascular System/Blood Vessels - hawthorn, garlic and ginkgo
- Respiratory System - mullein and coltsfoot
- Digestive System - chamomile and lemon balm
- Glandular System - panax ginseng
- Bowel/Urinary System - corn silk for the bladder; yellow dock for the bowel.
- Reproductive System - Women: black cohosh, false unicorn root. Men: saw palmetto and damiana.
- Nervous System - oats and St. John's wort.
- Musculo-Skeletal System - aloe vera, oatstraw, sarsaparilla
- Skin - cleavers, nettles, and red clover; and calendula, St. John's wort oil or cream for scarring.
- Immune System - nettles, cleavers, red clover.
- Drug and Liver detoxification - milk thistle seed.

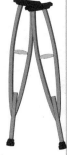

When you return home:

Eat a very nutritious diet. Include frequently:

- AloeLife ALOE GOLD drink, one 8-oz. glass daily.
- A potassium broth (page 167), vegetable drink (page 168), or hot tonic (page 170).
- A protein drink such as Nature's Life SUPERGREEN PRO 96, or Nutri-Tech ALL ONE multi drink.
- Plenty of fresh fruits and vegetables. *Have a green salad every day.*
- Organ meats and/or sea vegetables for vitamin B$_{12}$ and new cell growth.
- Brown rice and other whole grains with tofu for protein complementarity and more B vitamins.
- Yogurt and other cultured foods for friendly intestinal flora.

Some foods interfere with medications. Dairy products and iron supplements interfere with some antibiotics. Acid fruits (oranges, pineapples and grapefruit) may inhibit the action of penicillin and aspirin. Avocados, bananas, cheese, chocolate, colas and fermented foods interfere with monoamine oxidase (MAO), a drug used for depression and hypertension. Avoid fatty foods before and after surgery; they slow nutrient assimilation.

Clean the body and vital organs, to counteract infection. Include daily for one month:

- High potency, multi-culture compound such as DOCTOR DOPHILUS, or Natren TRINITY with meals.
- Crystal Star LIV-ALIVE™ capsules, tea or extract.
- Crystal Star GINSENG/REISHI MUSHROOM extract to overcome toxicity and provide deep body tone.
- Bovine cartilage capsules, 6 daily, or colloidal silver, 1 teasp. for 1 week, then $^1/_2$ teasp., to fight infection.
- Enzyme therapy such as Rainbow Light DETOX-ZYME or Prevail VITASE.
- Fresh carrot juice, or one can of BE WELL juice daily.

Build up the body tissues. Include daily for one month:

- Futurebiotics VITAL K or other food source absorbable potassium liquid.
- Crystal Star SYSTEMS STRENGTH™ drink, and/or BODY REBUILDER™ with ADR-ACTIVE™ capsules.
- Vitamin C with bioflavonoids and rutin 500mg only, with pantothenic acid 1000mg.
- Carnitine 250mg with CoQ$_{10}$, 60mg 3x daily as antioxidants.
- Zinc 30-50mg or Flora VEGE-SIL to help rebuild tissue.
- Co-enzymate B complex sublingual, 1 tablet 3x daily, or Nature's Bounty B$_{12}$ INTERNASAL GEL.
- Enzymatic Therapy LIQUID LIVER capsules, or Crystal Star CHLORELLA /GINSENG extract.
- AloeLife ALOE SKIN GEL or Crystal Star ANTI-BIO™ gel to heal skin and scars.

Other recovery and recuperation information:

- If you are taking antibiotics, take them with bromelain for better effectiveness, and supplement with B Complex, Vitamin C, Vitamin K and calcium.
- If you are taking diuretics, add Vitamin C, potassium and B complex, to strengthen kidneys.
- If you are taking aspirin, take with vitamin C for best results.
- If you are taking antacids, supplement with Vitamin B$_1$ and/or calcium.
- If your surgery involved bone and cartilage, take Crystal Star MINERAL SPECTRUM™ capsules 4 daily.
- If you smoke, add Vitamin C 500mg, E 400IU, beta-carotene 50,000IU and niacin 100mg.
- If you are considering chelation therapy, remember that it works in your body like a magnet collecting heavy metals and triglycerides. It is not recommended if you have weak kidneys; too many toxins are dumped into the elimination system too fast, putting unneeded stress on a healing body. Consider FORMULA 1 by Golden Pride.

Normalizing The Body After Chemotherapy & Radiation

Chemotherapy and radiation treatments are widely used by the orthodox medicine for several types, stages and degrees of cancerous growth. While some partial successes have been proven, the effects of both treatments are often worse than the disease in terms of healthy cell damage, body imbalance, and reduced immunity. Doctors and therapists recognize the drawbacks to chemotherapy, but under current government and insurance restrictions, neither they nor their patients have alternatives.

Only surgery, chemotherapy, radiation and a few extremely strong drugs are approved by the FDA in the United States for malignant disease. The cost for these treatments is beyond the financial range of most people, who, along with physicians and hospitals must rely on health insurance to pay the expense. Medical insurance will not reimburse doctors or hospitals if they use other healing methods. Thus, exorbitant medical costs and special interest regulations have bound medical professionals, hospitals, and insurance companies in a vicious circle where no alternative or new measures may be used to control cancerous growth. Everyone, including the patient, is caught in a political web where it all comes down to money instead of health. This is doubly unfortunate, since there is advanced research and health care choice easily available in Europe and other countries to which Americans are denied access.

Scientists admit that current treatments have been pushed to their limits. But new testing and research are extremely expensive. The vast majority of the funds provided by the National Cancer Act support research to improve the effectiveness of *existing* therapies - radiation, surgery and chemotherapy. This practice is easier and cheaper, but it leaves patients with the same three therapies, just a more precise use of them. Even when a new treatment is substantiated, there is no reasonable investment certainty that government (and therefore health insurance) approval can be obtained through the maze of red tape and politics.

Some of this is changing as cancer patients refuse to become victims of their medical system as well as the disease. The American people are demanding access, funding and insurance approval for alternative health techniques and medicines. Slowly, state by state, especially in the western states, legislators and regulators are listening, health care parameters are expanding, and insurance limitations are becoming more inclusive.

Conventional medicine rarely treats cancer as a systemic illness, defining it only by location and symptomology. It's the way lab science and left brain thinking work, breaking everything down into one-for-one causes and effects, assaying, isolating, identifying.... and as a consequence, hardly ever looking at the whole person or the whole picture.

By contrast, alternative healers regard cancer as an unhealthy body whose defenses can no longer destroy abnormal cells. Most naturopaths believe that a healthy body with strong immune response does not develop cancer, and that cancer is a reflection of the body as a whole rather than a localized disease in one particular part. Alternative therapists seek to strengthen the immune system of the cancer patient, and generally shun highly toxic modalities, such as radiation and chemotherapy. Instead, they employ a multifaceted, non-toxic approach, incorporating treatments which rely on bio-chemistry, metabolic, nutritional, and herbal therapies, and immune enhancement.

☿

HELP YOUR BODY MINIMIZE DAMAGE, AND REBUILD ITS STRENGTH AFTER CHEMOTHERAPY AND RADIATION.
For three months after chemotherapy or radiation, take the following daily:
- Crystal Star SYSTEMS STRENGTH™ broth daily - 1 TB. in hot water.
- CoQ$_{10}$ capsules, 60mg 3x daily, and/or germanium 150mg daily.
- Vitamin C crystals with bioflavonoids, $1/4$ teasp. in liquid every hour, about 5 to 10,000 mg daily.
- GINSENG/REISHI MUSHROOM extract 2x daily, or 2 cups Crystal Star GINSENG 6 SUPER™ TEA.
- 800mcg folic acid daily to normalize DNA synthesis, especially if methotrexate has been used in your treatment. (Ask your doctor.)
- An herbal anti-inflammatory as needed for swelling - turmeric (curcumin), or Crystal Star ANTI-FLAM™.
- HAWTHORN or GINKGO BILOBA extract, 30 drops daily under the tongue as a circulatory tonic.
- A liver support and strength capsule or tea, such as Crystal Star LIV-ALIVE™ tea or capsules.
- Floradix HERBAL IRON, 1 teasp. 3x daily, or Crystal Star ENERGY GREEN™ drink.
- Aloe vera concentrate, like Aloe Life ALOE GOLD for detoxification and to ease nausea.
- Keep your diet about 60 percent fresh foods for the first month after chemotherapy.
- Co-enzymate B complex sublingual, 1 tablet 3x daily for hair regrowth.
- Exercise with a morning sun walk and some stretches on rising and retiring.
- Practice good relaxation techniques so that you stay optimistic and cheerful.

Section Two

HERBS HAVE A UNIQUE HEALING SPIRIT

AMERICANS ARE REDISCOVERING HERBAL HEALING WITH ENTHUSIASM. USING HERBS FOR HEALING BRINGS US BACK TO ONE OF THE BASICS OF LIFE. HERBS GIVE YOU RESPECT FOR THE WONDERS OF OUR PLANET. THEY ARE HIGHLY COMPLEX, INTELLIGENT PLANTS....LIVING MEDICINES....ONE OF THE POWERS OF THE UNIVERSE.

Herbal healing exemplifies universal truth at its highest level. It is both a science and an art, with qualities we would all like to represent, and the ones we value most in ourselves. In a very grasping world, they are always giving. They show us how health care ought to be....conscious of the whole person, easy to use, gentle, safe, inexpensive, always available, and able to handle any problem.

Herbs work better together than they do by themselves, and they bring people together because they help us care for each other.

Herbal medicines are products for problems. They can be used in the first line of defense against disease. I find that except for emergency or life-threatening situations, herbs deserve a place in your primary care for healing.

Herbs work integrally with each person's body. Each of us can draw from an herb's wonderful complexity the properties we need in order to heal.

Although herbs respond to scientific methods, they are much more than a scientific, or even a natural healing system. Their healing work goes on automatically, whether it is analyzed or not. Our bodies know how to use the body balancing nutrients of herbs without our brains having to know why.

Like all great realities of nature, there is so much more than we shall ever know.

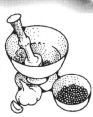

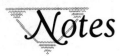

Notes

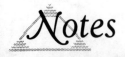

Notes

Herbal Healing Today

Medical science is changing fast. How does the tradition of herbal healing fit in? Herbal medicines have been meeting people's medical needs for thousands of years. Clearly, American consumers are increasing their use of herbs as natural complements to drugs and drugstore medicines.

In many ways in America, and indeed around the world, we are in a time of paradigm shift....especially in the global approach to healing. As our world grows undeniably smaller, people are interacting more, and changing long-held beliefs.

We are coming to see the Earth as an intelligent being, evolving and growing. Mankind is also evolving and growing. Unfortunately pathogenic organisms that cause disease, are changing, too - often replicating at enormous rates. Both organisms and diseases are becoming more virulent, and our immune defenses are becoming weaker.

The latest scientific drugs aren't the answer. In fact, it seems that new drugs are becoming less effective against pathogens like powerful viruses, instead of more effective. Recent research shows that even the newest, most powerful antibiotics hardly survive a year before the microbe they were designed to arrest, develops, mutates and grows stronger against them.
It's a good example of a non-living agent like a drug trying to control a living thing.

While we must be respectful of all ways of healing, most of us don't realize we have a choice. All the advances made by modern medicine still don't address chronic diseases or disease prevention very well.

I call today's allopathic medicine "heroic medicine" because it was developed largely in wartime for wartime emergencies. But this type of medicine often hits the body with a heavy hammer, preventing it from being able to rebuild against slow-growing, degenerative diseases. Nor can drugs help the body by stimulating its immune response. In fact, most drugs, and all surgeries, create body trauma along with their corrective benefits.

Immune strength is where natural, complementary medicines, like herbs and homeopathic compounds are important. Each of us is so individual; our healing supports need to be able to work with us in our own way for permanent health. Natural remedies involve the cooperation of our own bodies in the healing that takes place. Herbs let your body do its own work better.

Herbal medicines are part of a larger picture, because they are worldwide, alive, big enough and intelligent enough to grow along with us.

I have long believed that herbs are a path to the universe - an eye of the needle through which we can glimpse the wonders of creation and what it's really all about. God shows us his face in herbs, because they seem almost miraculous in their benefits to mankind.

HERBS CAN PERHAPS POINT OUT A PATH FOR US ON HOW WE MIGHT GROW AND CHANGE IN A BIG WORLD THAT IS BECOMING A GLOBAL VILLAGE. WE KNOW WE CAN COUNT ON THE SAFETY AND EFFICACY OF HERBS IN WAYS THAT THE LATEST DRUG CAN NEVER ACHIEVE. WE KNOW THAT THEY REACH OUT TO US WITH THEIR MARVELOUS COMPLEXITY AND ABILITIES TO HELP US ADDRESS THE HEALTH PROBLEMS OF TODAY, JUST AS THEY ADDRESSED ANCIENT ONES. HERBS MAY BE OUR BEST HOPE TO BRING THE BALANCE BACK BETWEEN THE HEALING FORCES AND DISEASES.

Herbs are without a doubt...UNIVERSAL. They do not discriminate, but embrace humans of all sorts and animals of all kinds, with their benefits. While it seems, on a day-to-day basis that we are hopelessly divided - in the end we are all one. Our hopes and dreams are the same.

Herbs help us care for each other. They grow eyes on our hearts.
Today, in the natural healing world, I see an astonishing thing happening. Herbs may indeed be a force to bring us together. We may be able to use the diverse, world-wide herbal healing knowledge for the good of us all.

Herbal medicines of the old traditions, such as the Ayurvedic philosophy, Native American herbs and rainforest medicines, long thought to work only for the people of their own cultures, are beginning to be used by grateful people everywhere. Even the strong tribal traditions, once so entirely separate, are sharing and combining their knowledge and their herbs.

 Integration is most seen in herbal formulas rather than in the ancient traditional practices....in the way they are being combined, and how they are being used. Rainforest culture herbs and Native American formulas are good examples.

We in the West are learning how to use time-honored Ayurvedic herbs, both in combination with our own herbs, and for our own health problems.

The West is also beginning to use Chinese and Rainforest herbs successfully for Western diseases, even though the healing tradition that originally used them comes from a different viewpoint.

Native American cleansing herbs and techniques such as herbal smudging and therapeutic sweating are also being used to help relieve modern pollution problems.

On a recent trip to the Orient, I could see that herbal ideas and formulas are going both ways, as Western herbs flow east to Oriental healers.

If man, an intelligent being, is changing, might not herbs, intelligent plants, be changing, too?
Herbs are so highly complex. And filled with such long memory. They have intelligently adapted to the Earth's changes as we have, and over the millennia, they have always interacted with man.
Perhaps they are moving along the universal continuum with us.... always available for us, with a highly complex structure able to match our own increasing complexity of need.

The following pages contain a short review of the world's great healing philosophies; how they work, and how they can better help us to understand and use herbal medicine today.

Tucked away in a quiet corner of every life are wounds and scars.

If they were not there, we would not need Healers.

Nor would we need one another.

Traditional Chinese Medicine

Traditional Chinese herbal medicine has a 5,000 year legacy. From its earliest history, Chinese medicine has been bound up with nature - the earth and sea, the seasons and climate, plants and animals. Because of the strongly held Chinese belief that the human body is a microcosm of the grand cosmic order, and the forces at work in man are the same as those of the universe, all the elements of the earth are significant in traditional Chinese healing. Unity with nature is actually a belief held throughout all civilizations in the history of the world, right up to the time of modern, scientific thought, which sees everything as separate and unrelated, instead of all one.

The basic premise of Chinese herbal medicine revolves around the belief in an essential life-force, called qi. Qi (pronounced "chee") is an ineffable, but vital energy in all things, including man. The food and drink we consume and the air we breathe are the most important factors for human qi. Digestion and breathing extract qi from food and air and transfer it to the body. When these two forms of qi meet in the bloodstream, they make human-qi, which circulates through the body as vital energy. The quality, quantity and harmonious balance of your qi determines your state of health and span of life.

Conditions which can upset the balance of qi are climatic factors, emotions, phlegm congestion and stagnant blood. Because variables that affect qi, like the weather and seasonal changes are not controlled by man, paramount importance is placed on diet and breathing exercises, variables that man *can* control.

Qi is further affected by the condition of the organs which absorb it. If the stomach and lungs are not functioning properly, they cannot extract and absorb the qi's vital energy in sufficient quantity, so the entire body suffers. When a person becomes ill, Chinese herbal doctors first look to the patient's lifestyle and habits for things that might affect qi. Many qi-deficient conditions can be corrected with the powerful tools of lifestyle, breathing and hygiene changes.

Demystifying Chinese herbs by learning and understanding how the herbs are used, gives us new opportunities to obtain more healing tools. Chinese herbal healers learn largely from empirical observation, with little faith in rigid systems drawn from abstract theories, like those we have in the West. They look to observation by sight, hearing and smell, to touch and to questioning the patient for diagnosis confirmation. Disease is viewed as an imbalance of two opposing energies, yin and yang, in the major body systems. Disease factors fit into conformations and stages for better understanding and control.

Chinese herbal medicine also recognizes qi as an important part of medicinal plants. Herbs are thought to possess specific parallel characteristics with humans. The qi energy of certain herbs has a natural affinity for certain parts of the human body and the ability to work effectively with them to restore vital energy. Body balance is the goal as natural functions are steered back toward the direction of harmony. Chinese herbal treatment always works with the opposite herb characteristic to the human problem. For example, a fever is treated with cooling herbs, a cold is treated with heating herbs.

Modern drugs treat "excess syndromes," usually having the effect of inhibiting a physiologic function. Chinese herb formulas resolve "deficiency syndromes," by promoting physiologic functions.

Although most of the bio-chemical constituents of Chinese herbs have long been known, the real healing ability of an herbal medicine depends on the integration and complexity of its components. A prescription for a Chinese remedy may contain four to twelve herbs, or more. The complex aspects of the formulas make them hard to understand for the Westerner, used to the "one solution for one problem" principle. But traditional Chinese herbal formulas aim for broad spectrum healing and normalizing results - to balance hormones, regulate blood components, enhance immune function, reduce inflammation and improve digestion.

Ayurveda

Ayurveda, "the science of life," is considered the world's most ancient existing medical system. Practiced for 6,000 years, it is even older than traditional Chinese herbalism. Originating on the Indian sub- continent, Ayurveda is a holistic tradition that emphasizes body-mind synergy and spiritual health. It has been called the first form of preventive medicine. It is a science for those who want to optimize energy and develop greater powers of awareness as well as for those who are ill.

As in Chinese medicine, Ayurveda believes in universal life energy force, called qi in Chinese and prana in Ayurveda. The force is expressed in bi-polar terms, yin-yang in Chinese medicine, and Shiva-shakti in Ayurveda. Diseases, medicinal herbs, diet elements and therapies are also classified bi-polarly, into "warm or cool," and "strong or weak," etc. Still widely practiced in India, Ayurveda is enjoying a strong revival in the West.

Its chief aim is longevity and a rejuvenative quality of life, by optimizing energy balance and the body's own self-repair mechanisms. Its method of healing seeks mind/body harmony, and involves detoxification, diet, natural therapies and herbs dependent on body type. An Ayurvedic treatment usually includes music, yoga, herbs, massage, steams, facials and aromatherapy.

Ayurveda is a highly personalized system; each individual's health requirements are seen as unique and ever changing. Healing is accomplished by determining the balance of energy patterns that exist in each person's nature, along with the specific imbalances that arise due to time and circumstances, like the effects of age, climate or lifestyle.

But, Ayurvedic medicine is much more than just a reaction to disease using natural remedies. It stresses disease prevention through health-promoting substances, and includes many elements that address emotional, intellectual and spiritual well-being as well as physical health.

THE KEY ELEMENTS OF AYURVEDA INCLUDE THE FOLLOWING:

1 **Body Typing according to the tridosha** is the most fundamental principal of Ayurvedic healing. Ayurveda considers that each person is a unique balance of physical, emotional, spiritual and mental traits called doshas, expressed in three great elements - water (Kapha), fire (Pitta), and air (Vata). Each dosha regulates many functions in the mind-body system, and most people are not just one type, but have elements of each, (usually one of the doshas predominates at birth). Changes in the doshas occur with age and season, keeping the balance of the three factors dynamic, and a person's overall health is thought to hinge on the interrelationships and transformations of these three forces by the food, water, sunlight and air that he or she takes in. Disease results when the balance of one or more dosha is disturbed - one's dominant dosha being the one that most often becomes unbalanced.

Here is a short summary of how the different doshas work:

• **Vata** represents the elements of space and air, controlling any form of movement in the body including blood circulation, digestion, breathing, the movement of nerve impulses, etc. Vata people are usually taller or shorter than average, thin in build, and have difficulty holding weight. They tend to run dry and cold, with high activity but low stamina. Digestion and metabolism are average. They are mentally creative, restless, nervous and moody. They are most affected by fear and anxiety; their greatest strength is quick response and adaptability.

• **Pitta** represents the elements of water and fire, governing metabolism and biochemical processes responsible for the transformation of food, air, and water into the body physiology. Pitta types are usually average in build, with ruddy, bright or lustrous complexions. They possess strong appetites, good digestion and circulation, and generally run warmer than other people. Mentally they are intelligent, sharp, aggressive and ambitious. They are prone to anger and irritability; their strength is courage and fearlessness.

• **Kapha** represents the elements of earth and water, influencing the formation and structure of tissues, muscles, bones, and sinews. Kapha individuals are usually large-boned and stockier than average. They put on weight easily, have slow digestion and metabolism, and are also slower but steadier in their movements and responses. Psychologically they are prone to attachment; their strength is calm, contentment and stability.

[2] **Herbal Therapy** - Ayurvedic herbal formulas are known for their rejuvenative powers. Much of its vast, documented herbal legacy has been scientifically validated. The drugs reserpine for hypertension, digitalis for heart stimulation, and aloe vera all stem from Ayurvedic treatments. New research is being conducted on herbal formulas for tumor reduction, and on anti-inflammatory compounds such as Boswellia for arthritis. Gum Guggul extract is widely recognized for controlling weight and cholesterol levels.

As in Chinese medicine, the aim is always body balance for Ayurveda, which believes that people are prone to the diseases that are the same nature as their predominant element, which tends to be too high. Air-types usually suffer from nervousness, pain or bone diseases; fire-types suffer from fever, infection and blood disorders involving an increase in body heat; water-types develop congestive disorders with an excess of watery mucus. Herbal formulas are prescribed to balance body types, rather than just making use of the properties of the herb.

SOME WELL-KNOWN AYURVEDIC HERBALS:
- *Triphala* - a laxative formula consisting of the fruit of three tropical trees is one of the best aids for restoring the tone of the colon. It is less likely than other herbal laxatives to cause dependency.
- *Guggul* - a resin like myrrh, is used for coronary heart disease because of recent scientific research showing its value in reducing cholesterol. It is also widely used for arthritis, diabetes, and for chronic fevers.
- *Ashwagandha* - "Indian ginseng," is used to reduce anxiety, give strength, and improve sexual function. Although energizing, ashwagandha also helps promote sleep, calming the nerves.
- *Gotu Kola* - an Ayurvedic nervine counters nerve pain, clears the senses, combats negative emotions, cleanses the liver, and removes toxins from the blood. It is an important aid to mental clarity and calm.
- *Chyavan Prash* - an herbal jelly based on the Amla fruit, the highest natural source of vitamin C, strengthens the blood and counters debility. It is recommended for all types as a general tonic.

[3] **Diet** - Ayurveda recommends a highly nutritive, vegetarian diet, including whole grains, beans, cooked vegetables, nuts and dairy products, with combinations of spices like Indian curries. It does not recommend raw food diets except for periods of body cleansing. Foods are classified by their effects on the doshas, and diets are tailored to the patient's body type and individual imbalances. Diet is thought to be a major means of affecting body balance, so the eating atmosphere should be peaceful and the menu balanced. One should eat only when the previous meal has been completely digested, and rest briefly after the meal. Iced foods and drinks should be avoided.
- **Vata**, air-types, need heavier, richer foods predominating in sweet, sour and salty tastes, with more nuts and dairy products, and grains like wheat and oats, along with spices to insure proper digestion.
- **Pitta**, fire-types require cooling foods predominating in sweet, bitter and astringent tastes, including some raw food, and limiting the amount of salt, spices and sour articles in the diet.
- **Kapha**, water-types do best with a light diet dominant in pungent, bitter and astringent tastes, using a lot of spices, and many vegetables, but avoiding sugar, dairy, nuts and oily food.

[4] **Behavior and Lifestyle** - patients are asked to follow daily and seasonal routines that will help them better integrate with the biological rhythms of nature. An Ayurvedic physician may prescribe panchakarma, a program, of herbal steam treatment, internal purification therapies and oil massages.

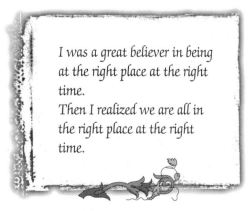

I was a great believer in being at the right place at the right time.
Then I realized we are all in the right place at the right time.

Native American Herbalism

Native Americans have always lived close to nature, and from earliest times have relied on its healing plants. Indeed, Native Americans were almost disease-free before the arrival of the Europeans. They had a firm understanding of the science of illness, and many of their traditional medical practices were as good as or better than those of their European counterparts.

Native Americans had a keen knowledge of anatomy; they practiced personal hygiene and sophisticated childbirth methods, understood the antiseptic value of plant juices and oils, tied off arteries to prevent blood loss, pulled teeth, and used complex pain killers. Health care was a normal part of life, and all family members were taught first aid techniques and how to cure common ailments from herbs stored at home. If these were not enough, tribal healers, who had a greater knowledge of plant medicines and supernatural powers, could be easily accessed as specialists to deal with life-threatening emergencies and serious problems, including advanced psychotherapy. Even today, Native American healing techniques have a strong spiritual component that strengthens people so they can face the travail of their sickness.

Native Americans had no word for medicine as we know it. To them, medicine involved a whole array of healing ideas and sensations, not just remedies. The general concern in medical matters was, of course, for the health and well-being of individuals or groups of individuals, but it was believed that health was a gift from the supernatural powers, and an outcome of correct living.

In contrast to the sharp Euro-American division between medicine and religion, Native Americans believed that health was holistic, and that well-being, medicine, and religion were all intertwined. They understood that everything depended on everything else, and felt that living and non-living environments flowed together in a giant circle supported and connected by a spirit world. Native American medicine is often symbolized by large, round medicine wheels or sacred circles.

Medicine men and women, though called "healers" were really shaman healers. They were powerful figures, intermediaries between man and the forces of nature. They cured the sick, controlled the weather, foretold the future, could bring success in war and hunting, communicated with and received news about those who were far away, found and restored those who were lost or captured by enemies, overthrew witches and evil spirits, and publicly demonstrated their powers in awe-inspiring ways.

In fact, Native American healing practices were so closely bound to spiritual beliefs that treatment of physical symptoms was never isolated from the spirituality of the patient. Herbs were used to treat specific body ailments but were seldom considered effective without ceremonies for spirits.

Many drugs we commonly use today came from our Native Americans heritage. Their contribution to present-day medicines includes salicin (the major ingredient in aspirin), syrup of ipecac (an emetic), quinine, morphine, curare, cocaine, atropine, scopolamine, hyoscyamine, and hundreds of lesser-known drugs that have been chemically duplicated and are now on drugstore shelves.

Most herbal healing compounds were quite complex and far-reaching...in order to address many parts of a problem, both its cause and effect. A Stomach Tea, from the famous Chief Two Moons Meridas for example, had thirteen herbs: *senna, coriander seed, gentian root, juniper berry, centaury, calamus root, buckthorn bark, ginger, cascara sagrada, pale rose buds, anise seed, lavender flowers, and fennel seed.*

His Female Tea contained *squaw vine, motherwort, chamomile, cramp bark, uva ursi, ginger, helonias root, celery seed, aletris, Mexican saffron, cascara sagrada, cornflowers, and black haw bark.*

His Rheumatism Tea used eleven herbs: *wintergreen, yellow dock, black cohosh, uva ursi, birch bark, bittersweet twigs, cascara bark, buckbean, coriander seed, burdock root, and buchu leaves.*

And his Tonic Tea contained fourteen herbs: *fennel seed, dandelion root, licorice root, sarsaparilla, senna leaves, cascara sagrada, sassafras bark, clover tops, juniper berries, chamomile, Mexican saffron, elder flowers, blue malva flowers, and calendula flowers.*

Today, modern herbalists are turning to many of these time-honored formulas.

Rainforest Herbal Healing
THE NEW SCIENCE OF ETHNOBOTANY

The last 20 years have witnessed a remarkable rediscovery in the West of plants as a source of pharmaceuticals. Interest started as a grassroots movement, with a huge rise in demand for herbal remedies in Europe and the Americas.... a demand that changed the focus of drug companies almost overnight. Today, over half of the top 250 pharmaceutical companies in the world have active research programs investigating the plant world for potential new drugs, compared with almost none 15 years ago.

The search for powerful medicinal plants has centered on the rainforests, where approximately one-half of the world's flowering plant species live. The rainforests of Central America are preeminent because they contain such a vast plant pharmacopoeia. To western medical science, the rainforest is a treasure box just beginning to be opened. The huge variety and many delivery systems of rainforest plants are still a great mystery for orthodox medicine. But both western herbalists and medical science are beginning to see that living medicines from rainforest herbs is one of the best answers for true, non-invasive healing. Rainforest herbs are so rich that often 6 or 7 biochemical drugs can be extracted from just one plant!

Yet rainforest conservation remains a critical issue. As more and more rainforests, the "Earth's lungs," are destroyed for economic development, everyone realizes that the health of the entire planet, and all its inhabitants is at risk. Many native medicines have already been wiped out, and native healers are aware that their heritage is threatened, both by the erosion of their own cultural traditions, and by the destructive environmental threat. Once again, education and information are the keys.

Understanding life in the rainforest and its relationship with humans is crucial to its preservation, *and to the health of over 80% of the world's population,* which still depends on plants for primary health care.

HOW CAN THE ETHNOBOTANICAL APPROACH HELP ALL SIDES?

Ethnobotany, the study of how native peoples use plants, is a complex mixture of sociology, anthropology, botany, ecology, and medicine. Western scientists are often amazed at the pharmacological knowledge of indigenous peoples. Traditional Shamanic medicine is more than just folklore and superstition. It is one the oldest forms of healing through mind/body communication. Shaman healers have been able for centuries to treat illnesses from colds to cancer.

Shamanic healers have incredible knowledge of the rainforest's ecosystem. When they discovered a remedy, it usually worked extremely well, and remained an integral part of their healing tradition for hundreds of years. The remedy was not tainted by the financial forces of modern medicine, nor was it subject to a constantly changing belief system like ours. While this profound knowledge is still largely unknown to modern science, some wise traditional healers are starting to educate doctors, pharmacists and botanists from around the world in an effort to benefit, perhaps even save, humanity.

Everyone feels that time is running out. We must shorten the period required to make a botanical drug available. Western drug research takes a decade or more to reach the market. We must honor and respect native healers who have known the plants intimately for centuries. If traditional rainforest healers agree to share their vast knowledge with western ethnobotanists, not only can understanding about the healing properties of various plants be increased, but an enormous amount of time can be saved without the trial and error method of mass screenings. The shaman's information, in effect, "prescreens" the plants, enabling identification of the best drug candidates without time-consuming random collection. Rainforest peoples will benefit as well, because their healing plants will become more economically valuable than real estate development. Everybody wins, including the rainforest and the planet.

Herbal Healing In Europe & The West

The medical path of Western Herbal Medicine has been a twisted one - influenced by religion, kicked around by warring politics, distorted by conflicting philosophies, and controlled by vested interests. Today, some truths stand firm, and the ageless wisdom behind many old remedies has withstood the tests of time. But many medical policies are still supported by politics and power. Although we think the great conflict of orthodox and alternative medicine is recent, the struggle between the two has been long and bloody.

WESTERN HERBALISM SEEMS ALWAYS TO HAVE BEEN BOUND UP WITH SCIENCE.

Hippocrates, a physician of Greece's Golden Age, stood at the beginning of western medicine as we know it. His system of medicine had one foot in scientific reason and the other in the power of Nature. Hippocrates theorized that the human body had four humors; blood, phlegm, yellow bile (choler), and black bile, and that illness resulted when one humor was out of balance with another. He believed that the healing resources of nature were all-powerful, and that the task of the physician was to help the healing process along rather than to take it over. Hippocrates' beliefs continued in mainstream medicine until the late 19th century - 2,300 years after he propounded them.

Western medical herbalism first seems to have come from a surgeon in the Roman armies of Nero, Dioscorides, who compiled the medicinal knowledge of the day into a volume known as De Materia Medica, still considered the prototype of herbal and pharmacopoeia materia medicas.

In the second century A.D., Galen, another Greek physician, brought a classification system to Hippocrates' concept of the four humors, evaluating all plant remedies in terms of their reaction *with* the patient's humors. Once a physician diagnosed a humor imbalance, he needed only to prescribe the proper medication to counteract it. The key to healing in the west became diagnosis, and the fitting of every health problem into a classification box....as indeed it is today.

Galen favored elaborate medicines compounded of many different ingredients rather than simple infusions of two or three herbs. He believed that the more complex a remedy, the better it was bound to be. His philosophy became the cornerstone for an elaborate and rigid system of medicine, where only a doctor had healing knowledge. The concept of "heroic medicine," man, intervening in body processes to fight against and overcome a disease, began in Galen's time. Over the years, procedures were used with increasing intensity to "whip" an illness.

The 500 year period of Europe's Dark Ages wasn't dark at all for herbal healing. Great medical advances were introduced by the Arabs who brought both alchemy and the pharmacy into Western practice, along with numerous new ointments, elixirs, pills, tinctures, suppositories, purgatives, cathartics and inhalations. Indeed, from the 12th century on, apothecaries swept over Europe. In the mid-16th century, a famous doctor, Paracelsus, today seen as the founder of chemical pharmacology, taught that alchemy and chemistry together were a way to unlock the secrets of Nature's healing plants. Paracelsus began the distillation of isolates - extracting the so-called "active principle" of the plant - claiming that the process was more potent and effective than the whole plant while still remaining safe. Both the alchemists of his day, and the chemists of ours, adhere to this belief. Even though pharmacies have been proven wrong on the safety of isolates more times than not, isolates remain popular with pharmaceutical companies because their manufacture can be patented and rigorously controlled.

As early as the 17th century, the battle began over-using costly, imported drugs rather than local plant remedies. Nicholas Culpeper, an English apothecary, tiring of the fact that virtually all plant medicines that existed in England were imported, created his own herbal handbook, the ENGLISH PHYSICIAN, in the 1650's. It became a popular herbal text then and is still popular today. (In 1990, there were some 42 different current editions on record.) Culpeper detailed the practical use of herbs rather than the theoretical, and gave a big boost to herb usage in England.

American herbalism, like America itself, is a melting pot of European herbs and traditions, and Native American herbs and traditions, with an overlay of American science and technology. Native Americans employed a holistic approach to healing; the first European settlers learned much, with great gratitude for their traditions. Yet, early in our history, the influence of science started medical practices which became very specialized and steered away from natural healing.

The American colonies also relied heavily on imported medicines. By the 1800s, both American and European medical schools favored prescription medicines. Herbal medicine was not taught, nor was there room for nature's healing powers. Most doctors were also apothecaries, and drug sales were often the only way they could keep solvent.

The western medical debate raged on for almost a century, between alternative healers, who relied, as they do today, on the healing power of nature and years of empirical experience and observation, and orthodox doctors who proceeded from theory to practice without stopping to consider the real results. Because alternative or "irregular" doctors undertook to restore body balance through detoxification means like sweating, vomiting and elimination, they were called "puke and steam doctors."

However, the name calling stopped in 1805, when an epidemic swept through the region of an herbalist named Samuel Thompson. He sweated his patients and gave them herbal healing mixtures. Conventional doctors bled their patients and administered calomel a mercury derivative. **Thompson lost none of the patients that he attended. The conventional physicians lost over half of theirs to the epidemic.**

Amazing results like this turned the debate in favor of herbal medicines and natural healing. Both the concept of Homeopathy (see page 13), and the Eclectic movement were introduced during this time. Eclectic physicians believed that medicines should be gentle, should consist of the direct action of single drugs, uncombined with others, and that there should be no "heroic" shocks to the system, no violent cathartics, emetics or blisters. Eclectic chemists worked to ensure that medicines remained pure and they engaged in the most detailed botanical studies ever performed, putting the Eclectics on the cutting edge of herbal medicine for more than 50 years.

In response to the popularity of "irregular" medical schools and movements, particularly in response to the people's enthusiasm for the new homeopathic movement, mainstream conventional doctors formed the American Medical Association (AMA), in 1847. It soon became underwritten by the pharmaceutical companies, who had a great deal to gain from its philosophy, and the whole vast, expanding medical/pharmaceutical industry of the United States formally turned its back on the plant world and looked to synthetic chemicals as its future.

By the turn of the 20th century, overwhelmed by the advancing growth of the AMA, herbal medicine went into a predictable decline. Chemists learned to synthesize some active plant constituents in the laboratory, standardizing and sterilizing drug doses, and stabilizing supplies. Surgery advanced, along with the discovery of antibiotics, especially during the emergency needs of the World Wars.

Today, conventional medicine's greatest accomplishments are technical ones, involving incredibly sophisticated orthopedics, burn treatment, cesarean section, resuscitation, microsurgery to attach severed limbs, heart-valve replacements and extraordinary feats like open-heart surgery. But, there is another side to the coin. Even with the best of intentions, modern medical intervention produces an astonishing amount of dysfunction, disability, and pain. The most rapidly spreading epidemic of the twentieth century is iatrogenic, or drug/doctor-caused disease. *Its annual victims are more numerous than traffic and industrial accidents combined.*

Americans take $19 billion worth of drugs each year. An expensive river of chemicals courses through our national veins. Many of these drugs are dangerous; many are ineffective in curing the condition for which they were prescribed. More than one million people a year (almost 5% of hospital admissions) end up in needing hospital care as a result of bad reactions to drugs. It is now common knowledge that X-rays increase cancer risk. Radiation from diagnostic X-rays contributes to blood disorders, tumors, diabetes, stroke, and cataracts. (In some cases, where the tissue being X-rayed is very delicate, such as the breasts, fibroids have been found in as little as three months.) Yet over 300 million of X-rays are ordered yearly as standard procedure, even without a specific medical need.

There are basic belief systems in modern medicine that are at the root of some of its problems.

- That a disease must be "interrupted" by surgical intervention or by drugs to restore health.
- That dietary habits are not related to symptoms or illnesses... a belief that is changing, yet is still held by many (especially scientists who maintain that the body identifies and uses the nutrients it needs, regardless of the source).
- That the primary work must be arresting and dealing with symptoms instead of addressing the cause of the problem.

Western medicine must evolve to do more good and less harm. Alternative or holistic medicine has been re-discovered to meet this need. Holistic health recognizes that our individual body parts are components of an integrated physical being, who has social, emotional, and spiritual levels, and that body balance and function is affected by a variety of factors like food, drink, exercise, emotions, and stress.

Nothing about a human being works in a vacuum. A weakness in the heart may also express a weakness of the other organs; an infection in a finger may indicate a polluted condition throughout the body; and improved nutrition and tonifying the body regularly leads to the improvement of many different symptoms.

Where is herbal healing going from here?

The winds of change are blowing once more as we sit before the new millennium. There is clearly an enormous rebirth of interest in the ways of Nature and holistic healing.

It is not a new idea. As you can see from this short discussion of the world's herbal philosophies, the holistic approach is the prevalent one in all societies except our own. Western herbal thought has taken a detour through technology. Yet useful knowledge has surfaced that otherwise might not have been found. We live in a time when holistic medicine can be supported by scientific studies, and scientific analysis can be validated by its relevance to human lifestyles.

If we can put aside the greed and politics that surround modern health care, I believe we are at another beginning where modern medical technology and the holistic approach can come together for the good of mankind.

A Practical Guide For Using Herbs Safely

*H*erbal medicines have been meeting people's medical needs for thousands of years. Although today, we think of herbs as natural drugs, they are really foods with medicinal qualities. Because they combine with our bodies as foods do, they are able to address both the symptoms and causes of a problem. As nourishment, herbs can offer the body nutrients it does not always receive, either because of poor diet, or environmental deficiencies in the soil and air. As medicine, herbs are essentially body balancers, that work with the body functions, so that it can heal and regulate itself.

Herbs work like precision instruments in the body, not like sledge hammers.
Herbal medicines can be broad-based for over all support, or specific to a particular problem.

Herbs provide a rich variety of healing agents, and most herbs, as edible plants, are as safe to take as foods. They have almost no side effects. Occasionally a mild allergy-type reaction may occur as it might occur to a food. This could happen because an herb has been adulterated with chemicals in the growing or storing process, or in rare cases, because incompatible herbs were used together. Or it may be just an individual adverse response to a certain plant. The key to avoiding an adverse reaction is moderation, both in formulation and in dosage. Anything taken to excess can cause negative side effects. Common sense, care, and intelligence are needed when using herbs for either food or medicine.

TWO-THIRDS OF THE DRUGS ON THE AMERICAN MARKET TODAY ARE BASED ON MEDICINAL PLANTS.
But modern herb-based drugs are not herbs; they are chemicals. Even when a drug has been derived from an herb, it is so refined, isolated and purified that only a chemical formula remains. Chemicals work on the body much differently than herbs do. As drugs, they cause many effects - only some of which are positive. Eli Lilly, a pharmaceutical manufacturer, once said "a drug isn't a drug unless it has side effects."
Herbs in their whole form are not drugs. Do not expect the activity or response of a drug, which normally treats only the symptoms of a problem. In general, you have to take more and more of a drug to get continuing therapeutic effect.
Herbal medicines work differently. Herbs are foundation nutrients, working through the glands, nourishing the body's deepest, basic elements, such as the brain, glands and hormones. Results will seem to take much longer. But this fact only shows how herbs actually work, acting as support to control and reverse the cause of a problem, with more permanent effect. Even so, some improvement from herbal treatment can usually be felt in three to six days. Chronic or long standing problems take longer, but herbal remedies tend to work more quickly with each new infection, and cases of infections grow fewer and further between. A traditional rule of thumb is one month of healing for every year of the problem.

Herbal combinations are not addictive, but they are powerful nutritional agents that should be used with care. **Balance is the key to using herbs for healing.** Every person is different with different needs. It takes a little more attention and personal responsibility than mindlessly taking a prescription drug, but the extra care is worth far more in the results you can achieve for your well-being.

As with other natural therapies, there is sometimes a "healing crisis" in an herbal healing program. This is known as the "Law of Cure," and simply means that you seem to get worse before you get better. The body may eliminate toxic wastes heavily during the first stages of a cleansing therapy. This is particularly true in the traditional three to four day cleansing fast that many people use to begin a serious healing program. Temporary exacerbation of symptoms can range from mild to fairly severe, but usually precedes good results. Herbal therapy without a fast works more slowly and gently. Still, there is usually some weakness as disease poisons are released into the bloodstream to be flushed away. Strength shortly returns when this process is over. Watching this phenomenon allows you to observe your body at work healing itself.....an interesting experience indeed.

HERBS WORK BETTER IN COMBINATION THAN THEY DO SINGLY.
LIKE THE NOTES OF A SYMPHONY, HERBS WORK BETTER IN HARMONY THAN STANDING ALONE.

There are several reasons why herbs work better in combination:

•   Each formula contains two to five primary herbs for specific healing purposes. Since all body parts, and most disease symptoms, are interrelated, it is wise to have herbs which can affect each part of the problem. For example, in a prostate healing formula, there would be herbs to dissolve sediment, anti-inflammatory herbs, tissue-toning and strengthening herbs, and herbs with antibiotic properties.

•   A combination of herbal nutrients encourages body balance rather than a large supply of one or two focused properties. A combination works to gently stimulate the body as a whole.

•   A combination allows inclusion of herbs that can work at different stages of need. A good example of this is an athlete's formula, where there are herbs for short term energy, long range endurance, muscle tone, glycogen and glucose use, and reduction of lactic acid build-up.

•   A combination of several herbs with similar properties increases the latitude of effectiveness, not only through a wider range of activity, but also reinforcing herbs that were picked too late or too early, or grew in adverse weather conditions.

•   No two people, or their bodies, are alike. Good response is augmented by a combination of herbs.

•   Finally, certain herbs, such as capsicum, lobelia, sassafras, mandrake, tansy, Canada snake root, wormwood, woodruff, poke root, and rue are beneficial in small amounts and as catalysts, but should not be used alone.

Herbs work better when combined with a natural foods diet. Everyone can benefit from an herbal formula, but results increase dramatically when fresh foods and whole grains form the basis of your diet. Subtle healing activity is more effective when it doesn't have to labor through excess waste material, mucous, or junk food accumulation. (Many congested people carry around 10 to 15 pounds of excess density.)

Interestingly enough, herbs themselves can help counter the problems of "civilization foods." They are rich in minerals and trace minerals, the basic elements missing or diminished in today's "quick-grow," over-sprayed, over-fertilized farming. Minerals and trace minerals are a basic element in food assimilation. Mineral-rich herbs provide not only the healing essences to support the body in overcoming disease, but also the foundation minerals that allow it to take them in!

Each individual body has its own unique, wonderful mechanism, and each has the ability to bring itself to its own balanced and healthy state. Herbs simply pave the way for the body to do its own work, by breaking up toxins, cleansing, lubricating, toning and nourishing. They work through the glands at the deepest levels of the body processes - at the cause, rather than the effect.

HERBS PROMOTE THE ELIMINATION OF WASTE MATTER AND TOXINS FROM THE SYSTEM
BY SIMPLE NATURAL MEANS. THEY SUPPORT NATURE IN ITS FIGHT AGAINST DISEASE.

HERE'S HOW TO TAKE HERBS CORRECTLY FOR THE MOST BENEFIT:
Herbs are not like vitamins.
•   Herbs are not isolated substances. There value is in their wholeness and complexity, not their concentration.

Herbs should not be taken like vitamins.
•   Vitamins are usually taken on a maintenance basis to shore up nutrient deficiencies. Except for some food-grown vitamins, vitamins are partitioned substances. They do not combine with the body in the same way as

foods or herbs do, and excesses are normally flushed from the system. Herbs combine and work with the body's enzyme activity; they also contain food enzymes, and/or proteolytic enzymes themselves. They accumulate in and combine with the body.

• **Taking herbs all the time for maintenance and nutrient replacement would be like eating large quantities of a certain food all the time.** The body would tend to have imbalanced nourishment from nutrients that were not in that food. This is also true of multiple vitamins. They work best when strengthening a deficient or weak system, not as a continuing substitute for a good diet.

• However, certain very broad-spectrum "superfood" herbs like the green grasses, sea plants, algae and bee products, and adaptogen tonics like ginsengs can be taken for longer periods of body balancing.

• Vitamins work best when taken with food; it is not necessary to take herbal formulas with food.

• **Unlike vitamins, herbs provide their own digestive enzymes for the body to take them in.** In some cases, as in a formula for mental acuity, the herbs are more effective if taken when body pathways are clear, instead of concerned with food digestion.

THERAPEUTIC HERBS WORK BEST WHEN USED AS NEEDED.
DOSAGE SHOULD BE REDUCED AND DISCONTINUED AS THE PROBLEM IMPROVES.

Herbal effects can be quite specific; take the best formula for your particular goal at the right time - rather than all the time - for optimum results. In addition, rotating and alternating herbal combinations according to your changing health needs allows the body to remain most responsive to their effects. Reduce dosage as the problem improves. Allow the body to pick up its own work and bring its own vital forces into action. If you are taking an herbal remedy for more than a month, discontinue for one or two weeks between months to let your body adjust and maintain your personal balance.

Best results may be achieved by taking herbal capsule combinations in descending strength: 6 the first day, 5 the second day, 4 the third, 3 the fourth, 2 the fifth, and 2 the sixth for the first week. Rest on the 7th day. When a healing base is built in the body, decrease to the maintenance dose recommended for the formula. Most combinations should be taken no more than 6 days in a row.

Take only one or two herbal combinations at the same time. When working with herbs and natural healing methods, address your worst problem first. Take the herbal remedy for that problem - reducing dosage and alternating on and off weeks as necessary to allow the body to thoroughly use the herbal properties. One of the bonuses of a natural healing program is the frequent discovery that other conditions were really complications of the first problem, and often take care of themselves as the body comes into balance. ·

Herb effectiveness usually goes by body weight, especially for children. Child dosage is as follows:

$^1/_2$ *dose for children 10-14 years*　　　　$^1/_4$ *dose for children 2-6 years*
$^1/_3$ *dose for children 6-10 years*　　　　$^1/_8$ *dose for infants and babies*

Herbs are amazingly effective in strengthening the body's immune response. But the immune system is a fragile entity, and can be overwhelmed instead of stimulated. Even when a good healing program is working, and obvious improvement is being made, adding more of the medicinal agents in an effort to speed healing can aggravate symptoms. Even for serious health conditions, moderate amounts are the way to go, mega-doses are not. Much better results can be obtained by giving yourself more time and gentler treatment. It takes time to rebuild health.

Your Herbal Medicine Choices
Whole-Herb Healing or Standardized Plant Constituents

Clearly, American health care consumers are increasing their use of herbs as natural alternatives to drugs. Standardizing separate herbal constituents for potency is becoming popular today as herbal manufacturers enter drug-oriented health care markets.

BUT WHAT IS SACRIFICED WHEN HERBAL CONSTITUENTS ARE "STANDARDIZED?"

It's a case of government regulations and orthodox medicine trying make herbal healing fit into a laboratory drug mold. Without question, Americans need safe, effective, alternative medicines. But this time the demand includes incredibly intricate, living medicines...medicines whose value lies in their complexity, and their ability to combine easily with the human body, not in their concentration or the potency of any one constituent. Standardization uses synthetic chemicals to peel away one or two so-called "active ingredients" out of dozens of constituents that make up a single herb. The result is an overly refined product that misses the full range of benefits offered by the natural herb.

As a naturopath and traditional herbalist, I believe that standardization short-changes the full spectrum of whole-herb healing. Throughout the ages and from many cultures and traditions, herbalists have effectively used whole herbs for whole bodies with immense success that rivals modern day allopathic medicine. There is tremendous value in the knowledge gained through empirical observation and interpretive understanding of real people with real problems and natural solutions.

Yet, in the modern health care world, laboratory yardsticks are the only measurements science understands or government approves. Herbal healing fell out of favor not because it was ineffective, or even because something better was discovered, but because scientific technology had little understanding of nature, and medical market economics had no incentive to investigate it. No one can "patent a plant."

Standardizing a so-called "active ingredient" in a drug-like approach neglects one of the main features of whole herbs. As naturally concentrated foods, herbs have the unique ability to address a multiplicity of problems simultaneously. In most cases, the full medicinal value of herbs is in their internal complexity. Single herbs contain dozens of natural chemical constituents working synergistically. It's why an herb is rarely ever known for just a single function. The evolutionary development of each herb has created a whole essence: the natural herb in correct and balanced ratios with all its constituents. Many of the constituents within a whole herb are unknown - even to modern science - and internal chemical reactions within and among herbs are even less understood.

CAN WE INTEGRATE HERBAL HEALING INTO SCIENTIFIC METHODOLOGY TO MAKE IT AVAILABLE TO EVERYBODY?

It's a question that's splitting herbal product providers apart. Standardization is seen by some companies, especially those whose main focus has been vitamins or other partitioned supplements, as a way for herb products to challenge the mainstream drug company monopoly, by measuring and assuring some "active constituents" of a plant for medicinal use.

Standardization is also considered a way to deal with FDA regulations that require drug measurability, and FDA guidelines that require so-called "active" ingredients to be stated on product labels. As herb companies begin to use structure, function and potency health claims, a way must be found to work with regulations that were never intended to deal with the complexities or broad-based effects of herbal healing.

Standardizing potency for only one or two extracted "active ingredients" for certain vested interests, attempts to use limited laboratory procedures to convince the AMA, the FDA and medical scientists of the value of herbal therapy. We must not fall into the same wrong-headed, self-defeating pit that occurred forty years ago, when the regulations for standardization of drugs nearly killed all herbal medicine.

We can't let ourselves forget that herbal healing is due not only to herbal bio-chemical properties, but also to their unique, wholistic effects, and most importantly, to their interaction with the human body.

HERBS HAVE REJUVENATIVE, TONIC QUALITIES ENTIRELY MISSED BY STANDARDIZATION. YET, QUALITY AND CONSISTENCY ARE A MAJOR CONCERN IN ASCERTAINING HERBAL EFFECTIVENESS. SOMEHOW, HERBALISTS AND HERBAL PRODUCT SUPPLIERS MUST INTEGRATE HERBAL TRADITIONS, ETHICAL COMMITMENTS, FDA REGULATIONS AND CONSUMER CONCERNS.

Here's what we lose when we try to standardize a complex medicinal plant.
• **Standardization attempts to isolate "active constituents" for a limited function.** For example, ginseng has become a popular ingredient in many herbal products. One laboratory test identified two of its 22 known constituents (called Rb1 and Rb2), in an attempt to isolate ginseng's functions as an anti-oxidant and for lowering cholesterol. Yet thousands of years of world-wide, well-documented experience show that ginseng has dozens of other actions that control disease and promote wellness, functions entirely missed by this test. Should we deny people the ultimate value and effectiveness of ginseng's activity simply because a laboratory hasn't tested for, or understood, every one of its functions yet?

• **Standardization fails to take advantage of the synergistic power of herbs in combination.** Standardizing one constituent within an herbal combination is risky because the whole balance of the compound is lost or changed. As a professional herbalist, I have been creating combination formulas since 1978. Combinations are used because, in most instances, they work more efficiently with multiple body functions. To make use of the full spectrum of healing possibilities, we combine ginseng, for example, with licorice. The resulting extract has synergistic benefits - exceptional body cleansing, nutrient assimilation support, and a significant role in balancing body sugar levels - **more than either of these herbs used alone.**

Since all body parts, and most disease symptoms, are interrelated, it is wise to have herbs which can affect each part of the problem. For example, Crystal Star's prostate healing formula contains herbs that help dissolve sediment, herbs with anti-inflammatory and antibiotic properties, and herbs to tone and strengthen tissue. The combination of herbal nutrients encourages overall body balance. A "standardized" supply of one or two constituents in a drug-like dose is not intended for this wholistic purpose.

Indeed, a good herbal combination will contain much more than even the **primary** whole herbs. It will include **secondary herbs** to soothe and help the body repair itself; **catalysts and transporter herbs** to carry active constituents into the body for optimal absorption and utilization, and **complementary herbs** to address side effects related to the main problem and balance body chemistry.

The interaction of constituents within a single herb is much like the supportive roles that secondary herbs, or catalysts and transporters perform in effective herbal combinations.

How do we assure ourselves that the herbs we buy have the medicinal qualities we want? How can we know that the herbs in the products we buy will work? Are the herbs on the label in there?
Here is the two-fold method used by Crystal Star Herbal Nutrition to assure that their products do the job.

Use the evidence of your senses and common sense. Here are checkpoints to use when buying medicinal herbs:
✔ Buy organically grown or wildcrafted (grown in their natural state) herbs whenever available. Buy fresh-dried, locally grown herbs whenever possible, to assure the shortest transportation time and freshest quality.
✔ When choosing unpackaged, loose herbs, rub a sample between your fingers, smell it and look at its color. Even in a dried state, the life and potency of an herb are easily evident.
✔ Buy the best herbs available. The experience and quality control methods at the growing/gathering/storage end of the herbal medicine chain are more costly, but they increase its healing abilities.
✔ When buying packaged herbs choose a product from a company that specializes in herbs. Herb companies live and breathe herbs and are generally regarded as having the highest level of herbal integrity. Be sure the product is tightly sealed and away from light and heat. Also, check the expiration date.
✔ Ask the supplement buyer at your local natural food store for the names of reputable herbal product manufacturers who have earned the trust of consumers for products that work.

The second part of the answer involves what I have come to trust.

A wise man once said that trust could settle every problem in the world right now. But, we're not talking about blind trust, or pie-in-the-sky trust. We're talking about common sense trust. All of us have to trust experts every day, to advise and inform us about things we don't know. We don't have to become physicists to use products that come from physics research, or mechanics in order to drive a car. Nor do we have to become herbal experts to avail ourselves of herbal medicines. It has been my experience that there are three things you can trust when you buy an herbal product in America today.

✓   You can trust the herb or herbal combination to do what its centuries old tradition says it will do.

✓   You can trust the vast majority of herbal product suppliers, most of whom are dedicated people, pledged to herbal excellence. In my opinion, their herbal knowledge and standards are worth more than chemical lab assays, many of which are incomplete, poorly done and expensive. A testimonial to this comes from a third party, non-profit lab that buys and tests health products for efficacy and quality. They have informed me that almost 100% of the traditional herbal products they review from open market samples contain what they say they contain.

✓   Finally, you can trust your natural food store. The typical herbal expert in a natural food store is in the job largely because of a commitment to the wonders of natural medicines, and a desire to share that commitment.

Just like you can't cheat an honest man, you can't cheat the honesty of herbs either. They will put out their truth no matter what. And to get the whole truth, I believe you have to use the whole herb. Here's why:

•   The so-called "active constituent" of a plant is only a part of the whole. Herbs, as whole foods have complex properties that combine with the body's enzyme activity. When an isolated constituent is used, a powerful but **unbalanced** reaction takes place, similar to eating refined sugar or taking a drug which works by overwhelming.

•   Standardizing one constituent for one plant denies the far greater benefits to be had from herbal combinations. Using a standardized herb is like using a "natural drug," with one property for one problem. Potentizing a single property only gives you part of the picture. It does a disservice to the plant's ability to work with other herbs. The whole herb offers wide latitude to work with several aspects and stages of a problem, and allows each person to draw benefits from the complexity of the whole combination. Herbs are living medicines. Just like our own bodies, they work best in their natural balance.

•   No laboratory can even begin to quantify all that whole natural plants have to offer us. They can make tomatoes in a lab today. But are they a food, or a fabrication? Most of us have tasted these tomatoes. Even judging by taste alone, the resemblance to an earth and sun grown tomato is pale. We need to keep reminding ourselves that herbs are so much more than a laboratory creation.

•   Standardization procedures allow the use of sub-standard materials. Since only one "active constituent" is measured, that constituent may be boosted with a concentration or isolate to reach the required standard, regardless of the quality of the herb itself. No one constituent, no matter how worthwhile, can do its healing job without the right stuff from the rest of the herb.

•   In their whole form, herbs, like foods, nourish the body with little danger of toxicity. Potentizing an herb to reach a certain standardized constituent makes it more drug-like, without the protection of the plant's natural gentleness and balance - a safety factor that means herbs can be used by everybody, not just herbal experts, without having to worry about harmful interactions. This is a consideration in today's litigious marketplace, where powerful substances carry more risk of abuse and consumer misuse. The slower, long term action of whole herbs is preferable for self-treatment.

•   Finally, standardization leaves no room for excellence, either in source of supply or in skillful preparation.

Herbs have a unique healing spirit. Herbs are intelligent plants - even thoughtful healers. They give the body a wealth of healing essences from which to choose. Science can only quantify, isolate and assay to understand. When we try to say that the standardized constituents are all there is to herbal healing, we lose. Herbs respond to scientific methods but an herbal compound is so much more than the sum of its parts. Herbs are a healing art that can teach your body what to do for its own wellness.

Herbs & Anatomy
Which Part Of Your Body Do You Want To Work On?

Herbal medicines can work for every body system, every body function and every body structure. There are even herbs for the mind and spirit. The ANATOMY & HERB CHARTS in this section graphically show just how all-encompassing herbs can be for your health and well-being. Herbs can also be quite specific; you can pinpoint a very small body area as easily as a large one to work on. The charts on these pages let you see at a glance just which herbs to use for which body part or system.

In general, herbs are very gentle, very subtle and very safe. A number of herbs listed on these charts can often be used together if two or more body areas have the same problem. Keep your combinations simple and direct if you decide to use more than one herb.

Blood   Bones

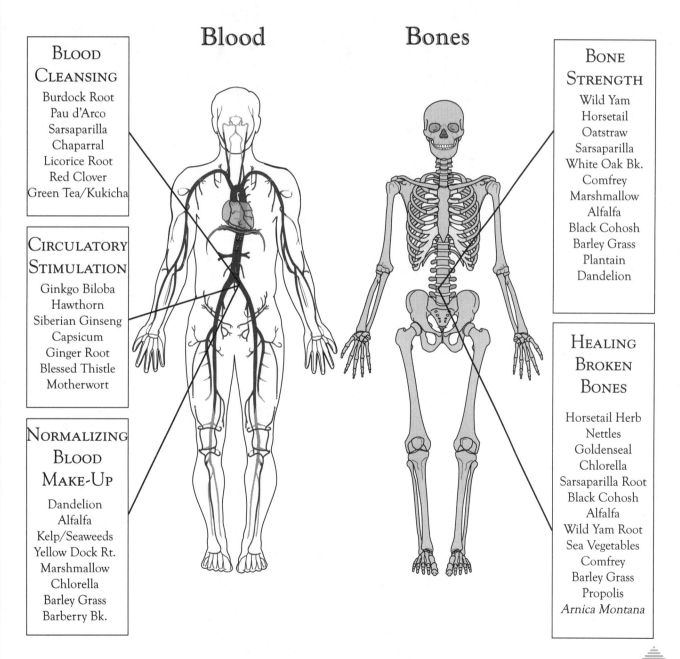

BLOOD CLEANSING
Burdock Root
Pau d'Arco
Sarsaparilla
Chaparral
Licorice Root
Red Clover
Green Tea/Kukicha

CIRCULATORY STIMULATION
Ginkgo Biloba
Hawthorn
Siberian Ginseng
Capsicum
Ginger Root
Blessed Thistle
Motherwort

NORMALIZING BLOOD MAKE-UP
Dandelion
Alfalfa
Kelp/Seaweeds
Yellow Dock Rt.
Marshmallow
Chlorella
Barley Grass
Barberry Bk.

BONE STRENGTH
Wild Yam
Horsetail
Oatstraw
Sarsaparilla
White Oak Bk.
Comfrey
Marshmallow
Alfalfa
Black Cohosh
Barley Grass
Plantain
Dandelion

HEALING BROKEN BONES
Horsetail Herb
Nettles
Goldenseal
Chlorella
Sarsaparilla Root
Black Cohosh
Alfalfa
Wild Yam Root
Sea Vegetables
Comfrey
Barley Grass
Propolis
Arnica Montana

Muscle & Tendons

Nerves

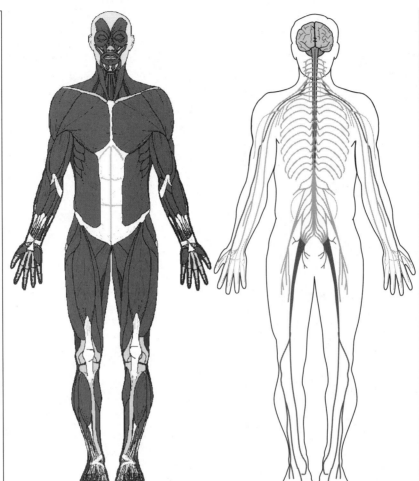

MUSCLE TONE

Sarsaparilla Root
Siberian Ginseng
Bee Pollen
Royal Jelly
Barley Grass
Suma
Sea Vegetables
Rosemary
Saw Palmetto
Damiana
Licorice Root
Alfalfa
Gotu Kola
Fo-Ti
Panax Ginseng
Scullcap
Horsetail Herb
Rose Hips
Spirulina
Evening Primrose
Chlorella
Bilberry
Wild Yam
Yarrow
Ginger Root
Capsicum

NERVE HEALTH

Gotu Kola
Scullcap
Oatstraw
Lady Slipper
Kava Kava
Black Cohosh
Chamomile
Rosemary
Siberian Ginseng
Barley Grass
Catnip
Eur. Mistletoe
Lobelia
Barley Grass
Dandelion
Pau d'Arco
Evening Primrose
Peppermint
Reishi Mushroom
Wood Betony
Black Haw
Nettles
Parsley Rt. & Lf.
Bee Pollen
Valerian Root
Watercress

Cardio-Pulmonary System

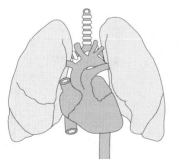

CARDIO-PULMONARY HEALTH

Hawthorn
Siberian Ginseng
Garlic
Capsicum
Sea Vegetables
Barley Grass
Chlorella
Bilberry
Ginger Root
Ginkgo Biloba
Motherwort
Evening Primrose
Scullcap

RESPIRATORY & BREATHING HEALTH

Marshmallow
Mullein
Ephedra
Fenugreek
Sarsaparilla Root
Pau d' Arco
Echinacea
Aloe Vera Juice
Royal Jelly
Lobelia
Barley Grass
Pleurisy Root
Comfrey

Respiratory Sinus System

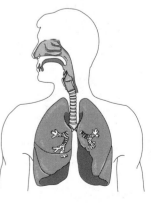

Digestive System

Elimination Systems

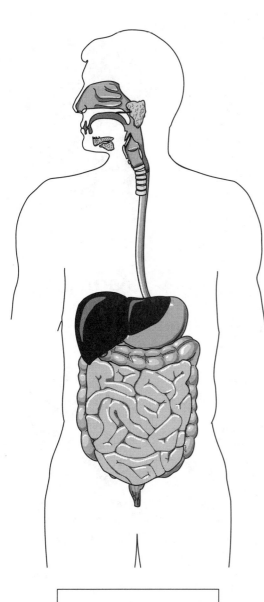

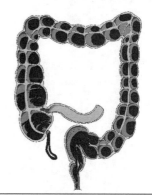

COLON HEALTH

Aloe Vera
Fennel Seed
Kelp/Sea Vegetables
Marshmallow
High Chlorophyll Herbs
Licorice Root
Butternut Bark
Flax Seed

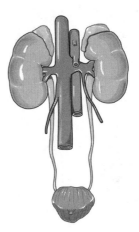

DIGESTIVE HEALTH

Ginkgo Biloba
Fenugreek Seed
Barley Grass
Goldenseal Root
Garlic
Ginger Root
Alfalfa
Licorice Root
Fennel Seed
Catnip
Capsicum
Kelp/Sea Vegetables
Slippery Elm

URINARY HEALTH

Dandelion
Uva Ursi
Parsley
Cornsilk
Watermelon Seed
Cleavers
Barley Grass
Alfalfa
Oregon Grape Root

Liver & Gallbladder

Heart & Arteries

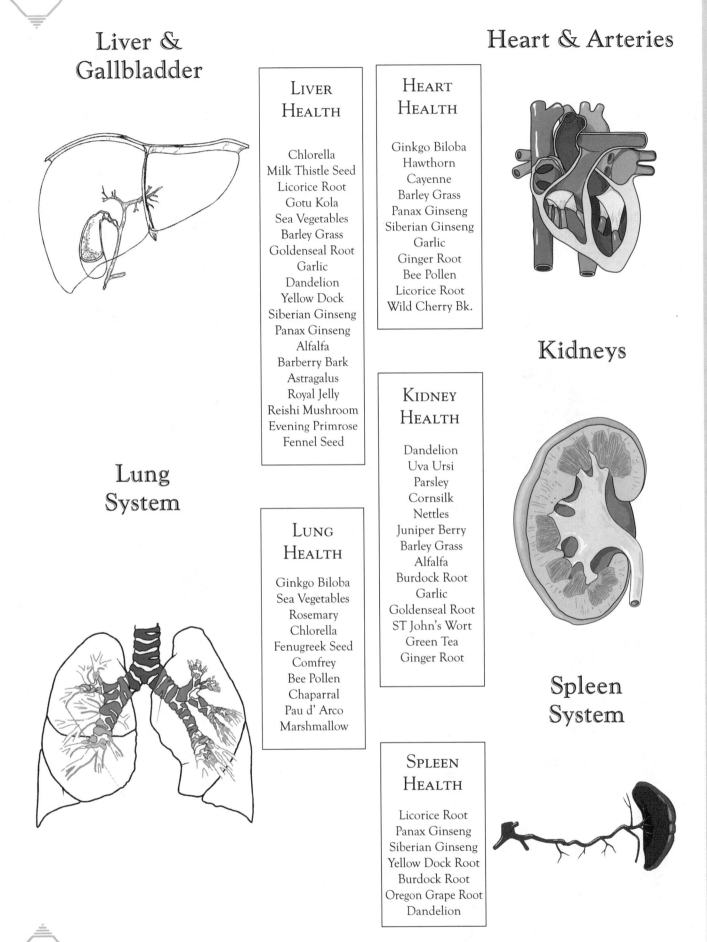

LIVER HEALTH

Chlorella
Milk Thistle Seed
Licorice Root
Gotu Kola
Sea Vegetables
Barley Grass
Goldenseal Root
Garlic
Dandelion
Yellow Dock
Siberian Ginseng
Panax Ginseng
Alfalfa
Barberry Bark
Astragalus
Royal Jelly
Reishi Mushroom
Evening Primrose
Fennel Seed

HEART HEALTH

Ginkgo Biloba
Hawthorn
Cayenne
Barley Grass
Panax Ginseng
Siberian Ginseng
Garlic
Ginger Root
Bee Pollen
Licorice Root
Wild Cherry Bk.

Kidneys

KIDNEY HEALTH

Dandelion
Uva Ursi
Parsley
Cornsilk
Nettles
Juniper Berry
Barley Grass
Alfalfa
Burdock Root
Garlic
Goldenseal Root
ST John's Wort
Green Tea
Ginger Root

Lung System

LUNG HEALTH

Ginkgo Biloba
Sea Vegetables
Rosemary
Chlorella
Fenugreek Seed
Comfrey
Bee Pollen
Chaparral
Pau d' Arco
Marshmallow

Spleen System

SPLEEN HEALTH

Licorice Root
Panax Ginseng
Siberian Ginseng
Yellow Dock Root
Burdock Root
Oregon Grape Root
Dandelion

The Endocrine System
HERBS FOR YOUR GLANDS

Adrenals

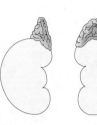

ADRENAL HEALTH

Royal Jelly
Bee Pollen
Licorice Root
Hawthorn
Astragalus
Sea Vegetables
Siberian Ginseng
Gotu Kola
Sarsaparilla Root

Ovaries

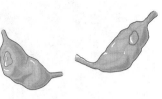

OVARY HEALTH

Dong Quai Root
Damiana
Ashwagandha
Wild Yam Root
Burdock Root
Sea Vegetables
Evening Primrose
Vitex
Sarsaparilla Root

Pituitary

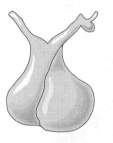

PITUITARY HEALTH

Royal Jelly
Sarsaparilla
Damiana
Dong Quai
Barley Grass
Horsetail Herb
Alfalfa
Oatstraw
Burdock Root
Licorice Root

Thymus

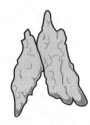

THYMUS HEALTH

Bee Pollen/Roy. Jelly
Evening Primrose
Panax Ginseng
Echinacea
Barley Grass
Fenugreek
Thyme
Rose Hips
Burdock Root
Licorice Root

Lymph

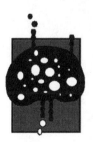

LYMPH HEALTH

Chaparral
Echinacea
Astragalus
Barberry Bark
Goldenseal Root
Yellow Dock Root
Garlic
Panax Ginseng
Burdock Root
Licorice Root
Green Tea

Thyroid

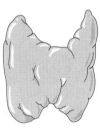

THYROID HEALTH

Sea Vegetables
Chlorella
Siberian Ginseng
Evening Primrose
Cayenne
Barley Grass
Mullein
Lobelia
Parsley
Sarsaparilla Root
Licorice Root

Pancreas

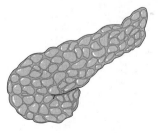

PANCREAS HEALTH

Juniper Berries
Dandelion
Licorice Root
Horseradish Root
Garlic

Testes

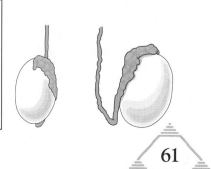

TESTICLE HEALTH

Panax Ginseng
Damiana
Licorice Root
Dandelion Root
Sarsaparilla

Mind & Spirit

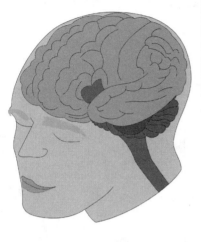

MIND/SPIRIT BALANCE

Ginkgo Biloba
Gotu Kola
Panax Ginseng
Sea Vegetables
Chlorella
Evening Primrose
Royal Jelly
Bee Pollen
Siberian Ginseng
Alfalfa
Rosemary
Sage

Skin System

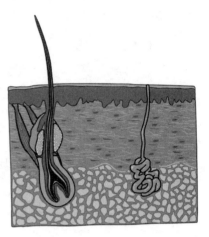

SKIN HEALTH

Evening Primrose
Dandelion
Rosehips
Chamomile
Royal Jelly

SKIN HEALING

Bee Pollen
Barley Grass
Horsetail
Panax Ginseng
Aloe Vera Gel

Vision System

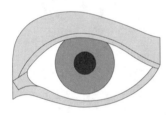

EYE HEALTH

Eyebright
Bilberry
Parsley Root
Aloe Vera
Calendula
Chaparral
Ginkgo Biloba
Burdock Root
Hawthorn
Yellow Dock Root
Barley Grass
Sea Vegetables

Hair Health

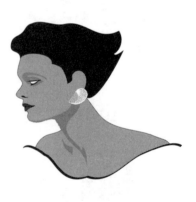

HAIR HEALTH

Rosemary
Jojoba Oil
Reishi Mushroom
Sea Vegetables
Sage

HAIR GROWTH

Horsetail
Oatstraw
Cayenne

Hearing System

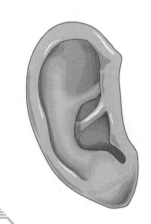

EAR HEALTH

Mullein
Ginkgo Biloba
Turmeric
Yellow Dock Rt.
Garlic
Sea Vegetables
Spirulina
Echinacea Root
Yarrow
Bayberry Bark
Lobelia

Nail Health

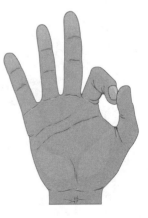

NAIL HEALTH

Horsetail
Nettles
Rosemary
Sage
Sea Vegetables
Oatstraw
Pau d' Arco
Evening Primrose
Garlic
Chamomile
Royal Jelly

Herbal Preparation & Delivery Methods

Today, hundreds of herbs are available at all quality levels. Worldwide communications and improved storage allow us to simultaneously obtain and use herbs from different countries and different harvests, an advantage ages past did not enjoy. However, because of the natural variety of soils, seeds, and weather, every crop of botanicals is unique. Every batch of a truly natural herbal formula will be slightly different, and offer its own unique benefits and experience.

There must be a firm commitment to excellence from growers and suppliers, because herbal combinations are products for problems. For therapeutic success, herbs must be BIO-ACTIVE and BIO-AVAILABLE.

If you decide to make your own herbal preparations, buy the finest quality you can find. There is a world of disparity between fairly good herbs and the best. Superior stock must go into a medicinal formula so that the herbal product can do its job correctly. Superior plants cost far more than standard stock, but their worth in healing activity is a true value for the health care customer.

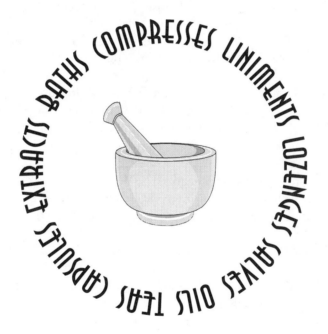

Which Preparation Form Should You Choose?

Whichever herbal preparation form you choose, it is generally more beneficial to take greater amounts at the beginning of your program, to build a good internal healing base, and to stimulate the body's own vital balancing force more quickly. As the therapeutic agents establish and build in the body, and you begin to notice good response and balance returning, less and less of the large initial doses should be taken, finally reducing the dosage to long range maintenance and preventive amounts.

"Parts" are a good way to set a common denominator for building an herbal compound. For individual use, one tablespoon is usually adequate as one part when using powdered herbs for filling capsules; one handful is common as one part for cut herbs in a tea or bath blend. (See HOW TO MAKE AN HERBAL EXTRACT for quantity information for an extract or tincture).

Herbs can be applied to almost any necessity of life. It is simply a matter of knowing their properties, how they work together and how to use them correctly. But herbs are foods, and your body knows how to use them. Give them time. Give yourself a good diet and some rest and relaxation for the best results.

*H*erbal teas are the most basic of all natural healing mediums; they are easily absorbed by the body as hot liquid. They are the least concentrated of all herbal forms, but many herbs are optimally effective when steeped in boiling water. The hot brewing water releases herbal potency and provides a flushing action that is ideal for removing toxic wastes that have been loosened and dissolved by the herbs. Although teas have milder and more subtle effects than capsules or extracts, they are sometimes the only way for a weakened system to accept therapeutic support, and often work synergistically with stronger medicinal forms to boost their value.

NOTE 1: The cutting of herbs for tea bags creates facets on the herb structure causing loss of essential volatile oils. Gently crumble leaves and flowers, and break roots and barks into pieces before steeping for best results.

NOTE 2: Medicinal teas may have bitter tasting properties. Where taste is unpleasant, mint, lemon peel, spices, or stevia (sweet herb), may be added to improve taste without harming therapeutic qualities.

TIPS ON TAKING HERBAL TEAS:

1 Use 1 packed small teaball to 3 cups of water for medicinal-strength tea. Use distilled water or pure spring water for increased herbal strength and effectiveness.

2 Bring water to a boil, remove from heat, add herbs and steep, covered, off heat; 10 to 15 minutes for a leaf/flower tea; 15 to 25 minutes for a root/bark tea. Keep lid closed during steeping so volatile oils won't escape.

3 Use a teapot of glass, ceramic or earthenware, not aluminum. Aluminum can negate the effect of the herbs as the metal dissolves into the hot liquid and gets into the body.

4 Drink medicinal teas in small sips throughout the day rather than all at once. One-half to 1 cup, taken 3 or 4 times over a day allows absorption of the tea, without passing before it has a chance to work.

❧ **An infusion** is a tea made from dried or powdered herb. Use directions above, or pour 1 cup of boiling water over 1 tablespoon of fresh herb, 1 teaspoon of dried herb, or 4 opened capsules of powdered herb. Cover and let steep 10 to 15 minutes. Never boil. A cold infusion can be made by simply allowing the herbs, especially powders, to stand in cool water for an hour or more.

❧ **A decoction** is a tea made from roots and barks. Use directions above, or put 2 tablespoons of cut herb pieces into 1 cup cold water. Bring to a light boil, cover, and simmer gently for 20 to 30 minutes. Strain. For best results, repeat the same process with the same herbs. Strain again and mix both batches.

❧ **"Sun tea"** is a cold infusion where herbs are put in a covered jar and allowed to stand in the sun.

❧ For an **herbal broth**, grind the dry ingredients in a blender. Mix 2 TBS. of dry mix to 2 cups hot water. Let flavors bloom for 5 minutes before drinking. Herbal broths are rich in minerals and enzymes. Add 1 teasp. BRAGG'S LIQUID AMINOS to each drink for a flavor/nutrient boost if desired. Sip over $1/2$ hour period for best assimilation.

*H*erbal capsules are generally four times stronger than teas, more concentrated in form, convenient to take, and bypass any herbal bitterness. Capsules can make both oil and water soluble herbs available through stomach acid and enzyme alteration. Freeze-dried powdered herbs, with all the moisture removed, are also available in capsules, and are four times more concentrated than regular ground herbs. As noted with herbal teas above, grinding herbs into powders creates facets on the whole herb structure causing potential loss of volatile oils. Effective potency for powdered herbs is six months to a year. (See page 53 for more information on how to take herbal capsules.)

*H*erbal extracts are 4 to 8 times stronger than capsules. They are effective used as a spray where all the mouth receptors can be brought into play, or as drops held under the tongue, that bypass the digestive system's acid/alkaline breakdown of substances. Their strength and ready availability make extracts reliable emergency measures. Small doses can be used repeatedly over a period of time to help build a strong base for restoring body balance. Holding an extract dose in the mouth as long as possible, 3 or 4 times daily, is effective for the first week of an acute condition. After this first week, the vital force of the body will often have been sufficiently stimulated in its own healing ability, and the dose may be reduced to allow the system to take its own route to balance. As with other forms of herbal mixtures, most extracts should be taken no more than 6 days in a row with a rest on the seventh day, before resuming, to allow the body to do its own work. As the body increases its ability to right itself, the amount, frequency and strength of the dosage should be decreased.

*H*erbal tinctures are also extractions, made using a 25% alcohol and water mixture as the solvent. Tinctures are generally extracted from individual herbs rather than compounds. When they **are** blended into a compound, each separately prepared tincture is added rather than made from the beginning as a compound. Commercial tinctures use ethyl alcohol, and may even be formed from fluid extracts, but diluted spirits are suitable for home use; vodka is ideal.

Extracts are more concentrated than tinctures, because they distill or filter off some of the alcohol. A tincture is typically a 1:10 or 1:5 concentration (10 or 5 units of extract come from 1 unit of herbs), while a fluid extract is usually 1:1.

Even stronger, *a solid or powdered extract* has the solvent completely removed. Powdered extracts are at least 4 times as potent as an equal amount of fluid extract, and 40 times as potent as a tincture. One gram of a 4:1 solid extract is equivalent to $1/_7$ of an ounce of a fluid extract, and $1^1/_2$ ounces of a tincture.

Note: Homeopathic liquid formulas are not the same as herbal tinctures or extracts, and their use is different.

HERE IS HOW TO MAKE A SIMPLE HERBAL EXTRACTION:

Alcohol, wine, apple cider vinegar, and vegetable glycerine are common mediums for extracting herbal properties for therapeutic use. Alcohol releases the widest variety of essential herbal elements in unchanged form, and allows the fastest sublingual absorption. Alcohol and water mixtures can resolve almost every relevant ingredient of any herb, and also act as a natural preserver for the compound. Eighty to one hundred proof (40-50%) vodka, is an excellent solvent for most plant constituents. It has long term preservative activity and is easily obtainable for individual use. The actual amount of alcohol in a daily dose is approximately $1/_{30}$ oz., but if alcohol is not desired, extract drops may be placed in a little warm water for 5 minutes to allow the alcohol to evaporate before drinking. Most extracts are formulated with 1 gram of herb for each 5ml of alcohol.

EXTRACT DIRECTIONS:

1. Put about 4 ounces dried chopped or ground herb, or 8 ounces of fresh herb, into a quart canning jar.
2. Pour about one pint of 80 to 100 proof vodka over the herbs and close tightly.
3. Keep the jar in a warm place for two to three weeks, and shake well twice a day.
5. Decant the liquid into a bowl, and then pour the slurry residue through several layers of muslin or cheesecloth into the bowl. Strain all the liquid through the layers once again to insure a clearer extract.
5. Squeeze out all liquid from the cloth. (Sprinkle solid residue around your houseplants as herb food. We have done this for years, and they love it.)
6. Pour the extract into a dark glass bottle. Stopper, seal tightly, and store away from light. An extraction made in this way will keep its potency for several years.

*H*erbal wine infusions are a pleasant, effective method of taking herbs, especially as digestive aids with meals, and as warming circulatory tonics by-the-spoonful in winter. The alcohol acts as a transport medium and stimulant to the bloodstream.

HERE IS HOW TO MAKE A SIMPLE WINE INFUSION. EITHER FRESH OR DRIED HERBS MAY BE USED:

• **Method 1:** For a warming winter circulation and energy tonic, pour off about $1/_4$ cup of a fortified wine, such as madeira, cognac or brandy. Place chosen herbs and spices in the wine and recork the bottle. Place in a dark cool place for a week or two. Strain off the solids, and combine the medicinal wine with a fresh bottle. Mix well, and take a small amount as needed for energy against fatigue.

• **Method 2:** For a nerve and brain tonic, steep fresh or dried herbs in a bottle of either white or red wine for about a week. Strain off herbs, and drink a small amount as needed.

*H*erbal syrups are well accepted by children, and can greatly improve the taste of bitter herbal compounds. They are also excellent treatment forms for throat coats and gargles, or bronchial, chest/lung infections. Syrups are simple and quick to make.

THERE ARE TWO SIMPLE WAYS TO MAKE AN HERBAL SYRUP:
• **Method 1:** Boil $^3/_4$ lb. of raw or brown sugar in 2 cups of herb tea until it reaches syrup consistency.
• **Method 2:** Make a simple syrup with $^3/_4$ lb. of raw sugar in 2 cups of water, boiling until it reaches syrup consistency. Remove from heat, and while the syrup is cooling, add an herbal extract or tincture - one part extract to three parts of syrup.

*H*erbal pastes and electuaries are made by grinding or blending herbs in the blender with a little water into a paste. The paste may then be mixed with twice the amount of honey, syrup, butter, or cream cheese for palatability and taste. Other electuaries (mediums that mask the bitter taste of medicinal herbs) include fresh bread rolled around a little of the paste, or peanut butter.

*H*erbal lozenges are an ideal way to relieve mouth, throat, and upper respiratory conditions. They are made by combining powdered herbs with sugar and a mucilaginous herb, such as marshmallow or slippery elm, or a gum, such as tragacanth or acacia. Both powdered herbs and essential herbal oils may be used. Proper mucilage preparation is the key to successful lozenges.

HERE'S HOW TO MAKE AN HERBAL LOZENGE:
• Soak 1-oz. of powdered mucilaginous herb (listed above) in water to cover for 24 hours; stir occasionally.
• Bring 2 cups of water to a boil and add the mucilage herb.
• Beat to obtain a uniform consistency and force through cheesecloth to strain.
• Mix with enough powdered herb to form a paste, and add sugar to taste. Or, mix 12 drops of essential peppermint oil (or other essential oil) with 2-oz. of sugar, and enough mucilage to make a paste.
• Roll on a board covered with arrowroot or sugar to prevent sticking. Cut into shapes and leave exposed to air to dry. Store in an airtight container.

External Use Preparations:

The skin is the body's largest organ of ingestion. Topical herbal mediums may be used as needed for all over relief and support.

*H*erbal baths provide a soothing gentle way to absorb herbal therapy through the skin. In essence, you are soaking in a diluted medicinal tea, allowing the skin to take in the healing properties instead of the mouth and digestive system. The procedure for taking an effective infusion bath is almost as important as the herbs themselves.

THERE ARE TWO GOOD THERAPEUTIC BATH TECHNIQUES:
• **Method 1:** Draw very hot bath water. Put the bath herbs in an extra large tea ball or small muslin bath bag, (sold in natural food stores). Steep in the bath until the water cools slightly and is aromatic, about 10-15 minutes.
• **Method 2:** Make a strong tea infusion on the stove as usual with a full pot of water. Strain and add directly to the bath. Soak for at least 30-45 minutes to give the body time to absorb the herbal properties. Rub the body with the solids in the muslin bag while soaking for best herb absorbency.

*H*erbal douches are an effective method of treating simple vaginal infections. The herbs are simply steeped as for a strong tea, strained off, and the liquid poured into a douche bag. Sit on the toilet, insert the applicator, and rinse the vagina with the douche. Use one full douche bag for each application. Most vaginal conditions need douching three times daily for 3 to 7 days. If the infection does not respond in this time, see a qualified health professional.

*H*erbal suppositories and boluses are an effective way to treat rectal and vaginal problems, acting as carriers for the herbal medicine application. Herbal compounds for suppositories generally serve one of three purposes; to soothe inflamed mucous membranes and aid the healing process, to help reduce swollen membranes and overcome pus-filled discharge, and to work as a laxative, stimulating normal peristalsis to overcome chronic constipation.

To prepare a simple suppository, mix about a tablespoon of finely powdered herbs with enough cocoa butter to make a firm consistency. Roll into torpedo shaped tubes about an inch long. Place on wax paper, and put in the freezer to firm. Remove one at a time for use, and allow to come to room temperature before using. Insert at night.

*H*erbal ointments and salves are semi-solid preparations, that allow absorption of herbal benefits through the skin. They may be made with vaseline, UN-Petroleum Jelly or cocoa butter for a simple compound; or in a more complex technique with herbal tea, oils and hardening agents such as beeswax, lanolin or lard.

To PREPARE A SIMPLE OINTMENT OR SALVE:
- **Method 1:** Warm about 6 oz. of vaseline, petroleum jelly or lanolin in a small pan with 2 TBS. of cut herbs; or stir in enough powdered herbs to bring the mixture to a dark color. Simmer gently for 10 minutes, stirring. Then filter through cheesecloth, pressing out all liquid. Pour into small wide-mouth containers when cool but still pliable.
- **Method 2:** This method is best when a carrier base is needed for volatile herbal oils, such as for chest rubs or anti-congestive balms, where the base itself is not to be absorbed by the skin. Steep herbs in water to make a strong tea. Strain off the liquid into a pan. Add your chosen oils and fats, such as almond, sesame, wheat germ, or olive, oils, and cocoa butter or lanolin fats (about 6-oz. total) to the strained tea.

Simmer until water evaporates, and the herbal extract is incorporated into the oils. Add enough beeswax to bring mixture to desired consistency; use about 2-oz. beeswax to 5-oz. of herbal oil. Let melt and stir until well blended. Add 1 drop of tincture of benzoin (available at most pharmacies), for each ounce of ointment to preserve the mixture against mold.

*H*erbal compresses and fomentations draw out waste and waste residue, such as cysts or abscesses via the skin, or release them into the body's elimination channels. Compresses are made by soaking a cotton cloth in a strong herbal tea, and applying it as hot as possible to the affected area. The heat enhances the activity of the herbs, and opens the pores of the skin for fast assimilation.

Use alternating hot and cold compresses to stimulate nerves and circulation. Apply the herbs to the hot compress, and leave the cold compress plain. Cayenne, ginger and lobelia are good choices for the hot compress.

Make an effective compress by adding 1 teasp. powdered herbs to a bowl of very hot water. Soak a washcloth and apply until the cloth cools. Then apply a cloth dipped in ice water until it reaches body temperature. Repeat several times daily.

Green clay compresses, for growths, may be applied to gauze, placed on the area, and left for all day. Simply change as you would any dressing when you bathe.

*H*erbal poultices and plasters are made from either fresh herbs, crushed and blended in a blender with a little olive or wheat germ oil, or dried herbs, mixed with water, cider vinegar or wheat germ oil into a paste. Either blend may be spread on a piece of clean cloth or gauze, and bound directly on the affected area. The whole application is then covered with plastic wrap to keep from soiling clothes or sheets, and left on for 24 hours. There is usually a great deal of throbbing pain while the poultice is drawing out the infection and neutralizing the toxic poisons. This stops when the harmful agents are drawn out, and signals the removal of the poultice. A fresh poultice should be applied every 24 hours.

Make a plaster by spreading a thin coat of honey on a clean cloth, and sprinkling it with an herbal mixture such as cayenne, ginger, and prickly ash, or hot mustard or horseradish. The cloth is then taped directly over the affected area, usually the chest, to relieve lung and mucous congestion.

*H*erbal liniments are used as warming massage mediums, to stimulate and relieve sore muscles and ligaments. They are for external use only. Choose heat-inducing herbs and spices such as cayenne, ginger, cloves and myrrh, and drops of heating oils such as eucalyptus, wintergreen and cajeput. Steep in rubbing alcohol for two to three weeks. Strain and decant into corked bottles for storage.

*H*erbal oils are used externally for massage, skin treatments, healing ointments, dressings for wounds and burns, and occasionally for enemas and douches. Simply infuse the herb in oil instead of water. Olive, safflower or almond oil are good bases for an herbal oil.

To make an herbal oil for home use:
- **Method 1:** Cut fresh herbs into a glass container and cover with oil. Place in the sun and leave in a warm place for three to four weeks, shaking daily to mix. Filter into a dark glass container to store.
- **Method 2:** Macerate dried, powdered herbs directly into the oil. Let stand for one or two days. Strain and bottle for use.

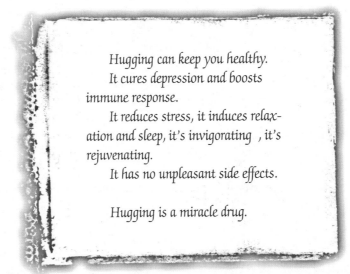

Hugging can keep you healthy.
It cures depression and boosts immune response.
It reduces stress, it induces relaxation and sleep, it's invigorating , it's rejuvenating.
It has no unpleasant side effects.

Hugging is a miracle drug.

The Herbal Medicine Garden

Growing your own herbal medicines is become increasingly popular as people get "back to the roots" of healing. From our experience in growing herbs for a gourmet kitchen, we see how easy herbs are to grow, and that many of our culinary favorites also have healing value. Because most herbs grow wild, an herb garden can be available to almost anyone. Herbs require minimal care, grow in tiny spaces, (virtually every herb will grow in a window box), and are so potent that a little goes a long way. Most herbs are drought resistant, evergreen or herbaceous perennials.

Here are a few tips on growing, harvesting and storing your own fresh medicinal herbs:

Herbs can help you get back to the basics, if you take care of their basics first. Good fertile soil structure is extremely important to the potency of herbal medicines, both for mineral and enzyme concentrations. If you don't have good soil, I strongly recommend enriching it before you plant. Add plenty of humus to either clay or sandy soil to improve soil structure and increase its fertility.

Most herbs are best planted in the fall, before the ground freezes, so they can establish a good root system in loose, well drained soil. If you live in extremely cold climates, where temperatures drop to and stay near zero, most herbs should be planted in early spring as soon as the ground can be worked. (I usually recommend window boxes for cold climates, and for basil anywhere, because you can extend your growing season so much longer.)

Carrot family herbs, like dill, fennel, chervil, coriander (cilantro) and parsley are easy to grow from seeds. Plant these herbs directly into the garden or pot in which they are going to grow because they don't like being transplanted. Annual herbs such as borage, and non-woody perennials like lemon balm, feverfew, chives, elecampane, pennyroyal or sweet violet usually reseed themselves. Woody perennial herbs, such as lavender, rosemary, and the thymes don't self-seed very well and produce far fewer offspring. And some plants, like mint and tarragons don't come up true from seed. They can only be propagated from cuttings or divisions. I recommend purchasing these from a good nursery.

Herbs are wonderful companion plants, not only for each other, but for other plants in your garden. They act as natural pesticides, enhance the growth and flavor of vegetables and help keep soil rich.

- Plant basil with tomatoes to improve flavor and growth, and to repel flies and mosquitoes. Don't plant basil near rue.
- Plant hyssop with cabbage and grapes to deter cabbage moths. Don't plant near radishes.
- Put a fresh bay leaf in storage containers of beans or grain to deter weevils and moths.
- Plant borage near tomatoes, squash and strawberries to deter tomato worms.
- Plant caraway to loosen compacted soil.
- Plant catnip to keep away flea beetles.
- Plant chamomile with cabbage and onions to improve flavor.
- Plant chervil with radishes to improve growth and flavor.
- Plant chives with carrots to improve growth and flavor.
- Plant dill with cabbage, but not near carrots.
- Plant gopher purge around your garden to deter burrowing pests.
- Plant horseradish in a potato patch to keep out potato bugs.
- Plant bee balm with tomatoes to improve growth and flavor.
- Plant lovage to improve health of most plants.
- Plant garlic near roses to repel aphids.
- Plant marjoram for more flavor of all vegetables.
- Plant mint for health of cabbage and tomatoes, and to deter white cabbage moths.
- Plant peppermint to deter moths and carrot flies.

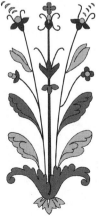

- Plant nasturtiums to deter white flies, cabbage moth, squash bugs.
- Plant rue with roses and raspberries to deter Japanese beetles.
- Plant sage to deter cabbage moths, beetles and carrot flies. Don't plant near cucumbers.
- Plant summer savory with beans and onions to improve flavor and deter cabbage moths.
- Plant tansy to deter flying insects, Japanese beetles, cucumber beetles, squash bugs and ants.
- Plant thyme to deter cabbage worms.
- Plant wormwood as a border to keep animals out of your garden.

You can harvest the leaves of medicinal herbs any time during the growing season as long as they look, smell and taste fresh. Avoid harvesting from plants that have begun to discolor, are buggy or diseased. Herbal flowers are best harvested before they are in full bloom.

 Harvest roots like burdock, dandelion and comfrey, in the spring and fall, when they are full of sap. Wait for a dry spell during rainy seasons because wet roots are difficult to dry and are not as concentrated in medicinal qualities. Look for roots that are fleshy, but not old-looking, woody or fibrous. Roots have to be fully developed, though; immature roots, don't have vital nutritional properties. I don't recommend harvesting roots or corms unless you are something of an expert, because drying and storing techniques are much more difficult, and roots may be contaminated or moldy inside without your being aware of it.

Harvest barks when you harvest roots, in the spring and fall when the sap is moving up and down the plant. Sassafras, birch, willow, oak and witch hazel are common tree barks valued for medicinal qualities.

Harvest seeds late in the day, after a few days of dry weather, to ensure that all plant parts are dry. Most herb seeds are brown or black when they're ready to harvest. Look for flower stalks that are dry and brown, and seed pods that have turned to brown, gray, or black. Cut off the entire seed head and place it in a large paper bag, cardboard box, or wooden bowl. Place only one kind of seed in each container, and label each container. Set seeds in a dry, warm place with good air circulation. Give them a few weeks of open-air drying before removing the seeds out of the pods or heads; then store them in airtight containers. Check seeds periodically for mold.

Drying herbs is the time-honored way of preserving their medicinal qualities. Harvesting herbs in the traditional way means cutting the stems with leaf, flower and all, tying the stalks in bundles and hanging them upside down in an attic or drying shed. I think a food dehydrator is by far the best way to dry herbs today. It provides you with a clean, thoroughly dried product, and it doesn't take up much space.

 Once dry, put the herbs in airtight, glass containers away from light and heat. I don't recommend either metal canisters or paper bags for medicinal herbs, because the qualities are either changed or lost.

Freezing fresh dried herbs retains their medicinal qualities very well. Here's how to do it.

Rinse the herbs and let them drain until dry. I usually strip the leaves off the stems, and snip them with kitchen shears for better storage and later use in teas. Lay the herb pieces in a single layer on baking sheets and freeze til rigid, about an hour. Pour the rigid herbs into small freezer plastic bags, press out air, seal, and return to the freezer.

To use, simply take out what you need, reseal, and return the rest to the freezer. It's so easy.

In California,
the Earth is so kind that you just
tickle her with a hoe
and she laughs with a harvest.

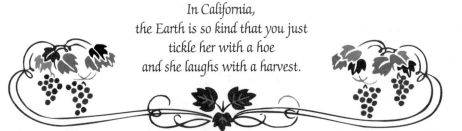

An Herbal First Aid Kit For Your Medicine Chest

An herbal first aid kit is a safe way to cope with everyday healing problems, and temporary or non-serious health conditions. It can handle many problems immediately and simply, save you hundreds of dollars in doctor bills, and keep you from a traumatic, time consuming visit to a medical clinic.

The choices in this kit are easy to use, inexpensive, gentle enough for children, effective for adults.

❧ **For colds, flu and chest congestion**: elder/yarrow/peppermint tea for sniffles; mullein oil for earaches, lavender or eucalyptus steams or hot ginger compresses for chest congestion, and an echinacea/goldenseal/myrrh combination as a natural anti-biotic.

❧ **For coughs, and sore throat:** loquat syrup or licorice/wild cherry/slippery elm tea for coughs, zinc source herbal extract for sore throat, herbal throat drops, aloe vera juice or tea tree oil gargle.

❧ **For cuts, wounds, scrapes and scars:** ginseng skin repair gel, pau d'arco/calendula gel, witch hazel compresses, comfrey/aloe salve, aloe vera gel, Deva Flowers First Aid Remedy extract, tea tree oil.

❧ **For fungal infections like athlete's foot, ringworm and nail fungus:** tea tree oil, grapefruit seed extract, black walnut extract, goldenseal/myrrh solution, pau d'arco/dandelion/gentian gel.

❧ **For minor bacterial and viral infections**: echinacea/golden seal/myrrh combination, white pine/bayberry capsules for first aid; osha root tea, usnea extract, St. John's wort/lomatium extract.

❧ **For rashes, itching, swelling from insect bites or other histamine reactions:** antihistamine marshmallow/bee pollen/white pine capsules, calendula/pau d'arco gel, comfrey/plantain ointment, tea tree oil, aloc vera gel, echinacea/St. John's wort/white willow capsules.

❧ **For pain, cramping and headache relief:** lavender compresses, black cohosh/scullcap extract, peppermint oil rubs, comfrey compresses, rosemary tea or steam, ginkgo biloba or feverfew extract.

❧ **For strains, sprains and muscle pulls:** White willow/St John's wort capsules or salve, Tiger Balm analgesic gel, Chinese white flower oil, tea tree or wintergreen/cajeput oil, and Fo-Ti (ho-shu-wu).

❧ **For periodic constipation and diarrhea:** fiber and herbs butternut/cascara capsules, senna/fennel laxative tea, milk thistle seed extract to soften stool, Ayurvedic Triphala formula, aloe vera juice.

❧ **For sleep aids for insomnia:** rosemary/chamomile/catnip, or passion flower/spearmint tea, hops/rosemary sleep pillow, wild lettuce/valerian extract, ashwagandha/black cohosh/scullcap capsules.

❧ **For calming stress and tension:** ginseng/licorice extract, rosemary/chamomile tea; Bach Flower Rescue Remedy drops, lemon balm/lemongrass tea, valerian/wild lettuce extract; chamomile aromatherapy.

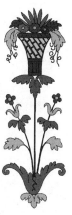

❧ **For indigestion, gas and upset stomach relief:** ginger tea or capsules; catnip/fennel tea; mint mix tea or extract, comfrey/pepsin capsules; aloe vera juice with herbs, spice mix tea or extract.

❧ **For eye infections and inflammations:** aloe vera juice wash, eyebright/parsley/bilberry capsules or wash, echinacea/goldenseal wash, chamomile/elder compress; witch hazel/rosemary solution.

❧ **For toothaches and gum problems:** tea tree oil, apply clove oil directly onto tooth or gums.

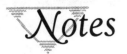

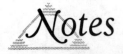

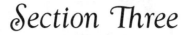

Section Three

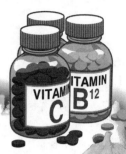

THE ALTERNATIVE HEALTH CARE ARSENAL

This invaluable section is an encyclopedia-style reference that details the storehouse of alternative health care options available to Americans today. While covering all aspects of natural healing, the real value of this section lies in the information about effective alternative remedies, products, and healing techniques that consumers can access for themselves. A wealth of information from the latest world-wide research and testing, empirical observation, and alternative specialist and practitioner recommendations is included.

The survey is structured in easy-to-use alphabet order - by name of substance, product, remedy or procedure. Over 350 entries are in this exhaustive survey.

Just Look It Up!

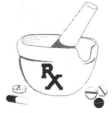

The Alternative Health Care Arsenal
Look It Up!

The alternative arsenal is an updated, exhaustive survey of the health care options available to Americans today. The value of this section lies in the information about effective alternative remedies, products, and healing procedures that consumers can access for themselves. Information from world-wide studies, empirical observation, and alternative specialist and practitioner recommendations is included.

The survey is structured in alphabetical order as an easy-reference guide. Access it by name of substance, product, remedy or procedure.

ACEROLA - derived from the ripe fruit of the cherry-like fruit of *Malpighia Glabra*, acerola is a rich source of vitamin and bioflavonoids. Used as an antioxidant and for its ascorbic acid content.

❖ ACIDOPHILUS CULTURE COMPLEX - including lactobacillus, bulgaricus, and bifida bacterium - beneficial bacteria that synthesize nutrients in the intestinal tract, counteract pathogenic micro-organisms and maintain healthy intestinal environment. Use for digestive maintenance and for friendly flora restoration after long courses of drugs.

❖ ACONITE - a homeopathic remedy for children's earaches. Helps the body deal with the trauma of sudden fright or shock. See HOMEOPATHIC REMEDIES on page 13.

❖ ACUPUNCTURE & ACUPRESSURE - see ALTERNATIVE HEALING TECHNIQUES, page 22.

❖ AGAR - a fibrous thickener in foods and cosmetics; derived from *Gelidiella Acerosa, a sea algae.*

❖ ALANINE - a non-essential amino acid which helps maintain blood glucose levels, particularly as an energy storage source for the liver and muscles. See also Amino Acids.

❖ ALGAE, GREEN & BLUE-GREEN, phyto-plankton - called perfect superfoods. See GREEN SUPERFOODS.

❖ ALLANTOIN - a cosmetic ingredient from the comfrey plant used as a skin protector and softener.

❖ ALOE VERA, *Aloe Barbadensis* - See GREEN SUPERFOODS.

❖ ALPHA HYDROXY ACIDS (AHA'S) - naturally occurring substances found in foods like apples, grapes, citrus fruit, sugarcane and sour milk, as well as in the body. AHAs work by dissolving the glue-like lipids holding cells together and can penetrate deep into the skin to loosen clingy bonds that clog and roughen skin. When top layers of skin are loosened and released they reveal a smoother complexion. Not all AHAs work the same. Glycolic acid from sugar cane acts the quickest and deepest, but can also be one of the most irritating. Lactic acid from sour milk is now often the AHA of choice because it doesn't penetrate as deeply and is not as irritating. Tartaric acid from grapes, malic acid from apples, citric acid from citrus, and new synthetics, work only on and near the skin surface. They take longer to show improvement, but do not sting, burn or redden the skin. Products advertised with high AHA percentage, carry no guarantee that they will work better - only faster. The real difference is in the pH level of the product. Quicker results can be achieved from a product **lower** on the pH scale (2.5pH) than a product higher on the pH scale (4.5pH). Products between 3pH and 4.5pH have more moisturizing effects.

❖ ALPHA-LINOLENIC ACID (LNA) - See FATS & OILS, page 193.

❖ ALPHA TOCOPHEROL - found in wheat germ, nut and seed oils, eggs, organ meats, oats and olives, helps prevent sterility, improves circulation, promotes longevity, prevents blood clots, prolongs life of red blood cells, strengthens capillary walls, helps the body utilize vitamin A, maintains integrity of cell membranes, and contributes to healthy skin and hair. Alpha tocopherol is an antioxidant, protecting healthy cells from destruction by free radicals, and as a result is a proven factor in the prevention of cardiovascular disease.

❖ **AMLA BERRY,** *Emblica Officinalis* - Indian gooseberry, one of the richest natural sources of bioflavonoid and vitamin C; each amla fruit contains up to 700mg of vitamin C. It is a natural ascorbate, synergistically enhanced by both bioflavonoid and polyphenols. Amla is revered for its anti-aging, immune enhancing properties. Since ancient times, it has been used as a rejuvenating, adaptive therapy, particularly indicated for anemia, asthma, bleeding gums, diabetes, colds, chronic lung disease, hyperlipidemia, hypertension, yeast infections, scurvy and cancer. Several studies show that amla protects against chromosome damage from heavy metal exposure.

❖ **AMINO ACIDS** - the building blocks of protein in the body - absolutely necessary to life, growth and healing. Protein is composed of, and depends upon the right supply of amino acids. There are 29 of them known, from which over 1600 basic proteins are formed, comprising more than 75% of the body's solid weight of structural, muscle, and blood protein cells. Amino acids are an important part of body fluids, antibodies to fight infection, and hormone/enzyme systems to regulate growth and digestion. Amino acids are also responsible for the growth, maintenance and repair of our bodies throughout our lives. They are sources of energy, play a vital role in brain function and mood elevation, are critical to rapid healing, and are buffering agents for proper acid/alkaline balance. The central nervous system cannot function without amino acids, because they act as neurotransmitters.

The liver produces about 80% of the amino acids it needs; the remaining 20% must be regularly obtained from our foods. But poor diet, unhealthy habits and environmental pollutants mean that the "essential amino acids", (those which the body cannot produce), are often not sufficient to produce the "non-essentials," (those formed by metabolic activity). This can be corrected by either increasing intake of protein foods or supplementation. A food-source, pre-digested supplement may often be taken in more quickly than dietary amino acids.

Specific amino acids produce specific pharmacological effects in the body, and can be used to target specific healing goals. Amino acids work well with other natural healing agents, such as herbs, minerals and anti-oxidant vitamins. The main amino acids are Alanine, Arginine, Aspartic Acid, Branch Chain Aminos, Carnitine, Cysteine, Cystine, GABA, Glutamic Acid, Glutamine, Glutathione, Glycine, Di-methyl-glycine, Histidine, Inosine, Lysine, Methionine, Ornithine, Phenylalanine, Taurine, Threonine, Tryptophan, Tyrosine. SEE REFERENCES BY NAME IN THIS SURVEY.

HERE ARE SOME TIPS FOR TAKING AMINO ACIDS EFFECTIVELY:
1. Take amino acids with extra water or other liquid for optimum absorption by the body.
2. If using an individual free form amino acid, add a full spectrum amino acid compound sometime during the same day for increased absorption and results.
3. Many free form aminos compete for uptake, take free forms separately from each other for best results.
4. Take individual free form amino acids with their nutrient co-factors for best metabolic uptake.
5. Take free form amino acids, except those for brain stimulation, before meals.

Note: The names of amino acids are often preceded by the letters "D," "L," or "DL." The prefixes are necessary because many biological compounds exist in nature in two forms that are identical, except that they are mirror images of each other (like your right and left hands). In most cases, only one of the forms is active in the body. "D" stands for "dextro" (right), "L" stands for "levo" (left). Sometimes the "D" form is active, such as D-glucose and D-alpha-tocopherol, sometimes the "L" form is active, such as L-carnitine, L-tryptophan, and L-lysine. Only the active form is usually available for sale, so whether the initial is stated or not, the product is the same.

❖ **AMINOPHYLLINE** - a theophylline-type extract of ephedra, is the primary ingredient in the latest effective spot reducing creams. Here's how aminophylline works. Fat cells are covered with little switches called beta-receptors. When the body needs energy, beta-receptors are stimulated to release a substance that activates fat for fuel, and then is neutralized. But, the type of cells for long term storage, that reside in a woman's thighs and upper arms, and on a man's belly, have only a few beta-receptors and consequently hang on to their fat stores. Prolonging fat release activity in these cells can result in one to two inches of fat loss from fat storage depots. Aminophylline's role in this process is to keep the fat releasing substance activated to prolong the mechanism of fat loss.

❖ **ANTI-NEOPLASTON THERAPY** - a relatively new cancer treatment developed by Dr. Stanislaw Burzynski. Antineoplastons consist of small peptides, components of protein, and peptide metabolites that are given orally or intravenously. They work by entering the cell and altering specific functions of the genes: Some activate the tumor suppressor genes that prevent cancer, while others turn off the oncogenes that force the cancer cell to divide uncontrollably. Antineoplastons cause cancerous cells to either revert to normal or die without dividing.

Burzynski first isolated the natural compounds from blood and urine in the early 1970's. He now synthesizes them at his own FDA regulated pharmaceutical lab. For complete information write to P.O. box 1770, Pacific Palisades, CA. 90272.

✢ **ANTIOXIDANTS** - one of today's bywords for a healthier, longer life. Increasing evidence shows that people live more vigorous, less-diseased lives when antioxidants are a part of their nutritional program. This is especially true if a person shows signs of premature aging, immune deficiency, allergy sensitivities, or is regularly exposed to environmental pollutants. Although oxygen is vital to our body functions, the presence of either too much or too little oxygen creates toxic by-products called free radicals. These highly reactive substances can damage cell structures so badly that immunity is impaired and DNA codes are altered, resulting in degenerative disease and premature aging. Specifically, free radical attacks are the forerunners of heart attacks, cancer, and opportunistic diseases such as HIV infection, candidiasis or chronic fatigue syndrome.

Antioxidants unite with oxygen, protecting the cells and other body constituents like enzymes from being destroyed or altered by oxidation. Antioxidant mechanisms are selective, acting against undesirable oxygen reactions but not with desirable oxygen activity. Anti-oxidants "scavenge" free radicals, neutralize their damage and render them harmless. A poor diet, inadequate exercise, illness and emotional stress result in a reduction of the body's system antioxidants.

See also Free Radicals.

Here are some anti-oxidants you can use for protective health care and healing:
* **Pycnogenol** - a highly active bioflavonoid extract from pine bark. Fifty times stronger than vitamin E, 20 times stronger than vitamin C, it is one of the few dietary antioxidants that readily crosses the blood-brain barrier to directly protect brain cells.
* **CoQ$_{10}$** - an essential catalyst co-enzyme for cellular energy in the body. Supplementation provides wide ranging therapeutic benefits. See Enzymes & Enzyme Therapy, pg. 30, for complete information.
* **Germanium** - A potent antioxidant mineral (stated as germanium sesqui-oxide), that detoxifies, blocks free radicals and increases production of natural killer cells. An interferon stimulus for immune strength and healing.
* **Ginkgo Biloba** - used therapeutically to combat the effects of aging, especially those involving memory acuity and circulation. Helps protect cells against damage from free radicals. Reduces blood cell clumping which leads to congestive heart disease.
* **Glutathione Peroxidase** - an antioxidant enzyme that scavenges and neutralizes free radicals by turning them into stable oxygen and H$_2$O$_2$, and then into oxygen and water. See Enzymes & Enzyme Therapy, pg. 30.
* **SOD, Super-Oxide Dismutase** - an anti-oxidant enzyme that works with catalase to scavenge and neutralize free radicals. See Enzymes & Enzyme Therapy, pg. 30.
* **Astragalus** - an herbal immune stimulant and body tonic, that enhances adrenal function. Vasodilating properties lower blood pressure, increase metabolism and improve circulation.
* **Methionine** - a free radical deactivator and "lipotropic" that keeps fats from accumulating in the liver and arteries. Protective against chemical allergic reactions.
* **Cysteine** - an antioxidant amino acid that works with vitamins C, E, and selenium to protect against radiation toxicity, cancer carcinogens, and free radical damage to skin and arteries. Stimulates white cell activity in the immune system. Aids in the body's uptake of iron. *Note:* Take vitamin C in a 3:1 ratio to cysteine for best results.
* **Egg lipids, egg yolk lecithin** - a powerful source of choline and phosphatides. Used in the treatment of AIDS and immune-deficient diseases. Refrigerate and take immediately upon mixing with water to retain potency.
* **Octacosanol** - a wheat germ derivative, used therapeutically to counteract fatigue and increase oxygen utilization during exercise and athletic sports.
* **L-Glutathione** - an amino acid that works with cysteine and glutamine as a glucose tolerance factor and anti-oxidant to neutralize radiation toxicity and inhibit free radicals. Cleanses the blood from the effects of chemotherapy, X-rays and liver toxicity.
* **Wheat Germ Oil** - extracted from the embryo of the wheat berry; rich in B vitamins, proteins, vitamin E, and iron. One tablespoon provides the anti-oxidant equivalent of an oxygen tent for 30 minutes.
* **GLA, Gamma Linoleic Acid** - obtained from evening primrose oil, black currant oil and borage seed oil. A source of energy for the cells, electrical insulation for nerve fibers, a precursor of prostaglandins which regulate hormone and metabolic functions.
* **Shiitake mushrooms** - produce a virus which stimulates interferon in the body for stronger immune function. Used in Oriental medicine to prevent high blood pressure and heart disease, and to reduce cholesterol.
* **Reishi Mushrooms (Ganoderma)** - a tonic that increases vitality, enhances immunity and prolongs a healthy life. Helps reduce the side effects of chemotherapy for cancer.
* **Tyrosine** - an amino acid formed from phenylalanine - a GH stimulant that helps build the body's store of adrenal and thyroid hormones. A source of quick energy, especially for the brain.
* **Di-Methyl-Glycine (commonly known as B$_{15}$)** - an energy stimulant, used chiefly by athletes for endurance and stamina. Sublingual forms are most absorbable. For best results, take before sustained exercise. *Note:* Too much DMG disrupts the metabolic chain and causes fatigue. The proper dose produces energy, overdoses do not.

Certain foods are also rich in anti-oxidant protection. Here are the main anti-oxidants in foods:

- **Selenium** - a component of glutathione. Protects the body from free radical damage and heavy metal toxicity. Food sources include bran, brewer's yeast, broccoli, cabbage, celery, corn, cucumbers, garlic, mushrooms, onions, wheat germ and whole grains.
- **Vitamin E** - a fat soluble anti-oxidant and immune stimulant whose activity is increased by selenium. Neutralizes free radicals against the effects of aging. An effective anticoagulant and vasodilator against blood clots and heart disease. Food sources include almonds, walnuts, apricots, corn, safflower oil, peanut butter, wheat germ.
- **Beta-carotene** - a vitamin A precursor, converting to vit. A in the liver as the body needs it. A powerful anti-infective and antioxidant for immune health, protection against environmental pollutants, slowing the aging process, and allergy control. Food sources include yellow and orange fruits and vegetables, and sea vegetables.
- **Vitamin C** - a primary preventive of free radical damage, and immune strength. Protects against infections, safeguards against radiation, heavy metal toxicity, environmental pollutants and early aging. Essential to formation of new collagen tissue, supports adrenal and iron insufficiency, especially when the body is under stress. Food sources include broccoli, grapefruit, kale, kiwi, oranges, potatoes, strawberries.

Note: The cancer-fighting potential of vitamins A, C, E, the trace mineral selenium, and beta carotene is enhanced when these anti-oxidant nutrients are taken together.

❖ **ANTI-CARCINOGENIC HERBS & FOODS** - anticarcinogens are any substances that prevent or delay tumor formation and development. Some herbs and foods with known anti-carcinogenic properties include panax ginseng, certain soy products, garlic, echinacea, goldenseal, licorice, black cohosh, wild yam, sarsaparilla, maitake mushroom and cruciferous vegetables.

❖ **ANTI-PARASITIC NUTRIENTS** - parasites are an extremely common and persistent ailment in countries around the globe. Like other biological creatures, parasites have adapted and become stronger in order to survive in the world, developing defenses against the drugs designed to kill them. In fact, most drugs commonly used to treat parasites not only lose effectiveness against new parasitic strains, but also cause a number of unpleasant side effects in the host. Herbal remedies, however, have been successfully used for centuries as living medicines against parasites, with little or no side effects. Natural antiparasitic herbs include black walnut hulls, garlic, pumpkin seed, gentian root, wormwood, butternut bark, fennel seed, cascara sagrada, mugwort, slippery elm and false unicorn.

❖ **APIS** - a homeopathic remedy consisting of macerated bee tincture. Relieves stinging after bee sting or insect bite See Homeopathic Remedies, page 13.

❖ **ARGININE** - a semi-essential amino acid which is a prime stimulant for growth hormone and immune response in the pituitary and liver. A specific for athletes and body builders, increasing muscle tone while decreasing fat. Promotes healing of wounds, blocks formation of tumors, and increases sperm motility. Helps lower blood serum fats, and detoxifies ammonia. Curbs the appetite, and aids in metabolizing fats for weight loss. Herpes virus, and schizophrenia can be retarded by "starving" them of arginine foods, such as nuts, peanut butter or cheese. Take with cranberry or apple juice for best results.

❖ **ARNICA** - a homeopathic remedy for pain relief and to speed healing, especially from sports injuries, like sprains, strains and bruises. May be used topically or internally. See Homeopathic Remedies page 13.

❖ **AROMATHERAPY** - see page Alternative Healing Techniques, pg. 33.

❖ **ARROWROOT** - powdered cassava herb, used as a thickener for sauces. A less processed substitute for cornstarch, arrowroot works without the digestive, elimination and vitamin loss cornstarch can cause.

❖ **ARSENICUM ALBUM** - a homeopathic remedy for food poisoning accompanied by diarrhea; for allergic symptoms such as a runny nose; for asthma and colds. See Homeopathic Remedies page 13.

❖ **ASPARTAME** - *Note:* FDA has received more complaints about adverse reactions to aspartame than any other food ingredient in the agency's history. See Sugar & Sweeteners in a Healing Diet, page 196.

❖ **ASPARTIC ACID** - a non-essential amino acid, abundant in sugar cane and beets; used mainly as a sweetener. A precursor of threonine, it is a neurotransmitter made with ATP that increases the body's resistance to fatigue. Clinically used to counteract depression and in drugs to protect the liver.

❖ ASTRAGALUS - a prime immune enhancing herb, it is a strong antiviral agent, working to produce extra interferon in the body. Astragalus can counteract immune-suppressing effects of cancer drugs and radiation. Vasodilating properties help significantly lower blood pressure, reduce excess fluid retention, and improve circulation. Chinese research indicates that astragalus is an anti-clotting agent in preventing coronary heart disease. Nourishes exhausted adrenals to combat fatigue. Also effective in normalizing the nervous system and hormone balance.

❖ AYURVEDA - See HERBAL HEALING PHILOSOPHIES, page 44.

BARLEY GRASS - See GREEN SUPERFOODS, page 183.

❖ BEE POLLEN - collected by bees from male seed flowers, mixed with secretion from the bee, and formed into granules. A highly bio-active, tonic nutrient rightly known as a "superfood." Completely balanced for vitamins, minerals, proteins, carbohydrates, fats, enzyme precursors, and all essential amino acids. Bee pollen is a full-spectrum blood building and rejuvenative substance, particularly beneficial for the extra nutritional and energy needs of athletes and those recuperating from illness. Often used as a pollen and spore antidote during allergy season, bee pollen also relieves other respiratory problems, like bronchitis, sinusitis and colds. Like royal jelly, pollen helps balance the endocrine system, with specific benefits for menstrual and prostate problems. The enzyme support in bee pollen normalizes chronic colitis and constipation/diarrhea syndromes. Recent research has shown that pollen helps counteract the effects of aging, and increases both mental and physical capability. Two teaspoons daily is the usual dose. Use only unsprayed pollen for therapeutic applications.

❖ BEE PROPOLIS - a product collected by bees from the resin under the bark of certain trees. As the first line of defense against beehive infective organisms, it is a natural antibiotic, antiviral and antifungal substance. In humans propolis stimulates the thymus gland to boost resistance to infection, and like all bee products, has strong antibiotic properties. It is also a powerful anti-viral, effective against pneumonia and similar viral infections. Propolis is rich in bioflavonoids and amino acids and a good source of trace minerals such as copper, magnesium, silicon, iron, manganese and zinc. It is high in B vitamins, C, E and beta-carotene.
Propolis has a wide range of therapeutic uses. It is used to treat stomach and intestinal ulcers. It speeds the healing of broken bones, and accelerates new cell growth. It is part of almost every natural treatment for gum, mouth and throat disorders. Research on propolis and serum blood fats has confirmed its reputation for lowering high blood pressure, reducing arteriosclerosis and lessening the risk of coronary heart disease. New testing shows preliminary healing effects on certain skin cancers and melanomas. Propolis is available in several medicinal forms: a concentrated application tincture for warts, herpes lesions or other sores, a lighter concentration to mix with liquids and take internally, and chewable lozenges for mouth and gum healing. Normal dosage is 300mg daily.

❖ BENTONITE - a natural clay substance used for internal cleansing and externally as a poultice or mask.

❖ BELLADONNA - a homeopathic remedy excellent for sudden fever or sunstroke, also childhood fevers, stomach spasms or restless sleep. See HOMEOPATHIC REMEDIES, page 13.

❖ BETA CAROTENE - a vitamin A precursor, converting to vit. A in the liver as the body requires. A powerful anti-infective and anti-oxidant for immune health, protection against environmental pollutants, the aging process, and allergy control. Supplementation protects against respiratory diseases and infections. Beta carotene helps prevent lung cancer, and in developing anti-tumor immunity. Food sources include green leafy vegetables, green pepper, carrots and other orange vegetables, dandelion greens and sea vegetables. See Vitamins.

❖ B COMPLEX VITAMINS - the B Complex vitamins are essential to almost every aspect of body function, including metabolism of carbohydrates, fats, amino acids and energy production. B Complex vitamins work together. While the separate B vitamins can and do work for specific problems or deficiencies, they should be taken as a whole for broad-spectrum activity. See Vitamins.

❖ BIOFEEDBACK - see ALTERNATIVE HEALING TECHNIQUES, page 25.

❖ BIOFLAVONOIDS - part of the vitamin C complex, bioflavonoids prevent arteries from hardening, lower cholesterol, and enhance blood vessel, capillary and vein strength. They protect connective tissue integrity, control bruising, internal bleeding and mouth herpes. Bioflavs stimulate bile production. They are anti-microbial against infections and inflammation.

B

One major study shows that bioflavonoids, when combined with enzymes and vitamin C, perform as well as anti-inflammatory drug prescriptions in reducing swelling. They retard cataract formation, and guard against diabetic retinopathy. The body does not produce bioflavonoids; they must be obtained from the diet. The strongest supplement form is quercetin. Food sources include blueberries, cherries, turmeric, ginger, alfalfa, the white pith of citrus fruits and certain herbs. See Vitamins.

✢ **BIOTIN** - a member of the B Complex family, necessary for metabolism of amino acids and essential fatty acids, and in forming immune anti-bodies. Needed for the body to use folacin, B_{12} and pantothenic acid. Naturally made from yeast, biotin supplements show good results in controlling hair loss, dermatitis, eczema, dandruff and seborrheic scalp problems. Improves glucose tolerance in diabetics. Research shows enhanced immune response for Candida Albicans and CFS. Those taking long term anti-biotics require extra biotin. Food sources include poultry, raspberries, grapefruit, tomatoes, tuna, brewer's yeast, salmon, eggs, organ meats, legumes and nuts. See Vitamins.

✢ **BORON** - a mineral which enhances the use of calcium, magnesium, phosphorus and vitamin D in bone formation and structure. Stimulates estrogen production to protect against the onset of osteoporosis. A significant nutritional deterrent to bone loss for athletes. Food sources include most vegetables, fruits and nuts.

✢ **BOSWELLIA** - *Boswellia glabra, Boswellia serrata* - an anti-inflammatory in Ayurvedic healing. The action of boswellia suppresses the proliferating tissue of inflamed areas and also prevents breakdown of connective tissue. Boswellia is effective in treating rheumatoid arthritis, osteoarthritis, low back pain, myositis, and fibrositis.

✢ **BOVINE TRACHEAL CARTILAGE** - a safe and effective anticancer, anti-inflammatory, wound healing agent. BTC is used to treat cancer, arthritis, rheumatism, acute and chronic skin allergies, and to accelerate the healing of wounds. BTC is a biological response modifier which activates and increases the ability of macrophages (white blood cells) to destroy bacteria and viruses. Paradoxically, BTC is a normalizer, stimulating the immune system in resisting cancer and viruses, but suppressing it in rheumatoid diseases. Standard dosage of BTC is 9 grams daily.

✢ **BRANCH CHAIN AMINO ACIDS** - Leucine, Isoleucine, Valine (BCAAs) - essential amino acids called the stress amino acids, they must be taken together in balanced proportion. Easily converted into ATP, critical to energy and muscle metabolism. Aid in hemoglobin formation, help to stabilize blood sugar and lower elevated blood sugar levels. Used to treat severe amino acid deficiencies caused by addictions. BCAAs show excellent results in tissue repair from athletic stress, rebuilding the body from anorexia deficiencies, and in liver restoration after surgical trauma.

✢ **BREWER'S YEAST** - See ABOUT PROTEINS AND A HEALING DIET, page 188.

✢ **BROMELAIN** - a naturally occurring enzyme derived from pineapple stems. As a nutritional therapy supplement, it is widely used to assist in the digestion of protein, to relieve painful menstruation, and to treat arthritis. Bromelain inhibits blood-platelet aggregation (clotting) without causing excess bleeding. It has become a popular internal sports injury medicine, to reduce bruising, relieve pain and swelling, and promote wound healing. It may also be used externally, as a paste applied to stings, to deactivate the protein molecules of insect venom. I highly recommend bromelain before and after surgery of all kinds to accelerate healing. Typically it is taken with meals as a digestive aid, or 30 minutes before or 90 minutes after a meal to help treat sports injuries. See also ENZYMES & ENZYME THERAPY, pg. 30.

✢ **BRYONIA** - a homeopathic remedy for the swelling and inflammation of arthritis when the symptoms are worse with movement and better with cold. Also for flu infections. See HOMEOPATHIC REMEDIES, page 13.

✢ **BUCKWHEAT** - a non-wheat grain, acceptable for candida diets. Known as kasha when roasted.

✢ **BURDOCK** - a nutritional, hormone-balancing herb, burdock is an important anti-inflammatory, antibacterial, antifungal and antitumor herb, with strong liver purifying and hormone balancing properties. A specific in all blood cleansing, detoxification and immune enhancing combinations, it has particular value for skin, arthritic, and glandular problems.

CALCIUM - the body's most abundant mineral. Every cell needs calcium to survive. Calcium is necessary for body synthesis of B_{12} and uses vitamin D for absorption. It works with phosphorus to build sound teeth and bones, with magnesium for cardiovascular health and skeletal strength. It helps blood clotting, lowers blood pressure, prevents muscle cramping, maintains nervous system health, controls anxiety and depression, and insures quality rest and sleep. It deters colon cancer and osteoporosis. Aluminum-based antacids, aspirin, cortisone, chemo-therapeutic agents, calcium channel blockers and some antibiotics, all interfere with calcium absorption. Antibiotics and cortico-steroids increase calcium needs. Calcium citrate has the current best record of absorbency. Good food sources include green vegetables, dairy products, sea vegetables, tofu, molasses and shellfish.

❖ **CALCAREA FLUOR** - a homeopathic cell salt used in the treatment of dilated or weak blood vessels, such as those found in hemorrhoids, varicose veins, hardened arteries and glands. See HOMEOPATHIC CELL SALTS, page 16.

❖ **CALCAREA PHOS** - a homeopathic cell salt used to strengthen bones, and help build new blood cells. Deficiency results in anemia, emaciation, poor digestion and slow growth. See HOMEOPATHIC CELL SALTS, page 16.

❖ **CALCAREA SULPH** - calcium sulphate - found in bile; promotes continual blood cleansing. When deficient, toxic build-up occurs in the form of skin disorders, respiratory clog, boils and ulcerations, and slow healing. Commonly used as a homeopathic cell salt. See HOMEOPATHIC CELL SALTS, page 16.

❖ **CAMPHOR OIL** - a mild antiseptic from the Cinnamonium camphora tree. Used in oily skin preparations.

❖ **CANOLA OIL** - See FATS & OILS.

❖ **CAPRYLIC ACID** - a short-chain fatty acid that has long been known for its antifungal effects. Effective against all candida species, caprylic acid helps restore and maintain a healthy balance of yeast. Caprylic acid is not absorbed in the stomach, making it an excellent choice for candida of the gut. Occurs naturally as a fatty acid in sweat, in the cow's and goat's milk, and in palm and coconut oil.

❖ **CAPSICUM** - increases thermogenesis for weight loss, especially when combined with caffeine herbs or ephedra. Works on the central system; gives the system a little cardiovascular lift by increasing circulation. Works as a catalyst to enhance the performance of other herbs in a formula.

❖ **CAROB POWDER** - a sweet powder with 45% natural sugars, made from the seed pods of a Mediterranean tree. It has a flavor similar to chocolate, but contains less fat and no caffeine.

❖ **CANTHARIS** - a homeopathic remedy for bladder infections and genito-urinary tract problems, especially if there is burning and urgency. Also good for burns. See HOMEOPATHIC REMEDIES, page 13.

❖ **CARNITINE** - a non-essential amino acid, it is a naturally occurring compound synthesized in the body, particularly from animal flesh (hence the name carnitine). Carnitine helps regulate fat metabolism by transporting fatty-acid molecules into the mitochondria of cells where they are "burned" to produce energy. Decreases ischemic heart disease by preventing fatty build-up, and providing muscle energy to the heart. Because of the role it plays in fat utilization, it helps prostaglandin metabolism and improves abnormal cholesterol and triglyceride levels. Carnitine speeds fat oxidation for weight loss, increasing the use of fat as an energy source. In addition, many weight-loss diets cause a problem called ketosis, the accumulation of ketones, fat waste products in the blood. Ketones cause the blood to become acidic, and lead to the loss of essential minerals. When uncontrolled, ketosis in excessive weight-loss diets or diabetes can be life-threatening. Carnitine encourages the proper metabolism of fats and prevents ketones from building up in serious dieters or diabetics.

❖ **CHAMOMILLA** - a homeopathic remedy for calming fussy children, when they are crying because of pain, especially for teething pain. An aid in drug withdrawal. See HOMEOPATHIC REMEDIES, page 13.

❖ **CHARCOAL, ACTIVATED** - a natural agent that relieves gas and diarrhea. An antidote for almost all poisons. ***Note: For any case of severe poisoning, phone the Poison Control Center 1-800-342-9293.

❖ **CHIROPRACTIC** - see ALTERNATIVE HEALING SYSTEMS, page 17.

❖ **CHLORELLA** - See GREEN SUPERFOODS, page 183.

❖ **CHLORINE** - naturally-occurring chlorine stimulates liver activity, bile and smooth joint/tendon operation. An electrolyte, it helps maintain acid/alkaline balance. Good food sources include seafoods, seaweeds and salt.

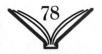

❖ **CHOLINE** - a lipotropic, B complex family member, choline works with inositol to emulsify fats. A brain nutrient and neurotransmitter that aids memory and learning ability, and is effective in retarding Alzheimer's disease and neurological disorders. It is used as part of a program to overcome alcoholism, liver and kidney disorders. New research indicates success in cancer management. Helps control dizziness, lowers cholesterol, and supports proper liver function.

❖ **CHROMIUM** - an essential trace mineral needed for glucose tolerance and sugar regulation. Chromium deficiency means high cholesterol, heart trouble, diabetes or hypoglycemia, poor carbohydrate and fat metabolism, and premature aging. Supplementation can reduce blood cholesterol levels, increase HDL cholesterol levels, and diminish atherosclerosis. Most effective as a biologically active form of GTF (chromium, niacin and glutathione), it helps control diabetes through insulin potentiation. For athletes, chromium is a healthy, safe way to convert body fat to muscle. For dieters, chromium curbs the appetite as it raises body metabolism. Good food sources include brewer's yeast, clams, honey, whole grains, liver, corn oil, grapes, raisins.

Chromium picolinate is an exceptionally bio-active source of chromium. It is a combination of chromium and picolinic acid, a natural substance secreted by the liver and kidneys. Picolinic acid is the body's best mineral transporter, combining with elements such as iron, zinc and chromium to move them quickly and efficiently into the cells. Chromium plays a vital role in sensitizing the body to insulin. Excess body weight in the form of fat tends to impair insulin sensitivity, making it harder to lose weight. Chromium picolinate also has other benefits. It builds muscles without steroid side effects, promotes healthy growth in children, speeds wound healing, and decreases proneness of plaque accumulation in the arteries. 200mcg of chromium picolinate appear to be the best dose.

❖ **COBALAMIN** - See Vitamin B_{12}. **Cyanocobalamin** may be made from sugar beets, molasses or whey. Used as a skin revitalizer, it improves the appearance of skin. Also used as a colorant.

❖ **COBALT** - an integral component mineral of vitamin B_{12} synthesis. Aids in hemoglobin formation. Good food sources are green leafy vegetables and liver.

❖ **COCONUT OIL** - See FATS & OILS, page 193.

❖ **Co-ENZYME Q10** - a vital enzyme catalyst in the creation of cellular energy. Found in rice bran, wheat germ, beans, nuts, fish and eggs, it is synthesized in the liver. The body's ability to assimilate food source Co-Q_{10} declines with age. Co-Q_{10} supplementation has a long history of effectiveness in boosting immunity, promoting natural weight loss, inhibiting aging and overcoming periodontal disease. Co-Q_{10} is successful in raising cardiac strength against angina, and is crucial in preventing and treating congestive heart and arterial diseases. It can reduce high blood pressure without other medication. The newest research at doses of 300mg for breast and prostate cancer protection and treatment is extremely encouraging.

Co-Q_{10} is similar chemically to vitamin E, and many of the symptoms of vitamin E deficiency can be corrected by taking Co-Q_{10}. Furthermore, vitamin E enhances the function of Co-Q_{10}, so the two taken in unison are a good choice. See ENZYMES & ENZYME THERAPY, page 30.

❖ **COLLAGEN** - the most abundant protein of the body, is responsible for maintaining the integrity of vein walls, tendons, ligaments, and cartilage. Collagen is similar to elastin and is the chief constituent in connective tissue. Connective tissue is dependant on nutrients from blood, so a healthy circulatory system aids in healthy skin, ligaments and tendons. (This is why smoking, a blood vessel constrictor, is so detrimental to connective tissue.) Exercise, a healthy diet and supplements like ginkgo biloba, cayenne and garlic work to keep the circulatory system functioning properly. Horsetail herb, high in silica, is an important trace mineral for connective tissue.

Vitamin C complex, especially with flavonoids like PCOs, supports collagen growth and structure and prevents collagen destruction. PCOs have the unique ability to crosslink collagen fiber, resulting in reinforcement of the natural crosslinking of collagen that forms the so-called collagen matrix of connective tissue. PCOs inhibit enzymatic cleavage of collagen by enzymes secreted by white blood cells during inflammation and microbes during infection.

❖ **COLLOIDAL SILVER** - pure metallic ionic silver held in suspension by the minute electrical charge of each particle. Probably the most universal antibiotic natural substance, consumable colloidal silver is not produced by a chemical process. It is tasteless, nonaddictive and nontoxic. Many forms of bacteria, viruses and fungi utilize a specific enzyme for their metabolism. Colloidal silver acts as a catalyst, to disable the enzyme. In fact, it has proven toxic to most species of fungi, bacteria, parasites, even many viruses. Most important, the bacteria, fungi and viruses do not seem to develop an immunity to silver as they do to chemical antibiotic agents.

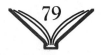

❖ **COPPER** - a mineral which helps to control inflammatory arthritis/bursitis symptoms. Aids in iron absorption, protein metabolism, bone formation and blood clotting. SOD (superoxide dismutase) is a copper-containing enzyme that protects against free radical damage. Helps prevent hair from losing its color. Copper deficiencies can be caused by mega-dose zinc therapy, or consuming excessive amounts of refined sugar. Deficiencies result in high cholesterol, anemia, heart arrhythmias and nerves. Excess copper sometimes results in mental depression.

❖ **CREAM of TARTAR** - is tartaric acid, a leavening agent in baking, helps incorporate egg whites. One half teasp. cream of tartar and $\frac{1}{2}$ teasp. Baking soda can be substituted for 1 teasp. baking powder.

❖ **CSA, CHONDROITIN SULFATE A** - an anti-inflammatory agent from bovine cartilage. May be used both topically and internally for a wide range of problems, from anti-aging, anti-stress, and anti-allergen uses for circulatory and orthopedic therapy. Also effective for cardiovascular disease and arthritis.

❖ **CURCUMIN** - a constituent of *curcuma longa*, curcumin is an extract of turmeric, the bright yellow spice used in curry. Curcumin is anti-inflammatory, affecting prostacyclin synthesis and relieving arthritic symptoms. It inhibits platelet aggregation to protect against thrombosis; its fibrinolytic activity controls the buildup of excess fibrin in blood vessels, which can lead to blood clots. Curcumin increases the secretion of bile and protects against blood cholesterol rise from eating fatty foods - a decided value in weight control. It is also a powerful, oil-soluble antioxidant which can protect essential fatty acids, and fight viruses. Curcumin inhibits tumor necrosis factor (TNF). TNF is a cytokine that can increase HIV replication in T-cells, as well as play a major role in many acute and chronic autoimmune diseases. Numerous studies have demonstrated the anti-cancer effect of turmeric and curcumin, inhibiting both the number of tumors and also tumor size.

❖ **CYSTEINE** - a semi-essential amino acid that works with vitamins C, E and selenium as an anti-oxidant to protect against radiation toxicity, cancer carcinogens, and free radical damage to skin and arteries. Stimulates white cell activity in the immune system. Plays an active role in healing treatment from burns and surgery, and renders toxic chemicals in the body harmless. Taken with evening primrose oil, cysteine protects brain and body from alcohol and tobacco effects. It is effective in preventing hangover. Used successfully in cases of hair loss, psoriasis, skin tissue diseases. Relieves bronchial asthma through breakdown of mucous plugs. Helps prevent dental plaque formation. Aids in body uptake of iron. Nutrient co-factors are vitamins B_6, C, B_{12}, magnesium and folacin. *Note:* Take vitamin C in a 3:1 ratio to cysteine for best results.

N-acetyl-L-cysteine, NAC - is an amino acid that acts as an antioxidant, and is a more stable, bio-available form of L-cysteine. NAC is also converted in the body to glutathione. Glutathione, a prime immune response enhancer, is a tri-peptide of the amino acids cysteine, glutamic acid, and glycine. It is currently being used in the treatment of HIV, because people with AIDS have a lowered amount of glutathione. NAC may itself be useful in treatments to enhance T-cell numbers. *Note: NAC is a powerful chelator of zinc and copper, and is capable of removing enough of these minerals from the body to produce deficiencies unless supplies are adequate.*

❖ **CYSTINE** - a semi-essential amino acid - the oxidized form of cysteine, and like it, promotes white blood cell activity and healing of burns and wounds. The main constituent of hair, and essential to formation of skin, cystine is cumulative in the body. It can sometimes be harmful to the kidneys, and should generally not be used clinically. Nutrient co-factors are vitamins B_6, C, B_{12}, magnesium and folacin.

*D*EAD SEA SALTS - obtained from the Dead Sea in Israel, are composed of potassium, chlorine, sodium, calcium and magnesium salts, and sulfur and bromine compounds. Used in detoxifying baths.

❖ **DEIONIZED WATER** - water treated to remove metallic ions, exposed to ultraviolet light to kill microorganisms, and filtered through a submicron filter to further remove impurities.

❖ **DHEA, dehydro-epiandro-sterone** - an abundant hormone in the body, naturally produced from cholesterol by the adrenals, with smaller amounts manufactured by the ovaries of women. It is part of an important activity cascade that ends in the making of estrogen and/or testosterone, depending on one's sex, or age. Cholesterol may be converted into progesterone or DHEA as the body requires. DHEA aids in maintaining muscle and skin tone, and bone health. It regulates the auto-immune mechanism, stimulating immune defenses to fight infections and monitoring over-reaction that might attack the body. It has thus proven helpful against lupus and rheumatoid arthritis. Recent research shows that HIV progression can be predicted by monitoring DHEA levels. DHEA stimulates T-cells by interfering with immune suppression. People with HIV do not develop full-blown AIDS until their adrenal output of DHEA drops.

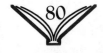

D

Supplementing DHEA is an effective therapy for post-menopausal women with osteoporosis who are low in DHEA, much the same as estrogen replacement. Other menopause symptoms are also relieved by DHEA, and breast cancer risk associated with synthetic estrogen replacement therapy (ERT) is greatly reduced; it may even be prevented by DHEA's immune support potential.

DHEA is of enormous interest today because it is called a youth hormone, an anti-aging substance that lowers serum cholesterol, reverses aging symptoms and promotes energy and libido. However, hormone balance and activity are highly individual in human bodies, so hormone test results are often inconclusive or contradictory. Recent studies show both good news and bad news, so there's a lot for you to consider. A U.C. San Diego School of Medicine study indicated that DHEA **did** act as a kind of youth drug, because older people felt better and had more energy when they took it, and there was a noticeable improvement in muscle and skin tone, as well as cardiovascular function. Another study showed that men with high levels of DHEA had half the incidence of heart disease as those with low levels. But, women with high DHEA levels had a **higher** risk of heart disease. Follow-up studies of the same patients were even more contradictory, and did not bear out the DHEA benefits in the long term.

Women who are **pre**-menopausal and have low levels of DHEA may develop breast cancer. Animal studies show that mice susceptible to breast cancer, do not develop it when treated with DHEA. Their immune systems improve, and treated mice outlive untreated ones. Women given DHEA have also seen their cholesterol levels drop.

DHEA has few side effects, but if you take too much, it suppresses your body's ability to make its own. People who use it and have good results usually have to take it for the rest of their lives to continue the results. Adult acne is a common side effect, as is excess facial and body hair. DHEA dosage falls between 5-15mg for women and 10-30mg for men. Most physicians today give it with a combination of estrogen, progesterone, and testosterone.

DHEA is not currently known to be made by plants, but the DHEA that is available in supplement form is produced from plant sterols (wild yam) by chemical synthesis. While the idea that wild yam acts as a precursor to DHEA in the body is being disregarded by researchers who have not been able to unravel all the actions of this complex plant, the fact that wild yam is used to manufacture synthetic DHEA and also progesterone might give us a clue as to why it works so well for women's hormone problems that involve progesterone.

❖ **DLPA, DL-PHENYLALANINE** - an amino acid which is a safe, effective pain reliever and anti-depressant with an endorphin effect for arthritis, lower back and cerebro-spinal pain. Increases mental alertness, and improves the symptoms of Parkinson's disease. Normal therapeutic dose is 500-750mg. Contra-indications: avoid DLPA if you have high blood pressure, are pregnant, or diabetic. See Amino Acids.

❖ **DNA** - *deoxyribonucleic acid*, is the substance in the cell nucleus that genetically codes amino acids, and determines the type of life form into which a cell will develop. Derived from fish sperm, DNA is used as a natural skin revitalizer to increase the oxygen uptake of the skin and increase circulation. Repeated exposure to radiation can cause DNA breakdown as well as free-radical damage. Optimal nutrition and antioxidants help to prevent DNA damage. Chemotherapy and radiation therapy work to destroy cancers, but also tend to mutate normal cell DNA.

E DTA, *(ethylenediamine tetra-acetic acid)* - used in chelation therapy to remove toxic, clogging minerals from the circulatory system - particularly those that impair membrane function and contribute to free radical damage. EDTA puts these minerals into solution where they can be excreted by the kidneys.

❖ **EGG OIL** - fat-soluble emollients and emulsifiers extracted from eggs. Provides protection against dehydration and has lubricating, anti-friction properties when rubbed on the skin.

Egg powder is used in many cosmetics including shampoos, creams, face masks, and bath preparations to make the hair more cohesive and manageable. Egg albumin is used in facial masks to give the characteristic tight feeling.

Egg Replacer is a combination of starches and leavening agents used to replace those qualities of eggs in baking. It is a vegetarian product, cholesterol free.

❖ **ELASTIN** - protein in connective tissue that is similar to collagen and is the chief constituent in connective tissue. Connective tissue receives its nutrients from blood, so a healthy circulatory system will aid in the health of skin, ligaments and tendons. Smoking can be very detrimental to connective tissue because it constricts the blood vessels. Exercise, a healthy diet and supplements like ginkgo biloba, cayenne and garlic work to keep the circulatory system functioning properly. Vitamins and minerals are important nutrients for connective tissue and the body can easily use them from herbs. Horsetail herb is high in silica, an important trace mineral for connective tissue. Vitamins A (and or beta-carotene, a vitamin A precursor), B, C, and D are essential for connective tissue health.

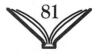

❖ **ELECTROLYTES** - ionized salts in the blood, tissue fluids and cells, transporting electrical "operating" energy throughout the body, so it can work. Electrolytes include salts of sodium, potassium and chlorine, and are essential to cell function and body pH balance. But they are easily lost through perspiration and fluid elimination, so regular replacement is necessary from drinking electrolytic fluids. When electrolytes are low, we tire easily. When they are adequate, we almost instantly experience more energy. Electrolyte drinks are especially beneficial for athletes and those doing hard physical work.

❖ **EMOLLIENTS** - a mixture of oils, are the heart of moisturizers. They help soften and smooth the skin, reduce roughness, cracking and skin irritation, and retard the fine wrinkles of aging. They do this by coating the skin with a film and retarding evaporation of water. Glycerine, an emollient, actually attracts water to the skin surface.

❖ **EMULSION** - a substance formed when two or more non-mixable liquids are mixed so thoroughly together that they appear to be homogenized. Most oils form emulsions with water.

❖ **ENERGIZERS & STIMULANTS, NATURAL** - the most common reason for taking stimulants is fatigue, both mental and physical. Stimulants increase the action of a system or metabolic process to create a sense of well-being, exhilaration, and self-confidence. They relieve fatigue and drowsiness. The downside to many stimulants is tolerance, dependency, nervousness, and restlessness. There may be difficulty in concentrating and after-effect headaches. Increasing the strength of a stimulant can increase the toxicity and/or dependency potential. Taken too often, even natural stimulants can drive a body system to exhaustion. In battling fatigue, natural energizers have great advantages over chemically processed stimulants. They have more broad-based activity so that they don't exhaust a particular organ or body system. They can be strong or gentle for individual needs. At correct dosage, they are nutrient supportive rather than depleting. Specific remedies for fatigue can be classified under central nervous system stimulants, metabolic enhancers, and adaptogens.

The following list takes a quick look at natural stimulants and what they do. See individual nutrient entries for more information about their properties, activity and benefits.

Central Nervous System (CNS) stimulants act by affecting the cerebral cortex and the medulla of the brain. Most contain either natural caffeine, naturally-occurring ephedrine, or certain free-form amino acids. In general, these substances promote alertness, energy, and a more rapid, clearer flow of thought. They also act as respiratory stimulants. Most central nervous system stimulants should be used for short-term energy needs. Long term use can result in a net loss of energy to the system. Most stimulants, even natural ones, should also be avoided during pregnancy. The tiny body of the fetus cannot handle the systemic excitation.

EXAMPLES OF COMMON, FOOD AND HERB SOURCE CENTRAL NERVOUS SYSTEM STIMULANTS:
- **Coffee and caffeine** - America's most popular stimulant. See CAFFEINE, page 202.
- **Guaraña** - a rich, natural source of rainforest guaranine, for long, slow endurance energy without coffee's heated hydrocarbons that pose health problems.
- **Glutamine** - converts readily into 6-carbon glucose; an excellent nutrient and energy source for the brain. Improves memory retention, recall, sustained concentration, and alertness. Improves mental performance in cases of retardation, senility, and schizophrenia. Increases libido and helps overcome impotence. See Amino Acids.
- **Kola Nut** - a natural caffeine without heated hydrocarbons. Allays hunger, combats fatigue.
- **L-Phenylalanine** - a Tyrosine precursor that works with vitamin B_6 as an antidepressant and mood elevator on the central nervous system. Successful in treating manic, post-amphetamine, and schizophrenic depression. Aids in learning and memory retention. A thyroid stimulant that helps curb the appetite by increasing the body's production of CCK. See Amino Acids.
- **Tyrosine** - builds adrenaline and thyroid stores. Rapidly metabolized as an antioxidant in the body; effective as a source of quick energy, especially for the brain. Safe therapy for depression, hypertension, in controlling drug abuse and aiding drug withdrawal. Increases libido. A growth hormone stimulant. See Amino Acids.
- **Yerba Mate** - a South American stimulant and rejuvenating herb that contains no caffeine. Naturally lifts fatigue and provides broad range nutrition to body cells. Rich in vitamins A, E, C and B (especially pantothenic acid), with measurable amounts of chlorophyll, calcium, potassium, iron, magnesium and manganese. Protects against the effects of stress. Helpful in opening respiratory passages to overcome allergy symptoms. In addition to its inherent benefits, yerba maté is a catalyst substance that increases the healing effectiveness of other herbs.
- **Ephedra** - a CNS stimulant that contains the biochemicals ephedrine and pseudoephedrine. Acts as an energy tonic to strengthen and restore body vitality. A natural bronchodilator and decongestant for respiratory problems. Used in many weight loss formulas for its ability to increase thermogenesis. Ephedra is also a cardiac stimulant and should be used with caution by anyone with high blood pressure. See Ephedra.

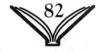

- **Ginkgo Biloba** - a primary brain and mental energy stimulant. Increases both peripheral and cerebral circulation through vasodilation. A good stimulant choice for older people who suffer from poor memory and other aging-related CNS problems. Causes an increase in acetylcholine levels, and therefore the ability to better transmit body electrical impulses. Best results are achieved from the extract. See Ginkgo Biloba.
- **Damiana** - a mild aphrodisiac, synergistic with other energy herbs in stimulating libido. A specific in a combination to treat frigidity in women and impotence in men. Also a mild anti-depressant tonic.
- **Yohimbe** - a hormone stimulant, effective in the production of testosterone. A strong aphrodisiac affecting both the male impotence and female frigidity. An effective bodybuilding and athletic formula herb where more testosterone production is desired. Note: Avoid if there is high blood pressure or heart arrythmia.

Metabolic Enhancers improve the performance of existing biochemical pathways by providing catalysts and co-factors for system support. They do not stress or deplete the body. Examples of metabolic enhancers include co-enzyme factors like B vitamins, fat mobilizers like L-carnitine, electron transporters such as CoQ-10, lactic acid limiters like inosine and gamma oryzonal (GO), and tissue oxygenators like Di-Methyl-Glycine (B_{15}).

EXAMPLES OF METABOLIC ENHANCERS:
- **Ginger** - a warming circulatory stimulant and body cleansing herb, ginger is useful in all formulas where circulation to the extremities is needed, such as arthritis. Ginger helps in all lung/chest clearing combinations, in digestive system stimulants and stomach alkalizers for clearing gas, in promoting menstrual regularity and cramping relief, and for all kinds of nausea, motion sickness and morning sickness. It may be used directly on the skin as a compress to stimulate venous circulation. Other uses include catalytic action in nervine and sedative formulas, as a gargle and sore throat syrup, as a diaphoretic to remove toxic wastes, and to stimulate kidney activity.
- **Capsicum** - increases thermogenesis for weight loss, especially when combined with xanthine herbs. It increases circulation, and is used as a central system catalyst to enhance the performance of other herbs in a formula.
- **Bee Pollen** - an energizing, nutritive substance known as a "superfood." See Bee Pollen & Royal Jelly.
- **Royal Jelly** - supplies key nutrients for energy, mental alertness and a general feeling of well-being. Enhances immunity and deep cellular health. One of the world's richest sources of pantothenic acid to combat stress, fatigue and insomnia. See Bee Pollen & Royal Jelly.
- **Green Tea** - is rich in flavonoids with anti-oxidant and anti-allergen activity. It is a beneficial fasting tea, providing energy support and clearer thinking during cleansing. It contains polyphenols (not tannins as commonly believed) that act as anti-oxidants, yet do not interfere with iron or protein absorption. As with other anti-oxidants from plants, such as beta carotene and vitamin C, green tea substances work at the molecular level, combatting free radical damage to protect against degenerative diseases. See Tea.
- **Rosemary** - an anti-oxidant herb and strong brain and memory stimulant. A circulatory toning agent, and effective nervine for stress, tension and depression.
- **CoQ$_{10}$** - an essential catalyst co-enzyme for cellular energy in the body. Supplementation provides wide ranging therapeutic benefits. See ENZYMES & ENZYME THERAPY, pg. 30.
- **DMG - Di-Methyl-Glycine, B$_{15}$** - a powerful anti-oxidant and energy stimulant. DMG is a highly reputed energizer and stimulant whose effects can be attributed to its conversion to glycine. See Amino Acids.

Adaptogens are herbal regulators that help the body handle stress and maintain vitality. They are more for long term revitalization than immediate energy. They are rich sources of strengthening nutrients such as germanium, and steroid-like compounds that provide concentrated body support. They increase the body's overall immune function with broad spectrum activity, rather than specific action. They promote recovery from illness and may be used synergistically with other tonic herbs to build strength. They are particularly beneficial in restoring the endocrine, nervous, digestive, muscle, and hepatic systems.

EXAMPLES OF ADAPTOGEN HERBS:
- **Panax Ginseng,** including Oriental red and white, and American Ginseng, is the most broad spectrum of all adaptogenic herbs. Beneficial to total health and capable of stimulating both long and short term energy. Ginseng has measurable amounts of germanium, provides energy to all body systems, is a stimulant for brain and memory centers, helps to lower cholesterol, and regulate sugar use in the body, promotes regeneration from stress and fatigue, and rebuilds foundation strength. Panax is rich in phyto-hormones for both men and women's problems, a circumstance that may be responsible for its long tradition as an aphrodisiac.

In fact, recent studies show that ginseng may be a source of testosterone production for men, and may be a protective factor for breast cancer in women because of its phyto-estrogen content. Ginseng benefits are cumulative in the body. Taking this herb for several months to a year is far more effective than short term doses. See Panax Ginseng.

- **Siberian Ginseng,** (Eleuthero) - a long-term energy tonic for the adrenal glands and circulatory health.
- **Schizandra** - synergistic with eleuthero against stress, weight gain and sports fatigue. Supports sugar regulation, and liver function and strength. Helps correct skin problems through better digestion of fatty foods.
- **Astragalus** - a superior tonic and strong immune enhancing herb. Provides therapeutic support for recovery from illness or surgery, especially from chemotherapy and radiation. Nourishes exhausted adrenals to combat fatigue. Helps normalize nervous, hormonal and immune systems. See Astragalus.
- **Suma** - an ancient herb with modern benefits for overcoming fatigue, and hormonal imbalance. Used to re-build the system from the ravages of cancer and diabetes.
- **Gotu Kola** - a brain and nervous system restorative. Especially effective after illness or surgery, it is also a tissue and circulatory toner.
- **Fo-Ti, (Ho-Shou-Wu)** - a flavonoid-rich herb with particular success in longevity formulas. A cardiovascular strengthener, increasing blood flow to the heart.
- **Tienchi** - a Japanese ginseng-type herb, used as a cardiac and blood tonic - particularly for athletes. Helps dissolve blood clots and circulatory obstructions.
- **Reishi** - an adaptogen mushroom for deep immune support, anti-cancer and anti-oxidant protection, liver regeneration and blood sugar regulation. Excellent for recovery from illness. See Reishi Mushroom.
- **Germanium** - use as organic sesquioxide. A potent adaptogen that detoxifies, blocks free radicals and increases natural killer cell production. An interferon stimulus for immune strength and healing. See Germanium.
- **Burdock** - a hormone balancing herb with antibacterial, antifungal and antitumor properties. A specific in all blood cleansing and detoxification combinations; an important anti-inflammatory and anti-infective.

❖ **ENFLEURAGE** - the time-consuming, expensive technique of making fine perfumes from delicate flowers, such as roses and orange blossoms that cannot be steam distilled. Glass trays are lined with lard, and scattered with flowers picked early in the morning. The next day the flowers are removed from the fat and replaced with fresh ones. The cycle is repeated for 4 to 5 weeks. The lard is then scraped from the trays and mixed with alcohol. When the alcohol is removed by distillation, a highly scented essential oil, or "absolute," is left behind.

❖ **ENZYMES** - see ENZYMES & ENZYME THERAPY, page 30.

❖ **EPHEDRA, Ma Huang** - used in Traditional Chinese Medicine for more than 5,000 years, few herbs have been as misunderstood as the classic herb Ma Huang. Commercially cultivated for its therapeutic properties longer than any other medicinal plant, ma huang has now become one of the most controversial herbs in America today. A wonderful bronchodilator, ma huang is used for colds and flus, fever, chills, headache, edema, bronchial asthma, lack of perspiration, nasal congestion, aching joints and bones, and coughs and wheezing.

Some of these uses for ma huang are approved by American FDA in over-the-counter (OTC) drugs, but Western manufacturers also use it for energy and diet products which are not FDA approved. Concerns over the potency and safety of this herb, especially its isolated alkaloids have prompted increased regulatory scrutiny. Ma huang contains a total of 0.5 to 2.5 percent of several ephedra alkaloids, with ephedrine comprising between 30 and 90% of total alkaloids. Ephedrine is a potent isolate; it excites the sympathetic nervous system, causes vasoconstriction and cardiac stimulation, and produces effects similar to those of adrenaline, raising blood pressure, and causing dilation of the pupils. In large doses ephedrine causes nervousness, insomnia, dizziness, palpitations and skin flushing.

The whole ephedra plant, which most knowledgeable herbalists use, is quite safe and gentle, especially in combination with other herbs. It is used as a primary anti-asthmatic, bronchodilator, hypertensive, and peripheral vasoconstrictor.

❖ **ESCIN** - a saponin occurring in the seeds of the horse chestnut tree, Aesculus hippocastanum. Used externally to reduce swelling and increase skin tissue tone by increasing circulation and encouraging flexibility.

❖ **ESSENTIAL FATTY ACIDS, Linoleic Acid, Alpha Linoleic Acid, Gamma Linoleic Acid, Linolenic Acid, and Arachidonic Acid** - See FATS & OILS, page 193.

❖ **ESSIAC** - an herbal tea formula of the Ojibway Indians, made famous by Rene Caisse for treating cancer, and being popularly rediscovered today. The name "Essiac" is actually an anagram of her last name "Caisse." The formula consists of sheep sorrel, burdock root, turkey rhubarb and slippery elm bark.

❖ **ESTROGEN** - natural estrogens are conjugated hormones, including estradiol, estrone, and estriol, thought to be formed with the involvement of the adrenals and the pituitary, especially after menopause.

- **Estradiol:** a steroid produced by the ovary and possessing estrogenic properties. Found in the urine of pregnant women and mares, and in the urine of stallions, the latter two serve as sources of the commercial product. Estradiol is converted to estrone in the body when taken orally.
- **Estrone:** an estrogen produced by the ovaries and by conversion of estradiol. This is a hormone thought to be linked to breast cancer.
- **Estriol:** believed to be a "good" estrogen (non-cancer-facilitating). Phyto-estrogens (plant estrogens) are thought to be close in chemical makeup to estriol.

*F*ERRUM PHOS - a homeopathic cell salt used to treat colds and flu, inflammation and nausea. It is a biochemical remedy for the first stages of inflammations and infective wounds. See HOMEOPATHIC CELL SALTS, page 16.

❖ FLAX SEED OIL - see ESSENTIAL FATTY ACIDS & OMEGA-3 OILS, page 194.

❖ FLUORINE - as calcium fluoride, (not sodium fluoride as is added to drinking water), a mineral which increases bone strength, reduces sugar-caused acidity in the mouth, and tooth decay.

❖ FOLIC ACID, Folacin - a B vitamin which plays an important role in the synthesis of DNA, enzyme production and blood formation. Essential for division and growth of new cells, it is an excellent supplement during pregnancy (800mcg daily) to guard against spina bifida and neural tube defects. It prevents anemia, helps control leukemia and pernicious anemia, and is effective against alcoholism, and even some precancerous lesions. It is absolutely necessary to counteract the immuno-depression state following chemotherapy with MTX. Folic acid can reduce homocysteine levels. Homocysteine tends to thicken the blood and facilitates the conversion of LDL (bad cholesterol) into free radical particles. Folacin deficiency results in malabsorption problems such as Crohn's disease and sprue. Aluminum antacids, oral contraceptives, alcohol, long-term antibiotics and anti-inflammatory drugs increase the need for folic acid. Good food sources include green leafy vegetables, organ meats, peas, brewer's yeast, broccoli, fruits, soy foods, chicken, brown rice, eggs and whole grains.

❖ FREE RADICALS - unstable fragments of molecules produced from oxygen and fats in cell membranes. Free radicals result when high energy chemical oxidation reactions in the body get out of control. Atoms and molecules consist of protons, neutrons and electrons, which normally come in pairs. Electron pairs form chemical bonds which hold all molecules together. A free radical contains an unpaired electron. In this unbalanced state, the free radical is stimulated to combine with other molecules, and in combination is capable of destroying an enzyme, a protein, or a complete cell. This destruction causes chain reactions that result in the release of thousands more free radicals stimulating accumulation of age pigment, damaging protein structures, and impairing fat metabolizing enzymes.

The body normally produces some free radicals in its ordinary metabolic breakdown of organic compounds. Indeed, some are released to fight bacteria during immune response. But as with most activities in nature, the body also produces the necessary substances (in this case the antioxidant enzymes superoxide dismutase, catalase, and glutathione peroxidase) to deactivate them. Free radicals can be caused by exposure to everything from radiation to rancid oils, including food additives and chemicals, heavy metal pollutants, UV sunlight, and fast foods.

SPECIFIC ANTIOXIDANT DEPLETERS ARE:
- Infections from viruses, bacteria, or parasites.
- Trauma from surgery, injury, inflammation, and wound healing.
- Burns, and exposure to excessive heat or cold.
- Smoking or passive exposure to cigarette smoke. Excessive alcohol and/or addictive drug intake.
- Exposure to toxic chemicals, like pesticide residues and household chemicals.
- Exposure to radiation, including excessive UV rays from sunlight.
- Cytotoxic drugs, such as the anticancer drug Adriamycin.
- Oxidant drugs that steal electrons, such as acetaminophen (Tylenol).
- Consumption of nitrites, nitrates and other food additives.
- Dietary lack of antioxidant-rich foods.
- Intense exercise on an antioxidant-deficient diet.

Some dietary substances make free radicals more likely to occur. Polyunsaturated fats, like sunflower, corn and soy oils, found in salad dressings and many "junk foods" can lead to excessive free radical production. A low-fat diet reduces the damage of oxidation by free radicals. Also, iron and copper, beneficial in small quantities, increase free radical production when ingested in large amounts.

Since we know that cell damage is at least partially responsible for the effects of aging, is involved in cancer, plays a triggering role in some forms of heart disease, and is an integral part of eye diseases like cataracts and macular degeneration, it seems likely that antioxidants which block excessive oxidation, should help prevent these conditions.

However, because we live in a polluted environment, it is increasingly doubtful that our bodies receive enough nutrients through normal food intake to meet our antioxidant needs. Zinc, carotenes and B vitamins work synergistically with antioxidants. Vitamins C and E, and a small protein called glutathione, act as anti-oxidants themselves. Herbs, such as garlic, ginkgo biloba, rosemary and the ginsengs are also rich in anti-oxidants.

❖ **FRUCTOSE** - See SWEETENERS IN A HEALING DIET, page 196.

GABA - **Gamma-Aminobutyric Acid** - a non-essential amino acid, useful in treating brain and nerve dysfunctions, such as anxiety, depression, nerves, high blood pressure, insomnia, schizophrenia, Parkinson's and Alzheimer's diseases, and ADD in children. GABA acts as a natural tranquilizer, improves libido, and along with glutamine and tyrosine, helps overcome alcohol and drug abuse. Used with niacinamide, it is a relaxant.

❖ **GARLIC** - a therapeutic food with antibiotic, antifungal, antiparasitic and antiviral activity. Used extensively for disease prevention; internally against infection of all kinds; externally for eye, ear, nose and throat infections, and because of its thiamine content, to prevent mosquito and insect bites. Garlic has a measurable amount of germanium, an antioxidant for endurance and wound healing.

❖ **GELSEMIUM** - a homeopathic remedy for chronic lethargy. See HOMEOPATHIC REMEDIES, page 13.

❖ **GENESTEIN** - See SOY FOODS IN A HEALING DIET, page 207.

❖ **GERMANIUM** - an anti-oxidant mineral which should be used as organic sesquioxide. Acts as an anticancer agent, particularly where there is tumor metastasis, by activating macrophages and increasing production of killer cells. An interferon stimulus for immune strength. Facilitates oxygen uptake, detoxifies and blocks free radicals. Effective for viral/bacterial and fungal infections, osteoporosis, arthritis, heart, blood pressure and respiratory conditions. Studies show success with leukemia, HIV, and brain, lung, pancreatic and lymphatic cancers. Good food sources include chlorella, garlic, tuna, oysters, green tea, reishi mushroom, aloe vera, ginseng, leafy greens.

❖ **GINGER** - a flavorful, aromatic, spicy herb. Both fresh and dried ginger root have therapeutic properties for digestive, hypertension, headaches and other problems. There is an easy way to have fresh ginger on hand without spoilage. Peel fresh roots, chop in the blender, put in a plastic bag, and freeze. Ginger thaws almost immediately. In less than 10 minutes, it's ready for use.

❖ **GINKGO BILOBA** - the leaf extract of an ancient Chinese tree, used therapeutically to combat the effects of aging. It improves circulation throughout the body, helps send more blood and oxygen to the brain for increased memory and mental alertness, and protects the brain against mental disorders that can cause senility. Ginkgo is effective for vertigo, dizziness and ringing in the ears. As an anti-oxidant, it protects the cells against damage from free radicals, and reduces blood cell clumping which can lead to congestive heart disease. Helps return elasticity to cholesterol-hardened blood vessels. Reduces inflammation in the lungs leading to asthmatic attack.

❖ **GINSENG, PANAX** - the most effective adaptogen of all tonic herbs, Panax ginseng, and its American brother, Panax Quinquefolium are being intensively studied today, especially in athletic and medical sciences. Since scientific research is incredibly expensive, the wealth of testing being done on ginseng gives you an idea of its importance in the minds of researchers around the world.

We list here only a small sampling of modern scientific validation of the benefits of this ancient healing plant.

Ginseng aids treatment for cardiovascular disorders, including heart attack, and heart disease. In clinical trials on patients with high blood pressure, ginseng tea helped produce a steady, consistent reduction in blood pressure. The average drop was 23 in the blood pressure of patients with a systolic pressure above 140.

Ginseng is able to benefit deep hormone balance for both men and women, a reasonable explanation for its long reputation as an aphrodisiac. Yet, it is unique in its activity on each sex, working with the needs and qualities of the opposite male and female systems. A smart plant indeed!

G

- **For men,** ginseng has a long tradition as a reproductive restorative. While ginseng won't make a man a SUPER-MAN, recent tests show that it is the only herb to clinically test as a source of phyto (plant) testosterone. Ginseng seems to increase sperm count and seminal vesicle weight, and supports key gland functions like the adrenals and prostate. Ginseng's anti-oxidant qualities help cardiovascular performance not only for sexual energy, but for sports and workouts... important for a man's outlook.

- **For women,** ginseng has hormone balancing benefits, notably those that guard against breast cancer, endometriosis, and hormone driven problems. Ginseng has an estrogen-like effect due to the chemical similarity of ginsenosides and natural steroidal hormones. It can exert the estrogen effect on the vaginal mucosa, enough to prevent thinning of the vaginal walls associated with menopause, and also to prevent general menopause discomfort. It affects a woman's brain and mental energy through hypothalamus stimulation.... and may be a factor in turning a woman's attention to love-making. Ginseng also has distinct, anti-oxidant cardiovascular benefits for women.

Ginseng polysaccharides protect against gastric ulcers induced by hard alcohol. Anyone who regularly drinks hard liquor is almost surely damaging the stomach lining. Ginseng may be a good preventive medicine choice.

Ginseng demonstrates an insulin-like effect on sugar regulation, stimulating sugar removal.

Ginseng shows therapeutic activity against recurrent, severe viral infections and syndromes, like HIV and other immune deficient diseases, according to recent Russian studies.

Ginseng has powerful, intercellular antioxidant substances, particularly in regard to its anti-aging capabilities, free radical neutralization and immune enhancement.

Ginseng stimulates many parts of the immune system, including phagocyte action, antibody response and natural killer cell activity. It modifies cytokine production, strengthens the immune properties of cellular connective tissue, enhances interleukin and balances red and white blood cell count .

Ginseng stimulates RNA synthesis in bone marrow cells, and has anti-toxic effects against radiation, heavy metals, and airborne pollutants.

Ginseng plays a definitive role in normalizing skin cancer cells! This may be a boon to all the world as the ozone layer thins and thins, exposing all of us to harmful UV rays. It also protects against aging skin and early wrinkling.

Ginseng offers long term mental and psychological benefits. European experiments with ginseng and the elderly show clear improvement for mental outlook states, raising spirits, and improving optimism and attitude. Ginseng is regularly recommended for depression and insomnia in Europe.

Ginseng assists memory, concentration, alertness, and improved learning ability, too. It is currently being tested for Alzheimer's disease, and I myself have seen evidence that ginseng helps in Alzheimer's cases.

Ginseng is the quintessential herb for stress - the very thing people need to handle the growing pressure in their lives today. Stress is anything that lessens vitality, and it's the single greatest factor in the promotion of disease. Beyond its specific abilities, ginseng **superbly** helps us to deal with stress.

Ginseng is being studied for its ability to inhibit the growth and formation of liver cancer cells, one of the most difficult cancers to overcome. Tests show that ginseng stimulates protein synthesis and converts cancer cell characteristics both functionally and morphologically to those resembling normal liver cells, a process induced by a **single ginsenoside!**

While scientific experiments go on, we can buy and use this safe remedy during its testing, something impossible with drugs. Taking ginseng for several months to a year is far more effective than short term doses.

❖ **GLA, Gamma Linoleic Acid -** obtained from evening primrose oil, black currant, and borage seed oil. A source of energy for the cells, electrical insulation for nerve fibers, a precursor of prostaglandins which regulate hormone and metabolic functions. Therapeutic use is wide ranging from control of PMS and menopause symptoms, to help in nerve transmission for M.S. and muscular dystrophy.

❖ **GLANDULAR EXTRACTS, RAW -** the organs and glands communicate biochemically to the body through micro-nutrients and polypeptides. Gland therapy is based on the premise that glandular substance is biologically active in humans, and that "like cells help like cells." Current research shows that it is valid, effective and safe. Only minute amounts of raw animal glandulars are required to support and normalize a particular organ or gland in a human body. For serious diseases, such as cancer, that debilitate organs and glands, this type of cell therapy can be very helpful in augmenting the body's own substance so that it can better heal itself.

Predigested, soluble gland tissue can provide all the benefits of whole fresh glands. Freeze-dried, de-fatted, dehydrated concentrates are also available and effective. The highest quality of preservation is obviously essential, since heat processing or salt precipitation render the glands useless. Every gland seems to be stimulated by a particular amino acid that enables it to function more effectively. So a combination of a raw glandular and a harmonizing amino acid provides the human gland with more ability to produce its hormone secretions.

THE MOST ESSENTIAL GLANDULARS

- **Raw Adrenal** - stimulates and nourishes exhausted adrenals. Reduces inflammation and increases body tone and endurance without synthetic steroids. Helps protect against chronic fatigue syndrome and candida albicans by normalizing metabolic rate. Increases resistance to allergic reactions and infections associated with poor adrenal function. Works to control both hypoglycemic and diabetic reactions, and menopause imbalance effects.

- **Raw Brain** - improves brain chemistry. Helps prevent memory loss, chronic mental fatigue, and senility onset. Encourages better nerve stability and restful sleep. Beneficial support during alcoholism recovery.

- **Raw Female Complex**, (usually including raw ovary, pituitary, uterus) - re-establishes hormonal balance, especially between estrogen and progesterone. Helps regulate the menstrual cycle, and stimulates delayed or absent menstruation. Normalizes P.M.S. symptoms, and controls cramping. Indicated for low libido and infertility.

- **Raw Heart** - improves heart muscle activity and reduces low density lipoproteins in the blood.

- **Raw Kidney** - aids in normalization of kidney/urinary disorders, and improves waste filtering functions. Helps normalize blood pressure. Maintains body fluid and acid/alkaline balance.

- **Raw Liver** - helps restore the liver from abuse, disease and exhaustion. Improves metabolic activity, and filtering of wastes and toxins like alcohol and chemicals. Aids fat metabolism. Increases healthy bile flow and glucose regulation. Supplementation is effective for jaundice, hepatitis, toxemia and alcoholism.

- **Raw Lung** - supports lungs against respiratory dysfunctions like asthma, emphysema, bronchitis and pneumonia.

- **Raw Male Complex,** (contains raw orchic, pituitary, and prostate), re-establishes hormonal balance, especially of testosterone/progesterone/estrogen. Helps normalize the functions of diseased or damaged male organs. Supports male body growth and fat distribution. Improves sperm count, virility, and chances of fertilization.

- **Raw Mammary** - helps heal breast/nipple inflammation. Controls profuse menstruation, period pain, and normalizes too-frequent cycles, especially at the onset of menopause. Supports insufficient milk during lactation.

- **Raw Orchic** - helps increase male sexual strength and potency by stimulating testosterone production and building sperm count. Also beneficial against male depression and low blood sugar. Supplementation can bring noticeable improvement in male athletic performance.

- **Raw Ovary** - normalizes estrogen/progesterone balance. Helps correct endometrial misplacement and overgrowth, P.M.S. symptoms and menstrual cramping. Supports hormone production slow down during menopause.

- **Raw Pancreas** - the pancreas is a triple function gland producing pancreatin for digestion, and insulin and glucagon for glucose metabolism and balanced blood glucose levels. Pancreas glandular supports enzyme secretions for fat metabolism, hormone balance, food assimilation, and keeps intestinal immune response strong.

- **Raw Pituitary** - the "master gland," stimulates overall body growth through electrolyte metabolism in the ovaries, testes, adrenals and skin. Plays a major role in reproduction, estrogen secretion, blood sugar metabolism, kidney function, skin pigmentation, water retention, and bowel movements. Helps overcome hypoglycemia and infertility. Effective for athletes in controlling body stress, sugar balance and fatigue.

- **Raw Spleen** - aids in the building and storage of red blood cells to promote strength and good tissue oxygenation. As a lymph organ, filters injurious substances from the bloodstream. Increases absorption of calcium and iron. Supplementation enhances immune function by increasing white blood cell activity.

- **Raw Thymus** - stimulates and strengthens the immune system against foreign organisms and toxins. Supplementation helps activate T-cells in the spleen, lymph nodes and bone marrow. Minimizes problems that occur from aging, since the thymus gland normally shrinks with age. (Zinc supplementation helps regenerate thymic tissue.)

- **Raw Thyroid** - supports energy production and helps regulate metabolism and circulation, and controlling obesity and sluggishness caused by thyroid deficiency. Helps mental alertness, hair, skin and reproductive/sexual problems. Works synergistically with tyrosine and natural iodine. (Be sure to use a compound that is thyroxin-free.)

- **Raw Uterus** - helps menses dysfunctions like amenorrhea, habitual abortion, infertility and irregular periods. Acts as a preventive against inflammation and infection of the cervical canal and vagina. Aids in calcium use for bone and muscle. Improves tissue growth and repair. Helps overcome birth control side effects.

✢ **GLUTAMIC ACID** - a non-essential amino acid, important for nerve health and function, and in metabolizing sugars and fats. Over 50% of the amino acid composition of the brain is represented by glutamic acid and its derivatives. It is a prime brain fuel because it transports potassium across the blood/brain barrier. Helps correct mental and nerve disorders, such as epilepsy, muscular dystrophy, mental retardation, and severe insulin reaction.

✢ **GLUTAMINE** - a non-essential amino acid that converts readily into 6-carbon glucose, a prime nutrient and energy sources for the brain. Supplementation rapidly improves memory retention, recall, concentration, and alertness. Glutamine helps mental performance in cases of retardation, senility, epileptic seizure and schizophrenia. It reduces alcohol and sugar cravings, protects against alcohol toxicity, and controls hypoglycemic reactions.

❖ **GLUTATHIONE** - a non-essential amino acid, works with cysteine and glutamine as a glucose tolerance factor and anti-oxidant to neutralize radiation toxicity and inhibit free radicals. Assists white blood cells in killing bacteria. Helps detoxify from heavy metal pollutants, cigarette smoke, alcohol and drug (especially PCP) overload. Cleans the blood from the effects of chemotherapy, x-rays and liver toxicity. Works with vitamin E to break down fat and protect against stroke, kidney failure and cataract formation. Stimulates prostaglandin metabolism.

• **GLYCERINE, VEGETABLE** - a naturally-occurring substance, today extracted from coconut, it is metabolized in the body like a carbohydrate, not a fat or oil, and is used regularly in natural cosmetics as a smoothing agent.

• **GLYCINE** - a non-essential amino acid which releases growth hormone when taken in large doses. Converts to creatine, to retard nerve and muscle degeneration, and is thus therapeutically effective for myasthenia gravis, gout, and muscular dystrophy. A key to regulating hypoglycemic sugar drop, especially when taken upon rising.

• **Di-Methyl-Glycine, DMG,** once commonly known as B_{15}, is a powerful antioxidant and energy stimulant. Used successfully to improve Down's Syndrome and mental retardation cases, and to curb craving in alcohol addiction. DMG is a highly reputed energizer whose effects can be attributed to its conversion to glycine. Successfully used as a control for epileptic seizure, with notable therapeutic results for atherosclerosis, rheumatic fever, rheumatism, emphysema and liver cirrhosis. For best results, take sub-lingually before sustained exercise. *Note:* Too much DMG disrupts the metabolic chain and causes fatigue. The proper dose produces energy, overdoses do not.

❖ **GRAPEFRUIT SEED EXTRACT** - a multipurpose, natural antibiotic, for bacterial, viral and fungal infections, against yeast infections, like candida albicans and vaginal infections, moderate parasitic infestations, dysentery, for cuts, gingivitis, strep and sore throat, ringworm, ear infections, nail fungus, dandruff and wart removal.

❖ **GREEN SUPERFOODS** - See GREEN SUPERFOODS & HEALING, page 183.

❖ **GREEN TEA, BANCHA GREEN TEA** - See BLACK & GREEN TEAS & HEALING BENEFITS, page 200.

❖ **GUAR GUM** - an herbal product that provides soluble digestive fiber and absorbs undesirable intestinal substances. Used therapeutically to lower cholesterol, and to flatten the diabetic sugar curve.

❖ **GUM GUGGUL** - an Indian gum resin herb from the mukul myrrh tree, it is used as a natural alternative to drugs for reducing cholesterol. In Ayurvedic healing it is used for rheumatism, nervous diseases, tuberculosis, urinary disorders and skin diseases. Guggulipid, an extract of guggul, is credited with the ability to lower both cholesterol and triglyceride levels because it increases the liver's metabolism of LDL cholesterol. In addition to lowering lipid levels, guggulipid prevents the formation of atherosclerosis and aids in regressing pre-existing atherosclerotic plaques. Guggulipid helps inhibit platelet aggregation and promotes fibrinolysis, implying that it may also prevent the development of a stroke or embolism. Also successful in treating acne vulgaris.

❖ **GUM TRAGACANTH** - an herbal emulsifier and gel used in cosmetics and toothpastes.

❖ **GUIDED IMAGERY** - See ALTERNATIVE HEALTH CHOICES, page 26.

❖ **GYMNEMA SYLVESTRE** - See SUGAR & SWEETENERS IN A HEALING DIET, page 196.

*H*DLs & LDLs (High and Low Density Lipoproteins) - water-soluble, protein-covered bundles, that transport cholesterol through the bloodstream, and are synthesized in the liver and intestinal tract. Bad cholesterol, (LDL) carries cholesterol through the bloodstream for cell-building needs, but leaves excess behind on artery walls and in tissues. Good cholesterol, (HDL) helps prevent narrowing of the artery walls by removing the excess cholesterol and transporting it to the liver for excretion as bile.

❖ H_2O_2, **HYDROGEN PEROXIDE,** *Food Grade* - Much controversy has surrounded the use of Food Grade Hydrogen Peroxide for therapeutic, anti-infective and anti-fungal health care. Our experience with this source of nascent oxygen has been successful in many areas, but a great deal of that success is predicated on the **way** H_2O_2 is used. Proper medicinal directions are very specific as to dosage and ailment. Read the bottle label carefully before embarking on a program that includes H_2O_2. Food Grade H_2O_2 is available in two refrigerated forms: hydrogen dioxide (hydrogen peroxide), mainly for external use or magnesium dioxide (magnesium peroxide), for internal use.

The internal product is formulated by Dr. Donsbach and can be purchased at health food stores or by calling 800-423-7662. It contains less oxygen but is much more palatable and more stable.

Both compounds form a stable substance which we know as oxygen. The 3% dilute solution may be used internally for serious complaints where higher tissue oxygen is needed to control disease growth. Response has been good for asthma, emphysema, arthritis, candida albicans, Epstein-Barr virus, certain cancerous growths, and degenerative conditions such as HIV infections. Other applications for a 3% dilute solution include fungal conditions, as a douche for vaginal infections, and as an enema or colonic solution during detox cleansing. It may be used as a mouthwash, skin spray, or on the skin to replace the skin's acid mantle that has been removed by soap.

Oxygen baths are valuable detoxifying agents, and noticeably increase body energy and tissue oxygen uptake. About 1 cup H_2O_2 per bath produces significant effect for 3 to 7 days. Oxygen baths are stimulating rather than relaxing. Other therapeutic benefits include body pH balance and detoxification, reduction of skin cancers and tumors, clearing of asthma and lung congestion, arthritis and rheumatism relief, and conditions where increased body oxygen can prevent and control disease. Add $1/_2$ cup sea salt and $1/_2$ cup baking soda for extra benefits.

HERE ARE SOME COMMON GUIDELINES:

• H_2O_2 is not for health maintenance use. It should be taken only if there is a specific need. Once improvement is noticed, the use of H_2O_2 should be discontinued. If you need to take H_2O_2 for more than 12 days orally or more than 60 days externally, contact a wholistic physician for a custom protocol.

• Like many antibiotics, H_2O_2 will also kill friendly bacterial culture in the digestive tract. When taking H_2O_2 orally, you should replace the intestinal flora (acidophilus, bifidus, and bulgaricus) by eating cultured foods, or taking a culture supplement, about 2 hours after taking H_2O_2. If taking H_2O_2 orally results in nausea or a bloated feeling discontinue oral use.

• Do not use 35% H_2O_2 if you have had a heart or liver transplant.

See HOME TESTS & PROTOCOLS in the Appendix for how to use H_2O_2 safely and effectively.

✤ **HERBAL WRAPS** - the best European and American spas use herbal wraps as restorative body-conditioning techniques. Wraps are also body cleansing methods that may be used to elasticize, tone, alkalize and release body wastes quickly. They should be used in conjunction with a short cleansing program, and 6-8 glasses of water a day to flush out loosened fats and toxins. Crystal Star makes two wraps for home use: TIGHTENING & TONING™ wrap to reduce cellulite deposits, and improve muscle, vein and skin tone; and ALKALIZING ENZYME™ wrap to replace and balance important minerals, enhance metabolism and alkalize the body. (Enzyme wraps are an important part of every spa program in Japan.)

✤ **HESPERIDIN** - a chemical present in orange and lemon peel; increases capillary strength.

✤ **HISTIDINE** - a semi-essential amino acid in adults, essential in infants. Histamine is formed from histidine, a precursor to good immune response, to effective defense against colds, respiratory infections, and for countering allergic reactions. It has strong vasodilating and hypotensive properties for cardio-circulatory diseases, anemia and cataracts. Abundant in hemoglobin and a key to the production of both red and white blood cells. Synthesizes glutamic acid, aids copper transport through the joints, and removes heavy metals from the tissues, making it successful in treating arthritis. Histidine raises libido in both sexes. See Amino Acids.

✤ **HOMEOPATHIC CELL SALTS** - See HOMEOPATHIC REMEDIES, page 13.

✤ **HYDROLYZE** - a chemical process in which the decomposition of a compound is resolved into a simpler compound by water. Hydrolysis also occurs in the digestion of foods. The proteins in the stomach react with water in an enzyme reaction to form peptones and amino acids.
• **Hydrolyzed Animal Elastin** - the hydrolyzed animal connective tissue used in emollients and creams.
• **Hydrolyzed Milk Protein** - moisturizer made of protein extracted from milk.
• **Hydrolyzed Vegetable Protein** - the hydrolysate (liquefication) of vegetable protein.

✤ **HYPERTHERMIA, CLINICAL** - see Overheating Therapy, page 29.

✤ **HYPNOTHERAPY** - see ALTERNATIVE HEALTH CHOICES, page 28.

✤ **HYPOALLERGENIC** - a term for cosmetics meaning less likely to cause an allergic reaction. Hypoallergenic cosmetics are made without the use of common allergens that most frequently cause allergic reactions. Some people may still be sensitive to these products.

*I*GNATIA - a homeopathic female remedy to relax emotional hypertension; especially during times of great grief or loss. See HOMEOPATHIC REMEDIES, page 13.

✣ INOSINE - a non-essential amino acid that stimulates ATP energy release. Inosine helps provide muscle endurance when the body's own glycogen reserves run out. Take on an empty stomach with an electrolyte drink before exercise for best results.

✣ INOSITOL - part of the B-complex family, a sugarlike crystalline substance found in the liver, kidney and heart muscle; also present in most plants. Deficiency is related to loss of hair, eye defects and growth retardation.

✣ IODINE - a mineral which exerts an antibiotic-like action and also prevents toxicity from radiation. A key component of good thyroid function and proper metabolism, necessary for skin, hair and nail health, and for wound healing. White blood cells absorb iodine from the blood and use it to enhance their pathogen killing capacity. Iodine also prevents mucous buildup. Iodine deficiency results in goiter, hypothyroidism, cretinism, confused thinking, and menstrual difficulties. Good food sources are seafoods and sea vegetables.

✣ IRON - a mineral which combines with proteins and copper to produce hemoglobin to carry oxygen throughout the body. Iron deficiency results in fatigue, muscle weakness and anemia. Iron strengthens immunity, and is a key to wound healing. It is important for women using contraceptive drugs and during pregnancy. It keeps hair color young, eyes bright, the body strong. Vitamin C-rich foods like tomatoes, lemon juice, vinegar and citric acid greatly enhance iron absorption. However, free, un-bound iron is a strong pro-oxidant, and can be toxic at abnormally high levels. Iron overload is linked to some cancers, heart disease, diabetes, arthritis and endocrine dysfunction. Using herbal or food source iron supplements avoids the problem altogether. Food sources include molasses, cherries, prunes, leafy greens, poultry, liver, legumes, peas, eggs, fish and whole grains. Herb sources are alfalfa, bilberry, burdock, catnip, yellow dock root, watercress, sarsaparilla and nettles.

✣ ISOPROPYL ALCOHOL - an antibacterial, solvent, and denaturant, it is prepared from propylene, obtained from petroleum. Ingestion or inhalation of large quantities of the vapor may cause headache, nausea, vomiting or coma. Can be fatal if ingested - even small doses.

*J*OJOBA OIL - oil extracted from the beanlike seeds of the desert shrub, *Simondsia Chinensis*. A liquid wax used as a lubricant and a substitute for sperm oil, carnauba wax and beeswax. Mexican and American Indians have long used the bean's oily wax as a hair conditioner and skin lubricant.

*K*ALI MUR - potassium chloride, a homeopathic remedy for inflammatory arthritic conditions. Deficiency results in glandular swelling, skin scaling, and excess mucous discharge. See HOMEOPATHIC REMEDIES, page 13.

✣ KALI PHOS - potassium phosphate, (body deficiency is characterized by intense odor from the body). A homeopathic remedy to treat mental problems such as depression. See HOMEOPATHIC REMEDIES, page 13.

✣ KALI SULPH - potassium sulphate, a homeopathic cell salt that carries oxygen for the skin. Deficiency causes a deposit on the tongue, and slimy nasal, eye, ear and mouth secretions. See HOMEOPATHIC REMEDIES, page 13.

✣ KEFIR - a cultured milk product, it comes plain or fruit-flavored, and may be taken as a liquid or used like yogurt or sour cream. Kefir provides friendly intestinal flora. Use the plain flavor, cup for cup as a replacement for whole milk, buttermilk or half and half; fruit flavors may be used in sweet baked dishes.

• **Kefir Cheese** - an excellent cultured replacement for sour cream or cream cheese in dips and other recipes, kefir cheese is low in fat and calories, and has a slightly tangy-rich flavor that really enhances snack foods. Use it cup for cup in place of sour cream, cottage cheese, cream cheese or ricotta.

✣ KOMBUCHA MUSHROOM - is actually a colony of yeast and bacteria. To prepare it, a mixture of black tea and sugar is brewed and a Kombucha "mother" (starter) is added. The B vitamin-rich environment allows the bacteria to convert to a type of vinegar, which is really an amino acid and enzyme-rich, digestive "tea." Proponents of kombucha claim that it is a panacea for almost any disease. People use kombucha for weight loss because it contains caffeine, and helps both liver and gallbladder work more efficiently. Others say it helps bronchitis, asthma and muscle aches and pains. One study found the tea contained a strong antibacterial, effective against antibiotic-resistant strains of Staphylococcus.

If you decide to use kombucha tea, start with about 2-oz. a day; do not exceed 8-oz. a day. People with uric acid problems or gout should limit their use, because the active yeasts contain significant amounts of nucleic acid which increase levels of uric acid in the blood. Use for diabetics is controversial because kombucha contains 3-4% simple sugars. If there is mold contamination floating on the surface, or the mushroom falls apart when handled, discard the tea entirely.

❖ KUZU - a powdered thickening root for Japanese dishes and macrobiotic diets. Superior for imparting a shine and sparkle to stir-fried foods and clear sauces. A dairy alternative in cooking.

*L*ACHESIS - a homeopathic remedy for premenstrual symptoms that improve once menstrual flow begins. For menopausal hot flashes. See HOMEOPATHIC REMEDIES, page 13.

❖ LACTIC ACID - a by-product of the metabolism of glucose and glycogen, present in blood and muscle tissue. Also present in sour milk, beer, sauerkraut, pickles, and other foods made by bacterial fermentation. It is used in cosmetic products to exfoliate skin.

❖ LACTASE - an enzyme normally produced in the small intestine, lactase supplements can be taken before or with meals that include dairy to aid in digestion. See Lactose below.

❖ LACTOBACILLUS - there are several types of lactobacilli, including L. acidophilus, L. bifidus, L. caucassus, and L. bulgaricus. These are all beneficial bacteria that synthesize nutrients in the intestinal tract, counteract pathogenic microorganisms and maintain a healthy intestinal environment. Lactobacillus organisms are delicate creatures and are readily destroyed by noxious chemicals and drugs, particularly chlorine and antibiotics. In fact a single long course of antibiotics can destroy most bowel flora, leading to the overgrowth of yeasty pathogenic organisms, like candida albicans, which are resistant to antibiotics. Even eating antibiotic-laced meats and dairy products leads to an insidious decline in the number of Lactobacillus organisms within the human body.

Skin disorders, chronic candidiasis, irritable bowel syndrome and other intestinal disorders, hepatitis, lupus and heart disease are all associated with a Lactobacillus deficiency. Top food sources include yogurt, kefir, miso, tempeh and uncooked sauerkraut.

❖ LACTOSE - milk sugar present in the milk of mammals. An estimated 50 million Americans are lactose intolerant, meaning they are unable to digest lactose. These people have a deficiency in the enzyme lactase. (See above.) When there is a lack of sufficient lactase, the unabsorbed lactose migrates to the colon, where it becomes fermented by intestinal bacteria and causes gastrointestinal problems.

❖ LANOLIN - also known as wool fat or wool wax is a product of the oil glands of sheep. Chemically a wax instead of a fat, lanolin is a natural emulsifier that absorbs and holds water to the skin.

❖ LECITHIN - a phospholipid (fat-like substance) produced in the liver, and present in some foods. Lecithin consists mostly of phosphatidyl choline, found in cell membranes, needed to maintain the surface tension of cells, and to control the flow of nutrients and wastes both in and out of cells. There is a high concentration of lecithin in heart cells and in the sheathing around the brain, spinal cord and nerves. Lecithin supplements come from high phosphatide soy or egg products, they are low in fat and cholesterol and can help thicken ingredients without using dairy foods.

Lecithin may be substituted for one-third of the oil in recipes for a healing diet. Two teaspoons daily may be added to almost any food to increase phosphatides, choline, inositol, potassium and linoleic acid. Lecithin is a natural emulsifier. Just as a detergent breaks down fat globules to be washed away by water, lecithin breaks down fat particles, an emulsifying action that is essential to the body's control of cholesterol and triglyceride levels. Lecithin reduces large, dangerous LDL cholesterol globules, and elevates smaller, healthier HDL particles.

For the brain, lecithin is a major source of phosphatidyl choline, for mental and nerve function. Choline has long been recognized as the direct precursor of acetylcholine, the neurotransmitter essential for memory. Acetylcholine deficiency is commonly associated with Alzheimer's disease and other degenerative senile conditions that involve memory and neurological abnormalities. Supplemental lecithin significantly increases choline levels.

❖ LEDUM - a homeopathic remedy for bruises. May be used following arnica treatment to fade the bruise after it becomes black and blue. See HOMEOPATHIC REMEDIES, page 13.

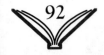

L.

❖ **LEMON,** *Citrus Limon* - rich in vitamin C and potassium, a traditional tonic for increasing salivary and gastric secretions, currently used to dissolve gallstones, and now showing promising anticancer properties.

❖ **LINOLEIC ACID** - See FATS & OILS, page 193.

❖ **LITHIUM** - an earth's crust trace mineral used clinically as lithium arginate. Successful in treating manic-depressive disorders, ADD in children, epilepsy, alcoholism, drug withdrawal, and migraine headaches. New research shows therapeutic success with malignant lymphatic growths, arteriosclerosis and chronic hepatitis. Overdoses can cause palpitations and headaches. Good food sources include mineral water, whole grains and seeds.

❖ **LUTEIN** - a nutrient from carotenoids like alpha-carotene, beta-carotene, cryptoxanthin, lutein, lycopene and zeaxanthin. Carotenoids are found in spinach, kale and other fruits and vegetables. Lutein is not converted to vitamin A, like beta-carotene, but it does serve as a potent antioxidant. Of all the carotenoids, lutein and zeaxanthin lend the most support to the eyes. Lutein and zeaxanthin make up the yellow pigment in the retina and appear to specifically protect the macula. A Harvard study reported that people eating the most lutein and zeaxanthin foods were most likely to have healthy retinas and maculae. Lutein and zeaxanthin supplements are now available.

❖ **LYCOPODIUM** - a homeopathic remedy that helps to increase personal confidence. Also favored by estheticians to soothe irritated complexions and as an antiseptic. See HOMEOPATHIC REMEDIES, page 13.

❖ **LYSINE** - an essential amino acid, is a primary treatment for the herpes virus. May be used topically or internally. High lysine foods, such as corn, poultry and avocados should be added if there are recurrent herpes breakouts. Helps rebuild muscle and repair tissue after injury or surgery. Important for calcium uptake for bone growth, and in cases of osteoporosis, and in reducing calcium loss in the urine. Helps the formation of collagen, hormones and enzymes. Supplementation is effective for Parkinson's disease, Alzheimer's and hypothyroidism.

MAGNESIUM - the critical mineral for osteoporosis and the skeletal system. Necessary for good nerve and muscle function, healthy blood vessels and balanced blood pressure. Athletes need extra magnesium for endurance. An important part of tooth and bone formation, heart and kidney health, and restful sleep. Counteracts stress, nerves, irregular heartbeat, emotional instability and depression. Calms hyperactive children. Supplementation helps alcoholism, diabetes, and asthma. Deficiency results in muscle spasms, cramping, gastro-intestinal disturbances and sometimes fibromyalgia. Magnesium is absorbed more readily from foods than high-dose supplements. Good food sources include dark green vegetables, seafood, whole grains, dairy foods, nuts, legumes, poultry, hot, tangy spices, cocoa.

❖ **MAGNESIUM PHOS** - a homeopathic remedy for abdominal cramping or spasmodic back pain; particularly for menstrual cramps. See HOMEOPATHIC REMEDIES, page 13.

❖ **MANGANESE** - a mineral which nourishes brain and nerve centers, aids in sugar and fat metabolism, and is necessary for DNA/RNA production. Dozens of enzymes are dependent upon manganese for optimal activity. The enzymes involved in cholesterol synthesis are manganese dependent, as are those involved in the formation of cartilage and bone. Mucopolysaccharides, substances necessary for the formation of strong connective tissues, cannot be produced if there is manganese deficiency. Manganese is also involved with SOD (Super-oxide dismutase) protection against free radical damage, enhancing immune response. Manganese helps eliminate fatigue, nerve irritability and lower back pain. Reduces seizures in epileptics. Deficiencies result in poor hair and nail growth, loss of hearing, and poor muscle/joint coordination. **Tranquilizer drugs deplete manganese.** The citrate form absorbs the best. Good food sources include blueberries, ginger, rice, eggs, green vegetables, legumes, nuts and bananas.

❖ **MELATONIN** - a hormone secreted cyclically by the pineal gland to keep us in sync with the rhythms of the day and the seasons. One of the best benefits of melatonin is its ability to help with the effects of jet lag. Melatonin has become popular for antioxidant effects as well. **Certain protective functions give it an anti-aging reputation:**
1 Oxidation is one of the reasons we age; melatonin helps protect the body from free radical damage.
2 Reduced immune function is another aging factor, as the thymus (our immune stimulating gland) shrinks, and lowers our ability to generate T-cells. Melatonin is believed to slightly reverse shrinkage of the thymus, enabling it to produce more infection-fighting T-cells. Melatonin also enhances antibody production.
3 Some studies have shown that a nightly melatonin supplement can boost the performance of immune systems compromised by age, drugs or stress, during sleep.

Here are some melatonin facts:

- Breast and perhaps prostate cancer, hormone driven cancers, may be involved with a deficiency of melatonin. When melatonin is deficient in the body, breast and prostate cancer risk is high.

- Melatonin dampens the release of estrogen. In fact, high melatonin levels can temporarily shut down the reproductive system. This is the theory basis for a new contraceptive combining a "high" dose (75mg) of melatonin with progestin. The new drug is called B-Oval.

- Melatonin decreases the size of the prostate gland. (A melatonin deficiency allows it to grow.) This is good news for older males with enlarged prostate. But melatonin supplementation can greatly decrease sex drive and actually shrink gonads - certainly an unwanted effect.

- Melatonin may also be indicated in low-tryptophan diseases, such as anorexia, hypertension, manic depression, Cushing's disease, schizophrenia, and psoriasis, because tryptophan is the raw material for melatonin.

We know that every drug has side effects, and this is true of melatonin. Here is information for you to consider.

- Once melatonin supplementation begins, the body tends to shut down its own production of the hormone.

- Melatonin is not recommended for persons under 40, unless for a short term, specific purpose, such as a temporary sleep disorder or jet lag.

- High levels of melatonin can be found in delayed puberty, narcolepsy, obesity, and spina bifida.

- Some medications raise or lower melatonin levels. Beta blockers suppress melatonin levels. Serotonin stimulants, such as 5-hydroxy-tryptophan (5-HT) or chlorpromazine (an antipsychotic), raise melatonin levels.

For all its popularity, I don't believe melatonin is the wonder drug of our age. We should use careful consideration before jumping into long term melatonin supplementation. Hormones are incredibly delicate substances. They have long-ranging, deep effects that we don't yet fully understand. Many synthetic hormone and hormone replacement drugs are detrimental to health and hormone balance. I think we will find that taking a hormone contraceptive drug that eventually shuts down the reproductive system is asking for trouble.

If you decide to take melatonin as a protective measure against breast or prostate cancer, I recommend a small protective dose...about .1-.3mg at night. Give your body a chance to use the supplementation and make its own hormone by stopping for a month or two. You can always resume if needed.

Some empirical observation also indicates that, unless you have a sleep disorder, melatonin can actually disrupt sleep patterns. If you are taking melatonin for anti-aging effects, for instance, you might find that a side effect is a lessening quality of sleep. Other natural anti-oxidant, immune protective choices that don't carry the hormone risk of melatonin, are panax ginseng, ginkgo biloba or garlic.

❖ **METHIONINE** - an essential amino acid - an antioxidant and free radical deactivator. A major source of organic sulphur for healthy liver activity, lymph and immune health. Protective against chemical allergic reactions. An effective "lipotropic" that keeps fats from accumulating in the liver and arteries, thus keeping high blood pressure and serum cholesterol under control. Effective against toxemia during pregnancy. An important part of treatment for rheumatic fever. Supports healthy skin and nails and prevents hair loss.

❖ **MILK** - see Dairy Products in a Healing Diet, page 190.

❖ **MINERALS & TRACE MINERALS** - the building blocks of life, minerals are the most basic of nutrients, the bonding agents in and between you and food - allowing the body to absorb nutrients. Minerals are needed by everyone for good health and an active life. They are especially necessary for athletes and people in active sports, because you must have minerals to run. All the minerals in the body comprise only about 4% of body weight, but they are responsible for major areas of human health. Minerals keep the body pH balanced - alkaline instead of acid. They are essential to bone formation, and to the digestion of food. They regulate the osmosis of cellular fluids, electrical activity in the nervous system, and most metabolic functions. They transport oxygen through the system, govern heart rhythm, help you sleep, and are principle factors in mental and emotional balance. Trace minerals are only .01% of body weight, but even deficiencies in these micronutrients can cause severe depression, P.M.S. and other menstrual disorders, hyperactivity in children, sugar imbalances (hypoglycemia and diabetes), nerve and stress conditions, high blood pressure, osteoporosis, premature aging, memory loss and the ability to heal quickly.

Minerals are important. Hardly any of us get enough.

Minerals cannot be synthesized by the body, and must be regularly obtained through our foods or mineral baths. Minerals from plants and herbs are higher quality and more absorbable than from meat sources. They work optimally with the body's enzyme production for assimilation. A diet of refined foods, red meats, caffeine and fatty foods, inhibits mineral absorption. A high stress lifestyle that relies on tobacco, alcohol, steroids, antibiotics and other drugs contributes to mineral depletion. To make matters worse, many minerals and trace minerals are no longer sufficiently present in our fruits and vegetables. They have been leached from the soil by chemicals used in commercial farming today, and by pesticide sprays used on the produce itself. Even foods that still show acceptable amounts of minerals have lower quality and quantity than we believe, because most measurements were done decades ago when sprays and pesticides were not as prolific as they are now.

Although it is more available, organically grown, unsprayed produce is difficult to obtain on a regular, high quality basis. Plant minerals from herb sources have become one of the best, most reliable ways to get valuable mineral benefits. Herbal minerals are balanced, whole foods that the body easily recognizes and uses. Herbal minerals can be used as healing agents and to maintain body nutrient levels. Unlike partitioned or chemically-formed supplements, minerals from herbs are cumulatively active in the body, forming a strong, solid base.

Minerals can really give your body a boost. Your best mineral choices are to eat organically grown produce whenever possible, and to take a high quality herb or food-source mineral supplement.

❖ **MOCHI** - is a chewy rice "bread" made from sweet brown rice. It is baked very hot, at 450° and puffs up to a crisp biscuit that can be used in a variety of delicious ways. It is acceptable for candida albicans diets.

❖ **MOLYBDENUM** - a metabolic mineral, necessary in mobilizing enzymes. New research is showing benefits for esophageal cancers and sulfite-induced cancer. Molybdenum amounts are dependent on good soil content. Good food sources include whole grains, brown rice, brewer's yeast and mineral water.

❖ **MUCOPOLYSACCHARIDES** - See polysaccharides.

❖ **MUSHROOMS** - *There are four main mushroom species with specific healing properties:*
   • **Shiitake** - often called oyster mushrooms when fresh, they are usually sold dry. These mushrooms have also been linked to cures for cancers and tumors. They apparently produce a virus which stimulates interferon in the body. Use them frequently - just a few each time. A little goes a long way.
   • **Reishi** - a rare mushroom from the Orient, now cultivated in America. Reishi, or ganoderma, increases vitality, enhances immunity and prolongs a healthy life. It is a therapeutic anti-oxidant used for a wide range of serious conditions, including anti-tumor and anti-hepatitis activity. It reduces the side effects of chemotherapy. New research shows success against chronic fatigue syndrome. Reishi helps regenerate the liver, lowers cholesterol and triglycerides, reduces coronary symptoms and high blood pressure, and alleviates allergy symptoms.
   • **Poria Cocos** - an American and Chinese mushroom, reduces and regulates excess water retention; purifies body fluids and prevents build-up of toxins.
   • **Maitake** - contains a polysaccharide that is immune boosting against tumor activity, especially hormone driven cancers. Maitake may also help CFS, diabetes, hepatitis, HBP, HIV infections, obesity and arthritis.

NEEM OIL - **Azadirachta Indica** - a tropical tree related to mahogany, used medicinally for centuries, now being rediscovered by the alternative health industry. Recent scientific study validates the traditional uses of neem, including skin care, treatment of bacterial and viral infections and immune system enhancement. Numerous studies show neem to be versatile, effective against skin and dental disease, funguses and viruses, pathogenic bacteria and parasites, fever, allergies, inflammation, ulcers, tuberculosis, cardiovascular problems and even as a spermicide.

❖ **NATRUM MUR** - sodium chloride - regulates the moisture within the cells. Deficiency causes fatigue, chills, craving for salt, bloating, profuse secretions from the skin, eyes and mucous membranes, excessive salivation, and watery stools. See HOMEOPATHIC REMEDIES, page 13.

❖ **NATRUM PHOS** - sodium phosphate, regulates the acid/alkaline balance, catalyses lactic acid and fat emulsion. Imbalance is indicated by a coated tongue, itchy skin, sour stomach, loss of appetite, diarrhea and flatulence. See HOMEOPATHIC REMEDIES, page 13.

❖ **NATRUM SULPH** - sodium sulphate - an imbalance produces edema in the tissues, dry skin with watery eruptions, poor bile and pancreas activity, headaches, and gouty symptoms. See HOMEOPATHIC REMEDIES, page 13.

❖ **NUX VOMICA** - a homeopathic remedy for gastrointestinal problem. A prime remedy for hangover, recovering alcoholics, drug addiction and migraine prevention. See HOMEOPATHIC REMEDIES, page 13.

O

OCTACOSANOL - a wheat germ derivative, used therapeutically to counteract fatigue and increase oxygen use during exercise and athletic performance. Antioxidant properties are helpful for muscular dystrophy and M.S.

✧ **OMEGA-3 & OMEGA-6 FATTY ACIDS** - See FATS & OILS, page 193.

✧ **ORNITHINE** - a non-essential amino acid that works with arginine and carnitine to metabolize excess body fat, and with the pituitary gland to promote growth hormone, muscle development, tissue repair, and endurance. It is an excellent aid to fat metabolism through the liver; builds immune strength, and helps scavenge free radicals.

✧ **OPCs, Oligomeric Proanthocyanidin Complexes** - a class of bioflavonoids composed of polyphenols. Generally extracted either from grape seeds or white pine bark, these potent antioxidants destroy free radicals, activity widely accepted in slowing the aging process and enhancing immune response. Free radicals also weaken cell membranes, cause inflammation, genetic mutations, and contribute to major health problems such as cancer and cardiovascular disease. Increasing evidence shows that people live more vigorous, less-diseased lives when OPCs are a part of their nutritional program. This is especially true if a person shows signs of premature aging, immune deficiency, allergy sensitivities, or is regularly exposed to environmental pollutants. A "side effect" of proanthocyanidin activity is the inhibition of histamine production, which allows the body to better defend against LDL-cholesterol.
    • **Pycnogenol** - a trade name for pine bark OPCs, pycnogenol is a concentrated, highly active bioflavonoid and antioxidant. It helps the body resist inflammation, and blood vessel and skin damage caused by free radicals. It strengthens the entire arterial system and improves circulation. OPCs from herbs do more than protect, they also help repair, reducing capillary fragility, and restoring skin smoothness and elasticity. Pycnogenol is used in Europe as an "oral cosmetic," because it stimulates collagen-rich connective tissue against atherosclerosis and helps joint flexibility in arthritis. It is used against diabetic retinopathy, varicose veins and hemorrhoids. It is one of the few dietary anti-oxidants that crosses the blood-brain barrier to directly protect brain cells.
    • **Grape seed extract** - highly bio-available proanthocyanidin bioflavonoids....a prime antioxidant. Studies show PCOs from grape seed extract scavenge free radicals 50% more effectively than vitamin E, and 20% more effectively than vitamin C. Vitamin E scavenges harmful free radicals in fatty environments of the body; Vitamin C scavenges free radicals in the watery environments. Grape seed extract scavenges free radicals in both environments, and does so more efficiently.
Vitamin C activity is vastly increased with all proanthocyanidins, especially strengthening collagen in the blood vessels, and increasing the resiliency of capillaries. German studies show OPCs possess a unique ability to bind to collagen structures as well as inhibit collagen destruction. Blood vessel strength is enhanced by as much as 140% after OPC supplementation. Capillaries become more elastic and circulation noticeably improves. By lessening the fragility of blood vessels, OPCs prevent the synthesis of compounds that promote capillary fragility, easy bruising and varicose veins. Tests on grape seed extract are leading to speculation that it's properties were the primary anti-carcinogen in the world famous "grape cure" against cancer widely used in the early part of this century.

THE DEMONSTRATED BENEFITS FROM OPCs FROM HERBS INCLUDE:
    • an extremely potent free radical scavenger, with tumor inhibiting properties.
    • an arteriosclerosis antidote, with free radical scavenging from the mutation of cells.
    • strengthens capillary/vein structure, reducing fragility to help prevent bruising and varicose veins.
    • anti-allergy properties, protective against early histamine production.
    • specifically aids vascular fragility associated with diabetic retinopathy.
    • reduces venous insufficiency, especially for restless legs and lower leg blood volume.
    • improves skin elasticity, and enhances cell vitality through improved circulation.
    • fights inflammation and improves joint flexibility.
    • helps PMS symptoms.

✧ **OSCILLOCOCCINUM** - a homeopathic remedy for flu. See HOMEOPATHIC REMEDIES, pg. 13.

✧ **OVERHEATING THERAPY (HYPERTHERMIA)** - See OVERHEATING THERAPY, page 29. NOTE: SIMPLE OVERHEATING THERAPY MAY BE USED IN THE HOME. IT STIMULATES THE BODY'S IMMUNE MECHANISM, WITHOUT THE STRESS OF FEVER-INDUCING DRUGS.

PABA - **Para-Aminobenzoic Acid** - a B Complex family member and component of folic acid, PABA has sun- screening properties, is effective against sun and other burns, and is used in treating vitiligo, (depigmentation of the skin).

P

Successful with molasses, pantothenic and folic acid in restoring lost hair color. New research shows success against skin cancers caused by UV radiation (lack of ozone-layer protection). Good food sources are brewer's yeast, eggs, molasses, wheat germ. See Vitamins.

✤ **PANTOTHENIC ACID** - See vitamin B₅.

✤ **pH** - the scale used to measure acidity and alkalinity. pH is hydrogen, or "H" ion concentration of a solution. "p" stands for the power factor of the H ion. pH of a solution is measured on a scale of 14. A neutral solution, neither acidic nor alkaline, such as water, has a pH of 7. Acid is less than 7; alkaline is more than 7.

✤ **PHENYLALANINE** - an essential amino acid; a tyrosine precursor that works with vitamin B₆ on the central nervous system as an anti-depressant and mood elevator. Successful in treating manic, post-amphetamine, and schizophrenic-type depression (check for allergies first). Aids in learning and memory retention. Relieves menstrual, arthritic and migraine pain. A thyroid stimulant that helps curb the appetite by increasing the body's production of CCK.
Contra-indications: phenylketonurics (elevated natural phenylalanine levels) should avoid aspartame sweeteners. Pregnant women and those with blood pressure imbalance, skin carcinomas, and diabetes should avoid phenylalanine. Tumors and cancerous melanoma growths have been slowed through dietary reduction of tyrosine and phenylalanine. Avoid if blurred vision occurs when using.

✤ **PHOSPHORUS** - the second most abundant body mineral. Necessary for skeletal infrastructure, brain oxygenation, and cell reproduction. Increases muscle performance while decreasing muscle fatigue. Excessive antacids deplete phosphorus. Good food sources include eggs, fish, organ meats, dairy products, legumes, nuts and poultry.

✤ **PHOSPHATIDYL CHOLINE** - a natural part of lecithin, phosphatidyl choline is an essential component of cell membranes. Its emulsifying action is essential to the body's control of cholesterol and triglyceride levels. Phosphatidyl choline helps maintain the "fluidity" of cellular membranes and plays a critical role in all membrane-dependent metabolic processes. The emulsifying action of phosphatidylcholine is often used to increase the absorption of fat-soluble vitamins and herbs.

✤ **PHOSPHATIDYL SERINE, PS** - a brain cell nutrient, that rapidly absorbs and readily crosses the blood-brain barrier. PS helps activate and regulate proteins that play major roles in nerve cell functions and nerve impulses. Studies show that PS may help maintain or improve cognitive ability such as memory and learning, especially for Alzheimer's patients. PS effectively helps individuals maintain mental fitness, with the benefits persisting even four weeks after PS is stopped. Common foods have insignificant amounts of PS, and the body produces only limited amounts. Until recently, concentrated PS was available only as a bovine-derived product with potential safety problems. The new concentrated, safe-source PS is derived from soybeans.

✤ **PHYTOCHEMICALS** - the substances in plants that have specific pharmacologic action. Also known as nutraceuticals, pharmafoods and phytonutrients. The actions of phytochemicals are predictable in much the same way as pharmaceuticals, but they are natural constituents of foods. The best way for your body to utilize phytochemicals is to ingest the plant source in its whole form.
  • **Anti-carcinogen substances** - phytochemicals that prevent or delay tumor formation. Some herbs and foods with known anticarcinogens include: ginseng, some soy products, garlic, echinacea, goldenseal, licorice, black cohosh, wild yam, sarsaparilla, maitake mushroom and cruciferous vegetables.
  • **Phytohormones** - research in plant chemistry shows that many plants contain substances with hormonal actions. Plant hormone phyto-chemicals are very similar to human hormones and capable of binding to hormone receptor sites in the human body. Unlike synthetic hormones, plant hormones show little or no adverse side effects. Some food plants and herbs that have phytohormone activity include soy, licorice root, wild yam, sarsaparilla root, dong quai, damiana and black cohosh.
  • **Phytoestrogens** - plant estrogen hormones remarkably similar to human estrogen hormones. Especially important in hormone-driven cancers, phytoestrogens bind to estrogen receptor sites in the body without the negative side effects of synthetic estrogens or even excess body estrogens. Recent studies show phytoestrogens inhibit the proliferation of both estrogen-receptor positive and negative breast tumor cells. Some plants with phytoestrogenic activity include dong quai, panax ginseng, licorice, fennel, alfalfa and red clover.
  • **Phytoprogesterones** - plant progesterone hormones similar to human progesterone. Progesterone participates in almost every physiological process. Biochemically, it provides the material out of which all the other steroid hormones (such as cortisone, testosterone, estrogen and salt-regulating aldosterone) can be made. Progesterone's simple molecular structure allows it to balance either an excess or deficiency of other hormones. As a precursor to estrogen, its tremendous increase

during pregnancy serves to stabilize the hormone adjustment and growth of both mother and child. This is especially visible in muscle tissue, such as the uterus, the heart, the intestines and the bladder. Less visibly, progesterone normalizes gland processes for both men and women. When progesterone is deficient, there tends to be hypoglycemia, often combined with obesity. Some phyto-progesterone sources include sarsaparilla, licorice root and wild yam.

• **Phyto-testosterone,** or plant testosterone, is a similar substance to the androgen or male hormone found in both men and women. It may help accelerate growth in tissues and stimulate blood flow, as well as the balance of secondary sexual characteristics. Testosterone is essential for normal sexual behavior and the occurrence of male erections. Yet, few people realize that testosterone determines sex drive in both sexes. The body's production of testosterone decreases and in some cases, changes its structure with age. Ginseng is the only herb known to stimulate production of testosterone in the body.

✣ **PHYTOSOMES** - a new form of botanical technology, the phytosome process enhances and intensifies the power of certain herbal compounds. A phytosome is created by binding flavonoid molecules from herbs to molecules of phosphatidyl choline from lecithin. The union becomes a completely new molecule that is better used by the body. Phytosomes are similar to the liposomes composed of phosphatidyl choline widely used in cosmetics.

ABOUT PHYTOSOME ABSORBABILITY: Phytosomes can deliver liposomes from plants directly into the body. The phytosome process works synergistically, both providing extra phosphatidyl choline and magnifying the power of an herbal compound in its absorption through the skin.

✣ **PODOPHYLLUM** - a homeopathic remedy which helps diarrhea. See HOMEOPATHIC REMEDIES, page 13.

✣ **POLYSACCHARIDES** - long chains of simple sugars, plant polysaccharides have long been used in healing, particularly in stimulating the immune system. Aloe, green tea, echinacea, astragalus and maitake mushroom contain large amounts of polysaccharides.

• **Mucopolysaccharides** - polysaccharides that form chemical bonds with water. They form an important constituent of connective tissue, supporting and binding together the cells to form tissues, and the tissues to form organs. Mucopolysaccharides, especially in the form of Chondroitin Sulphate A (CSA), are beneficial in the prevention and reversal of coronary heart disease. CSA is also anti-inflammatory, anti-allergenic, and anti-stress. It has been used successfully in treating of osteoporosis and in accelerating recovery from bone fractures.

✣ **POTASSIUM** - an electrolyte mineral in body fluids, potassium balances the acid/alkaline system, transmits electrical signals between cells and nerves, and enhances athletic performance. It works with sodium to regulate the body's water balance, and is necessary for heart health against hypertension and stroke, (people who take high blood pressure medication are vulnerable to potassium deficiency), muscle function, energy storage, nerve stability, and enzyme and hormone production. Potassium helps oxygenate the brain for clear thinking and controls allergic reactions. Stress, hypoglycemia, diarrhea and acute anxiety or depression generally result in potassium deficiency. A potassium broth (page 167) from vegetables is one of the best natural healing tools available for cleansing and restoring body energy. Good food and herb sources are fresh fruits, especially kiwis and bananas, potatoes, sea vegetables, spices like coriander, cumin, basil, parsley, ginger, hot peppers, dill weed, tarragon, paprika and turmeric, lean poultry and fish, dairy foods, legumes, seeds and whole grains.

✣ **PROBIOTICS** - a category of dietary supplements consisting of beneficial microorganisms, including Lactobacillus, Bifidobacteria, and Streptococcus termophilus. Probiotics compete with disease-causing microorganisms in the gastrointestinal tract. They are responsible for several activities, including the manufacturing of B vitamins like biotin, niacin, folic acid and pyridoxine (B_6), improving digestion, combatting vaginal yeast infections, and killing harmful bacteria by changing acid/alkaline balance and depriving the harmful bacteria of nutrients they need.

✣ **PROPYL PARABEN** - a preservative used in natural cosmetics. Used medicinally to treat fungus infections. Less toxic than benzoic or salicylic acids. Always used with Methyl Paraben.

✣ **PROSTAGLANDINS** - a vital group of hormone-like substances derived from essential fatty acids (EFA's) that regulate body functions electrically. EFA's control reproduction and fertility, inflammation, immunity and communication between cells. Prostaglandins balance the body's essential fatty acid supply. Foods like ocean fish, sea foods, olive, safflower, or sunflower oils, and herbs like evening primrose and flax oils all affect prostaglandin balance. Conversely, excess saturated fats in the body, especially from fatty animal foods, inhibit both prostaglandin production and proper hormone flow.

✢ **PSYLLIUM HUSKS** - a lubricating, mucilaginous, fibrous herb, with cleansing and laxative properties. Acts as a "colon broom" for chronic constipation; effective for diverticulitis; a lubricant for ulcerous intestinal tract tissue.

✢ **PULSATILLA** - a homeopathic remedy for child allergies and infections. See HOMEOPATHIC REMEDIES, page 13.

✢ **PYCNOGENOL** - a trade name for pine bark OPCs. See OPCs.

✢ **PYRIDOXINE** - see vitamin B_6.

QUERCETIN - a powerful bioflavonoid and cousin of rutin, quercetin is isolated from blue-green algae. Its primary therapeutic use has been in controlling allergy and asthma reactions, since it suppresses the release and production of the two inflammatory agents that cause asthma and allergy symptoms - histamines and leukotrienes. Always take quercetin with bromelain for best bioavailability and synergistic anti-inflammatory activity.

✢ **QUINOA** - an ancient Inca supergrain, containing complete protein from amino acids, and good complex carbohydrates. It is essentially gluten-free, light and flavorful, and can be used like rice or millet.

RAW GLANDULAR EXTRACTS - See Glandulars.

✢ **REFLEXOLOGY** - see YOUR ALTERNATIVE HEALTH CARE CHOICES, page 20.

✢ **RETIN-A** - a prescription drug for treating acne, fine lines and hyperpigmentation, Retin-A is a vitamin A derivative, available, through prescription in five strengths and in cream, gel or liquid form. Retin-A works by decreasing the cohesiveness of skin cells, causing the skin to peel. Because it is a skin irritant, *other* irritants (like extreme weather, wind, cosmetics, or soaps) can cause severe irritation. Many people are sensitive to Retin-A.
Note: Alpha Hydroxy Acids (AHAs) are an alternative, but should also be used cautiously. See Alpha Hydroxy Acids.

✢ **RHUS TOX** - a poison ivy derivative; used homeopathically for pain and stiffness in the joints and ligaments when the pain is worse with cold, damp weather. See HOMEOPATHIC REMEDIES, page 13.

✢ **RIBOFLAVIN** - see vitamin B_2.

✢ **ROYAL JELLY** - the milk-like secretion from the head glands of the queen bee's nurse-workers. RJ is a powerhouse of B vitamins, calcium, iron, potassium and silicon; it has enzyme precursors, a sex hormone and the eight essential amino acids. In fact, it contains every nutrient necessary to support life. It is a natural antibiotic, stimulates the immune system, supplies key nutrients for energy and mental alertness, promotes cell health and longevity, and is effective for a wide range of health benefits. It is one of the world's richest sources of pantothenic acid, known to combat stress, fatigue and insomnia, and is a necessary nutrient for healthy skin and hair. It has been found effective for gland and hormone imbalances that reflect in menstrual and prostate problems. The highest quality royal jelly products are preserved in their whole, raw, "alive" state, which promotes ready absorption by the body. As little as one drop of pure, extracted fresh royal jelly can deliver an adequate daily supply.

SALICYLIC ACID - occurs naturally in wintergreen leaves, sweet birch, and white willow. Synthetically prepared, it is used in making aspirin, and as a preservative in cosmetics. It is antipyretic (anti-itch) and antiseptic. In medicine, it is used as an antimicrobial at 2 to 20% concentration in ointments, powders, and plasters. It can be absorbed through the skin, but large amounts may cause abdominal pain and hyperventilation.

✢ **SATURATED & UNSATURATED FATS** - see FATS & OILS, page 193.

✢ **SAUNA HEAT THERAPY** - a sauna is another way to use overheating therapy principles. A long sauna not only induces a healing, cleansing fever, but also causes profuse therapeutic sweating. The skin, in overheating therapy, acts as a "third kidney" to eliminate body wastes through perspiration. Although it is possible to make a do-it-yourself sauna, the procedure is cumbersome. Professional saunas are available in every health club and gym as part of the membership, and the new home-installed models are not only adequate but reasonable in price.

HERE ARE SOME OF THE HEALTH BENEFITS OF A DRY SAUNA:

1. speeds up metabolism.
2. inhibits the replication of pathogenic organisms.
3. stimulates activity of all vital organs and glands.
4. supports the body's immune system and accelerates its healing functions.
5. dramatically increases the detoxifying and cleansing capacity of the skin.
6. a proven jump-start technique for a weight loss program, especially for sugar cravers.

For optimum skin cleansing and restoration, take a sauna once or twice a week. Finish each sauna with a cool shower and a brisk rubdown to remove toxins that have been eliminated through the skin.

NOTE: ALTHOUGH INDUCED FEVER IS A NATURAL, CONSTRUCTIVE MEANS OF BIOLOGICAL HEALING, SUPERVISION AND ADVICE FROM AN EXPERT PRACTITIONER ARE RECOMMENDED. A HEART AND GENERAL VITALITY CHECK IS ADVISABLE. ALSO SOME PEOPLE WHO ARE SERIOUSLY ILL LOSE THE ABILITY TO PERSPIRE, AND THIS SHOULD BE KNOWN BEFORE USING OVERHEATING THERAPY. Reduce time in the sauna if there is redness or skin irritation that persists over a week.

❖ **SEA VEGETABLES** - including arame, bladderwrack, dulse, hijiki, kelp, kombu, nori, sea palm, and wakame are foods with superior nutritional content. They are rich sources of proteins, carbohydrates, anti-oxidants, minerals and vitamins, especially healing carotenes. They are good alkalizers for the body, and can be used in place of salt or other seasonings. Sea vegetables are the mainstay of iodine therapy. See ABOUT SEA VEGETABLES & IODINE THERAPY, pg. 204 for more information on healing properties from food sources.

❖ **SELENIUM** - a component of glutathione and powerful antioxidant, selenium protects the body from free radical damage and heavy metal toxicity. An anticancer substance and immune stimulant, it works with vitamin E to prevent fat and cholesterol accumulation in the blood. It protects against heart weakness and degenerative diseases. It enhances elasticity of skin tissue. A deficiency results in aging skin, liver damage, increased oxidation, hypothyroidism, and in severe cases, digestive tract cancers. The most effective supplement source is selenomethionine from organic sources. Good food sources include brewers yeast, sesame seeds, garlic, tuna, kelp, wheat germ, oysters, fish, organ meats, organically grown vegetables, nuts and mushrooms.

❖ **SEPIA** - a homeopathic remedy for treating herpes, eczema and hair loss. See HOMEOPATHY, page 13.

❖ **SHARK CARTILAGE** - contains a biologically active protein that strongly inhibits the development of new blood vessel networks (angiogenesis). Angiogenesis is a primary cause of rheumatoid arthritis and increased tumor growth in cancers. Other health conditions which are dependent on angiogenesis blood supply may also be corrected somewhat by shark cartilage: eye diseases like diabetic retinopathy, macular degeneration, and neo-vascular glaucoma; lupus erythematosus; inflammatory bowel diseases like Crohn's disease; scleroderma; yeast diseases like candida enteritis; cancers like Kaposi's sarcoma and most solid tumors; plus skin disorders such as eczema and psoriasis.

Because of its efficient inhibition on the formation of new capillary networks, there are some contra-indications for this nonprescription, over-the-counter product: a pregnant woman should not supplement with shark cartilage because she **wants** capillary growth for her fetus. A person with heart disease or peripheral vascular disease should avoid shark cartilage since new capillaries are desirable. Shark cartilage is unsuitable for anyone suffering from liver dysfunction or disabling kidney disease. The daily therapeutic dosage is between 20 and 90 gm daily; the course of therapy often runs from six to nine months. Use under a practitioner's care if possible. Large amounts of shark cartilage can cause gastric upset - it's perhaps wise to take smaller dosages throughout the day.

❖ **SILICA,** *silicon dioxide* - a chemical compound of silicon and oxygen, silica comprises a large percent of the earth's crust and mantle, is the main ingredient of rocks and is the major constituent of sand. There is some confusion about the words "silica" and "silicon," both of which are available as supplements in health food stores. Silicon is the elemental silicon mineral that is found in man, animals and plants. Silica is generally silicon dioxide, the most abundant silicon compound.

Silica gel contains hydrogen, oxygen and silicon, one form of which is an agent used to absorb moisture. We've all seen small packets of it in containers for certain foods and in the bottles of our supplements as a desiccant. Quartz consists solely of silica. Silica gel is derived from quartz crystals. Some silica supplements are water-soluble extracts of the herb horsetail. Others are derived from purified algae.

In addition to the well-known benefits of maintaining healthy hair, skin and nails, and for calcium absorption in the early stages of bone formation, silica/silicon is needed for flexible arteries, and plays a significant role in the prevention of cardiovascular disease. Beneficial food sources include husks of grain, seeds, green leafy vegetables - particularly barley, oats, millet, whole wheat, red beets, asparagus, Jerusalem artichokes, parsley, bell peppers, sunflower seeds and horsetail herb.

❖ **SILICEA, silica** - a homeopathic cell salt essential to the health of bones, joints, skin, and glands. Deficiency produces catarrh in the respiratory system, pus discharges from the skin, slow wound healing, and offensive body odor. Very successful in the homeopathic treatment of boils, pimples and abscesses, for hair and nail health, blood cleansing, and rebuilding the body after illness or injury. See Homeopathic Cell Salts, page 13.

❖ **SILICON** - a mineral responsible for connective tissue growth and health. Prevents arteriosclerosis. Necessary for collagen synthesis. Regenerates body infrastructure, including the skeleton, tendons, ligaments, cartilage, connective tissue, skin, hair and nails. Silicon supplementation may actually bring about bone recalcification.

Silicon counteracts the effects of aluminum on the body and is important in the prevention of Alzheimer's disease and osteoporosis. Silicon levels decrease with aging and are needed in larger amounts by the elderly. Beneficial food sources include whole grains, horsetail herb, well water, bottled mineral water and fresh vegetables.

❖ **SODIUM** - an electrolyte that helps regulate kidney and body fluid function. Involved with high blood pressure only when calcium and phosphorous are deficient in the body. Works as an anti-dehydrating agent. Beneficial food sources include celery, seafoods, sea vegetables, cheese, dairy products.

❖ **SORBITOL** - a humectant. Gives a velvety feel to skin. Used as a replacement for glycerin in emulsions, ointments, embalming fluid, mouthwashes, toothpastes, various cosmetic creams and cosmetics. First found in the ripe berries of the mountain ash; it also occurs in other berries and in cherries, plums, pears, apples, seaweed and algae. Used in foods as a sugar substitute. Medicinally used to reduce body water and for intravenous feedings. If ingested in excess, it can cause diarrhea and gastrointestinal disturbances.

❖ **SOY FOODS** - see Soy Foods & Therapeutic Benefits, page 207.

❖ **SPIRULINA** - see Green Superfoods, page 183.

❖ **STEVIA REBAUDIANA,** *"sweet herb"* - see Sugar & Sweeteners in a Healing Diet, page 196.

❖ **SULPHUR** - the "beauty mineral" for smooth skin, glossy hair, hard nails and collagen synthesis. It is critical to protein absorption. Good food sources include eggs, fish, onions, garlic, hot peppers and mustard.

❖ **SUPER OXIDE DISMUTASE (SOD)** - an enzyme, SOD prevents damage caused by the toxic oxygen molecule known as superoxide. Manganese and zinc, in particular, stimulate production of SOD. Many experts do not believe that antioxidant enzyme levels in cells can be increased by taking antioxidant enzymes like SOD orally. Human tests with SOD do not appear to increase the levels of SOD in the blood or tissues. See also Antioxidants.

T**AURINE** - a non-essential amino acid, taurine is a potent anti-seizure nutrient. A neurotransmitter that helps control hyperactivity, nervous system imbalance after drug or alcohol abuse, and epilepsy. Normalizes irregular heartbeat. Helps prevent circulatory and heart disorders, hypoglycemia, hypothyroidism, water retention and hypertension. Aids in lowering cholesterol levels. Found in high concentrations in bile, mother's milk, shark and abalone. Supplementation is necessary for therapy.

❖ **TEAS** - see Black & Green Teas For Healing, page 200.

❖ **THIAMINE** - see Vitamin B$_1$.

❖ **THREONINE** - an essential amino acid - works with glycine to aid in overcoming depression, and neurologic dysfunctions such as genetic spastic disorders and M.S. Works with aspartic acid and methionine as a lipotropic to prevent fatty build-up in the liver. Helps to control epileptic seizures. An immune stimulant and thymus enhancer. Important for the formation of collagen, elastin and enamel.

❖ **THUYA** - a homeopathic remedy for warts and sinusitis. See Homeopathic Remedies, page 13.

❖ **TRITICALE** - a hybrid flour of wheat and rye berries, containing the best properties of both and higher in protein than either.

❖ **TRYPTOPHAN** - an essential amino acid and precursor of the neurotransmitter serotonin, which is involved in mood and metabolism regulation. It is a natural, non-addictive tranquilizer for restful sleep, and an effective anti-depressant. It is used successfully to decrease hyperkinetic, aggressive behavior, migraine headaches, and schizophrenia, to counteract compulsive overeating (by raising serotonin), smoking effects (by producing natural niacin) and alcoholism. It raises abnormally low blood sugar, and reduces seizures in petit mal epilepsy.

NOTE: AT THE TIME OF THIS WRITING, SUPPLEMENTAL TRYPTOPHAN IS STILL EMBARGOED AS AN OVER-THE-COUNTER NUTRIENT BY THE FDA, EVEN THOUGH IT NOW APPEARS IN SEVERAL PRESCRIPTION SLEEP-AID DRUGS, AND IS A SAFE NUTRIENT. A CLOSELY RELATED ALTERNATIVE CALLED 5-HTP PROVIDES THE BODY BUILDING BLOCKS TO SUPPORT AND REGULATE SEROTONIN. IT IS NOW BEING USED IN PLACE OF TRYPTOPHAN BY THE PUBLIC FOR SLEEP, DEPRESSION AND MIGRAINES AND APPEARS TO BE SAFE AT NORMAL DOSAGES. I WOULD CONSULT A PHYSICIAN IF YOU ARE ALSO TAKING MAO INHIBITORS.

❖ **TYROSINE** - a semi-essential amino acid, and growth hormone stimulant formed from phenylalanine, tyrosine helps to build the body's natural store of adrenaline and thyroid hormones. It rapidly metabolizes as an anti-oxidant throughout the body, and is effective as a source of quick energy, especially for the brain. It converts to the amino acid L-Dopa, making it a safe therapy for depression, hypertension, and Parkinson's disease, for controlling drug abuse and aiding drug withdrawal. It appears to increase libido and low sex drive. It helps reduce appetite and body fat in a weight loss diet. It produces melanin in the body for skin and hair pigment. Note: Tumors, cancerous melanomas and manic depression have been slowed through dietary **reduction** of tyrosine and phenylalanine.

UMEBOSHI PLUMS - pickled Japanese apricots with alkalizing, bactericide properties; part of a macrobiotic diet.

❖ **UREA**, *carbamide* - used in yeast food and wine production, also to "brown" baked goods such as pretzels. Commercial urea consists of colorless or white odorless crystals that have a cool, salty taste. Today it is widely used as an antiseptic in antiperspirants and deodorants, mouthwashes, shampoos, lotions and other such products.

VANADIUM - a mineral cofactor for several enzymes. Deficiency linked to heart disease, poor reproductive ability, and infant mortality. Good food sources include whole grains, fish, olives, radishes, vegetables.

❖ **VINEGAR** - brown rice, balsamic, apple cider, herb, raspberry, ume plum - vinegars have been used for 5000 years as healthful flavor enhancers and food preservers. As part of condiments, relishes or dressings, they help digest heavy foods and high protein meals. The most nutritious vinegars for health are not overly filtered, and still contain the "mother" mixture of beneficial bacteria and enzymes in the bottle. They look slightly cloudy.

❖ **VITAMINS** - organic micro-nutrients that act like spark plugs that "tune up" the body, and keep it functioning at high performance. You can't live on vitamins; they are not pep pills, substitutes for food, or components of body structure. They stimulate, but do not act as, nutritional fuel. As catalysts, they work on the cellular level, often as co-enzymes, regulating body metabolic processes through enzyme activity, to convert proteins and carbohydrates to tissue and energy. Most vitamins cannot be synthesized by the body, and must be supplied by food or supplements. Excess amounts are excreted in the urine, or stored by the body until needed. Yet, even with their minute size and amounts in the body, vitamins are absolutely necessary for growth, vitality, resistance to disease, and healthy aging. It is impossible to sustain life without them. Even small deficiencies can cause big problems. Unfortunately, it takes weeks or months for signs of most vitamin deficiencies to appear because the body only slowly uses its supply. Even when your body is "running on empty" in a certain vitamin, problems may be hard to pinpoint, because the cells usually continue to function with decreasing efficiency until they either receive proper nourishment or suffer irreversible damage. **x**Vitamins fill nutritional gaps at the deepest levels of the body processes. Regenerative changes in body chemistry usually require as much time to rebuild as they did to decline. As we age, vitamins can be valuable aids to health both body and mind. Indeed, vitamins can help us to go beyond average health to optimal health. In most cases, after a short period of higher dosage in which a good nutrient foundation may be built, a program of moderate amounts over a longer period of time brings about better body balance and more permanent results; and a little goes a long way.

Vitamin RDA's were established by the National Academy in the fifties as a guideline for the nutrient amounts needed to prevent severe deficiency diseases. Today, because of poor dietary habits, over-processed foods, and agri-business practices, most health professionals recognize that supplemental amounts are needed for adequate nutrition and health.

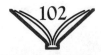

Even as basic as the RDA recommendations are, not one dietary survey has shown that Americans consume anywhere near the RDA amounts in their normal daily diets. A recent large USDA survey of the food intake of 21,500 people over a three day period showed that not a single person consumed 100% of the RDA nutrients. Only 3% ate the recommended number of servings from the four food groups. Only 12% ate the RDA for protein, calcium, iron, magnesium, zinc or vitamins A, C, B_6, B_{12}, B_2, and B_1. Moreover, the study noted that trying to change long-held dietary habits and ignoring supplementation as an option, left much of the American population at nutritional risk.

PEOPLE MOST AFFECTED BY VITAMIN DEFICIENCIES INCLUDE:
- Women with excessive menstrual bleeding who may need iron supplements.
- Pregnant or nursing women who may need extra iron, calcium and folic acid.
- The elderly, many of whom do not even eat two-thirds of the RDA for calcium, iron, vitamin A or C. In addition, the elderly take more than 50% of all medication prescriptions in the U.S. Since 90 out of the 100 most prescribed drugs interfere with normal nutrient metabolism, it is becoming a sad fact that many older people don't absorb even very much of the nutrition that they do eat.
- Everyone on medications that interfere with nutrient absorption, digestion or metabolism.
- People on weight loss diets with low total calorie intake.
- People at risk for heart and circulatory blockages, and those at risk for osteoporosis.
- People who have recently had surgery, or suffer from serious injuries, wounds or burns.
- People with periodontal disease.
- Vegetarians, who may not receive enough calcium, iron, zinc or vitamin B_{12}.

HERE ARE THE MOST IMPORTANT VITAMINS AND WHAT THEY CAN DO FOR YOU:
- **Vitamin A** - fat soluble vitamin, requiring fats and zinc as well as other minerals and enzymes for absorption. Dietary vitamin A comes from both plant and animal sources. The type found in animals is vitamin A, while plants contain beta carotene, which is two vitamin A molecules bound together by a chemical bond. Animals cannot make vitamin A, they get it from eating plants. Vitamin A counteracts night blindness, weak eyesight, and strengthens the optical system. Supplementation lowers risk of many types of cancer. Retinoids inhibit malignant transformation, and reverse pre-malignant changes in tissue. Vitamin A is particularly effective against lung cancer. It is also an anti-infective that builds immune resistance. It helps develop strong bone cells, a major factor in the health of skin, hair, teeth and gums. Deficiency results in eye dryness and the inability to tear, night blindness, rough, itchy skin, poor bone growth, weak tooth enamel, chronic diarrhea, frequent respiratory infection. The adrenal and thyroid glands are also highly sensitive to a decline in vitamin A levels. Good food sources include fish liver oils, seafood, dairy products, peaches, peppers, cantaloupe, winter squash, pumpkin, dark leafy greens, yams, sweet potatoes, liver, watermelon, fruits and eggs. Note: Avoid high doses of Vitamin A during pregnancy.

- **VITAMIN B_1 - Thiamine** - known as the "morale vitamin" because of its beneficial effects on the nervous system and mental attitude. Promotes proper growth in children, aids carbohydrate utilization for energy, and supports the nervous system. Enhances immune response. Helps control motion sickness. Wards off mosquitos and stinging insects. Pregnancy, lactation, diuretics and oral contraceptives require extra thiamine. Smoking, heavy metal pollutants, excess sugar, junk foods, stress and alcohol all deplete thiamine. Deficiency results in insomnia, fatigue, confusion, poor memory, and muscle coordination. Naturally-occurring thiamine is a rather delicate compound and is readily inactivated by cooking and/or chlorine. One way to prevent thiamine loss while cooking is to add acidic substances, such as lemon juice or vinegar to the cooking medium. Good food sources include asparagus, brewer's yeast, brown rice and whole grains, beans, nuts, seeds, wheat germ, organ meats and soy foods.

- **VITAMIN B_2, Riboflavin** - a vitamin commonly deficient in the American diet. Necessary for energy production, and for fat and carbohydrate metabolism. Helps prevent cataracts and corneal ulcers, and generally benefits vision. Promotes healthy skin, especially in cases of psoriasis. Helps protect against drug toxicity and environmental chemicals. Pregnancy and lactation, red meat, excess dairy consumption, prolonged stress, sulfa drugs, diuretics and oral contraceptives require extra riboflavin. Deficiency is associated with alcohol abuse, anemia, hypothyroidism, diabetes, ulcers, cataracts, and congenital heart disease. Good food sources include almonds, brewer's yeast, broccoli, dark green leafy vegetables, eggs, wild rice, mushrooms, yogurt, organ meats and caviar.

- **VITAMIN B_3, Niacin** - a vitamin with a broad spectrum of functions, including energy production, cholesterol metabolism, sex hormone synthesis and good digestion. Niacin is essential for fat metabolism, helping to mobilize fat from adipose tissue so that it can be burned as energy. It prevents the buildup of cholesterol in the liver and arteries. Niacin is

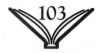

involved in the synthesis of the myelin sheath, the protective fatty covering of the nerves. It promotes healthy skin and nerves, and relieves acne, diarrhea and gastrointestinal conditions, migraines and vertigo attacks. Deficiency results in dermatitis, headaches, gum diseases, sometimes high blood pressure, and negative personality behavior with mental depression. However, because niacin can rapidly open up and stimulate circulation, (a niacin flush is evidence of this), it can act quickly to reverse deficiencies and disorders. Niacin is synergistic with chromium, via glucose tolerance factor (GTF) to improve blood sugar regulation for diabetes and hypoglycemia. The amino acid tryptophan may be regarded as a form of niacin, since, if niacin stores are depleted, it is readily converted into the vitamin. Good food sources include almonds, avocados, brewer's yeast, fish, organ meats, legumes, bananas, whole grains, cheese, eggs and sesame seeds.

- **VITAMIN B$_5$, Pantothenic Acid** - an antioxidant vitamin vital to proper adrenal activity, pantothenic acid is a precursor to cortisone production and an aid to natural steroid synthesis. It is important in preventing arthritis and high cholesterol. It fights infection by building antibodies, and defends against stress, fatigue and nerve disorders. It is a key to overcoming postoperative shock and drug side effects after surgery. Pantothenic acid inhibits hair color loss. Deficiency results in anemia, fatigue and muscle cramping. Individuals suffering from constant psychological stress have a heightened need for B$_5$. Good food sources include brewer's yeast, brown rice, poultry, yams, organ meats, egg yolks, soy products and royal jelly.

- **VITAMIN B$_6$, Pyridoxine** - a key factor in red blood cell regeneration, amino acid/protein metabolism, and carbohydrate use. A primary immune stimulant, shown in recent studies to have particular effect against liver cancer. Supplementation inhibits histamine release in the treatment of allergies and asthma. Supports all aspects of nerve health including neuropsychiatric disorders, epilepsy and carpal tunnel syndrome. Works as a natural diuretic, especially in premenstrual edema. Controls acne, promotes beautiful skin, alleviates morning sickness, and is a key to anti-aging. Protects against environmental pollutants, smoking and stress. Oral contraceptives, thiazide diuretics, penicillin and alcohol deplete B$_6$. Deficiency results in anemia, depression, lethargy, nervousness, water retention, and skin lesions. Good food sources include bananas, brewer's yeast, buckwheat, organ meats, fish, avocados, legumes, poultry, nuts, rice bran, brown rice, wheat bran, sunflower seeds and soy foods.

- **VITAMIN B$_{12}$, Cyano Cobalamin** - an anti-inflammatory and analgesic that works with calcium for absorption. A primary part of DNA synthesis and red blood cell formation. Involved in all immune responses. A specific in blocking sulfite-induced asthma. New research shows success in cancer management, especially in tumor development. Energizes, relieves fatigue, depression, hangover, and poor concentration. Supplied largely from animal food sources, B$_{12}$ is often deficient for vegetarians, and deficiency can take five or more years to appear after body stores have been depleted. Deficiency results in anemia, nervous system degeneration, dizziness, heart palpitations, and unhealthy weight loss. Long term use of cholesterol-lowering drugs, oral contraceptives, anti-inflammatory and anti-convulsant drugs deplete B$_{12}$. Good food sources include cheeses, poultry, sea vegetables, yogurt, eggs, organ meats, brewer's yeast and fish.

- **VITAMIN C, Ascorbic Acid** - a primary factor in immune strength and health. Protects against cancer, viral and bacterial infections, heart disease, arthritis and allergies. It is a strong antioxidant against free radical damage. Supplementation helps reduce cancer risk. Safeguards against radiation poisoning, heavy metal toxicity, environmental pollutants and early aging. Accelerates healing after surgery, increases infection resistance, and is essential to formation of new collagen tissue. Vitamin C controls alcohol craving, prevents constipation, lowers cholesterol, and is a key factor in treatments for diabetes, high blood pressure, male infertility, and in suppressing the HIV virus. Supports adrenal and iron insufficiency, especially when the body is under stress. Relieves withdrawal symptoms from addictive drugs, tranquilizers and alcohol. Aspirin, oral contraceptives, smoking and tetracycline inhibit vitamin C absorption and deplete C levels. Supplementation should be considered if these things are part of your life-style. Deficiency results in easy bruising and bleeding, receding gums, slow healing, fatigue and rough skin.

Note: The new metabolite form of vitamin C, Ester C™ is biochemically the same as naturally metabolized C in the body. It is both fat and water soluble, and non-acid. Uptake of Ester C is absorbed twice as fast into the bloodstream, and excreted twice as slowly as ordinary vitamin C. Good food sources include citrus fruits, green peppers, papaya, tomatoes, kiwi, potatoes, greens, cauliflower and broccoli.

- **VITAMIN D** - a fat soluble "sunlight vitamin," works with vitamin A to utilize calcium and phosphorus in building bone structure and healthy teeth. The term "vitamin" D is actually a misnomer, vitamin D is in reality a hormone, since it can be synthesized in the human body, specifically in the skin. When light rays strike the skin, they provoke the synthesis of vitamin D from cholesterol. As little as a half hour of sunshine per day may fulfill an individual's vitamin D needs. Helps in all eye problems including spots, conjunctivitis and glaucoma. Helps protect against colon cancer. Air pollu-

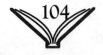

tion, anti-convulsant drugs and lack of sunlight deplete Vitamin D. Deficiency results in nearsightedness, psoriasis, soft teeth, muscle cramps and tics, slow healing, insomnia, nosebleeds, fast heartbeat and arthritis. Good food sources include cod liver oil, yogurt, cheese, butter, herring, halibut, salmon, tuna, eggs and liver.

• **VITAMIN E** - an active fat soluble antioxidant and important immune stimulating vitamin. An effective anticoagulant and vasodilator against blood clots and heart disease. Retards cellular and mental aging, alleviates fatigue and provides tissue oxygen to accelerate healing of wounds and burns. Works with selenium against the effects of aging and cancer by neutralizing free radicals. Beneficial for even the chronic so-called incurable diseases such as arthritis, lupus, Parkinson's disease and multiple sclerosis. The most cell protecting form seems to be E succinate (dry E). Improves skin problems and texture. Helps control baldness and dandruff. Deficiency results in muscle and nerve degeneration, anemia, skin pigmentation. Good food sources include almonds, leafy vegetables, salmon, soy products, wheat germ/wheat germ oil and organ meats.

• **VITAMIN K** - a fat soluble vitamin necessary for blood clotting, vitamin K is synthesized in the liver but is also produced in the intestinal organisms. Thus, drugs which alter or destroy beneficial intestinal bacterial flora, such as antibiotics and cortisone, are a primary cause of vitamin K deficiency. Vitamin K reduces excessive menstruation. Helps heal broken blood vessels in the eye. Aids in arresting bone loss and post-menopausal brittle bones. Helps in cirrhosis and jaundice of the liver. Acts as an antiparasitic for intestinal worms. Good food sources: seafoods, sea vegetables, dark leafy vegetables, liver, molasses, eggs, oats, crucifers and sprouts.

*W*HEAT GERM & WHEAT GERM OIL - wheat germ is the embryo of the wheat berry - rich in B vitamins, proteins, vitamin E, and iron. It goes rancid quickly. Buy only in nitrogen-flushed packaging. Wheat germ oil is a good vitamin E source and body oxygenator. One tablespoon provides the anti-oxidant equivalent of an oxygen tent for 30 minutes.

❖ **WHEAT GRASS** - See GREEN SUPERFOODS, page 183.

*Z*INC - a co-enzyme of SOD that protects against free radical damage, zinc is essential to formation of insulin, and to maintaining immune strength, gland, sexual and reproductive health. Helps prevent birth defects, enhances sensory perception, accelerates healing. Zinc is a brain food that helps control mental disorders and promotes mental alertness. Stress causes a rapid depletion of tissue zinc levels. Individuals with a high stress lifestyle or those recovering from injury may need to increase zinc levels in their diet. Certain drugs, notably alcohol, diuretics, cortisone and antacids significantly impair zinc absorption. The picolinate form is the most absorbable. Good food sources include crab, herring, liver, lobster, oysters, turkey, poppy seed, caraway seeds, brewer's yeast, eggs, mushrooms, wheat germ, sunflower and pumpkin seeds.

You will never find time for anything.

If you want time you have to make it.

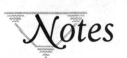

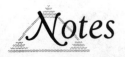

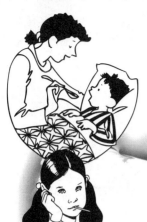

Section Four

Lifestyle Healing Programs
For People With Special Needs

CERTAIN GROUPS OF PEOPLE HAVE SPECIAL LIFESTYLE THERAPY REQUIREMENTS.

• **If you are pregnant,** your diet needs are different, your nutritional supplement and herbal choices may have to be modified, your exercise regimen will have to change at least temporarily, and you'll have special health problems to address.

• **If you are in your golden years,** your health maintenance diet and exercise needs change as your metabolism and glandular functions change. Herb and nutritional supplement choices may need a different focus to fight the symptoms of aging, and immune respone enhancement becomes far more important.

• **If you are an athlete,** active sports enthusiast or body builder, you are probably using nutrients at a far greater rate than most people, and more than likely need far more herbal or nutritional supplementation. Normal dosage is usually not enough, either, for an athlete's higher metabolic needs.

• **If you are a kid, children's health** requirements are different than an adult's. Childhood diseases are often singular to children; your immune systems will probably need much less stimulation. Certain natural remedies seem to just work better for small people in their childhood years.

Finally...
• **If you are a family pet,** you probably know how wonderful Mother Nature's remedies can be for your health problems. But you may not have access to the remedies or your mom may not be around to help. The special natural therapies for animals in this section may be just the ticket for you.

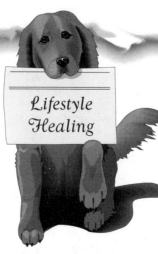

Lifestyle
Healing

Having A Healthy Baby
Optimal Pregnancy Choices

Pre-conception Planning:

In America today, one in six married couples of child-bearing age has trouble conceiving and completing a successful pregnancy. Preconception planning has become important because neither our environment with its toxic pollutants, our diets full of fast foods, or our stressful lifestyles are conducive to successful child conception.

Poor nutrition and stress seem to be at the base of most fertility problems. For men, the main hindrances are zinc deficiency, too much alcohol, and tobacco; for women, prime inhibitors are anxiety, emotional stress, severe anemia, and hormonal imbalance. There is a link between infertility and vitamin C deficiency in both sexes.

DIET IS AN ALL-IMPORTANT KEY TO SUCCESSFUL CONCEPTION:

We know that the body does not readily allow conception without adequate nutrition. Nature tries in every way possible to insure the survival and health of a new life. Gland and hormone health, the basis of reproductive health, is so primary and so potent that it must receive good nutrition for conception. Conscious attention needs to be paid by both prospective parents to a healthy diet and lifestyle for at least six months before trying to conceive.

A "virility nutrition" program for a man usually includes a short cleansing diet, then zinc-rich foods, some fats, some meat and other protein rich foods, some sweets and dairy foods, and plenty of whole grains. Unless grossly overweight, a man should not be on a weight loss diet during preconception. Studies show that fasting or severe food limitation has a direct impact on the testicles. A poorly balanced diet also inhibits hormone formulation and reduces testicle response to hormone secretions. A man may see increased potency and sexual vigor within the first two weeks of diet improvement.

A woman uses food more efficiently and does not have so much need for an initial cleansing fast, so a "fertility nutrition" program for a woman usually includes plenty of salads, greens and lighter foods; less fat, no meats except seafoods, very low sugars, and a smaller volume of whole grains and nuts. A women should normalize her body weight before conception. Overweight women are at higher risk of developing toxemia and high blood pressure during pregnancy. Severely underweight women run the risk of premature birth and low birth weight babies. A woman's fertility rise may take 6 to 18 months after her diet change.

Both men and women should avoid fatty, fried foods or reduce their fat intake to between 8% and 10% of the diet. (This is good for your sex life, too.) Low-fat, fresh produce, whole grains, seafoods, turkey and chicken provide minerals, protein, fiber and complex carbohydrates to build gland functions quickly, while avoiding cholesterol. Reduce or avoid full fat dairy foods, sugary foods, foods made from chemicals, and meats that are regularly laced with nitrates and/or hormones, like red meats, and smoked, cured and processed meats like bologna.

LIFESTYLE HABITS ARE IMPORTANT, TOO.

Avoid or reduce consumption of tobacco, caffeine, and alcohol. (Moderate wine is ok until conception.) Get light exercise, and morning sunshine every day possible. Take alternating hot and cold showers to stimulate circulation and glandular secretions throughout the body. Apply alternating hot and cold compresses to the abdomen or scrotum to increase circulation to the reproductive areas.

I find relaxation techniques like massage therapy sessions, and deep breathing exercises, especially during long walks together, are very beneficial.

VITAMINS, MINERALS AND HERBS CAN HELP, TOO.

See "DO YOU WANT TO HAVE A BABY?" by Linda Rector-Page for extensive, complete nutritional supplement recommendations for both men and women trying to conceive a child.

Diet - Optimal Eating For Two During Pregnancy:

A woman's body changes so dramatically during pregnancy and childbearing that her normal daily needs change. The body takes care of some needs through cravings. During this one time of life, the body is so sensitive to its needs, that the cravings you get are usually good for you. We know that every single thing the mother does or takes in affects the child. Good nutrition for a child begins before it is born, even before it is conceived. The absence of certain nutrients during the early months of pregnancy can result in birth defects. New research shows that when a child reaches adulthood, his or her risk for heart disease, cancer, and diabetes can be traced to poor eating habits of the parents as well as genetic proneness. The highly nutritious diet suggestions in this section will help build a healthy baby, minimize the mother's discomfort, lessen birth complications, and reduce excess fatty weight gain that can't be lost after birth.

A highly nutritious diet will help you remember the pleasures of childbearing with less discomfort or risk of complications. It will help prevent miscarriage and high blood pressure, and aid in instances of toxemia, fluid retention, constipation, hemorrhoids and varicose veins, anemia, gas and heartburn, morning sickness and general system adjustment. After pregnancy, a good diet is important for sufficient breast milk, reducing post-partum swelling, and for healing tissues and stretch marks.

Promise yourself and your baby that at least during the months of pregnancy and nursing, your diet and lifestyle will be as healthy as you can make it. A largely vegetarian diet of whole foods provides optimum nutrition for pregnancy. Many staples of a lacto-vegetarian, seafood and poultry diet are nutritional powerhouses, such as whole grains, leafy greens, fish, turkey, eggs, legumes, nuts, seeds, green and yellow vegetables, nutritional yeast, bananas and citrus fruits. You can base your pregnancy diet on these foods with confidence that the baby will be getting the best possible nutrition.

HERE ARE THE KEYS:
- Protein is important. Most experts currently recommend 60 to 80 grams of protein daily during pregnancy, with a 10 gram increase every trimester. Eat a high vegetable protein diet, with whole grains, seeds and sprouts, with fish, seafood or turkey at least twice a week. Take a protein drink several times a week for optimal growth and energy.

The following is a proven example: *Mix $^1/_2$ cup raw milk, $^1/_2$ cup yogurt, the juice of one orange, 2 TBS. brewer's yeast, 2 TBS. wheat germ, 2 teasp. molasses, 1 teasp. vanilla, and a pinch cinnamon.* Even though protein requirements increase during pregnancy, it is the quality of the protein, not the quantity that prevents and cures toxemia.
- Have a fresh fruit or green salad every day. Eat plenty of soluble fiber foods like whole grain cereals and vegetables for regularity. Eat complex carbohydrate foods like broccoli and brown rice for strength.
- Drink plenty of healthy fluids - pure water, mineral water, and juices throughout the day to keep the system free and flowing. Carrot juice at least twice a week is ideal. Include pineapple and apple juice.
- Eat folacin rich foods, such as fresh spinach and asparagus for healthy cell growth.
- Eat carotene-rich foods, such as carrots, squashes, tomatoes, yams, and broccoli for disease resistance.
- Eat zinc-rich foods, such as pumpkin and sesame seeds for good body formation.
- Eat vitamin C foods, such as broccoli, bell peppers and fruits for connective tissue.
- Eat bioflavonoid-rich foods, such as citrus fruits and berries for capillary integrity.
- Eat alkalizing foods, such as miso soup and brown rice to combat and neutralize toxemia.
- Eat mineral-rich foods, such as sea veggies, leafy greens, and whole grains for baby building blocks. Especially include silicon-rich foods for bone, cartilage and connective tissue growth, and for collagen and elastin formation; brown rice, oats, green grasses and green drinks.
- Eat small frequent meals instead of large meals.

Note: See COOKING FOR HEALTHY HEALING by Linda Rector-Page for a complete, detailed pregnancy diet.

THERE ARE IMPORTANT DIET WATCHWORDS YOU SHOULD KNOW DURING PREGNANCY AND NURSING:
- Don't restrict your diet to lose weight. Low calories often mean low birth weight for the baby. Metabolism becomes deranged during dieting, and the baby receives abnormal nutrition that can impair brain and nerve development. Even if you feel you are gaining too much, a healthy diet is full of nutritious calories (not empty calories), that you can lose easily after nursing. Until then, you are still eating for two.

- Don't restrict food variety. Eat a wide range of healthy foods to assure the baby access to all nutrients. Avoid cabbages, onions, and garlic. They sometimes upset body balance during pregnancy. Avoid red meats. Most are full of nitrates, hormones and other chemicals the baby can't eliminate.
- Don't fast - even for short periods where fasting would normally be advisable, such as constipation, or to overcome a cold. Food energy and nutrient content will be diminished.
- Avoid all processed, refined, preserved and colored foods. Refrain from alcohol, caffeine and tobacco.
- Avoid X-rays, chemical solvents, CFCs such as hair sprays, and cat litter. Your system may be able to handle these things without undue damage; the baby's can't. Even during nursing, toxic concentrations occur easily.
- Don't smoke. Avoid secondary smoke. The chance of low birth weight and miscarriage is twice as likely if you smoke. Smoker's infants have a mortality rate 30% higher than non-smoker's. Nursing babies take in small amounts of nicotine with breast milk, and become prone to chronic respiratory infections.

About Breast Feeding

Unless there is a major health or physical problem, mother's breast milk should be the only food for the baby during the first six months of life. Despite all the claims made for fortified formulas, nothing can take the place of breast milk for the baby's health and ongoing well-being. The first thick, waxy colostrum is extremely high in protein, fats (which are needed for brain and nervous system development), and protective antibodies. A child's immune system is not fully established at birth, and the antibodies are critical, both for fighting early infections and in creating solid, balanced, immune defenses that will prevent the development of allergies. The baby who is not breast-fed loses nature's "jump start" on immunity. He/she faces life with health disadvantages that can last a lifetime.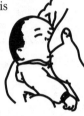

Breast-fed babies have a lower instance of colic and other digestive disturbances than bottle-fed babies, a fact attributed to bifidobacteria, the beneficial micro-organisms that make up 99% of a healthy baby's intestinal flora. Their growth is intensified by mother's milk. They are extremely important for protection against salmonella food poisoning and other intestinal pathogens. Bifidobacteria also produce lactic and acetic acids that inhibit the growth of yeasts and toxic amines from amino acids.

If there is simply no way to breast feed your baby, goat's milk is a better alternative than either chemically made formulas or cow's milk, both of which result in a higher risk of allergy development.

- **During labor:** Take no solid food. Drink fresh water, or carrot juice; or suck on ice chips.
- **During lactation:** Add almond milk, brewer's yeast, green drinks and green foods, avocados, carrot juice, goats milk, soy milk and soy foods, and unsulphured molasses, to promote milk quality and richness.
- **During weaning:** Drink papaya juice to slow down milk flow.

Supplements Help Nutritional Deficiencies During Pregnancy:

Illness, body imbalance, even regular maintenance supplementation need to be handled differently than your usual healing approach, even if your method is holistically oriented. A mother's body is very delicately tuned and sensitive at this time, and imbalances can occur easily. Mega-doses of anything are not good for the baby's system. Dosage of all medication or supplementation should almost universally be less than normal to allow for the infant's tiny systemic capacity. Dosage should be about half of normal. Ideal supplementation should be from food-source complexes for best absorbability.

- Avoid all drugs during pregnancy and nursing - including alcohol, tobacco, caffeine, MSG, Saccharin, X-rays, aspirin, Valium, Librium, Tetracycline, and harsh diuretics. Even the amino acid L-Phenylalanine can adversely affect the nervous system of the unborn child.
- Especially stay away from recreational drugs - cocaine, PCP, marijuana, meth-amphetamines, Quaaludes, heroin, LSD and other psychedelics.

HERE ARE SOME SUPPLEMENTS THAT CAN HELP YOU DURING PREGNANCY:

• Try a body building, whole green drink. The ingredients should be unrefined and have whole cell availability for maximum health support. A green drink is a good nutritional "delivery system" during pregnancy because it is so quickly absorbed with so little work by the body. Crystal Star's ENERGY GREEN™ drink mix or capsules contains green vegetables, grasses and herbs full of absorbable, potent chlorophyllins, complex carbohydrates, minerals, trace minerals, proteins, and amino acids. It combines the best building and energizing qualities of herbs with the stabilizing, rejuvenating qualities of rice and bee pollen, and the oxygen and iodine therapy benefits of land and sea greens.

• Take a good prenatal multi-vitamin and mineral supplement, such as Rainbow Light PRE-NATAL; especially starting six to eight weeks before the expected birth. Clinical testing has shown that mothers who took nutritional supplementation during pregnancy were far less likely to have babies with neural tube and other defects.

• Take a food source multi-mineral supplement (not just calcium) that will be absorbed well by both you and the baby, such as MEZOTRACE SEA MINERALS, or Crystal Star MINERAL SPECTRUM™ capsules for good body building blocks. Recent studies show that beta-carotene 10,000mg, with vitamin C 500mg, niacin 50mg, and liquid herbal iron are better for skeletal, cellular and connecting tissue development than calcium supplements.

• Take extra folic acid, 800mcg daily to prevent neural tube defects. Timing is essential. Supplemental folic acid after the first three months of fetal development cannot correct spinal cord damage.

• Bioflavonoids are necessary for both mother and child. Recent tests show that over 50% of women who habitually miscarry have low levels of vitamin C and bioflavonoids. As an integral part of the natural vitamin C complex, bioflavonoids offer a broad spectrum of healthful activity. Since they often occur naturally with vitamin A and rutin, bioflavs are best known for enhancing vein and capillary strength, and for helping to control the bruising and internal bleeding experienced in hemorrhoids and varicose veins. But support goes to even deeper body levels.

Bioflavonoids also play a key role in new collagen production, with tightening and toning activity for skin elasticity. They can minimize skin aging and wrinkling, especially because of pregnancy stretching. Recent research indicates that supplemental bioflavonoids are important in the control of excess fatty deposits. Think of bioflavonoids as a "tissue tonic" because of their ability to support and maintain tissue tone integrity. Herbal and citrus sources are a wonderful way to get them. A good natural bioflavonoid-source compound will also be fiber-rich for regularity - a definite advantage during prenatal care! Take bioflavonoids 1000mg with vitamin C daily, or an herbal supplement, such as Crystal Star BIOFLAVONOID, FIBER & C SUPPORT™ drink.

Note: **BILBERRY** extract is one of the single richest sources of herbal flavonoids in the botanical world. It is especially helpful for pregnant women suffering from distended veins, hemorrhoids, weak uterine walls, and toxemia. It is gently effective for both mother and child at a time when strong supplementation is inadvisable.

• Take vitamin B_6-50mg for bloating, leg cramps and nerve strength, as well as to prevent proneness to glucose intolerance and seizures in the baby.

• Take kelp tablets, 4-6 daily, or Crystal Star IODINE/POTASSIUM SOURCE™ capsules, for natural potassium and iodine. Too little of these minerals mean mental retardation and poor physical development.

• Take natural vitamin E 200-400IU, or wheat germ oil capsules, to help prevent miscarriage and reduce baby's oxygen requirement, lessening the chances of asphyxiation during labor.

• Take zinc 10-15mg daily, (or get it from your pre-natal multi-mineral). Zinc deficiencies often result in poor brain formation, learning problems, low immunity, sub-normal growth and allergies in the baby.

IMPORTANT SUPPLEMENTATION WATCHWORDS:

• **During the last trimester:** Rub vitamin E or wheat germ oil on the stomach and around the vaginal opening each night to make stretching easier and skin more elastic. Begin to take extra minerals as labor approaches.

• **During labor:** Take natural vitamin E and calcium/magnesium to relieve pain and aid dilation.

• **During nursing:** Nutritional supplements that were used during pregnancy, such as iron, calcium, B vitamins or a prenatal multiple, should be continued during nursing. Indeed, they may be slightly increased for optimum nutrition if the mother has not recovered normal strength. Breast milk is a filtered food supply that prevents the baby from overdosing on higher potencies. Apply vitamin E oil to alleviate breast crusting.

• Take EFA's, (Omega-3 flax oil, borage seed or evening primrose oils), for baby's brain development.

• Take calcium lactate with calcium ascorbate vitamin C for collagen development.

Herbs For A Healthy Pregnancy

Herbs have been used successfully for centuries to ease the hormone imbalances and discomforts of stretching, bloating, nausea and pain of pregnancy, without impairing the development or health of the baby. Herbs are concentrated mineral rich foods that are perfect for the extra growth requirements of pregnancy and childbirth. They are easily-absorbed and nonconstipating. A developing child's body is very small and delicate. Ideal supplementation should be from food source complexes for best absorbability. Herbs are identified and accepted by the body's enzyme activity as whole food nutrients, lessening the risk of toxemia or overdose, yet providing gentle, easy nutrition for both mother and baby. Herbs are good and easy for you; good and gentle for the baby.

Important Note: Early pregnancy and later pregnancy must be considered separately with herbal medicinals. If there is any question, always use the gentlest herbs.

DURING PREGNANCY:

• Many women, because of morning sickness and general body imbalance, prefer teas as a way to take in balancing nutrients during pregnancy. Take two daily cups of red raspberry tea, Crystal Star MOTHERING TEA™, a red raspberry blend, or Mother Love TEA FOR TWO. Each is safe, high in iron, calcium and other minerals, strengthening to the uterus and birth canal, effective against birth defects, long labor and afterbirth pain, with uterine toning properties for a quicker return to normal.

• Iodine rich foods are a primary deterrent to spinal birth defects. Take kelp tablets, or Crystal Star IODINE/POTASSIUM SOURCE™ capsules, or try the OCEAN THERAPY SPRINKLE food sprinkle on page 204.

• Many pregnant women need extra calcium and iron. Herbal sources can be the best way to get these minerals because they are absorbable through the body's own enzyme system, they are rich in other naturally-occurring nutrients that encourage the best uptake and use by the body, they provide an optimum-use bonding agent between the body and other foods it is taking in, and they are gentle and easily usable.

• During the 1st and 2nd trimester, take a mineral-rich pre-natal herbal compound for gentle, absorbable minerals and toning agents to elasticize tissue and ease delivery. A broad spectrum herbal capsule compound, rich in the extra minerals needed during pregnancy might contain herbs like red raspberry, nettles, oatstraw, alfalfa, yellow dock root, fennel, rosemary and vegetable acidophilus.

Certain herbs are excellent sources of absorbable calcium and iron, minerals that are easily depleted during pregnancy. Crystal Star CALCIUM SOURCE™, a calcium-rich compound of herbs, includes magnesium for optimum uptake, and is rich in naturally-occurring silica to help form healthy tissue and bone; IRON SOURCE™, an absorbable, non-constipating herbal iron compound has measurable amounts of calcium and magnesium, with naturally-occurring vitamins C and E for iron uptake; and SILICA SOURCE™, an organic silica from oatstraw and horsetail herb is a prime factor in collagen production, and formation of connective and interstitial tissue.

• During the last trimester, a broad range herbal mineral compound, such as Crystal Star MINERAL SPECTRUM™ capsules, has highly absorbable plant minerals for health maintenance. Five weeks before the expected birth date, an herbal formula to aid in hemorrhage control and and uterine muscle strength for correct presentation of the fetus might contain herbs like red raspberry, pennyroyal, false unicorn, black cohosh, squaw vine, blessed thistle, lobelia leaf, and bilberry.

DURING LABOR:

• Take Medicine Wheel LABOR TINCTURE drops, or Crystal Star CRAMP BARK COMBO™ extract to ease contraction pain. Put 15 to 20 drops in water and take in small sips as needed during labor. Take BACK TO RELIEF™ capsules for afterbirth pain, an analgesic formula that works on the lower back and spinal block area.

• For false labor, drink 4 to 6 cups catnip/blue cohosh tea to renormalize. If there is bleeding, take 2 capsules each cayenne and bayberry, and get to a hospital or call your midwife.

DURING NURSING:

- Add 2 TBS. brewer's yeast to your diet, along with red raspberry, marshmallow root, or Crystal Star MOTHERING TEA™ to promote and enrich milk.
- Take Vitex extract or Mother Love MORE MILK to promote an abundant supply of mother's milk.
- Fennel, alfalfa, red raspberry leaf, cumin, or fenugreek teas help keep the baby colic free.
- For infant jaundice, use Hyland's *BILIOUSNESS* tabs.

DURING WEANING:

- Take parsley/sage tea to help dry up milk.

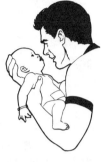

HERBS TO USE DURING PREGNANCY:

In general, take herbs in the mildest way, as hot, relaxing teas, during pregnancy.

- **Red raspberry** - the quintessential herb for pregnancy. Raspberry is an all around uterine tonic. It is anti-abortive to prevent miscarriage, antiseptic to help prevent infection, astringent to tighten tissue, rich in calcium, magnesium and iron to help prevent cramps and anemia. It is hemostatic to prevent excess bleeding during and after labor, and facilitates the birth process by stimulating contractions.
- **Nettles** - a mineral-rich, nutritive herb, with vitamin K to guard against excessive bleeding. It improves kidney function and helps prevent hemorrhoids.
- **Peppermint** - may be used after the first trimester to help digestion, soothe the stomach and overcome nausea. Contains highly absorbable amounts of vitamin A, C, silica, potassium and iron.
- **Ginger root** - excellent for morning sickness; has lots of necessary minerals.
- **Bilberry** - a strong but gentle astringent, rich in bioflavonoids to fortify vein and capillary support. A hematonic for kidney function and a mild diuretic for bloating.
- **Burdock root** - a mineral-rich, hormone balancing herb. Helps prevent water retention and baby jaundice.
- **Yellow dock root** - improves iron assimilation; helps prevent infant jaundice.
- **Dong quai root** - a blood nourisher, rather than a hormone stimulant. Use in moderation.
- **Echinacea** - an immune system stimulant to help prevent colds, flu and infections.
- **Chamomile** - relaxes for quality sleep, and helps digestive and bowel problems.
- **Vitex** - normalizes hormone balance for fertility. Discontinue when pregnancy is realized.
- **False unicorn, black and blue cohosh** - for final weeks of pregnancy only, to ease and/or induce labor.
- **Wild yam** - for general pregnancy pain, nausea or cramping; lessens chance of miscarriage.

HERBS TO AVOID DURING PREGNANCY:

Medicinal herbs should always be used with common sense and care. Especially during pregnancy, some herbs are not appropriate. The following list includes contra-indicated herbs.

- **Aloe vera** - can be too laxative. We have found George's ALOE VERA JUICE to be very gentle.
- **Angelica and rue** stimulate oxytocin that causes uterine contractions.
- **Barberry, buckthorn, rhubarb root, mandrake, senna and cascara sagrada** are too strong as laxatives.
- **Buchu and juniper** are too strong diuretics.
- **Coffee** - too strong a caffeine and heated hydrocarbon source - irritates the uterus. In extremely sensitive individuals who take in excessive amounts, may cause miscarriage or premature birth.
- **Comfrey** - pyrrolizide content (carcinogen) cannot be regulated or controlled for an absolutely safe source.
- **Ephedra, Ma Huang** - too strong an anti-histamine if used in extract or capsule form. It is gentle enough as a tea to relieve bronchial and chest congestion.
- **Horseradish** - too strong for a baby.
- **Goldenseal, lovage, mugwort and wormwood** are emmenagogues that causes uterine contractions.
- **Male fern** - too strong a vermifuge.
- **Mistletoe, tansy and wild ginger** are emmenagogues that causes uterine contractions.
- **Pennyroyal** - stimulates oxytocin that can cause abortion. May be used in the final weeks of pregnancy.
- **Yarrow and shepherd's purse** are strong astringents and mild abortifacients.

PREVENTING SIDS, SUDDEN INFANT DEATH SYNDROME:

If the baby has a weak system, or poor tissue or lung development (signs that it is a candidate for SIDS) give a weak ascorbate vitamin C, or Ester C with bioflavonoids solution in water daily. Routinely feeding babies iron-fortified weaning foods to prevent anemia may increase the risk of SIDS, according to the British Medical Journal. New evidence indicates that infant pillows filled with foam polystyrene beads cause the baby to inhale toxic gases and suffocate. Smoking increases the risk of SIDS. Even if the baby is merely in the room where smoking has occurred, its risk of dying from SIDS can increase 800%! Some new research shows that low doses of carnitine during the last trimester can help protect the baby from SIDS.

Bodywork For Two

•   Get some mild daily exercise, such as a brisk walk for fresh air, oxygen and circulation. Take an early morning, half hour sun bath when possible for vitamin D, calcium absorption and bone growth.

•   Consciously set aside one stress-free time for relaxation every day. The baby will know, thrive, and be more relaxed itself.

•   If you practice reflexology, do not press the acupressure point just above the ankle on the inside of the leg. It can start contractions.

•   Rub cocoa butter, vitamin E oil or wheat germ oil on the stomach and around the vaginal opening every night to make stretching easier and the skin more elastic.

•   Get adequate sleep. The body energy turns inward during sleep for repair, restoration and fetal growth.

Special Problems During Pregnancy

Dosage of any medication, orthodox or natural, should be less than normal to allow for the infant's tiny system. The following section contains effective natural products that may be used without harm.

•   **AFTERBIRTH PAIN** - take Crystal Star MOTHERING TEA™ or BACK TO RELIEF™ capsules, especially after a long labor, to tone and elasticize uterus and abdomen for quicker return to normal. For post-partum tears and to heal sore perineal muscles, use a sitz bath with 1 part uva ursi, 1 part yerba mansa rt., and 1 part each comfrey leaf and root. Simmer 15 minutes, strain, add 1 tsp. salt, pour into a large shallow container; cool a little. Or use MOTHER LOVE'S SITZ BATH or CRAMPBARK COMPLEX. Sit in the bath for 15-20 minutes 2x daily.

•   **ANEMIA** - take a non-constipating herbal iron, such as Floradix LIQUID IRON, yellow dock tea, or Crystal Star IRON SOURCE™ caps. Have a green drink often, such as apple/alfalfa sprout/parsley juice, Green Foods BETA CARROT, or Crystal Star ENERGY GREEN™. Add vitamin C and E to your diet, and eat plenty of dark leafy greens.

•   **BREASTS** - for infected breasts: 500mg Vitamin C every 3 hours, 400IU vitamin E, and beta-carotene 10,000IU daily. Get plenty of chlorophyll from green salads, green drinks, or green supplements such as chlorella, Crystal Star ENERGY GREEN™ drink or Green Foods GREEN MAGMA.
-for caked or crusted breasts: simmer elder flowers in oil and rub on breasts. Wheat germ oil, almond oil and cocoa butter are also effective, or use Mother Love's PREGNANT BELLY SALVE.
-for engorged breasts during nursing: apply ice bags to the breasts to relieve pain; or use a marshmallow root fomentation with 1/2 cup powder to 1 qt. water. Simmer 10 minutes. Soak a cloth in mixture and apply to breast.

•   **CONSTIPATION** - use a gentle fiber laxative, (Yerba Prima COLON CLEANSE, or Crystal Star CHO-LO FIBER TONE™), or an herbal laxative such as HERBALTONE. Add fiber fruits, like prunes and apples to your diet.

•   **FALSE LABOR** - catnip tea or red raspberry tea will help. See also MISCARRIAGE page in this book.

•   **GAS & HEARTBURN** - usually caused by an enzyme imbalance. Take papaya or bromelain chewables or papaya juice with a pinch of ginger, or comfrey/pepsin tablets.

- **HEMORRHOIDS** - BILBERRY extract, Crystal Star HEMR-EASE™ capsules or Mother Love RHOID BALM (Use any of these combinations effectively mixed with cocoa butter as a suppository.)

- **INSOMNIA** - take a liquid or herbal calcium supplement, like Crystal Star CALCIUM SOURCE™ capsules or extract, with chamomile tea. Nervine herbs like scullcap and passion flower also help. Try Crystal Star RELAX™ caps.

- **LABOR** - For nausea during labor, take ginger tea or miso broth, or Alacer EMERGEN-C with a little salt. For labor pain, take crampbark extract, lobelia, scullcap or St. John's wort extract in water. For nerve pain, apply St. John's wort oil to temples and wrists and rosemary/ginger compresses. For post-partum bleeding, take shepherd's purse or nettles tea. For sleep during long labor, use scullcap tincture (scullcap may be used throughout labor for relaxation.) Hydrate with cool drinks during labor even if there is nausea. Take bromelain to relieve pain and swelling after episiotomy.

- **MORNING SICKNESS** - use homeopathic IPECAC and NAT. MUR, add vitamin B_6 50mg. 2x daily, sip mint tea whenever queasy, and see MORNING SICKNESS program in this book.

- **MISCARRIAGE** - for prevention and hemorrhage control, drink raspberry tea every hour with $^1/_4$ teasp. ascorbate vit. C powder added, and take drops of hawthorn or lobelia extract every hour. See the MISCARRIAGE PREVENTION program in this book for complete information.

- **POST-PARTUM SWELLING & DEPRESSION** - use homeopathic ARNICA. Make a post-partum cordial with 4 slices of dong quai rt., $^1/_2$ oz. false unicorn rt., 1 handful nettles, $^1/_2$ oz. St. John's wort extract, 1 handful motherwort herb, $^1/_2$ oz. hawthorn berries, and 2 inch-long slices of fresh ginger. Steep herbs in 1 pint of brandy for 2 weeks, shaking daily. Strain, add a little honey if desired. Take 1 teasp. daily as a tonic dose. Cordials and teas are more effective than capsules for post-partum healing.

- **STRETCH MARKS** - Apply wheat germ, avocado, sesame oil, vitamin E, or A D & E oil. Take vitamin C 500mg. 3 to 4 times daily for collagen development. See STRETCH MARKS program in this book.

- **SWOLLEN ANKLES** - use BILBERRY extract in water.

- **TOXEMIA, Eclampsia** - toxemia is caused by liver malfunction and disease. The liver simply cannot handle the increasing load of the progressing pregnancy. There is a marked reduction in blood flow to the placenta, kidneys and other organs. Severe cases result in liver and brain hemorrhage, convulsions and coma. Toxemia is indicated by extreme swelling, accompanied by high blood pressure, headaches, nausea and vomiting.)
    Take several green drinks such as apple/alfalfa sprout/parsley or Green Foods GREEN MAGMA for a "chlorophyll cleanout." Add vitamin C 500mg every 3 to 4 hours, 10,000IU beta-carotene, BILBERRY extract in water, and B Complex 50mg daily. Apply Transitions PROGEST CREAM as directed. Enzymatic Therapy MUCOPLEX and DGL have also been helpful, as has iodine therapy via daily kelp tablets.

- **UTERINE HEMORRHAGING** - Take bayberry/cayenne capsules, and get to professional help immediately. Take bilberry extract daily with strengthening herbal flavonoids for tissue integrity. Use angelica tea for uterine contractions or Mother Love's SHEPHERD'S PURSE extract.

- **VARICOSE VEINS** - Take vitamin C 500mg. with bioflavonoids and rutin, 4 daily; or bilberry extract 2x daily in water; or butcher's broom tea daily (also helpful for leg cramps during pregnancy). Take and apply Crystal Star VARI-TONE™ caps and VARI-VAIN™ roll-on gel directly to swollen veins.

Note: Baby diapers are a huge cause for concern for parents who are ecologically minded, and for people who live or play on America's coastlines where they are being dumped. Most diapers are still non-biodegradable, disposable toilets for babies, and most are impregnated with chemical polymer salts to absorb and control moisture. Our planet needs special help in this area. I recommend recycling diapers through a diaper service, or your own washing machine, or at the very least, using all-cotton TUSHIES, a disposable diaper available in health food stores that uses an all natural cotton and wood pulp blend instead of chemicals in its padding.

Alternative Healing Options For Children

*U*nless unusually or chronically ill, a child is born with a well-developed, powerful immune system. He or she often needs only the subtle body-strengthening forces that nutritious foods, herbs or homeopathic remedies supply, rather than the highly focused medications of allopathic medicine which can have such drastic side effects on a small body.

The undeniable ecological, sociological and diet deterioration in America during the last fifty years has had a marked effect on children's health. Declining educational performance, learning disabilities, mental disorders, drug and alcohol abuse, hypoglycemia, allergies, chronic illness, delinquency and violent behavior are all evidence of declining immunity and general health.

You can get a lot of help from the kids themselves in a natural health program. Kids don't want to be sick, they aren't stupid, they don't like going to the doctor any more than you do. They often recognize that natural foods and therapies are good for them. Children are naturally immune to disease. A nutritious diet and natural supplements help keep them that way.

Diet Help For Childhood Diseases

THREE DIET PROGRAMS ARE INCLUDED: A short liquid detox cleanse for rapid toxin elimination, a raw foods purification diet for body cleansing during the beginning and acute stages of an illness, and an optimal whole foods maintenance diet for disease prevention.

Diet is the most important way to keep a child's immunity and defense mechanisms working. Pathogenic organisms and viruses are everywhere. But they aren't the major factor in causing disease if the body environment is healthy. Well-nourished children are usually strong enough to deal with infection in a successful way. They either do not catch the "bugs" that are going around, contract only a mild case, or develop strong healthy reactions that are short in duration, and get the problem over and done with quickly. This difference in resistance and immune response is the key to understanding children's diseases.

A wholesome diet can easily restore a child's natural vitality. Even children who have eaten a junk food diet for years quickly respond to a diet of fresh fruits, vegetables, whole grains, low fats and sugars. I have noted great improvement in as little as a month's time. A child's hair and skin takes on new luster, they fill out if they are too skinny, and lose weight if they are fat. They sleep more soundly and regularly. Their attention spans markedly increase, and many learning and behavior problems diminish or disappear.

Keep it simple. Let them help prepare their own food, even though they might get in the way and you feel like it's more trouble than it's worth. They will have a better understanding of good food, and are more likely to eat the things they have a hand in fixing. Keep only good nutritious foods in the house. Children may be exposed to junk foods and poor foods at school or friend's houses, but you can build a good, natural foundation diet at home. For the time that they are at home, they should be able to choose only from nutritious choices.

Kids have extraordinarily sensitive taste buds. Everything they eat is very vivid and important to them. The diet program we offer in this section has lots of variety, so they can experiment and find out where their own preferences lie. There are plenty of snacks, sandwiches, fresh fruits, and sweet veggies like carrots - all foods children naturally like.

Diet and nutritional therapy for most common childhood diseases, including measles, mumps, chicken pox, strep throat and whooping cough, is fairly simple and basic - a short liquid elimination fast, followed by a fresh light foods diet in the acute stages.

A Short, Liquid Detox Cleanse for Childhood Diseases: *24 to 72 hours*

• Start the child on cleansing liquids as soon as the disease is diagnosed to clean out harmful bacteria and infection. Give fruit juices such as apple, pineapple, grape, cranberry and citrus juices, or give Crystal Star FIRST AID TEA FOR KIDS™. The juice of two lemons in a glass of water with a little honey may be taken once or twice a day to flush the kidneys and alkalize the body.

• Alternate fresh fruit juices throughout the day with fresh carrot juice, bottled mineral water, and clear soups. A potassium broth or veggie drink (pages 167-168) should be taken at least once a day. Encourage the child to drink as many healthy cleansing liquids as she/he wants. Light smoothies are special favorites with kids. No dairy products should be given.

• Offer herb teas throughout the cleanse. Make them about half the strength as those for an adult. Children respond to herb teas quickly, and they like them more than you might think. Just add a little honey or maple syrup if the herbs are bitter.

The following teas are effective for most childhood diseases:
- elder flowers with peppermint to induce perspiration
- catnip/chamomile/rosemary tea to break out a rash
- mullein/lobelia or scullcap as relaxants
- catnip, fennel and peppermint for upset stomachs
- Crystal Star COFEX TEA™ for sore throats
- Crystal Star X-PECT-T™ to help bring up mucous
- Crystal Star FIRST AID™ TEA for warming against chills
- Crystal Star ECHINACEA EXTRACT drops in water every 3 to 4 hours to keep the lymph glands clear and able to process infective toxins.

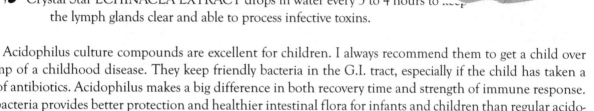

• Acidophilus culture compounds are excellent for children. I always recommend them to get a child over the hump of a childhood disease. They keep friendly bacteria in the G.I. tract, especially if the child has taken a course of antibiotics. Acidophilus makes a big difference in both recovery time and strength of immune response. Bifido-bacteria provides better protection and healthier intestinal flora for infants and children than regular acidophilus strains. Natren LIFE START, Solaray BABY LIFE, or DR. DOPHILUS powder, work very well for children. Use about 1/4 teasp. at a time in a glass of water or juice three to four times daily.

BODYWORK THERAPIES ARE ESPECIALLY GOOD FOR CHILDREN, BECAUSE THE PATHWAYS IN THEIR BODIES ARE SO CLEAR.
• A gentle enema should be given at least once during the detox cleanse to clear the colon of impacted wastes that hinder the body in its effort to rid itself of diseased bacteria. A catnip tea enema is effective and safe for children.

• Oatmeal baths help neutralize rashes coming out on the skin. Hydrotherapy baths, (pg. 177) help induce cleansing perspiration, but the child should be watched closely all during the bath to make sure he or she is not getting too hot. Make up a big pot of calendula or comfrey tea for the bath water. Rub the child's body with calendula or tea tree oil, or Tiger Balm to loosen congestion after the bath.

• Hot ginger/cayenne compresses applied to affected or sore areas stimulate circulation and defense mechanisms, to rid the body more quickly of infection. Alternate them with cold, plain water compresses.

• Herbal steam inhalations, such as eucalyptus or tea tree oil, or Crystal Star RSPR TEA™ in a vaporizer help to keep lungs mucous free and improve oxygen uptake.

• Golden seal, myrrh, yellow dock, black walnut, yarrow, or Crystal Star ANTI-BIO™ phyto-therapy gel, may be patted onto sores, scabs and lesions with cotton balls to help heal and soothe.

Fresh Foods Purification Diet For Children's Diseases: *A 3 day diet.*

This diet may be used for initial, acute and chronic symptoms when a liquid detox is not desired, or following a liquid cleanse after the acute stage has passed. The child's body will continue cleansing, and the addition of solid foods will start to rebuild strength. Dairy products, except for yogurt should be avoided. This diet should last about three days depending on the strength and condition of the child.

On rising: give citrus juice with a teaspoon of acidophilus liquid, or $1/4$ teasp. acidophilus powder;
 or a glass of lemon juice and water with honey or maple syrup.
Breakfast: offer fresh fruits, such as apples, pineapple, papaya or oranges. Add vanilla yogurt or soymilk if desired.
Mid-morning: Give a vegetable drink, a potassium broth, (page 167-168) or fresh carrot juice. Add $1/4$ teasp.
 ascorbate vitamin C or Ester C crystals.
Lunch: give fresh raw crunchy veggies with a yogurt dip; or a fresh veggie salad with lemon/oil or yogurt dressing.
Mid-afternoon: offer a refreshing herb tea, such as licorice or peppermint tea, or Crystal Star FIRST AID TEA
 FOR KIDS™ to keep the stomach settled and calm tension;
 or another vegetable drink with $1/4$ teasp. vitamin C added.
Dinner: give a fresh salad, with avocados, carrots, kiwi, romaine and other high vitamin A foods; and/or a cup of
 miso soup or other clear broth soup.
Before bed: offer a relaxing herb tea, such as chamomile or scullcap tea, or Crystal Star GOOD NIGHT TEA™.
 • Add $1/4$ teasp. ascorbate vitamin C or Ester C crystals; or a cup of Organic Gourmet MISO broth for strength
and B vitamins.

Note: **It is important to incorporate fresh, enzyme-rich foods in the diet of your children. The cleansing drinks and broths in this section may be used as part of a nourishing, healthy diet as well as for purification. If you have a vegetable juicer, you can make fresh juices. The following is a basic idea for a very nourishing mixed vegetable juice. There are many variations that you can use. Juicing some carrot, some sunflower greens and some other greens is a basic concept to use.**

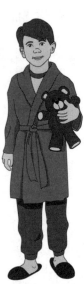

❧ GREEN DRINK FOR KIDS
Make it in a juicer. Make it easy. Use fresh veggies that your child likes most.

Be sure to use green leafy vegetables like spinach, sunflower greens and lettuces.
I find kids like baby veggies a lot. Add baby bok choy, baby carrots and sprouts.
Don't forget sweet tasting veggies like cucumbers, celery and tomatoes.

❧ ENERGY SOUP FOR KIDS
*A liquid salad for kids. Add avocado for creaminess, with a little broth or water,
 and add tamari sauce or Bragg's LIQUID AMINOS for taste.*

$1/4$ CUP CELERY
$1/4$ CUP FRESH PEAS
1 CUP SALAD GREENS, like BOK CHOY, DANDELION, LETTUCES and SPINACH
$1/2$ to 1 CUP SPOUTS like SUNFLOWER GREENS, ALFALFA or MUNG BEAN SPROUTS
 • Blender blend with $1/2$ cup water, then add half an avocado for creaminess. Season to taste.

❧ HEALING FRUIT SMOOTHIE
Always use fresh fruit (organic if possible), for this drink, not canned or frozen.

Blend 1 BANANA and PEELED ORANGE with some unpasteurized apple juice. Add half a papaya or mango if available, or one-quarter of a fresh pineapple.

Here are some effective supplements you can give your child during the fresh foods diet. I recommend continuing to give them until the child is symptom free.

•   A vitamin/mineral drink, such as NutriTech ALL-ONE, or 1 teasp. liquid multi-vitamin in juice, such as Floradix CHILDREN'S MULTIVITAMIN or Prevail MULTI-VITAMIN/MINERAL FOR CHILDREN.

•   Continue with your acidophilus choice. Add vitamin A & D in drops if desired, and ascorbate vitamin C or Ester C crystals in juice.

•   Continue with the therapeutic herbal teas you found effective during the liquid cleanse, especially Crystal Star FIRST AID TEA FOR KIDS™.

•   Use a mild herbal laxative, like HERBALTONE, in half dosage to keep the child eliminating regularly.

•   Use garlic oil drops or open garlic capsules into juice or water for natural anti-biotic activity; or give Crystal Star ANTI-BIO™ CAPS or EXTRACT in half dosage.

BODYWORK IS A GOOD CHOICE FOR CHILDREN THROUGHOUT ANY ILLNESS.
Continue with herbal baths, washes and compresses to neutralize and cleanse toxins coming out through the skin. Give a soothing massage before bed. Get some early morning sunlight on the body every day possible for regenerating vitamin D.
When the crisis has passed, and the child is on the mend with a clean system, begin an optimal nutrition diet, like the one below, to prevent further problems, and increase general health and energy.

❖

An Optimal Whole Foods Diet For Children

The best health and disease prevention diet for children is high in whole grains and green veggies for minerals, vegetable proteins for growth, and complex carbohydrates for energy. It is low in fats, pasteurized dairy foods and sugars, (sugars inhibit release of growth hormones), and avoids fried foods. It is also very easy on you, the parent. Once children are shown the foods that will give them health and energy they can fix a lot of these simply prepared foods on their own. Make sure you tell and graphically show your child what junk and synthetic foods are. We find over and over again that because of TV advertising and peer pressure, kids often really don't know what wholesome food is, and think they are eating the right way.

Vitamins and minerals are important for a child's physical, emotional and mental growth, and for a healthy immune system. A child's normal immune defenses are strong. If a child is eating well, with lots of green veggies, and few sugars, refined foods or dairy products, he or she may not need extra supplementation. However, because much of our growing soils are depleted, and most of our foods are sprayed or gassed, many vitamins, minerals and trace minerals are no longer sufficiently present in our foods; supplementation is often needed for good body building blocks, and to enable children to think, learn and grow at optimum levels. The most common deficiencies are calcium, iron, B_1, and vitamins A, B Complex and C.

Use SUPERFOODS for kids! These concentrated nutrients, so popular with adults today (check out the many superfoods listings in this book), are just as good in healthy diet programs for children. They can be added into, or sprinkled on, other foods to increase the nutritional content of the meal. And superfood supplements can get some great nutrients into fussy eaters. SYSTEMS STRENGTH™ drink mix is a potent vegetarian blend of sea vegetables, herbs, and foods like miso, soy protein, brewer's yeast, and brown rice which can be added to soups, sauces, and even salad dressings. Another superfood kids like is bee pollen, a highly bio-active, tonic nutrient often called "nature's complete nutrition," because it is so full of balanced vitamins, minerals, proteins, carbohydrates, fats, enzyme precursors, and all essential amino acids. It has a sweet flavor which works well sprinkled on cereals, or added to smoothies. A half teaspoon of bee pollen granules is a good amount to use for children.

HERE ARE SOME OTHER DIET TIPS TO HELP KEEP YOUR CHILD HEALTHIER AND HAPPIER:

We know it's a lot easier said than done to change old dietary patterns to more healthful eating....for anybody, but especially for kids. One good way to start is to make sure you find something delicious to replace whatever is being taken away.

FOR EXAMPLE:

• If you want to include more wholesome foods, like fruits and vegetables, start with *food forms that children naturally go for* - like dried fruit snacks, and smoothies for fruits. Sandwiches, tacos, burritos and pitas can hold vegetables. Most kids like soup.... another good place to add vegetables. Let them add sauces or flavors they like.

• If you want to include more whole grains in a child's diet, start by keeping only whole grains in the house. Kids love bagels, and there are lots of healthy choices. Pastas come in a wide variety of whole grain options. Brown or basmati rice is *much tastier than white rice* if your kid is a "rice kid." Stuffing is already a big favorite with kids - make sure it's whole grain. Popcorn is a healthy snack. (Season it with tamari or a healthy season blend rather than gobs of butter and salt.)

• If you want to add healthy cultured foods to your child's diet, start by keeping a good assortment of yogurt flavors with fruit for snacks in the fridge. Offer delicious kefir cheese for snack spreads instead of sour cream.

• If you want to reduce the amount of sugar your child is consuming, go to your health food store for a wide variety of delicious, sugar-free snacks. Granolas and oatmeal with toppings can replace sugar-filled cereals. Offer dried fruit, too. Almost every kid likes raisins.

• If you want to reduce the amount of meat and heavy dairy proteins your child is eating, keep good plant protein available. Kids like tofu and grain burgers, especially with their favorite trimmings. Most kids like beans, too - look for healthy chili blends. Keep peanut butter, and nuts and seeds, like almonds, sunflower seeds and pumpkin seeds around the house for snacks; recommend them as toppings for everything from soup or salad crunchies to smoothies and desserts. (Seeds and nuts give kids unsaturated oils and essential fatty acids, too.) Eggs are a good protein choice for kids...one of Nature's perfect foods that's gotten a bad rap. Most kids like deviled eggs, and eggs are great in healthy honey custards, another kid favorite.

• If you want to add more fish and seafood to a child's diet, start with a favorite like shrimp, tuna fish or salmon.

• If you want to encourage your child to drink more water, instead of carbonated sodas or sweetened drinks, keep plenty of natural fruit juices and flavored mineral water around the house.

Your presence as a loving parental authority is a powerful influence. Have the whole family sit together and eat healthfully as often as possible to establish good eating habits for your children.

A sample diet might look like the one below. It's optimally healthy, and it's been kid-tested for taste.

On rising: offer a protein drink such as NutriTech ALL-ONE, especially if the child's energy or school performance level is poor, or if a weak system is constantly leading to chronic illness, (a child's body must have protein to heal), or 1 teaspoon liquid multi-vitamin in juice, such as Floradix CHILDREN'S MULTI-VITAMIN/MINERAL.

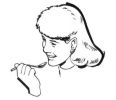

Breakfast: have a whole grain cereal with apple juice or a little yogurt and fresh fruit;
and/or whole grain toast or muffins, with a little butter, kefir cheese or nut butter;
add eggs, scrambled or baked or soft boiled (no fried eggs);
or have some hot oatmeal or puffed kashi with a little maple syrup, and yogurt.

Mid-morning: whole grain crackers with kefir cheese or dip, and a fruit juice;
and/or some fresh fruit, dried fruit, or fruit leathers with yogurt or kefir cheese;
or fresh crunchy veggies with peanut butter or a nut spread;
or dried fruit, sugar-free candy bar, or a healthy trail mix, stirred into yogurt.

Lunch: have a fresh veggie, turkey, chicken or shrimp salad sandwich on whole grain bread, with low fat cheese and mayonnaise. Add whole grain or corn chips with a low fat dip;
or a bean soup with whole grain toast, and a small salad or crunchy veggies with garbanzo spread;
or a baked potato with a little butter and kefir cheese, and a small green salad with Italian dressing;
or a vegetarian pizza on a chapati or whole grain crust;
or whole grain spaghetti or pasta with a light sauce and parmesan cheese;
or a Mexican bean and veggie, or rice burrito with a natural salsa or a little kefir cheese topping.

Mid-afternoon: have a sparkling juice and a dried fruit candy bar; or fresh fruit or fruit juice, or a kefir drink;
or a hard boiled egg and some whole grain chips with a veggie or low fat cheese dip;
or some whole grain toast and peanut butter or other nut butter.

Dinner: have a pizza on a whole grain, chapati or egg crust, with veggies, shrimp, and low fat cheese topping;
or whole grain or egg pasta with vegetables and a light tomato/cheese sauce;
or a baked Mexican quesadilla with low fat cheese and some steamed veggies or a salad;
or some roast turkey with cornbread dressing and a salad; or a tuna casserole with rice, peas and waterchestnuts.
Before bed: a glass of apple juice or a little soy milk or flavored kefir.

Note: See COOKING FOR HEALTHY HEALING, by Linda Rector Page, for a complete optimal Children's Diet for Childhood Disease Control, and for a Healthy Vegan Diet For Infants & Toddlers.

Here are some tips for optimizing your child's nutritional health for the long term:
If your child needs more nutrition than she/he is receiving from diet, daily supplements might include:
• Acidophilus, in liquid or powder - give in juice 2 to 3x daily for good digestion and assimilation. Nature's Path FLORA-LYTE, Natren LIFE START, Solaray BABY LIFE, or DR. DOPHILUS are excellent for children.

• Vitamin C, or Ester C in chewable or powder form with bioflavonoids; give in juice, $^1/_4$ teasp. at a time 2x daily. If chewable wafers are chosen, use 100mg, 250mg, or 500mg potency according to age and weight of the child.

• A sugar-free multi-vitamin and mineral supplement daily, in either liquid or chewable tablet form. Some good choices are from Floradix, Prevail, Solaray and Mezotrace.

Note: Exercise is the key to health, growth and body oxygen. Don't let your kid be a couch potato, or a computer junkie. Encourage outdoor sports and activity every day possible, and make sure she/he is taking P. E. classes in school. Exercise is one of the best "nutrients" for both body and mind of kids.

About Herbal Remedies For Healing Children

A child's body responds very well to herbal medicines. Children are naturally born with a well-developed immune system, and this resistance ability is a key factor in understanding childhood diseases. They often only require the subtle, body strengthening forces that herbs or homeopathic medicines supply. Highly focused allopathic medications can have drastic side effects on a small body. We have found that children drink herbal teas, take herbal drops, syrups and homeopathic medicines much more readily than you might think. The remedies and methods listed in this section are building, strengthening and non-traumatic to a child's system.

Most herbal remedies can be taken as needed, then reduced and discontinued as the problem improves. Herbal effects can be quite specific; take the best formula for your particular need at the right time - rather than all the time - for optimum results. In addition, rotating and alternating herbal combinations according to the changing health state of the child allows the body to remain most responsive to herbal effects. Reduce dosage as the problem improves - allowing the body to pick up its own work and bring its own vital forces into action.

Use only one or two herbal combinations at the same time when working with a child's system. Choose the herbal remedy that addresses the worst problem first, reducing dosage and alternating on and off weeks as necessary to allow the body to thoroughly use the herbal properties. One of the bonuses of a natural healing program is the frequent discovery that other conditions were really complications of the first problem, and often take care of themselves as the body comes into balance.

Let herbs gently rebuild health. Even when a good healing program is working, and obvious improvement is being made, adding more of the remedy in an effort to speed healing can aggravate symptoms and bring about worse results!

Herbal remedy effectiveness usually goes by body weight. Base dose decisions on weight for both adults and children. Child dosage is as follows:
$^1/_2$ dose for children 10 - 14 years
$^1/_3$ dose for children 6 - 10 years
$^1/_4$ dose for children 2 - 6 years
$^1/_8$ dose for infants and babies

SPECIAL NOTES:

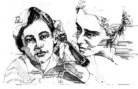

- Do not use honey in teas for children less than one year old. Honey has been linked with infant botulism, which can be life threatening.

- Do not use aspirin for a child's viral infection. Aspirin given during a viral infection is linked to the development of Reye's syndrome, a dangerous liver disease in children. Aspirin is also known as a common cause of childhood allertgies.

- Antibiotic drugs can be tough on a small child's system, especially over a long period of time. Question your doctor if an antibiotic prescription seems automatic, particularly if your child has a viral infection.

Here are some specific traditional remedies for children's problems.
Conditions not listed below have their own specific page in the "AILMENTS" section of this book.

- **ALLERGIES** - (see how to determine specific allergies in the DIAGNOSTICS section of this book, page 445.) General dietary and healing guidelines include:

&Common allergen foods include dairy, wheat, eggs, chocolate, nuts, seafood and citrus fruits. Try eliminating one at a time for a few weeks and watch to see if there is improvement. Eliminate dairy foods and cooked fats and oils because they thicken mucous and stimulate an increase in mucous production.

&Give lots of water to thin secretions and ease expectoration. Use Crystal Star ALLR-HST™ tea as needed, or a fenugreek/thyme/nettles tea, to help restore breathing capacity and dry out sinuses. Use Crystal Star ADRN™ extract in water, to support adrenal function. Use an herbal combination of echinacea, goldenseal and garlic 2 to 3 times daily, for 5 to 7 days to boost immunity and clear the lymph system. Essential fatty acids help regulate the inflammatory response. Use flaxseed oil for children, and mix into foods like salad dressing or in place of butter.

&Supplements for childhood allergies might include: (be sure to give in childhood amounts.)
- Beta-carotene to help heal irritated mucous membranes. One dose per day during allergy season.
- Vitamin C with bioflavonoids acts as an anti-inflammatory. One dose, 3x daily for two weeks.
- Calcium/magnesium for overreactive nerves. Use a ratio of 250mg calcium to 125mg magnesium.

- **ASTHMA** - Use flax oil to help regulate inflammatory response (see allergies) and Crystal Star ASTH-AID™ tea for bronchodilating effect. Use lobelia tea as a mild muscle relaxant. Use a B-vitamin complex with extra pantothenic acid or 1 TB. bee pollen granules, or Crystal Star ADRN™ extract in water daily for adrenal support. Use milk thistle extract in water daily as a liver-cleansing bile stimulant. B_{12} deficiency is linked to some types of childhood asthma - check with a nutritionally oriented physician and consider adding sea vegetables to the child's diet. Astragalus extract in water helps strengthen the lungs; use for 2 weeks of each month for six months after an asthma attack (do not use during a fever or infection). (See ASTHMA in the AILMENTS section of this book for extended information.)

- **BITES & STINGS** - for common bites from mosquitoes, fleas, gnats, etc. Seek immediate medical attention for poisonous bites from black widow spiders, brown recluse spiders or other serious bites. Apply B & T *SSSTING STOP* CREAM for pain and itch. (May also be used as a repellent). Use TEA TREE OIL on the bite, and give vitamin C 100-500mg. chewables every 4-5 hours to neutralize poison. A CAL-LYTE combination from Nature's Path helps relieve pain and calm nerves. Crystal Star GINSENG SKIN CARE GEL™ is helpful as an anti-inflammatory. Use vitamin B_1 as a natural insect repellent, 100mg 2x daily.

- **BRONCHITIS** - go on a mucous cleansing liquid diet to reduce congestion. Refer to Diet Help For Childhood Diseases - a Short Liquid Elimination Fast in this section. See the general chapter on DETOXIFICATION for recipes for effective juices and broths. After the liquid diet, give your child only fresh foods for a day; then follow the Optimal Whole Foods Diet for Children. Avoid dairy products, sweets and fried foods which continue mucous formation.

&Supplements for childhood allergies might include: (be sure to give in childhood amounts.)
- Vitamin C with bioflavonoids for anti-inflammatory properties; beta-carotene to aid mucous membranes.
- Zinc to boost the immune system (ZINC SOURCE™ drops from Crystal Star are especially effective.)
- Herbal remedies include thyme, mullein or plantain tea every 3 or 4 hours. Chamomile/honey tea helps curb bronchial inflammation.
- Crystal Star BRNX™ extract encourages respiratory tract drainage and stimulates immune response.
- Prevail CHILDREN'S DEFENSE FORMULA, and B & T *Cough & Bronchial Syrup* are also useful.

- **BRUISES** - use a cold compress (ice inside a towel) immediately. Leave ice on for 5 to 10 minutes - then off for 15 minutes. Repeat cycle 3 to 5 times to reduce swelling. Use vitamin C with bioflavonoids to help restore integrity of blood vessel walls. Homeopathic Arnica 30x or 9c eases pain and prevents bruise from becoming larger.

- **BURNS (minor)** - if your child receives a serious burn, seek medical assistance. Minor burns can be helped by applying TEA TREE OIL or Crystal Star ANTI-BIO GEL™ which promote healing of burns. Vitamin C and bioflavonoids, beta-carotene, zinc (be careful not to exceed the recommended dosage with zinc), and B Complex 25 to 50mg. with extra niacin 100mg to support healing.

- **CHEST CONGESTION** - see BRONCHITIS on preceding page for diet recommendations. Herbal steam inhalations with eucalyptus oil, tea tree oil, or Crystal Star RESPR™ TEA help keep lungs mucous free and improve oxygen uptake. Hydrotherapy baths with calendula flowers or strong comfrey tea infusions will induce cleansing perspiration and neutralize body acids. Peppermint and raspberry tea are effective liquids. Apply a soothing chest rub with TIGER BALM, WHITE FLOWER or calendula oil to loosen congestion after a bath.

- **COLDS** - refer to the general COLDS chapter for tailoring the child's diet for healing (a liquid diet during the acute stage, with green drinks etc.), Use Crystal star BIOFLAVONOID FIBER & C SUPPORT™ drink for nasal congestion during the day, and 2 TBS. each lemon juice and honey with 1 teasp. fresh grated ginger at night, for anti-inflammatory properties, Crystal Star ZINC SOURCE™ DROPS boost immune response, COLD SEASON DEFENSE™ caps help shorten and soften symptoms, and FIRST-AID TEA FOR KIDS™ helps normalize a child's body.

- **COLIC** - if you are nursing, watch your diet carefully. Sometimes mother's milk is acid from stress or diet. Avoid cabbage, brussel sprouts, onions, garlic, yeast breads, fried and fast foods. Refrain from red meat, alcohol, refined sugar and caffeine until the child's digestion improves. Use goat's milk instead of cow's milk, if possible. To promote healthy bacteria in the gastrointestinal tract, Solaray BABYLIFE for infants, Hyland's *COLIC* tabs, or Natren LIFE START $1/_4$ teasp. in water or juice 2-3x daily. Give a dilute B Complex liquid in water once a week. Give papaya or apple juice, or small doses of papaya enzymes. Give the baby an morning sunbath for vitamin D. Give a catnip enema once a week, or as needed for gas release. Never give honey to babies less than 1 year old. Effective teas include chamomile and lemon balm.

- **CONSTIPATION** - increase the amount of fiber and fluid in the child's diet, with more fresh vegetable salads, fresh fruits, spring water, herbal teas, juices and soups. Soak raisins in senna tea and feed to young children for almost instant relief; use Crystal Star FIBER & HERBS CLEANSE™ for older children. Give weak licorice or mullein tea and molasses in water, 2 times daily. A gentle catnip enema will effectively clear the colon of impacted waste.

- **CRADLE CAP** - if you are nursing, avoid eating refined sugar which supports bacteria and yeast. Use FLORA-LYTE by Nature's Path, or BABYLIFE by Solaray for infants to foster healthy flora. Massage in vitamin E or jojoba oil for 5 minutes. Leave on 30 minutes, then brush scalp with soft baby brush and shampoo with TEA TREE or aloe vera shampoo. Repeat twice weekly. Use a comfrey root tea. Apply to infant's scalp or dry skin area, and let air dry. Symptoms usually disappear within 10 days. Cradle cap may be a biotin deficiency. Take biotin -1000mcg while nursing; the baby will receive the necessary amount through breast milk.

- **CUTS** - apply TEA TREE OIL or Crystal Star ANTI-BIO GEL™ as an antiseptic healing agent. Use a calendula ointment, or AloeLife ALOE SKIN GEL or B & T *CALIFLORA* GEL every 2 or 3 hours. Use Crystal Star GINSENG SKIN REPAIR™ GEL, then apply vitamin E oil at bedtime. Apply B & T *ARNIFLORA* GEL for swelling.

- **DIAPER & SKIN RASH** - give plenty of water to help dilute urine acids. Mix comfrey, golden seal and arrowroot powders with aloe vera gel and apply. Or use calendula ointment, liquid lecithin, or a vitamin A, D & E oil. Expose the child's bottom to morning sunlight for 20 minutes for vitamin D nutrients. Wash diapers in water with 1 teasp. of tea tree oil. Try Mother Love GREEN SALVE. Avoid petroleum jelly. Use talc-free powders from the health food store.

- **DIARRHEA** - to prevent dehydration give frequent small sips of water. Offer broths, diluted apple juice and herbal teas. To give intestines a chance to settle and heal avoid dairy products during diarrhea and for two weeks. Use foods that are easily digested such as pureed brown rice (B vitamins), bananas, dry cereal, crackers, toast, and cooked vegetables and grains.

Give a supplement to help restore healthy flora. like Nature's Path bFLORA-LYTE, BABYLIFE by Solaray or ACI-DOPHILUS PLUS by NEC. Give carob powder in apple juice every 3 hours; offer apples every day. Give slippery elm tea in a little juice, or peppermint tea twice daily. Feed plenty of brown rice and yogurt for B complex vitamins and friendly intestinal flora. Red raspberry, chamomile, thyme teas, and Crystal Star FIRST AID TEA FOR KIDS™ are also helpful.

• **EARACHE** - offer plenty of liquids (water, soups, herbal teas and diluted fruit juices). Avoid dairy foods which thicken and increase mucous, making it difficult for the ear to drain. Use mullein essence, or Mother Love Mullein Flower EAR OIL, or garlic oil (antibacterial) ear drops directly in the ear. Or mix vegetable glycerin and witch hazel, dip in cotton balls and insert in the ear to draw out infection. Give lobelia extract drops in water or juice for pain. Use an echinacea and goldenseal combination for clearing the infection. See also EAR INFECTIONS, page 291.

• **FEVER** - a child's moderate fever is usually a body cleansing and healing process - a result of the problem, a part of the cure. (See a doctor if fever is high.) The diet should be liquids only - diluted fruit or vegetable juices, herb teas, such as peppermint and raspberry, water and broth for at least 24 hours until fever breaks. Catnip tea and catnip enemas can help moderate a fever. Hyland's homeopathic remedies for fever, *ACONITUM NAPELLUS* and *BRYONIA ALBA* are effective for kids. Use echinacea and goldenseal for immune-boosting effects. See FEVER page 301 for more information.

• **FLU & INFLUENZA** - during the acute stage give only liquid nutrients - fresh vegetable juices and green drinks, hot broths and steamy chicken soup to stimulate mucous release. Refer to Diet Help For Childhood Diseases - a Short Liquid Elimination Fast. Also see recipes for juices, broths, tonics, etc. in the general chapter on DETOXIFICATION for recipes. During the recuperation stage: follow a vegetarian, light "green" diet, such as the Raw Foods Purification Diet For Children's Diseases in this chapter. Anti-viral herbal remedies include: garlic, echinacea, yarrow, St John's wort, osha root, bee propolis and una de gato. Use Crystal Star ANTI-VI™ for anti-viral properties, ZINC SOURCE™ extract for immune boosting zinc, and ANTI-BIO™ and vitamin C with bioflavonoids to help overcome inflammation. Colloidal Silver has proven toxic to many viruses as well as bacteria, fungi and parasites.

• **GAS & FLATULENCE** - unhealthy food choices, poor food combinations, eating too fast and not chewing food well are the main reasons for gas in kids. Improve digestion to stop it. See the FOOD COMBINING CHART on page 452 and the Optimal Children's Diet in this section. A plant based digestive enzyme, such as Prevail VITASE or Dr. Green's POWER-PLUS Food Enzymes by Herbal Products & Development, can be helpful. Use FLORA-LYTE by Nature's Path, BABYLIFE by Solaray or Natren LIFE START to restore beneficial bacteria. Soak anise dill or carraway seed, or chamomile in water or juice and strain off. Give 1 to 2 TBS. of liquid every 4 hours until digestion rebalances.

• **HEADACHES** - calcium and magnesium can help calm muscles and relax blood vessels - Use CAL-LYTE from Nature's Path. Crystal Star ASPIR-SOURCE™ is effective against pain in the frontal and facial areas. It is especially good for children's head pains, such as toothache, earaches, sore throats, etc. Take two at a time for children. Feverfew and a VALERIAN/WILD LETTUCE extract may also be helpful.

• **INDIGESTION** - give chamomile, fennel or catnip tea, or a little ground ginger and cinnamon in water. Use soy milk or goat's milk instead of cow's milk for digestibility. Give a teaspoon of acidophilus liquid before meals to build healthy flora. Also see above, Gas & Flatulence.

• **JAUNDICE** - since this is mainly an infant condition, give a tiny amount of low-dose vitamin E oil on the tip of your finger, or a diluted lemon water with maple syrup.

• **MUMPS** - the salivary and parotid glands are involved and cause pain when chewing or swallowing. So during acute stage give only liquid nutrients - fresh fruit juices, except citrus or acidic foods, fresh vegetable juices, green drinks, hot broths, chicken or vegetable soups. A good tea to alleviate pain in swallowing: heat 1 qt. apple juice with 8-10 cloves. Strain and cool. Anti-viral herbs include: garlic, echinacea, yarrow, St John's wort and osha root. Use Crystal Star ANTI-VI™ for anti-viral properties; give Crystal Star ANTI-BIO™ extract in water or Burdock tea every few hours to clear the lymph glands, and to help overcome the infection and inflammation. Make sure the child gets plenty of rest and sleep.
  ☙Supplements for childhood mumps might include: (*be sure to give in childhood amounts.*)
    - Extra vitamin C with bioflavonoids acts as an anti-inflammatory. One dose, 3x daily for two weeks.
    - COLLOIDAL SILVER can help fight the mumps virus.

- **PARASITES & WORMS** - Eliminate refined sugar and carbohydrates from the diet. (See the Optimal Whole Foods Diet for Children in this chapter.) High fiber foods such as grains, raw vegetables, and especially greens aid in treatment and help with prevention. Use a probiotics supplement like FLORA-LYTE by Nature's Path, or BABYLIFE by Solaray. Give raisins soaked in senna tea to cleanse the intestines or use Crystal Star FIBER & HERB CLEANSE™ capsules in child dosage. Garlic is a natural antiparasitic; use a garlic enema 2 to 3x a week. Give chlorophyll liquid, wormwood tea or herbal pumpkin oil tablets (by Hain). Colloidal Silver may also be effective. See the PARASITES page in this book for more information.

For **HEAD LICE** - tea tree oil is effective. Use 25 drops in 1 pint of water. Rub the mixture into your child's head 3 times daily; rinse hair after third application. Goldenseal tincture or strong goldenseal tea can be added as an additional rinse. Comb hair with a fine-toothed comb to remove lice and eggs. Garlic helps fight head lice infestation.

- **RINGWORM** - tea tree oil is a strong botanical antifungal effective against ringworm. Use undiluted on affected area. Continue applications until rash goes away. Use Crystal Star FUNGEX GEL™ or BLACK WALNUT extract on affected area. Use the homeopathic remedy Sulphur 30x or 9c, three times daily, for three days. (Use at least one hour before or after using tea tree oil because the oil may cancel the effectiveness of the homeopathic remedy). Boost immune strength with an echinacea, goldenseal, and burdock root combination three times a day for ten days.

- **SINUS PROBLEMS** - Refer to Diet Help For Childhood Diseases - a Short Liquid Elimination Fast. Also see recipes for juices, broths, tonics, etc. in the general DETOXIFICATION chapter. A short three day cleansing liquid diet will help clear mucous congestion. Use Crystal Star ANTI-BIO™ drops or goldenseal liquid drops to overcome infection and inflammation, and FIRST AID CAPS™ for vitamin C and anti-oxidant activity 2-3 times daily each for a week. Use Crystal Star X-PEC-TEA™ to release mucous buildup in the head and chest.

- **SORE THROAT** - Use Crystal Star ZINC SOURCE™ drops or give Crystal Star COFEX™ TEA as a throat coat at night for almost immediate relief. Give echinacea and goldenseal, or Crystal Star ANTI-VI™ or ANTI-BIO™ to overcome infection. Give pineapple juice 2-3x daily for natural enzyme therapy. Mild zinc lozenges and licorice sticks or tea are effective. Give Vitamin C with bioflavonoids to help ease inflammation in the throat and to fight infection.

- **SLEEPLESSNESS** - avoid stimulant foods like refined sugars, chocolate, and foods containing caffeine. Use CAL-LYTE™ from Nature's Path for the calming effects of calcium and magnesium. Use homeopathic CALMS FORTE by Hylands. Give Crystal Star RELAX CAPS™ or GOOD NIGHT™ tea, or WILD LETTUCE/VALERIAN extract. Passion flower, skullcap and chamomile teas are effective.

- **TEETHING** - Rub gums with honey, a little peppermint oil, or a few drops of lobelia tincture. Give weak catnip, fennel or peppermint tea to soothe. Add a few daily drops of A, D & E oil to food. Licorice root powder (2 pinches) made into a paste can help soothe inflamed gums. Use *KIDS TLC* by B & T for teething. (See TEETHING page in this book for more information.)

- **THRUSH FUNGAL INFECTION** - Give probiotics, like Nature's Path FLORA-LYTE or Natren LIFESTART, by mouth, and use as a rectal suppository, and vitamin C 100mg. or Ester C chewable. Thrush may be caused by widespread antibiotic use. Give garlic extract drops in water, squirt a pricked garlic oil cap in the mouth or give KYOLIC by Wakunaga. Colloidal silver is also effective.

- **WHOOPING COUGH** - Give Crystal Star ANTI-SPZ™ and ANTI-BIO™ capsules, ZINC SOURCE™ drops and VALERIAN/WILD LETTUCE extract. Use B & T *COUGH & BRONCHIAL syrup* or thyme extract in water. Give Vitamin C with bioflavonoids $1/4$ tsp. every hour until stool turns soupy, as an ascorbic acid flush. Give marshmallow root, slippery elm bark, or osha root tea to soothe the throat and respiratory tract, or lobelia extract. Apply hot ginger/garlic compresses to the chest, and use a eucalyptus steam at night. Give a liquid diet during acute stage with plenty of juices, broths and pure water.

- **WEAK SYSTEM** - Build strength with a good diet. See the Optimal Whole Foods Diet For Children in this chapter. Give a broth of Crystal Star SYSTEMS STRENGTH™ drink daily. Add a mineral supplement like Nature's Path TRACE-LYTE. Add 1 teasp. nutritional yeast for B vitamins and protein, and to assure increased absorption of protein. Hyland's BIOPLASMA is a good general homeopathic remedy. Give an apple or carrot juice daily. Include a daily chewable vitamin C wafer as a preventive against disease exposure.

A BRIEF MEDICINE CHEST LIST FOR KIDS:

❧TEA TREE OIL - For infections that need antiseptic or antifungal activity - including mouth, teeth, gums, throat, ringworm, fungus, etc. Effective on stings, bites, burns, sunburns, cuts, and scrapes.

❧RESCUE REMEDY - For respiratory problems, coughing, gas, stomach ache, constipation and digestive upset. A rebalancing calmative for emotional stress and anxiety.

❧KIDS KIT from Hylands Homeopathic - A first aid kit with gentle, all-purpose remedies.

❧FIRST AID TEA FOR KIDS™ - Crystal Star's gentle, all-purpose tea that addresses many childhood problems. A cleansing, detoxifying, body-balancing blend that may be taken as needed for infant jaundice and teething pain; for a fever in hot water to induce a cleansing sweat; for stomach aches, diarrhea and a generally over-acid condition, when the child is whine-y and sickly.

❧To help prevent contagious disease after exposure, give 1 cayenne capsule 3x a day, 2 chewable vitamin C 500mg. wafers 3x a day, and a cup of roasted dandelion root tea daily - for 3 or 4 days.

TO VACCINATE OR NOT TO VACCINATE YOUR CHILD..... it depends on the vaccination - some have serious side effects for sensitive individuals, like the flu vaccination; some can wear off and allow a more serious disease to develop as an adult, like the chicken pox vaccination (a childhood case of chicken pox confers lifetime immunity). My own sense is that most vaccines as they exist today, unnaturally stimulate and imbalance the immune system, eventually allowing many more immunological disorders, such as M.S., lupus, chronic fatigue syndrome, and Candida and Herpes infections.

When Should You Call A Doctor?

Herbal and nutritional remedies are wonderful for most common childhood health problems, but sometimes your child may need strong medicine. Here are the signs that tell you to call a doctor:

•If your child has a chronic stuffy nose and thick discharge that doesn't go away.

•If a fever persists longer than 3 days or returns after 3 days, or is unusually high.

•If a cold doesn't clear up and a rash or honking cough develops after 7 days of a cold.

•If your child shows respiratory distress such as rapid breathing, gasping, wheezing, pale or bluish skin color.

•If your child is recovering from chicken pox or flu virus, and goes into prolonged, heavy vomiting with a fever followed by drowsiness, fatigue and confusion, He or she may have Reyes Syndrome, a rare disease linked to aspirin reaction in children. Other symptoms include agitation, delerium, seizures, double vision, speech impairment, hearing loss and coma. Brain damage and death can result if the child does not get emergency treatment of intravenous glucose and electrolytes within 12 to 24 hours after vomiting starts.

•If your child breaks a bone, or gets a deep, blood-gushing gash.

"A baby makes love stronger ,
days shorter, nights longer,
bankroll smaller,
home happier,
clothes shabbier,
the past forgotten,
and the future worth living for.

Aging
How To Slow Down The Clock Naturally

It's happening to everybody, most of the time faster than we'd like. But even though the hourglass tells us we're older, the passage of time isn't really what ages us. It's the process that reduces the number of healthy cells in the body. Whenever the gold and silver years begin for you, it's when the fun begins, when hectic family life quiets down, financial strains and needs ease, business retirement is here or not far off, and we can do the things we've always wanted to do but never had time for - travel, art, music, a craft, gardening, writing, quiet walks, picnics, more social life...... doing what we want to do, not what we have to do. We all look forward to the treasure years of life, and picture ourselves on that tennis court, bicycle path or cruise ship, healthy and enjoying ourselves. But, there's a catch - our freedom comes in the latter half of life, and many of us don't age gracefully in today's world.

The concept of anti-aging has become popular in the 1990's. There are so many interesting things to do and see in the world..... without enough time to do them. We all want to extend our life spans with the best health possible. *Fortunately, youth is not a chronological age.* It's good health and an optimistic spirit. Human life span is at least 20 to 30 years longer than most of us actually live today. It's astonishing to realize that we are living only two-thirds of the years our bodies are capable of!

There is a paradox about aging: **Life expectancy lengthens as you age.** The average American child born in 1993 has a life expectancy of 75.4 years. But average life expectancy at 85 years is six more years. The longer you live, the longer your total expected life span becomes. **Age is not the enemy.... illness is.**

Our cells don't age; they're sloughed off as their efficiency diminishes, to be replaced by new ones. When the body is given the right nutrients, cell restoration may continue for many years past current life expectancy. Environmental pollutants, a long standing diet of chemical-laced, refined foods, vitamin and mineral deficiencies, overuse of prescription drugs and antibiotics, all prevent our seniority dreams from becoming a reality. Eighty percent of the population over 65 years old in industrialized nations is chronically ill, usually with arthritis, heart disease, diabetes or high blood pressure. A negative outlook can dampen the natural optimism of our minds and spirits, too, if we let stress rule our lives.

Human lifespan can be increased. Youthfulness can be restored from the inside, by strengthening lean body mass, metabolism, and immune response with good nutrition, regular exercise, fresh air, and a positive outlook. **A balanced life is the key to long life.** While cell life is largely genetically controlled, disease is usually the result of diet, lifestyle or environment. We can do something about these things.

Slower aging means a better memory with no senility, better skin with fewer wrinkles, a strong heart, bones and immune response, flexible joints and muscles, a good metabolic rate and a healthy sex life, (organ and endocrine activity keeps your whole body youthful).

Regular aerobic exercise, like a brisk daily walk, prolongs fitness at any age. Exercise helps maintain stamina, strength, circulation and joint mobility. Stretching out every morning limbers the body, oxygenates the tissues, and helps clear it of the previous night's waste and metabolic eliminations. Stretches at night before you retire help insure muscle relaxation and a better night's rest.

Don't worry. Be happy. Think positive to stay young. There is no question that the subtle energies of the mind effect the body. A pessimistic outlook on life depresses not only your personality, but your immune response. Science is validating the "mind/body connection" today in terms of the body's ability to heal. An optimistic, well-rounded, loving life needs friends and family. Regular contact is important for you and for them. Doing for, and giving to others at the stage of your life when there is finally enough time to do it graciously, makes a world of difference to your spirit.

Are you aging faster than you want to?

Here's a questionnaire to ask yourself in a quiet moment when you can really take a look at yourself and your life. Don't be overly harsh. We all have health and physical imperfections. But an honest look can help to identify areas where action can be taken to slow down some of aging's effects.

1. Has your skin lost elasticity? Does it seem thinner? Does it bruise easier? Do bruises last longer?
2. Do you have age spots (liver spots) on your face, neck, hands or arms?
3. Does your skin have some vitiligo (white spots with loss of pigment)?
4. Are you wrinkling in your face (more than just smile lines), and or hands?
5. Are your gums receding slightly? Are your teeth cracking or chipping?
6. Do you have tiny red capillary spots on your face, arms, chest or legs?
7. Are there recent nodular growths on your face, nose, hands or chest?
8. Is there beginning to be a tilt forward of your head and neck? (Check your mirror.)
9. Do your joints ache? Are they starting to become deformed? Is your joint mobility reduced?
10. Do you have a tendency to shuffle instead of stride while walking? Is your spine stiff?
11. Are there ridges on your fingernails? Do your nails crack easily? Are they discolored?
12. Has there been a decline in your vision? Do you have floaters in your eyes?
13. Do you suffer from macular degeneration, retinopathy, or loss of peripheral vision?
14. Are the mucous membranes in your nose, sinuses, mouth, or vagina, dry?
15. Do you have one bowel movement or less per day?
16. If you are a man, is your hairline receding or balding? If you are a woman, are you experiencing massive hair loss, or rapid hair graying?
17. Do you experience heart arrhythmia, or rapid heartbeat? Are you more and more easily fatigued?
18. Do you suffer from gradual hearing loss? Does conversation sound garbled?
19. Are your hands, feet, arms, legs, face, and ears constantly chilled?
20. Are you becoming increasingly vulnerable to injuries (sprains, strains, bruises, cuts, etc.)?
21. Is your recovery time becoming longer after a cold, flu or other infections?

Here are the lifestyle factors that affect aging the most. Start your anti-aging campaign with these.

1. Smoking, especially heavy smoking (a half pack or more per day); or living with a heavy smoker.
2. Drinking six or more drinks per week or having been a heavy drinker for more than 5 years.
3. Consuming large amounts of refined sugars, either as foods or as food additives every day.
4. Eating deep fried foods on a regular basis. Regular consumption of nitrated and/or preserved meats.
5. Currently working closely, or a history of working closely, with volatile petrochemicals.
6. Exposure to excessive amounts of sunlight without protection.

Longevity begins with a good diet.

A healthy diet rich in nutrients is the center piece of a vibrant long life. Indeed, your diet must be optimally nourishing as the years pass. A good diet improves health, provides a high level of energy, maintains harmonious system balance, keeps memory and thinking sharp, staves off disease, and contributes to a more youthful appearance. The aging process slows if you have a good internal environment.

Some dietary practices accelerate aging. Excessive eating is one of them. Nutrition quality, not quantity, is the key. The per capita calorie consumption in America is astronomically high, nearly twice that of primitive societies who live closer to Nature's provisions. Research documents that moderate food intake helps retard the aging process, and may extend lifespan as much as ten years. Consciously undereat as you age. You need fewer calories for good body function. Optimum body weight should be some 10 to 15 pounds less than in the 20's and 30's.

Your skin is a barometer of how rapidly you are aging. Americans often marvel at how elderly people from non-Western societies have such beautiful, youthful skin. The diet of these individuals is relatively free of the additives and preservers so prevalent in the American diet. Toxic food substances like refined or hydrogenated oils, refined sugars, inorganic iron, nitrates, synthetic additives, and excess caffeine and tobacco are aging factors.

HERE ARE THE BEST FOODS FOR ANTI-AGING. INCLUDE THEM IN YOUR DIET REGULARLY.

🐚 **Fresh fruits and vegetables!** Fresh produce gives you the most vitamins, minerals, fiber and enzymes. Plants have the widest array of nutrients and are the easiest for the body to use. Enzyme-rich fruits and vegetables are an essential link in our stamina and energy levels. **Eat organically grown foods when possible** to insure higher nutrient content and avoid toxic sprays. **Have a green salad every day!**

🐚 **Fresh fruit and vegetable juices.** Juices offer quick absorption of high-quality nutrients, especially antioxidants, which protect the body against aging, heart disease, cancer, and degenerative conditions. Juices provide increased energy levels and nutrition in the most easily digestible form.

🐚 **Sea vegetables.** Sea vegetables have superior nutritional content. They transmit the energies of the ocean as a rich source of proteins, complex carbohydrates, vitamins, minerals, trace minerals, chlorophyll, enzymes and fiber. In fact, sea vegetables contain all the necessary elements for life, many of which are depleted in the earth's soil. Sea plants convert inorganic ocean minerals into organic mineral salts that combine with amino acids. Our bodies use this combination as an ideal way to get usable nutrients for body structure building blocks. Sea plants are almost the only non-animal source of vitamin B_{12} for cell growth and nerve function. In this era of processed foods and iodine-poor soils, sea vegetables and sea foods stand almost alone as potent sources of natural iodine. Sea vegetables are delicious. Some are salty, like kelp and bladderwrack; some are sweet, like wakame, kombu and sea palm; some are tangy like nori, arame and hijiki. They may be crushed or snipped into soups and sauces, used as toppings on salads or casseroles. If you add sea vegetables, no other salt is needed, an advantage for a low salt diet.

🐚 **Whole grains, nuts, seeds and beans** are good sources of protein and essential fatty acids. They are building, warming and high in fiber and minerals for good assimilation. Sprouted seeds, grains, and legumes are some of the healthiest foods you can eat. They are living nutrients that can go directly to your cells. Include some of these foods every day to assure regular passing of toxic body wastes and a free-flowing system.

Soaked and roasted flax, sesame, sunflower, pumpkin, almonds, and chia are our favorite nuts and seeds. A flour blend of amaranth, buckwheat, whole wheat, rye, oats and rice makes a nutty, healthy flour. Legumes (beans) should be part of a healthy diet, because they supply nourishing, low fat calories and protein, but they get harder to digest as you age. Soak and then cook them well, and combine them in a meal with grains to form a "complete protein."

🐚 **Eat cultured foods for friendly digestive flora.** Yogurt tops the list, but there are a host of other healthy "cultures"....kefir and kefir cheese, miso, tamari, tofu, tempeh, even a glass of wine at the evening meal to promote better nutrient assimilation in the digestive system. Raw sauerkraut, rich in lactobacillus acidophilus, is especially good for boosting friendly bacteria. (Make sure the kind you buy isn't processed with alum.)

🐚 **Have fish and fresh seafoods two to three times a week,** to enhance thyroid and metabolic balance.

🐚 **Drink plenty of pure water every day to keep your body hydrated and clean.** Take gentle herbal tonics and green drinks often to keep the system clear and immunity strong.

🐚 **Keep your system alkaline** with green drinks, green foods, miso, and grains like rice.

🐚 **Lower fats and oils** to about 2 to 3 tablespoons a day - from unsaturated vegetable sources.

🐚 **Eat poultry, other meats, butter, eggs, and dairy in moderation.** Avoid fried foods, excess caffeine, red meats, highly seasoned foods, refined and chemically processed foods altogether.

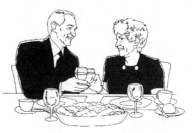

Plant Enzymes Are The Key To Anti-Aging

Enzymes are the cornerstone of anti-aging, because they support strong immune system health and provide the active food antioxidants which fight free-radicals. Replenishing our enzymes helps us maintain health, implement healing, and build bodies which resist disease and premature aging. In fact, Dr. Edward Howell, a founder of enzyme therapy said that "the very length of life is tied to the increased use of food enzymes because they decrease the rate of body enzyme exhaustion."

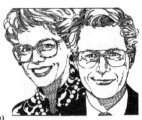

Enzymes operate on both chemical and biological levels. They are the single most important factor that powers our bodies, the workhorses that drive metabolism which puts to use the nutrients we take in. The biological level has been called life energy or vital force, because without the life energy of enzymes we would be a pile of lifeless chemical substances.

Enzyme depletion and aging go hand in hand. Each of us is born with a battery charge of body enzyme energy at birth. The faster you use up this enzyme supply - the shorter your life. Enzymes are used up in normal metabolism and in healing from illness. But enzymes are wasted haphazardly throughout life by the use of alcohol, drugs, chemical-laced food, overcooked food which has no enzymes, and harmful environmental chemicals. As we get older our internal enzymes become depleted. Unless we do something to stop the one-way-flow out of the body of enzyme energy, our digestive and eliminative capacities weaken, obesity, and chronic illness set in and lifespan shortens.

Nature intended us to eat a largely plant-based diet, rich in fresh foods. The refining of food and fast-heat cooking methods have rendered the modern diet enzyme-deficient. Because enzymes are so heat-sensitive, they are the first to be destroyed during cooking, pasteurization, canning, microwaving, fast food processing, or heating above 118 degrees Fahrenheit. Enzyme rich foods, like fresh fruits and vegetables and whole grains, bring into our bodies not only enzymes but the full array of all plant nutrients. Enzyme rich foods assure us the main components of anti-aging - adequate amounts of antioxidants to fight free radicals, and nutrients to keep our immune systems strong.

Eating food devoid of enzymes means the pancreas and the liver have to use their enzyme stores. As a result, reserve enzymes for metabolic processes are pulled from their normal work, to digest food. But even this substitute measure does not make up for the missing enzymes that should be in our food, because without food enzymes the body can't break the food down correctly to deliver nutrients to the blood. So we end up with undigested food in the blood. White blood cell immune defenses are pulled from their jobs to take care of all the undigested food, so the immune system takes a dive.

Eating enzyme rich foods or taking plant-based enzyme supplements takes care of this unhealthy cascade of reactions before it ever starts. Any enzymes left over after the digestion process go on to be used by the body as metabolic enzymes, which run our bodies and contribute to healing.

I believe that your optimal choice for enzymes is from a good diet. It is not necessary to always eat raw, live foods. But it is important to have a large percentage of the overall diet be enzyme rich. If you don't feel you get enough fresh foods, or you need extra enzyme concentration for healing through enzyme therapy, plant based, food enzyme supplements are the next best choice.

See ENZYMES & ENZYME THERAPY, page 30 for more information.

"I didn't come to be told I'm burning the candle at both ends," said a patient to his doctor.
"I came for more wax."

Herbs Can Help Slow The Effects Of Aging

Since ancient times, people have searched for the Fountain of Youth. The answer may have been available all along in the youth-extending nutrients of herbs and superfoods.

Herbs have wide ranging properties, and far reaching possibilities as health restoratives. They can help with almost every aspect of human need as we age, Herbs assist the body in normalizing its functions and adapting to stress. Herbs have antioxidant properties which prevent body components from destruction by free radicals. Herbal superfoods have potent, whole essence nutritional content that can address both the symptoms and causes of a problem. Herbs are full of food-source vitamins, minerals, phytochemicals, and powerful enzymes that make them easy to digest and absorb. Certain herbs are specifics for better memory, strong gland and metabolic activity, smoother skin, stamina, endurance, and good organ and muscle tone.

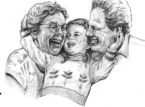

The two main causes of aging are **1) cell and tissue damage** caused by free radicals that aren't neutralized when the body lacks antioxidants; **2) reduced immune response** that puts the body at risk for disease-causing stress and environmental toxic reactions.

Herbal therapy is a premier agent for both of these aging actions.
- Anti-oxidant herbs quench and neutralize free radicals, energize and tone.
- Adaptogen herbs strengthen immunity, and equip the body to handle stress.

Free radicals play a key role in the deterioration of the body. They are highly active compounds produced when fat molecules react with oxygen. Although they're involved in normal metabolic breakdown, our bodies experience excesses of these cell damagers from air pollutants, tobacco smoke, rancid foods and hydro-carbons. After years of free radical assaults, cells become irreplaceably lost from major organs, like the lungs, liver, kidneys, and brain. When the cells of the nervous system are attacked, for instance, senile dementia or Alzheimer's disease results. Cell damage to connective tissue results in loss of skin tone and elasticity, and degenerative aging affects, like atherosclerosis and arthritis.

Lowering the fat in your diet is the single most beneficial step you can take to reduce free radical damage. A high fat diet depresses the body's antioxidant enzyme response to free radical attacks.

HERE ARE SOME POTENT HERBAL ANTIOXIDANTS TO REDUCE AND NEUTRALIZE FREE RADICALS:
- **Pine bark, and grapeseed** contain powerful **proanthocyanidins (OPCs or PCOs)**, concentrated, highly active bioflavonoids. Fifty times stronger than vitamin E, 20 times stronger than vitamin C, they are one of the few dietary antioxidants that readily crosses the blood-brain barrier to protect brain cells and aid memory. PCOs help protect against cancer, heart disease, are good anti-inflammatories and strengthen capillaries.
- **Ginkgo biloba** is used worldwide to combat the effects of aging. It protects the cells against damage from free radicals, reduces blood cell clumping which leads to congestive heart disease, improves memory and brain activity, restores blood circulation, helps improve hearing and vision functions and fights allergic reactions. It is currently being tested for its affects in strengthening memory function against Alzheimer's disease.

Ginkgo is a biological super tree! The species has survived almost unchanged for over 150 million years and is so hardy that a solitary ginkgo was the only tree to survive the atomic blast in Hiroshima! This tree is still alive today, standing near the epicenter of the blast, a testament to ginkgo's remarkable ability to survive.
- **Shiitake mushrooms** support stronger immune response. They promote vitality and longevity, and are especially valuable as a treatment for systemic conditions related to aging and sexual dysfunction. In Oriental medicine, shiitake are used to prevent high blood pressure and heart disease, and to reduce cholesterol.
- **Reishi mushrooms,** *ganoderma*, are tonic herbs that increase vitality and enhance immunity. They also lower cholesterol and high blood pressure, combat bacteria and viruses, and may help prevent cancer and aid in the treatment of chronic fatigue syndrome, ulcers, and heart disease.
- **Astragalus** is a strong immune enhancer, adrenal stimulant and body tonic, with vasodilating properties that lower blood pressure, increase metabolism and improve circulation. I have found it to be a specific in liver dysfunction and respiratory problems that involve allergies.
- **Alfalfa** is rich in chlorophyll, which helps to heal damaged tissue and promotes the growth of new tissue. It is one of the oldest fatigue remedies known and in general builds up the body, restoring health and vitality.

- **GLA, Gamma Linoleic Acid**, obtained from evening primrose oil, black currant oil and borage seed oil, is a source of cell energy, electrical insulation for nerves, and precursor of prostaglandins which regulate hormone and metabolic functions.
- **Ashwagandha** has significant antimicrobial properties, strengthening the immune system and countering infections. The immune stimulating properties contribute to anti-cancer and anti-tumor activity. It is an energy builder and rejuvenating herb, providing stable vigor and vitality. Ashwagandha is regarded as an ideal energy tonic for vegetarians, providing stamina that people often associate with meat.
- **Echinacea** activates the immune system with both anti-bacterial and anti-viral properties. It is one of the most effective herbal prescriptions for the prevention and treatment of colds and flu infections that I know.
- **Hawthorn** is bioflavonoid-rich, and adept at conteracting the damaging effects of free radicals on the cardiovascular system. Hawthorn helps make the heart a more efficient pump, increasing output of blood from the heart and decreasing resistance from the blood vessels.
- **Licorice** has immune-enhancing properties that increase the overall number of lymphocytes, and the activity of killer T-cells. It is antiviral and antibacterial, with powerful antioxidant properties. New testing indicates it may even have cancer-inhibiting properties
- **Wheat germ oil** - one tablespoon provides the antioxidant equivalent of an oxygen tent for 30 minutes.

HERBAL ADAPTOGENS ARE SUBSTANCES WITH TONIC, ANTI-STRESS ACTIONS. THEY INCREASE RESISTANCE TO ADVERSE INFLUENCES BY HELPING THE BODY ADAPT OR NORMALIZE. HERBS LIKE ASTRAGALUS, REISHI MUSHROOMS AND ASHWAGANDHA ALREADY MENTIONED IN THE ANTIOXIDANT SECTION ARE ALSO ADAPTOGENS.

Here are some effective herbal adaptogens:

- **Panax Ginseng**, (red, white and American ginsengs) are the most effective of all adaptogen herbs. Beneficial to total health, stimulating both long and short term energy, ginseng has measurable amounts of germanium, provides energy to all body systems, promotes regeneration from stress and fatigue, and rebuilds foundation strength. A central nervous system stimulant that also enhances improved sleep, ginseng is nourishing to reproductive and circulatory systems. Red ginseng is especially beneficial for men since it promotes testosterone production. White and American Ginsengs help stimulate the brain and memory centers for women as well as men. Ginseng benefits are cumulative in the body. Taking ginseng for several months to a year is far more effective than short term doses.
- **Siberian Ginseng,** (eleuthero) is a long term tonic that supports the adrenal glands, circulation and memory.
- **Schizandra** is synergistic with eleuthero for anti-stress, weight loss and sports endurance formulas. It supports sugar regulation and liver function. It helps keep aging skin healthy through better digestion of fatty foods.
- **Suma** is an ancient herb with modern results for overcoming fatigue, and hormonal imbalance. Used to rebuild the system from the ravages of cancer and diabetes.
- **Gotu Kola** is a brain and nervous system restorative. Considered an elixir of life and a longevity herb in Chinese medicine, it is a primary nerve and deep body healer after illness. Gotu kola has therapeutic applications for the skin, cellulite, wound repair, burns, helps inhibit scar formation and varicose veins.
- **Fo-Ti, (Ho-Shou-Wu)** is a flavonoid-rich herb with special success in longevity formulas. It is a cardiovascular strengthener, increasing blood flow to the heart.
- **Burdock** is a highly nutritional, hormone balancing herb - antibacterial, antifungal and antitumor. It is a strong liver purifying and hormone balancing herb, with particular value for skin, arthritic, and glandular problems. It is a specific in all blood cleansing and detoxification combinations.
- **Bilberry** is a bioflavonoid-rich herb that helps keep connective tissues healthy and strengthens small blood vessels and capillaries, factors that keep skin youthful and free of wrinkles.
- **Pau d'arco** may be taken over a long period of time to give greater vitality, build up immunity to disease, strengthen cellular structure and help eliminate pain and inflammation.
- **Cayenne** is a central system and circulation stimulant, a key to healing. When the body and organs are properly stimulated, they will heal, cleanse and begin to function normally. Cayenne also helps the digestion when taken with meals, arouses all the secreting organs and improves metabolism, a definite advantage for anti-aging.

Note: **Consider Crystal Star AGELESS VITALITY™ with extraordinary anti-aging, antioxidant, adaptogen activity.**

The Importance of Vitamins, Minerals & Superfoods As You Age

Vitamins, minerals and superfoods offer a potent source of nutrients to deal with the body-aging realities of today's environment. Mineral depleted soils mean we get less of important minerals. Strong chemical substances everywhere expose our bodies to unhealthy toxins. Many of these pollutants decrease the available oxygen we receive from the air. Fortifying our diets with supplements and superfoods strengthens our ability to function in a world which makes it tough to be healthy. Vitamins, minerals and superfoods optimize your healing potential.

Note: In addition to the information offered here about vitamins, minerals and superfoods as they relate to aging, be sure to check THE ALTERNATIVE ARSENAL chapter for broader data.

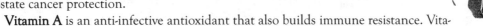

ONCE AGAIN, ANTI-OXIDANTS ARE THE KEY TO ANTI-AGING.

Here are some important anti-aging antioxidant vitamins and amino acids:

•   **CoQ10** - the body's ability to assimilate food source CoQ10 declines with age. Supplementation provides therapeutic benefits, in the areas of gum disease, and breast and prostate cancer protection.

•   **Vitamin A** is an anti-infective antioxidant that also builds immune resistance. Vitamin A strengthens the optical system, counteracting night blindness. Supplementation lowers risk of many types of cancer, particularly lung cancer. Retinoids inhibit malignant transformation, and reverse premalignant changes in tissue. It helps develop strong bone cells, and is a major factor in the health of skin, hair, teeth and gums. By improving the stability of tissue in cell walls it helps to prevent premature aging and senility.

•   **Carotenes, beta, alpha and lycopene,** are powerful anti-infectives and anti-oxidants for immune health, protection against environmental pollutants, slowing the aging process, and allergy control. New testing indicates carotenes may be a key in preventing several kinds of cancer, and in developing anti-tumor immunity.

•   **Vitamin C** is a primary antioxidant for preventing free radical damage, boosting immune strength and maintaining health. Vitamin C helps protect against viral and bacterial infections, cancer, heart disease, arthritis and allergies. It safeguards against radiation, heavy metal toxicity, environmental pollutants and early aging. It is essential to formation of new collagen tissue. It accelerates healing after surgery and increases infection resistance.

•   **Bioflavonoids** prevent arteries from hardening, enhance blood vessel, capillary and vein strength. They protect connective tissue and control bruising. They help lower cholesterol, and stimulate bile production. Bioflavonoids are anti-microbial against infections. The strongest supplementation form is quercetin.

•   **Vitamin E** is an anticoagulant and vasodilator against blood clots and heart disease. It retards cellular and mental aging, alleviates fatigue and works as an anti-aging antioxidant with selenium by neutralizing free radicals.

•   **L-Glutathione** is an antioxidant amino acid that works to neutralize radiation toxicity and inhibit free radicals. It also cleans the blood from the effects of chemotherapy, X-rays and liver toxicity.

•   **L-Cysteine** is an antioxidant amino acid that works to protect against radiation toxicity, carcinogens, and free radical damage to skin and arteries.

•   **Tyrosine** is an amino acid formed from phenylalanine, a growth hormone stimulant that helps build the body's natural store of adrenalin and thyroid hormones. It is a source of quick energy, especially for the brain.

•   **Methionine** is an antioxidant free radical de-activator and "lipotropic" that keeps fats from accumulating in the liver and arteries. Protective against chemical allergic reactions.

Here are the most important antioxidant minerals:

•   **Germanium** (organic), is a potent anti-oxidant mineral that detoxifies, blocks free radicals and increases production of natural killer cells. It is an interferon stimulus for immune strength and healing, and strong anti-viral properties. Germanium is a powerful healing agent, using the body's own immune resources to ameliorate even severe food intolerances like candida albicans. A lack of cellular oxygen (hypoxia) is one of the most common causes of cell injury and disease. The key to the many benefits of germanium is its ability to increase tissue oxygenation.

•   **Selenium** is an antioxidant trace mineral that protects the body from free radical damage and heavy metal toxicity. It is an anti-cancer agent that helps prevent fat and cholesterol accumulation in the bloodstream, and protects against heart weakness. Deficiency results in aging skin, liver damage, increased oxidation, hypothyroidism, and in severe cases, digestive/eliminative tract cancers. Most effective supplement source is selenomethionine.

•   **Zinc** is a powerful antioxidant mineral that helps limit the amount of free radicals the body naturally produces, such as superoxide and malondialdehyde (MDA). Zinc is essential for tissue repair and is important for immune system response, especially for respiratory problems and allergies.

Superfoods are becoming widely popular as anti-aging factors. Superfoods include green, and blue-green algae, like chlorella and spirulina, green grasses like barley and wheat grass, sprouts and alfalfa. Superfoods like aloe vera, royal jelly and bee pollen are extra rich sources of essential, concentrated nutrients. Even though you may be adding more salads and vegetables to your diet, uncertainty about the nutritional quality of produce that is grown on mineral depleted soils and heavily sprayed, has established a solid role for the nutrient-richness of superfoods. Superfoods contain thousands of enzymes for digestion and absorption. The small molecular proteins and high chlorophyllins in these plants can be absorbed directly into the cell membranes. We have found the incredible claims about their valuable benefits to have substance and truth.

See Green Superfoods in the HEALING FOODS & DIETS section for information about specific superfoods.

SUPERFOOD SUPPLEMENTS CONTAIN A COMBINATION OF GREEN GRASSES, ALGAES, HERBS, AND OTHER HIGH NUTRIENT SUBSTANCES. WE RECOMMEND:
- SYSTEMS STRENGTH™ by Crystal Star contains superfoods from land and sea, herbs, enzymes and amino acids. The blend is designed for extra energy and strength as well as for rebuilding a weakened, recovering system.
- ENERGY GREEN™ by Crystal Star is designed for detoxification to restore and energize body systems.
- GREEN MAGMA by Green Foods Corporation is powdered juice from young barley leaves.
- GREEN ESSENCE by Green Foods - juice from barley, vegetables, shiitake mushroom, lecithin and more.
- PRO-GREENS by NutriCology contains several green superfoods, herbs and other nutrients.
- EASY GREENS by Transitions is a high density whole food and herb concentrate.

BEE PRODUCTS SHOULD BE PART OF YOUR ANTI-AGING PICTURE:
- **Bee pollen** has been used as a food source, energy builder and health restorer since ancient times. Bee pollen is a full-spectrum blood building and rejuvenative substance. Recent research shows that pollen helps counteract the effects of aging, and increases both mental and physical capability.
- **Royal jelly,** contains every nutrient necessary to support life. It is a natural anti-biotic, stimulates the immune system, deep cellular health and longevity, and supplies key nutrients for energy, mental alertness and general well-being.

Note: See bee pollen and royal jelly in the ALTERNATIVE ARSENAL section for more information about these superfoods.

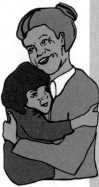

About Melatonin & DHEA

Two hormones, melatonin and DHEA, have recently become widely publicized for anti-aging.

Melatonin is an antioxidant hormone secreted cyclically by the pineal gland to keep us in sync with the rhythms of the day and the seasons. Melatonin sets our internal biological clock that governs our sleep/wake cycles or rhythms. One of the best benefits of melatonin is its ability to help with the effects of jet lag. Melatonin has become popular for other hormone effects as well.

SOME OF MELATONIN'S PROTECTIVE FUNCTIONS GIVE IT AN ANTI-AGING REPUTATION:

[1] Oxidation is one of the reasons we age; melatonin helps protect the body from free radical damage.

[2] Reduced immune function is another aging factor, as the thymus (our immune stimulating gland) shrinks, and lowers our ability to generate T-cells. Melatonin is believed to reverse shrinkage of the thymus a little, enabling it to produce more infection-fighting T-cells. Melatonin also enhances antibody production.

[3] Some studies have shown that a nightly melatonin supplement can boost the performance of immune systems compromised by age, drugs or stress, during sleep.

As a synthetic hormone in its supplement form, there is increasing wariness about melatonin. Pharmaceutical-grade melatonin is synthesized from methylated serotonin. Melatonin can also be naturally derived from glandular material. This is frowned upon by the FDA because of possible contamination of the glandular material, which comes from slaughterhouse animals. Even were this acceptable, it takes a huge number of pineal glands from cows or sheep to produce adequate amounts.

Most reports on melatonin's safety relate to short-term use. The safety of its long-term use, both in terms of dosage, and condition-specifics has not been established. We should use careful consideration before jumping into long term melatonin supplementation. Hormones are incredibly delicate, yet incredibly powerful biological compounds. They act in extremely tiny doses. One milligram, the smallest commercially available dose is three times higher than the normal amount in the body. Many synthetic hormone and hormone replacement drugs are detrimental to health and hormone balance.

Here are some melatonin facts for you to consider:

• Breast and perhaps prostate cancer, hormone driven cancers, may to be involved with a deficiency of melatonin. When melatonin is deficient in the body, breast and prostate cancer risk is high.

• Melatonin dampens the release of estrogen. In fact, high melatonin levels can temporarily shut down the reproductive system. This is the theory basis for a new contraceptive combining a "high" dose (75mg) of melatonin with progestin. The new drug is called B-Oval.

• Melatonin decreases the size of the prostate gland. (A melatonin deficiency allows it to grow.) This is good news for older males with enlarged prostate. But melatonin supplementation can greatly decrease sex drive and actually shrink gonads - certainly an unwanted effect.

• Melatonin may also be indicated in low-tryptophan diseases, such as anorexia, hypertension, manic depression, Cushing's disease, schizophrenia, and psoriasis, because tryptophan is the raw material for melatonin, becoming serotonin, and then through the body's enzyme action, melatonin.

We know that every drug has side effects, and this is true of melatonin. Here is information for you to consider.

• Once melatonin supplementation begins, the body tends to shut down its own production of the hormone.

• Melatonin is not recommended for persons under 40, unless for a temporary sleep disorder or jet lag.

• Some medications raise or lower melatonin levels. Beta blockers suppress melatonin levels. Serotonin stimulants, such as 5-hydroxy-tryptophan (5-HT) or chlorpromazine (an antipsychotic), raise melatonin levels.

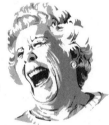

If you decide to take melatonin as a protective measure against breast or prostate cancer, take a small safeguard dose...about 3mg at night. Give your body a chance to use the supplementation and make its own hormone by stopping for a month or two. You can always resume if needed. Natural anti-oxidant, immune protective choices that don't carry the hormone risk of synthetic melatonin, are panax ginseng, ginkgo biloba or garlic.

DHEA, (dehydro-epiandrosterone), is sometimes called the mother of hormones because it is used by the body to manufacture other hormones, such as estrogen, testosterone, progesterone, and corticosterone. DHEA is of enormous interest today because it is called a youth hormone. It has been touted as an anti-aging substance that lowers serum cholesterol, reverses aging symptoms and promotes energy and libido.

DHEA regulates the auto-immune mechanism, stimulating immune defenses to fight infections and monitoring over-reaction that might attack the body. It has thus proven helpful against lupus and rheumatoid arthritis. Recent research has shown the importance of DHEA in the prevention of cancer, heart disease, and Alzheimer's disease.

DHEA supplements are effective for post-menopausal women with osteoporosis who are low in DHEA, much the same as estrogen replacement. Other symptoms of menopause are also relieved, and cancer risk associated with estrogen replacement is greatly reduced; it may even be prevented by DHEA's immune potential.

DHEA has few side effects, but if you take too much, it suppresses your body's ability to make its own. People who use DHEA and have good results usually have to take it for the rest of their lives to continue the results. Adult acne is a common side effect, as is excess facial and body hair. DHEA dosage falls between 5-15mg for women and 10-30mg for men.

Dioscorea (wild yam), contains diosgenin which some researchers think help the body help the body produce its own DHEA.

🐍 *For more information on these two hormone substances, see* THE ALTERNATIVE ARSENAL *in this book.*

Exercise Is An Important Anti-oxidant For Anti-aging

Exercise does not have to be complicated. Simple mild stretches every morning can oxygenate your tissues, limber your body, and help clear it of the previous night's waste. Stretches at night before bed help insure muscle relaxation and better rest. There are so many ways to bring exercise into your life: yoga, dance, sports like tennis or sailing, aerobic exercise, swimming, bike riding or hiking.

There are two keys to maintaining regular exercise. Find something that you like, because that's something you'll do on a long term basis; and switch around your exercise activities so you don't get bored. Take an aerobics class one day, swim the next, play tennis on the weekend, etc.

HERE ARE THE ADVANTAGES OF REGULAR EXERCISE FOR AN ANTI-AGING LIFESTYLE:
* Exercise improves blood circulation and the body's ability to use oxygen for physical energy.
* Exercise helps reduce the risk for heart attacks and cancer.
* Exercise greatly contributes to weight control by fanning the metabolic fires.
* Exercise contributes to the reduction of stress and tension. Exercise encourages relaxation.
* Exercise stimulates hormone production in men and women.
* Exercise contributes to strength and endurance. Inactivity contributes to fatigue.
* Weight bearing exercises trigger bone mineralization to help prevent osteoporosis.
* Exercise helps agility and joint mobility.

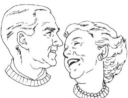

Take a walk every day, especially after your largest meal, for better circulation, energy, strength, stress reduction and enzyme function. Walking exercises both your body and your brain. Walking is an "anti-oxidant nutrient," because it helps keep your immune system in good working order. Exercise makes the most difference in the least fit, and the most elderly. Raising the heart rate just 20 beats per minute can markedly decrease blood pressure.

Get a therapeutic massage once a month. Use it like a monthly tune-up to refresh the body, calm the nerves, release stress, and restore immune function.

Relaxation Techniques Slow The Aging Process

Meditation isn't just for gurus. Everybody is beginning to see its value. In fact, just about everyone gets into a state of meditation several times a day. Being caught up in the moment, living in the present, digging in the garden, playing with a child, watching a sunset or indulging in the peaceful bliss of a shower. They're all forms of meditation. Intentionally finding a quiet spot, relaxing and taking in some deep breaths can do a world of good for an anti-aging life-style.

Deep breathing is one of the simplest ways to relax. It gives profound positive physiological and psychological effects. Deep, relaxed breathing takes away stress, induces relaxation, makes aches and pains vanish, composes the mind, increases energy levels, lowers blood pressure, heightens awareness, improves mood, and helps us access creativity by restoring your "battery charge."

Here is a simple breathing exercise to do when you are tense, your sense of well-being will change for the better.
* Take a deep, full breath. Exhale it. Slowly. Slowly.
* Take another deep, full breath. And let it out slowly.
* And again. Exhale slower than you inhale.
* Maintain a nice, quiet rhythm, exhaling more slowly than you inhale.

*Do not complain about growing old.
Not everyone is granted that privilege.*

Optimizing Exercise & Sports Performance
Getting The Most Out Of Your Exercise Choices

Regular exercise is an integral part of good health. It's not just for athletes anymore. A sedentary lifestyle has the same effect on heart disease risk as smoking a pack of cigarettes a day! We all know that exercise speeds results in weight loss and heart recovery, but regular exercise also helps a healing program. It strengthens the whole body - muscles, nerves, blood, glands, lungs, heart, brain, mind and mood. It increases metabolic rate, muscle mass, tissue oxygen uptake, respiratory and circulatory vigor, and increases the enzymes in the body that help burn up fat.

Good metabolism is optimized by exercise. An interesting feature of metabolism is brown fat activity. Brown fat is metabolically very active and is different from yellow fat (the kind you can see deposited around your body). Brown fat is bound to the skeleton and is filled with tiny, brown-colored, mitochondria and cytochromes, chemical power-houses that produce energy in our cells. Brown fat is thermogenically responsive, so that when we take in excess calories, our body compensates in part by producing more body heat to burn them off instead of storing them as yellow fat. Brown fat activity explains in part why some people can overeat and stay slim and other people gain weight easily.

For most of us, brown fat becomes less active and less thermogenically responsive as we age. Instead of calories being burned off, they get stored as yellow fat. Keeping brown fat active and thermogenically responsive is the key to weight control as you age. The two major factors that cause low brown fat activity are lack of aerobic exercise that increases your lung capacity and elevates your heart rate, and poor diet. Putting on weight and not exercising causes lean muscle tissue to break down, leaving you flabby, with less energy and ultimately, with even less brown fat activity to burn calories.

A daily, thirty minute, aerobic walk, breathing deeply, for even a mile a day ($\frac{1}{2}$ mile out, $\frac{1}{2}$ mile back) makes a big difference to brown fat activity. And it's almost a necessity for long term health. Deep exhalations release metabolic waste along with CO_2; deep inhalations flood the system with fresh oxygen. The circulatory system is cleansed, heart strength and muscle tone are improved. Think of sunlight on your body as *heliotherapy,* adding natural Vitamin D for skin and bone health.

A low fat diet with whole grains, fresh vegetables, moderate protein increases brown fat activity. A fatty, high protein diet, (like the average American diet) tends to prevent brown fat from being thermogenically responsive. Even if you didn't reduce your calorie intake, but added aerobic exercise, you would still lose weight and increase body tone.

Besides losing muscle mass, we also lose about 1% of bone mass every year if we don't exercise, and this can begin as early as age 35. An exercise program that includes weight bearing exercises such as walking, running, and cycling, increases both muscle and bone mass. Aerobic exercise is the key to long-term weight and stress control, reduced cholesterol, and a stronger heart. It also stimulates antibody production, enhancing immune response. Aerobic exercise is easy, and as available as your front door.

In addition to **a daily walk, or light jog, dancing** is great aerobic exercise. Legs and lungs both show rapid improvement, not to mention the fun you have. Any kind of **dancing** is a good workout, and the breathlessness you feel afterward is the best sign of aerobic benefit. **Swimming** works all parts of the body at once, so noticeable definition improvement comes quickly with regular swimming. Just fifteen to twenty steady laps, three or four times a week, and a more streamlined body is yours.

Aerobic exercise classes are easily available. They are held every day, everywhere, at low prices, with good music and spirit-raising group energy. Workout clothes look great on both men and women. They are comfortable, permit deep breathing, and make you feel good about your body even when you are not exercising.

If your schedule is so busy that you hardly have time to breathe, let alone exercise, but still want the benefits of bodywork, there is an all-in-one aerobic exercise. It has gotten resounding enthusiasm and response rates for aerobic activity and muscle tone - **all in one minute.** The exercise sounds very easy, but is actually very difficult, and that is why it works so well. You will be breathless (the sign of an effective aerobic workout) before you know it.

Simply lie flat on your back on a rug or carpet. Rise to a full standing position any way you can, and lie down flat on your back again. That's the whole exercise. Stand and lie down, stand and lie down - for one minute. Typical repetitions for most people with average body tone are six to ten in 60 seconds. Record time for an athlete in top competitive condition is about 20-24 times in a minute. Be very easy on yourself. Repeat only as many times as you feel comfortable and work up gradually. It is worth a try because it exercises muscles, lung capacity and circulatory system so well, but don't overdo it.

Whatever exercise program you choose for yourself, make rest a part of it. Work out harder one day, go easy the next; or exercise for several days and take two days off. It's better for body balance, and will increase energy levels when you exercise the next time. After a regular program is started, exercising four days a week will increase fitness level; exercising three days a week will maintain fitness level; exercising two days a week will decrease a high fitness level. But any amount of exercise is better than nothing at all.

Every exercise helps. Vigorous physical exercise is the most efficient way to burn yellow fat. Choose those that work for you conveniently and easily. Every series of stretches and exercises you do tones, elasticizes, shapes and contours your skin, connective tissue and muscles.

Eating For Energy & Performance

Nutrition is the most important factor for exercise or sports performance, at any level.

Body building is 85% nutrition. Eating junk foods pays the penalty of poor performance. Athletic excellence cannot be achieved by just adding anabolic supplements of any kind to an inferior diet. The only e f -fective action is optimal nutrition. Good nutrition helps eliminate fluctuating energy levels, abnormal fatigue, and susceptibility to injury or illness. A regular, long-term, optimally nutritious diet is the basis for high performance; not protein or even carbo-loading before an event.

Exercise is an integral part of good nutrition, too. We have all experienced the fact that exercise eases hunger. You are thirsty after a workout as the body calls for replacement of water and lost electrolytes, but not hungry. One of the reasons rapid results are achieved in a body streamlining program is this phenomenon. Not only do muscles become toned, heart and lungs become stronger, and fats lost, but the body doesn't call for calorie replacement right away. Its own glycogens lift blood sugar levels and provide a feeling of well being. **Exercise becomes a nutrient in itself.**

Sixty-five to seventy-five percent of a high performance diet should be in unrefined, clean-burning complex carbohydrates. Complex carbohydrates like those from whole grains, pasta, vegetables, rice, beans and fruits, are the key to strength and endurance for both the athlete and the casual body builder. They improve performance, promote storage of muscle fuel, and are easily absorbed without excess fats.

Twenty to twenty-five percent should be in high grade proteins from whole grains, nuts, beans, raw dairy prod-ucts, tofu and other soy foods, yogurt, kefir, eggs, and some occasional poultry, fish, and seafood. Vegetable protein is best for mineral absorption and bone density. Strength and muscle mass decline if you are getting too little protein. However, eating excess protein, especially from red meats, creates a condition that hampers performance. Excess amino acids from too much protein causes the formation of toxic ammonia in the body. The body then protects itself by converting ammonia into less toxic urea and excretes it via the kidneys. Too much protein can also overload the kidneys (you feel this in lower back pain) and poison the blood.

About 10 to15% of a high performance diet should be in energy-producing fats and oils necessary for glycogen storage. The best fats are from unrefined, mono-or polyunsaturated oils, a little pure butter, nuts, low fat cheeses, and whole grain snacks.

Your remaining diet fuel should be liquid nutrients; fruit juices for natural sugars, mineral waters and electrolyte replacement drinks for potassium, magnesium and sodium, and plenty of pure water. When the body senses lack of water, it will naturally start to retain fluid. Waste and body impurities will not be filtered out properly, and the liver will not metabolize stored fats for energy. Six to eight glass of water a day are a must, even if you don't feel thirsty. It often takes the sensory system time to catch up with actual body needs.

There are special foods that can give an athlete the edge in strength and stamina. "Superfoods" are effective, highly concentrated, bio-available, nutrients. Athletic success and intense exercise require a strong immune system. Superfoods strengthen and enhance immunity. Green superfood blends contain concentrates of spirulina, alfalfa, chlorella, barley grass, blue-green algae and wheat grass. Bee pollen and royal jelly are rich in essential nutritional elements. Aged garlic has valuable properties for the athlete, providing anti-fatigue effects (prevention of exhaustion and promotion of recovery), and anti-stress effects (enhancing the body's ability to adapt to stress), with potent anti-oxidants (for free radical protection).

Three Strength Diets: Sports Nutrition, High Energy, Competition

Nutrition for body strength enhances endurance capabilities, speed and focus. Strength nutrition assists with injury prevention and repair, and body stress reduction, with the ability to absorb and carry more oxygen, replace ATP, remove lactic acid, and improve electrolyte balance. For the serious athlete, strength nutrition can create the edge that can make the difference between winning and losing, especially in the last burst of energy for peak performance.

HERE ARE THREE STRENGTH NUTRITION DIETS TO CHOOSE FROM:

The **HIGH ENERGY, ACTIVE LIFE STYLE DIET** is targeted for people who lack consistent daily energy and tire easily, and those who need more endurance and strength for hard jobs or long hours. It is also for weekend sports enthusiasts who wish to accomplish more than their present level of nutrition allows.

The **MODERATE AEROBIC DIET** is for people who work out 3 to 4 times a week. It emphasizes complex carbohydrates for smooth muscle use, and moderate fat and protein amounts. Complex carbohydrates also produce glycogen for the body, resulting in increased energy and endurance.

The **HIGH PERFORMANCE / TRAINING DIET** concentrates on energy for competitive sports participation, and long range stamina. For the serious athlete, and for those who are consciously body building for higher workout achievement, this diet is a good foundation for significantly improved performance. Sports tests show that adjusting the diet before competition can increase endurance 200% or more - well worth consideration.

Athletes' nutritional needs are considerably greater than those of the average person. Normal RDAs are far too low for high performance or competition needs. Consult a good sports nutritionist, or knowledgable person at a health food store or gym to determine your specific supplement requirements. The important consideration is not body weight, but body composition.

Each of the three diets can be useful to the serious, performing athlete. Competitive training and a training diet alone cannot insure success. Rest time, and building energy reserves are also necessary to tune the body for maximum efficiency. When not in competition or pre-event training, extra high nutrient amounts are **not** needed, and can be hard for the body to handle. A reduced density diet is better for maintenance tone, and can be easily increased for competitive performance.

The next 2 pages include a Food Exchange List and a Food Amounts Chart by Diet so you can adjust individual needs.

Food Exchange List

Any food listed in a category may be exchanged one-for-one with any other food in that category. Portion amounts are given for a man weighing 170 pounds, and a woman weighing 130 pounds.

GRAINS, BREADS & CEREALS: One serving is approximately one cup of cooked grains, such as brown rice, millet, barley, bulgur, kashi, couscous, corn, oats, and whole grain pasta;

or one cup of dry cereals, such as bran flakes, Oatios, or Grapenuts;

or three slices of wholegrain bread; or three six-inch corn tortillas; or two chapatis or whole wheat pita breads;

or twelve small wholegrain crackers; or two rice cakes.

VEGETABLES:

Group A: One serving is as much as you want of lettuce (all kinds), Chinese greens and peas, raw spinach and carrots, celery, cucumbers, endive, sea vegetables, watercress, radishes, green onions and chives.

Group B: One serving is approximately two cups of cabbage or alfalfa sprouts;

or $1^1/_2$ cups cooked bell peppers and mushrooms;

or one cup cooked asparagus, cauliflower, chard, sauerkraut, eggplant, zucchini or summer squash;

or $^3/_4$ cup cooked broccoli, green beans; onions or mung bean sprouts;

or $^1/_2$ cup vegetable juice cocktail, or cooked brussels sprouts; or 8 to 10 water chestnuts.

Group C: One serving is approximately $1^1/_2$ cups cooked carrots;

or one cup cooked beets, potatoes, or leeks;

or $^1/_2$ cup cooked peas, corn, artichokes, winter squash or yams;

or one cup fresh carrot or vegetable juice.

FRUITS: One serving is approximately one apple, nectarine, mango, pineapple, peach or orange;

or 4 apricots, medjool dates or figs; or half a honeydew or cantaloupe;

or 20 to 24 cherries or grapes; or one and a half cups strawberries or other berries.

DAIRY FOODS: One serving is approximately one cup of whole milk, buttermilk or full fat yogurt, for 3mg. of fat;

or one cup of low-fat milk or yogurt, for 2gm. of fat;

or one cup of skim milk or non-fat yogurt, for less than 1gm. of fat;

or one ounce of low fat hard cheese, such as swiss or cheddar;

or $^1/_3$ cup of non-fat dry milk powder.

POULTRY, FISH & SEAFOOD: One serving is approximately 4-oz. of white fish or fresh salmon, skinned for 3gm. of fat;

or four ounces of chicken or turkey, white meat, no skin for 4gm. of fat;

or one cup of tuna or salmon, water packed for 3gm. of fat;

or one cup of shrimp, scallops, oysters, clams or crab for 3 to 4gm of fat.

I recommend avoiding red meats. These include all beef, carved, ground, corned or smoked, such as luncheon meat; veal, lamb, pork, sausage, ham, bacon, and wild game. They are high in saturated fats and cholesterol, and unsound as a use of planetary resources. Many have been injected with hormones and antibiotics.

HIGH PROTEIN MEAT & DAIRY SUBSTITUTES: One serving is approximately four ounces of tofu (one block);

or $^1/_2$ cup low fat or dry cottage cheese; or $^1/_3$ cup ricotta, parmesan or mozzarella;

or one egg; or $^1/_2$ cup cooked beans or brown rice.

FATS & OILS:

One serving is approximately one teaspoon of butter, margarine or shortening for 5gm. of fat;

or one tablespoon of salad dressing or mayonnaise for 5gm. of fat;

or 2 teaspoons of poly-unsaturated or mono-unsaturated vegetable oil for 5gm. of fat.

The following foods are very high in fat and the amounts listed are equivalent to 1 fat serving on the diet chart. Use sparingly.

2 tablespoons of light cream, half and half, or sour cream; 1 tablespoon of heavy cream;

$^1/_8$ slice of avocado; $^1/_4$ cup of sunflower, sesame, or pumpkin seeds.

10 almonds, cashews or peanuts; 20 pistachios or Spanish peanuts; 4 walnut or pecan halves;

Food Amounts Chart By Diet

Servings should be scaled up or down to fit your individual weight and type of active diet. For complete sports, training and energy diets, see "Cooking for Healthy Healing" 2nd Edition by Linda Rector Page.

Daily Diet for Men Approx. 170 pounds			Daily Diet for Women Approx. 130 pounds		
High Energy, Active Life Diet Calories 2800 Protein 17% Carbos 70% Fat 13%	**Moderate Aerobic Diet** Calories 3250 Protein 20% Carbos 65% Fat 15%	**Training & Competition Diet** Calories 3950 Protein 23% Carbos 65% Fat 12%	**High Energy, Active Life Diet** Calories 2000 Protein 17% Carbos 70% Fat 13%	**Moderate Aerobic Diet** Calories 2200 Protein 20% Carbos 65% Fat 15%	**Training & Competition Diet** Calories 2750 Protein 23% Carbos 65% Fat 12%
6 whole grain servings	7 whole grain servings	8 whole grain servings	4 whole grain servings	4 whole grain servings	6 whole grain servings
Group A vegetables - all you want	Group A vegetables - all you want	Group A vegetables - all you want	Group A vegetables - all you want	Group A vegetables - all you want	Group A vegetables - all you want
Group B vegetables - 6 servings	Group B vegetables - 6 servings	Group B vegetables - 7 servings	Group B vegetables - 4 servings	Group B vegetables - 4 servings	Group B vegetables - 6 servings
Group C vegetables - 6 servings	Group C vegetables - 6 servings	Group C vegetables - 8 servings	Group C vegetables - 3 servings	Group C vegetables - 4 servings	Group C vegetables - 5 servings
5 fruit servings	5 fruit servings	6 fruit servings	3 fruit servings	`4 fruit servings	4 fruit servings
3 dairy servings	4 dairy servings	4 dairy servings	2 dairy servings	3 dairy servings	3 dairy servings
2 poultry or seafood servings	4 poultry or seafood servings	5 poultry or seafood servings	1 poultry or seafood servings	1 poultry or seafood servings	3 poultry or seafood servings
5 fat servings	5 fat servings	6 fat servings	3 fat servings	3 fat servings	3 fat servings

Supplements & Herbs For Exercise, Bodybuilding & Sports Performance

Strength training supplements are good for both the serious and casual athlete. They can help build muscle tissue, maintain low body fat, and improve strength and endurance when the body is under the stress of a workout series. Supplements optimize recuperation time between workouts, are a proven adjunct to fitness and muscle growth, and speed healing from sports-related injuries. Antioxidants have become a byword for sports performance, because antioxidant supplementation helps maintain the body's defenses against exercise-induced free radicals to combat injury and speed muscle recovery.

How you take training supplements is as important as what you take. Your program will be more productive if you balance supplements between workout days and rest days. Muscle growth occurs on rest days as the body uses the workout you have been giving it. Obtain increased enhancement by taking vitamins, minerals, and glandulars on your rest days. Take proteins, amino acids, anabolics and herbs on workout days, before the workout.

Herbal supplements can be efficient partners in your exercise program. Herbs act as concentrated food nutrients for body building. They offer extra strength for energy and endurance. Herbs have been used by athletes from ancient times. Yarrow and other herbs were used by the gladiators to help heal flesh wounds. Chinese and Japanese warriors and wrestlers have used herbs to increase endurance and strength from pre-history to the present. In Russia, Germany, Japan, and Korea, herbs are extremely popular with sports enthusiasts and athletes. American athletes are just beginning to see the value of herbs for a winning body.

Here are a few popular, available herbs you can use for your exercise program. Herbal supplements work better in combination, and they work best when taken on exercise days, either in the morning with a protein drink, or 30 minutes before exertion.

• **ANTIOXIDANT HERBS FOR AEROBIC SUPPORT:** Siberian ginseng, ginkgo biloba, barley grass, spirulina, chlorella, American and Chinese panax ginseng, rosemary, white pine bark, Crystal Star ANTI-OXIDANT™ extract.

• **ADAPTOGEN HERBS FOR BODY STRESS:** American and Chinese panax ginseng, Chinese astragalus, schizandra, ashwaganda, fo-ti, Siberian ginseng, damiana, Crystal Star ACTIVE PHYSICAL ENERGY™ extract.

• **ANTI-INFLAMMATORY HERBS FOR INJURIES:** Turmeric and white willow, Crystal Star ANTI-FLAM™ extract and caps, BACK TO RELIEF™ extract.

• **ENERGY STIMULANTS:** guarana, ginkgo biloba, damiana, green tea, yerba mate, Crystal Star SUPER MAN'S ENERGY TONIC™, HIGH PERFORMANCE™ caps, HIGH ENERGY™ tea, or RAINFOREST ENERGY™ caps.

• **STAMINA & ENDURANCE HERBS:** Siberian ginseng, sarsaparilla, wild yam, schizandra, spirulina, American and Chinese panax ginseng, fo-ti, Crystal Star HIGH PERFORMANCE™ caps.

• **ADRENAL TONIC HERBS:** licorice, panax ginseng, Crystal Star ADRN-ACTIVE™ or GINSENG/LICORICE extracts.

• **BLOOD TONIC & BLOOD CLEANSING HERBS:** wheatgrass, chlorella, spirulina, barley grass, yellow dock, sarsaparilla and goldenseal, Crystal Star ENERGY GREEN™ drink, SYSTEMS STRENGTH™ drink or caps.

• **CIRCULATION ACTIVATING HERBS:** ginkgo biloba, cayenne, ginger, Crystal Star HEARTSEASE CIRCU-CLEANSE™.

• **METABOLIC ENHANCING HERBS:** sarsaparilla, licorice rt., bee pollen, royal jelly, panax ginseng, green tea, Crystal Star MALE PERFORMANCE™ caps and THERMO-CITRIN GINSENG™ caps and extract.

• **ANABOLIC STIMULANT HERBS:** suma, Crystal Star GINSENG 6 SUPER CAPS™.

• **MUSCLE RELAXERS FOR SORENESS:** valerian, passion flower, Crystal Star STRESSED OUT™ extract.

• **WORKOUT RECOVERY & NERVE STRENGTH HERBS:** sarsaparilla, Crystal Star BODY REBUILDER™.

• **MINERAL-RICH HERBS:** yellow dock root, barley grass, dandelion, Crystal Star MINERAL SPECTRUM™ caps, POTASSIUM/IODINE SOURCE™ and CALCIUM SOURCE™ capsules.

Note: Mineral balance is critical for an athlete at any level. Macro and trace minerals are built into every bio-chemical reaction of athletic movement, from energy, to digestion, to utilization of vitamins and protein, to nerve transmission, muscle contraction, the regulation of metabolism, cholesterol levels, and blood sugar. Athletes regularly become deficient in minerals and can benefit greatly by replacing electrolytes (the ionized mineral salts found in body fluids) lost after workouts. TRACE-LYTE by Nature's Path is a true electrolyte formula.

A Word About Steroids

As the standards of excellence rise in sports and competition, the use of steroids is increasing. Steroid enhancement has spread beyond the professional and Olympic arenas to dedicated weight lifters, body builders and team players at all levels. The dangers of synthetic steroids far outweigh any advantages. Steroid use leads to wholesale destruction of glandular tissue, stunted growth from bone closure in males, testicle shrinkage, low sperm counts with sterility noticeable after only a few months of use, enlargement and tenderness of the pectorals, weakening of connective tissue, jaundice from liver malfunction, circulation impairment, and adverse side effects of hostile personality behavior and facial changes. **Can Herbal Steroids do the sports enhancement job?**

Although there are no magic bullets for energy, endurance and healing of sports injuries, there are plant-derived steroids called phytosterols that **do** have growth activity similar to that of free form amino acids and anabolic steroids. Amino acids from sources such as herbs, and foods high in amino acids, can act as steroid alternatives to help build the body to competitive levels without chemical steroid consequences. These "natural steroids" help release growth hormone, promote ammonia and acid detoxification, stimulate immunity and liver regeneration. They maximize potential, promote fast recuperation, increase stamina, and support peak performance. Testing still needs to be done on the herbs for anabolic effectiveness, especially on steroid strengths in normal herbal dosage form. Nevertheless, they may still be used with confidence in body building and endurance formulas.

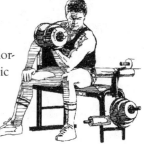

THE MOST WELL-KNOWN OF THESE HERBS ARE:
- **Damiana,** a mild aphrodisiac and nerve stimulant.
- **Sarsaparilla Root,** *Smilax,*, coaxes the body to produce greater amounts of the anabolic hormones, testosterone and cortisone. A blood purifier for nitrogen-based waste products such as uric acid. Speeds recovery time after workouts.
- **Saw Palmetto,** a urethral toning herb that increases blood flow to the sexual organs.
- **Siberian and Panax Ginsengs**, adaptogens for over-all body balance and energy.
- **Wild Yam,** an anti-spasmodic that prevents cramping. Contains disogenin, a phyto progesterone.
- **Yohimbe,** a testosterone precursor for body building, and potent aphrodisiac for both male and female.

Supplementing Your Individual Exercise Requirements

The following pages detail three separate supplement and herb programs tailored for 1) a high energy active lifestyle, 2) a moderate aerobic workout, and 3) high performance and competitive training needs.

1) SUPPLEMENTS AND HERBS FOR THE HIGH ENERGY DIET:

Use Superfoods! This is one of the best ways to supercharge your diet for energy. Here are some to try:
- Crystal Star SYSTEMS STRENGTH™ - superfoods from land and sea.
- Crystal Star ENERGY GREEN DRINK™ - a concentrated, body-building, whole green drink with herbs.
- PLANT POWER by Herbal Products and Development.
- NutriCology PRO-GREENS contains several green superfoods, herbs and other nutrients.
- Green Foods GREEN ESSENCE is powdered juice from young barley leaves and vegetables.
- Wakunaga KYO-GREEN is a superfood with young barley leaves, wheat grass, chlorella, and kelp.
- POWER-PLUS Food Enzymes by Herbal Products & Development. Enzymes play a key role in the utilization of vitamins and minerals. They are also a major factor in healing and repair.
- A good B complex daily, 100 to 125mg with extra B_{12} 2000mcg.
- MEZOTRACE - sea bottom mineral and trace mineral complex.
- Bioforce GINSAVENA extract tablets for men; Floradix HERBAL IRON LIQUID for women; or use HEMA-LYTE Iron by Nature's Path with electrolytes for total absorption.
- Effective herbal energizers include Crystal Star ADRN-ACTIVE™ caps with BODY REBUILDER™ caps, and IRON SOURCE™ caps or extract for women; SUPER MAN'S ENERGY TONIC™, SIBERIAN GINSENG extract or GINSENG 6 SUPER CAPS™ for men. HIGH ENERGY TEA™ and FEEL GREAT™ caps and tea are effective for both sexes; ANTI-OXIDANT HERBS™ caps contain phyto-antioxidants for long range resistance support.

2) SUPPLEMENTS AND HERBS FOR THE MODERATE AEROBICS WORKOUT:

Start with superfoods for deep body strength, and faster recovery. See previous page for suggestions.

MINERALS: You need minerals to run - for bone density, speed and endurance; as anabolic enhancers.
•Potassium/magnesium/bromelain - relieves muscle fatigue/lactic acid buildup.
•Cal/mag/zinc with boron - to prevent muscle cramping and maintain bone integrity.
•Chromium picolinate, 200mcg - for sugar regulation and glucose energy use.
•Zinc picolinate, 30-50mg. daily for athletes - for immunity, healing of epithelial injuries.
•Crystal Star MINERAL SPECTRUM™, IRON and CALCIUM SOURCE™ extract and capsules.
•CAL-LYTE or HEMA-LYTE Iron, electrolytes by Nature's Path for strong muscles and absorption.

VITAMINS: Anti-stress factors for muscles, nerves and heart.
•B Complex, 100mg. or more - for nerve health, muscle cramping, carbohydrate metabolism.
•Vitamin C, 3000mg. daily w. bioflavs. and rutin. Take 5 minutes before exercise to help put into resistant areas.
•Lewis Labs BREWER'S YEAST - chromium fortified, to simulate protein synthesis.

ANTIOXIDANTS: To increase oxygen use in blood, tissues and brain.
•CoQ$_{10}$ - a catalyst co-enzyme factor to produce and release energy.
•KYOLIC SUPER FORMULA 105 by Wakunaga combines several potent antioxidants.
•ENERGY FUEL by NutriCology - energy production, cardio-protective, improves oxygenation.
•UniPro LIQUID DMG - offers energy and reduces lactic acid build-up in the muscles.

GLANDULARS: Growth gland and hormone stimulation.
•Pituitary, 200mg - the master gland, for upper body development.
•Adrenal, 500mg - Country Life ADRENAL w/ TYROSINE, Crystal Star ADR-ACTIVE™ phyto-glandular support.
•Liver, 400mg - for fat metabolism, Enzymatic Therapy LIQUID LIVER with SIB. GINSENG.

TESTOSTERONE SUPPORT: As part of a natural anabolic program for increased male muscle hardness.
•Crystal Star ACTIVE PHYSICAL ENERGY™ with panax ginseng.
•Muira Pauma Bark (potency wood) and sarsaparilla (smilax) herbs.

STIMULANTS: for quick, temporary, energy.
•Siberian ginseng extract
•Crystal Star ACTIVE PHYSICAL ENERGY™, HIGH PERFORMANCE™ caps, or HIGH ENERGY™ tea.

FREE FORM AMINO ACIDS: Activators to increase body structure and strength. (Don't forget bee pollen.)
•Arginine/Ornithine/Lysine, 750mg, to burn fats for energy, Glutamine, strong growth hormone release.
•Anabol Naturals GH RELEASERS and MUSCLE OCTANE, AMINO BALANCE.
•AmeriFit WOMEN'S FITNESS PAK, pre-digested amino acids - easily absorbed for better performance.
•Carnitine, 500mg. - to strengthen heart and circulatory system during long exercise bouts.
•Inosine, 1000mg. - to reduce workout stress and kick in glycogen for extra edge performance.
•Branched Chain Complex, BCAAs - for ATP energy conversion, endurance improvement.

ENZYMES: To process fuel nutrients for most efficient body use.
•Rainbow Light ADVANCED ENZYME SYSTEM.
•POWER PLUS Enzymes by Herbal Products & Development.

PROTEIN/AMINO DRINKS: Mainstays for muscle building, weight gain, energy and endurance.
•Twin Lab AMINO FUEL - effective twice daily for endurance energy.
•Twin Lab GAINERS FUEL 1000 - for maximum weight gain.
•Nature's Life SUPER PRO 96 green protein.
•Champion LEAN GAINER - low-fat weight gainer.

FAT BURNERS: Metabolize blood and body fats, and enhance muscle growth.
•Bricker Labs EN-DURO, Advanced Research FAT BURNERS with L-Carnitine.
•SLIM-LYTE 1200 by Nature's Path with chromium to burn fat, not muscle tissue.

SPORTS BARS: Rich sources of carbohydrates, protein and fiber
•Power Foods POWER BARS.
•Nature's plus SPIRUTEIN ENERGY BARS and SOURCE OF LIFE ENERGY BARS.

SPORTS DRINKS/ELECTROLYTE REPLACEMENTS: Use after exertion to replace body minerals
•Champion Nutrition CYTOMAX, Alacer MIRACLE WATER, Knudsens RECHARGE and Twin Lab ULTRA FUEL.
•Anabol Naturals CARBO SURGE and Nature's Path TRACE-LYTE liquid electrolytes.

RECOVERY ACCELERATION: for muscles, ligaments, tendons.
•Proteolytic Enzymes - break down scar tissue build-up and shortens recovery time after injury.
•Crystal Star BODY REBUILDER™ capsules.
•Wakunaga KYOLIC SUPER FORMULA 103.
•NutriCology GERMANIUM 150mg.
•Bromelain/Papain 500mg - for muscle and ligament repair and strength.

3) SUPPLEMENTS AND HERBS FOR THE COMPETITION AND TRAINING NEEDS OF THE SERIOUS ATHLETE:
Choices For Training days; before you work out:

SUPER PROTEIN DRINKS:
•Champion PRO-SCORE 100, PHOSPHAGAIN or MYOPLEX PLUS PRECISION by EAS, Twin Lab AMINO FUEL and CREATINE FUEL PLUS, AmeriFit EGG PROTEIN.

OXYGENATORS / ANTIOXIDANTS:
•CoQ$_{10}$ 60mg, UniPro LIQUID DMG or Muscle Masters SMILAX + DMG, KYOLIC SUPER FORMULA 105, HEMA-LYTE Iron by Nature's Path with electrolytes, Nutricology GERMANIUM 150mg to protect the thymus.

FREE FORM AMINO ACIDS: to increase workout performance - full spectrum pre-digested or individual
•Arginine/ornithine/lysine, to metabolize fats, carnitine to strengthen muscle activity, inosine to reduce workout stress; or Anabol Naturals ANABOLIC AMINO BALANCE, AMINO GH RELEASERS or HI-TEST MUSCLE OCTANE.

NATURAL ANABOLIC STEROIDS:
•Natural Health 100% NATURAL STEROIDS, Champion MET MAX, Champion MUSCLE-NITRO, (BCAAs) - for ATP energy conversion, Radiant Life SUMAX 5 derived from the herb suma, has shown to be as effective as the illegal synthetic steroid, dianabol, but without the side effects. Also has liver protection and detox properties, is anti-cholesterol and immune stimulating. 10mg per capsule / dosage 3 to 8 caps per day depending upon intensity of training. Highly recommended.

TESTOSTERONE SUPPORT: to increase muscle hardness
•Nature Health RAW TESTOSTEROL drops, Source Naturals YOHIMBE 1000mg caps. **(Use with great caution.)** Crystal Star ACTIVE PHYSICAL ENERGY™ with panax ginseng, raw orchic extract, approx. 6 to 10x strength.

FAT BURNERS:
•Richardson Labs ULTRA CITRALEAN, advanced thermogenic formula, CUT-UP PLUS by Bricker Labs, premium Carnitine and Chromium fat-burner, MAXIMAL BURNER by Bricker Labs - nutritional fat burner with HCA.

ENZYMES:
•POWER-PLUS Enzymes by Herbal Products Development, ADVANCED ENZYME SYSTEM by Rainbow Light.

HERBS:
•Crystal Star GINSENG ACTIVE PHYSICAL ENERGY™, HIGH PERFORMANCE™ or SUPERMAN'S ENERGY TONIC™, Richardson Labs ENERGIA for both women and men, BioSource GINSAVENA for increased glandular activity.

RECOVERY ACCELERATION:
•Champion CORTISTAT-PS to reduce cortisol levels and inflammation during a "burning" workout.

In between workout sessions, take natural power bars for an energy boost, such as Power Foods POWER BARS, Champion SNAC-BAR, or SUPER HEAVYWEIGHT BARS, Hoffman ULTRA FUEL BARS or DIET FUEL BAR by Twin Labs.

After your work out, take an electrolyte replacement to bring lost minerals and energy back faster: TRACE-LYTE Electrolyte Formula by Nature's Path, Knudsen RECHARGE drink, Alacer's MIRACLE WATER.

REST DAY SUPPLEMENTS CHOICES:

SUPERFOODS:
•PLANT POWER by Herbal Products and Development, Bee pollen, completely balanced for vitamins, minerals, proteins, enzyme, and all essential amino acids, KYOLIC by Wakunaga, anti-fatigue and immune enhancement.

SUPER DRINKS:
•Champion HEAVYWEIGHT GAINER and POWER CREATINE drinks, Twin Labs CREATINE FUEL PLUS.

VITAMINS:
•Energen STRESS PAK, Dibencozide B_{12}, B Complex 150mg, ESTER-C with minerals/electrolytes.

MINERALS:
•Nature's Path TRACE-LYTE, Chromium picolinate, 500mcg, Twin Labs MEGA CHROMIC FUEL, Richardson Labs CHROMA SLIM PLUS or CHROMA SLIM FOR MEN.

ENZYMES:
•POWER-PLUS Enzymes by Herbal Products & Development, ADVANCED ENZYME SYSTEM by Rainbow Light, VITASE DIGESTION FORMULA by Prevail, Bromelain 500mg., or bromelain with minerals.

REST DAYS AMINO ACIDS:
•Tyrosine/arginine/tryptophan/glycine/ornithine, needed in multigram doses to stimulate GH release, GKG by EAS - designed especially for athletes who train with weights; may support the volume of muscle cells by preserving their most abundant amino acids (glutamine and taurine).

HERBS:
•Crystal Star ADRN-ACTIVE™ extract or GINSENG 6 SUPER TEA™, MINERAL SPECTRUM™ extract.

LIPIDS:
•Twin Labs LIPOTROPIC FUEL
•Beta Sitosterol, 2 to 4 daily - to keep blood fats and cholesterol low, and circulation clear.

Bodywork Watchwords for Body Building, Training & Competition:

•**Cross train.** Besides your major sport or activity, supplement it with auxiliary exercise such as dancing, bicycling, jogging, walking, or swimming and aerobics. This balances muscle use and keeps heart and lungs strong. Unless you are a serious, competitive athlete, make **body tone** your goal.

•**Recuperation time is essential for optimum growth and strength**. Muscles do not grow during exercise. They grow during rest periods. Alternate muscle workouts with rest days. Exercise different muscle sets on different days, resting each set in between. Move joints in their full range of motion during weight training for optimum flexibility.

•**Deep breathing is important.** Lung capacity is a prime training factor. Muscles and tissues must have enough oxygen for endurance and stamina. Breathe in during exertion, out as you relax for the next rep. Vigorous exhaling is as important as inhaling for the athlete, to expel all carbon dioxide and increase lung capacity for oxygen.

•**Stretch out before and after a workout** to keep cramping down and muscles loose. Get some morning sunlight on the body every day possible for optimal absorption of nutrient fuel.

•**No pain does not mean no gain.** Your exercise doesn't have to hurt to be good for you. Once you work up to a good aerobic level and routine, you don't need to push yourself ever harder to benefit.

•**Water is important.** Good hydration is necessary for high performance, cardiovascular activity and overheating. Take an electrolyte replacement drink after a workout or anytime during the day.

•**Weight training is beneficial for both sexes.** Women do not get a bulky, masculine physique from lifting weights. They have low levels of testosterone, which influences their type of muscle development.

How much fat are you burning?

Check your heart rate to see how many fat calories you're burning during your workout. If your heart rate is 70% of maximum, you are burning 20% fat of the total calories per hour/exercise time. If your heart rate is 45% of maximum, you are burning 40% fat of the total calories per hour/exercise time. **More fat is burned in low intensity activities** because you can take in the extra oxygen needed to burn fat - more than twice as much as carbohydrates per fat gram. (If you reduce maximal effort, you will need to exercise longer to burn the fat.)

A study of young men and women on stationary bikes at 70% maximal effort took 30 minutes to burn 300 calories; 65 of the calories came from fat. At 45% of maximal effort it took 48 minutes to reach 300 total calories, but 133 of the calories burned was fat.

Calorie burning choices for your exercise program:

Aerobic Dancing - 300-700 calories per hour
Calisthenics - 360 calories per hour
Cross Country Skiing - 350-1,400 calories per hour
Cycling - 200-850 calories per hour
Jumping Rope - 480-1,000 calories per hour
Racquet Ball or Tennis - 350-1,000 calories per hour
Rowing - 180-1,120 calories per hour
Running - 400-1,300 calories per hour
Stretching - 60-120 calories per hour
Swimming - 380-850 calories per hour
Walking - 240-430 calories per hour
Water Aerobics - 180-880 calories per hour
Weight Training - 260-480 calories per hour

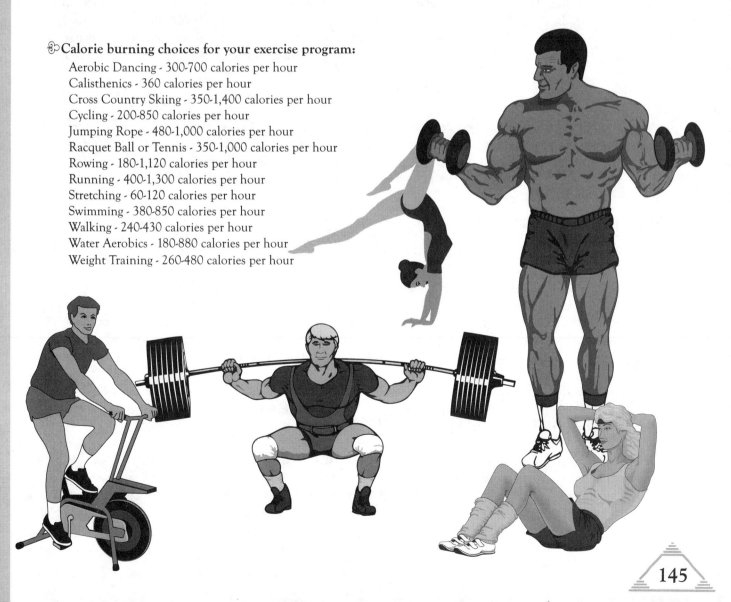

Alternative Healing Options For Pets

Cats and dogs usually need more nutrition than is found in common commercial animal foods. Most pet foods are derived from low quality ingredients rejected for human consumption. Pet foods that are advertised as "Complete and Balanced" are regularly based on uncertain minimum nutrition requirements designed only for *adequate* health, not optimal health. We have come to accept canned and dried foods as being normal, but many vitamin and mineral nutrients are lost through "mixmaster" processing that relies heavily on chemical additives to make the food palatable, and the shelf life long. Veterinarians today are seeing an abundance of premature and chronic health problems that seem to stem from substandard, low quality, processed foods.

Chemical additives (many known to be toxic) can be legally included in animal foods. Some of the worst offenders, present in virtually every supermarket pet food include: sodium nitrite, red dye #40, BHA, BHT, MSG, sodium metabisulfite, artificial flavorings, propylene glycol, and ethoxyguin. Salt is used as a preservative in pet foods, which can irritate the intestines and contribute to high blood pressure and heart disease in pets. Sugar is a frequent additive, and causes animal problems like hypoglycemia, overweight, nervousness, cataracts, tooth decay, arthritis, and allergies, because sugar drains nutrients from the body.

Animals need the life energy of fresh foods just like humans. Their bodies rely on enzymes even more than ours, It's the reason some animals, even some breeds, tend to eat waste excrement - for the enzymes. Besides being the driving force behind all life processes, enzymes are responsible for keeping internal systems working (in animals and humans), and a lack of sufficient enzymes promotes degenerative disease. Almost all pet food is cooked, pasteurized, canned or microwaved, which means most enzymes are destroyed. Uncooked, whole foods contain enzymes, as well as vitamins, minerals and chlorophyll, so it is important to add some fresh greens and vegetables to an animal's diet.

Remember - your busy schedule affects your *whole* family, including your pets. Provide good nutrition for your cat or dog with a wholesome, preservative-free dry kibble as a base, and supplement it with meat and veggies, (leftover fresh salad is just fine). Herbs, homeopathic medicines and high quality natural supplements can help maintain pet health.

Diet For Healthy Dogs & Cats

Cats and dogs thrive on the healthy foods that are good for people. A whole grain, additive-free kibble, a little meat and plenty of fresh water are basic. (*Note: Cats need more meat, and do better with fresh meat. If you have an indoor cat, you need to make up for their inability to catch fresh mice or birds, and offer them uncooked meat.*) Most pets need some fresh vegetables every day, too. Greens keep their systems clean and healthy. We've all seen our pets chewing on grass. Mix greens with a little fish, raw liver and kidney, chicken, low-ash canned or dry food (use meat free of chemicals, and organic vegetables if possible). Most animals like salad greens, cucumbers, green peppers, carrots, green onions, parsley, celery and vegetable juice. Both dogs and cats like oatmeal, too.

I recommend the chemical-free pet foods found in health food stores. Several veterinarians that use natural healing methods on pets and advise us for this book, feel that many of today's pet ailments are a result of chemical-laced foods and environmental pollutants....just like people.

Note: Animals like people, can become addicted to particular foods if they have been given them for long periods of time. Some animals will make quick adjustments to diet improvements; for others, you may need to introduce new foods gradually. You might try a water fast for a particularly finicky pet until it's hungry enough to try the new diet.

HERE ARE SOME ANIMAL DIET WATCHWORDS:
- Give them some dairy foods. Most animals like cheese, yogurt, kefir and cottage cheese and goat's milk.
- A little fruit is OK occasionally to loosen up a clogged system, but give sparingly. Most animals like raisins, coconut, cantaloupe and apples.
- Have fresh water available all day long. Animals need plenty of liquids.
- A good sample meal for general health can be made up all at once and divided between feedings.
  Mix lightly: 1 small can fish or poultry, 4TBS. whole grain kibble, 3 teasp. brewer's yeast, 1 raw egg,
  1 cup chopped vegetables, a little broth or water to moisten. THEY'LL LOVE IT.
- Don't give junk foods, refined foods, or candy to your pets. They are even worse for their smaller, simpler systems than they are for you.

Cats and dogs need slightly different diets. If you make your pet's food from scratch, the following knowledge is good to have.

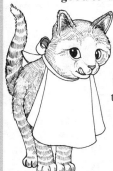

•**Key foods for cats** to provide sustained energy with the correct proportions of proteins and carbohydrates include liver, bone meal, sea vegetables, whole grains, rice and vegetables. Add some wheat bran or corn germ or oatmeal, vegetable oil and leafy greens at least three times a week.
Note: vegetarian humans should know that cats need the amino-acid taurine found in meat and fish. Without taurine, a cat may develop heart problems and possibly go blind. If liver is used, be aware that if it is more than 10% of a cat's diet (too much vitamin A), this can lead to distorted bones, gingivitis, tooth problems and stiff joints. Raw fish and raw egg whites contain an enzyme, thiaminase which inactivates Vitamin B_1, which animals need to repel fleas and mosquitos.

•**Key foods for dogs** need to be easily digestible, and based on high quality proteins and whole grains. Dog foods should be low in saturated fat. Contrary to popular advertising, dogs do not need meat as an essential part of their diet. Their quality protein can come from eggs, soy foods and low fat dairy products, as well as occasional fish or poultry. Dogs tolerate a vegetable diet better than cats because dogs are able to synthesize sufficient quantities of taurine. *Note*: Make sure your dog's diet doesn't consist of your leftover table scraps (especially spicy foods like cold pizza). The animal won't get the nutritional balance it needs.

REMEMBER:
- Both puppies and kittens need twice the nutrients and calories as adult animals.
- Pregnant and nursing females need more protein, vitamins and minerals.
- Older animals need very digestible foods, less fat and less vitamins, minerals, proteins and sodium.

Herbs and Other Supplements For A Healthy Pet

Food source supplements are good for animals. Wheat germ oil, spirulina, kelp, brewer's yeast, bran and lecithin are all good for keeping animals in tip top condition. Homeopathic remedies are good for animals, too, both in liquid and tablet form. They are effective, gentle, non-toxic, and free of side effects. They heal without harming.

Crystal Star has three highly beneficial food and herbal supplements for animals.

•HEALTHY LIFE ANIMAL MIX™ is a delicious food sprinkle packed with nutrients for a shiny coat and eyes, for healthy gums and teeth, for good temperament, regularity, immune strength and freedom from fleas and ticks. HEALTHY LIFE™ gives animals the valuable benefits of concentrated greens to keep the blood strong, the body regular and the breath and stomach sweet. It is rich in carotenes for natural immune strength. HEALTHY LIFE™ is high in antioxidants such as vitamin C and E to help control arthritis and dysplasia symptoms, and helps prevent damage from rancid fats or poor quality foods. It is full of natural enzymes for easier digestion and regularity. All kinds of animals love it, from hamsters to horses. Some of them (including our own) won't eat without it!

HEALTHY LIFE ANIMAL MIX™ is rich in chlorophyll foods. Chlorophyll is a cell stimulator, red blood builder, rejuvenator, and an internal antiseptic. Chlorophyll helps relieve respiratory troubles, discomforts in the sinus and lungs and is helpful for heart conditions.

•AR-EASE FOR ANIMALS™ eases stiff joints, and increases mobility in animals, especially larger dogs.

• SYSTEMS STRENGTH™ drink is an advanced healing combination for animals as well as people. It is a complete food-source mineral supplement, for basic body building blocks, to balance the acid/alkaline system, regulate body fluid osmosis and electrical activity in the nervous system, and to aid in digestion and regularity. SYSTEM STRENGTH™ is a rich chlorophyll and green-vitamin source, with large amounts of plant beta-carotene, B vitamins, choline, essential fatty acids with GLA, DGLA and linoleic acid, and octacosonal for tissue oxygenation. It is a vigorous source of usable proteins and amino acids. It has almost twice the amount of protein as a comparable amount of wheat germ. It is an exceptional source of alkalizing enzymes for good assimilation and digestion.

We have found it to be rapidly restorative for animal systems. Even sick or injured animals seem to know instinctively that it is good for them, and will eagerly take it as a broth from an eye dropper if they can't eat any other way.

(See ingredients and dosage listing for the above combinations in the back of this book.)

• BARLEY DOG by Green Foods Corp. is a powdered barley grass supplement. The high nutrient formula also contains garlic, brown rice and nutritional yeast.

• PET-ALOE by Pharm-Aloe, whole leaf aloe vera pet crumbles can be mixed into daily meals. The formula includes organically grown aloe vera, yucca, vitamins and minerals. It appears to be an immune system stimulator.

• PET-LYTE by Nature's Path is an aqueous solution of trace minerals for energy and balance.

Keep TEA TREE OIL and RESCUE REMEDY as first aid remedies for emergencies on hand for your pets. These natural medicinals can handle many minor emergencies, and even some major problems. All are effective and non-toxic. Tea Tree Oil is a natural, broad-spectrum antiseptic and fungicide. Tea tree oil can be used on cuts, abrasions, infections, painful sores, burns, insect bites, stings, fungus infections like ringworm and other skin conditions. In most cases the oil can be used full strength, however it may be diluted (one part tea tree to ten parts olive oil) for sensitive skin. Avoid contact with the animals eyes or other mucous membranes.

Bodywork For A Healthy Pet

• Brush and comb your animals often. It keeps their coats shiny, circulation stimulated, and they love the attention. (Brush cats gently; their skin is very sensitive.)

• Use Nature's Path SKIN-AIDE, a 5-herb blend with minerals for skin nutrients.

• Use DERMA-DREAM by Halo, Purely For Pets, as a natural healing skin salve.

• Avoid commercial, chemical-impregnated flea collars. They often have DDT or a nerve gas in them that is potentially toxic to pet, owner and environment. Use a mild shampoo with essential herbal oils for your pet. The oils interfere with the insect's ability to sense the moisture, heat and breath of the animal.

• Sprinkle cedar shavings around your animal's sleeping place to keep insects away and to make the area smell nice.

• Give your pet plenty of fresh air, exercise and water.

• Give your pets lots of love and affection. It is always the best medicine for health and happiness. They need it as much as you do.

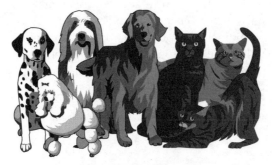

Nutritional Healing For Animals

Except in emergency situations, an optimal diet should be the key concern for natural animal healing. A wholesome diet with a greens supplement (as discussed on the previous pages) needs to be at the base of every healing program. If commercial, highly processed foods continue to be used as the major part of the diet, the problem will be harder to turn around. Many animal health problems are actually caused by poor diets. If possible, use meats without hormones or nitrates and also organically grown veggies.

ANEMIA:
- Give a diet high in protein, iron, and vitamin B_{12}. Add green vegetables for iron, minerals and enzymes. Add some beef liver occasionally for protein, B complex, B_{12} and iron.
- Give nutritional yeast flakes, sprinkled on food; or Nature's Path TOTAL-LYTE, an electrolyte yeast formula that insures good protein absorption.
- Mix about $^1/_2$ teasp. kelp into food for sea minerals and trace minerals.
- Give 500 to 2,000mg vitamin C, depending on size of animal.

ARTHRITIS:
- Avoid giving refined and preserved foods, especially white flour and sugar. Reduce red meat and canned foods. Add green and raw foods, particularly grated carrots, beets and celery.
- Make a barley grass or alfalfa tea, and add to animal's drinking water.
- Give 2 teasp. cod liver oil, 100-200IU vitamin E daily, 2 to 8 alfalfa tablets, and $^1/_4$ teasp. sodium ascorbate, Ester C powder, or vitamin C crystals daily. If you open vitamin C capsules, depending on the size and age of animal, give 250 to 2,000mg a day. (a puppy - 250mg, a great dane - 2,000mg).
- Apply Boswellia Creme to affected area.
- Give Crystal Star AR-EASE FOR ANIMALS™; or SYSTEMS STRENGTH™ broth mix, $^1/_2$ teasp. daily.
- Give shark cartilage (dose by weight); give continually until no evidence of the problem.

BAD BREATH:
- Feed more fresh foods, less canned processed foods. Snip fresh parsley into food at each meal.
- Sprinkle a little spirulina powder or Green Foods BARLEY DOG or BARLEY CAT on food.
- Give Dr. Goodpet GOOD BREATH homeopathic remedy.

BLADDER INFECTION / INCONTINENCE:
- Put the animal on a liquid diet for 24 hours of vegetable juices and broths - no solid foods, plenty of water.
- Give vitamin C 250mg twice daily, B Complex 10 to 20mg daily, magnesium 100mg daily for a week.
- Vitamin E 100IU daily for a month, then decrease to 400IU once a week.
- Use Wysong URETIC cat food for cat bldder infections and blockage.

CANCERS / LEUKEMIA / MALIGNANT TUMORS:
- Avoid commercial foods; use as much fresh, unprocessed foods as the animal will accept.
- Give vitamin C as sodium ascorbate powder, $^1/_4$ teasp. twice daily for larger animals and cats with leukemia, or Alacer EMERGEN-C in water. As tumor starts to shrink, decrease to a small daily pinch.
- Give Crystal Star SYSTEM STRENGTH™ broth 2 to 3x daily, $^1/_4$ cup or as much as animal will take.
- Shark cartilage, give continually until no evidence of the problem.
- Apply Crystal Star GINSENG SKIN REPAIR GEL™ or ANTI-BIO™ gel to tumorous areas.
- Give vitamin E 200IU daily, and apply vitamin E oil locally if there is a tumor or malignancy.
- Give NU-PET PLUS from Biogenetics as directed.
- Dilute a goldenseal/echinacea extract to $^1/_2$ strength. Give $^1/_4$ teasp. daily.
- ALOE VERA juice, 2 to 3 teasp. daily; apply aloe vera gel if tumor is visible.

COAT & SKIN HEALTH:
- Add lecithin granules, 2 teasp. cod liver, or Crystal Star HEALTHY LIFE MIX™ to food daily.
- Give vitamin E 100IU daily. Apply E oil or jojoba oil to affected skin areas.
- Add 1 teasp. Spirulina or kelp powder to food daily. Use SKIN-AIDE by Nature's Path.
- Give Dr. Goodpet SCRATCH-FREE to curb itching and dry hot spots.

CONSTIPATION:

- Add more greens and veggies to the diet; mix $^1/_2$ teasp. to 1 TBS. bran to each meal; decrease canned food.
- Add Crystal Star HEALTHY LIFE MIX™ for soluble food fiber.
- Mix a little garlic powder with 1 TB. olive oil and add to food.
- Exercise the animal more often. Let it outside more often for relief.
- Give aloe vera juice, 2 to 3 teasp. daily.

CUTS & WOUNDS:

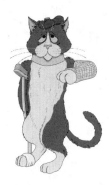

- Apply a goldenseal/myrrh solution, or comfrey salve.
- Apply vitamin E oil. Give vitamin E 100IU daily. Give RESCUE REMEDY for trauma.
- Apply calendula ointment, or DERMA-DREAM by Halo, Purely For Pets, healing salve.
- Apply aloe vera gel and give desiccated liver tabs or powder in food daily.
- Give vitamin C crystals (as sodium ascorbate if possible) $^1/_4$ to $^1/_2$ teasp. in a cup of water. Apply directly, and give internally throughout the day.

DEHYDRATION:

- This is a major emergency for cats. Check for dehydration by pulling up the scruff of the neck. If skin is slow to return, animal is dehydrated. Take to a vet as soon as possible.
- Make a comfrey tea, or Crystal Star SYSTEM STRENGTH™ broth immediately. Force feed if necessary about 2-oz. an hour. Mix a little bran, tomato juice and sesame oil. Feed each hour until improvement.
- Try to feed green veggies; especially celery, lettuce and carrots for electrolyte replacement. Once the crisis has passed, add kelp, spirulina or a green drink to the diet.
- PET-LYTE by Nature's Path is liquid minerals in electrolyte solution.
- Check for worms, often a cause of dehydration.
- Give the animal lots of love and attention. Dehydration is often caused by depression. The animal simply curls up and will not eat or drink anything. Bach Flower RESCUE REMEDY is excellent in this case.

DIABETES:

- Strictly avoid sugar-containing foods, especially soft moist animal foods that come in cellophane bags - (very high in sugar, preservatives and artificial colors)
- Lower fat intake. (Use good oils, $^1/_2$ teaspoon cod liver oil/alternate with a vegetable oil).
- Certain foods are beneficial for diabetes. It is good to emphasize in your selections:
  - Grains to use are millet, rice, oats, cornmeal, and rye bread.
  - Vegetables to use are green beans (pods contain hormonal substances closely related to insulin), dandelion greens, alfalfa sprouts, corn, parsley, onion, and garlic to reduce blood sugar.
  - Alkalizing foods like grated raw vegetables, and fermented milk products like yogurt, to help counter overacidity due to the disordered metabolism of diabetes.
  - Sprinkle nutritional yeast on food; add $^1/_2$ teasp. to 1 TB. lecithin in granular or liquid form.
- Add vitamin C - 500 milligrams to 2000mg daily depending on animals size - divide into 2 or more doses.

DIARRHEA:

- Diarrhea is often caused by spoiled food, non-food items, worms or harmful bacteria. Put the animal on a short 24 hour liquid diet with vegetable juices, broths, and lots of water.
- Give yogurt, acidophilus liquid or brewer's yeast at every feeding until diarrhea ends.
- Sprinkle crushed activated charcoal tablets on food; use Dr. Goodpet DIAR-RELIEF remedy.
- Give aloe vera juice, 2 to 3 teasp. daily.

DISTEMPER:

- If the problem is acute, put the animal on a short liquid diet with vegetable juices, broths.
- Give vitamin C crystals (sodium ascorbate if possible), $^1/_4$ teasp. mixed in water, divided throughout the day, in an eye dropper if necessary. If there is severe vomiting and loss of fluids, give some vitamin C liquid every hour. Give Dr. Goodpet CALM STRESS homeopathic remedy to calm vomiting.
- Add $^1/_2$ dropperful B complex liquid and 1 teasp. bonemeal to food daily.
- Give a dilute (1 drop extract in 2 teasp. water) goldenseal/myrrh, or echinacea solution.
- Give yogurt or acidophilus liquid to rebuild friendly flora; add Green Foods BARLEY DOG to diet.
- Give fresh garlic, or a garlic/honey mixture daily. Give raw liver or liver tablets several times a week.
- Add brown rice and bran to daily food for B vitamins and system tone.

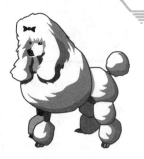

ECZEMA:

- Give zinc 25mg internally, and apply zinc ointment to infected areas.
- Mix cottage cheese, corn oil, vitamin E oil, and brewer's yeast. Give 1 TB. daily. Or give 1 teasp. cod liver oil mixed with 1 TB. garlic powder daily.
- Give Green Foods BARLEY DOG daily. Apply solution locally to sores.
- Reduce meat and canned foods. Add fresh veggies and greens to the diet.
- Use SKIN-AIDE (Pet Aid) by Nature's Path for healing and rebuilding the skin.

EAR MITES:

- Use NATURAL HERBAL EAR WASH by Halo, Purely For Pets and follow directions. This product is a soothing blend of herbal extracts in a witch hazel base. Prevents infection, heals abrasions, promotes healthy cell formation and eliminates ear wax and odors.
- Apply TEA TREE OIL regularly, or Crystal Star ANTI-BIO GEL™; or make a homemade oil treatment:
- #1 Combine $1/2$ oz. olive oil and 400IU vitamin E from a capsule in a $1/2$-oz dropper bottle. At room temperature, put a dropperful in each ear, massage ear canal, then let animal shake its head. Gently clean out ear (not deep into ear) with cotton swab. Repeat for 3 days. Let ear rest for 3 days. This mixture smothers many of the mites and starts a healing process inside ear.
- #2 Grind about 1-oz dried or 2-oz fresh thyme and rosemary and combine with $1/2$ cup olive oil - let sit in a sunny windowsill or on top of a water heater to rest for 3 days. Shake mixture a few times a day to help extract essential oils. Strain mixture into a 1 oz dropper bottle and add 400IU vitamin E. Once a day for 3 days put warmed mixture in each ear as above. Let ear rest for 10 days. Repeat herbal oil treatment for 3 days to catch any mites that may have hatched from eggs.

EYE & EAR INFECTION:

- 1 teasp. cod liver oil, and vitamin E 100IU to the diet. Cod liver oil and E oil may also be applied locally.
- Give goat's milk daily in food, and apply with cotton balls to the eye.
- Use NATURAL HERBAL EAR WASH by Halo Purely For Pets. An effective soothing blend of herbal extracts in a witch hazel base. It prevents infection, heals abrasions, promotes healthy new cell formation, and eliminates ear wax and odors; ANITRA'S HERBAL EYEWASH KIT by Halo, Purely For Pets for eye infections.
- Use Dr. Goodpet EYE-C homeopathic remedy for eyes, EAR RELIEF for ears.
- Give homeopathic *Nat. Mur* in early stages; *Silicea* in later stages to arrest cataract development.
- Apply an eyebright herb tea or Crystal Star EYEBRIGHT HERBAL™ tea to infected area.

FLEAS / TICKS / MITES: *Give floppy-eared pets a weekly ear inspection for mites and ticks.*

- Give fresh garlic, or mix $1/2$ teasp. garlic powder and 1 teasp. nutritional yeast and sprinkle on food.
- Use CLOUD-NINE HERBAL DIP by Halo, Purely For Pets.
- Have your dog swim in the ocean, or give him a seaweed bath.
- String eucalyptus buds around animal's neck, and/or strew round sleeping area. Add rosemary and bay leaves; sprinkle with cedar oil. Or put eucalyptus, pennyroyal, and citronella oils on pets collar. Or grind these herbs into a powder and sprinkle on pet and sleeping area.
- Rub rosemary, myrrh oil, or tea tree oil directly on animal's coat between shampoos. Stuff a pillow with rosemary, pennyroyal, eucalyptus and mint leaves, and place on animal's bed.
- Sprinkle Crystal Star HEALTHY LIFE MIX™ on food. Use Dr. Goodpet FLEA RELIEF homeopathic remedy.
- Give $1/2$ of a 100mg vitamin B_1 tablet daily to ward off insects.
- Apply tea tree oil directly on the insect to kill it. As an alternative to chemical dips, add a few tea tree oil drops to pet's regular shampoo. Leave on 3 to 5 minutes before rinsing.
- Apply jojoba oil on the bitten place to heal it faster.

House treatments:

- Vacuum carpets and bare floors. For carpet infestation, the most effective solution is inorganic salts (sodium bo rate). Use only 100% pure borates such as TERMINATOR by Canine Care Inc. This product is non-toxic, safe to use around children & pets, highly effective and outlasts toxic insecticides.
- Use carpet and bedding sprays containing citronella, eucalyptus, tea tree oil, and lemon grass oils. (Make your own up if possible; chemical foggers and sprays can be very toxic to people and pets).
- Natural pyrethrum powders are safe unless they contain additives.

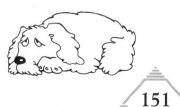

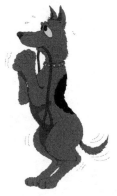

GAS & FLATULENCE:
- Give alfalfa tabs, spirulina, or Green Foods BARLEY DOG at each feeding.
- Sprinkle a pinch of ginger powder on food at each feeding.
- Give comfrey, chamomile or peppermint tea daily.

GUM & TOOTH PROBLEMS:
- Apply a dilute goldenseal/myrrh or propolis solution to gums.
- Give Green Foods BARLEY DOG. Apply a liquid solution directly.
- Give a natural fresh foods diet, adding crunchy raw veggies and whole grains.
- Apply vitamin E oil, tea tree oil, or calendula oil to gums.
- Rub vitamin C - a weak solution of ascorbate crystals in water on the gums.

HIP DYSPLASIA & LAMENESS (See also ARTHRITIS):
- Mix 1 teasp. sodium ascorbate, or Ester-C crystals in water and give throughout the day, every day.
- Mix 1 teasp. bonemeal powder in 1 c. tomato juice, with 1 teasp. bran and $\frac{1}{2}$ teasp. sesame oil. Give daily.
- Give Crystal Star AR-EASE FOR ANIMALS™ daily, or NU-PET PLUS for pets from Biogenetics as directed.
- Give shark cartilage, as directed, continually until no evidence of the problem.

INTESTINAL & STOMACH PROBLEMS:
- Put animal on a short liquid fast for 24 hours, with water, broth and green juices to clear intestines. Then feed yogurt or liquid acidophilus and fresh foods for 2-3 days. Give comfrey tea in the water bowl.
- Give Crystal Star HEALTHY LIFE MIX™ with $\frac{1}{2}$ teasp. extra garlic powder daily.
- Give garlic, mullein/myrrh extract, or echinacea or black walnut extract diluted in water, or mugwort tea.

MANGE & FUNGAL INFECTION:
- Put drops of tea tree oil in the animal's shampoo; use every 2 or 3 days. Use tea tree oil directly on infected areas - by itself or diluted with olive oil.
- Apply PAU D' ARCO salve, zinc ointment and fresh lemon juice to relieve area.
- Use Dr. Goodpet CALM STRESS remedy.
- Apply dilute echinacea tincture, or goldenseal/echinacea/myrrh water solution to affected areas daily. Also sprinkle on food. Add bonemeal powder to food to ease tension and curb frantic licking.
- Apply SKIN-AIDE by Nature's Path for skin healing and rebuilding, or Crystal Star FUNG-EX GEL™.
- Give 1 teasp. lecithin granules daily. Mix 2 teasp. cod liver oil with 1 TB. brewer's yeast and 2 teasp. desiccated liver powder. Give daily.

OVERWEIGHT:
- Reduce canned and saturated fat foods. Increase fresh foods, whole grains and organ meats.
- Give Crystal Star HEALTHY LIFE MIX™ for fiber without calories.
- Add more exercise to the animal's life.

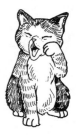

PREGNANCY & BIRTH:
- Give red raspberry tea daily during the last half of gestation for easier birth.
- Give daily spirulina tabs or powder for extra protein.
- Give desiccated liver tabs, extra bonemeal, and cod liver oil daily.
- Give extra vitamin C 100mg chewable, and vitamin E 100IU daily.

RESPIRATORY INFECTIONS & IMMUNE STRENGTH:
- Put animal on a short liquid diet for 24 hours to cleanse the system, with vegetable juices, broths and water. Offer comfrey tea to flush toxins faster.
- Give Crystal Star HEALTHY LIFE MIX™ for immune strength. COFEX TEA™ for dry hacking cough.
- Give Crystal Star SYSTEM STRENGTH™ broth 2 to 3 times daily, about $\frac{1}{4}$ cup, or what the animal will take.
- Add 1 teasp. bee pollen, vitamin E 100IU, and $\frac{1}{4}$ teasp. vitamin C (as sodium ascorbate if possible) dissolved in a cup of water to diet.
- Add 2 to 4 garlic tablets and 6 alfalfa tablets to the daily diet.
- Give Green Foods BARLEY DOG or BARLEY CAT.

WORMS & PARASITES:
- Build up parasite immunity with Crystal Star HEALTHY LIFE MIX™, as directed daily.
- Put the animal on a short 24 hour liquid fast with water to weaken the parasites. Then give Crystal Star VERMEX CAPS™ as directed with charcoal tabs in water or an electuary for 3 to 7 days. Repeat process in a week to kill newly hatched eggs.
- Mix $^1/_2$ teasp. garlic powder and a pinch of cloves; sprinkle on food daily until worms are gone. Then, give spirulina or Green Foods BARLEY DOG or BARLEY CAT for a month after worming to rebuild immune strength.
- Garlic, mullein/myrrh blend; echinacea or black walnut extract diluted in water, or mugwort tea.

Note: Acupuncture has been a very successful alternative treatment for animals - especially in cases of arthritis, hip dysplasia, asthma, epilepsy, cervical-disk displacements and chronic infections.

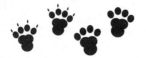

About Animals & Toxic Substances

There is a wide range of substances that are harmful or lethal to animals. They include pesticides from lawn and garden products, rat poison, commercial flea killers, herbicides like Round-Up, and others. House cleaning products and disinfectants, building and decorating hazards, like paint and outgassing from synthetic carpets are toxic when you're only 12 inches off the ground. They are hazardous to small pets that have to live so close to them. Animals can get into things that humans leave in the reach of the pets they love. Many household substances are also harmful to humans. Use products that are environmentally safe as a general rule.

Many people are unaware of plant poisoning. Laurel, commonly used in dried flower arrangements, Christmas mistletoe, poinsettias, jimson weed, and oleander can cause death in a pet. Dogs who love to dig and chew the bulbs of the hyacinth can experience convulsions.

I recommend the medicine-chest information from The National Animal Poison Control Center, University of Illinois College of Veterinary Medicine, 2001 S. Lincoln Ave., Urbana , IL 61801. It's a good idea to call them before you have an emergency at 217-333-2053. This organization is the first animal-oriented poison center in the United States. They provide advice to animal owners who suspect pesticide, drug, plant, metal and other poisonous exposures and who are in a panic and can't get to a veterinarian immediately. The phones are answered by licensed veterinarians and board-certified veterinary toxicologists.

Emergency calls go to 1-900-680-000 (there is a charge) or 1-800-548-2423 (credit cards, no charge).

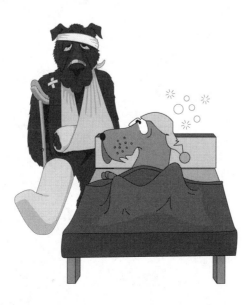

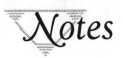

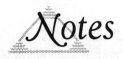

The Details Of
Detoxification & Cleansing

DETOXIFICATION IS BECOMING NECESSARY FOR EVERYBODY. NO ONE IS FREE FROM THE ENORMOUS AMOUNT OF ENVIRONMENTAL TOXINS ASSAULTING US IN THE WORLD TODAY; NO ONE IS IMMUNE TO EVERY UNHEALTHY LIFESTYLE OPTION. HOW DO WE REMAIN HEALTHY IN A DESTRUCTIVE ENVIRONMENT?

This section discusses detoxification in detail - including the signs that your body needs a good cleansing, and the types of detox programs you can use to best suit your individual needs.

It defines a good detoxification program, how it works in the body, and the benefits you can expect.

Step by step instructions are included for the initial diets, supplements, and herbs you'll need, along with tried and true watchwords that can give you the best results.

DETOXIFICATION PROGRAMS ARE INCLUDED FOR:
- Colon and bowel cleansing
- Bladder and kidney cleansing
- Lung and mucous congestion cleansing
- Liver and organ cleansing
- Blood cleansing - for heavy metal toxicity, serious immune deficient diseases, and alcohol and drug addictions

A Basic Guide To Detoxification
Body Cleansing Is Becoming Necessary For Everybody

There's no doubt about it. Americans are immersed in synthetic, often toxic substances. Every system of the body is affected, from deep level tissue damage to sensory deterioration.

Today, people are exposed to chemicals on an unprecedented scale. Industrial chemicals and their pollutant by-products, pesticides and additives in our foods, heavy metals, anesthetics, residues from all kinds of drugs, and environmental hormones are trapped within the human body in greater concentrations than at any other point in history.

Many chemicals are so widely spread that we are unaware of them. But they have worked their way into our bodies faster than they can be eliminated, and are causing allergies and addictions in record numbers. And these things don't even count the secondary smoke, caffeine and alcohol overloads, or daily stress that are an increasing part of our lives.

More than 2 million synthetic substances are known, 25,000 are added each year, and over 30,000 are produced on a commercial scale. Only a tiny fraction are ever tested for toxicity. A lot of them come to us on the winds from developing countries that have few safeguards in place.

Because the molecular structure of many chemical carcinogens interacts with human DNA, long term exposure can result in metabolic and genetic alteration that affects cell growth, behavior and immune response. New research by the World Health Organization implicates toxic environmental chemicals in 60 to 80% of all cancers.

Studies also link pesticides and pollutants to hormone dysfunctions, psychological disorders, birth defects, still births and now breast cancer. The wide variety of toxic substances means that every system of the body is affected - from deep level tissue damage to sensory deterioration.

As toxic matter saturates our tissues, and anti-oxidants and minerals in vital body fluids are reduced, immune defenses are thrown out of balance. Vitality is overwhelmed and eventually disease begins. Circumstances like this have become the prime factor in today's immune compromised diseases like candidiasis, lupus, fibromyalgia, chronic fatigue syndrome, and cancer.

Chemical oxidation is the other process that affects body degeneration and allows disease. The oxygen that "rusts" and ages us also triggers free radical activity, a destructive cascade of incomplete molecules that damages DNA and other cell components. And if you didn't have a reason to reduce your fat intake before, oxygen combines with fats in body storage cells to speed up the free radical deterioration process.

How do you know if you need to detoxify? Almost everybody does. It's one of the best ways to remain healthy in a destructive environment. Not one of us is immune to environmental toxins, and most of us can't escape to a remote, pristine habitat. We **can** take a closer look at our own air, water and food, and keep an ever watchful eye on the politics that control our environment. Legislation on health and the environment follows two pathways in America today...the influence of business and profits, and the demands of the people for a healthy environment and responsible stewardship of the Earth.

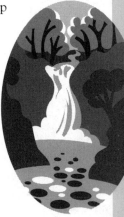

I believe we are in a paradigm shift in humanity's time on the planet. For millions of years, the Earth has controlled its own destiny. But humans have risen in intelligence and command, to challenge the universe - even the Earth and the stars.

In the last few decades we have become dangerously able to harm the health of our planet, even to the point of making it uninhabitable for life. We must develop further and take even larger steps... not the steps of rulers or challengers, but those of cooperation and support.

The analogy to atomic power is clear. *Fission is great, but fusion is greater.*

The well-being of the world depends on the cooperation of mankind and the Earth together, to save it for us all. It starts with ourselves. We can take positive steps to keep our own body systems in good working order, so that toxins are eliminated quickly.

Our bodies are clearly created as self-cleaning, self-healing mechanisms. Internal detoxification is an ongoing process performed on a daily basis. Just as our hearts beat nonstop and our lungs breathe automatically, so our metabolic processes continually dispose of wastes and poisons. Detoxification is the body's natural process of eliminating or neutralizing toxins, by the liver, the kidneys, urine, feces, exhalation, and perspiration. If you keep immune response high, elimination regular, circulation sound, and stress under control, your body can handle a great deal of toxicity and regularly prevent disease.

Yet body systems and organs that were once completely capable of detoxification are now so overloaded that they are largely unable to purify us of the daily poisons that assault us. So poisons build and build in our systems, and eventually result in disease.

In the past, detoxification was used either clinically for recovering alcoholics and drug addicts, or individually as a once-a-year mild "spring cleaning" for general health maintenance. Today, a regular detoxification program two or three times a year can make a big difference in the way your body performs. In fact, it might be the missing link for preventing chronic opportunistic diseases like cancer, candida, chronic fatigue, arthritis, diabetes and obesity.

Most people eat too much animal protein, fat, caffeine, alcohol, and chemicalized foods that inhibit optimum cell function. Even if your diet is good, a cleanse can restore body vitality against environmental toxins. Detoxification is becoming necessary not only for health, but for the quality of our lives.

HERE ARE SOME SIGNS THAT YOU MAY NEED TO DETOXIFY:
- If you get frequent, unexplained headaches or back pain,
- if you have chronic respiratory problems, sinus problems or asthma,
- if you have abnormal body odor, bad breath or coated tongue,
- if you have food allergies, poor digestion, or constipation with chronic intestinal bloating, or gas.
- if you have brittle nails and hair, psoriasis, adult acne, or unexplained weight gain over 10 pounds,
- if you have joint pain, or arthritis,
- if you are depressed and irritable, and always out of energy,
- if you have unusually poor memory and chronic insomnia.

HERE ARE SOME OF THE BENEFITS YOU CAN EXPECT FROM A BODY CLEANSE:
- Your digestive tract is cleansed of accumulated waste and fermenting bacteria.
- Liver, kidney and blood purification take place, impossible under ordinary eating patterns.
- Mental clarity is enhanced, impossible under chemicals and food additive overload.
- Dependency on habit-forming substances, such as sugar, caffeine, nicotine, alcohol and drugs, is reduced as the blood stream is purified.
- Bad eating habits are often turned around, and the stomach has a chance to reduce to normal size for weight control.

✤A good detox program should be in 3 stages .... cleansing, rebuilding and maintaining.

HERE ARE THE STEPS FOR TAILORING A DETOXIFICATION PROGRAM TO YOUR SPECIFIC NEEDS.

First consider what you really need to do. A detox is essentially cleansing the body of waste deposits, so you aren't running with a dirty engine or driving with the brakes on.
- Do you need a mild spring body cleansing?
- Do you need to eliminate drug residues?
- Does your body need to normalize after a disease or hospital stay?
- Do you need a jump start for a healing program?
- Do you need a specific detox program for a serious health problem?

Next, consider the time factor. How much time can you take out of your busy life style to focus on a cleansing program? 24 hours, 2 or 3 days, or up to ten days? It's important to allot your time ahead of time, so that all the processes of the cleanse can be completed.

Do you always have to fast? A few days without solid food can be a refreshing and enlightening experience about your lifestyle. A short fast increases awareness as well as energy availability for elimination. Your body will become easier to "hear." It can tell you what foods and diet are right for your needs via cravings, such as a desire for protein foods, or B vitamins or minerals, for example.

Kind of like a "cellular phone call," body cravings are natural bio-feedback.

Fasting works by self-digestion. During a cleanse, the body decomposes and burns only the substances and tissues that are damaged, diseased or unneeded, such as abscesses, tumors, excess fat deposits, and congestive wastes. Even a relatively short fast accelerates elimination, often causing dramatic changes as masses of accumulated waste are expelled. Live foods and juices literally pick up dead matter from the body and carry it away.

You will be very aware of this if you experience the short period of headaches, fatigue, body odor, bad breath, diarrhea or mouth sores that commonly accompany accelerated elimination. However, digestion usually improves right away as do many gland and nerve functions.

The second part of a good cleansing program is rebuilding healthy tissue and restoring body energy. This phase allows the body's regulating powers to become active with obstacles removed, so it can rebuild at optimum levels. A rebuilding diet emphasizes fresh and simply prepared foods. It should be very low in fat, with little dairy, and no fried food. Avoid alcohol, caffeine, tobacco, and sugars. Avoid meats except fish and sea foods. Supplements and herbal aids may be included for specific needs.

The final part of a good cleansing program is keeping your body clean and toxin-free - very important after all the hard work of detoxification. Modifying lifestyle habits to include high quality nutrition from both food and supplement sources is the key to a strong resistant body.

A diet for health maintenance should rely heavily on fresh fruits and vegetables for fiber, cooked vegetables, grains and seeds for strength and alkalinity, sea foods, soy foods, eggs, and low fat cheeses as alternate sources of protein, and lightly cooked sea foods and vegetables with a little dinner wine for circulatory health. A personalized group of supplements and herbal aids, as well as exercise and relaxation techniques, should be included.

Cleansing also helps release hormone secretions that stimulate immune response, and encourage a disease-preventing environment. After a cleanse, the body starts rebalancing, energy levels rise physically, psychologically and sexually, and creativity begins to expand. You start feeling like a "different person" - and of course you are.

Your outlook and attitude change, because through cleansing and improved diet, your actual cell make-up has changed.

You really are what you eat.

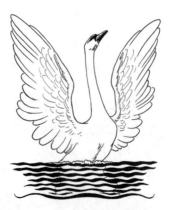

Different Types Of Detoxification Programs

$\mathcal{T}$here are several effective types of cleanses you can tailor to your specific needs. Unless you are addressing a serious illness, or recovering from a long course of drugs or chemical therapy, you should consider a detoxification cleanse twice a year, especially in the spring, summer or early fall, when sunlight and natural vitamin D can offer the body an extra boost.

A mild "spring cleanse" is important in a naturally healthy lifestyle. Even though we exercise during the winter to keep our bodies trim, most people still feel at an energy low during cold seasons. And there is no question, much to the dismay of many of us, that fall and winter are the most difficult times of the year to lose and control our weight. Our bodies still reflect the ancient seasonal need to harbor more fat for warmth and survival.

In the days when people were closer to nature than we are today, the great majority farmed the land from spring to fall, and lived lives of demanding physical labor. Winter was a time of inactivity, with a natural tendency towards rest. Food supplies stored in the autumn lost much of their nutrition. Even in modern times, many days without sunshine and vitamin D mean that our bodies are less able to utilize nutrients properly. And cold weather prompts people to consume heavier, fattier, comfort foods.

Winter weather illnesses like colds and flu leave us with an accumulation of toxins. Heavy winter clothing, especially thick waterproof coats, hinder deep breathing and perspiration, and contribute to clogged body functions. When spring finally arrives, our metabolism livens up. Warmer weather tends to lower appetites and prompts more activity and movement. It's easier to stimulate cleansing processes. New, green food sources, with their metabolism-stimulating effects, abound from the first tender shoots of herbs and leafy vegetables. Cleansing, antioxidant-rich herbs promote a feeling of new life and restored well-being. It's time to go on a spring cleanse.

A "spring cleaning" is actually a very light diet, focusing on digestion and the intestines to help eliminate accumulated wastes, and improve body functions. A good length for a spring or summer cleanse is 2 or 3 days or a long weekend. A weekend is enough time to fit comfortably into most people's lives, and it doesn't become too stressful on the body. The best way is to start on Friday night with a pre-cleansing salad, then follow with a cleansing diet like the one in this book, and end with a light Monday morning fruit bowl. Amplify the purifying effect with a stimulating, circulation bath.

A three to ten day healing cleanse focuses on more ambitious detoxification, and it's often a good choice for those who are addressing serious health problems. I recommend using this type of detox for only 10 days at any one time. Cleansing for more than ten days may dredge up deep seated toxins (like DDT) that when released can result in concentrated amounts that the body can't handle, especially if it is in a weakened state. Body stress may also increase to the point where healing stops, defeating the purpose of the cleanse.

If you want to go on a longer detox schedule, break it up into several segments of 7 to 10 days each, and adjust your target areas for specific health problems.

A long 4 day weekend is an ideal starting time for many people, even for relatively serious problems. Remember, a detox and cleanse is just the beginning of your healing program. Don't overdo it. Efficient, yet gentle herbal aids to cleansing can go a long way to accelerating the process, and shortening the time frame.

As with other cleanses, a longer detox involves a pre-fasting meal, aimed at tee-ing your body up for increased elimination. It moves into a juice fast accompanied with supplements, plenty of water, some exercise and stress-reduction techniques. Arranging the order and types of juices, supplements, exercise and bodywork choices vary depending on specific needs.

A 24 hour cleanse can be a good answer if you need a cleanse, but your busy life won't allow you to set aside even a few days. People always tell me how busy their lives are. Even a short cleanse seems like too much time.

"Beginning" is usually the hardest part of a cleanse. You have to set aside a block of time, gather all the ingredients for your diet, alter eating times and patterns; in essence change your lifestyle and that of those you live with for a while. This is very difficult to do for many people, and can delay a needed program.

A 24-hour detox is a juice and herbal tea cleanse that lets you go on with your normal activities, and "jump start" a healing program. Even though it's quick, without the depth of vegetable juices needed for a major or chronic problem, it's often enough, is definitely better than no cleanse at all, and it will make a difference in the speed of healing. Even if your program is only going to consist of lifestyle changes aimed at better health, a 24 hour cleanse can point you in the right direction.

- Start the night before with a green leafy salad to give your bowels a good sweeping. Dry brush your skin before you go to bed to open your pores for the night's cleansing eliminations.
- Then take the next 24 hours for fresh juices, pure water, and a long walk during the day.

On rising: take a glass of 2 fresh squeezed lemons, 1TB. maple syrup and 8-oz. of pure water.
Midmorning: take a glass of cranberry juice from concentrate.
Lunch: take a glass of fresh apple juice, or apple/alfalfa sprout juice with 1 packet of chlorella or Green Foods GREEN MAGMA granules dissolved in it.
Midafternoon: take a cup of Crystal Star CLEANSING & PURIFYING™ TEA or MEDITATION™ TEA.
Dinner: take a glass of papaya/pineapple juice to enhance enzyme production, or another glass of apple juice with 1 packet SUN CHLORELLA or Green Foods GREEN MAGMA granules.
Before bed: have a cup of mint tea, or 1 teasp. Organic Gourmet's NUTRITIONAL YEAST extract or MISO soup in a cup of hot water for relaxation and strength the next day.

•The next morning, break your fast with fresh fruits and yogurt. Eat light, raw foods during the day, and have a simply prepared, low fat dinner that night.

Take a seaweed or mineral bath in the morning and one before you go to bed. Add some favorite beauty/cleansing treatments like a facial, a pedicure, manicure and deep hair conditioning during your bath. Get a full eight hours of rest that night, and start the next morning as the first day of a healthy diet change aimed at restoring your optimum health.

A 7 day brown rice cleanse is an effective option to a juice cleanse. It's based on macrobiotic principles, and is effective for dropping a few quick pounds and balancing your body when it's feeling low in energy or out-of-sorts. The diet is simple, easy to take, and easy to fit in with your lifestyle.

1 Simply drink 2 to 3 glasses of mixed vegetable juices throughout the day whenever you like. Use the "Personal Best Juice" recipe on page 168 of this book, or something like Knudsen's Very Veggie Juice, or even regular V-8 juice. Don't eat any solid food during the day.
2 Have steamed brown rice and mixed vegetables for an early dinner. Any blend of your favorite vegetables is fine. Have at least a cup of rice and several cups of vegetables.
3 Add any non-fat seasonings to your own taste. NO butter or oil dressings.

That's all there is to it. Follow this diet for 6 days. Results in weight, body definition and body chemistry change are noticeable almost immediately. You need the six days to set up an ongoing body balance. Then ease yourself into a good, on-going healthy diet. Try not to let the "reward mode" trigger a binge on fats and sugars.

Much of the time your body will crave the healthy nutrients it needs. You can watch for these. It's interesting!

Detoxification Diets For Specific Body Needs

*Y*our diet is the place to start a cleanse. The modern diet has too many animal proteins, fats, caffeine, alcohol, and chemicals for our bodies to function very well. A poor diet with over-processed food, fried foods, and clogging, low-fiber food, sets the stage for toxic build-up. Not only is nutrition low, but a diet of these foods doesn't have the necessary enzymes for good digestion, nor the fiber to assist in proper elimination. Here are five body systems that need cleansing most.

The Colon Elimination Cleanse: *a 3 to 10 day liquid diet*

A colon elimination cleanse is something most of us need. The bowel and colon are essential to body detoxification. Just like a city, our bodies deteriorate if our sewage systems aren't cared for. When colon health is compromised, there is greater release of toxins from the bowel into the bloodstream, causing diseases, organ dysfunction and accelerated aging. Constipation is usually a chronic problem, and while body cleansing progress can be felt fairly quickly with a diet change, it takes from three to six months to rebuild bowel and colon elasticity with good systole/diastole action. The rewards of a regular, energetic life are worth it.

Elements causing colon toxicity come from three basic areas:

1 **Slow elimination time.** Constipation contributes to toxicity. Slow bowel transit time allows wastes to become rancid, and then recirculate through the body. Blood capillaries lining the colon wall absorb these poisons into the bloodstream, exposing all body tissues and organs to the toxins, lowering overall performance of body functions, and setting the stage for health problems. Bowel transit time should be approximately twelve hours. Over 80% of all human ailments, including headaches, skin blemishes, senility, bad breath, fatigue, arthritis and heart disease can be attributed to a congested colon. Waste overload can become a breeding ground for parasite infestation, too. A nationwide survey reveals that one in every six people has parasites living somewhere in the body.

2 **Synthetic chemicals in food and environmental pollutants.** A clean, strong system can metabolize and excrete many of these, but when the body is weak or constipated, they are stored as unusable substances. As more and different chemicals enter the body they tend to inter-react with those that are already there, forming second generation chemicals far more harmful than the originals. Evidence in recent years shows that most colon cancer is a direct result of accumulated toxic waste. Colon cancer is the second leading cancer in the United States today, only slightly behind lung cancer in men and breast cancer in women. Colitis, irritable bowel syndrome, diverticulosis, ileitis and Crohn's disease, are all signs of poor waste management. And they're on the rise. Over 100,000 Americans have a colostomy every year! An incredible fact.

3 **The most common signal of toxic bowel overload is poor digestion.** Our rich diet of meats, refined foods, salt and sugar, means we get a lot of grease and little fiber. Food fiber's importance comes from its ability to move food through the digestive system quickly and easily, but the Standard American Diet causes a glue-y state that can't be efficiently processed by the intestines. You can picture this if you remember the hard paste formed by white flour and water when you were a kid. Foods are simply crammed into the colon and never fully excreted.

A high fiber, whole foods diet is both cure and prevention for waste elimination problems. It seems like so much media attention has been focused on high fiber foods for so long, that everybody in America would have changed their diet to a more colon-health oriented pattern. This is simply not the case. Most diet attention has been targeted at reducing fat at all costs, often at the expense of a healthy, fiber-rich diet. Even a gentle, gradual change from low fiber, low residue foods helps almost immediately. In fact, a gradual change is better than a sudden, drastic about-face, especially when the colon is inflamed.

THE PROTECTIVE LEVEL OF FIBER IN THE DIET IS EASILY MEASURED:
- The stool should be light enough to float.
  - Bowel movements should be regular, daily and effortless.
  - The stool should be almost odorless, signalling decreased bowel transit time.
  - There should be no gas or flatulence.
  Good policy: Make a mental note of your colon health every time you have a bowel movement to prevent problems.

What are the signs that you might need a colon cleanse?

Look for reduced immunity, tiredness, coated tongue, bad breath, body odor, mental dullness and sallow skin.

If your cholesterol numbers are too high, a colon cleanse is a good choice because it increases absorption of cholesterol-lowering foods and also helps you lose colon congestive weight. **You can easily combine a colon cleanse with a cholesterol cleanse.** Add a fiber-rich supplement such as Crystal Star CHO-LO-FIBER TONE™ for easy fiber, appetite suppression, and acidophilus to restore friendly digestive flora.

Bowel elimination problems are often chronic, and may require several rounds of cleansing. This cleanse may be done all at once or in periods of five days each.

Anyone with a sensitive colon should heal the colon before cleansing it. A very gentle herbal formula like Crystal Star BWL-TONE IBS™ would be a good choice. Avoid a colon cleanser that contains senna or psyllium husks if you have a sensitive or irritated bowel.

HERE ARE SOME BRIEF POINTERS TO GIVE YOU THE BEST RESULTS FOR YOUR COLON CLEANSE:

•A colonic irrigation is a good way to start a bowel cleanse. Grapefruit seed extract is very effective, especially if there is colon toxicity along with constipation. (Dilute to 15 to 20 drops in a gallon of water.) Or take a catnip or diluted liquid chlorophyll enema every other night during the cleanse. *Note:* Enemas may be given to children. Use smaller amounts according to size and age. Allow water to enter very slowly; let them expel when they wish.

•Drink six to eight glasses of water daily during a colon cleanse.

•Be sure to take a brisk walk for an hour every day to help keep your elimination channels moving.

•Take several long warm baths during your cleanse. A lower back and pelvis massage and dry skin brushing will help release toxins coming out through the skin.

The night before you begin.....

•Take a gentle herbal laxative, such as HERBALTONE tablets, AloeLife FIBER MATE powder or Crystal Star LAXA-TEA™. Herbal combinations provide cleansing, tonifying activity to cleanse efficiently and gently.

•Soak dried figs, prunes and raisins in water to cover; add 1TB. unsulphured molasses, cover, leave overnight.

The next day....

On rising: take Nature's Secret SUPERCLEANSE tablets in juice or water;
  or 1 heaping teasp. Crystal Star CHO-LO FIBER TONE™ DRINK MIX (either flavor) in water.

Breakfast: discard dried fruits from their soaking water and take a small glass of the liquid.

Mid-morning: take 2 TBS. AloeLife ALOE GOLD concentrate in a glass of juice or water.

Lunch: take a small glass of potassium broth or essence (page 167); or a glass of fresh carrot juice.

Mid-afternoon: take a large glass of fresh apple juice; or an herb tea such as alfalfa, fennel, or red clover;
  or Crystal Star CLEANSING & PURIFYING™ tea to enhance elimination and provide energy support.

About 5 o' clock: take another small glass of potassium broth or essence; or another fresh carrot juice;
  or a vegetable drink (page 168), or Green Foods GREEN ESSENCE, or Crystal Star ENERGY GREEN™ drink.

Supper: take a large glass of apple juice or papaya juice.
  (Note: Break the fast with a small raw foods salad on the last night of the cleanse.)

Before Bed: repeat the herbal body cleansers that you took on rising, and take a cup of mint tea.

Suggested herbal aids for the bowel elimination cleanse:

•Take 4 to 6 Crystal Star FIBER & HERBS COLON CLEANSE™ caps daily, to help increase systole/diastole activity of the colon, and tone bowel tissue during heavy elimination.

Note: Drugstore laxatives aren't really body cleansers. They offer only temporary relief, are usually habit-forming, destructive to intestinal membranes and don't even get to the cause of the problem. They enable the bowels to expel debris because the colon becomes so irritated by the laxative that it expels whatever loose material is around.

After the initial bowel cleansing program, the second part of a colon health system is rebuilding healthy tissue and body energy. This stage takes 1 to 2 months for best results. It emphasizes high fiber through fresh vegetables and fruits, cultured foods for increased assimilation and enzyme production, and alkalizing foods to prevent irritation while healing. Avoid refined foods, saturated fats or oils, fried foods, meats, caffeine or other acid/mucous forming foods, such as pasteurized dairy products.

The Bladder/Kidney Cleanse: *a 3 to 5 day liquid diet.*

Kidney function is vital to health. The kidneys are largely responsible for the elimination of waste products from protein breakdown (such as urea and ammonia). If the movement of salts, proteins or other bio-chemicals goes awry, a whole range of health problems arises, from mild water retention to major kidney failure, and mineral loss. Concentrated protein wastes can cause chronic inflammation of the kidney filtering tissues (nephritis), and can overload the bloodstream with toxins, causing uremia. Naturopaths emphasize the importance of ample, high-quality water for kidney health. Dehydration is the most common stress on the kidneys. Body purification systems operate efficiently only if the volume of water flowing through them is sufficient to carry away wastes. Drink 6 to 8 glasses of water or other cleansing fluids daily for kidney health.

But your bladder and kidneys do more than just remove water wastes. They are part of a complex process that maintains body fluid stability. Urinary controls are involved with the brain, hormones, and receptors all over the body. They are smart controls that register what your body needs in the way of fluids. So sometimes they remove very little salt or water, at other times they remove a lot.

A bladder and kidney cleanse is simple, and usually works right away. A three to five day cleanse can often clear out toxic infection quickly. If you have chronic lower back pain, irritated urination, frequent unexplained chills, fever, or nausea, and fluid retention, you may be feeling the inflammation of a kidney infection. A gentle, natural, kidney cleansing course might be just the thing to keep you from getting a full-blown kidney or bladder infection.

HERE ARE SOME BRIEF POINTERS TO GIVE YOU THE BEST RESULTS FOR YOUR KIDNEY CLEANSE:
- Drink 10 glasses of bottled water each day of your cleanse.
- Avoid dietary irritants on the kidneys, such as coffee, alcohol, and excessive protein.
- Herbal supplements provide excellent support for a kidney cleanse. Take them as liquids for best results.
- Take a liquid green supplement daily, such as Green Foods GREEN ESSENCE, or Sun CHLORELLA.
- Apply wet, hot compresses on the lower back to speed cleansing; or take alternating hot and cold sitz baths.

The night before you begin....
- Take a cleansing herb tea, such as oatstraw, cornsilk, or Crystal Star BLDR-K™ TEA. This tea may also be used throughout the cleanse. Add $^1/_4$ teasp. ascorbate C crystals to the tea every time you take it.

The next day....
On rising: take a glass of lemon juice and water, with 1 teasp. acidophilus liquid;
    or 3 teasp. cranberry concentrate in a small glass of water with $^1/_4$ to $^1/_2$ teasp. ascorbate C crystals;
    or 2 TBS. cider vinegar in a glass of water with 1 teasp. honey.
Breakfast: have a glass of watermelon juice, or another glass of cranberry juice with $^1/_4$ teasp. vitamin C crystals;
    or a glass of organic apple juice with $^1/_4$ teasp. high potency acidophilus complex powder.
Mid-morning: take 1 cup of watermelon seed tea. (Grind seeds, steep in hot water 30 minutes, add honey);
    or a potassium broth or essence (page 167), with 2 teasp. Bragg's LIQUID AMINOS;
    or a cup of Crystal Star BLDR-K™ tea.
Lunch: have a vegetable drink (page 168), or Sun CHLORELLA, or Crystal Star ENERGY GREEN™ in water;
    or a glass of carrot juice, or carrot/beet/cucumber juice, every other day.
Mid-afternoon: take a cup of healing herb tea, such as parsley/oatstraw, plantain tea, or cornsilk tea;
    or Crystal Star BLDR-K™ TEA;
    or another cup of watermelon seed tea.
    Dinner: have another carrot juice, with 1 teasp. liquid chlorophyll or spirulina added;
        or another cranberry juice with $^1/_4$ teasp. ascorbate vitamin C crystals added.
    Before Bed: take a glass of papaya or apple juice with $^1/_4$ teasp. high potency acidophilus powder.

- After your cleanse, add sea foods and sea vegetables, whole grains and vegetable proteins. Continue with a morning green drink or Crystal Star GREEN TEA CLEANSER™ for the rest of the month.
- Kidney healing foods include garlic and onions, papayas, bananas, watermelon, sprouts, leafy greens and cucumbers. Take some of these frequently during the rest of the month. Avoid heavy starches, red and prepared meats, dairy products (except yogurt or kefir), refined, salty, fatty and fast foods. They all inhibit kidney filtering.
- Take hot saunas to release toxins and excess fluids, and to flush acids out through the skin.
- For kidney stones, see OLIVE OIL FLUSHES under the Liver Cleansing Liquid Diet in this book.

161

The Mucous Congestion Cleanse: *a 3 to 7 day liquid diet.*

A lung and mucous congestion cleanse can help if you have chronic colds, allergies or asthma. We tend to think of body mucous as a bad thing. But the same mucous, that obstructs our breathing during a sinus infection, asthma or a cold, also protects our tissues. Excess mucous may be a sign that the body is trying to bring itself to health.

Human beings take about 22,000 breaths a day, and along with the oxygen, we take in dirt, pollen, disease germs, smoke and other pollutants. Mucous gathers up these irritants as they enter the nose and throat, protecting the mucous membranes that line the upper respiratory system.

Your body systems together. It may seem, as we discuss its different parts and processes, that they are not wholly related. Extra pressure of disease or heavy elimination on one part of the body puts extra stress on another. Support for the kidneys, for example, takes part of the waste elimination load off the lungs so they can recover faster. Similarly, promoting respiratory health also helps digestive and skin cleansing problems. The lungs, though, are on the front line of toxic intake from viruses, allergies, pollutants, and mucous-forming congestives. Our own lung health is the reason we need to care for the vital lungs of the earth through rainforest preservation.

A program to overcome any chronic respiratory problem is usually more successful when begun with a short mucus elimination diet. This allows the body to rid itself first of toxins and accumulations that cause congestion before an attempt is made to change eating habits.

HERE ARE SOME BRIEF POINTERS TO GIVE YOU THE BEST RESULTS FOR YOUR EXCESS MUCOUS CLEANSE:

• Herbal supplements are a good choice during a mucous and congestion cleanse. They act as premier broncho-dilators and anti-spasmodics to open congested airspaces. They can soothe bronchial inflammation and cough. They have the ability to break up mucus. They are expectorants to remove mucus from the lungs and throat.

• Drink 8 to 10 glasses of water daily to thin mucous and aid elimination.

• Take 10,000mg ascorbate vitamin C crystals with bioflavonoids daily the first three days; just dissolve $\frac{1}{4}$ teasp. in water or juice throughout the day, until the stool turns soupy, and tissues are flushed. Take 5,000mg daily for the next four days.

• Take a brisk, daily walk. Breathe deep to help lungs eliminate mucous.

• Take an enema the first and last day of your fasting diet to thoroughly clean out excess mucous.

• Apply wet ginger/cayenne compresses to the chest to increase circulation and loosen mucous.

• Take a hot sauna or a long warm bath with a rubdown, to stimulate circulation.

The night before....

Mash several garlic cloves and a large slice of onion in a bowl. Stir in 3 TBS. of honey. Cover, and let macerate for 24 hours, then remove garlic and onion and take only the honey/syrup infusion - 1 teaspoon, 3 times daily.

The next day....

On rising: take 2 squeezed lemons in water with 1 TB. maple syrup.

Breakfast: take a glass of grapefruit, or pineapple, or cranberry-apple juice.

Mid-morning: have a glass of *fresh* carrot juice with 1 teasp. Bragg's LIQUID AMINOS added;
or a cup of a congestion clearing tea, such as Crystal Star X-PECT™ tea, an expectorant to aid mucous release, or RESPR TEA™, an aid in oxygen uptake.

Lunch: have a mixed vegetable juice, like V-8, or a potassium broth or essence (page 167).

Mid-afternoon: have a veggie drink (page 168), or a packet of Sun CHLORELLA granules in water;
or a greens and sea vegetable mix, such as Crystal Star ENERGY GREEN™ drink.

Supper: take a glass of apple juice or papaya/pineapple juice.

Before retiring: take a hot broth with 1 teasp. Organic Gourmet NUTRITIONAL YEAST extract for relaxation and strength.

To break your fasting cleanse....

For best results, have a small fresh salad on the last night of the cleanse. Begin eating the next day with small simple meals. Have toasted wheat germ or muesli, or whole grain granola for your first morning of solid food, with a little yogurt, apple, or pineapple/coconut juice. Take a small fresh salad for lunch with Italian or lemon/oil dressing. Have a fresh fruit smoothie during the day. Fix a baked potato with butter and a light soup or salad for dinner. Avoid pasteurized dairy products, heavy starches and refined foods that are a breeding ground for continued congestion.

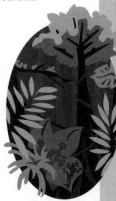

The Liver Cleanse: *a 3 day liquid diet.*

Be good to your liver! Your life depends on it. The health and vitality of the body depend to a large extent on the health and vitality of the liver. It is the body's most complex organ - a powerful chemical plant that converts everything we eat, breathe and absorb through the skin into life-sustaining substances. The liver is a major blood reservoir, forming and storing red blood cells, and filtering toxins at a rate of a quart of blood per minute. Blood flows directly from the gastrointestinal tract to the liver, so it can neutralize or alter some of the toxic substances before they are distributed to the rest of the body through the blood. Blood also keeps returning to the liver, processing toxins again and again so that most are altered by the time they are excreted by the bile or kidneys. It makes undeniable good sense to keep your liver in good working order.

A healthy liver produces natural antihistamines to keep immunity high. It can deal with a wide range of toxic chemicals, drugs, alcohol, solvents, formaldehyde, pesticides and food additives. With the acknowledgment that most of us are continually assailed by toxins in our food, water and air, it is generally realized that none of us has a truly healthy liver. The good news is that the liver has amazing rejuvenative powers, and continues to function when as many as 80% of its cells are damaged. Even more remarkable, the liver regenerates its own damaged tissue.

A liver and organ cleanse can get to the bottom of a lot of health problems. A clean liver is vital for the body to even begin to heal itself. I recommend a short liver cleanse and detoxification twice a year in the spring and fall to maximize its abilities, using the extra vitamin D from the sun to help. See the liver health pages in this book if your liver is seriously toxic; a complete liver renewal program can take from three to six months.

Do you need a liver cleanse?

Body signals that your liver needs some TLC include great fatigue, unexplained weight gain, depression or melancholy, mental confusion, sluggish elimination system, food and chemical sensitivity, PMS, jaundiced skin and/or liver spots on the skin, repeated nausea, dizziness and dry mouth.

HERE ARE SOME BRIEF POINTERS FOR THE BEST RESULTS IN A DETOX PROGRAM TO OVERCOME ADDICTIONS:

•Take the strain off your liver by eliminating red meats, concentrated fats and oils (except for essential oils), refined sugars, preservatives, food dyes and additives.

•Eat plenty of vegetables. Have a green, leafy salad every day.

•Good liver function is dependent on the amount and quality of oxygen coming into the lungs. Exercise, air filters, time spent in the forest and at the ocean, and early morning sunlight are important.

•Get adequate rest and sleep during a liver cleanse. The liver does some of its most important work while you sleep!

•Reducing dietary fat is crucial for liver health and regeneration.

•Drink six to eight glasses of bottled water every day to encourage maximum flushing of liver tissues.

HERE IS A 3 DAY " SPRING CLEANING" LIVER CLEANSE AND DETOXIFICATION DIET:

On rising: take 2 TBS. cider vinegar in water with 1 teasp. honey, or 2 TBS. lemon juice in water.

Breakfast: take a glass of potassium broth, or carrot/beet/cucumber juice, or organic apple juice.

Mid-morning: take a veggie drink (See Therapeutic Drinks, Juices, Tonics & Broths in this chapter),
 or Sun CHLORELLA or Green Foods GREEN MAGMA, or Crystal Star ENERGY GREEN™ in water.

Lunch: have another glass of organic apple juice or fresh carrot juice.

Mid-afternoon: have a cup of peppermint tea, pau d'arco tea, or Crystal Star LIV-ALIVE TEA™;
 or Crystal Star SYSTEMS STRENGTH drink™ or another green drink.

Dinner: have another glass of organic apple juice, or another potassium broth.

Before bed: take another glass of lemon juice or cider vinegar in water. Add 1 teasp. honey or royal jelly.

A TARGET SUPPLEMENT PROGRAM ACCELERATES LIVER DETOXIFICATION.

Except for the following suggestions, supplements affect the cleansing process, and should not begin until after heavy cleansing is over.

•Ascorbate vitamin C crystals, $\frac{1}{4}$ to $\frac{1}{2}$ teasp. at a time in aloe vera juice.

•One teasp. high quality royal jelly may be added to any cleansing liquids for increased benefits.

•Use 15 MILK THISTLE SEED EXTRACT drops in water. Milk Thistle contains some of the most potent liver protecting substances known. The components of this herb stimulate protein synthesis, increasing the production of new liver cells to replace damaged old ones.

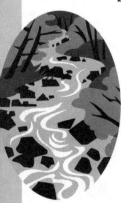

The Blood Purifying Cleanse: *a 3 to 7 day diet.*

Your blood is your river of life. The health of your blood is critical. The blood must supply oxygen to the body's sixty trillion cells, transport nutrients, hormones and wastes, warm and cool the body, ward off invading micro-organisms, seal off wounds and much more. It is the chief neutralizing agent for bacteria and toxic wastes. Many diseases are the result of blood toxins, and will benefit from a healthy blood supply. Although not immediately obvious, toxins ingested in sub-lethal amounts can eventually add up to disease-causing amounts. Slow viruses that lead to nerve diseases like M.S. can enter the cells and remain dormant for years, mutating and feeding on toxic substances, then reappear in a more dangerous form. While the body has its own self-purifying complex for maintaining healthy blood, the best way to protect yourself from disease is to keep those cleansing systems in good working order.

Many naturopaths recommend that serious blood cleansing programs be accompanied by a liquid juice diet. Vegetable and fruit juices stimulate rapid, heavy waste elimination, a process that can generate mild symptoms of a "healing crisis." A slight headache, nausea, bad breath, body odor and dark urine occur as the body accelerates release of accumulated toxins. Five to 10,000mg. of ascorbate Vitamin C is recommended daily during serious cleansing, to help keep the body alkaline, encourage oxygen uptake, and promote collagen development for new healthy tissue. Vitamin C should be added especially if you are detoxifying from alcohol or drug overload.

HERE ARE SOME OF THE REASONS YOU MIGHT NEED A BLOOD CLEANSE:

❖ **Heavy metal poisoning** has become a major health problem of modern society. Numerous studies indicate a strong relationship between heavy metal storage in the body, childhood learning disabilities and criminal behavior. If you served in Vietnam, if your work puts you in contact with petro-chemicals, if you live near a congested highway, or in a crop-dusting fly-way, check yourself for the following symptoms of heavy metal/ chemical toxicity:

- a deep, choking cough
- depression, memory loss and unusual insomnia
- schizophrenic behavior, seizures, periodic black-outs
- sexual dysfunction
- black spots on the gums, bad breath/body odor, unusual, severe reactions to foods and odors
- loss of hand/eye coordination, especially in driving

Include daily in your diet to release heavy metals....

Brown rice, miso soup, a glass of aloe vera juice and a glass of fresh carrot juice. Include artichokes to promote the flow of bile, the major pathway for chemical release from the liver. High sulphur foods like garlic, onions and beans are important. Other foods should be organically grown as much as possible.

Note: Do not go on an all-liquid diet when trying to release heavy metals or chemicals from the body. They enter the bloodstream too fast and heavily for the body to handle, and will poison you even more.

An effective herbal remedy course should include ECHINACEA ROOT 100% extract or PAU D' ARCO/ECHINACEA extract, 3 times daily, an herbal green drink such as chlorella or spirulina, or Crystal Star's ENERGY GREEN™ drink, and a compound like Crystal Star HEAVY METAL™ caps to help neutralize and release hazardous chemicals.

A strong, accompanying supplement program should include anti-oxidants like OPCs from grape seed or pine bark extract, Co-Q$_{10}$, beta carotene, vitamin C (5 to 10,000mg. daily), and cysteine, a heavy metal chelator.

See HEAVY METAL POISONING, page 387 in this book.

❖ **Serious immune deficient diseases** can benefit from a blood purifying diet to boost compromised immunity. There is usually a great deal of blood toxicity, fatigue and lack of nutrient assimilation in serious degenerative conditions. A liquid fast is *not recommended*, since it is often too harsh for an already weakened system. The initial diet should, however, be as pure as possible, in order to be as cleansing as possible - totally vegetarian - free of all meats, dairy foods, fried, preserved and refined foods, and above all, saturated fats. This diet may be followed for 1 to 2 months, or longer if the body is still actively cleansing, or needs further alkalizing. The diet may also be returned to when needed, to purify against relapse or additional symptoms.

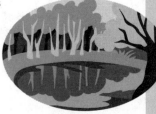

HERE ARE SOME BRIEF POINTERS TO GIVE YOU THE BEST RESULTS FOR YOUR BLOOD PURIFYING CLEANSE:

•Produce should be fresh and organically grown when possible. The investment in a good juicer is well worth it.

•Take a colonic irrigation or a Nature's Secret SUPERCLEANSE once a week to remove infected feces.

•Overheating therapy speeds up metabolism and inhibits replication of the invading virus. See page 178.

•Avoid canned, frozen prepackaged foods, and refined foods with colors, preservatives and flavor enhancers.

•Avoid sodas, artificial drinks, concentrated sugars, and sweeteners. Avoid all fried foods of any kind.

•Unsweetened mild herb teas and bottled mineral water (6 to 8 glasses) are recommended throughout each day, to hydrate, alkalize, and keep the body flushed of toxic wastes. See specific recommendations in the diet.

•For optimum results, $^{1}/_{2}$ teasp. ascorbate vitamin C crystals with bioflavonoids may be added to any drink.

•Sprinkling $^{1}/_{2}$ teasp. Natren TRINITY lactobacillus powder in any juice, or over any cooked food, makes a big difference to your body chemistry change.

•Exercise daily in the morning, if possible. Aerobic oxygen intake alone can be an important nutrient.

HERE IS A DETOXIFYING DIET THAT CAN HELP PURIFY THE BLOOD SO THAT IMMUNE RESPONSE FUNCTIONS BETTER:

On rising: take 2 to 3 TBS. cranberry concentrate in 8 oz. water with $^{1}/_{2}$ teasp. ascorbate vitamin C crystals, or use a green tea blood cleansing formula, such as Crystal Star GREEN TEA CLEANSER™;
or cut up a half lemon with skin and blend in the blender w. 1 teasp. honey, and 1 cup distilled water;
and $^{1}/_{2}$ teasp. Natren TRINITY in 8-oz. aloe vera juice.

Breakfast: have a glass of fresh carrot juice, with I TB. Bragg's LIQUID AMINOS added, and whole grain muffins
or rice cakes, or cereal or pancakes with kefir cheese or yogurt, and fresh fruit;
or a cup of soy milk or plain yogurt mixed in the blender with a cup of fresh fruit, walnuts, and $^{1}/_{2}$ teasp. Natren TRINITY in 8 oz. aloe vera juice.

Mid-morning: take a weekly colonic irrigation. On non-colonic days, take a potassium broth or essence, page 167, with 1 TB. Bragg's LIQUID AMINOS, and $^{1}/_{2}$ teasp. ascorbate vitamin C crystals; and another fresh carrot juice, or pau d'arco tea with $^{1}/_{2}$ teasp. Natren TRINITY.

Lunch: have a green leafy salad with lemon/flax oil dressing; add sprouts, tofu, avocado, nuts and seeds;
or have an open-face sandwich on rice cakes or a chapati, with soy or yogurt cheese and fresh veggies;
or a cup of miso soup with rice noodles or brown rice; or steamed vegetables with brown rice and tofu;
and pau d'arco tea or aloe vera juice with $^{1}/_{2}$ teasp. ascorbate vitamin C and $^{1}/_{2}$ teasp. Natren TRINITY.

Mid-afternoon: have another carrot juice with 1 TB. Bragg's LIQUID AMINOS;
and a green drink, such as SUN CHLORELLA, GREEN MAGMA or Crystal Star ENERGY GREEN™.

Dinner: have a baked potato with Bragg's LIQUID AMINOS or lemon/oil dressing and a fresh salad;
and another potassium broth, or black bean or lentil soup;
or fresh spinach or artichoke pasta with steamed vegetables and a lemon/flax oil dressing;
or a Chinese steam/stir fry with shiitake mushrooms, vegetables and brown rice;
or a tofu and veggie casserole with yogurt or soy cheese.

Before Bed: take another 8 oz. glass of aloe vera juice with $^{1}/_{2}$ teasp. ascorbate vitamin C with bioflavs;
and another carrot juice, or papaya juice with $^{1}/_{2}$ teasp. Natren TRINITY lactobacillus powder.

Because such vigorous treatment is necessary, supplementation is desirable during a blood purifying cleanse.

•Anti-oxidants, such as germanium, 100 to 150mg with astragalus, Vitamin E 1000IU with selenium 200mcg., CoQ_{10} 180mg. daily can strengthen white blood cell and T-cell activity. Take with Quercetin and bromelain 500mg 3x daily, for auto-immune reactions, and potent digestive enzymes, such as Rainbow Light DETOX-ZYME capsules.

•Egg yolk lecithin, highest potency, for active lipids that make the cell walls resistant to attack.

•Acidophilus culture complex with bifidus - refrigerated, highest potency, 3 teasp. daily, with biotin 1000mcg.

•Aloe vera juice, like AloeLife ALOE GOLD concentrate in water daily, to block virus spreading from cell to cell.

•Shark liver oil or cartilage, and echinacea or pau de arco extract, $^{1}/_{2}$ dropperful 3x daily, to stimulate production of interferon, interleukin and lymphocytes.

•Carnitine 500mg daily for 3 days. Rest for 7 days, then take 1000mg for 3 days. Rest for 7 days. Take with high Omega-3 fish or flax oils, 3 to 6 daily, and EVENING PRIMROSE OIL 1000mg 3x daily.

•Centipede KITTY'S OXYGEL, rubbed on the feet morning and evening. Alternate use, one week on and one week off. *Note:* A simple blood-color test monitors blood improvement. Make a small, quick, sterilized razor cut on your finger. If the blood is a dark, bluish-purplish color it is not healthy. A bright red color indicates healthy blood.

•Crystal Star LIV-ALIVE™ capsules and LIV-ALIVE™ Tea to detoxify the liver, along with St. John's wort extract or Crystal Star ANTI-VI™ Extract for anti-viral activity.

Blood Purifying To Overcome Addictions

❖ **Overcoming addictions and alcohol abuse** experiences far more success when treatment is begun with a blood purifying cleanse. Follow-up studies indicate that as many as 75% of patients are still sober after one year when they first follow a detoxification program. A detox diet is positive support therapy in successful recovery from drug, alcohol, nicotine or concentrated sugar addictions. The overwhelming majority of habitual drug and controlled substance users suffer from malnutrition, metabolic upset and nutritional imbalances. When these conditions are corrected, the need to get high by artificial means is sharply diminished.

The following diet not only helps purify toxic blood, but helps rebuild a depleted system. It is rich in vegetable proteins, high in minerals (especially magnesium for nerve stress), with Omega-3 oils, vitamin B and C source foods, and antioxidants. Regeneration takes time.... sometimes up to a year to detoxify and clear drugs from the blood.

HERE ARE SOME BRIEF POINTERS FOR THE BEST RESULTS IN A DETOX PROGRAM TO OVERCOME ADDICTIONS:
- •Eat magnesium-rich foods - green leafy and yellow vegetables, citrus fruits, whole grain cereals, fish, legumes.
- •Eat potassium-rich foods - oranges, broccoli, green peppers, seafoods, sea vegetables, bananas, tomatoes.
- •Eat chromium-rich foods, such as brewer's yeast, mushrooms, whole grains, sea foods and peas.
- •Eat some vegetable protein at every meal. Get some exercise every day.
- •Take kudzu caps. New research on kudzu for over-consumption of alcohol shows a reduction in alcohol intake.
- •Avoid smoking and secondary smoke. Tobacco increases craving for all drugs.

HERE IS A DETOXIFYING DIET THAT HELPS PURIFY THE BLOOD SO THAT IMMUNE RESPONSE CAN FUNCTION BETTER:
On rising: take a superfood drink such as Be Well Juice, to give energy and control morning blood sugar drop:
add 1 teasp. each in a glass of apple or orange juice - glycine powder, spirulina, sugar-free protein powder, brewer's yeast;
or take a sugar free high protein drink such as Nature's Life Super Green PRO 96;
or a concentrated mineral drink, such as Crystal Star SYSTEMS STRENGTH™ DRINK.
Breakfast: make a concentrated food mineral mix to shore up mineral depletion: 1 teasp. each: sesame seeds, toasted wheat germ, unsulphured molasses, bee pollen granules, and brewer's yeast. Sprinkle some on any of the following breakfast choices: fresh fruit with yogurt or kefir cheese topping, or oatmeal or kashi pilaf with a little yogurt and maple syrup, or a whole grain cereal, muesli or granola with apple juice or fruit.
Mid-morning: have a veggie drink (page 168), Sun CHLORELLA or Green Foods GREEN ESSENCE drink, or Crystal Star ENERGY GREEN™ drink;
and a whole grain muffin or corn bread with kefir cheese, and a small bottle of mineral water.
Lunch: have a fresh veggie salad with cottage cheese, topped with nuts, seeds and crunchy noodles;
or a high protein sandwich on whole grain bread, with avocados, low-fat cheese, and greens;
or some oriental fried rice and miso soup with sea vegetables;
or a seafood salad with a black bean or lentil soup.
Mid-afternoon: have a hard boiled egg with mayonnaise or yogurt, and some whole grain crackers;
and another bottle of mineral water, or herb tea, such as Crystal Star HIGH ENERGY™ tea.
Dinner: have a vegetable casserole with tofu, or chicken and brown rice;
or an oriental stir-fry with noodles and vegetables, and miso soup;
or a whole grain pasta with steamed vegetables and a green salad.
Before bed: have a cup of Organic Gourmet SAVORY SPREAD yeast broth, or apple or papaya juice.

ADDITIONAL SUPPLEMENTS TO HELP OVERCOME ADDICTIONS:
- •Take ascorbate vitamin C crystals, $^1/_4$ to $^1/_2$ teasp. in water 3x daily (5 to 10,000mg.), or to bowel tolerance as an antioxidant and detoxifying agent, with Solaray CHROMIACIN to restimulate circulation. Take vitamin E as an antioxidant to strengthen adrenals and restore liver function.
- •Take a full spectrum, pre-digested amino acid compound, 1000mg daily to rebuild from a low protein diet.
- •Take a mega potency Stress B Complex daily, 100-150mg to overcome deficiencies.
- •Take glutamine 500mg and tyrosine 500mg daily to help reduce drug cravings, or Crystal Star WITHDRAWAL SUPPORT™ extract. Use Crystal Star DEPRESS-EX™ extract to help overcome drug-related depression.
- •Take EVENING PRIMROSE OIL or high Omega-3 flax oil to stimulate prostaglandin production.
- •Take a complete herb source multi-mineral/trace mineral, such as Mezotrace SEA MINERAL COMPLEX, or Crystal Star MINERAL SPECTRUM™ capsules, or MINERAL SPECTRUM™ extract.

Drinks For Detoxification

Detoxification drinks are targeted at neutralizing the effects of pesticides, environmental pollutants and heavy metals, as well as toxins from the overuse of drugs, caffeine and nicotine. Foods for cleansing juices should be organically grown, and juiced fresh for best results. Fresh food materials retain the full complement of food nutrients, to help stabilize and maintain the acid/alkaline balance of the body.

- **Fresh fruits and fruit juices** eliminate wastes quickly and help reduce cravings for sweets.
- **Fresh vegetable juices** carry off excess body acids, and are rich in vitamins, minerals and enzymes that satisfy the body's nutrient requirements with less food.
- **Chlorophyll-rich juices**, with foods like spirulina, chlorella, and barley grass also have anti-infective properties. Since chlorophyll has a molecular structure close to human plasma, (only the central magnesium or iron molecule are different) so body availability is excellent. They help clear the skin, cleanse the kidneys, and clean and build the blood.
- **Herb teas and mineral drink mixes** during a cleansing diet provide energy and cleansing at the same time, without having to take in solid proteins or carbohydrates for fuel.

Mother Nature is drastically cleaning house during a detox cleanse. You may eliminate accumulated poisons and wastes quite rapidly, causing headaches, slight nausea and weakness as the body purges. These reactions are usually only temporary, and disappear along with the waste and toxins. New healthy tissue starts building right away when the detoxification juices are taken in. Our bodies are designed to be self-healing organisms. Healing is allowed to occur through cleansing. Hormone secretions stimulate the immune system during a cleanse to set up a disease defense environment.

NOTE: ANY OF THE DRINKS, JUICES, TONICS AND BROTHS IN THIS SECTION CAN BE A PART OF YOUR LIQUID INTAKE DURING CLEANSING OR ILLNESS.

❧ POTASSIUM JUICE

The single most effective juice for cleansing, neutralizing acids, and rebuilding the body. It is a blood and body tonic to provide rapid energy and system balance.

For one 12-oz. glass:

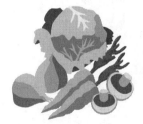

Juice in the juicer
3 CARROTS	$\frac{1}{2}$ BUNCH SPINACH
3 STALKS CELERY	$\frac{1}{2}$ BUNCH PARSLEY

- Add 1 to 2 teasp. Bragg's LIQUID AMINOS if desired.

❧ POTASSIUM ESSENCE BROTH

If you do not have a juicer, make a potassium broth in a soup pot. While not as concentrated or pure, it is still an excellent source of energy, minerals and electrolytes.

For a 2 day supply:

Cover with water in a soup pot
3 to 4 CARROTS	$\frac{1}{2}$ BUNCH PARSLEY
2 POTATOES, with skins	$\frac{1}{2}$ HEAD CABBAGE
1 ONION	$\frac{1}{2}$ BUNCH BROCCOLI
3 STALKS CELERY	

- Simmer covered 30 minutes. Strain and discard solids.
- Add 2 teasp. Bragg's LIQUID AMINOS, or 1 teasp. miso. Store in the fridge, covered.

Green Drinks, Vegetable Juices & Blood Tonics

Green drinks are chlorophyll rich. The molecular composition of chlorophyll is so close to that of human hemoglobin that these drinks can act as "mini-transfusions" for the blood, and tonics for the brain and immune system. They are an excellent nutrient source of vitamins, minerals, proteins and enzymes. They contain large amounts of vitamins C, B_1, B_2, B_3, pantothenic acid, folic acid, carotene and choline. They are high in minerals, like potassium, calcium, magnesium, iron, copper, phosphorus and manganese. They are full of enzymes for digestion and assimilation, some containing over 1000 of the known enzymes necessary for human cell response and growth. Green drinks also have anti-infective properties, carry off acid wastes, neutralize body pH, and are excellent for mucous cleansing. They can help clear the skin, cleanse the kidneys, and purify and build the blood.

Green drinks and vegetable juices are potent fuel in maintaining good health, yet don't come burdened by the fats that accompany animal products. Those included here have been used with therapeutic success for many years. You can have confidence in their nutritional healing and regenerative ability.

Note: A high quality juicer is the best way to get all the nutrients from vegetable juices. A blender or food processor gives only moderate results, but is definitely better than nothing at all. Use organically grown produce whenever possible.

❧ PERSONAL BEST V-8

A high vitamin/mineral drink for body balance. A good daily blend even when you're not cleansing.
For 6 glasses:

6 to 8 TOMATOES, or 4 C. TOMATO JUICE
$^1/_2$ GREEN PEPPER
2 STALKS CELERY with leaves
$^1/_2$ BUNCH PARSLEY

3 to 4 GREEN ONIONS with tops
2 CARROTS
$^1/_2$ SMALL BUNCH SPINACH, washed
2 LEMONS peeled, or 4 TBS. LEMON JUICE

•option.... Add 2 teasp. Bragg's LIQUID AMINOS and $^1/_2$ teasp. ground celery seed

❧ KIDNEY FLUSH

A purifying kidney cleanser and diuretic drink, with balancing potassium and other minerals.
For four 8 oz. glasses:

4 CARROTS
4 BEETS with tops
4 CELERY STALKS with leaves

1 CUCUMBER with skin
8 to 10 SPINACH LEAVES, washed

•option.... Add 1 teasp. Bragg's LIQUID AMINOS

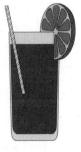

❧ HEALTHY MARY COCKTAIL TONIC

A virgin mary is really a healthy green drink when you make it fresh.
For 4 drinks:

3 CUPS WATER
2 TOMATOES
1 GREEN ONION with tops

1 SLICE GREEN PEPPER
1 STALK CELERY
12 SPRIGS FRESH PARSLEY

•Add 1 TB. crumbled, dry SEA VEGGIES, such as WAKAME or DULSE, or 1 teasp. KELP POWDER

❧ STOMACH/DIGESTIVE CLEANSER

For one 8 oz. glass:

Juice a half CUCUMBER with skin, 2 TBS. APPLE CIDER VINEGAR and a PINCH GROUND GINGER.
•Add enough cool water to make 8 oz.

❧ CARROT JUICE PLUS
For 2 large drinks:

Juice 4 CARROTS, $^1/_2$ CUCUMBER, 2 STALKS CELERY with leaves, and 1 TB. CHOPPED DRY DULSE.

❧ SKIN CLEANSING TONIC
Deep greens to nourish, cleanse and tone skin tissue from the inside.
For 1 drink:

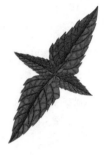

1 CUCUMBER with skin $^1/_2$ BUNCH FRESH PARSLEY
1 TUB (4-OZ.) ALFALFA SPROUTS   3 to 4 SPRIGS FRESH MINT

❧ EVER GREEN ENZYME DRINK
A personal favorite for taste, mucous release and enzymatic action.
For 1 drink:

Juice 1 APPLE, cored, 1 TUB (4 OZ.) ALFALFA SPROUTS, $^1/_2$ FRESH PINEAPPLE skinned/cored, 3 to 4
    SPRIGS FRESH MINT and 1 teasp. SPIRULINA or CHLORELLA GRANULES.

❧ SPROUT COCKTAIL
This high protein juice is particularly good for ending a fast.
For 2 drinks:

Juice 3 cored APPLES with skin, 1 TUB (4 oz.) ALFALFA SPROUTS and 3 to 4 SPRIGS fresh MINT.

Cleansing Fruit Drinks

Fruits are wonderful for a quick system wash and cleanse. Their high water and sugar content speeds up metabolism to release wastes quickly, have an alkalizing effect on the body and help reduce cravings for sweets. However, because of their rapid metabolism, pesticides, sprays and chemicals on fruits can enter the body rapidly. Eat organically grown fruits whenever possible. Wash fruit well if commercially grown. Fruits and fruit juices have their best nutritional effects when taken alone. Eat them before noon for best energy conversion and cleansing benefits.

❧ BLOOD BUILDER
A blood purifying drink with iron enrichment.
For 4 large drinks:

Juice 2 BUNCHES of GRAPES, or 2 CUPS GRAPE JUICE, 6 ORANGES, or 2 CUPS ORANGE JUICE,
    and 8 LEMONS peeled, or 1 CUP LEMON JUICE. Stir in: 2 CUPS WATER and $^1/_4$ CUP HONEY.

❧ ENZYME COOLER
An intestinal balancer to help lower cholesterol, cleanse intestinal tract, and allow better assimilation of foods.
For 2 large drinks:

Juice 1 APPLE, cored, or $^1/_2$ CUP APPLE JUICE, 2 LEMONS, peeled, or $^1/_4$ CUP LEMON JUICE, and 1
    PINEAPPLE, skinned and cored, or $1^1/_2$ CUPS PINEAPPLE JUICE.

❧ STOMACH CLEANSER & BREATH REFRESHER

A body chemistry improving drink.
For 2 drinks:

1 BUNCH GRAPES, or 1 CUP GRAPE JUICE   I BASKET STRAWBERRIES
3 APPLES cored, or 1 CUP APPLE JUICE   4 SPRIGS OF FRESH MINT

❧ DIURETIC MELON MIX

A good morning drink with diuretic properties. Take on an empty stomach - 3 to 5 glasses daily.
For 1 quart:

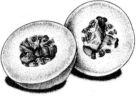

Juice 3 CUPS WATERMELON cubes
2 CUPS PERSIAN MELON CUBES
2 CUPS HONEYDEW CUBES

❧ GOOD DIGESTION PUNCH

Natural sources of papain and bromelain for enzyme activity, and ginger to break up excess stomach acids.
For 2 drinks:

Juice 1 PAPAYA, peeled and seeded, 1 PINEAPPLE, skinned and cored, or 1 to 2 ORANGES, peeled and
$\frac{1}{4}$" SLICE FRESH GINGER, or $\frac{1}{4}$ teasp. cardamom powder.

Note: Other good cleansing fruit juices include black cherry juice for gout conditions; cranberry juice for bladder and kidney infections; grape and citrus juices for high blood pressure; watermelon juice for bladder and kidney malfunction, celery for nerves, and apple juice to overcome fatigue.

Cleansing Broths & Hot Tonics

Clear broths are a very satisfying form of nutrition during a cleansing fast. They are simple, easy, inexpensive, can be taken hot or cold, and provide a means of "eating" and being with others at mealtime without going off a liquid program. This is more important than it might appear, since solid food, taken after the body has released all its solid waste, but before the cleanse is over, will drastically reduce the diet's success. Broths are also alkalizing, and contribute toward balancing body pH.

Hot tonics are neither broths nor teas, but unique hot combinations of vegetables, fruits and spices with purifying and energizing properties. The ingredients provide noticeable synergistic activity when taken together - with more medicinal benefits than the single ingredients alone. Take them morning and evening for best results.

❧ PURIFYING CLEAR BROTH

Rich in potassium and minerals.
For 6 cups:

Saute in 2 TBS. OIL   Add:
$\frac{1}{4}$ CUP CHOPPED CELERY   6 CUPS RICH VEGETABLE STOCK
$\frac{1}{4}$ CUP DAIKON RADISH   2 TBS. FRESH SNIPPED LEMON PEEL
$\frac{1}{2}$ CUP BROCCOLI chopped   2 teasp. BRAGG'S LIQUID AMINOS
$\frac{1}{4}$ CUP CHOPPED LEEKS $\frac{1}{4}$ CUP SNIPPED PARSLEY
$\frac{1}{4}$ CUP GRATED CARROTS
• Heat for 1 minute, then serve hot.

ᕲ RICE PURIFYING SOUP

A good start to a macrobiotic cleansing diet.
For 6 cups:

Toast in a large pan until aromatic, about 5 minutes, $^2/_3$ CUP LENTILS, $^2/_3$ CUP SPLIT PEAS, $^2/_3$ CUP BROWN RICE.

Add and cook over low heat for 1 hr. stirring occasionally
2 CLOVES MINCED GARLIC	1 CARROT CHOPPED
1 ONION CHOPPED	1 STALK CELERY, chopped
3 CUPS WATER	1 teasp. CAYENNE
3 CUPS ONION OR VEGGIE BROTH	$^1/_2$ teasp. PEPPER and $^1/_2$ teasp. GINGER POWDER

ᕲ ONION & MISO BROTH

A therapeutic broth with antibiotic and immune-enhancing properties.
For 6 small bowls of broth:

Saute 1 CHOPPED ONION in $^1/_2$ teasp. SESAME OIL for 5 minutes until aromatic.
Add 1 STALK CELERY WITH LEAVES, and saute for 2 minutes.
Add 1 QUART WATER or VEGETABLE STOCK. Cover and simmer 10 minutes.
Add 3 to 4 TBS. LIGHT MISO. Remove from heat.
Add 2 GREEN ONIONS with tops, and whirl in the blender.

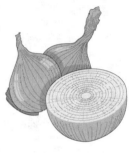

ᕲ PURIFYING DAIKON & SCALLION BROTH

A clear cleansing drink with bladder flushing activity.
For one bowl:

Heat gently together for 5 minutes, 4 CUPS VEGETABLE BROTH, ONE 6" PIECE DAIKON RADISH, peeled and cut into matchstick pieces, and 2 SCALLIONS, with tops.
Stir in 1 TB. TAMARI, or 1 TB. BRAGG'S LIQUID AMINOS, 1 TB. FRESH CHOPPED CILANTRO and a PINCH of PEPPER.

ᕲ ONION/GARLIC BROTH

A therapeutic broth with antibiotic properties to reduce and relieve mucous congestion.
For 1 bowl:

Sauté 1 ONION and 4 CLOVES GARLIC in $^1/_2$ teasp. SESAME OIL until very soft.
Then whirl in the blender with a little vegetable broth. Take in small sips.

ᕲ COLD DEFENSE CLEANSER

Make this broth the minute you feel a cold coming on. Drink in small sips for best results.
Heat gently for 2 drinks:

$1^1/_2$ CUPS WATER	1 TB. HONEY
1 teasp. GARLIC POWDER	$^1/_2$ teasp. CAYENNE
1 teasp. GROUND GINGER	3 TBS. BRANDY
1 TB. LEMON JUICE	

❧ COLDS & FLU CONGESTION TONIC

This drink really opens up nasal and sinus passages fast. Very potent.
For 2 drinks:

Toast in a dry pan until aromatic, 4 CLOVES MINCED GARLIC, $\frac{1}{4}$ teasp. CUMIN POWDER, $\frac{1}{4}$ teasp. BLACK PEPPER and $\frac{1}{2}$ teasp. HOT MUSTARD POWDER
- •Add 1 TB. FLAX OIL and stir in. Toast a little more to blend.

Then add I CUP WATER, 1 CUP COOKED SPLIT PEAS or 1 CUP FROZEN PEAS, 1 teasp. TURMERIC, $\frac{1}{2}$ teasp. SESAME SALT, 1 TB. FRESH CILANTRO or $\frac{1}{2}$ teasp. GROUND CORIANDER.
- •Simmer gently for 5 minutes, and whirl in blender.

❧ REVITALIZING TONIC

A good drink for addiction purifying program or any kind of hangover. Effective hot or cold. Works every time.
Enough for 8 drinks:

Mix in the blender:

48 OZ. KNUDSEN'S SPICY VEGGIE JUICE
2 STALKS CHOPPED CELERY
1 BUNCH PARSLEY, chopped
$1\frac{1}{2}$ CUPS WATER
$\frac{1}{2}$ teasp. FENNEL SEEDS

1 CUP MIXED CHOPPED ONIONS
2 TBS. CHOPPED FRESH BASIL, or 2 teasp. dried
2 teasp. HOT PEPPER SAUCE
1 teasp. ROSEMARY LEAVES
1 teasp. BRAGG'S LIQUID AMINOS

- •Pour into a large pot. Bring to a boil and simmer for 30 minutes. Use hot or cool.

❧ STOMACH & DIGESTIVE CLEANSER

For one 8-oz. glass:

Whirl in the blender, 1 APPLE cored, 2 TBS. ALOE VERA JUICE and $\frac{1}{4}$ teasp. GROUND GINGER.
- •Add enough WATER to make 8-OZ.

❧ MINERAL RICH ENZYME BROTH

Perfect for enzyme therapy.
For 6 cups of broth:

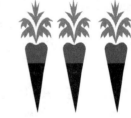

Put in a large soup pot with $1\frac{1}{2}$ QTS. WATER.
3 SLICED CARROTS
1 CUP FRESH PARSLEY, chopped
1 LARGE ONION, chopped

2 POTATOES
2 STALKS CELERY with tops

- •Bring to a boil; reduce heat; simmer for 30 minutes. Strain and add 1 TB. Bragg's LIQUID AMINOS.

❧ WARMING CIRCULATION STIMULANT

For 4 drinks:
1 CUP CRANBERRY JUICE
1 CUP ORANGE JUICE
4-6 CARDAMOM PODS
4 TBS. RAISINS
1 teasp. VANILLA

2 TBS. HONEY
4-6 WHOLE CLOVES
1 CINNAMON STICK
4 TBS. ALMONDS chopped

- •Heat all gently for 15 minutes. Remove cloves, cardamom and cinnamon stick. Serve hot.

Herb Teas For Detoxification

Herb teas and high mineral drinks during a liquid diet can provide energy and cleansing without having to take in solid proteins or carbohydrates for fuel. Herbal teas are the most time-honored of all natural healing mediums. Essentially body balancers, teas have mild cleansing and flushing properties, and are easily absorbed by the system. The important volatile oils in herbs are released by the hot brewing water, and when taken in small sips throughout the cleansing process, they flood the tissues with concentrated nutritional support to accelerate regeneration, and the release of toxic waste. In general, herbs are more effective when taken together in combination than when used singly. (See page 64 for the way to take herb teas for therapeutic results.)

A tea combination for blood cleansing might include: Red Clover, Hawthorn, Pau d'Arco, Nettles, Sage, Alfalfa, Milk Thistle Seed, Echinacea, Horsetail, Gotu Kola, and Lemon Grass.

A tea combination for mucous cleansing might include: Mullein, Comfrey, Ephedra, Marshmallow, Pleurisy Root, Rose hips, Calendula, Boneset, Ginger, Peppermint, and Fennel Seed.

A tea combination for cleansing the bowel and digestive system might include: Senna Leaf, Papaya Leaf, Fennel Seed, Peppermint, Lemon Balm, Parsley Leaf, Calendula, Hibiscus, and Ginger Root.

A tea combination for gentle bladder and kidney flushing might include: Uva Ursi, Juniper Berries, Ginger Rt., and Parsley Leaf.

A tea combination for clearing sinuses might include: Marshmallow, Rose hips, Mullein, and Fenugreek.

Simple Medicinal Tea Blends For Healing Diets

Use one small packed tea ball for 2 to 3 cups of tea.

A RELAXING TEA For STRESS & HEADACHES
2 PARTS ROSEMARY   1 PART CATNIP
2 PARTS SPEARMINT or PEPPERMINT   1 PART CHAMOMILE

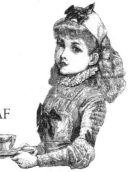

A DIURETIC TEA For GENTLE BLADDER FLUSHING
2 PARTS UVA URSI   1 PART GINGER
2 PARTS JUNIPER BERRIES   1 PART PARSLEY LEAF

A DECONGESTANT TEA For CHEST & SINUSES
2 PARTS MARSHMALLOW ROOT   2 PARTS ROSE HIPS
2 PARTS MULLEIN LEAF   2 PARTS FENUGREEK SEED

AN ENERGIZING TEA For FATIGUE
2 PARTS GOTU KOLA   2 PARTS RED CLOVER
2 PARTS PEPPERMINT   1 PART CLOVES

A DIGESTIVE TEA For GOOD ASSIMILATION
2 PARTS PEPPERMINT   2 PARTS HIBISCUS
1 PART PAPAYA LEAF   1 PART ROSEMARY

Superfood Mineral Drinks

Superfood drinks are formulated with the wonderful, new concentrated food forms available today for premium nutrition. They offer the body basic building blocks to balance the acid/alkaline system, regulate body fluid osmosis and electrical activity in the nervous system, and to aid in digestion and regularity. They are vigorous sources of minerals, proteins, enzymes, antioxidants and amino acids with whole cell availability.

❧ MINERAL-RICH AMINOS DRINK

This is an easy, short version of the Crystal Star Herbal Nutrition SYSTEM STRENGTH™ drink. It is a complete, balanced food-source vitamin/mineral supplement that is rich in greens, amino acids and enzyme precursors. A superior drink to use after a long illness or a hospital stay.
Enough for 8 drinks:

Make up a dry batch in the blender, then mix about 2 TBS. powder into 2 cups of hot water for 1 drink. Let flavors bloom for 5 minutes before drinking. Add 1 teasp. Bragg's LIQUID AMINOS to each drink if desired. Sip over a half hour period for best assimilation.

4 to 6 PACKETS MISO CUP SOUP POWDER (Edwards & Son Co. makes a good one)
1 TB. CRUMBLED DRY SEA VEGETABLES (Kombu, Wakame or Sea Palm)
$1/_2$ CUP SOY PROTEIN POWDER
1 PACKET INSTANT GINSENG TEA
2 TBS. BEE POLLEN GRANULES
1 teasp. SPIRULINA or CHLORELLA GRANULES
1 TB. BREWER'S YEAST FLAKES
1 teasp. ACIDOPHILUS POWDER
2 TBS. FRESH PARSLEY LEAF or 1 teasp. dried
1 teasp. BRAGG'S LIQUID AMINOS

❧ MINERAL-RICH ENERGY DRINK

This is an easy, simplified version of the Crystal Star Herbal Nutrition ENERGY GREEN™ drink. It is rich in chlorophyllins, with substantial amounts of plant beta carotene, B vitamins, choline, essential fatty acids with GLA, DGLA and linoleic acid, and octacosanal for tissue oxygenation. It contains complex carbohydrates, complete minerals, trace minerals, proteins, and a full-spectrum amino acid complex. This drink may be used to detoxify, alkalize, and energize. It is a good choice for an over-eater's diet during weight loss.
Enough for 4 drinks:

Mix in the blender, then mix about 2 TBS. into 2 cups of hot water for 1 drink. Let flavors bloom for 5 minutes before drinking.

$1/_2$ CUP AMAZAKE RICE DRINK
$1/_2$ CUP OATS
2 TBS. BEE POLLEN GRANULES
1 PACKET INSTANT GINSENG TEA GRANULES
2 TBS. GOTU KOLA HERB
1 TB. DANDELION LEAF
1 TB. CRUMBLED DULSE
2 PACKETS BARLEY GRASS or CHLORELLA GRANULES
2 TBS. ALFALFA LEAF
1 teasp. VITAMIN C CRYSTALS with BIOFLAVONOIDS
  •Add 1 teasp. LEMON JUICE for flavor if desired.
  •Add 1 teasp. BRAGG'S LIQUID AMINOS to each drink if desired.

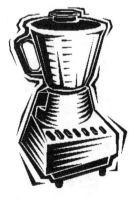

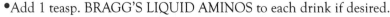

SUPER FOOD MINERAL-RICH ALKALIZING ENZYME DRINK

This blend is an exceptional source of minerals, trace minerals and enzymes for good assimilation and digestion, and for all cell functions. It helps alkalize body pH for better body balance.

Enough for 8 drinks:

Put the following vegetables in a pot with $1\frac{1}{2}$ quarts of cold water. Simmer for 30 minutes. Strain, and take hot or cold.

2 POTATOES, chunked
1 CUP FRESH PARSLEY LEAVES
1 CUP ONION, chunked
1 CUP CARROTS, sliced
1 CUP SLICED CELERY with LEAVES
- •Add 2 TBS. soaked flax seed or oat bran if there is chronic constipation of poor peristalsis.
- •Add 1 teasp. BRAGG'S LIQUID AMINOS to each drink if desired.

NON-DAIRY MORNING PROTEIN DRINK

You must have protein to heal, and the new breed of light, vegetarian protein drinks are a wonderful way to get protein without meat or bulk or excess fat. These drinks obtain protein from several sources so that a balance with carbohydrates and minerals is achieved, and a real energy boost felt.

For 2 drinks:

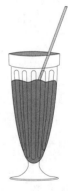

1 CUP STRAWBERRIES or KIWI, sliced
1 BANANA, sliced
1 CUP PAPAYA or PINEAPPLE, chunked
8-OZ. SOFT TOFU or 1 CUP AMAZAKE RICE DRINK
2 TBS. MAPLE SYRUP
1 CUP ORGANIC APPLE JUICE
1 teasp. VANILLA
1 TB. TOASTED WHEAT GERM
$\frac{1}{2}$ teasp. GINGER POWDER

THE DRINKS AND JUICES IN THIS SECTION ARE FOR THE INITIAL CLEANSING PHASES. SEE COOKING FOR HEALTHY HEALING BY LINDA RECTOR PAGE FOR COMPLETE DETOX DIETS AND RECIPES.

We need to give each other stretching space -- the room to respond and react in a variety of ways, according to our personalities and character. We need to stop anticipating the ideal in our lives and start living with the real---which is always checkered with failure and imperfection as well as with success and wonder.

Bodywork Techniques For Detoxification

Therapeutic baths: Clinics and spas are famous all over the world for their mineral, seaweed and enzyme baths. The skin is the body's largest organ of ingestion, and can assimilate the valuable nutrients from a therapeutic bath in a pleasant, stress-free way. Bathe at least twice daily during a cleanse to remove toxins coming out through the skin. The procedure for taking an effective healing bath is important. In essence, you are soaking in an herbal tea, where the skin takes in the healing nutrients instead of the mouth and digestive system.

There are two good ways to take a therapeutic bath:

1. Draw very hot bath water. Put the herbs, seaweeds, or mineral crystals into a large teaball or muslin bath bag. Add mineral salts directly to the water. Steep until water cools and is aromatic.

2. Make a strong tea infusion in a large teapot, strain and add to bath water.

- Soak as long as possible to give the body time to absorb the healing properties. Rub the body with the solids in the muslin bag during the bath for best results.
- All over dry skin brushing before the bath for 5 minutes with a natural bristle brush will help remove toxins from the skin and open pores for better assimilation of nutrients.
- After the bath, use a mineral salt rub, such as Crystal Star LEMON BODY GLOW™, a traditional spa "finishing" technique to make your skin feel healthy for hours.

Note: Food grade 35% H_2O_2 may be used as a detoxifying bath to increase tissue oxygen via the skin. Use $1^1/_2$ cups to a tub of water; or, add $^1/_2$ cup H_2O_2, $^1/_2$ cup sea salt, and $^1/_2$ cup baking soda to bath, and soak for $^1/_2$ hour.

A seaweed bath is a great way to get iodine therapy.

Seaweed baths are Nature's perfect body/psyche balancer, and they're an excellent way to take in iodine therapy. Remember how good you feel after an ocean walk? Seaweeds purify and balance the ocean; they can do the same for your body. Noticeable rejuvenating effects occur when toxins are released from body tissues. A hot seaweed bath is like a wet-steam sauna, only better, because the sea greens balance body chemistry instead of dehydrating it. The electrolytic magnetic action of the seaweed releases excess body fluids from congested cells, and dissolves fatty wastes through the skin, replacing them with depleted minerals, especially potassium and iodine. Iodine boosts thyroid activity, so food fuels are used before they can turn into fatty deposits. Vitamin K in seaweeds aids adrenal regulation, meaning that a seaweed bath can help maintain hormone balance for a more youthful body.

Here is how to take a seaweed bath:

If you live near the ocean, gather kelp and seaweeds from the water, (not the shoreline) in clean buckets or trash cans, and carry them home to your tub. If you don't live near the ocean, dried sea vegetable leaves are available in most herb sections of health food stores. Crystal Star packages dried seaweeds, gathered from the San Juan Islands, in a made-to-order HOT SEAWEED BATH™. Whichever form you choose, run very hot water over the seaweed in a tub, filling it to the point that you will be covered when you recline. The leaves will turn a beautiful bright green. The water will turn rich brown as the plants release their minerals. Add an herbal bath oil if desired, to help hold the heat in and pleasantly scent the water. Let the bath cool enough to get in. As you soak, the gel from the seaweed will transfer onto your skin. This coating increases perspiration to release toxins from your system, and replaces them by osmosis with minerals. Rub your skin with the sea leaves during the bath to stimulate circulation, smooth the body, and remove wastes coming out on the skin surface. When the sea greens have done their therapeutic work, the gel coating dissolves and floats off the skin, and the leaves shrivel - a sign that the bath is over. Each bath varies with the individual, the seaweeds used, and water temperature, but the gel coating release is a natural timekeeper for the bath's benefits. Forty five minutes is usually long enough to balance the acid/alkaline system, encourage liver activity and fat metabolism. Skin tone, color, and circulatory strength are almost immediately noticeable from iodine and potassium absorption. After the bath, take a capsule of cayenne and ginger to put these minerals quickly through the system.

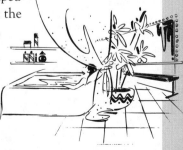

*H*ot & cold hydrotherapy helps open and stimulate the body's vital healing energies. Alternating hot and cold showers, are effective in many cases for getting the body started on a positive track toward healing. Spasmodic pain and cramping, circulation, muscle tone, bowel and bladder problems, system balance, relaxation, and energy all show improvement with hydrotherapy. The form of hydrotherapy included here is easy and convenient for home use.

•Begin with a comfortably hot shower for three minutes. Follow with a sudden change to cold water for 2 minutes. Repeat this cycle three times, ending with cold. Follow with a full or partial massage, or a brisk towel rub and mild stretching exercises for best results.

*H*erbal body wraps: The best European and American spas use herbal wraps as restorative body-conditioning methods. Wraps are also body cleansing techniques that can be used to elasticize, tone, alkalize and release body wastes quickly. They should be used in conjunction with a short cleansing program, and 6-8 glasses of water a day to flush out loosened fats and toxins. Crystal Star makes two wraps for home use: TIGHTENING & TONING™ wrap to improve muscle, vein and skin tone, and ALKALIZING ENZYME™ wrap to replace and balance important minerals, enhance metabolism and alkalize the system. (Follow directions enclosed with these products to use them correctly.)

*C*ompresses are used during a cleanse to draw out waste and waste residues, such as cysts or abscesses through the skin, and to release them into the body's elimination channels. Use alternating hot and cold compresses for best results. Apply the herbs to the hot compress, and leave the ice or cold compress plain. We regularly use cayenne, ginger and lobelia effectively for the hot compresses.

•Add 1 teasp. powdered herbs to a bowl of very hot water. Soak a washcloth and apply until the cloth cools. Then apply a cloth dipped in ice water until it reaches body temperature. Repeat several times daily.
•Green clay compresses are also effective toxin-drawing agents for growths, and may be applied to gauze, placed on the area, covered and left for all day. Simply change as you would any dressing when you bathe.

*E*nemas are a very important therapeutic aid to a congestion cleansing regimen. They increase the release of old, encrusted colon waste, encourage discharge of parasites, freshen the G.I. tract, and make the whole cleansing process easier and more thorough. Enemas should be used during both mucous and colon cleansing diets for optimum results. They are particularly helpful during a healing crisis, or after a serious illness or drug-treated hospital stay to speed healing. Even some headaches and inflammatory skin conditions can be relieved with enemas.

•Herbs are effective in enema and compress solutions for use during a cleanse. The addition of herbs in the enema water serves to immediately alkalize the bowel area, help control irritation and inflammation, and provide local healing activity where there is ulceration or distended tissue.

•We recommend three herbs regularly for enemas - catnip and pau d'arco, (use 2 cups of very strong brewed tea to 1-quart of water), and liquid chlorophyll, (use 3 TBS. to 1-quart water) or spirulina, (2 TBS. powder to 1-quart water). Catnip is effective for stomach and digestive conditions, and for childhood diseases. Pau d'arco is used to balance the acid/alkaline system, as in chronic yeast and fungal infections. Chlorophyll-source herbs are successful for blood and bowel toxicity.

Herbs are helpful for specific-use enemas. Use 2 cups of strong brewed tea to 1 qt. of water per enema.
•Garlic helps kill parasites and cleanse harmful bacteria, viruses and mucous. Blend six garlic cloves in two cups cold water and strain. For small children, use 1 clove garlic to 1 pint water.
•Pau d'arco is effective for body chemistry imbalances, especially immune deficient diseases.
•Lobelia helps for food poisoning, especially when vomiting prevents antidotal herbs being taken by mouth.
•Aloe vera heals tissues in cases of hemorrhoids, irritable bowel and diverticulitis.
•Lemon juice internal wash, to rapidly neutralize an acid system, cleanse the colon and bowel.
•Acidophilus powder helps relieve gas, yeast infections, and candidiasis. mix 4 oz. powder in 1 qt. water.

Coffee enemas have become somewhat of a standard in natural healing for liver and blood related cancers.

Caffeine used in this way stimulates the liver and gallbladder to remove toxins, open bile ducts, encourage increased peristaltic action, and produce necessary enzyme activity for healthy red blood cell formation and oxygen uptake. Use 1 cup of regular strong brewed coffee to 1 qt. water.

Fresh wheatgrass juice enemas stimulate the liver to cleanse.

Wheatgrass enema nutrients are absorbed by the hemorrhoidal vein, just inside the anal sphincter, and enter the portal circulation to the liver. Wheatgrass increases the peristaltic action of the colon, and attracts waste and old fecal matter like a magnet to be eliminated from the body. Wheatgrass juice tones the colon and is absorbed into the blood, adding oxygen and energy to the body.
- Use pure water for an initial enema rinse of the colon.
- Then use about a cup of pure water with 4 ounces of fresh wheatgrass juice.
- Hold the juice for ten minutes, or more, or a bit of time if you can, and massage colon area.
- Expel when necessary.

Here's how to take a colonic enema for detoxification:

Place the enema solution (at a temperature comfortable to the body) in a water bag, and hang or hold about 18 inches higher than the body. Attach colon tube, and lubricate with vaseline or vitamin E oil. Expel a little water from the tube to let out air bubbles. Lying on the left side, slowly insert the tube about 18 inches into the colon. Never use force. Rotate tube gently for ease of insertion, removing kinks, so liquid will flow freely. Massage the abdomen, or flex and contract stomach muscles to relieve any cramping. When all solution has entered the colon, slowly remove the tube and remain on the left side for 5 minutes. Then move to a knee-chest position with the weight of the body on the knees and one hand. Use the other hand to massage the lower left side of the abdomen for several minutes.

Massage releases encrusted fecal matter. Roll onto the back for another 5 minutes, massaging up the descending colon, over the transverse colon to the right side, and down the ascending colon. Then move onto the right side for 5 minutes, so that each portion of the colon is reached. Get up and quickly expel fluid into the toilet. Sticky grey or brown mucous, small dark incrusted chunks, or tough ribbon-like pieces are frequently loosened and expelled during an enema. These poisonous looking things are usually the obstacles and toxins interfering with normal body functions. The good news is that they are no longer in you. You may have to take several enemas before there is no more evidence of these substances.

*H*erbal implants are concentrated solutions for more serious health problems, such as colitis, arthritis or prostate inflammation. Prepare for the implant by taking a small enema with warm water to clear out the lower bowel, so you to hold the implant longer.
- Mix 2 TBS. of your chosen herbal powder, such as spirulina, or wheat grass in $1/2$ cup water. Lubricate the tip of a syringe with vaseline or vitamin E oil, get down on your hands and knees and insert the nozzle into the rectum. Squeeze the bulb to insert the mixture, but do not release pressure on the bulb before it is withdrawn, so the mixture will stay in the lower bowel. Hold as long as you can before expelling.

*O*verheating therapy stimulates a slight fever in the body, is a powerful natural healing tool against serious disease. Fever is a natural defense and healing force of the immune system, created and sustained by the body to rid itself of harmful pathogens and to restore health. The high body temperature speeds up metabolism, inhibits the growth of the harmful virus or bacteria, and literally burns the invading organism with heat.

Fever has long been known to be an effective, protective healing measure against colds and simple infections, even against serious diseases such as cancer and leukemia. Today, artificially induced fevers are used in many biological, holistic clinics for treating acute infectious diseases, arthritic conditions, skin disorders and much more. The newest research indicates that AIDS and related syndromes are also responding to blood heating. (See ALTERNATIVE HEALING METHODS in this book for more about clinical hyperthermia.)

A moderate, natural version may be effectively used in the home. It has the beneficial effect of stimulating the body's immunological mechanism, without the stress of fever-inducing drugs.

Here's how to take an overheating bath:

1. Do not eat for two hours before treatment. Empty bladder and colon if possible.

2. Obtain a good thermometer so that water temperature can be correctly measured. The bath temperature must be monitored at all times.

3. Use as large a tub as possible. Plug the emergency outlet to raise the water to the top of the tub. The patient must be totally covered with water for therapeutic results - with only nose, eyes and mouth left uncovered. Start slowly running water at skin temperature. After 15 minutes raise temperature to 100 degrees, then in 15 minutes to 103 degrees. Although the water temperature is not high, when the patient is totally covered, no heat escapes from the body and its temperature will rise to match that of the water, creating a slight healing fever.

4. The length of the treatment should be about 1 hour. If the patient is ill, constant supervision is necessary. The patient's pulse should not go over 130 or 140. Watch the patient's reactions closely. If he or she experiences discomfort, raise to a sitting position for 5 minutes.

5. Gentle massage with a skin brush during the bath is helpful in stimulating circulation. It helps bring the blood to the surface of the skin, and relieves the heart from undue pressure.

*S*auna heat therapy is another way to use the overheating therapy principles. A long sauna not only induces a healing, cleansing fever, but also causes profuse therapeutic sweating. The skin, in overheating therapy, acts as a "third kidney" to eliminate body wastes through perspiration.

As with the overheating therapy bath above, a sauna speeds up metabolism, and inhibits the replication of pathogenic organisms. All vital organs and glands are stimulated to increased activity. The body's immune system is supported and its healing functions accelerated. The detoxifying and cleansing capacity of the skin is dramatically increased by profuse sweating.

It is possible to make a do-it-yourself sauna, but the procedure is cumbersome. Professional saunas are available in every health club and gym as part of the membership, and the new home-installed models are not only adequate but reasonable in price. For optimum skin cleansing and restoration, take a sauna once or twice a week. Finish each sauna with a cool shower and a brisk rubdown to remove toxins that have been eliminated through the skin.

Note: Overheating and iodine therapy are two of the most effective treatments in natural healing. Induced "fever" is a natural, constructive means the body also uses to heal itself. Yet, these methods are powerful and should be used with care. If you are under medical supervision for heart disease or high blood pressure, a heart and general vitality check is advisable. Also some people who are seriously ill lose the ability to perspire, and this should be known before using overheating therapy. Check with your physician to determine if overheating therapy from a sauna or a seaweed bath is all right for you.

> *Today is a very important day. You are exchanging today for a day of your life. You can waste it...or use it for good. When tomorrow comes, today will be gone forever, leaving in its place what you have traded it for.*
>
> *Use it for gain and not loss, for good and not evil, for right and not wrong, for success and not failure. Use it for the best that is in you so that you will never regret the price you have paid for this day.*

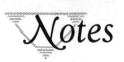

Notes

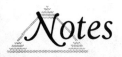

Section Six

Food & Diet Choices
That Affect Healing

CLEARLY, YOUR DIET IS THE BASIS FOR GOOD HEALTH AND OPTIMUM HEALING.
Recent research on neutraceuticals and phytonutrients in our foods shows a wealth of evidence to support the fact that our diets can heal as well as nourish us.

Diet improvement is a major weapon against disease, from the common cold to cancer. Whole food nutrition allows the body to use its built-in restorative and repairing abilities. A healthy diet can intervene in the disease process at many stages, from its inception to its growth and spread.

However, foods aren't equal in their healing abilities, and certain foods don't contribute to healing activity at all. This section can help you sort out the facts about foods, especially the foods and food categories that are making news today.

We'll consider both food options that help, and food options that hinder the healing process:
- Fresh fruits and vegetables
- Green superfoods
- Water's healing effects
- Protein for healing
- Dairy foods and healing
- Fats and oils
- Sugars and sweeteners
- Sea vegetables and iodine therapy
- Green and black teas
- Wines
- Soy foods
- Salts and seasonings

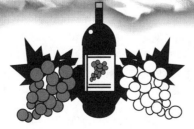

Fresh Fruits & Vegetables & Healing

Fruits and vegetables are a major weapon against disease. Whole food nutrition allows the body to use its built-in restorative and repair abilities. Even if your genetics and lifestyle are against you, your diet still makes a tremendous difference in your health and healing odds. Fresh fruits and vegetables can accelerate body detoxification, and help normalize body chemistry. It's one of the reasons I emphasize a detoxification diet as part of a disease control program.

Fruits and vegetables are full of neutraceuticals, the substances in plants that have pharmacologic action. Also known as phytochemicals and phytonutrients, the actions of neutraceuticals are predictable in much the same way as pharmaceuticals, but they are natural constituents of foods.

Fresh fruits and vegetables can even intervene in the cancer process at many stages, from its inception to its growth and spread. For example, we know that certain body chemicals must be "activated" before they can initiate cancer cell growth. Foods can block the activation process. Food chemicals in cells can determine whether a cancer-causing virus or a cancer promoter, like excess estrogen, will turn tissue cancerous. Yet even after cells have massed into structures that may grow into tumors, food compounds can intervene to stop further growth. Phyto-chemicals found in cruciferous vegetables, for instance, can remove carcinogens from the body. Others actually shrink the patches of precancerous cells. Antioxidant foods can snuff out carcinogens, nip free radical cascades in the bud, even repair some cellular damage.

Although far less powerful at later stages, diet can still influence the metastasis or spread of cancer. Wandering cancer cells need deficient conditions in which to attach and grow. Healthy food nutrients can foster a favorable environment, so even after cancer is diagnosed, the right foods may help prolong your life. The best way for your body to utilize phytochemicals is to ingest the plant source in its whole form.

Fresh fruits are nature's way of smiling. Fruits are wonderful for a quick system wash and cleanse. Their high natural water and sugar content speeds up metabolism to release wastes rapidly. Fresh fruit also has an alkalizing effect in the body, and is high in vitamins and nutrients. The easily convertible natural sugars in fruit transform into quick energy that speeds up the calorie burning process.

But these advantages are only true of fresh fruits. With fruit, the way that you eat it is as important as what you eat. Fruits have their best healing and nutritional effects when eaten alone or with other fruits, as in a fruit salad, separately from grains and vegetables. With a few exceptions, both fruits and fruit juices should be taken before noon for best energy conversion and cleansing benefits.

Cooking fruits changes their properties from alkalizing to acid-forming in the body. This is also true of sulphured, dried fruit, and the combination of fruits with vegetables or grains. When you eat fruit in any of these ways, digestion slows down because the fruits stay too long in the stomach, and gas forms, because the fruit sugars become more concentrated, resulting in fermentation instead of assimilation.

New studies on fruits and their usefulness indicates amazing benefits. Some researchers are even calling citrus fruits a total anti-cancer package, because citrus possesses every class of natural substances (carotenoids, flavonoids, terpenes, limonoids, coumarins) that neutralize chemical carcinogens. One analysis found that citrus fruits possess fifty-eight known anti-cancer compounds, more than any other food!

Like medicinal herbs, the phytochemical compounds in citrus fruits act more powerfully as a whole than any of the separate anticancer compounds they contain. One phytochemical, found in whole oranges, is the powerful antioxidant glutathione, a confirmed disease combatant. When chemically extracted, orange juice loses its glutathione concentrations. Oranges are the highest of all foods by far in glucarate, another cancer-inhibitor. Beta-carotene and vitamin C compounds in citrus fruits are well-documented for their healing ability.

Eat organically grown fruits whenever possible. The pesticides from sprayed fruits can enter the body very rapidly because of quick fruit sugar metabolism.

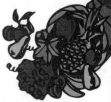

Fresh vegetables are Nature's "superfoods." Massive new research is validating what natural healers have known for decades. The more fruits and vegetables you eat, the less your risk of disease. Even for cancer, people who eat plenty of vegetables have half the risk of people who eat few vegetables.

Most studies show that even small to moderate amounts of vegetables make a big difference. Eating certain fresh vegetables twice a day, instead of twice a week, can cut the risk of lung cancer by 75%, even in smokers. One National Cancer Institute spokesman said it is almost mind-boggling, that ordinary fruits and vegetables could be so effective against such a potent carcinogen as cigarette smoke.

The evidence is so overwhelming that some researchers are beginning to view fruits and vegetables as powerful preventive "drugs" that could substantially wipe out the scourge of cancer. What an about-face this has been for cancer study!

The healing power of vegetables works both raw and cooked. It is not always true that raw vegetables are better. Even though several fragile anticancer agents, like indoles and vitamin C, are destroyed by heat, a little heat makes beta carotene more easily absorbed. I frequently recommend lightly cooked vegetables because their action is gentler, especially if your body is very ill or your digestion is impaired.

> What is a serving of fresh fruits or vegetables? One serving is about $1/2$ cup of cooked or chopped raw fruit or vegetables; 1 cup of raw leafy vegetables; 1 medium piece of fruit, or 6-ounces of fruit juice or vegetable juice. Only 10% of Americans eat that much every day.

A wealth of recent research shows just how valuable the phytochemicals in fruits and vegetables are against disease. Here is some of the latest reasons they should be the basis for your healing diet:

• **Garlic and Onions** contain more than 30 different anti-carcinogens, such as quercetin and ajoene. Such compounds can block the most feared cancer-causing agents like nitrosamines and aflatoxin, linked specifically to stomach, lung and liver cancer. In the county where Georgia's Vidalia onions are grown, the stomach cancer rate is only half that of other Georgia counties, and only one-third that of the rest of the United States.

Garlic and onions defend cells against damage by oxidizing agents and heavy metals. Their sulphur-containing compounds inhibit the growth of staphylococcus, streptococcus and salmonella. Garlic particularly fights candida albicans yeast.

Garlic suppresses cholesterol synthesis in the liver, lowering serum cholesterol by reducing LDL cholesterol while maintaining high density lipoproteins at normal levels. It lowers blood pressure, by decreasing peripheral vascular resistance. Garlic also lowers triglycerides, blood fats associated with increased risk of heart attacks. Garlic reduces the tendency of blood to clot, and helps to dissolve existing clots, preventing heart attacks and strokes. It may even reverse arterial blockages caused by atherosclerosis.

Harvard scientists have immunized mice against some cancers by putting onions in their drinking water. Mice who eat garlic have 75% fewer colon tumors. Even when the mice were given agents that cause cancers like breast cancer, not a single one who ate the garlic compound got cancer. A new German study shows that garlic compounds are toxic to malignant cells, destroying the cells very like the way chemotherapy does. The potent garlic compound, *ajoene*, was three times as toxic to malignant cells as to normal cells. Interleukin from garlic is one of the biological response modifiers that boost immune macrophages and T-lymphocytes that destroy tumor cells. Garlic also discourages colon cancer by working as an antibiotic against certain infective bacteria identified with colon cancer.

• **Green leafy vegetables** exhibit extraordinarily broad cancer protective powers. A recent Italian study showed protection from the risk of most cancers. Greens have many different antioxidants, including beta carotene, folic acid, and lutein, a little-known antioxidant that scientists think may be as potent as beta carotene against cancer. Choose the darkest green vegetables. The darker green they are the more cancer-inhibiting carotenoids they have.

• **Antioxidants in foods** like wheat germ, soy, yellow, orange and green vegetables, green tea, citrus fruits, and olive oil help normalize pre-cancerous cells, and neutralize cancer-causing free radicals.

• **Genistein** found in soybeans and to a lesser extent cabbage family vegetables, inhibits angiogenesis, and deters proliferation of cancer cells especially in hormone-related cancers. See Soy & Healing, page 207.

- **Vitamin C (ascorbic acid)**, rich in foods like citrus fruits, cherries, tomatoes, green peppers, strawberries, kale, parsley, hot red peppers and broccoli, offers both immune support and anti-oxidant protection. Ascorbic acid aids in production of collagen, maintains capillary integrity and contributes to healthy teeth and gums. Vitamin C aids iron absorption, promotes wound healing, and assists in the production of interferon to enhance immune response and T-cell production.

- **Beta carotene,** found in red, yellow and dark green vegetables and fruits, is another important antioxidant. Beta carotene protects against cancer, stroke and cataracts, enhances the immune system, lowers serum cholesterol, and protects against heart disease by preventing oxidation of LDL cholesterol. Beta carotene can destroy human tumor cells by multiple mechanisms. It reduces proliferation of cancer cells, reduces free-radical activity in cancerous cells and accelerates enzyme activity to fight cancer. It even stimulates immune response to directly kill tumor cells, so that if a tumor forms, it is substantially smaller than a tumor not exposed to beta carotene. Recent Harvard studies show that beta carotene has a direct toxic effect on human squamous carcinoma cells from solid tumors, performing as a chemotherapy agent. Research from Tufts University shows that beta carotene changes into a substance called retinoic acid which is being used to treat bladder cancer, with considerable success.

- **Lycopene,** a carotenoid found in tomatoes, red grapefruit, apricots and watermelon works as an antioxidant to inhibit the oxidation of LDL cholesterol to its atherogenic form - a factor in cardiovascular disease. Low blood lycopene is associated with a higher risk of pancreatic cancer and lung cancer. Other lycopene studies show promise against prostate cancer.

- **Phytic acid**, an anti-oxidant substance from rye, wheat, rice, lima beans, sesame seeds, peanuts and soybeans, appears to prevent colon cancer and enhance natural killer cell activity.

- **Soluble fiber** from whole grains, fruits and vegetables absorbs excess bile and improves intestinal bacteria.

- **Folic acid,** found in whole wheat and wheat germ, leafy vegetables, beets, asparagus, fish, sunflower seeds, and citrus fruits are critical to normal DNA synthesis so healthy cells stay healthy.

- **Sulforaphane** found in cruciferous vegetables plus mustard and horseradish, induces protective phase II enzymes, which detoxify carcinogens and eliminate them from the body. Sulforaphane delays onset of cancer, and inhibits the size and number of tumors.

- **3 indole carbinol** from cruciferous vegetables, also induces phase II enzymes which neutralize toxic carcinogens (see above). It increases the activity of glutathione S-transferase, to enhance pathways for the removal of carcinogens. 3 Indole carbinol is believed to be valuable in the prevention of breast cancer. Men who regularly consume cruciferous vegetables have a substantially lower risk of colon cancer compared to men who eat little or none.

- **Ellagic acid** found in walnuts, berries, grapes, apples, tea and pomegranates, demonstrates anti-tumor activity. It inhibits lung and skin tumors by interfering with certain carcinogens. Belonging to the polyphenol group of healing food factors, like those in red wine and green tea, ellagic acid also inhibits nicotine-induced lung tumor genesis.

May you enter heaven an hour before the devil knows you've gone.
_____Old Irish Proverb.

Green Superfoods & Chlorophyll

Green foods are rich sources of essential nutrients. We are all adding more salads and green vegetables to our diets. But, because of the great concern for the nutritional quality of produce grown on mineral depleted soils, green superfoods, such as chlorella, spirulina, alfalfa, barley and wheat grass are becoming popular. They are nutritionally more potent than regular foods, and are in my opinion, the best of the food-source antioxidants for healthy healing.

Green, and blue-green algae, (phyto-plankton), have been called perfect superfoods. They have abundant, high quality, digestible protein, fiber, chlorophyll, vitamins, minerals and enzymes. They are the most potent source of beta carotene available in the world today, and the richest food sources of vitamin B_{12}. The amino acids in blue green algae are virtually identical to those needed by the human body. Their protein yield is greater than soy beans, corn or beef. They are the only foods sources, other than mother's milk, of GLA, (gamma-linolenic acid), an essential fatty acid. Deficiencies in GLA contribute to obesity, heart disease, and PMS. Phytoplankton are used therapeutically to stimulate immune response, improve digestion, detoxify the body, enhance growth and tissue repair, accelerate healing, protect against radiation, help prevent degenerative disease and promote longer life.

- **Chlorella** contains a higher concentration of chlorophyll than any other known plant. It is a complete protein food, with all the B vitamins, vitamin C and E, and many minerals actually high enough to be considered supplementary amounts. The cell wall material of chlorella has a particularly beneficial effect on intestinal and bowel health, detoxifying the colon, stimulating peristaltic activity, and promoting the growth of friendly bacteria. Chlorella is effective in eliminating heavy metals, like lead, mercury, copper and cadmium. Antitumor research shows it is an important source of beta carotene in healing. It strengthens the liver, the body's major detoxifying organ, so that it can rid the body of infective agents that destroy immune defenses. It reduces arthritis stiffness, lowers blood pressure, relieves gastritis and ulcers. Its rich nutritional content has made it effective in weight loss programs, both for cleansing ability, and to maintain muscle tone during lower food intake. But its most important benefits come from a combination of molecules that biochemists call the Controlled Growth Factor, a unique composition that provides a noticeable increase in sustained energy and immune health. The list of chlorella benefits is long and almost miraculous, from detoxification to energy enhancement, to immune system restoration.

- **Spirulina** is the original green superfood, an easily produced algae with the ability to grow in both ocean and alkaline waters. It is ecologically sound in that it can be cultivated in extreme environments which are useless for conventional agriculture. It can be cultivated on small scale community farms, doubling its bio-mass every two to five days, in such a variety of climates and growing conditions that it could significantly improve the nutrition of populations currently on the brink of starvation. Research has shown that spirulina alone could double the protein available to humanity on a fraction of the world's land, while helping restore the environmental balance of the planet. Acre for acre, spirulina yields 20 times more protein than soybeans, 40 times more protein than corn, and 400 times more protein than beef. It is a complete protein, providing all 21 amino acids, and the entire B complex of vitamins, including B_{12}. It is rich in beta carotene, minerals, trace minerals, and essential fatty acids. Digestibility is high, stimulating both immediate and long range energy.

The Green Grasses

Green grass is the only vegetation on earth that can give sole nutritional support to an animal from birth to old age. Grasses have the extraordinary ability to transform inanimate elements from soil, water and sunlight into living cells with nutrient energy. They contain all the known mineral and trace mineral elements, a balanced range of vitamins and hundreds of enzymes for digestion. The small molecular proteins in grasses can be absorbed directly into the blood for cell metabolism. They are highly therapeutic from the chlorophyll activity absorbed directly through the cell membranes.

Green grasses are some of the lowest-calorie and most nutrient-rich edibles on the planet, and some of the most overlooked and underused. Since the cause of most illness is the lack of sufficient, necessary nutrients, flooding the tissues with live, organic nourishment from grasses can have a powerful effect on strengthening the body's immune response against disease.

Barley, wheatgrass and alfalfa are helpful for high blood pressure, obesity, diabetes, gastritis, ulcers, pancreas and liver problems, asthma, eczema, hemorrhoids, skin problems, fatigue, anemia, constipation, breath and body odor and the odor of infection. They are especially effective for oral inflammations, bleeding gums, osteomyelitis (chronic bone marrow inflammation), burns, athlete's foot and cancer. Wheat and barley grasses are also good for bones because they are rich sources of vitamin K, a nutrient that helps maintain normal bone metabolism. Taking in nutrients from grasses enhances the feeling of well-being while simultaneously improving energy and stamina.

- **Barley grass** has a wide range of concentrated vitamins, minerals, enzymes, proteins and chlorophyllins - eleven times the calcium of cow's milk, five times the iron of spinach, and seven times the amount of vitamin C and bioflavonoids as orange juice. One of its most important contributions to a vegetarian diet is 80mcg of vitamin B_{12} per hundred grams of powdered juice. Research on barley grass shows encouraging results for DNA damage repair and delaying aging. Barley juice powder contains anti-viral properties, and neutralizes heavy metals like mercury. It is an ideal food-source anti-inflammatory for healing gastro-intestinal ulcers, hemorrhoids, and pancreas infections. According to Dr. Kubota of the Tokyo Pharmacy Science University, "barley grass is an ideal anti-inflammatory medication, with effects measurably stronger than steroid and non-steroid drugs. It has few if any side effects."

- **Alfalfa** is one of the world's richest mineral-source foods, pulling up earth minerals from root depths as great as 130 feet! A green superfood, it is an excellent source for liquid chlorophyll, with a balance of organic chemical and mineral constituents almost identical to human hemoglobin. Alfalfa is a body cleanser, infection fighter and a natural deodorizer, not only because of its chlorophyll content, but also because it's a rich source of fiber. It is a good spring tonic, eliminates retained water, and relieves urinary and bowel problems. It is a restorative, helping to treat recuperative cases of narcotic and alcohol addiction. It is used therapeutically for arthritis, intestinal and skin disorders, liver problems, breath and body odor, and even cancer.

Today, herbalists use alfalfa to encourage blood-clotting, because of its high content of vitamin K. It is also used to treat bladder infections, all colon disorders, anemia, hemorrhaging, diabetes and most recently as an aid in normalizing estrogen production.

- **Wheat grass** has curative powers for treating cancerous growths and other degenerative diseases, when taken as a fresh liquid. Fifteen pounds of fresh wheatgrass has the nutritional value of 350 pounds of vegetables. We have seen particular success with wheat grass rectal implants in colon cancer cases. Wheat grass helps cleanse the blood, organs and gastrointestinal tract, and is recommended as a way to stimulate metabolism and enzyme activity. Wheat grass also normalizes the thyroid gland, which may be helpful in correcting obesity problems.

As with all the green grasses, the primary benefit of wheat grass is its chlorophyll content. Its ability to provide protection from carcinogens comes from chlorophyll's ability to strengthen cells, detoxify the liver and blood, and chemically neutralize pollutants. Chlorophyll helps humans, as it does plants, to resist harm from the destructive effects of air pollution, X-rays and radiation, and especially from carbon monoxide in vehicle emissions. Wheat grass has beneficial external effects as well. Its ointment has been used to successfully treat such disorders as skin ulcers, impetigo and itching.

- **Aloe vera** has long been known as an effective skin moisturizer and healer for cuts, sunburn, bruises, insect bites, skin sores, acne, eczema and burns in gel form, aloe juice is now becoming widely known for its digestive, soothing laxative properties, and as a specific for colon problems and liver disease. Aloe vera has excellent transdermal properties, allowing it to penetrate deep skin levels. It is becoming a necessity in doctor's pre-op and post-op healing instructions, because it is a natural antiseptic and astringent for infections, both internal and external. It is a natural oxygenator, increasing the body's uptake of oxygen. Research is indicating even more wonderful healing results from this superfood - for arthritis, skin cancers, hemorrhoids and varicose veins. Aged aloe vera juice is even being widely used in AIDS treatment to block the HIV virus movement from cell to cell.

About Chlorophyll

The most therapeutic ingredient of the green grasses, and indeed all the super green foods, is chlorophyll. Chlorophyll is the pigment that plants use to carry out the process of photosynthesis. It absorbs the light energy from the sun, and converts it into earth and plant energy. This energy is transferred into our cells and blood when we consume live, fresh greens. Chlorophyll is in all fresh green plants, but is particularly rich in the green and blue-green algae, wheat grass, barley grass, parsley, and alfalfa.

Chlorophyll is the basic component of the "blood" of plants. The chlorophyll molecule is remarkably similar to human hemoglobin in composition, except that it carries magnesium in its center instead of iron. Consuming chlorophyll-rich foods helps the body to build red blood cells, which carry oxygen to every cell. In essence, eating any of the green superfoods is almost like giving yourself a little transfusion to help treat illness, enhance immunity and sustain well-being. They have a synergistic effect when added to a normal diet. The green superfoods are valuable in almost all of the healing diets.

Chlorophyll is recommended for anemia fatigue and for a calming activity on the nervous system. It is helpful in insomnia, exhaustion and nervous irritability. It is used beneficially for skin ulcers, and helps in coping with deep infections, skin disorders, and dental problems, such as pyorrhea.

Because of its detoxifying and anti-bacterial qualities, chlorophyll has proven to be a valuable remedy in the treatment of colds, rhinitis, inner-ear infections and inflammation.

Chlorophyll is a primary aid for the detoxification of organs, particularly the liver. It helps to neutralize and remove drug deposits from the body, purify the blood and counteract acids and toxins in the system. Even the medical community is seeing chlorophyll as a possible means of removing heavy metal buildup, because it can bind with several toxins, including heavy metals, and help eliminate them.

Chlorophyll is easily digested, yet it is rich in vitamin K, which is necessary for blood clotting. It is used by naturopathic physicians for women with heavy menstrual bleeding as well as for anemia. Vitamin K also helps form a compound in the urine that inhibits growth of calcium oxalate crystals (common kidney stones), so chlorophyll may help with this very painful condition.

A new U.S. Army study revealed that a chlorophyll-rich diet doubled the lifespan of animals exposed to lethal radiation, and chlorophyll is now being considered (since the days of Agent Orange and Gulf War Syndrome) as a protective against some chemical warfare weapons.

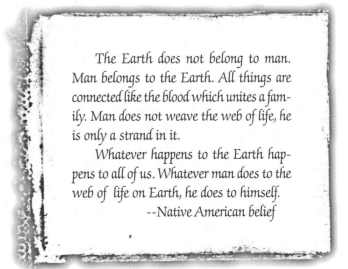

The Earth does not belong to man. Man belongs to the Earth. All things are connected like the blood which unites a family. Man does not weave the web of life, he is only a strand in it.

Whatever happens to the Earth happens to all of us. Whatever man does to the web of life on Earth, he does to himself.

--Native American belief

Water Is Essential To A Healing Diet

Water is the basis of life. Water is second only to oxygen in importance for health. It makes up 65 to 75% of the body, and every cell requires water to perform its essential functions. Water maintains system equilibrium, lubricates tissues, flushes wastes and toxins, hydrates the skin, regulates body temperature, acts as a shock absorber for joints, bones and muscles, adds needed minerals, and transports nutrients, minerals, vitamins, proteins and sugars for assimilation. It is the most crucial of all nutrients for survival. A human being can live for weeks without food but only for days without water.

When the body gets enough water, it works at its peak. Fluid and sodium retention decrease, gland and hormone functions improve, the liver breaks down and releases more fat, and hunger is curtailed. Water deficiency is related to a number of ailments including chronic constipation, hemorrhoids, varicose veins, urinary tract infections and kidney stones.

Yet, despite the fact that water is conveniently available in America, dehydration is as common here as it is in dry regions of the world, probably because Americans are not very conscious of the health practice of drinking plenty of water on a daily basis. Even when their fluid intake is normal, many Americans are deficient in essential fatty acids (EFAs). Severe EFA deficiency in the body opens the door to dehydration, because fatty acids act as cellular glue to prevent excessive fluid loss, particularly from the skin.

Poor water quality is also a problem in many areas of the U.S. Most tap water today is chlorinated, fluoridated, and treated to the point where it can be an irritating, disagreeable fluid instead of a healthful drink. City tap water may contain as many as 500 different disease-causing bacteria, viruses and parasites. Fluoridated water increases absorption of aluminum from deodorants, pots and pans, etc. by 600%, a possible concern for Alzheimer's disease. Chemicals and heavy metals used by industry and agriculture find their way into our ground water, adding more pollutants. Some tap water is now so bad, that without the enormous effort our bodies use to dispose of these chemicals, we would have ingested enough of them to turn us to stone by the time we were thirty! These concerns keep many individuals from drinking tap water. I recommend keeping plenty of good bottled water near at hand. Tap water purifiers or a purifier on your fridge water are other easy solutions for making your water consumable.

Water waste is removed by the kidneys, **through which the entire blood supply passes and is filtered fifteen times each hour.** If the body becomes overheated, our 2 million sweat glands begin perspiration, which is 99% water. Blood heat evaporates the sweat, cooling the body and keeping the internal organs at a constant temperature. A minimal but consistent loss of water occurs during the processes of breathing and tearing. Moisture is breathed out from the nasal passages and the lungs. Tiny tear ducts carry a liquid solution to the upper eyelids, which lubricate the eyes 25 times every minute. The tears then pass down to the nose, where they evaporate.

Approximately 3 quarts of replacement water is needed by the body each day under normal conditions. Strenuous activity, a high climate temperature, or a diet too high in salt may increase this requirement. Metabolic water is produced as part of the food digestion process, yielding as much as a pint per day. Foods can provide up to $1^1/_2$ quarts. For example, fruits and vegetables are more than 90% water. Even dry foods like bread are about 35% water.

Other healthy liquids beside water count as replenishment. Plain or carbonated cool water is the best way to replace lost body fluid, but unsweetened fruit juices diluted with water or seltzer, and vegetable juices should also be considered. Alcohol and caffeine-containing drinks are counter-productive in replacing water loss because of their diuretic activity. Drinks loaded with dissolved sugars or milk increase water needs instead of satisfying them. Commercial sodas leach several minerals from the body.

It is possible to consume too much water. Some over-enthusiastic people may feel that if ten glasses is good, twenty glasses, or even gallons, is better - on a *daily* basis. But drinking this much makes the body become "waterlogged," severely depressing electrolyte count. Purified water, such as distilled or reverse osmosis techniques compound the problem.

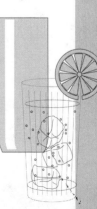

Eight to ten 8-ounce glasses of water is a sufficient daily amount. If you are physically active or working under hot weather conditions and need to consume a lot of liquids, replace your electrolytes with electrolyte drinks like Alacer EMERGEN-C, or supplements, like Bragg's LIQUID AMINOS in water.

Pay conscious attention to getting enough water because thirst is not a reliable signal that your body needs water. Thirst is an evolutionary development designed to indicate severe dehydration. The sense of thirst (as well as sleep, appetite, satiety, and sexual responses) is controlled by a part of the forebrain called the hypothalamus. You can easily lose a quart or more of water during activity before thirst is even recognized. The thirst signal also shuts off before you have had enough for well-being.

♒

Water is critical to a good detoxification program. Add half a squeezed lemon for the best cleansing effects. For a healing program, several types of water are worth consideration.

♈ **Mineral water** comes from natural springs with varying mineral content and widely varying taste. The naturally occurring minerals are beneficial to digestion and regularity. In Europe this form of bottled water has become a fine art, but in the U.S., it is not tested for purity except in California and Florida.

♈ **Distilled water** can be either from a spring or tap source; it is "de-mineralized" so that only oxygen and hydrogen remain. Distilling is accomplished by reverse osmosis, filtering or boiling, then converting to steam and recondensing. It is the purest water available, and ideal for a healing program.

♈ **Sparkling water** comes from natural carbonation in underground springs. Most are also artificially infused with CO_2 to maintain a standard fizz. This water is an aid to digestion, and is excellent in cooking to tenderize and give lightness to a recipe.

♈ **Artesian well water** is the Cadillac of natural waters. It always comes from a deep pure source, has a slight fizz from bubbling up under rock pressure, and is tapped by a drilled well. Artesian water never comes in contact with ground contaminants.

♒

Note: Beyond buying bottled water, you can also take steps as an individual to conserve water and diminish pollution of ground water supplies:
- Use biodegradable soaps and detergents.
- Don't use water fresheners in your toilet bowls.
- Avoid pouring hazardous wastes such as paints, solvents, and petroleum based oils into drains or sewers.
- Use natural fertilizers such as manure and compost in your garden.
- Avoid using non-biodegradable plastics and polystyrene.
- Conserve water with conscious attention to what you really need for a shower, a bath, laundry or cooking.

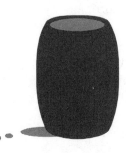

About Protein & A Healing Diet

*Y*ou must have protein to heal. Next to water, protein is the body's most plentiful substance. It is the major source of building material for muscles, blood, skin, hair, nails, and internal organs, including the heart and brain. It is of primary importance for the growth and development of body tissues and for blood clotting. Protein and its precursors, amino acids, work at the deepest hormonal level of the body controlling basic body functions like growth, sexual development, and metabolism. At even more basic levels, enzymes, necessary for immune function and antibody response, are also formed from protein. Protein also helps regulate body chemistry and fluid balance.

Protein is a source of energy, providing 4 calories of heat per gram of protein. However, this energy function is spared when sufficient fats and carbohydrates are present in the diet. So protein that is not used for building tissue or energy may be converted by the liver and stored as fat in the body tissues.

Protein requirements differ according to your nutritional status, body size, and activity level. The traditional rule of thumb for protein requirements is to simply divide body weight by 2; the result will indicate the approximate number of grams of protein required each day.

Protein deficiency leads to abnormalities of growth and tissue development. Hair, nails, skin and muscle tone are especially affected. A child whose diet is protein deficient may not attain his potential height. Extreme protein deficiency in children can even be fatal, and at the very least results in disease vulnerability, stunted mental and physical growth, loss of hair pigment, and inflamed joints. In adults, protein deficiency results in low stamina, mental depression, poor resistance to infection, and slow wound healing. Loss of body protein can occur as a result of stresses like surgery, wounds, or prolonged illness. At times of high stress, you might want to consume extra protein to rebuild worn-out tissues.

However, the protein deficiency health threat has been over-emphasized in wealthy countries, and today, most Americans take in too much protein for good health. Protein does not burn cleanly, it leaves behind nitrogen waste that the body must metabolize and eliminate. This can be especially taxing to the liver and kidneys, so too much protein is harmful to persons with kidney disease or diabetes. Further, excessive protein irritates the immune system and keeps it in a state of overactivity. Too much protein may cause fluid imbalance, so that calcium and other minerals are lost through the urine. Large amounts of animal protein actually contributes to osteoporosis, heart disease and certain cancers.

As it occurs naturally, vegetable protein is high fiber, complex carbohydrate-rich food, high in vitamins and minerals with little or no fat. Vegetarians have much less heart disease, lower blood pressure and osteoporosis, and much less risk of cancer than those who eat meats regularly. While animal protein has been shown to increase cholesterol deposits, vegetable protein lowers them.

Yet, human health thrives on a balanced diet. Even an excessively strict vegetarian diet can endanger health because amino acids and vitamin B_{12} are so easy to lose. Vegetarians who eat neither eggs nor milk products are encouraged to eat plenty of legumes and grains to insure sufficient amino acids. **Black Beans** in particular, are an excellent source of absorbable protein that can also alkalize an over-acid system. Synergistic vegetable protein combinations are black beans and rice, beans and tortillas, or whole wheat flat bread and stew or soup made from a variety of legumes.

Here are some vegetable protein sources to consider for your healing diet:
Along with grains and legumes, soy foods are high protein vegetarian foods. Other good sources include the blue-green algas, spirulina and chlorella, brewer's yeast, wheat germ, nuts, seeds and their butters. Dark green, leafy vegetables, like kale and chard, and cruciferous vegetables, like broccoli and cauliflower, have easily assimilated protein content.

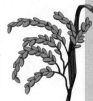

- **Brewer's Yeast** is an excellent source of protein, B vitamins, amino acids and minerals. It is one of the best-immune-enhancing supplements available in food form. Because it is chromium-rich, brewer's yeast can be a key food factor in significantly improving blood sugar metabolism, and in substantially reducing serum cholesterol. It helps speed wound healing through an increase in the production of collagen. It has antioxidant properties to allow the tissues to take in more oxygen for healing. Its B vitamin and mineral content improves both skin texture and blemishes. (Try brewer's yeast for a nourishing natural facial mask.) Brewer's yeast is *not* the same as candida albicans yeast.

- **Sprouts** are ideal for a natural source of protein that also helps the body cleanse itself. Besides protein, sprouts are rich in almost every nutrient, vitamins (especially vitamins A, B-complex, C, D and E), enzymes, essential fatty acids, and minerals, (including iron, potassium, magnesium, phosphorus, calcium, zinc and chromium, all of which are natural antioxidants that strengthen the immune system and protect the body from toxic chemical buildup. Sprouts are cholesterol free, and the few calories they have come from the simple sugars they contain that make them a quick source of energy.

About Red Meat & A Healing Diet

Eating red meats puts us a step away from environmental harmony. Human digestive systems are not easily carnivorous. The body has to struggle to transmute red meat energy. Eating red meat is a lot like extracting oil out of the ground. It often costs more to get the oil out than it is worth on the market. Thus meat protein, which the body can use, is often cancelled out by the length of digestion time, and after-dinner lethargy, because a disproportionate amount of energy goes to the task of assimilation. Frequent intake of red meat's highly concentrated protein can also create toxicity from unused nitrogens, that are hard for the elimination system to cope with or excrete. A common example of this is the frequent instance of kidney stone formations in heavy red meat eaters.

Animals are also closer to us on the bio-scale of life. They experience fear when killed. They don't want to be eaten. Unlike eating plants, there is no uplifting transmutation of energy. Instead our bodies become denser, with more internal fermentation and body odor. In addition to avoiding red meats for humanitarian reasons, and an awareness of what meats do to the body, the red meats available today are shot through with hormones and slow-release antibiotics, and preserved with nitrates or nitrites. All these are passed into your body at the dinner table. The stockyard animals we eat now are often sick and over medicated, and their meat is tainted, chemicalized and adulterated. Red meat is the biggest diet contributor to excess protein levels and saturated fat. No one argues that less fat in the diet is healthier, or that saturated fats are the most harmful. Avoidance of red meat considerably reduces dietary saturated fat and concentrated calories. Cooked red meats are acid-forming in the body, and when red meat is cooked to well-done can create chemical compounds capable of causing many diseases.

Finally, meat eating promotes more aggressive behavior - a lack of gentleness in personality, and arrogance. From a spiritual point of view, red meat eating encourages ties to the material things in life, expansion of territory, and the self-righteous intolerance that makes adversaries.

People who do not eat red meats have a well documented history of lower risk for heart disease, obesity, diabetes, osteoporosis, and several types of cancer. These people also play an active role in conserving precious water, topsoil, and energy resources that are wasted by an animal-based diet. Avoiding red meats has become one of the most important things you can do for your own health and that of the planet.

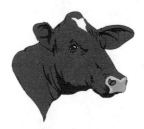

Dairy Foods In A Healing Diet

airy products interfere with the cleansing/healing process because of their density and high satu rated fats. Cow's milk in particular has clogging, mucous forming properties. Pasteurized milk is a relatively dead food as far as nutrition is concerned. Even raw milk can be difficult to assimilate for someone with allergies or respiratory problems. I recommend that dairy foods be avoided during a cleansing diet.

For almost 25% of Americans, dairy intolerance causes allergic reactions, poor digestion, and abnormal mucous build-up. The human system in general does not easily process cow's milk, cream, ice cream or hard cheese, tending to throw off excess from these foods. The unused dairy usually turns to mucous, causing cumulative strain and clogging on eliminative organs.

Women do not handle building foods, such as dairy products, as well as men. Their systems back up more easily, so less dairy may mean easier bowel movements. Many female problems, such as fibrous growths, bladder, and kidney ailments can be improved by avoiding dairy foods. Even people with no noticeable sensitivity to dairy products report a rise in energy when they stop using them as main foods.

Children can be especially susceptible to dairy food reactions. Besides childhood allergies, cow's milk can cause loss of iron and hemoglobin in infants by triggering blood loss from the intestinal tract. Some research also shows that iron absorption is blocked by as much as 60% after dairy products are consumed in a meal. Heavy consumption of milk, especially by small children, may result in vitamin D toxicity.

Contrary to advertising, dairy products are not even a desirable source of calcium. Absorbability is poor because of pasteurizing, processing, high fat content, and an unbalanced relationship with phosphorus. Hormone residues and additives from cattle-raising practices also mean that calcium and other minerals are incompletely absorbed. In cattle tests, calves given their own mother's milk that had first been pasteurized, didn't live six weeks!

Many vegetables, nuts, seeds, fish and sea vegetables contain calcium that is easier for the body to assimilate. Soy cheese, tofu, soy milk, and nut milks may all be used in place of dairy products. Kefir and yogurt, although made from milk, don't have the assimilation problems of dairy products. Unless lactose intolerance is very severe, these foods do not cause a lactose reaction, and are beneficial to healing because of their friendly bacteria cultures. They offer rich quality without the downside of rich dairy.

Dairy foods aren't a very usable source of protein for humans, either. Cow's milk contains proteins that are harmful to our immune systems, because they are absorbed into the blood undigested, provoking an immune response. Repeated exposure to these proteins disrupts normal immune function and may lead to disease. Fish and chicken proteins are much less damaging; plant proteins pose the least hazard.

Because dairy is a tremendous mucous producer it is often a burden on the respiratory, digestive and immune systems. Removing dairy from the diet has been shown to shrink enlarged tonsils and adenoids, a sign of immune system relief. Doctors experimenting with dairy-free diets often report a marked reduction in colds, flus, sinusitis, and ear infections.

When using dairy foods, purchase low-fat or non-fat products, and goat's milk, raw milk and raw cheeses instead of pasteurized. Full fat dairy foods are clearly not good if there is lactose intolerance or if you are on a mucous cleansing diet.

For building and maintenance diets, consider most dairy products as good for taste, but questionable for nutrition. A little is fine - a lot is not. Some small changes in cooking habits and point of view are all it takes - mostly a matter of not having these products around the house, and substituting in your favorite recipes with dairy free alternatives. (See individual listings in this section.) Reduced dairy intake usually means some weight loss, too, and lower blood pressure and cholesterol levels. Soon, you won't feel deprived at all. Just remember the easy weight you'll lose by not eating saturated dairy.

See **COOKING FOR HEALTHY HEALING** by Linda -Page, for delicious, healthy, non-dairy recipes that can be used on almost any healing plan without sacrificing richness or taste.

Here's how specific dairy foods can affect your healing diet:

• **Butter** - Surprise! Butter is okay in moderation. Although a saturated fat, butter is relatively stable, and like raw cream, is a whole, balanced food, used by the body better than its separate components. When butter is needed, use raw, unsalted butter, not margarine or shortening. Don't let it get hot enough to smoke. If less saturated fat is desired, use clarified butter. Simply melt the butter and skim off the top foam. Let it rest a few minutes and spoon off the clear butter for use. Discard whey solids that settle to the bottom, and the foam. Soy margarine is an acceptable vegan alternative in baking.

• **Eggs** - More good news! "Eggsperts" are finally realizing what many of us in the whole foods world have long known. Although high in cholesterol, eggs are also high in balancing lecithins and phosphatides, and do not increase the risk of atherosclerosis. Nutrition-rich fertile eggs from free-run chickens are a perfect food. The difference in fertile eggs and the products from commercial egg factories is remarkable; the yolk color is brighter, the flavor is definitely fresher, and the workability in recipes is better. The distinction is very noticeable in poached and baked eggs, where the yolks firm up and rise higher. Eggs should be lightly cooked for the best nutrition, preferably poached, soft-boiled, or baked, never fried. Eggs are concentrated protein; use them with discretion.

• **Cheese** - Unfortunately for cheese lovers, the saturated fats in cheese make it difficult for a healing diet to succeed. Dairy fats challenge both digestion and metabolism. Commercial cheeses, even though labeled "natural," contain bleaches, coagulants, emulsifiers, moisture absorbants, mold inhibitors, and rind waxes and dyes that visibly leak into the cheese itself. Many restaurant and pizza cheeses add synthetic flavorings, coloring and preservatives. Processed cheese foods obtain their texture from hydrogenated fats rather than natural fermentation. Even if you are not on a healing diet, limit cheese consumption to small amounts of low-fat and raw cheeses which provide usable proteins, with good mineral balance ratio. Today, low sodium and low fat cheeses are made in almost every type of cheese, and are a better choice for a healing program. Raw mozzarella, farmer cheese, ricotta and cheddar are superior in taste and health value to pasteurized cheeses, which have higher salts and additives.

-**Rennet-free cheeses** use a bacteria culture, instead of calves' enzymes to separate curds and whey.

-**Goat cheese (chevre) and sheep's milk cheese (feta)** are both lower in fat than cow's milk cheeses, and are more easily digested. There is a world of difference in taste. Real mozzarella cheese is made from buffalo milk - low fat and absolutely delicious! Raw, fresh cream cheese is light years ahead of commercial brands with gums, fillers and thickeners.

• **Yogurt** is a good intestinal cleanser that helps balance and replace friendly flora in the G.I. tract. Even though yogurt is dairy in origin, the culturing process makes it a living food, and beneficial for health. Most yogurts contain the beneficial bacteria Lactobacillus bulgaricus and Streptococcus thermophilus. Some brands have Lactobacillus acidophilus added. Yogurt is better tolerated than milk, even by those with a deficiency in the enzyme lactase, because yogurt seems to stimulate lactase activity: Bacterial fermentation elements that occur in yogurt actually substitute for the missing enzyme lactase. Yogurt can lower cholesterol and raise HDLs (protective lipoprotein) levels. Calcium is more readily absorbed in the presence of fermented cultures, like yogurt and cultured buttermilk. Yogurt boosts blood levels of gamma interferon, a component of the immune system that rallies killer cells to fight infections. Yogurt kills the bacteria which causes most ulcers and gastritis.

To use yogurt instead of milk in cooking, mix equal parts of yogurt with water, chicken or vegetable broth, white wine or sparkling water, and use cup for cup instead of milk in cooking.

-**Yogurt cheese** is very easy to make, much lighter in fat and calories than sour cream or cream cheese, but with the same richness and consistency. See COOKING FOR HEALTHY HEALING by Linda Rector Page for how to make fresh yogurt cheese.

-**Lowfat cottage cheese** is a cultured dairy product, beneficial for those with only slight lactose intolerance. It is a good substitute for ricotta, cream cheese, and processed cottage cheese foods that are full of chemicals. Mix with non-fat or low fat plain yogurt to add the richness of cream or sour cream to recipes without the fat.

• **Almond Milk** is a rich, non-dairy liquid that may be used for cream soups, sauces, gravies and protein drinks. Use 1 to 1 in place of milk in baked recipes, sauces or gravies. For 1 cup almond milk: place 1 cup blanched almonds in a blender; add 2 to 4 cups water, depending on the consistency desired. Add 1 teasp. honey; whirl until smooth.

- **Sesame tahini** is a rich, creamy ground sesame seed butter. Tahini may be used as a dairy replacement in soups and dressings or sauces without the cholesterol and all the protein. Mixed with water to milk consistency, it may be used as a milk substitute in baking. It can be used in healthy candies and cookies, and on toast in place of peanut butter. It is an excellent complement to greens and salad ingredients. Mix tahini with oil and seasonings for salad toppings.

❧

Apart from how dairy foods affect a healing diet, there are several issues surrounding dairy foods and how they influence good health.

[1] There is a whirlwind of controversy about recombinant bovine growth hormone, rBGH or rBST. The hormones increase milk production, but since America *always has surplus milk supplies, as well as long standing dairy subsidies,* it's hard to see why any American dairy farmer would use such a potentially harmful hormone in order to get even more surplus milk.

Much is still unknown about the long-term effects of rBGH. Increased rates of mastitis infections in rGBH cows leads to increased use of antibiotics to treat the mastitis. This inevitably leads to higher levels of antibiotics in the milk, additives already questioned by both scientists and concerned consumers. We all know, doctors around the world are losing the battle against the onslaught of new drug-resistant bacterial infections. Even moderate use of antibiotics in animal feed can result in antibiotic resistance in animal bacteria, and the transfer of that resistance to human bacteria.

[2] Pesticides seem to concentrate in the milk of both farm animals and humans. A study by the Environmental Defense Fund found widespread pesticide contamination of human breast milk among 1,400 women in forty-six states. The levels of contamination were twice as high among the meat-and-dairy-eating women as among vegetarians.

[3] Consumption of cow's milk has been associated with insulin-dependent diabetes. The milk protein bovine serum albumin (BSA) somehow leads to an autoimmune reaction in the pancreas and ultimately impairs its ability to produce insulin. Research suggests that a combination of genetic predisposition and exposure to lots of cow's milk in the diet may lead to juvenile diabetes.

[4] Ovarian cancer rates parallel dairy-eating patterns around the world. The culprit seems to be galactose, the simple sugar broken down from the milk sugar lactose. In tests, animals fed galactose go on to develop ovarian cancer. Women with this cancer often have trouble breaking down galactose. In fact, about 10% of the U.S. population lacks the enzymes to metabolize galactose. Only a series of enzyme tests can tell you whether you lack these enzymes (unlike lactose intolerance, in which there are clear signs of digestive upset). Yogurt, cheese, and other fermented dairy products are the richest sources of galactose.

[5] A 1989 study linked the risk of developing non-Hodgkin's lymphoma with the consumption of cow's milk and butter. A growing consensus among scientists shows that dairy proteins play a major role in the genesis of this cancer of the immune system. High levels of the cow's milk protein beta-lactoglobulin have been found in the blood of lung cancer patients as well.

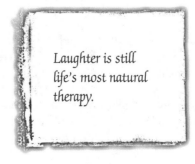

Laughter is still life's most natural therapy.

Fats & Oils In A Healing Diet

We all know that there is a direct relationship between the quantity of fat we consume and the quality of health we can expect. During this century, Americans have increased their intake of fat calories by over 33%. The link between high salt and fat intake on health has also become clear. Excess salt inhibits the body's capacity to clear fat from the bloodstream. The debate about fat has filled the American media for a decade, yet much of the information is contradictory and inaccurate. This section should simplify the confusion, especially as it relates to choices made for a healing diet.

WHAT IS THE DIFFERENCE BETWEEN SATURATED AND UNSATURATED FATS?

All foods contain saturated and unsaturated fats in varying proportions. The difference is in molecular structure, with animal foods being higher in saturated fat, and except for palm and coconut oil, vegetable foods being higher in unsaturated fat. Saturated fats are solid at room temperature, as in butter or meat fat. They are the culprits that clog the arteries, and lead to heart and degenerative disease. Unsaturated fat, (mono or polyunsaturated) is liquid at room temperature, as in vegetable or nut oils. Although research supports unsaturates as helping to reduce serum cholesterol, just switching to unsaturated fats without increasing dietary fiber will not bring about improvement. In fact, consuming moderate amounts of both kinds of unsaturated fats, coupled with a high fiber diet will benefit most people.

WHAT IS THE DIFFERENCE BETWEEN POLY-UNSATURATED AND MONO-UNSATURATED FATS?

Poly-unsaturated vegetable oils are the chief source for the "essential fatty acids" (linoleic, linolenic and arachidonic) so necessary to proper cell membrane function, balanced prostaglandin production and other metabolic processes. Good poly-unsaturates include sunflower, safflower, sesame oil, and flax oil, one of the best sources of essential fatty acids.

-Olive oil is a mono-unsaturated fat that reduces the amount of LDL in the bloodstream. Research shows that it is even more effective in this process than a low fat diet. Another oil high in mono-unsaturated fats is canola or rapeseed oil.

-Canola oil has 10% Omega-3 fatty acids, and half the amount of saturated fat found in other vegetable oils.

ARE ALL VEGETABLE OILS UNSATURATED FATS?

All vegetable oils are free of cholesterol, but most commercial cooking oils contain synthetic preservatives and are heavily refined, bleached and deodorized with chemical solvents. Unrefined oils are mechanically pressed, filtered and bottled. They are the least processed and the most natural. They have some sediment, and a taste of the raw vegetable. (Cold pressing applies only to olive oil.) The highest quality vegetable oils are rich in fatty acids and essential to health in their ability to stimulate prostaglandin levels.

Solvent-extracted oil is a second pressing from the first pressing residue. Hexane is generally used to enable the most efficient extraction, and even though small amounts of this petroleum chemical remain, it is still considered an unrefined oil. Refined oils go through several other processing stages, such as degumming, which keeps the oil from going rancid quickly, but also removes many nutrients, including vitamin E. Refined oils are de-pigmented through charcoal or clay, clarified through deodorizing under high heat, and chemically preserved. Refined oil is clear, odorless, and almost totally devoid of nutrients.

Note: Natural, unrefined oils are fragile and become rancid quickly. They should be stored in a dark cupboard or in the refrigerator. Purchase small bottles if you don't use much oil in your cooking.

WHAT ARE HYDROGENATED FATS?

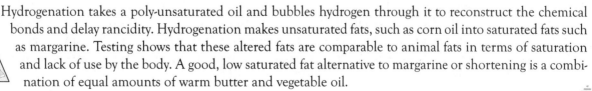

Hydrogenation takes a poly-unsaturated oil and bubbles hydrogen through it to reconstruct the chemical bonds and delay rancidity. Hydrogenation makes unsaturated fats, such as corn oil into saturated fats such as margarine. Testing shows that these altered fats are comparable to animal fats in terms of saturation and lack of use by the body. A good, low saturated fat alternative to margarine or shortening is a combination of equal amounts of warm butter and vegetable oil.

WHAT ARE ESSENTIAL FATTY ACIDS?

The essential fatty acids, linoleic acid, alpha linoleic acid, gamma linoleic acid, linolenic acid, and arachidonic acid, are major components of all cell membranes; without them the membranes are unable to function. EFAs convert into prostaglandins, hormone-like cell messengers, that are instrumental in energy production, vital to circulatory health, and integral to good metabolism.

The brain, when its water weight is removed, **consists primarily of EFAs.** Mental symptoms which arise from severe EFA deficiency include attention deficit disorder (ADD), violent behavior, memory loss, autism, mental retardation, anxiety/depression syndromes, headaches and seizures. EFAs function as components of nerve cells, cell membranes, and hormone-like substances known as prostaglandins. Because linoleic acid and alpha-linolenic acid form entirely different prostaglandins, researchers have found that manipulating the type of dietary oils a person ingests can dramatically alter body function and, in some cases, treat disease. A diet rich in plant foods results in low levels of saturated fat and relatively higher levels of essential fatty acids.

Ailments associated with EFA deficiency include eczema, dermatitis, psoriasis, lupus, hair loss, heart disease, diabetes, arthritis, loss of mental acuity and memory, senility, Crohn's disease, I.B.S., teen-age and adult acne and respiratory diseases like asthma.

Food oils, such as those found in supermarkets, are traditionally regarded as top dietary sources of essential fatty acids. However, this is true only of those oils processed by cold-pressing methods. Commercial oils contain such a large number of contaminants and are so heavily processed that they can no longer be regarded as optimal sources of EFAs.

WHAT ARE OMEGA-3 & OMEGA-6 FATTY ACIDS?

Omega-3 oils are a family of fatty acids high in EPA (eicosapentaenoic acid), DHA (dihomogammalinolenic acid), and GLA (gamma linoleic acid). They include cold water fish oils, walnut oil, canola oil, wheat germ oil, evening primrose oil and flax oil. Research has indicated that treatments for P.M.S., high blood pressure and rheumatoid arthritis benefit from the use of these fatty acids. Omega-3 oils are also a specific for the 30% of America's population who need to lower serum cholesterol levels.

Clinical results show a long list of benefits for Omega oils - smoother skin, smoother muscle action, stronger cardiovascular performance and better digestive function. They provide fuel for the heart, help prevent blood clotting and reduce high blood fats of all kinds. In weight loss diets, Omega-3 oils eliminate binging and food addiction, help to burn fats and increase stamina by supporting good liver function. They also help overcome food allergies, promote clearer thinking, and improve stamina.

Alpha-linolenic acid (LNA), is the Omega-3 essential fatty acid found in flax oil. Other Omega-3s, such as DHA and EPA, found in fish oils, are synthesized from LNA in the body.

Omega-6 oils are a group of fatty acids high in linoleic and arachidonic acids, and include sesame, sunflower, safflower and corn oil. Along with Omega-3 fatty acids, they stimulate the formation of prostaglandins. They also inhibit the over-production of thromboxane, a substance in the body that promotes clotting. Because blood tends to clot in narrowed arteries, and is the major cause of heart attacks, prostaglandins are essential to health.

Linoleic acid is the Omega-6 essential fatty acid that is found abundantly in almost all vegetable oils, particularly seed oils. Linoleic acid is a polyunsaturated fat, and along with alpha-linolenic acid, is "essential" to human body function.

Both Omega-3 and Omega-6 fatty acids help in the development and correct body balance of prostaglandins. Prostaglandins are produced by every cell in the body, and control such things as reproduction and fertility, inflammation reactions, immunity and cell communications. While primitive man lived on roughly equal amounts of Omega-6 and Omega-3, the dietary ratio for modern man is between 10 and 20 parts Omega-6 to 1 part Omega-3, a highly imbalanced ratio.

WHAT KIND OF LIPIDS ARE CHOLESTEROL AND TRIGLYCERIDES?

Lipid is an inclusive term for a group of fats and fat-like substances essential to human health. Lipids are found in every cell, and are integral to membrane, blood and tissue structure, hormone/prostaglandin production, and nervous system functions. **Triglycerides** are dietary fats and oils used as fuel by the body, and as an energy source for metabolism. Phospholipids are fats such as lecithin and **cholesterol**, vital to cell membranes, nerve fibers and bile salts, and for sex hormones.

Lipids are dynamic in the body. Even stored fat is not an inert mass, but active. A good example of highly active fat is a type of fat called brown adipose tissue or BAT. BAT has a very high metabolic rate capable of burning large amounts of calories, stimulating thermogenesis, and assisting weight control.

Cholesterol is a type of fat that travels through the bloodstream bound to two types of lipoproteins. Low-density lipoproteins (LDLs) are richest in cholesterol. Too much LDL cholesterol in the body is related to heart disease. High-density lipoproteins (HDLs) clear fat away from artery walls and return it to the liver for excretion. Cholesterol is vital for many important functions of the body and is found in all body tissues. It is essential in the production of nerve tissue, bile, many hormones and vitamin D. The liver and brain make about *1.5 gm.* of cholesterol every day to insure the body has enough of it. About 10 percent of the dry weight of the brain is cholesterol. *Reduced consumption of cholesterol spurs the body to increase production of it.* Lower than normal levels are correlated with anemia, acute infection, autoimmune disorders and excess thyroid function.

Triglycerides are a group of fats stored in the connective tissues. Excess triglycerides develop into a fat stomach or fat thighs. They also serve as a reserve for fuel energy, surrounding vital organs, giving them support and cushioning them from physical trauma. Refined flour, sugar, soda, alcohol and coffee elevate triglyceride levels in the blood and thus, add excess weight. Lower than normal triglyceride levels may indicate liver dysfunction.

WHAT ARE HIGH DENSITY LIPO-PROTEINS (HDLs) AND LOW DENSITY LIPO-PROTEINS (LDLs)?

Lipoproteins are water-soluble, protein-covered bundles, that transport cholesterol through the bloodstream, and are synthesized in the liver and intestinal tract. "Bad cholesterol," LDL, or low density lipoproteins, carries cholesterol through the bloodstream for cell-building needs, but leaves behind any excess on artery walls and in tissues. "Good cholesterol," HDL, or high density lipo-proteins, helps prevent narrowing of the artery walls by removing the excess cholesterol and transporting it to the liver for excretion as bile.

WHAT IS THE STORY ON COCONUT OIL AND OTHER TROPICAL OILS?

Coconut oil, a much maligned tropical oil, long under attack by the American Soybean Association, is making a comeback for its taste and therapeutic value. Coconut oil contains medium chain triglycerides (MCT's), the form of fatty acids occurring in vegetable and palm kernel oils. MCT's are easily digested. In fact, some practitioners use a formula containing MCT's from coconut oil for patients with malabsorption problems who cannot digest conventional fats. A formula containing MCT's can also be a lifesaver for premature babies.

Common misconceptions of coconut oil are that it raises blood cholesterol, causes heart disease and obesity. However, coconut oil does not raise blood cholesterol in a normal diet, nor does it, by itself, cause heart disease. Polynesian islanders, who get most of their fat calories from coconut oil have an exceedingly low rate of heart disease. Coconut oil is less likely than other oils to cause obesity, because the body easily converts it into energy rather than depositing its calories as body fat. In addition, coconut oil, like mother's milk, contains a component that is antimicrobial. Coconut oil users who dwell primarily in the tropics, an ideal environment for parasites, are protected from infections. Coconut oil is a premier natural emollient, supremely lubricating to the skin and hair.

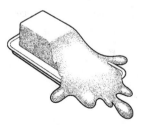

Sugars & Sweeteners In A Healing Diet

*J*s the bad health rap on sugar too extreme? Sugar in America is synonymous with fun, good times and snacking. Our culture instills the powerful urge for sweetness from an early age. Americans eat a lot of it. It's a food that we eat to "cope" in times of stress and tension.

We know that sugar offers quick energy, helps metabolism, and provides "closure" to digestive processes. A little sugar can actually suppress appetite, reducing the likelihood of overeating. It's the reason we traditionally eat sweet things at the end of a meal. Sugar can also improve the taste of complex carbohydrate foods which are better for you than fatty foods. And new research is beginning to show that some of the current caveats about sugar have been overstated. In regard to weight gain, for instance, the sugar in most snacks and desserts is a less-fattening culprit than fat. Fat not only contributes more calories, but the calories are metabolized differently in the body, causing more weight gain than sugar.

However, sugar can be a major interference in a healing program. Refined sugar is sucrose, the ultimate naked carbohydrate - stripped of all nutritional benefits. Sugars include raw, brown, turbinado, yellow D, sucanat, and white sugar. All sugars can be addictive, and most add nothing but calories to your body. Like a drug or alcohol, sugar affects the brain first, offering a false energy lift that eventually lets you down lower than when you started.

There's no question that excessive sugar consumption can have detrimental health effects. Regular sugar intake plays a negative part in a host of common diseases, like diabetes, hypoglycemia, heart disease, high cholesterol, obesity, nearsightedness, eczema, psoriasis, dermatitis, gout, indigestion, yeast infections, and tooth decay. It also provides a breeding ground for dangerous staph infections.

Sugar needs insulin for metabolism - a process that promotes the storage of fat. Metabolized sugar is transformed into fat globules, and distributed over the body where muscles are not very active, such as on the stomach, hips and chin. Every time you eat sugar, some of those calories become fat instead of energy.

Too much sugar upsets body mineral balances, particularly draining away calcium, and overloading the body with acid-ash residues that are responsible for much of the stiffening of joints in arthritis. Sugar ties up and dissolves B vitamins, producing an over-acid condition in the body. Skin, nerve and digestive problems result. Excess sugar depresses immune response and resistance to disease, a proven fact for those with diabetes and hypoglycemia, and also for people with high triglycerides and high blood pressure.

Products and substances that affect body sugar regulation can have major impact, both good and bad, on a healing program. Glucose is the main sugar in the blood and brain. Under ideal conditions, glucose is released into the bloodstream slowly to maintain blood sugar at the optimum level. Yet the inability to properly process glucose, affects millions of Americans. At least twenty million of us suffer from diabetes (high blood sugar) or hypoglycemia (low blood sugar). While seeming to be opposite problems, these two conditions really stem from the same cause - an imbalance between glucose and oxygen in the body. Poor nutrition is a common cause of both disorders, and both can be improved with a high mineral, high fiber diet, adequate usable protein, small frequent meals, and regular mild exercise.

If you have a sugar imbalance condition, there must be diet and lifestyle change for there to be a real or permanent cure. Alcohol, caffeine, refined sugars and tobacco must be avoided.

Hypoglycemia is one of the most widespread disorders in industrialized countries today. It is a direct effect of excess consumption of refined sweets, low fiber foods, and other processed carbohydrates. Excess sugar can cause the pancreas to flood the body with insulin, taking too much sugar from the blood and creating hypoglycemia. Hypoglycemia is marked by dozens of unpleasant symptoms, including fatigue, confusion, depression, anxiety, unconsciousness or, in the worst case, death. Chronic hypoglycemia often precedes diabetes.

Diabetes is also a "civilization" disease resulting from too much sugar, refined carbohydrates and caffeine. When carbohydrates are not used correctly, too little balancing insulin is produced, and blood sugar levels stay too high. The pancreas becomes damaged, so glucose cannot enter the cells to provide body energy. Instead, it accumulates in the blood, resulting in symptoms from mental confusion to coma.

Note: Even though poor blood sugar metabolism is the *cause* of both diabetes and hypoglycemia, the different *effects* of each problem call for specific modifications. Faster body response can be attained by approaching low blood sugar and high blood sugar diets separately. See Diabetes and Hypoglycemia pages in this book.

Here are some sugar substitutes for you to consider on a healing diet:

Just because you follow a sugar-free diet doesn't mean you have to give up good taste or the comforts of sweetness. Whole food sweeteners, such as honey, molasses, maple syrup, fruit juice or barley malt can satisfy the sweet need. They can be handled and metabolized easily by the body in its regular processes.

Recent clinical testing with crystalline fructose, and the herbs stevia rebaudiana and gymnema sylvestre, have produced some scientific good news for sugar reaction disorders. These substances may be seen as blood sugar balance heros, especially in the effort to control sugar intake and sugar cravings, but they do not eliminate hypoglycemia or diabetes reactions. Only diet improvement along with regular exercise can make a permanent difference.

• **Crystalline fructose** is a commercially produced sugar with the same molecular structure as that found in fruit. It is called fruit sugar, but is usually refined from corn starch. It is low on the glycemic index, meaning that it releases glucose into the bloodstream slowly. Fructose produces liver glycogen rapidly making it a more efficient energy supply than other sweeteners. It is almost twice as sweet as sugar, so less is needed for the same sweetening power. New information indicates it may also stimulate raised blood fat levels and might contribute to heart disease.

Fructose can be the sweetener of choice in a weight loss diet. In clinical tests before meals, subjects who drank liquids sweetened with fructose ate 20 to 40% fewer calories than normal, more than compensating for the 200 calories in the fructose. Those who drank liquids sweetened with table sugar ate 10 to 15% fewer calories; those who drank liquids sweetened with NutraSweet or aspartame ate the same amount of calories as normal. Fructose also seems to make eaters pick foods with less fats. In dental health studies, less dental plaque was reported with fructose than with sugar. Products labeled fructose can be pure fructose, 90% fructose or high fructose corn syrup (55% fructose), which contains a high percentage of glucose that needs insulin to be metabolized. It seems there are advantages to fructose, but if you are hypoglycemic or diabetic, fructose is still sugar and should be used carefully.

• **Stevia rebaudiana**, known as "sweet herb," is a South American sweetening leaf. It is totally non-caloric, and approximately 25 times sweeter than sugar when made as an infusion with 1 tsp. leaves to 1 cup of water. Two drops of the infusion equal 1 teaspoon of sugar in sweetness. In baking, 1 teaspoon of finely ground stevia powder is equal to 1 cup of sugar.

Stevia has been used as a natural sweetener in South America for over 1500 years, and clinical studies indicate it is safe to use even in cases of severe sugar imbalance. In the 1970's, the Japanese refined the sweet glycosides out of the stevia leaf, creating a product called Stevioside, 300 times sweeter than sugar. Stevioside is currently in use as a non-calorie sweetener in South America and the Orient where it enjoys a 41% share of the food sweetener market. While Stevioside does not affect blood glucose levels and is a good sweetener for both diabetics and hypoglycemics, it *does not retain* the extraordinary healing benefits of stevia leaves and extract. Research shows that stevia can actually regulate blood sugar. (In South America, stevia is sold as an **aid** to people with diabetes and hypoglycemia.) Stevia helps lower high blood pressure but does not affect normal blood pressure. Stevia is an effective aid in weight loss and control because it contains no calories, while significantly increasing glucose tolerance and inhibiting glucose absorption. People whose weight loss problems stem from a craving for sweets benefit most from stevia supplements, reporting that it decreases their desire for sugary foods. Many users also report that stevia tea reduces desire for tobacco and alcoholic beverages.

A facial mask of water-based stevia extract effectively smoothes out skin wrinkles while healing skin blemishes, including acne. A drop of the extract may be applied directly on a blemish outbreak. Today, stevia is returning to the market after a long FDA import ban which was heavily influenced by Nutrasweet™ politics. Many experts say that stevia may soon be regarded as one of the best and certainly the most "good for you" sweetener on earth.

- **Gymnema sylvestre** is an herb that reduces blood sugar levels after sugar consumption. Gymnema has a molecular structure similar to that of sugar that can block absorption of up to 50% of dietary sugar calories. Both sugar and gymnema are digested in the small intestine, but the larger molecule of gymnema cannot be fully absorbed. Therefore, taken before sugar, the gymnema molecule blocks the passages through which sugar is normally absorbed, and fewer sugar calories are assimilated. A person who eats a 400 calorie, high sugar dessert only absorbs 200 of the sugar calories. The remaining sugar is eliminated as waste. Gymnema has obvious uses for hyperinsulinism. Take with GTF Chromium for best results.

    A taste test shows how gymnema works. Taste something sweet, then swish a sip of gymnema sylvestre tea in your mouth. Now taste something sweet again. You will not be able to taste the sugar, because gymnema blocks the taste of the sugar in your mouth in much the same way it blocks sugar in digestion.

- **Amazake** is a pudding-like, whole-grain sweetener made from organic brown rice. The rice is cooked, then injected with koji, the Aspergillus enzyme culture that is also used in miso, shoyu and rice vinegar. It is about 21% sugar, mainly glucose and maltose, and is high in carbohydrates and other nutrients, including vitamin B and iron.

- **Barley malt or rice syrups** are mild, natural sweeteners made from barley sprouts, or rice and water cooked to a syrup. Only 40% as sweet as sugar, barley malt's blood sugar activity is a slow, complex carbohydrate release in the body that does not imbalance insulin levels. Brown rice syrup is derived by culturing rice with enzymes.

- **Blackstrap molasses** is the leftover sludge after sucrose extraction in the sugar making process. Rich in minerals and vitamins, molasses has more calcium, ounce for ounce than milk, more iron than eggs, and more potassium than any other food. The amounts of B vitamins, pantothenic acid, iron, inositol and vitamin E make it an excellent treatment for restoring thin and fading hair.

    -**Sorghum molasses** is concentrated juice of sorghum, a cereal grain, similar to molasses but with lighter flavor.

- **Corn syrup** is commercial glucose from chemically purified cornstarch with everything removed except the starch. Most corn syrup also contains added sugar syrup because glucose is only half as sweet as white table sugar. It is highly refined and absorbed into the bloodstream very quickly.

- **Date sugar** is ground, dried dates, and can be used like brown sugar. It contains the same nutrient values as dried dates, and is about half as sweet as white sugar. To use in baking, mix with water and then add to the recipe to prevent burning. Good as a sweet topping after removing from the oven or stove.

- **Fruit juice concentrate** is a highly refined product containing about 68% soluble sugar, with the percentage of fructose to glucose or sucrose varying depending on the fruit used (most commonly grapes).

- **Honey** is a natural sweetener with proven bioactive, antibiotic and antiseptic properties. Honey is a mixture of sugars formed from nectar by the enzyme, invertase, present in the bodies of bees. Along with its sweetening power, honey contains all the vitamins and enzymes necessary for the proper metabolism and digestion of glucose and other sugar molecules. Honey is almost twice as sweet as sugar and should be avoided by those with candidiasis and diabetes, and used with great care by those with hypoglycemia. Honey is naturally about 38% fructose, 31% glucose, 18% water, 9% other sugars and 2% sucrose. Flavors vary according to the flower source.

- **Maple syrup** is concentrated from the sap of sugar maple trees. It takes 30 to 40 gallons of sap to make one gallon of syrup. Unless it is labeled pure maple syrup, it probably is mixed with corn syrup to cut its cost and also might contain other additives. **Maple sugar** is crystallized maple syrup which has been concentrated.

- **Sucanat** is the trade name for a sweetener made from dried granulated cane juice, available in health food stores. The average sugar content is 85%, with the complex sugars, vitamins, minerals, amino acids and molasses retained. Use 1 to 1 in place of sugar. It is still a concentrated sweetener. Use carefully if you have sugar balance problems.

- **Turbinado sugar** is raw sugar that has been refined by washing in a centrifuge. Surface molasses is removed in the washing process. It has gone through the same refining process as white sugar, just short of the final extraction of molasses, and is essentially the same as white sugar.

The following chart can help you convert your favorite recipes from sugar to natural sweeteners. If you have serious blood sugar problems, such as diabetes or hypoglycemia, consult the appropriate pages in this book, or your healing professional, about the kind and amount of sweets your body can handle.

SWEETENER SUBSTITUTION AMOUNTS ARE FOR EACH CUP OF SUGAR:

Substitute Sweetener	Amount	Reduce Liquid in the Recipe
•Fructose	$^1/_3$ to $^2/_3$ cup	....
•Maple Syrup	$^1/_3$ to $^2/_3$ cup$^1/_4$ cup	....
•Honey	$^1/_2$ cup	$^1/_4$ cup
•Molasses	$^1/_2$ cup	$^1/_4$ cup
•Barley or Rice Syrup	1 to $1^1/_4$ cups	$^1/_4$ cup
•Date Sugar	1 cup	....
•Sucanat	1 cup	....
•Apple/Other Fruit Juice	1 cup	$^1/_4$ cup

What about Aspartame, Nutrasweet and Equal? We get lots of these chemical sweeteners in our food today.

The FDA has received more complaints about adverse reactions to aspartame than any other food ingredient in the agency's history. **Aspartame** combines the two amino acids phenylalanine and aspartic acid. Both have neurotransmitter activity. Aspartame is 200 times sweeter than sugar, and has been linked to sugar use problems, such as PKU seizures (phenylketonuria), high blood pressure, headaches, insomnia and ovarian cancer and brain tumors. (A recent study showed that the more NutraSweet was consumed, the more likely tumors were to develop.) There are immediate, serious reactions to aspartame.....severe headaches, extreme dizziness, throat swelling, allergic effects, and retina deterioration. The retina damage is attributed to methyl alcohol, a substance released when aspartame breaks down. Aspartame has also been linked to brain damage in fetuses.

Aspartame's major brand names, NutraSweet and Equal, have taken the place of saccharin in pre-prepared foods and drinks, and that means we get a lot of it. Be careful of these sweeteners if you have sugar sensitivities. Fortunately, adverse effects are reversible when consumption is stopped. Pregnant and lactating women, very young or allergy-prone children, and those with PKU, should avoid aspartame products. Dangerous side effects are worsened when NutraSweet is used hot or in cooking.

Here are some of the chemical sweeteners you'll see on food labels. Beware of them if you have sugar-related health problems.

•**Dextrose,** a monosaccharide, is found in most plants but is often synthetically derived from cornstarch.

•**Lactose,** milk sugar, is a disaccharide sweetener used mainly in infant foods and baked goods. Lactose intolerant people experience gastrointestinal disturbances after consuming lactose.

•**Maltose,** or malt sugar, is a disaccharide that is often synthetically derived from corn syrup.

•**Sorbitol,** derived from corn, is absorbed slowly and is used in many foods designed for diabetics because it needs little, if any, insulin. It does not promote tooth decay, but can cause diarrhea.

•**Saccharin** is made form petroleum and toluene, a petroleum-based solvent used to prevent knocking in gasoline engines. The substance is intensely sweet and calorie free, but has been liked to bladder cancer. The FDA tried to ban saccharin in 1977, but relented under pressure from consumers and industry. It is now sold with a warning label.

•**Raw sugar** is a granulated sugar obtained by evaporating sugar cane juice. It is 98% sucrose.

•**Xylitol,** from birchwood chips, has been shown to reduce cavities by neutralizing the acids in the mouth.

Is it possible to eat a healthy diet that won't stimulate over-production of insulin and will allow normal blood sugar activity? Can we keep hunger under control all day, and lose weight without starving?

A diet that keeps insulin levels low means fewer calories are turned into fat and more are burned for energy, resulting in a loss of body weight. A low glycemic diet is a good answer, both for blood sugar regulation and for a sugar craver's diet. I recommend whole, natural foods, especially whole grains and fresh vegetables, which have a low-glycemic index. They don't elevate blood sugar after a meal like high-glycemic index, or sugary foods, which put blood sugar on a roller coaster.

The Benefits Of Green Tea For Healing

All black, green and Oolong teas come from *thea sinensis,* an evergreen shrub that ranges from the Mediterranean to the tropics, and from sea level to 8000 feet. Tea leaves can be harvested every 6 to 14 days depending on the area and climate; a plant will yield for 25 to 50 years. The kind of tea produced is defined by the manner in which the leaves are processed. For green tea, the first tender leaves of spring are picked, then partially dried, rolled, steamed, crushed and dried again with hot air. Oolong tea leaves have been allowed to semi-ferment for an hour. Black teas are partially dried, rolled on tile, glass or concrete, and fermented for 3 hours to strengthen aroma and flavor, and reduce bitterness. Black teas are often scented during fermentation with fresh flower blossoms or spices. Green tea leaves are not fermented, but instead are steamed or dried after harvest.

Both green tea and black tea possess enzymes with the ability to help the body modify potentially toxic components, and make it easier for them to be excreted. Both black and green teas contain enough naturally-occurring fluoride to prevent tooth decay. Both contain polyphenols (not tannins as commonly believed) that act as antioxidants, yet do not interfere with iron or protein absorption.

But for health benefits, green tea is seen as superior to black because it contains larger amounts of vitamins, including twice as much vitamin C and more than twice the amount of high bioflavonoid activity as black tea. Regular consumption of green tea may meet the human daily requirements for bioflavonoids with very bioactive availability. Green tea leaves are enzyme-active for asthma or weight loss and cleansing. Green tea is a vasodilator and smooth muscle relaxant in cases of bronchial asthma. It is a beneficial fasting tea, providing energy support and clearer thinking during cleansing.

Here are some of the health benefits of green tea:

Long popular as an aid to longevity, the broad spectrum of healthful benefits of green tea has been validated by modern science, with an astounding catalog of curative applications. The polyphenol compounds in green tea provide many of the beneficial effects. They can lower cholesterol and protect against cancer by stopping enzymes that produce cancer-causing substances. A tea substance called EECG epigallocatechin gallate), has been identified with a formidably high level of free-radical-scavenging, or anti-oxidant activity. EECG is 200 times more powerful as an anti-oxidant than vitamin E as a free radical scavenger against DNA destroying attacks. During fermentation, black tea loses its EECG entirely during fermentation, as well as other beneficial polyphenols. Research at the American Health Foundation in New York indicates that green tea's protective anti-carcinogens "prevent the activation of carcinogens so that free radicals never form."

Green tea has been used since antiquity for body cleansing and eliminating pollutants, to combat mental fatigue as well as colds and flu. It produces healthful benefits for digestion and the nervous system, facilitates cardiovascular function by stabilizing blood lipids, and helps lower blood pressure. Tea catechins in green tea are potent inhibitors of platelet aggregation, which could lead to atherosclerosis. Those who consume green tea daily have stable, low blood cholesterol levels.

Green tea has antibacterial qualities, discovered 5,000 years ago by the Chinese, who used it to purify water. The most abundant compounds in green tea provide a wide range of antimicrobial actions against carcinogenic bacteria, such as *streptococcus mutans.* Streptococcus mutans is a typical bacterium found in the mouth and is a common cause of tooth decay. This bacterium can cause serious illness if it establishes in normally sterile parts of the body, like the heart valve.

Green tea may reduce the risk of several forms of cancer induced by environmental carcinogens. Particular research has been done in Japan on stomach, skin and lung cancers, where people who drink a large amount of strong green tea have a low incidence of these cancers. Both black and oolong tea also contain some of the same cancer-preventive compounds, but green tea contains the highest and most effective levels. Interestingly, this Japanese study showed that there was little reduction in any of these cancers for those who smoked, even though they drank green tea.

Other research in Japan, however, is showing that several cups of green tea on a regular daily basis *are* effective in reducing lung cancer death rates even in men who smoked two packs of cigarettes a day. Smoking is far more prevalent in Japan than in the U.S., but the instance of lung cancer is much lower; many researchers see green tea as a protection against disease for the smoker.

Green tea shows good results, in a Rutgers study, against skin cancer. As the ozone layer thins, and UV radiation increases, skin cancers have multiplied throughout the world. Drinking green tea daily before and during exposure to harmful ultraviolet light showed much less susceptibility for skin damage.

The National Cancer Institute also reports that green tea provides a protective effect against esophageal cancer. Today, researchers are studying green tea as protection against radiation damage, and against oral cancer. Other new studies include arthritic and rheumatism treatment. The future for green tea indeed looks bright.

Tea nomenclature can be confusing. Names like oolong, black or jasmine tea refer to how the tea was processed. Names such as Assam, Darjeeling or Ceylon, etc., refer to the country or region where the tea was grown. Names such as pekoe, orange pekoe, etc., refer to the leaf size.

- **Bancha Leaf** - the tender spring leaves of the Japanese tea plant, containing unprocessed, bioactive caffeine for mental clarity and weight loss, and theophylline for asthmatic conditions. Bancha is the green tea with the best therapeutic properties.
- **Kukicha Twig** - a smooth, roasted Japanese tea, made from the twigs and stems rather than the leaves of the tea plant. Containing much less caffeine and acidic oils than the leaves, this tea is a favorite in macrobiotic diets for its blood cleansing qualities, high calcium content, and roasted mellow flavor.
- **Darjeeling** - the finest, most delicately flavored of the black Indian teas.
- **Earl Grey** - a popular hearty, aromatic black tea that has been sprayed with bergamot oil.
- **English Breakfast** - a connoisseur's rich, mellow, fragrant black tea with Chinese flavor. It is a combination of Assam flowery orange pekoe and Ceylon broken orange pekoe.
- **Ceylon** - a tea grown in Sri Lanka with a intense, flowery aroma and flavor.
- **Irish Breakfast** - a combination of Assam flowery orange pekoe and Ceylon orange pekoe.
- **Jasmine** - a black tea scented with white jasmine flowers during firing.
- **Lapsang Souchong** - a fine black tea with a strong, smoky flavor.
- **Oolong** - a delicate tea with complex flavor, semi-fermented and fired in baskets over hot coals.

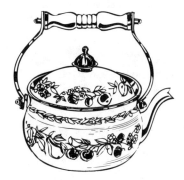

Caffeine & A Healing Diet

Like most of mankind's other pleasures, there is good news and bad news about caffeine. Moderate use of caffeine has been hailed for centuries for its therapeutic benefits. Every major culture uses caffeine in some food form to overcome fatigue, handle pain, open breathways, control weight and jump-start circulation. Caffeine is a plant-derived neutraceutical - a part of both foods and medications; coffee, black tea, colas, sodas, chocolate and cocoa, analgesics such as Excedrin, and over-the-counter stimulants such as Vivarin, all contain caffeine. Taking aspirin or an herbal pain reliever with a caffeine drink increases the pain relieving effects.

There is solid evidence for the effects of caffeine on mental performance, clearer thinking, and shortened reaction times. Caffeine stimulates serotonin, a brain neurotransmitter produced by tryptophan, that increases the capacity for intellectual tasks, and decreases drowsiness. In modest doses, it improves mood and increases alertness by releasing adrenaline into the bloodstream. It mobilizes fatty acids into the circulatory system, facilitating greater energy production, endurance and work output. It has a direct potentiating effect on muscle contraction for both long and short-term sports and workout activity.

Caffeine promotes enhanced thermogenesis, the conversion of stored body fat to energy, so the benefits of caffeine for weight loss have long been known. Recent research shows that overweight dieters have subnormal heat production during dieting as the body reacts to lower food intake and metabolic changes. After eating, obese and post-obese people respond to caffeine with greater thermogenesis.

You don't need a lot of caffeine to get the positive advantages. Even relatively small, commonly consumed, doses of caffeine significantly influence calorie use by the body. One recent study showed that a single dose of 100mg of caffeine (the amount in one cup of coffee) increased metabolic rate almost 4% for two to three hours! When the same amount of caffeine was consumed at two-hour intervals for 12 hours, metabolic rate increased 8 to 11%. While these increased metabolic rates seem small, monitoring over several months shows steady, substantial reduction in body weight.

The same study also indicated that low doses of caffeine are a good choice for weight control after initial weight loss, by keeping metabolism optimally active, and calorie-burning efficient.

Caffeine's health problems are also well known - headaches and migraines, irritability, digestive problems, anxiety and high blood pressure. As an addictive stimulant, caffeine can have drug-like activity, causing jumpiness and nerves, heart disease and heart palpitations. Like any other addiction, caffeine is difficult to overcome, but if you have caffeine-related health problems, it is worth going through the temporary withdrawal symptoms. Improvement in the problem condition is often noticed right away after cutting out caffeine.

In excessive amounts, caffeine can produce oxalic acid in the system, causing health problems waiting to become diseases. It can lodge in the liver, restricting proper function, and constrict arterial blood flow. It leaches B vitamins from the body, particularly thiamine (for stress control). It depletes some essential minerals, including calcium and potassium. (Moderate amounts do not cause calcium depletion or contribute to bone loss.)

Excessive caffeine affects the glands, particularly exhausting the adrenals, and causes other hormonal imbalances to the point of becoming a major factor in breast cancer risk and uterine fibroids in women, and prostate trouble in men. It has been indicated in PMS symptoms, bladder infections, and hypoglycemic/ diabetic sugar reactions.

However, the carcinogenic effects blamed on caffeine are thought to be caused by the roasting process used in making coffee, tea and chocolate.

Since decaffeinated coffee is *also* implicated in certain organ cancers, scientists are concluding that caffeine is not the culprit - the roasted hydrocarbons are.

SPECIFIC AREAS OF HEALTH AND THE EFFECTS OF CAFFEINE INCLUDE:
- **Caffeine and Pregnancy** - caffeine should be avoided during pregnancy. Like alcohol, it can cross the placenta and affect the fetus' brain, central nervous system and circulation. Recent studies show, however, that there is no relationship between moderate caffeine intake and infertility.
- **Caffeine and Heart Disease** - heavy coffee drinking (more than 4 cups a day), has been directly implicated in heart disease and high cholesterol. However, many early tests were flawed, because HDLs (good cholesterol) rose proportionately with LDLs so that risk of heart disease did not increase. Moderate caffeine does not appear to increase heart disease risk.
- **Caffeine and High Blood Pressure** - excessive caffeine can elevate blood pressure significantly and produce nervous anxiety. This is particularly true when caffeine is combined with phenyl-propanolamine, the appetite suppressant in commercial diet pills.
- **Caffeine and Ulcers** - caffeine stimulates gastric secretions, sometimes leading to a nervous, acid stomach or heartburn. However, it is the key "bitter" in the western diet, stimulating bile secretions needed for good digestion. Caffeine has not been linked to either gastric or duodenal ulcers.
- **Caffeine and Headaches** - caffeine causes headaches in some people - and causes withdrawal headaches when avoided after regular use. As a traditional remedy for temporary relief of migraines, the inherent niacin content of coffee increases when the beans are roasted.
- **Caffeine and PMS** - caffeine causes congestion through cellular overproduction of fibrous tissue and cyst fluids. However, low-dose caffeine intake can improve memory and alertness during the menstrual phase. Reducing, rather than avoiding caffeine during menses may offer the best of both worlds.
- **Caffeine and Sleep Quality** - caffeine consumed late in the day or at night jeopardizes the quality of sleep by disrupting brain wave patterns. It also means you will take longer to get to sleep.
- **Caffeine and Breast Disease** - the link between caffeine and breast fibroids is not official, but there is almost immediate improvement when caffeine intake is decreased or avoided.
- **Caffeine and Cancer** - recent world-wide studies on breast and bladder cancer have shown no cause relationship between these diseases and caffeine. However, the acidic body state promoted by caffeine is not beneficial to the healing process as the body works to alter its chemistry during healing.

There are foods to help break the caffeine habit: herb teas, delicious coffee substitutes such as Roma, carob treats instead of chocolate, plain aspirin in place of Excedrin, and energy supportive herbal pick-me-ups with no harmful stimulants of any kind. Use green tea and kola nut as bio-active forms of caffeine for weight loss and mental clarity. Neither has the heated hydrocarbons of coffee.

The following chart shows amounts of caffeine in common foods so you can make an informed choice.

CAFFEINE FOOD	APPROX. AMT. OF CAFFEINE
Coffee, one 5-oz. cup	
Decaf	4mg.
Instant	65mg.
Percolated	100mg.
Drip	125mg.
Tea, one 5-oz. cup	
Bag, brewed for 3 minutes	40mg.
Loose, black, brewed for 3 minutes	50mg.
Loose, green, brewed for 3 minutes	45mg.
Iced	30mg.
Colas, 12-oz. glass	45mg.
Chocolate/Cocoa, 5-oz. cup	5mg.
Milk chocolate, 1-oz	5mg.
Bittersweet Chocolate, 1-oz	30mg.

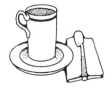

Sea Vegetables & Iodine Therapy

Sea vegetables have superior nutritional content. They transmit the energies of the sea to the body as a rich source of proteins, complex carbohydrates, minerals and vitamins. Ounce for ounce, along with herbs, they are higher in vitamins and minerals than any other food group. Sea vegetables are one of nature's richest sources of vegetable protein, and they provide full-spectrum concentrations of beta carotene, chlorophyll, enzymes, amino acids and fiber. The distinctive salty taste is not just "salt," but a balanced, chelated combination of sodium, potassium, calcium, magnesium, phosphorus, iron and trace minerals. They convert inorganic ocean minerals into organic mineral salts that combine with amino acids. Our bodies can use this combination as an ideal way to get usable nutrients for structural building blocks. In fact, sea vegetables contain all the necessary trace elements for life, many of which are depleted in the earth's soil.

Sea vegetables are almost the only non-animal source of Vitamin B_{12}, necessary for cell development and nerve function. Their mineral balance is a natural tranquilizer for building sound nerve structure, and proper metabolism. Their benefits for a healing diet rival the healing powers of their cruciferous cousins broccoli and cabbage.

Sea vegetables act as the ocean's purifiers, and they can perform many of the same functions for the human body, also largely made up of salt water. Sea plant chemical composition is so close to human plasma, that it can help balance the cells of the body. Sea vegetables help alkalize and purify the blood from the acid effects of a modern diet, allowing for better absorption of nutrients. They strengthen the body against disease, especially those caused by environmental pollutants. They reduce excess stores of fluid and fat, and work to transform toxic metals in the system (including radiation), into harmless salts that the body can eliminate. In fact, the natural iodine in sea vegetables can reduce by almost 80% the radioactive iodine-131 absorbed by the thyroid.

Japanese women have less than one-sixth the breast cancer rate of American women of similar age. Japanese women who live in rural areas have a much lower breast cancer rate than do Japanese women in urban areas. The determining factor seems to be diet. Japanese women living in rural areas routinely eat sea plants - a food uncommon in the diets of American and urban Japanese women who traditionally eat many processed foods. In animal studies, rats exposed to chemicals known to cause breast cancer were fed sea vegetables and were protected against getting cancer.

Sea vegetables are delicious, and convenient to buy, store, and use as needed in their sundried form. Store them in a moisture proof container and they will keep indefinitely. A wide variety of sea vegetables is available today, both in macrobiotic and regular quality. These include: Arame, Bladderwrack, Dulse, Hijiki, Irish Moss, Kelp, Kombu, Nori, Sea Palm, Spirulina, and Wakame. They may be crushed, chopped or snipped into soups and sauces, crumbled over pizzas, and used as toppings on casseroles and salads. If you add sea vegetables, no other salt is needed, an advantage for a low salt diet.

Preventive measures may be taken against iodine deficiency problems by adding just 2 tablespoons of chopped, dried sea vegetables to the daily diet.

Here is a delicious salad or soup topping blend to add sea veggies to your diet. Just barely whirl in the blender so there are still sizeable chunks. They will expand in any recipe with liquid, and when heated will return to a beautiful ocean green color.

OCEAN THERAPY SPRINKLE:
$^3/_4$ CUP chopped dried dulse
$^1/_4$ CUP chopped dried wakame
$^1/_4$ CUP chopped dried kombu
$^1/_4$ CUP chopped dried nori or sea palm
$^1/_2$ CUP toasted sesame seeds

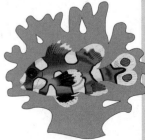

About Iodine Therapy & Healing

In this era of processed foods and iodine-poor soils, sea vegetables and sea foods stand almost alone as potent sources of natural, balanced iodine. Iodine is essential to life, since the thyroid gland cannot regulate metabolism without it. It is an important element of alertness, and rapid brain activity, and a prime deterrent to arterial plaque. Iodine is also a key factor in the control and prevention of many endocrine deficiency conditions prevalent today, such as breast and uterine fibroids, tumors, prostate inflammation, adrenal exhaustion, and toxic liver and kidney states. Sea vegetables have the ability to reduce tumors, to lower serum cholesterol, and to aid metabolism and digestion.

Thyroid hormones are made from iodine and the amino acid tyrosine. Iodine deficiency results in the development of goiter, an enlarged thyroid gland. When the level of the iodine is low in the diet and blood, it causes the thyroid gland to become quite large due to pituitary stimulation.

The recommended dietary allowance for iodine in adults is quite small, 150 micrograms. Few people in the United States are now considered iodine deficient, because the average American intake of iodine is estimated at over 600 micrograms per day from iodized salt. Yet the rate of goiter is still relatively high, at 6% of the population in some areas. It is believed that the goiter in these people is a result of impaired thyroid function from an excess of refined sugar, alcohol, fats and caffeine in the diet; or eating certain foods called goitrogens, which block iodine utilization.

Tests show that cruciferous vegetables like broccoli, cauliflower and cabbage, legumes like beans. Peas and peanuts, beets, carrots, spinach and nuts like almonds may cause a mild hypothyroid state when eaten raw. **Cooking neutralizes the thyroid-blocking components.** If you have a tendency to goiter or hypothyroidism, you might try eating these healthy foods cooked instead of raw.

Iodine deficiency has a profound effect on the health of the fetus early in conception. A woman wishing to become pregnant might consider taking an herbal iodine supplement while she is trying to conceive, rather than waiting until she realizes that she is pregnant. Most American women get sufficient iodine from fish and other ocean foods, but in developing, landlocked countries, where iodine is not plentiful in food, infants are often born with cretinism, which results in dwarfism, mental deficiency, puffy facial features and lack of muscle coordination.

Kelp tablets for pregnant women have shown some interesting results in terms of health for the mother, too.
- Hemoglobin count rose from 65% to 83%
- Decrease in the number and severity of colds
- Hair color and quality improved; fingernails grew stronger
- Capillary strength increased, with less bruising; skin complexion improved
- Arthritic conditions improved; eye conditions improved, especially iritis and cataracts
- Constipation lessened
- Sense of well-being increased

As a douche for vaginitis, iodine-rich herbs and sea vegetables are effective against a wide range of organisms, including trichomonas, candida, and chlamydia as well as nonspecific vaginal infections. A douching solution with one tablespoon of dried sea vegetables to 1 quart of water, used twice daily for 7 to 14 days, is effective against most organisms.

Iodine deficiency and hypothyroidism are clearly involved with a higher incidence of breast cancer. Women with low iodine levels often have symptoms relating to hyperplasia and fibrocystic disease of the breast. In clinical trials, precancerous lesions have even been corrected by iodine supplementation. Our own empirical evidence with herbal and sea plant iodine shows that it is very important in the treatment and prevention of fibrocystic breast disease (FBD), restoring pituitary, thyroid and adrenal functions, as well as having significant anti-inflammatory and anti-scarring effects. Specific iodine therapy treatment for these conditions is addressed on the ailment healing pages in this book.

A SEAWEED BATH IS A GREAT WAY TO GET IODINE THERAPY.

Seaweed baths are Nature's perfect body/psyche balancer, and they're an excellent way to take in iodine therapy. Remember how good you feel after a walk in the ocean? Seaweeds purify and balance the ocean; and they can do the same for your body.

Noticeable rejuvenating effects occur when toxins are released from your tissues. A hot seaweed bath is like a wet-steam sauna, only better, because the sea greens balance body chemistry instead of dehydrating it. The electrolytic magnetic action of the seaweed releases excess body fluids from congested cells, and dissolves fatty wastes through the skin, replacing them with depleted minerals, particularly potassium and iodine. And because iodine boosts thyroid activity, food fuels are used before they can turn into fatty deposits. Vitamin K, a precursor nutrient in seaweeds, aids adrenal regulation, meaning that a seaweed bath can also help maintain hormone balance for a more youthful body.

Note: See Bodywork Techniques For Detoxification & Cleansing, page 176 for how to take a seaweed bath:

Note: Overheating and iodine therapy are two of the most effective treatments in natural healing. They are powerful and should be used with care. If you are under medical supervision for heart disease or high blood pressure, check with your physician to determine if a seaweed bath is all right for you.

Sea vegetables are natural superfoods. Modern science is validating many of the traditional benefits of sea plants, particularly in relation to their algin content. Algin is responsible for the success of seaweeds in the treatment of obesity, asthma, atherosclerosis and as blood purifiers. Algin absorbs toxins from the digestive tract in much the same way that a water softener removes the hardness from tap water. Less toxins enter the circulatory system because of algin's activity.

While kelp and seaweeds contain certain compounds that directly counteract carcinogens, most researchers believe that sea plants primarily boost the body's immune system, allowing it to combat the carcinogens itself. In addition, because of their high antioxidant qualities, sea vegetables are effective toxin scavengers that can help detoxify both the digestive and eliminative tracts.

Dishonesty creates a failure force that manifests itself in many ways- often not apparent at the moment or to an outside observer.

Cheating affects the life of the cheater far more than the person he cheats.

Soy Foods In A Healing Diet

Soyfoods are nutritional powerhouses. Whether or not soy proves to be a magic bullet for pre-venting heart disease or curing cancer, it possesses many health-enhancing benefits. Soy pro-tein is comparable in quality to animal protein, which makes it an excellent alternative to meat or dairy products. Soy protein helps lower blood cholesterol. Numerous studies show that when animal protein in the diet is replaced by soy protein, there is significant reduction in both total blood cholesterol and LDL (bad) cholesterol. Adding as little as 25 to 50 grams of soy protein daily to the diet for 1 month can result in a cholesterol drop. Soy foods are rich in other essential nutrients, too, like calcium, iron, zinc and B vitamins.

Because low insulin levels mean that the liver manufactures less cholesterol, researchers theorize that the amino acids in soy which decrease the amount of insulin in the blood are responsible for lowering cholesterol. Soy also prevents oxidative damage to LDL cholesterol. The newest research indicates that oxidation of LDL cholesterol is the main culprit in the progressive hardening and blocking of arteries known as atherosclerosis. Since soy is high in antioxidant activity, researchers believe that these phyto-chemicals are thwarting oxidation of LDL cholesterol.

Soybeans possess at least five known anticancer agents. They are the richest source of protease inhibitors, which block or hinder the development of colon, oral, lung, liver, pancreatic and esophageal cancers. Soybean compounds also block formation of nitrosamines, which can lead to liver cancer. Two other soybean constituents, phytosterols and saponins, are strongly anticancer. Phytosterols help defeat colon cancer by inhibiting cell division and proliferation. Saponins can stimulate general immune response, destroy certain cancer cells, and slow or reverse the growth of cancerous skin cells.

Soy contains phytochemicals called isoflavones which contain beneficial disease-prevention properties, espe-cially for lowering the risk of hormone-related cancers. **Genistein**, a particular isoflavone, is abundant in soyfoods. Genistein works much like estrogen, functioning both as an estrogen, and as an estrogen blocker. Like many herbs, it seems to promote the positive actions of body estrogen while preventing many of its bad effects. There are a wealth of studies on genistein and its anticancer properties. It competitively binds to both estrogen receptors **and** progesterone receptors, preventing them from being available for tumor growth.

Genistein also inhibits angiogenesis, the formation of new blood vessels necessary for the nourishment of a growing tumor. One study found that pre-menopausal females who rarely ate soy foods had twice the risk of breast cancer compared to those who frequently ate soy foods. Tofu seems to be the soy food highest in both total isoflavones and genistein.

Not surprisingly, the Japanese, with low rates of cancer, eat five times more soy products than Americans While the typical U.S. diet yields 80 milligrams of phytosterols per day, the Japanese typically eat 400 milligrams a day. Western vegetarians eat about 345 milligrams of saponins a day. Ironically, nearly all of the soybeans raised in the United States go into animal feed. Most of the rest is shipped to Japan.

Soy's benefits for men's health and prostate diseases are the newest area to come under study. Research on 8,000 Hawaiian men with Japanese ancestry, found that the men who ate the most tofu had the lowest rates of prostate cancer.

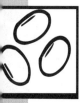

For women, there seems to be no question that including a serving a day of soy protein can lead to significant changes in the menstrual cycle, prolonging cycle length, and markedly suppressing the midcycle surge of gonadotrophins, luteinizing hormone and follicle-stimulating hormone - effects that appear to de-crease the risks of breast cancer. Genistein also helps maintain bone density, which decreases the risk of osteoporosis, and aids in reducing the uncomfortable side effects of menopause, especially the severity and frequency of hot flashes.

Here are some of the most common soy foods and how they can benefit a healing diet:

•**Miso** is a wonderful medicinal food made from fermented soybean paste. It is very alkalizing to the system, lowers cholesterol, represses carcinogens, helps neutralize environmental allergens and pollutants, lessens the effects of smoking, and provides an immune-enhancing environment.

Miso is a tasty base for soups, sauces, dressings, dips, spreads and cooking stocks, and a healthy substitute for salt or soy sauce. There are many kinds, strengths and flavors of miso, from chickpea (light and mild) to hatcho (dark, and strong). Natto miso is the sweetest, a mix of soybeans, barley and barley malt, kombu, ginger and sea salt. Unpasteurized miso is preferred for a healing diet, since beneficial bacteria and other enzymes, as well as flavor, are still intact.

Miso is very concentrated; use no more than $\frac{1}{2}$ to 1 teasp. of dark miso, or 1 to 2 teasp. of light miso per person. Dissolve in a small amount of water to activate the beneficial enzymes before adding to a recipe. Omit salt from the recipe if you are using miso.

•**Soy cheese** is made from soy milk, and is lactose and cholesterol free. The small amount of calcium caseinate (a milk protein) added allows soy cheese to melt. Mozzarella, cheddar, jack and cream cheese types are widely available. Use it cup for cup in place of any lowfat or regular cheese.

•**Soy ice cream, frozen desserts and soy yogurt** are available in a variety of flavors. **Soy mayonnaise** has also finally been developed with the taste and consistency of dairy mayonnaise.

•**Tamari** is a wheat-free soy sauce, lower in sodium and richer in flavor than regular soy sauce. Bragg's LIQUID AMINOS, an excellent, energizing protein broth, is also of the tamari family, but unfermented, lower in sodium, and containing 8 essential amino acids.

•**Tempeh** is a meaty, Indonesian fermented soy food, containing complete protein and all essential amino acids. It has a robust texture and mushroom-like aroma. Tempeh is also a predigested product due to the enzyme action in its culturing process, making it highly absorbable.

•**Soy milk** is nutritious, smooth, delicious, and versatile. Soy milk is vegetable-based, lactose and cholesterol free, with unsaturated or polyunsaturated fat. Soy milk contains less calcium and calories than milk, but more protein and iron. It adds a slight rise to baked goods. Use it cup for cup as milk for cooking; plain flavor for savory dishes, vanilla flavor for sweet dishes and on cereal.

•**Tofu** is a delicious soy food, made from soybeans, water, and nigari, a mineral-rich seawater precipitate. Combined with whole grains, tofu yields a complete protein, and provides dairy and egg richness without the fat or cholesterol, but with all the calcium and iron. As tofu's popularity has risen in America, so has the variety of ways you can buy, prepare and eat it. Fresh tofu has a light, delicate character that can take on any flavor perfectly, from savory to sweet. It comes firm-pressed in cubes, or in a soft, delicate form, or silken with a custard-like texture. It is smoked or pre-cooked in seasonings to give it a cheese-like flavor and firmness, or freeze-dried so that it can be stored at room temperature and reconstituted, (suitable for camping and travel). It comes in deep-fried pouches called age (pronounced "ah-gay") that are hollow inside for filling.

In addition to its culinary talents, tofu is a nutritionally balanced healing food, and a nutritionally adequate source of complex carbohydrates, minerals and vitamins. It is easy on the digestive system, full of soluble fiber, and a non-mucous-forming way to add richness and creamy texture to recipes.
*   Tofu is low in calories. Eight ounces has only 164 calories.
*   Tofu is rich in organic calcium. Eight ounces supplies the same amount of calcium as eight ounces of milk, but with far more absorbability.
*   Tofu is high in iron. Eight ounces supplies the same amount of iron as 2 oz. of beef liver or 4 eggs.
*   Tofu has high quality protein. Eight ounces supplies the same amount of protein as $3\frac{1}{4}$ oz. of beef, $5\frac{1}{2}$ oz. of hamburger, $1\frac{2}{3}$ cups of milk, or 2-oz. of regular cheese, or 2 eggs; but it is lower in fat than any of these.

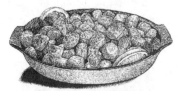

A Low Salt Diet & Healing

*I*n the past generation, Americans have consumed more NaCl than ever before; too much restaurant food, too many refined foods and too many animal foods. Most people are aware that excessive salt leads to heart disease, hypertension, and blood pressure problems. Too much salt means that circulation is constricted, kidneys retain too much body fluid, and migraines occur frequently. Like too much sugar, it's a cause of hyperactivity, aggressive behavior, and poor gland health.

Nutrition and medical documents are replete with the negative effects of salt. Yet, sodium is undeniably a necessary nutrient for optimal health; indeed it is essential to human existence. In ancient times, salt was so valuable that men traded it for its weight in gold. Today, modern medicine teaches us that salt is dangerous and that the public should avoid it. While it is true that certain individuals are salt-sensitive and must curb their intake, most Americans do not suffer ill effects from moderate salt intake in their diets.

Sodium resides in body fluids surrounding the cells, accompanied by its working partner mineral, potassium. Together sodium and potassium pump nutrients into the cells and waste products out of them, helping to nourish and clean every cell. The sodium-potassium relationship also keeps body fluid pressure stable, making sure you don't retain too much water and don't get dehydrated.

Adequate salinity is needed for good body tone, because sodium is necessary for muscles to contract. It is needed for strong blood, because without sodium, the body cannot use calcium. Sodium helps keep body pH in the proper balance because it transports nutrients and nerve impulses throughout the body. It keeps organs and glands healthy and produces hydrochloric acid, which allows us to digest our foods. Too little, or no sodium can lead to lack of vitality, stagnated blood and loss of clear thinking, because the brain depends on good circulation of fluids.

Signs of sodium deficiency include flatulence, diarrhea, nausea and vomiting. Tissue dehydration causes wrinkles and sunken eyes. Poor fluid circulation in the brain may cause confusion in breathing, irritability, heightened allergies and low blood pressure.

A salt free diet is obviously desirable for someone who eats too much salt. However, once the body's salinity normalizes, some salt should be brought back into the diet quickly. **LOW SALT, NOT NO SALT,** is best for a permanent way of eating. The average American adult consumes between 4,000 to 6,000 mg. a day. A therapeutic, sodium-restricted diet would range from 1,000 to 3,000mg a day. One teaspoon of salt has about 2,000 mg or 2 grams of sodium. Sodium-containing ingredients you may not recognize on a label as such include sodium caseinate, monosodium glutamate, trisodium phosphate, sodium bicarbonate and sodium sterol lactate.

While regular table salt is almost totally devoid of nutritional value, there are many other ways to get the good salts that the body needs. Tamari, soy sauce, miso, umeboshi plums, sea vegetables, sundried sea salt, herb salts and seasonings, sesame salt, and naturally fermented foods such as pickles, relishes and olives, all have enzymes and alkalizing properties that make salts usable and absorbable.

- **Sea salt** is a rich source of iodine, additive-free, and contains a plethora of minerals besides sodium.
- **Tamari** is a wheat-free soy sauce, lower in sodium and richer in flavor than soy sauce.
- **Bragg's LIQUID AMINOS** is an energizing protein broth, and contains valuable amino acids.
- **Miso** is a salty-tasting soy paste made from cooked, aged soybeans and sometimes grains.
- **Gomashio** is a mixture of sesame seeds and sea salt, a delicious staple in oriental cooking.

Wine As Part Of A Healing Diet?

Naturally fermented wine is more than an alcoholic beverage. It is a complex biological fluid possessing definite physiological values. Records dating back 4,000 years refer to the dietary and therapeutic uses of wine. It has been used as a food, a medicine, as part of various religious ceremonies and as an important element in social life.

Wine is still a living food, and can combine with, and aid the body like yogurt or other fermented foods. Many small, family owned wineries make chemical and additive free wines that retain inherent nutrients, including absorbable B vitamins, minerals and trace minerals, such as potassium, magnesium, organic sodium, iron, calcium and phosphorus. Wine is a vastly more complex product than beer or spirits; it is never boiled, so its biologically active compounds are not destroyed or altered by heat.

Wine is a highly useful drink for digestion, and in moderation, is a mild tranquilizer and sedative for the heart, arteries and blood pressure. Wine can free circulation, relieve pain and reduce acid production in the body. It is superior to tranquilizers or drugs for relief of nervous stress and tension. Its importance should not be overlooked in a weight loss program, because a glass or two of wine relaxes both mind and body. When you are relaxed, you tend to eat less.

Research indicates that drinking one or two glasses of wine per day can cut coronary heart disease risk by 50%, help prevent blood clot formation, and increase life span by reducing stress. Wine raises high-density lipoproteins (HDLs) in the blood, while decreasing low-density lipoproteins (LDLs) to help lower dangerous cholesterol levels.

Recent studies at U.C. Berkeley have shown that red wine is rich in the new class of polyphenols, powerful antioxidants that help neutralize free radicals which damage DNA, alter body chemistry and destroy cells outright. A new study on hepatitis A by the Epidemiology Journal shows that these polyphenols can even help prevent virus replication.

U.C. Davis research involves the wine compounds, tannins, quercetin and resveratrol, found in red wines. Their studies showed that tannin-rich red wine was able to reduce ADP-induced platelet aggregation and increase HDL cholesterol levels, suggesting that tannins may help protect against heart disease.

• Quercetin, a flavonoid that appears in red wine grapes and other dark fruits, may be one of the most powerful anticancer agents ever discovered, because of its ability to reverse tumor development by blocking the conversion of normal body cells to cancer cells. Quercitin activity is intensified by the wine fermentation process and by naturally-occurring flora in the intestinal tract. Quercetin improves pancreas function, and levels the release of insulin. It helps prevent some of the major complications of diabetes, including cataracts, diabetic retinopathy (blindness), neuropathy (nerve damage) and nephropathy (kidney damage). Since quercetin is an antioxidant and free radical scavenger, certain medical doctors are using quercetin in wine with HIV infections, because wine also relieves some of the pain and stress.

• Resveratrol is a natural compound in grapes that fights fungal disease, predominantly in red wines. Although alcohol in any form has been associated with a reduced risk incidence of heart disease, new studies suggest that something in wine in addition to the alcohol is responsible for its cholesterol - lowering benefits. Resveratrol may be that "something," or at least play a role in this healthful activity. Scientists believe it may be a key to wine drinkers' healthy cholesterol levels, and may also reduce other unhealthy fats circulating in the blood. Resveratrol also seems to prevent blood platelet aggregation, and reduce blood clotting in arteries narrowed by years of heavy fat consumption.

Note: Liquor other than wines is not recommended, even for cooking, when you are involved in a healing program. Although most people can stand a little hard liquor without undue effect, and alcohol burns off in cooking, the concentrated sugar residues won't help a recovering body.

Always use in moderation.

The Macrobiotic Diet

A MACROBIOTIC DIET is an effective method of improving body chemistry against cancer, and has for centuries been part of the natural healing tradition for cancer. In the Orient, where it originated, macrobiotics encourage body harmony and balance by teaching that health and vitality can be achieved through living in harmony with the universe.

Macro-biotic, or long life, stems from the Oriental philosophy that considers the seasons, climate, traditional culture, and a person's health condition and activity level in determining the way to eat. In America, macrobiotics has become popular as a therapeutic diet approach for serious and degenerative illness, because it detoxifies and alkalizes the body to protect it against chronic diseases. It is an effective technique because it works to alter body chemistry, not only acting as a toxin cleansing regimen, but also by helping to rebuild healthy blood and cells.

The macrobiotic way of eating is low in fat, non-mucous-forming, and rich in vegetable fiber and protein. It is stimulating to the heart and circulatory system through emphasis on Oriental foods such as miso, bancha green tea, and shiitake mushrooms. It is alkalizing with umeboshi plums, sea vegetables and soy foods. It is high in potassium, natural iodine, and other minerals and trace elements.

The most apparent difference between the macrobiotic system and other organic approaches is its reliance on whole grains. It suggests that at least half of the daily food intake be whole grain products, such as brown rice, whole wheat, oats, barley, millet, buckwheat, rye and corn. Other foods in order of their importance in a macrobiotic diet are vegetables, oil, nuts, fruits, fish and occasional eggs.

Although many macrobiotic followers prefer to avoid all animal foods, macrobiotics is not a vegetarian system and some fish is included. Other meats, refined grains, sugar and sweeteners (except rice syrup and barley malt in small amounts), most dairy products, infertile eggs, processed foods and beverages containing stimulants, are not part of a strict macrobiotic diet. Vegetables, both raw and cooked, make up 30% of the diet. Beans, sea vegetables and soups comprise 10 to 15%. Fruits and nuts are considered pleasure foods and are eaten only occasionally as desserts or snacks.

A macrobiotic diet's greatest benefit is that it is cleansing and strengthening at the same time, and offers a way of eating that is easily individualized for the environment, the seasons, and the constitution of the person using it.

However, a strict macrobiotic diet used over a long period of time, can be excessively stringent for a person living a busy, stressful life in today's polluted environment. A better way is to follow a strict macrobiotic diet for three to six months, and then to gradually move to a more modified macrobiotic diet. A light, modified macrobiotic diet does not follow a set pattern, but rather emphasizes the principles of macrobiotics with the flexibility of individual needs. One should still avoid refined foods, and foods with additives and preservatives on a modified macrobiotic diet. Brown rice, other whole grains, and fresh, in season foods, should still be the diet mainstays. Therapeutic foods, such as miso, bancha tea, shiitake and reishi mushrooms, sea plants, soy foods and umeboshi plums should be included regularly.

As we learn more about therapeutic ways of eating; macrobiotics, fruit cleansing diets, juice fasting, mono diets, etc., caution should be used if one is not in a controlled clinical environment. In their strict cleansing/ healing form, excessively limited diets should be used only as short term programs.

There must be balance to your diet. It is largely "civilization" foods and lack of balance that get us into trouble, that lower resistance to disease. A wide range of nutrients is necessary for cell growth, immunity and energy, for healing and strength, for endurance and stamina, for assimilation and body cleansing, and weight maintenance. For the best route to long term health, find out what foods have the elements you need in their natural state, and include them in your diet, raw or simply cooked, on a regular basis.

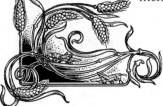

For more on this optimum way of eating, see
COOKING FOR HEALTHY HEALING, by Linda Rector-Page.

An Important Message About Your Health Care Responsibility

The material on the following pages is intended as an educational tool to offer information about alternative healing and health maintenance options available to the health care consumer today.

I believe we must be respectful of all ways of healing. The crisis intervention measures of drug therapy are sometimes needed to stabilize an emergency or life-threatening situation, but for long term well-being, disease prevention, and many common, self-limiting problems, diet improvement, exercise, and natural medicine choices make good sense. They are gentle, non-invasive, and in almost every case, free of any side effects.

The optional recommendations in this section are not intended as a substitute for the advice and treatment of a physician or other licensed health care professionals. In many cases, they may be used as adjuncts to professional care, to help shorten the time you may have to use drug treatment, and to help overcome any side effects.

Are there interactions between drugs and herbs? It is important to remember that herbs are foods, remarkably safe in their naturally-occurring state, and especially in combinations. They do not normally interact with drugs any more than a food would interact. However, be fair to your doctor and yourself. Discuss your alternative choices with your physician, and always inform your doctor or pharmacist of any other medication you are taking. Pregnant women are especially urged to consult with their health care provider before using any therapy.

I feel that education is the key to making wise health decisions. Part of the job of taking more command of your own health care is using your common sense, intelligence, and adult judgement based on the knowledge of your own body experiences. Ultimately, you must take the full responsibility for your choices and how you use the information presented here.

AILMENTS

IN ALPHABETICAL ORDER

Each ailment page consists of a four lifestyle therapy programs:
FOOD THERAPY, HERBAL THERAPY, SUPPLEMENT/SUPERFOOD THERAPY & BODYWORK

The programs can be approached in several ways, according to each person's needs. Many people choose a selection of remedies from among the therapy areas; some people pinpoint one or two areas.

Pick the suggestions that you feel instinctively strong about. They are invariably the best for you, and will be the easiest to incorporate into your lifestyle.

All the recommended therapies have been found effective, but every person has a different body and is a different individual. Healing response seems to accelerate when people select their own remedy programs.

• Bold print entries indicate the most successful, or most often used therapeutics.
• Where a method has also proven effective for children, a small child's face ☺ appears by the recommendation.
• Where a method has proven particularly successful for women, a female symbol ♀ appears by the recommendation.
• Where a method has proven particularly successful for men, a male symbol ♂ appears by the recommendation.

Refer to the ALTERNATIVE HEALTH CARE ARSENAL on page 72 for more information about any recommended healing agent.

All recommended doses are daily unless otherwise specified. Dosage listed is for the major time of healing, and is not to be considered as maintenance or long term.

For chronic conditions, the traditional rule of thumb is one month of natural healing therapy for every year you have had the problem.

No prescription is as valuable as knowledge.

Ailments Table of Contents

Check the Index for other ailment references.

Abscesses

Boils ✤ Carbuncles ✤ Suppurating Sores ✤ Dental Abscesses

Pus accumulation that forms due to infection, anywhere in the body - both externally and internally. Recurrent attacks of boils and abscesses indicate a depressed immune system.

Diet & Superfood Therapy

☙ Go on a short 1 to 3 day fresh juice diet (pg. 157), followed by a fresh foods cleansing diet for 2 weeks to remove toxins.

☙ Simmer flax and fenugreek seeds together until soft. Mash pulp. Apply to abscess as a compress.

☙ Mix fresh grated garlic or onion with lemon juice and apply directly.

☙ Eat yogurt, kefir, and acidophilus for friendly intestinal flora.

☙ Drink 6 to 8 glasses of pure water daily.

☙ Effective superfoods:
➤Crystal Star ENERGY GREEN™.
➤Green Foods GREEN MAGMA.
➤Propolis tincture - apply directly and take internally, twice daily.
➤AloeLife FIBERMATE powder daily to cleanse intestinal tract.
➤George's ALOE VERA JUICE each morning.

Herbal Therapy

☙ Jump start herbal program:
Crystal Star ANTI-BIO™ caps, 6 daily for 3 days, then 4 daily for one week;

with

➤CLEANSING & PURIFYING TEA™ for one week, or Aloe Life ALOE GOLD 2 TBS. in juice a.m. and p.m.
➤ANTI-FLAM™ caps as needed; and apply
➤ANTI-BIO™ gel or PAU D' ARCO/ECHINACEA™ extract directly.
❧

☙ Other effective herbal therapy:
➤ECHINACEA extract 3x daily. Apply Echinacea extract drops topically.
➤Crystal Star ZINC SOURCE™ extract with burdock root tea 2 cups daily.
➤BLACK WALNUT EXTRACT - take internally; apply directly.

☙ Effective topical applications:
➤Aloe Life ALOE SKIN GEL.
➤Tea tree oil or Thursday Plantation ANTISEPTIC CREAM.

☙ For dental abscesses:
➤Use sage tea mouthwashes twice daily, especially for dry socket abscesses.
➤Apply myrrh extract 2x daily.

Supplements

✍ Apply and take internally Nutribiotic GRAPEFRUIT SEED SKIN SPRAY, ointment, or extract capsules as needed.

✍ Colloidal silver - take internally as directed; apply directly.

✍ Dr. Diamond HERPANACINE capsules, 4-6 daily.

✍ Oceanic beta-carotene 100,000IU daily for one week, with vitamin E 400IU 2x daily or zinc 50mg daily;

or

➤Vitamin C ascorbate powder with bioflavs. 3 to 5 grams daily, with zinc 50mg 2x daily for 1 week; with garlic caps 8 daily.

✍ Add acidophilus to your diet if taking high dose courses of antibiotics for abscess infections.
➤Take DR. DOPHILUS caps 3x daily, with garlic caps, 2 caps 3x daily;

✍ Liquid chlorophyll - apply locally. Take internally, 3 teasp. daily.

Lifestyle Support Therapy

Squeezing a boil can force infectious bacteria into the bloodstream. Use hot compresses to bring boil to a head instead - 3 compresses, 3x daily.

☞ Take a catnip, aloe vera juice, or wheat grass juice erema every other day for 1 week to clean out toxins.

☞ Expose the area to early morning sunlight for 15 minutes a day.

☞ Effective topical applications:
➤Hot epsom salts compress - 2 TBS. salts to 1C. hot water to bring to a head.
➤Burdock or St. John's wort poultice.
➤Centipede KITTY'S OXY-GEL.
➤A green or white clay compress 3 times daily to bring to a head.

☞ For dental abscesses:
Homeopathic remedies are very successful. See a homeopathic professional.
➤*Belladonna* for throbbing pain.
➤*Bryonia* for acute inflammation.
➤*Pyrogenium* for undrained pus.
➤*Silicea* to increase pus drainage.
➤*Mercurius* for foul breath.
and

☞ Dissolve 10 acidophilus capsules in water and rinse your mouth out 3x daily.

Common Symptoms: *Inflammation and infection of the skin layers, along with swelling of the nearest lymph glands; suppuration with white, rather than clear drainage; weeping, pus-filled sores, often accompanied by chills and fever.*

Common Causes: *Toxicity of the system, especially the colon and blood; a low resistance condition following a staph infection, viral or bacterial infection; an infection of a hair follicle, especially under the arms.*

Acidity ✣ Acidosis
Restoring Balanced Body Chemistry

Over-acidity in the body tissues is one of the basic causes of many arthritic and rheumatic diseases. Stomach ulcers are almost always in the wings if the body is continually over acidic. Balanced body chemistry is vital to immune system maintenance and disease correction.

Diet & Superfood Therapy

A healthy body keeps large alkaline reserves to meet the demands of too many acid-producing foods. When these are depleted beyond a 3:1 ratio, health can be seriously threatened.

✷ Go on a short 24 hour (pg. 158) liquid diet to cleanse excess acid wastes.

✷Then, for the next 3 days, eat only fresh, raw foods to complete the body-alkalizing process. (Cooked foods increase acidity in the body.)

✷Then, eat a diet of 75% alkalizing foods, including fresh and steamed vegetables, sprouts, fruits and fruit juices, miso soups, brown rice, green drinks, ume plums, honey, etc.

✷Acid-forming foods should be no more than 25%. Avoid foods like coffee and caffeine-containing foods, meats, dairy foods (except yogurt or kefir), poultry, eggs, fish and seafoods, lentils, peanuts and legumes, cheeses, highly processed foods and most condiments.

✷Eat smaller meals. Chew slowly.

✷ Drink an 8-oz. blend of tomato juice, wheat germ, brewer's yeast and lecithin daily, or BeWell TOMATO juice. ♀
or

✷ Drink 1 to 2 glasses of cranberry juice daily, or BeWell CRANBERRY NECTAR juice. ♀

Herbal Therapy

☙ Jump start herbal program: Crystal Star FIBER & HERBS COLON CLEANSE™ caps to clean out acid waste;

along with

✷Ginger compresses on the kidneys to increase elimination of toxins; then for 3 weeks

✷Two IODINE/POTASSIUM™ caps daily for body chemistry balance; and

✷Two ginger caps with each meal, or Crystal Star AFTER-MEAL ENZ™ extract, avoiding yeasted breads, dairy foods, meats and sugars until condition clears.

☙ Other effective herbal therapy: ✷Planetary Formulas TRIPHALA tablets as directed.

☙ Effective teas: ☺
✷Catnip
✷Chamomile
✷Fennel seed ♀
✷Wisdom of the Ancients YERBA MATÉ tea.

Supplements

✷ Take ascorbate vitamin C crystals with bioflavonoids - 3000mg daily for 4 weeks.

✷ HCL Pepsin tabs after meals.
or
✷ High potency alkalizing enzymes, such as Prevail FIBER ENZYMES.

✷ B Complex 100mg with extra pantothenic acid 500mg, 2 daily.

✷ Future Biotics VITAL K PLUS, 2 teasp. daily.

✷ For kids:
✷Prevail VITASE for kids.
✷Orange Peel GREENS PLUS (good tasting).

✷Probiotics: Natren LIFE START or Professional Nutrition DR. DOPHILUS powder in the morning.

✷ Effective superfoods:
✷Crystal Star ENERGY GREEN™.
✷Green Foods BETA CARROT blend.
✷Salute ALOE VERA JUICE with ginger each morning.
✷Crystal Star SYSTEMS STRENGTH™ for minerals (especially potassium).
✷Solgar WHEY TO GO protein drink.

Lifestyle Support Therapy

Take the Acid/Alkaline Self Test on page 449 to check your body chemistry balance and progress.

☙ Get some mild exercise every day for body oxygen. A daily walk is a good choice, with deep breathing exercises.

☙ Have a little wine before dinner to relax and reduce body acid.

☙ Crystal Star ALKALIZING ENZYME BODY WRAP™ for almost immediate change in body pH.

☙ Reflexology point:

food assimilation

Common Symptoms: *Frequent skin eruptions that don't go away; sunken eyes with darkness around the eyes; rheumatoid arthritis; burning, foul-smelling stools and anal itching; chronic poor digestion; latent ulcers or ulcer flare-ups; bad breath and body odor; alternating constipation and diarrhea; insomnia; water retention; excessively low blood pressure; frequent migraine headaches.*

Common Causes: *Mental stress and tension; kidney, liver or adrenal malfunction; poor diet with excess acid-forming foods, such as caffeine, fried foods, tobacco, or sweets. Acidosis is often related to or caused by arthritis, diabetes or borderline diabetes. (Refer to those pages in this book.)*

Acne

Pimples * Blemishes

Acne is a hormone-related problem affected by the action of male testosterone on the sebaceous skin glands. Although teenage acne is extremely common (4 out of 5 teenagers develop it) adult acne is now more prevalent - a clear sign of our modern poor diet. Whiteheads (comedones) are plugs of oil and dead skin cells under the surface of the skin that block oil from flowing freely to the skin surface. They can either turn into blackheads (open comedones) when they reach the surface of the skin and are exposed to air, or in a more severe condition, can spread under the skin, rupture and expand the inflammation.

Diet & Superfood Therapy

♨ Go on a short 3 day liquid cleanse (pg. 157) to clean out acid wastes. Use apple, carrot, pineapple and papaya juices.
 ✱Then eat more fiber - especially from fresh foods. Have a salad every day. Add often to the diet: whole grains, green veggies, brown rice, fish, sprouts, low-fat dairy and apples.
 ✱Choose turkey, chicken and vegetable sources (beans, tofu, sprouts) for your protein instead of red meat.
 ✱Limit wheat germ, shellfish, kelp, cheese, citrus, eggs and salt, or foods with high iodine levels that may increase oil secretions.
 ✱Drink 6 glasses of pure water daily.
 ✱Avoid white flour or sugar, soft drinks, caffeine, fried foods, candy, especially chocolate, pasteurized dairy, hard cheese, nightshade plants like eggplant, peppers, tobacco, and tomatoes, peanut butter, and any foods with preservatives or additives.
 ✱Eliminate junk and fast foods!
 ✱Rub face with insides of papaya and cucumber skins to neutralize acid wastes.

♨ Effective superfoods:
 ✱Crystal Star ZINC SOURCE™ extract.
 ✱AloeLife FIBER-MATE drink, $\frac{1}{2}$ teasp.
 ✱Y.S. ROYAL/JELLY GINSENG drink.
 ✱Green Foods BETA CARROT blend.
 ✱Wakunaga KYO-GREEN.

Herbal Therapy

🌿 **Jump start herbal program:**
 Relieve inflammation and infection first with Crystal Star ANTI-BIO™ caps or extract, 4x daily for 1 week.
 ✱**Then take high potency royal jelly with ginseng 2 teasp. daily.** ♀ with ♂
 ✱Crystal Star BEAUTIFUL SKIN™ tea. Drink and apply with cotton balls, or BEAUTIFUL SKIN GEL™ with VITEX extract.
 ✱Take BEAUTIFUL SKIN™ caps for at least 3 months for skin clarity.

🌿 Other effective herbal therapy:
 ✱EVENING PRIMROSE OIL 4-6 daily, with Siberian ginseng or licorice tea daily, and pat on George's ALOE VERA JUICE.

🌿 Effective herbal applications:
 ✱Golden seal and myrrh solution.
 ✱Propolis tincture on sores. ◯
 ✱Stevia Extract drops - apply directly, esp. for adult acne.
 ✱Tea tree oil on sores 3x daily.
 ✱Beehive Botanicals PROPOLIS CREAM.

🌿 Use oilfree herbal-based cosmetics. Zia Cosmetics has a good program:
 ✱ALOE CITRUS WASH
 ✱CAMPHOR TREATMENT MASK
 ✱AROMATHERAPY ESSENTIAL OILS for oil control and to calm glands.

Supplements

✑ **For adult acne:**
 ✱**Dr. Diamond HERPANACINE capsules as directed.**
 ✱**Enzymatic Therapy DERMA-KLEAR cream, soap and cleanser, and AKNEZYME caps daily.**
 ✱Flora VEGE-SIL tabs, 3 daily.
 ✱**B Complex 100mg daily if acne is stress-caused (appearing around the chin).**

 Note: Mega-doses of vitamins often aggravate acne because too much iodine and vitamin E can stimulate the sebaceous glands to produce too much oil.
 ✱Add acidophilus and vitamin C to the diet if taking antibiotics for acne. Mix $\frac{1}{4}$ teasp. vitamin C crystals with 1 TB. acidophilus liquid and take 4x daily.

✑ **For teenage acne:**
 ✱**Dr. Diamond HERPANACINE caps.**
 ✱**Pancreatin after meals to digest oils.**
 ✱**1 TB. Omega-3 flax oil 2x daily. If there is scarring, add bromelain 500mg 2x daily.)**
 ✱Beta carotene 25,000IU 2x daily, with vitamin D 1000IU daily.

 ✱**For acne scars:** Place fresh pineapple on the scars for enzyme therapy, and take extra bromelain 750mg daily.

Lifestyle Support Therapy

🜂 Apply Marrix Health GENESIS H_2O_2 OXY-SPRAY to affected areas for 1 month. Do not squeeze. Whiteheads and blackheads come to the surface for elimination.
 ✱Apply Nutribiotic GRAPEFRUIT SEED extract to stop infected eruptions.

🜂 Wash affected areas with a mild hypoallergenic cleanser or tea tree or calendula soap. Exfoliate with a gentle, alkalizing scrub with AHAs.

🜂 **Steam face with Swiss Kriss Herbs, or with aromatherapy lavender essential oil or water, or eucalyptus and thyme.**
 ✱Apply a drop of lavender, lemon grass or tea tree oil to spots several times daily.

🜂 Get early morning sun on the face daily possible. Get fresh air and exercise daily, and plenty of rest to eliminate toxins.

🜂 Place alternating hot and cold cloths on affected area to bring up cleansing circulation.

🜂 **Rub on lemon juice or Aloe Life SKIN GEL at night. Wash in the morning.**

🜂 **Apply white clay or Crystal Star NATURAL CLAY TONING MASQUE and let dry 3x times daily to bring to a head; then use once a week.**

See also SKIN CARE pages in this book for more information.

Common Symptoms: Inflamed and infected pustules on the face, chest and back. Often itching and scarring from Cystic Acne in which fluid-filled cysts develop.
Common Causes: Gland (particularly pituitary), and hormone (particularly male) imbalance during teenage years, and before menstruation. Both teenage and adult acne are aggravated by a diet with lots of fatty foods, poor digestion of fats and essential fatty acid deficiency. Sugar-saturated skin is susceptible to acne, because a rise in blood sugar is multiplied by 5 when it gets to the skin. Poor liver function, poor elimination/constipation, heredity, some oral contraceptives, high oil cosmetics, emotional stress, and lack of green veggies.

Addictions

Alcohol Abuse ✳ Rehabilitation

As with other addictive practices, alcohol abuse is both brought on and marked by stress and depression, and often, a lack of confidence about one's self, or reason for one's life. As fatuous as it may seem, contentment, or purposely making a major life style change is sometimes the best medicine for changing body chemistry - and thus curbing the craving for alcohol effects.

Diet & Superfood Therapy

Cleanse the liver. No alcohol detox program will work without liver regeneration.

✤ Go on a short juice fast (pg. 157) to clean out alcohol residues.

🌿 Then follow the *HYPOGLYCEMIA DIET* in this book for 3 months. Take a daily protein drink, like Solgar WHEY TO GO to balance body chemistry and replace electrolytes quickly. Add 1 TB. Omega-3 flax seed oil during withdrawal stage.

🌿 Add plenty of mineral-rich foods to your diet for a solid nutritional foundation. 🌿 The continuing diet should be high in magnesium foods, like wheat germ, bran, brewer's yeast, whole grains and cereals, brown rice, green leafy vegetables, potatoes, miso, low-fat dairy, eggs and fish.

🌿 Avoid refined and fried foods, sugary or heavily spiced foods and caffeine. They aggravate alcohol craving.

🌿 Take Organic Gourmet NUTRITIONAL YEAST BROTH every night for B vitamins and to curb craving.

✤ Effective superfoods:
🌿 Crystal Star ENERGY GREEN™
🌿 Nappi PERFECT MEAL protein drink.
🌿 Revitalizing Tonic, page 172.
🌿 Nature's Life SUPER GREEN PRO.
🌿 Nutrex HAWAIIAN SPIRULINA drink.
🌿 Sun CHLORELLA, 1 pkt. daily.

Herbal Therapy

☙ Jump start herbal program:
Crystal Star WITHDRAWAL SUPPORT™ caps for several months, with EVENING PRIMROSE oil caps 24 daily.
or
🌿 CALCIUM SOURCE™ extract in water as a rapid calmative *with* GINSENG/ REISHI extract and spirulina 500mg.
or
🌿 LIV-ALIVE™ for detox, with ADR-ACTIVE™ caps and MENTAL INNER ENERGY™ caps or extract for energy support. ♀

☙ Other effective herbal therapy:
🌿 Country Life SHIITAKE/REISHI COMPLEX w. CHLORELLA.

🌿 Enzymatic Therapy KAVA-TONE to calm nerves.

✤ Effective extracts:
🌿 Passion flower to control craving
🌿 MILK THISTLE SEED for liver detox
🌿 Scullcap to calm nerves
🌿 Hops to regulate blood sugar
🌿 Panax ginseng to protect stomach lining. ♀
🌿 Homeopathic *Nux Vomica* or *Camomilla* at night before retiring.

Supplements

☙ Vitamin C - up to 10,000mg daily (or until stool turns soupy), ascorbate vit. C crystals with bioflavs - 1/4 tsp. at a time in juice through the day for at least 1 month.
with
🌿 5-Hydroxy-Tryptophan 50-100mg.

☙ Mega-vitamin therapy is effective:
🌿 To curb alcohol craving, take either combination below daily with meals for a month:
2 Glutamine 500mg.
2 Cysteine 500mg.
2 B Complex 100mg.
3 Ascorbate Vit. C 1000mg.
2 Niacinamide 500mg.
2 Zinc 50mg. ♂
or
3 Solaray CHROMIACIN
2 Twin Lab GABA Plus
3 Glutamine 500mg
2 Magnesium 400mg
Rainbow Light DETOX-ZYME caps ♀

☙ For nerve and withdrawal effects:
🌿 One raw brain glandular capsule, 500mg tyrosine, 500mg taurine, 250mg B₆, 100mg niacin and zinc 30mg. ♀
or
🌿 DLPA 750mg, Country Life B₁₅ 125mg, magnesium 500mg, B₆ 250mg, and L-Carnitine 500mg daily. ♀

Lifestyle Support Therapy

🌿 Acupuncture and massage therapy re-alignment are successful in curbing craving for alcohol.

🌿 Improved fitness and system oxygen are important. Get fresh air, sunlight and exercise every day.

🌿 Foot reflexology:

liver

🌿 Although it seems to state the obvious, avoid the places, people and circumstances that sharpen your desire to escape through alcohol. This usually means major life change and may seem impossible. But it almost always starts the road to lasting success and is often the only way. *Liver detoxification shortens withdrawal time significantly.*

🌿 Excessive drinking particularly affects men and their estrogen balance, through liver damage, often engendering enlarged breasts, reduced sex drive and beard growth, and shrunken testes.

Common Symptoms: *Alcohol dependence, and using alcohol for daily calories instead of food; short term memory loss; liver degeneration and disease; nervousness and poor coordination; high LDL cholesterol and blood sugar (there is a stress/sugar connection for both conditions); immune depression; poor enzyme production leading to poor fat and protein metabolism, and especially to mineral deficiency; anger, lack of emotional control, aggressive/compulsive behavior toward friends and family members.*

Common Causes: *Excessive intake of alcohol influenced by socio-psychological factors, genetic disorder, hypoglycemia because of too much refined, sugary food and too little fresh, high mineral foods; unrelieved daily stress, tension and emotional depression.*

See the LIVER DETOX program in this book for more information.

Addictions

Alcohol Poisoning & Toxicity Reactions ❋ Hangover

A high-stress, fast-paced, jet-lag lifestyle overloads your biochemical detox systems so that you get a steamroller effect the "morning after." Your body can't work adequately unless you give yourself a break. A hangover should be gone by five o'clock the next day. If it isn't, you probably have alcohol poisoning. There are effective natural means of reducing alcohol's damage to your body and brain, but the real idea is to reduce alcohol consumption below the toxicity level.

Diet & Superfood Therapy

❧ **Good food improves body stability:**
Eat vitamin B-rich, high fiber foods like brown rice and vegetables to soak up blood alcohol. Add cruciferous vegetables and soy foods to help the body detoxify.
➤No sugary foods or "hair of the dog" drinks; they seem to make you feel better but in reality drag out a hangover.

❧ **Here are 3 effective hangover tonics:**
➤Mix brewer's yeast, raw egg yolk, orange juice and cayenne pepper. Drink all at once - straight down.
➤Mix tomato juice, green and yellow onions, celery, parsley, hot pepper sauce, rosemary leaves, fennel seeds, basil, water, and Bragg's LIQUID AMINOS. Drink straight down.
➤Knudsen's VERY VEGGIE SPICY juice, V-8 juice, or the Revitalizing Tonic on pg. 172.

❧ **Effective superfoods:**
➤Crystal Star BIOFLAV., FIBER & C SUPPORT™ drink. **Excellent results within a half hour.**
➤Electrolyte replacement drink, such as Knudsen's RECHARGE.
➤AloeLIFE ALOE GOLD 2TBS. in juice
➤Lewis Labs BREWER'S YEAST, $^1/_4$ teasp. in water to alleviate nausea.

Herbal Therapy

➤ **Jump start herbal program:**
Before drinking, to minimize toxicity:
➤**Crystal Star ASPIR-SOURCE™ capsules, with 1 to 2 MENTAL INNER ENERGY™ capsules with kava kava.** ♀
or
➤**GINSENG 6 SUPER™ tea, for energy, with 2 to 6 kudzu caplets.** ♂
➤WITHDRAWAL SUPPORT™ caps.
➤EVENING PRIMROSE oil 1000mg.
➤Dragon Eggs SAGES GINSENG.
➤**Siberian ginseng extract in angelica root tea.**
➤Enzymatic Therapy KAVA-TONE.

➤ **Nervines and enzyme therapy after you drink:**
➤Cayenne/ginger capsules to settle stomach and relieve headache.
➤Scullcap tea to soothe nerves and oxygenate the brain.
➤BILBERRY extract to protect the liver.
➤MILK THISTLE SEED extract for liver support.

☞ Take a quick liver tonic if you think you have alcohol poisoning:
➤Steep for 20 minutes - hibiscus, cloves, allspice, and juice of 2 lemons in white grape or orange juice. Drink slowly.

Supplements

➥ **Before you drink to minimize toxicity to the brain:**
➤**Alacer EMERGEN-C with bioflavonoids** $^1/_2$ **teasp. in water with a vitamin B Complex 100mg capsule, zinc 30mg and DLPA** 750mg for withdrawal..
or
➤**Cysteine 500mg with 2 EVENING PRIMROSE OIL 500mg caps before drinking and before retiring.**

➥ **Anti-oxidants *with* B vitamins after you drink help end the misery.**
➤Unipro DMG liquid with Source Naturals CO-ENZYMATE B complex SL, or **Nature's Bounty internasal B$_{12}$.**
➤American Biologics INFLAZYME FORTE tablets, 2-4 between meals.
➤Glutamine 500mg with vitamin E 400IU and selenium 2x daily.
➤Homeopathic *Nux Vomica.*
➤Biotec CELL GUARD w. SOD 6 tabs.
➤**Source Naturals HANGOVER FORMULA.**

➥ **Hangover healing vitamin blend - take 1 each on the morning after:**
Flax seed or evening primrose oil
Vitamin B$_1$ 500mg
B$_2$ 100mg
B$_6$ 250mg
Emulsified A 25,000IU

Lifestyle Support Therapy

☞ Apply cold compresses to the head before and after a long hot shower, to wash off toxins coming out through the skin. (You wont believe what a difference this makes.) Or, take alternating hot and cool showers to stimulate circulation and eliminate blood alcohol.

☞ Take a sauna for 20 minutes. Scrub skin with a dry skin brush.
➤Get outside in the fresh air as soon as possible - the more oxygen in the lungs and tissues, the better.

☞ If your hangover doesn't go away, you may have alcohol poisoning. Take a catnip, chlorophyll or coffee enema, and the liver tonic on this page.
➤If the case is severe, you may need a stomach pump at an urgent care center.

☞ **Hand reflexology:**

liver

squeeze all around fingers for brain health

Common Symptoms: *Sensitivity to light, headache, eyeache, bad taste in the mouth, weakness and debility, shakiness, dull mind and senses, stomach queasiness, lethargy. Initial withdrawal symptoms include high anxiety, rapid pulse with tremors, hot flashes and drenching perspiration, dehydration, insomnia and sometimes hallucinations.*
Common Causes: *Alcohol poisoning from too much alcohol; liver exhaustion and consequent malfunction.*

Addictions

Drug Abuse ✤ Rehabilitation

Most people begin taking drugs to alleviate boredom and fatigue, or to relieve physical or psychological pain. In almost every case, nutritional health is severely compromised regardless of whether the drug being abused is a prescription or pleasure substance. Multiple depletions of critical nutrients like vitamins, minerals, essential fatty acids and enzymes set off addictive chain reactions. It takes a year or more to detoxify the blood of drugs. No program is successful against drug abuse without consistent therapy and awareness. Lifestyle therapy helps treat addictions successfully by minimizing the discomfort and maximizing the healing process on a continuing basis as you go about your life.

Diet & Superfood Therapy

Most addictive drugs create malnutrition. A healthy, wellbalanced diet is essential for overcoming substance abuse.

☙ **Healthy food is a key to body stability:**
—Include plenty of slow-burning complex carbohydrates from whole grains and fresh vegetables, and vegetable protein in your diet.
—Eliminate refined sugars, alcohol and caffeine from the diet. They aggravate the craving for drugs.

☙ Mix wheat germ and brewer's yeast in juice with 1 teasp. each, honey and Bragg's LIQUID AMINOS; take 2 teasp. of the mix daily. ♂ ♀

☙ The brain is dependent on glucose as an energy source. Drug withdrawals often mean blood glucose levels drop with the consequent results of sweating, tremor, palpitations, anxiety and cravings. ♀

☙ **Effective superfoods:**
—**YS ROYAL JELLY/GINSENG blend.**
—Long Life IMPERIAL TONIC with royal jelly and evening primrose oil. ♂
—Crystal Star SYSTEMS STRENGTH™ (especially for prescription drugs).

Herbal Therapy

☙ **A six-step herbal program:**
1) Normalize body chemistry:
—Crystal Star GINSENG SIX SUPER TEA™, WITHDRAWAL SUPPORT™ caps. or GINSENG/REISHI extract.
2) Clean out drug residues:
—Crystal Star HEAVY METAL™ or DETOX™ capsules 4 daily, and SUN CHLORELLA tabs with echinacea extract.
3) Detoxify the liver:
—Crystal Star LIV-ALIVE™ tea, or GREEN TEA CLEANSER™ with MILK THISTLE SEED extract.
4) Strengthen and relax the nerves:
—Crystal Star RELAX CAPS™ and/or VALERIAN/WILD LETTUCE™ extract.
5) Enhance circulation:
—Crystal Star HAWTHORN or GINKGO BILOBA extracts.
6) Increase available energy:
—Crystal Star GINSENG SIX SUPER ENERGY™ caps, or MENTAL INNER ENERGY™ extract or caps with ginseng.

☙ **Extra withdrawal support from herbs:**
—Rosemary tea for depression.
—Oatstraw tea as an anti-addictive.
—Chamomile for stress relaxation.
—Gotu kola for energy/nerve health.
—Scullcap to calm anxiety.
—Siberian ginseng for cocaine.
—GINKGO BILOBA for memory loss.

Supplements

☙ **Supplement your nervous and digestive systems:**
—Take Vitamin C crystals up to 10,000mg daily, with niacin 1000mg 3x daily, a full spectrum pre-digested amino acid compound 1000mg daily and a B Complex 150mg.
—Add **acidophilus** to replace friendly G.I. flora, **chromium** to help rebalance sugar levels, SOD or Solgar SOD INDUCERS to detoxify.

—Add Country Life RELAXER (GABA with taurine) and glutamine 500mg. ♂
—Add Enzymatic Therapy THYROID/TYROSINE caps,
and
—DLPA 750mg for withdrawal. ♀

☙ Enzyme therapy is important: use Prevail VITASE or Enzymatic Therapy MEGA-ZYME, or Rainbow Light ADVANCED ENZYME SYSTEM.

☙ **Effective drug withdrawal support:**
—Methionine for heroine.
—Tyrosine for cocaine.
—CoQ_{10} for prescription drugs.
—Atrium LITHIUM 5mg for uppers and depressants.
—B complex 100mg for LSD.

Lifestyle Support Therapy

Note: Strong drugs, from LSD to hard alcohol to nicotine to heroin can put you at higher risk for Alzheimer's disease due to microvascular blockage and cerebral dementia.

❧ Biofeedback, chiropractic and acupuncture techniques have a high success rate in overcoming drug addictions.

❧ Avoid smoking. It increases craving for drugs by stripping the body of stabilizing nutrients.

❧ Apply tea tree oil, or B&T *CALI-FLORA GEL* to ulcers in the nose.

❧ **Reflexology point:**

Drug spot is between the 2nd and 3rd toe on top of the foot.

Common Symptoms: *Metabolic disorders like low blood sugar, hypothyroidism, poor adrenal function, liver malfunction and depression; general irritability, fatigue, unusual drowsiness, shakiness, nervousness, disorientation, memory loss, wired feeling, anxiety and paranoia, headaches, sweating and cramps; palpitations; poor food absorption even when meals are good.*
Common Causes: *Addictive origins cover a broad spectrum of factors, ranging from inherited genetics, childhood social behavior patterns, poor nutrition, along with allergies to certain foods, and metabolic physiology.*

See the HYPOGLYCEMIA DIET, pg. 338, and "COOKING FOR HEALTHY HEALING" by Linda Rector-Page for a complete program.

Caffeine Addiction

Caffeine is one of the most widely used stimulant drugs in the world. It is found in coffee, tea, cocoa, chocolate and herbs such as cola nuts and yerba mate tea. It is a constituent of prescription medicines like Excedrin, Anacin, Vanquish and Bromo-seltzer. It is an ingredient of almost every appetite suppressant and many soft drinks. More than 80% of American adults use coffee, and almost everybody else gets caffeine in one of its other forms. There is good news and bad news about caffeine. See CAFFEINE & A HEALING DIET in this book, page 202. Clearly it is a quick energy pick-me-up, and a memory stimulant, but just as clearly, excessive use of caffeine (over 5 cups of coffee a day), can lead to anxiety, sleeplessness, increased blood sugar levels, rapid heartbeat, exhausted adrenals and increased tolerance to its effects - all the signs of addiction.

Here are some good ideas for successfully cutting down on caffeine without the agony of withdrawal:
• Drink a cup of energizing herbal tea instead of coffee, such as Crystal Star HIGH ENERGY™ tea (energy rise is rapid), or GINSENG SUPER SIX™ tea (slower, longer energy).
• Strengthen your adrenal glands with herbal formulas like Crystal Star FEM SUPPORT™ extract for women, or ADR-ACTIVE™ extract for men.
• Normalize your body chemistry with a ginseng adaptogen compound, that might contain herbs like Siberian ginseng, panax ginseng, ashwagandha, gotu kola and reishi mushroom.
• Take Natra-Bio homeopathic CAFFEINE WITHDRAWAL RELIEF, zinc 30mg. daily (caffeine leaches out body zinc stores), and add a B-Complex 100mg daily.

Prescription Drug Dependence

One of the most serious addictions today is the widespread attraction to prescription drugs - especially mood altering drugs like tranquilizers, anti-depressants and anti-psychotics. Others, like amphetamines, create an addictive high through a metabolic process similar to the effect of the body's endorphins.

Here are some signs that addiction is occurring: 1) The body builds up a tolerance to the drug, so that the user increases the dosage to a dangerous point. 2) There is a decreased desire to work, with inattentiveness, mood swings, restlessness, temper tantrums, crying spells, or all of the above. 3) There is unusual susceptibility to illness because the immune system has been weakened by the drug. 4) Withdrawal symptoms of headaches, insomnia, light sensitivity, hot flashes, diarrhea and disorientation occur when the individual stops the drug.

Some tranquilizers and anti-depressants can be replaced with herbal remedies to avoid dependence, but specific prescription information is necessary to make the withdrawal process straightforward and safe. A good holistic doctor or naturopath should be able to help you.

Three types of herbs are needed to wean yourself from addictive prescription drugs. They should include:
• **Nervines,** such as scullcap and passionflower, to relax and rebuild the nervous system.
• **Tonic adaptogens,** such as ginseng or chlorella to strengthen and normalize the body.
• **Liver detoxification herbs,** such as MILK THISTLE SEED extract, or turmeric (curcumin), so your body can run with a clean system.

About Marijuana Use

The use of marijuana is rising again in the U.S., this time with new propagation techniques that make THC content over **200%** greater than 20 or 30 years ago. We should be clear about what marijuana is and what it isn't. Marijuana is no longer the mildly euphoric 3 or 4 hour high of the 60s and 70s. It is addictive. Those who are dependent on it are either constantly thinking about it, under intoxication, or recovering from its influence. Both mental and physical health are clearly affected, especially in terms of blood sugar balance, muscle coordination, reaction time and emotional deterioration. Work habits suffer from lack of ambition and direction, family life and relationships suffer because of apathy and non-communication.

However, many casual marijuana users are not aware of new research about this drug. Largely because of its increased strength, many more people are experiencing exaggerated effects, such as acute anxiety, paranoia, incoherent speech, extreme disorientation and hallucinations lasting up to 12 hours. Marijuana also impairs the reproductive system, especially in terms of reduced male sperm count, both short term **and** long term memory, and depressed immune response (by as much as 40%). Marijuana smoke today contains the same health-damaging carcinogens as tobacco smoke, only now in much higher concentrations. Because its smoke is inhaled more deeply and held in the lungs longer than tobacco, it leads to severe lung damage. All the attendant diseases of nicotine smokers are now besetting marijuana smokers - especially chronic bronchitis, emphysema and lung cancer.

As with every addictive substance, marijuana withdrawal is characterized by anxiety, sleeplessness, tremors and chills. Simple nutrition and lifestyle changes can go a long way toward minimizing the discomfort and mental craving.
• Marijuana leaches B vitamins; make brown rice and broccoli mainstays of your diet during the withdrawal period. Follow the diet for HYPOGLYCEMIA (pg. 338) to control sugar cravings.
• Take a protein drink every morning, such as Nature's Life SUPER GREEN PRO-96, Nappi's THE PERFECT MEAL, or Crystal Star SYSTEMS STRENGTH™ drink.
• Take antioxidants like tyrosine and plenty of vitamin C with bioflavonoids, and herbal nerve relaxers such as rosemary aromatherapy, or Crystal Star RELAX CAPS™.

Adrenal Gland Health
Adrenal Exhaustion

Small glands resting on top of the kidneys, the adrenals are comprised of two parts: the medulla, which secretes adrenaline, and norepinephrine to help the body cope with stress by increasing metabolism; and the cortex, responsible for maintaining body balance, regulating sugar metabolism, and a complex array of steroid hormones, including cortisone, DHEA, aldosterone, progesterone, estrogen, and testosterone. Adrenal function is impaired by long term cortico-steroid drug use, because these drugs cause the adrenals to shrink in size.

Diet & Superfood Therapy

See DIET FOR HYPOGLYCEMIA in this book for more specifics.

♋ **A good diet is essential to adrenal health.** Eat small, instead of large meals, low in sugar and fats. Eat lots of fresh foods, cold water fish, brown rice, legumes and whole grains.

✽Add more potassium-rich foods such as sea vegetables, potatoes, fish, and avocados to your diet. Intake should be about 3 to 5 grams daily. Cut down on high sodium foods.

✽Avoid stimulants like hard liquor, tobacco and excess caffeine during healing. ✽Avoid fats, fried foods, red meats and highly processed foods.

♋ Make a fresh mix daily of flax seed, bran, miso broth and honey. Take some each morning to feed adrenals. Or, take 2 teasp. each brewer's yeast and wheat germ daily in fruit juice. ♋

♋ **Effective superfoods:**
✽Crystal Star IODINE/POTASSIUM SOURCE™ caps, SYSTEMS STRENGTH™ drink, or BIOFLAVONOID, FIBER & C SUPPORT™ drink.
✽Wakunaga KYO-GREEN drink.

Herbal Therapy

☙ **Jump start herbal program:**
Crystal Star ADR-ACTIVE™ capsules or ADRN™ extract, 2x daily with BODY REBUILDER™ caps to stimulate hormone rebalance.
✽Add high potency YS ROYAL JELLY with ginseng, 2 teasp. daily,
✽For women: add J.R.E. IOSOL drops or Crystal Star IODINE SOURCE™ extract as a potassium rich source.♀+
✽For men: add Crystal Star GINSENG/LICORICE ELIXIR™ extract 2x daily, or Siberian ginseng/astragalus capsules, 4 daily. ♂

☙ **Other effective herbal therapy:**
EVENING PRIMROSE oil 4-6 daily, with
✽Siberian ginseng or licorice tea daily.

☙ **Adrenal balancing teas:**
✽Licorice root
✽Hawthorn leaf, berry & flower
✽Gotu kola

☙ **Adrenal health extracts:**
✽ECHINACEA root
✽Panax ginseng root
✽MILK THISTLE SEED

Supplements

Adrenal nutrients include essential fatty acids, amino acids, pantothenic acid, vitamins E, A, C, and bioflavonoids, and the minerals zinc, selenium, potassium, manganese, chromium, and magnesium.

❧ Adrenal complex glandular, such as Country Life ADRENAL with TYROSINE or MAXI-B with TAURINE. ♂

❧ Enzymatic Therapy LIQUID LIVER w. SIBERIAN GINSENG. ♀

❧ **Pantothenic acid 500-2000mg daily. with B Complex 100mg and Tyrosine 500mg daily.** ♀

❧ American Biologics SUB-ADRENE, 5 drops daily.

❧ Ascorbate vitamin C 3000mg or Ester C 1500mg daily.

❧ High potency digestive enzymes, like Rainbow Light ADVANCED ENZYME SYSTEM, or Prevail VITASE to stimulate adrenal cortex production. ♂

❧ CoQ₁₀ 30mg 3x daily as an enzyme therapy antioxidant.

❧ Nutricology GERMANIUM 150mg.

Lifestyle Support Therapy

Take the Adrenal Self Test in the DIAGNOSTICS SECTION of this book for a quick look at your personal adrenal health.

☙ Massage therapy is effective in improving adrenal function. Most therapists use muscle testing to determine the degree and indications of the dysfunction and then work to clear the adrenal pathways.

☙ **Reflexology point:**

adrenals

☙ Moderate exercise, such as a daily walk benefits adrenal health.

☙ **The adrenals:**

adrenals
kidneys

See DIET FOR HYPOGLYCEMIA in this book for more specifics.

Common *Symptoms*: Lack of energy and alertness; a sense of being "driven" and anxious, followed by great fatigue, weakness and lethargy; poor memory, low blood pressure and poor circulation; moodiness and irritability; sugar dysfunctions (hypoglycemia and diabetes); low immunity; brittle nails, dry skin; food cravings, especially for sugar.

Common *Causes*: Continuing stress; extensive use of cortico-steroid drugs for arthritis, asthma, allergies, etc.; pituitary disease or T.B.; poor diet with too much sugar and refined carbohydrates; over use of alcohol and nicotine, or recreational drugs; too much caffeine; vitamin B and C deficiencies, especially during menopause years.

Adrenal Failure Syndrome

Adrenal insufficiency is suffered by tens of millions of Americans. Its incidence is rising every year largely due to worsening nutritional deficiencies from an over-processed food diet and chronic mental and emotional strain. The adrenal glands are the primary organs for fighting stress. They are responsible for warding off the ill effects of every conceivable mental and/or physical stressor. Emotional strain causes significant disruption of adrenal function. Anger is perhaps the most devastating stressor. Researchers have discovered that its negative effects on adrenal function are profound. Virtually all people with adrenal insufficiency also suffer from severe allergic tendencies, because the adrenals are the primary means for preventing or reversing allergic reactions. Adrenal failure is associated with hypoglycemia, too, because the adrenals exert potent control over blood sugar status. Their job is to prevent blood sugar levels from dropping suddenly as a result of stress. Generally, all individuals with weakened adrenal glands suffer from the symptoms of blood sugar imbalance syndromes like diabetes and hypoglycemia.

The adrenal glands are normally golf-ball size. As a result of poor nutrition and/or stress, they may become significantly enlarged - a condition known as cellular hypertrophy, in which the cells within the adrenal glands multiply excessively in an attempt to supply the body with the additional steroid hormones demanded to handle stress. The adrenals are painful when pressed if this is the case, and the heels are usually cracked and extremely dry.

A wide range of nutrients are required for adrenal steroid syn-hesis to proceed normally, so poor nutrition compromises this process. The nutrients include essential fatty acids (evening primrose oil 500mg is a good choice), amino acids, B vitamins (especially pantothenic acid 500-1000 mg daily or royal jelly as the richest food source), vitamin E, vitamin A, vitamin C with bioflavonoids, (Ester C is a good choice), zinc, selenium, potassium, manganese, chromium, and magnesium. Stress-reducing techniques along with improved nutrition usually result in regenerating exhausted adrenals, and a return to normal function, but if the stresses remain unabated and the nutritional deficits are neglected, the adrenal glands ultimately self-destruct and shrink, a condition known medically as atrophy of the adrenal cortex.

Addison's Disease

If adrenal atrophy becomes extreme, it may result in a potentially life-threatening condition called Addison's disease, where there is continual, severe adrenal exhaustion, and the adrenal glands are totally incapable of producing steroid hormones. Individuals suffering with this condition are unable to cope with stress of any kind. Even insignificant stresses can precipitate a noticeable decline in health. Addison's can be a lifelong disease. Seventy-five percent of cases are auto-immune related; approximately one in four Americans are affected. It is characterized by black freckles on the head and shoulders, unhealthy, anorexic weight loss, nausea, dehydra-ion due to vomiting and diarrhea, low blood sugar (hypoglycemia), and great apathy. There is usually abnormally dark brownish pigmentation of the skin, particularly on the knees, elbows, scars, skinfolds and palms. The hair darkens, and dark striations appear on the nails. Body hair decreases. Circulation is reduced, blood pressure is low and the person always feels cold. An acute state of Addison's may be life-threatening and begin as sudden loss of strength, severe abdominal pain, and kidney failure.

- A good diet is critical in overcoming Addison's disease. Alcohol, caffeine, tobacco, and highly processed foods must be avoided.
- Take Enzymatic Therapy ADRENAL CORTEX concentrate, with PITUITARY concentrate to stimulate and balance ACTH output.
- Take Lewis Labs brewer's yeast, 2TBS. daily, or brewer's yeast tablets, with extra B Complex 100mg and pantothenic acid 1000mg.
- Take royal jelly, 60,000 to 100,000mg or more, 2x daily; YS ORGANIC ROYAL JELLY with GINSENG is an excellent choice.
- Take licorice extract or Crystal Star GINSENG/LICORICE ELIXIR™, under the tongue or in water, 2x daily.

Cushing's Syndrome

A rare, dysfunctional disease caused by an overactive adrenal cortex, Cushing's syndrome is an opportunistic condition, allowed by immune suppression, and sometimes brought on by overdose of cortico-steroid drugs, (particularly those used for rheumatoid arthritis). It is also a metabolic disease that causes the formation of kidney stones. It is characterized by obesity in the stomach, face and buttocks, but severe thinness in the limbs. There is muscle wasting and weakness, poor wound healing, thinning of the skin leading to stretch marks and bruising. Peptic ulcers, high blood pressure, mental instability, and diabetes also accompany Cushing's. The face may get acne-like sores and the eyelids are often swollen. Cushing's appears in women five times more than men; there is scalp balding, yet excess body and facial hair (hirsutism), brittle bones, along with a wide variety of menstrual disorders.

Because of its rarity, our experience has been limited with this disease. The following protocols have been found helpful:

- A vegetarian diet should be followed, low in fat, sodium ard sugar. Add high potassium foods daily.
- Add green drinks, such as chlorella with germanium, and protein for healing or Crystal Star ENERGY GREEN™ drink regularly.
- Take potassium in large doses - particularly herbal potassiun drinks, such as Future Biotics VITAL K, 2 teasp. daily, or Crystal Star IODINE/POTASSIUM SOURCE™ capsules.
- Melatonin appears to be helpful; take 1 to 3 mg at bedtime for 1 to 3 months.

AIDS & HIV Infection

AIDS and related syndromes are the result of immune system breakdown, caused by HIV (human immunodeficiency virus). The body becomes unable to defend itself against infection. HIV is a retro-virus meaning it can affect DNA and T-cells. Infection occurs in stages: an asymptomatic state (when the disease is most often passed), an acute mononucleosis-like stage, a state with one or more AIDS-related complexes, and "full blown" AIDS. The protocols here are for people who have been diagnosed with HIV, but are asymptomatic; for people who have decided to reject orthodox AIDS treatment in favor of alternative methods, and for people who have tried orthodox medical treatment, but showed no improvement and decided to take charge of their own health with alternative techniques. If you decide to use a combination of orthodox and alternative treatments, be quite careful...ask a knowledgeable naturopath. Mixing natural products with the powerful drugs used for AIDS can be dangerous.

Diet & Superfood Therapy

Compromised nutrition is bound to immune dysfunction. Diet improvement is the primary step to preventing HIV infection from becoming full-blown AIDS.

There is a great deal of toxicity, fatigue and malabsorption in AIDS and related conditions. A liquid fast is therefore not recommended - it is too harsh for an already weakened system.

➥The diet should, however, have the highest possible nutrition. Intestinal chemistry and pH environment must be changed to optimize disease protection. A modified macrobiotic diet is ideal for high resistance and immune strength.

➥See recommendations for a beginning diet on page 211.

Take 3 glasses fresh carrot juice daily, and a potassium broth (pg. 167) every day for ongoing detoxification.
A good juicer is really necessary.

Other diet watchwords:
➥All produce should be fresh and organically grown when possible.
➥Eat plenty of foods with anti-parasitic enzymes: cranberries, pineapple, papaya.
➥No fried foods of any kind. Avoid concentrated sweeteners, and highly processed foods of all kinds.
➥Flush the body with 6 to 8 glasses of mild herb teas and bottled water daily. Add $1/2$ teasp. ascorbate vitamin C to each daily drink for optimum results.

Herbal Therapy

Plant anti-virals and antioxidants have been among the most effective treatments against HIV. The following herbs should be part of your initial program.

Concentrated aloe vera juice, like AloeLife ALOE GOLD, 2 to 4 TBS. daily to curb virus spread, with garlic extract caps 8 daily, and turmeric to inhibit TNF.

Nutricology CAR-T-CELL shark cartilage vials, 15ml under the tongue.

Crystal Star DETOX™ caps, ANTI-VI™ extract, GREEN TEA CLEANSER™, with LIV-ALIVE™ caps or extract, and ADR-ACTIVE™ caps.
➥HEARTSEASE/ANEMI-GIZE™ for stronger blood, and ANTI-BIO™ gel for KS lesions.

Effective anti-viral herbs:
➥Una da gato solution
➥St. John's wort extract proven effective against retro-viruses.

Effective immuno-modulators:
➥Siberian ginseng extract or Health Aid America SIBERGEN, with Enzymatic Therapy THYMU-PLEX caps.
➥Astragalus extract or capsules.
➥Reishi mushroom capsules.
➥**Maitake mushroom extract.**

Effective superfoods:
➥Sun CHLORELLA.
➥Crystal Star SYSTEMS STRENGTH™.
➥YS GINSENG/ROYAL JELLY drink.
➥Solgar WHEY TO GO.

Supplements

Supplementation is recommended at all stages of healing to improve intestinal environment, strengthen immunity and increase tissue oxygen.

Purifying supplements:
➥**Egg yolk lecithin. Active lipids help make cell walls virally resistant.**
➥American Biologics DIOXYCHLOR.
➥Enzymatic Therapy LIVA-TOX caps.

➥Vitamin C powder with bioflavonoids, 10-30g daily, injection or orally; and 300,000IU mixed carotenes to stimulate T-cell activity.

Rebuilding supplements:
➥NAC (N-acetyl-cysteine) as directed.
➥Carnitine 500mg 2x daily.
➥Co-enzyme B complex SL.
➥Natra-Bio THYMUS EXTRACT.

Effective anti-oxidants:
➥Nutricology germanium 150-200mg daily for interferon production.
➥CoQ_{10} 300mg daily.
➥Quercetin with bromelain 500mg 3x daily.
➥ **Bromelain for enzyme therapy** 1500mg daily.
➥OPCs from grape seed and white pine 100mg 4 daily.
➥Glutathione 50mg daily.

Effective enzymes:
➥Solgar SOD INDUCERS.
➥Natren BIFIDO FACTORS, highest potency acidophilus powder, 3 teasp. daily with biotin 1000mcg.

Lifestyle Support Therapy

It is absolutely necessary to detoxify the liver for holistic healing to be effective. See LIVER CLEANSING in this book.

Lifestyle practices to avoid HIV:
➥Practice safe sex.
➥Avoid anal intercourse.
➥Avoid needle-injected and all pleasure drugs.
➥Make sure any blood transfusion plasma has been tested for HIV virus.

Detoxification bodywork:
Remove infected feces from the intestinal tract. Take both a colonic and an enema implant with aloe vera, wheat grass or spirulina once a week until recovery is well underway.

Get fresh air and sunlight on the body every day. Get mild exercise daily, and plenty of rest. Do deep breathing exercises morning and evening, especially when recovering from pneumocystis.

Overheating therapy helps kill the virus. See pgs. 29 and 178 in this book.

Reflexology point:

liver

Is There Hope If You Are HIV "Positive?"

Testing "anti-body positive" does not mean that one **has** AIDS, only that one has been **exposed** to the HIV virus. Being HIV "positive" does not even mean that you will **develop** AIDS. It is a warning, not a sentence. Some research attests that only 60% of people diagnosed as HIV positive develop full-blown AIDS. Even more encouraging, the face of AIDS has changed dramatically just within the last half of 1996. New protease inhibitors from the medical world, coupled with a healthy diet, elimination of recreational drugs and responsible sexual behavior are presaging modifications in HIV status unheard of even a year ago. HIV positive people are recognizing that the destructive lifestyle factors leading to their diagnosis can be changed to prevent further re-infection, and that they can greatly improve their condition by choosing healthy lifestyle behavior and natural therapies that can help keep them symptom free.

What Does It Take To Survive AIDS?

You can co-exist with HIV and lead a normal life. Today there are hundreds of long term AIDS survivors who are free of HIV symptoms. In **every case that we know of,** the survivor consciously decided to take charge of his or her own life and healing. All energies were channeled into the therapies that the survivors thought were correct for themselves. They faced reality, acknowledged that there was no silver bullet, realized that the process would be long and hard, and that the battle would take a great deal of courage. Almost universally, AIDS survivors believe that they grew a great deal in their humanity, compassion and maturity by taking responsibility for such an enormous task. They also felt that they gained great strength, confidence and control of their lives - and indeed, have become the kind of person they always wanted to be.

A phenomenon of AIDS survival is the intense desire to reach out to other sufferers to share the experience through encouragement and hope. Here are some survival watchwords:
1] You cannot think or behave like a victim - you must fight for your life. There is no invariably fatal diagnosis - no mortal can decide when or if someone will die. **Expect favorable results for courageous lifestyle steps.** 2] You must take charge of your own healing. Educate yourself about alternative approaches and treatment - lifestyle therapy must be part of recovery. **Destructive life patterns must be stopped.** 3] Seek life re-inforcing, healing modalities. Avoid stress, learn to laugh, engage in some form of physical exercise, eliminate harmful drugs and alcohol; reduce red meat and sugar. 4] Seek the healing power of God and of Love. You are not alone - seek people and relationships that support your great effort. Have no fear of death - **look forward to your life.**

AIDS Risks & Symptoms You May Not Know

• It is relatively easy to transfer HIV virus through anal intercourse, more difficult through vaginal or oral sex. Enzymes in the saliva, friendly flora in the intestinal tract, and HCl in the stomach produce a hostile environment that destroys the virulence of HIV. There is no such protection in the colon. Suppression of the immune system is believed to occur when the HIV virus slips through the intestinal wall and into the bloodstream. Normal immune response is to attack the virus with macrophages that then die and are removed through the lymphatic system. These toxic wastes are finally dumped into the colon on its last leg of clearance from the body, but in an unprotected colon without friendly bacteria or good defensive pH environment, new HIV viruses hatch from the dead macrophages and multiply in the feces all over again, repeating the same cycle. The immune system cannot detect the virus in the colon and does not marshal its forces until the infection is in the bloodstream; often too late if immune defenses are exhausted.

• **HIV never stands alone as the only culprit in the AIDS connection. Immuno-suppression comes _before_ HIV. Syphilis is usually present in AIDS victims, as are parasites and other viruses that set the stage for AIDS and related conditions.** Parasites are also, many times, a co-factor in HIV development. If you are frequently diagnosed with a bacterial infection and treated with antibiotics that dont help, have your stool tested for parasites. If your lifestyle is immuno-suppressing, parasites can easily take hold, and they are becoming an epidemic in the U.S.

• You can continually re-infect yourself! The most destructive immune-suppressing lifestyle elements are continual exposure to HIV and other STDs through sexual excess and multiple sex partners, and excessive use of chemicals, drugs and alcohol.

• Hepatitis predisposes a person to AIDS, because the liver is so weakened it cannot play its part in resisting infection.

• Environmental factors, such as water, air and soil pollution are now full of chemicals that affect delicate immune balance. You must consciously make healthy choices for yourself.

• Symptoms can appear anywhere from 6 months to 3 years after infection. If you feel you are at risk, here are the early symptoms: swollen glands and lymph nodes in the neck area, armpits and groin; inability to heal even minor ailments like a small cut, bruise or cold; unusual fatigue; white patches in the mouth and trouble swallowing (thrush), nail ringworm fungus.

• Continuing symptoms mean that AIDS is undeniable: purplish blotches that look like hard bruises occurring on or under the skin, inside the mouth, nose, eyelids or rectum that do not go away (Kaposi's Sarcoma); swollen glands that never go away; persistent dry, hacking cough (unrelated to smoking) that doesn't go away; fevers and night sweats that last for days or weeks; severe, unexplained fatigue; persistent diarrhea; unexplained, rapid weight loss; visual disturbances; personality changes; memory loss, confusion and depression.

Addressing AIDS Related Syndromes

An HIV-weakened immune system is susceptible to "opportunistic" diseases that accompany AIDS and play a major role in the body's susceptibility to it. It eventually becomes overwhelmed by them. Many of these side-effect syndromes can be addressed with natural, lifestyle therapies.

❧ **PNEUMOCYSTIS CARINII (PCP)** - a rare form of pneumonia that develops with AIDS, is the leading cause of AIDS-related death, affecting over 70% of all AIDS cases. It is thought to be caused by a parasite. Natural protocols for PCP include: black carrot extract, (an anti-viral, anti-fungal and anti-bacterial with immune stimulating properties, 30 drops 4x daily, available from naturopaths that treat HIV), and/or colloidal silver as directed; Crystal Star SYSTEMS STRENGTH™ broth every morning until improvement; Matrix Health OXY-CAPS as directed and GENESIS OXY SPRAY rubbed on the feet morning and evening; Nutricology germanium 150mg daily for interferon production; Crystal Star ALRG-HST™ extract to ventilate the lungs and stimulate the liver to produce anti-histamines; Enzymatic Therapy MEGA-ZYME and LIVA-TOX to stimulate the pancreas to attack foreign protein in the blood; Enzymatic Therapy LIQUID LIVER and MILK THISTLE SEED extract to strengthen the liver; a potassium broth (page 167) with 2 to 4 drops Crystal Star IODINE THERAPY™ extract to increase cell metabolism; Ester C with minerals and bioflavonoids 5000mg for collagen production and healing of infected tissue; Natren BIFIDO FACTORS powder (rinse mouth 3x daily); Solaray quercetin with bromelain (QBC PLEX) 4x daily; YS ROYAL JELLY/GINSENG drink as a prime source of pantothenic acid; Aloe Life ALOE GOLD drink to rebuild immunity. *Note: vegetables in your diet should be lightly steamed rather than eaten raw, because the protozoan parasite thought to cause pneumocystis lives in the soil and is destroyed by heat.*

❧ **KAPOSI'S SARCOMA** - usually considered as being benign skin tumors, but when they accompany AIDS drugs, KS becomes a serious connective tissue cancer. (When the drugs are stopped, the lesions regress.) EBV and Cytomegalovirus are also involved. Natural protocols for KS include: Curcumin (turmeric) herbal combinations to inhibit tumor necrosis factor; Crystal Star ANTI-BIO™ gel with una da gato and ginseng *and* DETOX™ capsules; Nutricology CAR-T-CELL shark cartilage liquid vials, 15ml daily; astragalus extract; CoQ_{10} 300mg daily; PCOs from white pine or grape seed oil to restore interleukin 100mg 3x daily; AloeLife SKIN GEL applied directly to lesions; black carrot extract (see a clinical naturopath); maitake mushroom extract to increase production of macrophages and T-cells; Enzymatic Therapy ADRENAL CORTEX COMPLEX; Nutribiotic GRAPEFRUIT SEED EXTRACT and SKIN SPRAY as a healing antibiotic. A daily potassium broth (page 167) and Green Foods BETA CARROT are important for healing, along with the modified macrobiotic diet on the next page.

❧ **EPSTEIN-BARR VIRUS (EBV)** - a chronic fatigue disease of the herpes family, and a cause of mononucleosis. EBV lives and hides in the B-cells of your immune system, producing a variety of anti-bodies that react against your tissue cells and result in autoimmune disease. Symptoms are swollen lymph nodes, fevers, chills, severe fatigue, chronic sore throat, usually pneumonia. Natural protocols for HIV-related Epstein Barr include: black carrot extract and/or Crystal Star ANTI-VI™ extract to kill the virus; American Biologics DIOXYCHLOR; Natren BIFIDO FACTORS as a source of all-important micro-flora; AloeLife ALOE GOLD juice every morning; ashwagandha extract and Crystal Star ZINC SOURCE™ extract to strengthen immune response and counter infections and fever, Crystal Star ECHINACEA/PAU d'ARCO extract (see a clinical naturopath); and GINSENG/LICORICE ELIXIR™ to mobilize anti-bodies; Matrix Health OXY-CAPS and Crystal Star LIV-ALIVE™ caps with GENESIS OXY SPRAY rubbed on the feet twice daily; Crystal Star ENERGY GREEN™ drink to rebuild immune strength; Enzymatic LIQUID LIVER, or Crystal Star LIV-ALIVE™ caps with MILK THISTLE SEED extract *and* GINSENG/REISHI extract for 3 to 6 months; Enzymatic Therapy LYMPHO-CLEAR for lymph node swelling, and ADRENAL CORTEX COMPLEX.

❧ **WASTING SYNDROME** - malabsorption characterized by severe, unhealthy weight loss can be addressed with superfoods. Normalizing body fluid levels, calories and protein is critical to fighting infections and inflammation. In addition, many drugs for AIDS leach valuable nutrients from already weak bodies, making superfoods such as Nature's Life SUPER GREEN PRO-96 or Crystal Star SYSTEMS STRENGTH™ drink, or Solgar WHEY TO GO protein drink even more important. Natural protocols for HIV-related wasting syndrome include: Probiologics C-CAL/MAG for malabsorption, food allergies, healing of gastric membranes and leaky gut, and detoxifying lymph glands **(take with food)**; Chinese bitter melon to inhibit the virus and treat the gastrointestinal infection; Crystal Star GINSENG/LICORICE ELIXIR™ for digestion, sugar balance, and to inhibit virus replication; BeWell juice drinks provide quickly absorbable, complete carotenes to delay progression of wasting disease. Diet should concentrate on metabolic care, with large amounts of vegetable juices (especially potassium broth (page 167), yogurt, kefir and kefir cheese, and high sulphur foods like garlic and onions. Eat complex carbohydrate-containing foods first, protein foods last, and plenty of high fiber foods. Avoid absolutely: caffeine, (drink herbal teas), all pork and other fatty meats, enzyme-inhibiting foods like soy products and peanuts, table salt and sugary foods.

❧ **CYTOMEGALOVIRUS (CMV)** - a salivary, herpes-type virus, associated with Epstein Barr infection, CMV produces fever, low white blood cell count and fungal infections of the gastro-intestinal tract. Natural protocols for HIV-related Cytomegalovirus include: nettles extract; ashwagandha extract; Matrix Health GENESIS OXY-SPRAY rubbed on the feet twice daily; Enzymatic Therapy MEGA-ZYME to digest foreign proteins and PHYTO-BIOTIC 816 formula for parasitic infestation; acupuncture treatments with accompanying shiitake and maitake mushroom and astragalus extracts (or ASTRA-8 Chinese herb compound) to strengthen the body's major organs; Crystal Star MIGR-EASE™ extract with feverfew to reduce severe headaches; Enzymatic Therapy ADRENAL CORTEX COMPLEX; black carrot extract (from a clinical naturopath) or Crystal Star ANTI-VI™ extract with MILK THISTLE SEED extract.

❧ **HERPES SIMPLEX VIRUS** - AIDS-related herpes is activated and aggravated by UV sunlight; antioxidants have been shown to protect against this. See HERPES SIMPLEX page in this book.

The Holistic Approach to Overcoming HIV Infection and AIDS

Holistic therapies are showing more promise than ever for AIDS, and its related immune deficiency diseases. Alternative treatments have been enormous factors in showing that HIV infection and AIDS are no longer inevitably fatal as they once were. In fact, holistic programs are the key to causing symptoms to abate, in some cases even to gradually disappear. The advance of the virus itself has been slowed in many instances, and the quality of life has improved in some full-blown AIDS cases. As more people with these diseases see their own progress, return to work, and pick up their lives, more expertise is coming into the field via holistic physicians, homeopaths, naturopaths, chiropractors, therapists, nutritional counselors and others.

The following protocol is a well-received holistic therapy program that has achieved measureable success with AIDS and its attendant conditions. Doses are generally quite high in the beginning. They may be reduced as improvement is observed. Treatments may be used together or separately as desired by each individual, along with the recommendations of a competent professional who has personal case knowledge. Note: In almost every case, allergies and malabsorption should be addressed before alternative HIV treatment can succesfully begin. A good naturopath can help.

✿ DETOXIFICATION PROTOCOLS:
•Biogenetics BIOGUARD w. SOD, American Biologics DIOXYCHLOR, Enzymatic Therapy LIVA-TOX, or Crystal Star LIV-ALIVE™ caps with GREEN TEA CLEANSER™ for enzyme therapy.
•Ascorbate vitamin C crystals - use calcium ascorbate, or a mixed mineral ascorbate with bioflavonoids; to flush and detoxify the tissues. Take orally 10-20 teasp. daily for 2 to 3 weeks, then reduce to 10 grams twice a week. Mega-doses may be resumed as necessary. Intravenous dose, 100-150 grams daily for 2-3 weeks, reducing to 30 grams every week for maintenance.
•Detoxify with a weekly colonic to clean out toxic wastes from the colon. A colonic stimulates and normalizes organ, gland function and mental balance as well. Follow with a sauna.

✿ DIET:
•Change body pH with micro-flora - an acidophilus complex with bifidus, like Natren BIFIDO FACTORS, 3 teasp. daily. May apply acidophilus topically, too.
•Fresh vegetable juices - a good juicer is critical to potency. Take a potassium juice (page 167) twice daily with garlic extract and flax oil added. Chew DGL tablets to neutralize acids.
•Egg lipids from egg yolk lecithin - highest potency, such as Jarrow Corp., or Source Naturals EGGS ACT liquid.
•Drink plenty of distilled water every day.

✿ PHYTOBIOTIC HERBAL THERAPY:
•St. John's wort extract or Crystal Star ANTI-VI™ EXTRACT (50% St. John's Wort/50% Lomatium) and ANTI-BIO™ with echinacea, goldenseal and myrrh; and EVENING PRIMROSE oil.
•Aged aloe vera juice, 2-3 glasses daily, to found to block the virus spread, and to reduce herpes lesions. Take with black carrot extract 30 drops 4x daily to fight infection.
•Essiac tea 3x daily, Flora FLOR-ESSENCE extract, or Crystal Star CANSSIAC™ extract solution with panax ginseng.
•An immune system booster, with herbs like pau d'arco, echinacea root, astragalus, suma, Siberian ginseng, reishi mushrooms, schizandra berries, ligustrum, chaparral, goldenseal and garlic, to stimulate production of interferon, interleukin and lymphocytes; or 4-6 cups daily of the following immune restorative tea: prince ginseng roots, dry shiitake mushrooms and soaking water, echinacea angustifolia root, schizandra berries, astragalus, ma huang, pau d'arco bark, St. John's wort. Steep 30 minutes. (See Crystal Star GINSENG SUPER SIX™ TEA.)

✿ SUPERFOOD THERAPY:
•Propolis extract with Wakunaga KYO-Green garlic extract, or YS ROYAL JELLY/GINSENG drink.
•Sun CHLORELLA - 15-20 tablets or 2 packets of granules daily, or Green Foods GREEN ESSENCE or BETA CARROT.
•Solgar WHEY TO GO protein drink, OR Nature's Life SUPER GREEN PRO 96.
•Crystal Star ENERGY GREEN™ or SYSTEMS STRENGTH™ drinks.

✿ ANTIOXIDANT & ENZYME THERAPY:
•American Biologics SHARKILAGE 740mg - 1 cap for every 12 pounds of body weight for 3 weeks before meals then 4-6 caps daily - increases leukocytes and white blood cell activity.
•Carnitine - 500mg daily for 3 days. Rest for 7 days, then 1000mg for 3 days. Rest for 7 days. Take with high omega 3 flax oils, 3 to 6x daily, or evening primrose oil 500mg 3x daily.
•Germanium - highest potency 200mg. 6x daily, or 150mg sublingually, 4x daily, with astragalus capsules, 4 daily.
•CoQ₁₀ 300mg daily, Pycnogenol or grape seed PCOs, 50mg 4x daily, DMG sublingual (di-methyl-glycine), Glutathione 50mg 2x daily to overcome the side effects and nerve damage from AZT, and to strengthen white blood cell and T-cell activity. Take with Solaray QUERCETIN PLUS with bromelain 500mg 3x daily for respiratory improvement, and digestive enzymes, such as Enzymatic Therapy MEGA-ZYME with pancreatin.
•NAC - a stable form of L-cysteine that helps deactivate HIV, with glutathione 50mg 2x daily.
•Raw thymus and raw adrenal extracts - 1 tablet 3x daily or ¹/₂ dropperful 2 x daily.
•The body produces H₂O₂ naturally as part of its immune defenses. Change the cell environment with Bio-oxidation therapy (catalytic H₂O₂ with shark cartilage) by injection, (with a qualified practitioner only), or rub Matrix GENESIS OXY-SPRAY on the feet morning and evening. Alternate H₂O₂ use, 4 days on and one week off for best results.

✿ BODYWORK THERAPY:
•Overheating therapy - effective for inhibiting growth of the invading virus. Hydrotherapy - effective in re-stimulating circulation. Take a sauna or overheating bath. (see page 178.)
•Use implant-enemas with either supergreen foods such as chlorella or spirulina, or micro-flora, or Enzymatic Therapy PHYTO-BIOTIC HERBAL FORMULA.

Diet Defense Against HIV and AIDS

A high resistance, immune-building diet is primary to success in overcoming AIDS and related conditions. The intestinal environment must be changed to create a hostile site for the pathogenic bacteria (a protocol also effective against candida albicans and some types of cancer). The following liquid and fresh foods diet is for the ill person who needs drastic measures - a great deal of concentrated defense strength in a short time. It represents the first "crash course" stage of the change from cooked to living foods. It has been extremely helpful in keeping an HIV positive person free of symptoms, and in symptom recession during full-blown AIDS. Optimal diet improvement also helps prevent other attendant diseases associated with immune deficiency. The space in this book only allows for a "jump start" form of this diet. The complete program with supporting recipes, may be found in "COOKING FOR HEALTHY HEALING" by Linda Rector Page. See also the BLOOD CLEANSING DIET FOR IMMUNE DEFICIENT DISEASES in this book (pg. 164).

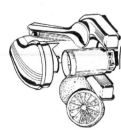

The suggested step-by-step program below is a modified, enhanced macrobiotic diet, emphasizing more fresh than cooked foods, and mixing in acidophilus powder with foods that **are** cooked to convert them to living nourishment with friendly flora. As with other immune-depressing viral diseases, pathogenic HIV bacteria live on dead and waste matter. For several months at least, the diet should be vegetarian, low in dairy, yeasted breads and saturated fats. Meats, fried foods, dairy products except yogurt and kefir, coffee, alcohol, salty, sugary foods, and all refined foods must be eliminated. Of course, all recreational drugs should be eliminated, as well as unnecessary prescription drugs. The ultra purity of this diet controls the multiple allergies and sensitivities that occur in the auto-immune state, yet still supplies the needs of a body that is suffering primary nutrient deprivation. For most people, this way of eating is a radical change, with major limitations, but the health improvement against HIV is excellent.

On rising: take 3 TBS. cranberry concentrate in 8-oz. of water with ¹/₂ teasp. ascorbate vitamin C crystals with bioflavonoids and ¹/₂ teasp. Natren BIFIDO FACTORS; or a Solgar WHEY TO GO protein drink.
    Take a brisk walk for exercise and morning sunlight.

Breakfast: have a glass of fresh carrot juice with 1 teasp. Bragg's LIQUID AMINOS, and whole grain muffins or rice cakes with kefir cheese; or a cup of plain yogurt blended with a cup of fresh fruit, sesame seeds, walnuts, or oatmeal, amaranth or buckwheat pancakes with yogurt and fresh fruit; and ¹/₂ teasp. Natren BIFIDO FACTORS or Alta Health CANGEST powder mixed in 8-oz. of aloe vera juice such as AloeLife ALOE GOLD.

Midmorning: take a weekly colonic. On non-colonic days, take a potassium broth or essence (page 167), with 1 TB. Bragg's LIQUID AMINOS and ¹/₂ teasp. ascorbate vitamin C crystals with bioflavonoids added; and have another fresh carrot juice, or pau d'arco tea, with ¹/₂ teasp. Natren BIFIDO FACTORS added.

Lunch: have a fresh green salad with lemon/flax oil dressing, with plenty of avocado, nuts, seeds and alfalfa sprouts; or an open-faced sandwich on rice cakes, or a chapati with fresh veggies and kefir cheese; or a cup of miso soup with rice noodles or brown rice, and some steamed veggies and tofu with millet or brown rice; and take a cup of pau d'arco tea or aloe vera juice with ¹/₂ teasp. ascorbate vit. C, and ¹/₂ teasp. Natren BIFIDO FACTORS added.

Midafternoon: have another carrot juice with Bragg's LIQUID AMINOS and ¹/₂ teasp. Natren BIFIDO FACTORS added; and a green drink such as Sun CHLORELLA, Green Foods GREEN ESSENCE, or Crystal Star ENERGY GREEN™, with ¹/₂ teasp. ascorbate vitamin C crystals and bioflavonoids added.

Dinner: have a baked potato with Bragg's LIQUID AMINOS, low-fat cheese or kefir cheese and a green salad, and black bean or lentil soup with ¹/₂ teasp. Natren BIFIDO FACTORS added; or a fresh spinach or artichoke pasta with steamed veggies and lemon/flax oil dressing; or a Chinese steam stir-fry with shiitake mushrooms, brown rice and vegetables. Sprinkle ¹/₂ teasp. Natren BIFIDO FACTORS or Alta Health CANGEST powder over any cooked food at this meal.

Before Bed: take a glass of aloe vera juice with ¹/₂ teasp ascorbate vit. C crystals and ¹/₂ teasp. Natren BIFIDO FACTORS; and a fresh carrot or papaya juice, or body chemistry balancing drink such as Crystal Star SYSTEMS STRENGTH™.

Note 1: Unsweetened mild herb teas and bottled water are recommended throughout the day for additional toxin cleansing and system alkalizing.
Note 2: For optimum results, add ¹/₂ teasp. ascorbate vitamin C powder with bioflavonoids to any drink throughout the day until the stool turns soupy.

The goal for overcoming HIV infection is staying strong. System strength greatly reduces the chances of succumbing to full-blown AIDS or to another infection. It allows you to survive while research for answers against the HIV virus goes on. In some cases, a strong person can develop resistance to the virus effects for many years.

Allergies

Multiple Chemical Sensitivities ✳ Environmental Illness ✳ Drug ✳ Contaminant Reactions

Multiple chemical sensitivities are multiplying. We're bombarded by chemical pollutants all our lives. More than 2¹/₂ billion pounds of pesticides are used in America every year! (300 million pounds in the home.) Repeated chemical exposures set off rampant free radical reactions, and our bodies react with an allergic response. Those making the news today, environmental illness, sick buildings, Gulf War syndrome, breast cancer, nerve damage, attention deficit disorder in children, latex and insecticide allergies, are just the latest in a growing list.

Diet & Superfood Therapy

❧ Go on a short 3 to 7 day liquid diet (pg. 157) to begin toxin release. Have one each daily:
  ✳a glass of fresh carrot juice
  ✳a potassium broth (pg.167)
  ✳**a cup of miso soup.**
  ✳Drink only bottled water.

❧ Then, eat organically grown foods as much as possible. Avoid canned foods. Avoid caffeine, which inhibits liver filtering function, and foods sprayed with colorants, waxes or ripening agents.
  ✳Eat legumes and sea vegetables to excrete lead.

❧ Have a bowl of high fiber cereal every morning. Eat plenty of fruits, veggies and whole grains for fiber protection. Sprinkle on brewer's yeast, toasted wheat germ and lecithin granules.

❧ **Effective superfoods:**
  ✳**Crystal Star ENERGY GREEN™** for detoxification and blood building.
  ✳Sun CHLORELLA or Green Foods GREEN MAGMA for detoxification.
  ✳Green Foods BETA CARROT blend.
  ✳**AloeLife ALOE GOLD juice.**
  ✳Solgar EARTH SOURCE GREENS & MORE drink.

Herbal Therapy

∨ **Jump start herbal program:**
  ✳**Detoxify the blood: Crystal Star DETOX™ caps with GREEN TEA CLEANSER™ or CLEANSING & PURIFYING™ TEA for 6 weeks.**
  ✳Support your liver: LIV-ALIVE™ tea or caps for 1 month to restore liver function. Then FIBER & HERBS COLON CLEANSE™ caps with MILK THISTLE SEED extract.
  ✳**Neutralize histamine reactions: ANTI-HIST™ caps and BITTERS & LEMON™ extract for enzyme therapy.**

∨ **Blood detoxification herbs:**
  ✳Garlic oil caps, 2-4 daily.
  ✳Dandelion/nettles caps, 6 daily.
  ✳Pau d'arco tea every 4 hours.

∨ **Herbal anti-inflammatories:**
  ✳**Crystal Star ANTI-FLAM™.**
  ✳**GRAPE-FRUIT SEED EXTRACT caps.**
  ✳**BILBERRY extract for quercetin.**

∨ **Neutralize allergens:**
  ✳Astragalus extract
  ✳Kelp 10 tabs daily, or Crystal Star IODINE THERAPY caps 4 daily.
  ✳Siberian ginseng extract caps.

Supplements

The right supplements can reinforce the body against chemical assault and help keep immune response intact.

✧ **Anti-oxidants are a key:**
  ✳Ascorbate vitamin C with bioflavonoids - 3-5000mg daily.
  ✳Vitamin E 400IU w/ selenium.
  ✳CoQ₁₀ 30mg 2x daily.
  ✳Beta/marine carotene 150,000IU.
  ✳Glutathione 50mg 3 daily.
  ✳Solgar SOD INDUCERS.
  ✳Golden Pride FORMULA ONE oral chelation with EDTA, 2 packets daily. ○

✧ A food grown multi-vitamin daily.
  Also:
  ✳B complex 100mg daily with extra B₆ 200mg and pantothenic acid daily.
  ✳Vitamin C 3000mg daily with bioflavonoids.
  ✳EVENING PRIMROSE or flax oil capsules, 500mg daily.

✧ **Glandulars reinforce the body at its deepest level:**
  ✳ **Enzymatic Therapy ADRENAL CORTEX COMPLEX and THYMU-PLEX caps as directed.**

✧ Biotec CELL GUARD, with S.O.D. and catalase, 6 daily. ○✛

Lifestyle Support Therapy

Use Coca's Pulse Test or muscle testing to identify allergens. (See page 445.)

☞ Acupuncture, chiropractic and massage therapy treatments seem to have the best results with chemical allergies.

☞ **You can take many steps to avoid contaminants in your life:**
  ✳Seek out trees. Plant them. Live around them. Trees produce oxygen and remove many pollutants from the air.
  ✳Avoid antacids; they interfere with enzyme production, and the ability of the body to carry off chemical residues.
  ✳Invest in an air filter.
  ✳Pay attention to unhealthy air alerts; stay indoors if you have chemical sensitivities. Don't exercise near freeways.
  ✳Avoid as much as possible: smoking and secondary smoke, pesticides and fungicides, phosphorus fertilizers, fluorescent lights, aluminum cookware and deodorants, electric blankets; microwave ovens, non-filtered computer screens.

☞ **Foot reflexology:**

liver

Common Symptoms: *Always feeling "low energy" and "under the weather" regardless of how much sleep one gets; abnormal metabolism; learning and behavior disabilities; skin rashes; chronic respiratory inflammation; ringing in the ears; nausea; diarrhea; headaches; low immune response.*

Common Causes: *Repeated exposure and sensitivity to toxic chemicals and environmental pollutants like auto exhaust; inherited tendency (affecting more women and children that men).*

See also CHEMICAL & CONTAMINANT POISONING in this book for more information.

Allergies

Seasonal Hayfever ❖ Allergic Rhinitis ❖ Respiratory Allergies

Respiratory allergies result from two main areas - environmental pollutants, such as asbestos and smoke fumes, and seasonal conditions, such as dust, pollen or spores. This type of allergic reaction often occurs when the body has an excess accumulation of mucous, which harbors environmental irritants. Common drugstore medications generally mask symptoms and also have a rebound effect - the more you use them, the more you need them. Steroid drugs for this type of allergy, if taken for long periods, do not cure, and often make the situation worse by depressing immune defenses, and impeding allergen elimination.

Diet & Superfood Therapy

Diet change and cleansing your internal environment is the single most beneficial thing you can do to control allergic rhinitis reactions.

☘ Begin with a short three to seven day cleansing diet (pg. 157) to get rid of excess mucous build-up, release allergens from the body, and pave the way for diet changes to have optimum effect.

❋Then start a diet with non-mucous-forming foods: fresh vegetables and fruits, whole grains, cultured foods like yogurt, high vitamin C foods like citrus and berries, and seafoods.

❋Drink more pure water to keep your system flushed.

❋Avoid refined, preserved and canned foods, sugary foods, caffeine, and fatty, mucous-forming foods during healing. This means dairy products.

☘ **Effective superfoods:**
❋Green drinks, like Nutri-Cology PRO GREENS or Crystal Star ENERGY GREEN™.
❋Crystal Star BIOFLAV., FIBER and C SUPPORT™ for absorbable C benefits.
❋YS ROYAL JELLY/GINSENG drink, a super source of pantothenic acid.
❋AloeLife FIBER-MATE as directed.

Herbal Therapy

☙ **Jump start herbal program:** Crystal Star ALRG™ and/or ANTI-HST™ caps, or ALRG-HST™ extract with ADR-ACTIVE™ caps as needed.
❋Then GINSENG/LICORICE ELIXIR™ or GINSENG/REISHI extract for 3 weeks, with RESPIR-TEA™, 2 cups daily.
and
❋Use Crystal Star ANTI-BIO™ caps as an anti-microbial and anti-inflammatory, or Zand DECONGEST HERBAL to control congestion.

☙ **Homeopathic remedies can help even acute attacks without side effects:**
❋Hyland's *HAYFEVER* tabs
❋BioForce *POLLINOSAN* tabs
❋BioForce *SINUSAN* tabs
❋Natra-Bio *BIO-ALLERS* oral homeopathic liquid, 3x daily. (When buying, specify for type of allergen.)
❋Similisan *EYE DROPS #1* and *NASAL SPRAY.*

☙ **Effective preventive herbs:**
❋Crystal Star ADR-ACTIVE™ extract.
❋Unsprayed bee pollen granules.
❋GINKGO BILOBA extract helps inactivate allergens.
  -❋EVENING PRIMROSE oil 4-6 daily.
  -❋Freeze-dried nettles caps.
  -❋Eyebright tea.

Supplements

If you are taking loratadine (Claritin) for allergies, it has been shown to cause liver tumors, including cancers.

❦ **Antioxidants are a key:**
❋**Quercetin 1000-2000mg daily with bromelain 500mg.**
❋**CoQ₁₀, 30mg 3x daily to reinforce defenses.**
❋Ascorbate Vitamin C or Ester C powder with bioflavonoids ¼-½ teasp. every 3 hours to flush and detoxify tissues; then reduce to 5000mg daily.
❋Nutricology GERMANIUM 150mg with B₁₂ SL 2500mcg daily.

❦ **Effective preventive supplements:**
❋B complex 100mg with extra pantothenic acid 500mg and B₆ 100mg 2x daily after meals, morning and evening. (Or use as a preventive measure before high risk seasons.)
❋Raw thymus and adrenal 3x daily.
❋Country Life ALLER-MAX CAPS with pycnogenol.
❋Enzymatic Therapy GARLINASE and THYMU-PLEX for immune support.
❋High potency royal jelly, 2 teasp. daily.

Lifestyle Support Therapy

Use Coca's Pulse Test or muscle testing to identify allergens. (See page 445.)

☙ Exercise is important to increase oxygen uptake. Take a daily walk with deep breathing exercises.

☙ Use relaxation techniques. Stress depresses immunity, aggravates allergies.
❋Acupuncture and chiropractic have both proven effective for allergies.

☙ Take 1tsp. fresh grated horseradish in a spoon with lemon juice. Hang over a sink to release great quantities of excess mucous fast.

☙ The obvious method of controlling allergy symptoms is to avoid allergens.
❋Stay indoors, esp. in the a.m. and exercise indoors on dry, windy days.
❋Invest in an air filter.

☙ Stop smoking and avoid secondary smoke. It magnifies allergies reactions.

☙ **Acupressure points:**
❋During an attack, press tip of nose hard as needed for relief.
❋Press hollow above the center of upper lip as needed.
❋Press underneath cheekbones beside nose, angling pressure upwards.

Common Symptoms: *Runny, watery, itchy nose and eyes; sneezing and coughing attacks; sore, irritated throat; chronic lung, bronchial and sinus infections; skin itching and rashes; asthma; frontal headaches; insomnia; menstrual disorders; hypoglycemia; learning disabilities.*

Common Causes: *Body sensitivity to pollen, spore, mold and other airborne allergens reacting with excess mucous and waste accumulation in the body; adrenal exhaustion; free radical damage lowering antihistamine levels and liver function; stress; hypoglycemia; candida albicans yeast overgrowth; EFA deficiency.*

For a complete diet to overcome allergies, see COOKING FOR HEALTHY HEALING by Linda Rector Page.

Allergies
Food Sensitivities & Intolerances

Food allergy - an antibody response to a certain food. Food intolerance - an enzyme deficiency to digest a certain food. This type of sensitivity is the fastest growing allergy group as people are more exposed to chemically altered, enzyme-depleted, processed foods. Without enzyme active foods, our bodies must assume all digestive responsibilities. This capacity eventually weakens, total food assimilation does not occur, and large amounts of undigested fats and proteins are left that the immune system treats as potentially toxic. It releases prostaglandins, leukotrienes, and histamines into the bloodstream to counteract the perceived threat, and allergy reactions occur. As the body's toxic burden increases it becomes increasingly less able to tolerate even small doses of an allergen.

Diet & Superfood Therapy

See "COOKING FOR HEALTHY HEALING" by Linda Rector Page for a complete diet program to overcome food allergies.

♠ Common allergy foods include wheat, dairy products, fruits, sugar, yeast, mushrooms, eggs, soy, coffee, corn and greens. Although some of these foods are healthy in themselves, they are often heavily sprayed, and in the case of animal products, secondarily affected by antibiotics and hormones.

♠ Go on a short 24 hour liquid diet (pg. 158) to clear the system of allergens. Then follow a diet emphasizing enzyme-rich fresh produce and grains.

—Take 2TBS. apple cider vinegar with honey at each meal to acidify saliva.
—Eat cultured foods, like yogurt to add friendly flora to the G.I. tract.
—Try a food rotation diet to eliminate suspected allergen foods, especially if Candida is involved.

♠ Effective superfoods:
—Crystal Star BIOFLAVONOID, FIBER & C SUPPORT™ drink daily to guard against leaky-gut syndrome.
—New Moon GINGER WONDER syrup to help block inflammation. ⊛
—Y.S ROYAL JELLY/GINSENG drink ♀

Herbal Therapy

♠ Jump start herbal program:
—Produce antihistamines: Crystal Star ANTI-HST™ caps or ALRG-HST™ extract.
—Reduce allergic reactions: GINSENG/REISHI extract.
—Cleanse the G.I. tract: Crystal Star BITTERS & LEMON CLEANSE™ extract or NatureWorks SWEDISH BITTERS with AFTER MEAL ENZ™ caps, for normalizing herbal enzymes.
—Take aloe vera juice, such as Aloe Falls ALOE GINGER JUICE.

♣ Omega-3 flax seed oil with meals for essential fatty acids (EFAs). ♀

♣ Herbal enzymes boost immunity and digestion:
—Dandelion root ♂
—Echinacea/golden seal root
—MILK THISTLE SEED

♣ Crystal Star CAND-EX™ capsules if the allergy is related to gluten foods. See also CANDIDA ALBICANS pages in this book - especially if there is unexplained weight gain from allergies.

♣ Herbs for adrenal support:
—Crystal Star FEM SUPPORT™ ♀
—Crystal Star GINSENG/LICORICE. ♂
—Siberian ginseng extract.

Supplements

✍ Quercetin Plus 400mg daily between meals with bromelain 500mg 3x daily for antioxidant activity and enzymes.

✍ Ester C up to 5000mg daily with bioflavonoids, and/or
—CoQ₁₀ 30mg 3x daily to help the liver produce antihistamines.

✍ A full spectrum digestive enzyme such as Rainbow Light DOUBLE STRENGTH ALL-ZYME or Alta Health CANGEST, or Prevail VITASE caps.
—or Source Naturals CO-ENZYMATE B with meals. ♀
—or Dr. DOPHILUS ¼ teasp. in liquid before meals. ⊛

✍ Liquid chlorophyll 1 teasp. 3x daily before meals. ♂

✍ For lactose intolerance:
—Lactaid drops or tablets.
—Nature's Plus SAY YES TO DAIRY.
—Country Life DAIRY-ZYME.
—NatraBio FOOD ALLERGY - DAIRY.
—Prevail DAIRY ENZYMES.

✍ For gluten intolerance:
—NatraBio FOOD ALLERGY - GRAIN.

Lifestyle Support Therapy

Use Coca's Pulse Test or muscle testing to identify allergens. (See page 445.)

☞ Food allergies are common in children; many childhood allergies are the result of feeding babies meats and pasteurized dairy foods before 10-12 months. Babies do not have the proper enzymes to digest these foods. Feed mother's milk, soy milk, or goat's milk for at least 8 months to avoid food allergies.

☞ Use a garlic/catnip enema to cleanse the digestive tract and balance colon pH.

☞ Reflexology point:

food assimilation

☞ One of the most insidious effects of food allergy is weight gain. Eliminate wheat from your diet to stop allergy-related weight gain.

See also FOOD POISONING page in this book for more information.

Common Symptoms: *The inability to eat normal amounts of a food; Crohn's disease; cyclical headaches; hypothyroidism; osteoarthritis; hypoglycemia; hyperactivity, irritability and flushing in children; excessively swollen stomach, gastrointestinal trouble; nausea or mental fuzziness after eating; palpitations, sweating, hives; puffiness around the eyes, unexplained obesity.*
Common Causes: *Eating chemically altered, sprayed, injected or processed foods that the body cannot handle; inherited food sensitivities; food additives such as nitrites, aspartame, MSG and sulfites; stress; fast-food diet; alkalosis with low gastric pH and enzyme deficiency; insufficient sleep; emotional trauma; chronic infections; a particular allergen food like gluten foods.*

Alzheimer's Disease

Senility ✳ Cerebral Atherosclerosis ✳ Loss of Memory ✳ Dementia

The growing number of people living into their 80's and 90's is evolving into a population of people who suffer from significant loss of memory, thought and language. Alzheimer's disease, a serious health problem, is now a common condition in the U.S. Many of those diagnosed are really victims of too many drugs, or have nutritional deficiencies that can be reversed. Although orthodox medicine has been unable to make a difference in this relentless disease, natural therapies have been successful in slowing the deterioration of brain function.

Diet & Superfood Therapy

A highly nutritious diet shows without question to be a deterrent to Alzheimer's onset.

✷ Excess meat protein and fat facilitate amyloid neurofiber tangle build-up. **Reduce them in your diet.** Alzheimer's has been linked to synthetic estrogens, such as those injected into certain red meats.

✷**Avoid red meats.** Eat organically grown foods (to avoid environmental estrogens as much as possible), with emphasis on brain foods like eggs, soy foods, sea vegetables, whole grains, seeds and fresh vegetables.

✷**The diet should be low in fats, salt, all meat, dairy with plenty of fiber.**

✷ Eat B vitamin foods, such as brown rice and other whole grains, brewer's yeast, molasses, liver, fish and wheat germ. (They block aluminum toxicity.)

✷ Eat tryptophan-rich foods, such as poultry, low-fat dairy products and avocados. There is almost always tryptophan deficiency in Alzheimer's disease.

✷ Make up a mix of lecithin granules, brewer's yeast, wheat germ oil, oat bran, flax oil and blackstrap molasses. Take 2 TBS. each morning with cereal or juice. ♀
✷Drink only bottled water.

Herbal Therapy

Phyto-hormones, especially from herbal sources like panax ginseng, may help memory retention in Alzheimer's.

☙ **Jump start herbal program:**
✷**Crystal Star MENTAL INNER ENERGY™ caps, and/or CREATIVI-TEA™** 2x daily; or GINSENG/REISHI extract.
✷ GINKGO BILOBA extract 2, 3x daily, and YS royal jelly 2-3 teasp. daily.
✷Crystal Star SILICA SOURCE™ extract in rosemary tea daily.

☙ **Herbal brain nutrients:**
-Solgar S.O.D. 2000units
-Ginseng/gotu kola caps 2 daily
-BILBERRY extract
-Dr. Chang's LONG LIFE TEA
-Wisdom of the Ancients tea
-EVENING PRIMROSE 500mg, 4 daily for needed EFAs.
-Siberian ginseng extract drops.
-Flora VEGE-SIL caps. ♀♂

☙ **Effective superfoods:**
✷Crystal Star SYSTEMS STRENGTH™ drink 3x weekly.
✷Green Foods WHEAT GERM extract.
✷Long Life IMPERIAL TONIC with royal jelly and evening primrose oil. ♀
-Y.S ROYAL JELLY/GINSENG drink. ♀

Supplements

Use pain killers and sleeping pills sparingly. They can leach acetyl-choline from brain tissues.

✑ **Phosphatidyl serine** 100mg 3x daily, for at least 3 months, or choline 650mg 3x daily for 3 to 6 months. **with**
✷CoQ$_{10}$, 60mg 2x daily.
✷OPCs 100mg daily.
✷Body Ammo DHEA as directed.
✷Source Naturals CO-ENZYMATE B$_{12}$ sublingual, and folic acid 400mcg. ♀

✑ Niacin therapy (flush free) 250-500mg. with
✷**Ethical Nutrients MAGNESIUM/ MALIC ACID.**
✷Ester C w/ bioflavonoids, up to 3000mg and Enzymatic Therapy THYMU-PLEX to improve T-cell count.

✑ **Amino acid therapy:**
✷**Lysine** 500-1000mg daily.
✷**L·Carnitine** 500mg or Twin Lab ACETYL CARNITINE.
✷Omega-3 flax oils 3x daily, pantothenic acid 1000mg, B$_6$ 100mg, and Floradix herbal iron for vit. B uptake.

✑ Chelation therapy is effective because it cleans up arterial pathways and detoxifies cells. Golden Pride FORMULA ONE. ♀

Lifestyle Support Therapy

Alzheimer's is aluminum related. Beware of fluoridated water. It increases absorption of aluminum from deodorants, pots and pans, etc. by over 600%.

✤ Get daily mild exercise and/or use hot and cold hydrotherapy for brain and circulation stimulation.

✤ Decrease prescription diuretics if possible. They leach potassium and nutrients needed by the brain.

✤ Avoid aluminum and alum containing products: cookware, deodorants, dandruff shampoos, anti-diarrhea compounds, canned foods, salt, buffered aspirin and analgesics, antacids, refined and fast foods, relishes, pickles, tobacco, etc. Read labels!

✤ **Reflexology brain pressure points:**
✷Squeeze all around the hand and fingers.
✷Pinch the end of each toe. Hold for 5 seconds.

✤ **Have silver amalgam dental fillings removed. They can cause mercury toxicity that releases into the brain, and affects brain health.**

Common Symptoms: *Loss of ability to think clearly or remember past or present facts, names, places, etc.; loss of touch with reality; confusion; impaired judgement; difficulty in completing thoughts or following directions; personality and behavioral change. In final stages, almost a return to infancy, communication is almost non-existent, feeding and elimination functions uncontrolled.*
Common Causes: *Poor or obstructed circulation; arteriosclerosis; anemia; decrease in hormones; lack of exercise, and body/brain oxygen; fluid accumulation in the brain; thyroid malfunction; aluminum toxicity; mercury toxicity from silver-amalgam dental fillings; inherited predisposition to mental illness; emotional shock and loss, such as the death of a spouse.*

A good sample diet would be the HYPOGLYCEMIA DIET in this book.

Anemia

Hemolytic * Iron-Deficiency * Folic Acid * Aplastic * Pernicious * Thalassemia * Sickle Cell

Hemolytic: vitamin B_{12} and/or folic acid deficiency causing red blood cells to be destroyed more quickly than they are replaced. *Iron-Deficiency:* a chronic condition caused by a lack of iron, or poor absorption of iron. *Thalassemia:* an inherited defect, usually affecting people of Mediterranean origin. *Sickle Cell:* an inherited abnormal hemoglobin defect among blacks. *Pernicious:* a heredity prone, auto-immune disease caused by a deficiency of vitamin B_{12}, affecting nerve and digestive systems; common among elderly people; *Folic acid:* caused by lack of folic acid. *Aplastic:* progessive bone marrow failure, generally caused by exposure to a chemical toxin.

Diet & Superfood Therapy

Good nutrition is a good remedy. Food and herbal iron sources are best for absorbability. Eat some fresh vegetables every day.

♨ Diet watchwords:

✻Eat iron-rich foods: liver, organ meats, figs, seafood, molasses, beets, brown rice, whole grains, poultry, eggs, grapes, raisins, yams, almonds, beans.

✻Eat manganese-rich foods, such as whole grains, greens, legumes, nuts, pineapples and eggs for iron uptake.

✻Eat cultured foods - yogurt, kefir, and soyfoods for friendly bacteria and B_{12}.

✻Eat potassium rich foods - broccoli, bananas, sunflower seeds, vegetables, whole grains, kiwi, dried fruits; or take a potassium broth with Bragg's LIQUID AMINOS until red blood count improves (pg. 167).

✻Eat vitamin C rich foods, such as citrus fruits, cruciferous vegetables, tomatoes and green pepper for iron absorption.

✻Avoid iron-depleting foods: sodas, caffeine, chocolate, red meat, cow's milk.

✻Mix brewer's yeast, molasses, wheat germ, sesame seeds, dry crushed sea veggies; take 2TBS. daily in food.

♨ Effective superfoods:

✻Nutricology PRO-GREENS.
✻Nature Care CHAWAN PRASH.
✻Beehive ROYAL JELLY/GINSENG.
✻Nature's Life SUPER GREEN PRO-96.

Herbal Therapy

♨ Jump start herbal program:

✻Crystal Star HEARTSEASE/ANEMI-GIZE™ capsules, and IRON SOURCE™ capsules or extract 3x daily until blood count improves.

or

✻ ENERGY GREEN™ drink daily, with POTASSIUM/IODINE™ caps, 2 daily, as a source of plant B_{12}.

and

✻AloeLife ALOE VERA JUICE to help stimulate bone marrow production and help digestion of protein.

✻ Planetary Form. TRIPHALA COMPLEX.

♨ Effective iron-enhancing teas:

✻Yellow dock
✻Pau d'arco
✻Red raspberry leaf
✻Dandelion root and leaf

♨ Effective iron-enhancing capsules:

✻Beet root
✻Spirulina/bee pollen, 6 daily. ♂
✻Kelp (especially during pregnancy). ♀

♨ Effective iron-enhancing extracts:

✻Siberian ginseng ♂
✻DONG QUAI/DAMIANA
✻Ginseng Co. CYCLONE CIDER
✻Solaray ALFA-JUICE caps. ♀

Supplements

❧ Nature's Bounty internasal gel B_{12}, or Solaray 2000mcg B_{12}.
✻Betaine HCL or American Biologics MANGANESE at meals for best uptake.
✻Multi-vitamin/mineral complex with copper, zinc and biotin.

❧ B Complex 100mg with extra pantothenic acid, B_6 100mg and biotin.

❧ **Absorbable iron supplements:**
✻Enzymatic Therapy LIQUID LIVER w. SIBERIAN GINSENG 2x daily. ♂
✻Nature's Secret ULTIMATE IRON. ☺
✻Floradix liquid iron 2x daily.
✻KAL folic acid w/ B_{12} and zinc 50mg to regain menstrual periods. ♀

❧ Take an iron supplement with digestive enzymes like Rainbow Light ADVANCED ENZYME SYSTEM, and an antioxidant, like germanium or vitamin C.

❧ **Sickle-cell anemia:** folic acid 800mcg, vitamin B_6 100mg 2x daily, zinc 50mg daily, and vitamin E 400IU 2x daily.

❧ **Thalassemia:** vitamin E 800IU with CoQ_{10} 30mg 3x daily.

❧ **Folic acid anemia:** Sun CHLORELLA 15-20 tabs daily and folic acid with iron.

Lifestyle Support Therapy

❧ Get some mild exercise daily to enhance oxygen uptake. Get morning sunlight every day possible for vitamin D.

❧ Avoid pesticides, sprays and fluorescent lighting that cause mineral leaching from the body.

❧ Poor food combining accounts for an amazing amount of iron deficiency. See the FOOD COMBINING CHART on page 452.

Common Symptoms: Overall weakness; dizziness and fainting; heart palpitations; shortness of breath; lack of libido; gastro-intestinal bleeding; ulcers; slow healing; fatigue; skin pallor; violent mood swings; irritability; spots before the eyes. *Secondary signs:* vision problems; apathy, brittle nails, poor appetite, hair loss, yellowish skin, headaches, dark urine, poor memory.
Common Causes: Recurring infections and diseases indicating low immunity and mineral deficiency; B_{12} and folic acid deficiency; pregnancy effect; rapid growth in childhood; poor diet or poor food assimilation; blood loss from an ulcer; parasites; excessive menstruation; lack of green vegetables; alcoholism.

Anxiety
Panic Disorder ✦ Phobias

Over 25 million Americans have suffered from an anxiety disorder at some time during their lives. It's more than just tension before a stressful confrontation, a public speech or an airline flight. It's long term, constant, debilitating anxiety so great that a person loses all reason and reality - that's a panic attack. Continued economic insecurity can generate this kind of fear, for instance. Anxiety and phobias (fear taken to extremes) are more than just frightening. They are closely tied to high blood pressure, heart spasms and fatal heart disease.

Diet & Superfood Therapy

Anxiety and prolonged stress in general, deplete the body of nutrients necessary to produce its own natural tranquilizers.

❧ **Diet watchwords:**
❋Eat simple, calming, comfort foods during the day to prevent a panic attack...brown rice, mashed potatoes, creamy yogurt, oatmeal, steamed vegetables, etc. Consider goat's milk instead of cow's milk.

❋Avoid caffeine, sugar, refined foods, fast foods, preserved foods (especially meats), salty foods and alcohol.

❧ **Eat:**
❋**Foods rich in calcium** for both stress and immune response: sesame seeds, almonds, soy foods, low fat dairy products, and dark, leafy greens.

❋**Foods rich in magnesium** to protect the nerves: kelp, wheat germ and bran, most nuts, soy foods.

❋**Foods rich in B vitamins** to support the adrenals and fuel the nerves: nutritional yeast, whole grains and brans, nuts, beans.

❋**Foods rich in vitamin C** for more active stress response: hot and sweet peppers, greens, broccoli, kiwi, acerola cherries. ❧

❧ **Effective superfoods:**
❋Crystal Star SYSTEMS STRENGTH™.
❋Organic Gourmet NUTRITIONAL YEAST or MISO broth before bed.
❋Green Foods BETA CARROT.

Herbal Therapy

❧ **Jump start herbal program:**
❋Crystal Star FEM SUPPORT™ extract with RELAX CAPS™. ♀♂
❋STRESSED OUT™ extract with ADR-ACTIVE™ caps for adrenal support. ♂
or
❋Kava kava or ashwagandha extract, like Enzymatic Therapy KAVA-TROL, and Swedish Institute AMANA. ♀♂
or
❋Bach Flowers RESCUE REMEDY.

❧ **Effective aromatherapy:**
❋Lavender oil
❋Chamomile oil or Rose oil
❋Apples and cinnamon
❋Sandalwood oil
❋Ylang Ylang oil

❧ Effective anxiety relief nervines:
❋Scullcap or passionflower extract
❋**Hawthorn for heart palpitations.**
❋St. John's wort extract
❋Valerian, or Crystal Star VALERIAN/WILD LETTUCE extract. ☺
❋Gotu Kola ♀

❧ **Tonic adaptogens:**
❋GINSENG/LICORICE ELIXIR™. ♂
❋DONG QUAI/DAMIANA extract. ♀
❋Crystal Star MENTAL INNER ENERGY™ with kava kava and panax ginseng.

Supplements

Avoid drugs of all kinds, even depression drugs like Prozac. Besides their unhappy side effects, they change your body chemistry, making you more at risk for a panic attack, and abnormal behavior.

Hypnotherapy has been extremely successful for panic attacks and anxiety.

◈ **Effective anti-stress supplements:**
❋**GABA 750-1000mg daily and as needed during an attack, to mimic valium effects without sedation.**
❋**5-Hydroxy-Tryptophan 50-100mg.** ◈ Enzymatic Therapy RELAX-O-ZYME, and BIO-K+ with magnesium.
❋Cal/Mag/Zinc, 4 at night.
❋L-Tyrosine 500mg a.m./p.m., between meals.

◈ B Complex 100mg, with extra B₆ 50mg, niacinimide 500mg, thiamine 500mg and taurine 500mg, 3x daily.

◈ **Effective homeopathic remedies:**
❋**Enzymatic Therapy ANTI-ANXIETY.**
❋Ignatia

◈ Phosphatidyl choline 1000mg 3x daily.

◈ Vitamin C 3000mg daily with bioflavonoids.

Lifestyle Support Therapy

☞ Most panic attacks, no matter what the cause, take place in the early hours of the morning, about 3 to 5 o'clock.

Here are some suggestions to put the 5 a.m. willys into perspective:
❋Get out of bed, turn on a TV show, take a shower; see the sun rising, and life going on. Get dressed and walk outside.

❋Stretch, get a little mild exercise, or walk your dog. There is a body chemical basis for fear, released in hormone secretions. Exercise oxygenates the body, replacing that function.

❋Think positive. Review a recent success, remind yourself of your talents and abilities, and all the advantages of your life.

❋You are not alone, no matter what situation you find yourself in or what mistakes you have made.

❋Don't let outside worries make you violent toward those you love, or against yourself, for instance, through a heart attack.

❋No matter what it is, it will pass.

☞ Relaxation techniques like a quiet bath, a massage therapy treatment, shiatsu, meditation or biofeedback can do wonders.

❋Deep breathing exercises are a natural tranquilizer: 1) exhale with a whoosh. 2) inhale through your nose slowly. 3) hold your breath for a count of six. 4) exhale with a whoosh. Repeat four more times.

See also DEPRESSION page in this book for more information.

Common Symptoms: "nerves" type attacks; ulcer or colitis attacks; irritability; high blood pressure; head and neck aches; loss of appetite; dizziness.
Common Causes: anxiety is the result of emotional and physical stress encountered in daily life - relationship difficulties, financial problems, job demands, traffic jams and our increasingly crowded and noisy environment. Fear is at the heart of all panic disorders.

Appendicitis
Chronic

Appendicitis is an inflammation of the appendix, a small 2 inch tube opening into the beginning of the large intestine. It is usually caused by blockage from a small, hard lump of fecal matter, which itself results from a fiber-deficient diet. The blockage stops the natural flow of fluids, unfriendly bacteria swarm in and inflamation and infection result. The suggestions on this page are for chronic, recurring appendicitis. Perforation and rupture of the organ is a major medical emergency, and you need emergency treatment. DON'T DELAY!

Diet & Superfood Therapy

♉ Go on a short vegetable juice diet (pg. 157) to clear and clean the intestine. Take one potassium drink (pg. 167) daily during this fast.

↝ Then, eat sweet fruits for a day to encourage healing.

↝ Then, resume a mild foods, simply cooked diet, and include a glass of carrot juice daily for 2 weeks.

♉ Make sure the diet is high in soluble fiber to help prevent attacks.

♉ Avoid refined and fried foods on a continuing basis.

♉ **Take no solid food or laxatives during an appendicitis flare-up.** ♉

♉ **Effective superfoods:**
 ↝**Crystal Star SYSTEMS STRENGTH™ drink for alkalinity and better food absorption.**
 ↝Crystal Star CHO-LO FIBER TONE™ drink to provide soluble fiber, or AloeLife FIBERMATE.
 ↝Nutricology PROGREENS.
 ↝Green Foods BETA CARROT.

Herbal Therapy

Chronic or grumbling appendicitis can be treated herbally with some success. Any hint of complications or deterioration of the condition must be taken seriously. Get to an emergency room.

↯ **Jump start: herbal program: Crystal Star ANTI-BIO™ capsules or extract every 2 hours to reduce infection.** ↝ANTI-FLAM™ extract to reduce inflammation.
 ↝CRAMPBARK COMBO HERBS™ extract to help reduce spasms.

↯ **ECHINACEA extract 4x daily after an attack for a month after an attack to keep the lymph glands flushed.**

↯ Make up the following formula as a strong tea, and sip as needed: 2 parts agrimony, 2 parts echinacea root, 1 part chamomile flowers, and 1 part wild yam root.
 or
 equal parts agrimony and calendula tea.

↯ Solaray TETRA CLEANSE or ALFA-JUICE capsules, or Yerba Prima COLON CARE SYSTEM after an attack for 6 days to clean the colon of infection.

Supplements

Take liquid supplements as much as possible to make it easier on your system.

↜ **Beta carotene 25,000IU 4x daily, with Liquid chlorophyll in water 3x daily.**

↜ Prof. Nutrition Dr. DOPHILUS lactobacillus powder ¹/₄ teasp. in water 4x daily.
 or
 Natren LIFE START powder for gentle, friendly bacteria and enhanced peristalsis. ⊛

↜ **Ester C or ascorbate vitamin C crystals ¹/₄ teasp. in water 4x daily.**

↜ Vitamin E 400IU 2x daily.

↜ Living Source STRESS MANAGEMENT COMPLEX multivitamin daily.
 and
 Rainbow Light ADVANCED ENZYME SYSTEM tablets at meals.

↜ Zinc picolinate 30mg daily.

Lifestyle Support Therapy

☙ Do not take high colonics or enemas during an attack.

☙ Keep the colon clean. Constipation is usually the cause of an attack. Use a mild catnip enema. ⊛

☙ **Use alternating hot and cold cayenne/ ginger compresses on affected area and along spine.**

☙ **Reflexology point:**

appendix

☙ Position of appendix in the body:

<u>The Appendix</u>

Large Intestine
Small Intestine
Appendix

Common Symptoms: *Early symptoms include colicky, central abdominal pain followed by nausea and vomiting; then pain shifting to the right lower abdomen as the inflammation spreads; intense, recurring sharp pain on the lower right side at the waist.*

Common Causes: *Poor diet, lacking in fiber and roughage; too many antibiotics; too many laxatives resulting in lack of peristalsis and friendly bowel flora; toxic build-up causing depressed immune response.*

Arteriosclerosis ❖ Atherosclerosis

Clogging & Hardening of the Arteries

Both arteriosclerosis and atherosclerosis block the flow of blood from the arteries to the heart, and damage the circulatory system. Atherosclerotic plaque is largely composed of cholesterol. It begins under the inner wall of the artery suggesting that a vitamin B_6 deficiency and a diet high in animal fats is the cause rather than cholesterol as previously thought. Arteriosclerosic plaque is the build-up of calcium on the inside of the artery walls. Both conditions are not only preventable, but reversable. Love and affection, both given and taken, really reduces heart and arterial problems.

Diet & Superfood Therapy

Follow the HEALTHY HEART DIET in this book. As a rule, vegetarians have healthier hearts and arteries.

❧ **Reduce dietary cholesterol.** Avoid saturated fat-containing foods, like red meats, full-fat dairy products, fried foods and refined, low fiber foods.

❧ Eat plenty of high fiber, whole grains, in the form of cereals, rather than bread or pasta, and lots of fresh greens.

✱Eat antioxidant-rich vegetables like broccoli, fresh fruits and greens. The risk of stroke from clogged arteries decreases by over 35% **for each increase of 3 fruit or vegetable servings per day.**

✱Take one cup daily of the following mix: 2 tsp. wheat germ, 2 tsp. honey, 1 TB. lecithin, in 1 cup fenugreek tea.

❧ Eat smaller meals, especially at night. Have a little wine at dinner; wine has an enzyme that breaks up blood clots.

✱Reduce coffee to 1 cup daily. ♂

❧ **Effective superfoods:**
✱**Nature's Secret ULTIMATE FIBER.**
✱Crystal Star CHO-LO FIBER TONE™, low cholesterol means clearer arteries.
✱Aloe Falls ALOE VERA GINGER JUICE, 1 8-oz. glass daily. ♂

Herbal Therapy

❧ **Jump start herbal program:**
Crystal Star HEARTSEASE/HAW-THORN™ capsules, and/or HEART-SEASE CIRCU-CLEANSE TEA™, a blood purifying tea with butcher's broom.
and
✱Flora VEGESIL as directed.

❧ **GINKGO BILOBA** extract to boost circulation and relieve claudication.
with
✱Sun CHLORELLA tabs 15-20 tabs or 1 packet daily, ♂
✱Solaray ALFAJUICE capsules. ♀

❧ Ginseng Co. CYCLONE CIDER liquid drops, or ginseng/cayenne caps daily.

❧ High omega-3 flax oil, 3 x daily, or EVENING PRIMROSE OIL caps, 4-6 daily for 1 month, then 3-4 daily.

❧ Butcher's broom or astragalus tea for a limited time to increase circulation.

Supplements

❧ **Golden Pride FORMULA ONE oral chelation therapy with EDTA.** ♂
✱Or, Enzymatic Therapy ORAL NUTRIENT CHELATES as directed, and CO-ENZYMATE B Complex with Carnitine 500mg daily. ♀

❧ **Niacin 500mg 2x daily with pancreatin 1400mg daily as a fat digestant.**

❧ Essential Life MULTI-NUTRIENT COMPLEX with copper, zinc and biotin.

❧ Phosphatidyl choline 1000mg daily. **with**
✱Chromium picolinate 2 daily to prevent plaque build-up.
✱Vitamin E 400IU w. selenium daily to relieve intermittant claudication.

❧ **Vitamin B₆ 50mg, 400mcg folic acid and 2000mcg B₁₂ with Betaine HCL, 3x daily to lower homocysteine levels.**

w **Effective anti-oxidants:**
✱PCOs from grape seed or white pine 100mg daily.
✱CoQ₁₀ 30mg 3x daily, or Sun Force CoQ₁₀ in flax oil.
✱**Zinc picolinate 30mg, daily.**
✱ **Ester C 3-5000mg daily with bioflavonoids and rutin.**

Lifestyle Support Therapy

❧ Stop smoking. Keep your weight down. Relax. The stress and tension from stressful life styles can cause big artery problems.

❧ Take a brisk walk daily. Aerobic exercise helps raise HDL levels. Then use a dry skin brush over the body to stimulate circulation.

✱Take an alternating hot and cold shower to increase blood circulation.

❧ **For arteriosclerotic retinopathy:** reduce fats, especially saturated fats from meats in your diet. Reduce sugar intake to help normalize blood sugar balance. Take garlic capsules daily to help normalize blood pressure levels.

Common Symptoms: *Poor circulation with cold hands and feet, and leg cramps; mild heart attacks; mental and respiratory deterioration; blurred vision; high blood pressure; sometimes impotence.*
Common Causes: *High risk factors include smoking, high cholesterol, high blood pressure, diabetes, too much saturated fat and refined food in the diet; vitamin B_6 deficiency; being overweight; stress; lack of aerobic exercise; too much caffeine and alcohol; excess salt.*

See also HEART DISEASE pages in this book for more information.

Arthritis

Connective Tissue Diseases

Arthritis is the country's number one crippling disease, affecting over 40 million Americans - 80% of the people over 50. It is not a simple disease in any form, affecting not only the bones and joints, but also the blood vessels, kidneys, skin, eyes and brain. Because its causes are rooted in lifestyle habits and wear-and-tear effects, conventional medicine has not been able to address arthritis with even a small degree of success. Natural therapies, based in lifestyle changes, however, do work extremely well, addressing the causes of arthritis while reducing pain and discomfort.

Diet & Superfood Therapy

Diet change is the single most beneficial thing you can do to control any kind of arthritis. A good, alkalizing diet can prevent or neutralize arthritis even in longstanding cases. See pages 158 & 159 for 2 brief cleansing/control diets.

❧ **Foods to add to your diet:** artichokes, cherries, cabbages, basic cereal grains, such as rice, oats and corn, cold water fish, fresh fruits, vegetables, leafy greens, garlic, onions, olive oil, sweet potatoes, squashes, eggs and parsley.

❧ **Foods to avoid:** refined foods, saturated fatty foods from meat and dairy products, wheat pastries and other high gluten foods that are also high in sugar, cholesterol and fat. Nightshade family foods such as peppers, eggplant, tomatoes and potatoes; mustard, salty foods, caffeine, colas, chocolate and highly spiced foods.

❧ **Arthritis V-8 Special: add to a bottle of** Knudsen's VERY VEGGIE JUICE, 4 TBS *each:* wheat germ, lecithin granules and brewer's yeast flakes. Take 8-oz. twice daily.

❧ **Effective superfoods:**
✒Crystal Star ENERGY GREEN™ drink and ZINC SOURCE™ drops. (If you take cortisone for arthritis, you are deficient in zinc.)
✒Sun CHLORELLA packets or tabs.
✒Wakunaga KYO-GREEN - take with glucosamine sulfate for 1 month. When symptoms are gone, continue with KYO-GREEN for 1 to 3 months.
✒Aloe Life ALOE GOLD drink.
✒Solgar WHEY TO GO™ protein.

Herbal Therapy

❧ **Jump start herbal program:**
Crystal Star AR EASE™ caps and/or tea, or GREEN TEA CLEANSER™, and 4 each LIV-ALIVE™ and ADR-ACTIVE™ caps daily with EVENING PRIMROSE OIL 1000mg 2 daily.
and apply
✒ANTI-FLO™gel with una da gato.
✒PRO-EST EASY CHANGE™ roll-on with GINKGO BILOBA extract daily to increase healthy circulation. ♀

❧ **Herbal anti-inflammatories:**
✒**Ginger 4 daily**
✒**Turmeric 4 daily**
✒**Ayurvedic Boswellin creme**
✒**Crystal Star ANTI-FLAM™ caps**
✒**Cayenne/ginger compresses**

❧ Solaray ALFA-JUICE caps, or liquid chlorophyll to help stimulate the body's own cortisone.

❧ **Effective ocean healers:**
✒Crystal Star HOT SEAWEED BATH™. ♀
✒Green-lipped mussel caps to reduce inflammation. ♂

✒Sea cucumber caps 1500-2000mg for 2 months to reduce inflammation.
✒**American Biologics SHARKILAGE.**

❧ **Effective desert healers:**
✒Alfalfa 10 daily, to alkalize the body
✒Yucca extract
✒Jojoba extract
✒Aloe vera gel and juice
✒Devil's claw root.

Supplements

❧ **Two supplement keys should be included in every arthritis program:**
✒**Quercetin Plus w/Bromelain, 2 daily to reduce swelling/inflammation.**
✒**Enzymatic Therapy GS COMPLEX or AR-MAX as directed, with THYMULUS to modulate the immune system.**

❧ **Adrenal therapy sources:**
✒YS royal jelly/ginseng 2 tsp. daily.
✒Enzymatic Therapy ADRENAL CORTEX COMPLEX as directed. ♀
✒American Biologocs SUB-ADRENE 3-5 drops 3x daily. ♀

❧ **Effective antioxidants:**
✒CoQ₁₀ 60mg 2x daily, with Carnitine 500mg 2x daily.
✒Grapeseed or white pine PCOs 50mg. 3x daily.
✒Ester C 500mg with bioflavonoids, up to 10 daily for collagen synthesis.

❧ **Effective anti-inflammatories:**
✒Country Life LIGA-TEND as needed; with B Complex 100mg daily. ♀
✒Am. Biologics INFLAZYME FORTE for pain and stiffness.
✒Prevail MOBILE. ♂
✒DLPA 750mg, or GABA as needed.
✒Omega-3 FLAX OIL 3x daily. Expect pain diminishment in 2 to 4 months.

❧ CAL/MAG CITRATE w. boron and vitamin D for uptake, and niacinimide to dilate blood vessels. ♀

Lifestyle Support Therapy

Note: High doses of aspirin, NSAIDS and cortisone for arthritic pain can hamper your body's ability to maintain bone strength.

☞ Avoid tobacco smoke. Tobacco is a nightshade plant. Note: The analgesic Motrin is also a nightshade derivative. It is an anti-inflammatory, but should not be used by nightshade-sensitive people.

☞ Massage therapy, hot and cold hydrotherapy, epsom salts baths, (see page 176), chiropractic treatments and overheating therapy (see page 178) are all effective.

☞ Apply Matrix Health GENESIS OXY-GEL to affected areas every 24 hours. Or take an arthritis elimination sweat (pg. 447).

☞ Use Crystal Star ALKALIZING ENZYME™ herbal wrap as directed.

☞ **Effective local applications:**
✒Transitions PRO-GEST cream. ♀
✒B & T TRIFLORA gel.
✒**Biochemics PAIN RELIEF lotion.**
✒**Aloe vera gel, a source of germanium.**
✒DMSO on clean skin as directed.
✒Bioforce ARNICA LOTION.

☞ To relieve pain, press the highest spot of the muscle between thumb and index finger. Press in the webbing between the two fingers, closer toward the bone that attaches to the index finger. Press into the web muscle, angling the pressure toward the bone of the index finger. Press for 10 seconds at a time.

See COOKING FOR HEALTHY HEALING by Linda Rector Page for a complete diet with recipes.

A 237

The Different Faces Of Arthritis

The term arthritis, meaning joint inflammation, refers to over 100 rheumatic diseases that attack joints and connective tissue. Over 40 million Americans are afflicted by one or more of these crippling rheumatic conditions. Other degenerative joint diseases include gout, lupus erythematosus, ankylosing spondylitis (arthritic spine), psoriatic arthritis (skin and nail arthritis), infective arthritis (bacterial joint infection) and rheumatism. Specific natural therapies for the most common types are offered on this page. See also the previous page for general help for arthritic problems.

❧OSTEOARTHRITIS, degenerative joint disease, is the most common form of arthritis. It most often appears in the weight-bearing joints like the knees, hips and spine, and in the hands, where there is much cartilage destruction followed by hardening and the formation of large bone spurs on the joints. The first signs of osteoarthritis show up as morning stiffness especially in damp weather, then pain in motion that worsens with prolonged activity. Osteoarthritis is a condition of age, (we see it in the creaking and cracking of joints on movement), because decades of use lead to degenerative changes in joints, and the decreasing ability of the body to repair itself. Although osteoarthritis affects more women than men, a man who is more than 20 pounds overweight doubles his risk of knee and hip arthritis. Repair ability can be greatly increased with body chemistry improvement. Food allergies almost always contribute to osteoarthritis symptoms, so a good body detox followed by a diet with plenty of fresh vegetables is the first place to start. (See next page.)

Standard drug therapy with aspirin or NSAIDS drugs like MOTRIN suppress pain and inflammation, but may actually promote the progression of the disease by damaging cartilage and inhibiting the ability of the body to maintain and repair normal collagen structures. Today, we know that osteoarthritis is repairable. Numerous studies have shown that **glucosamine sulfate (NAG)**, a natural body substance that stimulates the production of cartilage components works even better than NSAIDS drugs. The dose is 500mg 3x daily.

In addition to the general recommendations on the previous page, natural therapies specific to osteoarthritis include: cherries to take the bumps out of the knuckles by helping the body to eliminate acids; take with a mild herbal diuretic such as Crystal Star TINKLE CAPS™ to flush out released material. Crystal Star PRO-EST OSTEO-PLUS™ roll-on gel with wild yam, and FEM-SUPPORT™ with ashwagandha for women; Ayurvedic BOSWELLIA with zinc 50mg for men. Bitters herbs to stimulate bile and better digestion are important, such as BITTERS & LEMON CLEANSE™ extract and vitamin E with selenium 400IU daily. New: Biochemics PAIN RELEAF.
❧

❧RHEUMATOID ARTHRITIS affects more than 6 million Americans, the vast majority of them women. RA is a chronic, auto-immune, inflammatory disease whose primary target is the joint lining synovial membrane. When this connective membrane becomes inflamed, it invades and damages nearby bone and cartilage, resulting in pain, stiffness, loss of movement, and eventually destruction of multiple joints. Damage goes even further, because RA also causes inflammation of the blood vessels and the outer lining of the heart and lungs. Most RA sufferers also have digestive problems, great fatigue, anemia, ulcerative colitis, chronic lung and bronchial congestion, and liver malfunction. Common causes include calcium depletion, gland and hormone imbalance - especially adrenal exhaustion, prolonged use of aspirin or cortico-steroid drugs, that eventually impair the body's own healing powers; poor diet, lacking in fresh vegetables, and high in acid and mucous-forming foods; food allergens; auto-toxemia from constipation; inability to relax; resentments and a negative attitude toward life that lock up the body's healing ability.

In addition to the general recommendations on the previous page, some specific natural therapies for rheumatoid arthritis include Vita Carte BOVINE TRACHEAL CARTILAGE, Rainbow Light ADVANCED ENZYME SYSTEM full-strength pancreatic enzymes, PCOs from grape seed oil, CAPSAICIN and Tiger Balm rub-on cremes, hot sulphur and mud baths at your favorite spa, ginger caps, and bromelain 1500mg.

EVENING PRIMROSE OIL 500mg 4 to 6 daily, Nutricology PRO-GREENS drink with flax oil,
7

❧RHEUMATISM, rheumatism myalgia - an acidic condition, characterized by pain, muscle stiffness, and tenderness in soft-tissue structures, where excess acid settles in the joints causing pain and inflammation, and inhibits the production of natural cortisone in the body. (Cortisone feeds your adrenals and helps your body metabolize proteins.) Improve your body chemistry to relieve rheumatism.

Start with a sage cleansing tea, such as Crystal Star CLEANSING & PURIFYING™ tea. Add a glass of cider vinegar and water each morning. Then build your diet around low acid foods and foods that help to absorb acid, such as potatoes, turnips, green beans and root vegetables like carrots. Low acid fruits like white grape juice and apples can help to stimulate digestion. Alfalfa has a long tradition of success for rheumatism - eat alfalfa sprouts often, take alfalfa tablets or Solaray ALFA-JUICE caps, or Crystal Star ENERGY GREEN™ drink with alfalfa daily. Anti-rheumatics such as Enzymatic Therapy AR-MAX or Crystal Star AR-EASE™, anti-inflammatories, such as Enzymatic Therapy GS-Complex or Crystal Star ANTI-FLAM™ work for rheumatism. A long term musculo-skeletal support herbal formula might be Crystal Star SYSTEMS STRENGTH™, along with circulatory stimulants, such as cayenne/ginger capsules and Capsaicin rub on cream. A mild diuretic like Crystal Star TINKLE CAPS™ is helpful in removing rheumatism pain. Since muscle tension is often at the core of rheumatic aches, Crystal Star RELAX CAPS™ or ANTI-SPZ™ formulas are also recommended. Topical rub-on cremes for inflammation relief include wintergreen oil and PRD PAIN-FREE lotion.
❧

❧GOUT - a metabolic disorder that results in pain in the hands, knees and toe joints, sometimes produces arthritis as its primary symptom. Barley grass juice is a specific for gout. See GOUT in this book for more information.

Note: Dr. Donsbach's spa and clinic for arthritis comes highly recommended. You can investigate further. Call 1-800-359-6547. ❧

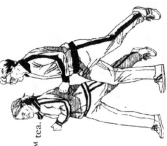

The following brief diet programs for arthritis may be used for several weeks to help detoxify the body and flush out inorganic mineral deposits. Small and subtle dietary changes are not successful in reversing arthritic conditions. Vigorous diet therapy is necessary. For permanent results, the diet must be changed to non-mucous and non-sediment-forming foods. See COOKING FOR HEALTHY HEALING, by Linda Rector Page for complete information and recipes.

Begin Your Arthritis Control Program With A Cleansing Diet

FOR 2 TO 3 DAYS:

On rising: take a glass of lemon juice and water; or a glass of fresh grapefruit juice. (Acidic foods like citrus fruits engender the production of enzymes that help alkalize the body.)

Breakfast: take a glass of potassium broth or essence (pg. 167); or a glass of carrot/ beet/cucumber juice.

Mid-morning: have apple or black cherry juice; or a green drink, such as Sun CHLORELLA, Green Foods GREEN ESSENCE, a drink from page 168, or Crystal Star ENERGY GREEN™ drink.

Lunch: have a cup of miso soup with sea veggies snipped on top, and a glass of fresh carrot juice.

Mid-afternoon: have another green drink, or Crystal Star GREEN TEA CLEANSER™; or an herb tea like alfalfa/mint, or Crystal Star CLEANSING & PURIFYING™ tea.

Dinner: have a glass of cranberry/apple, or papaya juice, or another glass of black cherry juice.

Before bed: take a glass of celery juice, or a cup of Organic Gourmet SAVORY SPREAD yeast extract broth; or a cup of miso soup.

Keep Arthritis Away With A Fresh Foods Diet

FOR 3 TO 4 WEEKS:

On rising: take a glass of lemon juice and water, or grapefruit juice; or a glass of apple cider vinegar in water with honey.

Breakfast: have a glass of cranberry, grape or papaya juice, or Crystal Star BIOFLAVONOID, FIBER & C SUPPORT™ drink; and fresh fruits like cherries, bananas, oranges and strawberries; and take 2 teasp. daily of the following mix. Two TBS. each: sunflower seeds, lecithin granules, brewer's yeast, wheat germ. Mix into yogurt, or sprinkle on fresh fruit or greens.

Mid-morning: take a glass of potassium drink (page 167); or a tea such as Crystal Star GREEN TEA CLEANSER™, or Green Foods BETA CARROT with 1 tsp. Bragg's LIQUID AMINOS added.

Lunch: have a large dark green leafy salad with lemon/oil dressing; and/or a hot veggie broth or onion soup; and/or some marinated tofu or tempeh in tamari sauce.

Mid-afternoon: have a cup of miso soup with sea veggies snipped on top; or a green drink, alfalfa/mint tea, or Crystal Star CLEANSING & PURIFYING™ tea.

Dinner: have a Chinese greens salad with sesame or poppy seed dressing; or a large dinner salad with soy cheese, nuts, tamari dressing, and a cup of black bean or miso soup; or some steamed vegetables and brown rice for absorbable B vitamins.

Before bed: have a cranberry or apple juice, or black cherry juice; or a cup of Organic Gourmet NUTRITIONAL YEAST or MISO extract broth; and/or celery juice.
Note: Make sure you are drinking 6 to 8 glasses of bottled mineral water daily to keep inorganic wastes releasing quickly from the body.

SUPPLEMENTS FOR THE FRESH FOODS DIET: As the body starts to rebuild with a stronger, more alkaline system, supplements may be added to speed this process along.
- Ascorbate Vitamin C powder and bioflavonoids in juice ($\frac{1}{4}$ teasp. four times daily) for interstitial tissue and collagen development.
- Omega-3 flax oil 3 teasp. daily. Add Rainbow Light ADVANCED ENZYME SYSTEM or Alta Health CANGEST for assimilation, and alfalfa tabs 6 to 10 daily to help alkalize the system.
- Crystal Star AR EASE™ caps as directed, and/or Quercetin with bromelain 500mg daily to aid the release of inorganic calcium and mineral deposits.
- Use DLPA 750 - 1000mg daily for pain relief.
- Use CAPSAICIN creme, or PRN PAIN FREE lotion as needed to help joint pain, flexibility and circulation.

Asthma

Allergic Breathing Disorder

Asthma has experienced almost a 50% rise in the decade between 1985 and 1995, mainly because of increased environmental pollutants. It now affects 3 percent of the U.S. population, about 15 million people. It is the leading serious, chronic illness among children under the age of ten, with a 2:1 ratio of boys to girls, and a death rate of about 5,000 kids yearly. Extrinsic or atopic asthma is an allergy-related condition, an antigen-antibody stimulation by foods or food additives. Intrinsic or bronchial asthma, is due to chemical toxicity, bronchial infection and emotional stress. Both types can appear at the same time.

Diet & Superfood Therapy

✿ Food sensitivities play a major part in asthma attacks. During an attack - eat only fresh foods. Include fresh apple or carrot juice daily.

✿ **Diet improvement is the key factor for maintaining control of asthma.**
➥Go on a short mucous cleansing liquid diet (see next page) for a week. **Then follow a non-mucous-forming, low salt diet for the next 3 months.** ➥Maintain a vegetarian diet as much as possible. Green leafy veggies provide needed magnesium.

✿ **Avoid all foods with sulfites and MSG. Avoid mucous-forming foods, such as pasteurized dairy products, meats, except fish and turkey, high gluten breads, and sugars. Avoid preserved foods, fried and fatty foods, oils and caffeine.**
➥Reduce salt and starchy foods. Asthma is common when salt intake is high.

✿ Make a syrup of pressed garlic juice, cayenne, olive oil and honey. Take 1 teasp. daily as a liver cleansing bile stimulant for fatty acid metabolism.

✿ **Effective superfoods:**
➥AloeLife ALOE FIBER MATE.
➥Crystal Star BIOFLAVS, FIBER & C™.
➥Klamath BLUE GREEN SUPREME.

Herbal Therapy

➥ **Jump start herbal program:**
Crystal Star ASTH-AID™ tea and capsules to clear the chest, and ANTI-HST™ caps or ALRG-HST™ for antihistamines.
with
➥**ADR-ACTIVE™ capsules or extract.**

➥ **Use Crystal Star ANTI-SPZ™ capsules as needed every hour to control spasmodic wheezing.** ➊
➥**X-PECT™ tea for mucous release.**

➥ For acute attacks: Lobelia extract under the tongue as needed, or sniff an anti-spasmodic oil like lavender, rosemary, or anise.

➥ **Two teas for chronic asthma:**
➥1 part each: ginger root, ephedra leaf, schizandra berries.
➥1 part each: bupleurum, fenugreek seed, gotu kola.

➥ Effective preventive herbals:
➥Green tea
➥Ayurvedic Coleus Forskholii
➥GINKGO BILOBA extract.
➥Reishi mushroom capsules
➥Lobelia as a chest muscle relaxant.

➥ **Take a catnip/garlic enema twice a week. Apply an onion poultice or hot ginger compress to the chest.** ➊

Supplements

✍ **Effective antioxidants:**
➥**Quercetin 1000-2000mg daily, with Bromelain 500mg, vitamin C 3000mg with bioflavs. and rutin, and magnesium 500mg.**
➥Vitamin E 400IU with selenium.
➥CoQ_{10} 60mg 2x daily.

✍ **Pantothenic acid therapy sources:**
➥High potency royal jelly 2 teasp. daily **(with caution if you are allergic to bee products).**
➥Pantothenic acid caps 1000mg, extra PABA 500mg and B_6 100mg.
➥B Complex 150mg daily with raw adrenal complex and/or raw thymus glandular 2x daily.

✍ Bioforce ASTHMA RELIEF drops. ➊

✍ **Magnesium/B_{12} therapy for kids:** ➊
Calcium 500mg/magnesium 250mg with Solaray B_{12}, 2000mcg every other day.
➥Use with vitamin C 1000mg and B complex 50mg for best results.

✍ Digestive enzymes help: Pancreatin, 1400mg before each meal to digest clogging fats and oils.

Lifestyle Support Therapy

Beware of aspirin if you are at asthma risk.

✿ Use eucalyptus oil, or food grade H_2O_2, 3% dilute solution in 8-oz. water in a vaporizer at night for relief and tissue oxygen. A twenty minute H_2O_2 bath also helps right away. See page 176 for instructions.

✿ Relaxation techniques have been very successful for asthma:
➥**Acupuncture, biofeedback, guided imagery and massage therapy are effective.**

✿ **Home health for asthma:** Avoid tobacco smoke, wood and gas stoves. Keep house temperature less than 70 degrees and humidity less than 55%. Launder in perfume-free, dye-free detergents. Vacuum often.
➥Keep indoor plants in your home as natural air filters.

✿ Massage and gently scratch the lung meridian from top of shoulder to end of thumb to clear chest of mucous. Massage between the shoulder blades.

✿ Do deep breathing exercises to increase lung capacity outdoors if air quality is acceptable. Before aerobic exercise, deplete the body of chemicals that induce asthma attacks by starting with a short warm up. Then take a walk, bicycle ride, or other exercise, exhaling strongly to expel toxins.

A 240

Common Symptoms: *Difficult breathing; choking, wheezing, coughing; difficulty in exhaling, often with heart palpitations. Colds are often accompanied by ear infections, a croupy cough. Accompanying hyperactivity in kids, high blood pressure in adults.*

Common Causes: *Food allergies, particularly to additives or preservatives, excess sugar, pasteurized dairy products, meats, wheat; adrenal exhaustion and imbalance; hypoglycemia; poor circulation and constipation; an increased toxic load from chemical environmental pollutants; sprayed produce; emotional stress or excessively cold air; low thyroid and adrenal exhaustion.*

See COOKING FOR HEALTHY HEALING by Linda Rector Page for a complete ASTHMA CONTROL diet.

LIQUID MUCOUS CLEANSING DIET FOR ASTHMA & RESPIRATORY DISEASE

A program to overcome asthma and other chronic respiratory problems is usually more successful when begun with a short mucous elimination diet. This allows the body to rid itself first of toxins, allergens and mucous accumulations causing congestion, and improve fatty acid metabolism in an attempt to change eating habits. Avoid eggs, shellfish, nuts, peanuts, and any food with additives, during your cleansing period because they can bring on an immediate allergy/asthma attack. Then avoid pasteurized dairy products, heavy starches and refined foods that are inherently a breeding ground for continued congestion. All respiratory problems will benefit from this way of eating. The first stage, a high vitamin C liquid diet, should be followed for 3 - 5 days at a time as needed for mucous release. It often produces symptomatic relief from respiratory problems in 24 to 48 hours.

On rising: take a glass of cranberry, apple or grapefruit juice; or lemon juice in hot water with 1 teasp. honey; or a glass of cider vinegar, hot water and honey.

Breakfast: take a hot potassium broth or essence (page 167), or Crystal Star SYSTEMS STRENGTH™ drink with 1 tsp. liquid chlorophyll, Sun CHLORELLA or Green Foods GREEN MAGMA. Add 2 garlic capsules, or 2 cayenne/ginger capsules and $^1/_4$ to $^1/_2$ teasp. ascorbate vitamin C or Ester C powder with bioflavonoids in water.

Mid-morning: have a glass of fresh carrot juice; and/or a cup of comfrey/fenugreek tea, or Crystal Star RESPR TEA™ or ASTH-AID TEA™.

Lunch: have a hot vegetable, miso or onion broth, or Crystal Star SYSTEMS STRENGTH™ drink; Add 2-3 more garlic capsules and $^1/_4$ to $^1/_2$ teasp. ascorbate vitamin C or Ester C powder with bioflavonoids in water.

Mid-afternoon: have a cleansing herb tea, such as alfalfa/mint or Crystal Star GREEN TEA CLEANSER™; or a green drink such as Sun CHLORELLA, or Crystal Star ENERGY GREEN™.

Dinner: have a hot veggie broth, potassium essence, or miso soup with sea veggies snipped on top; or another glass of carrot juice. Take 2-3 more garlic capsules, and $^1/_4$ to $^1/_2$ teasp. ascorbate vitamin C or Ester C powder in water.

Before bed: take another hot water, lemon and honey drink; or hot apple or cranberry juice.

Note 1: Salts should be kept low during this diet, but a little Bragg's LIQUID AMINOS can be added to any broth or juice for flavor.
Note 2: Drink six to eight glasses of bottled water or mineral water each day for best cleansing results.
Note 3: Add 1 teasp. acidophilus liquid, or $^1/_4$ to $^1/_2$ teasp. acidophilus powder to any broth or juice, and 1 teasp. high omega-3 flax oil.
Note 4: If you have a cold, include even more liquids than described above, such as hot broths, mineral water, fruit and vegetable juices, or a little brandy with lemon.

See "COOKING FOR HEALTHY HEALING" by Linda Rector Page for the complete diet.

Supplements for the Mucous Cleansing Diet

The most overlooked characteristic in treating asthma, especially childhood asthma, is whether chronic fungal or parasite infection is present. Most people with allergic breathing disorders have one of these conditions. If there are multiple allergies in conjunction with the fungal infection, treat it as if it were systemic - an una da gato formula is highly recommended. If parasites are present, consider an herbal pumpkin seed formula, or Crystal Star VERMEX™ combination.

• Ascorbate vitamin C or Ester C powder may be taken thoughout the day in juice or water, to bowel tolerance for tissue flushing and detoxification. Take up to 10,000mg daily for the first three days, then 5,000mg daily until the end of the liquid fast.

• Add EVENING PRIMROSE OIL 500 to 1000mg daily to improve fatty acid metabolism.

• Try to stay away from cortisone compounds that eventually weaken the immune system, and from over-the-counter drugs that often simply drive congestion deeper into the lungs.

Attention Deficit Hyperactivity Disorder

Learning Disabilities ❋ Minimal Brain Dysfunction ❋ Autism

Hyperactive behavior and Attention Deficit Disorder have been serious problems for children since the fifties. Hyperactivity seems to be the expression of either hypoglycemia or food allergies or both. Attention Deficit Disorder is slow learning caused by any or all of the learning disorders. Autism is almost a "mind-blind" condition, characterized by withdrawn behavior, lack of emotion and speech, extreme sensitivity to sound and touch. Autistic children have a brain malfunction that creates a barrier between them and the rest of the world. Children at greatest risk are male, with a history of family diabetes or alcoholism. Nutritional improvement and calming herbs are the cornerstones of successful treatment in overcoming hyperactivity.

Diet & Superfood Therapy

Diet improvement is the key to changing disordered brain chemistry. Results are almost immediately evident, generally within 1 to 3 weeks. When behavior normalizes, maintain the improved diet to prevent reversion.

❧ **Food sensitivities play a major part in attention disorders.**

❧ Use applied kinesiology to determine allergens, or test foods like milk, wheat, corn, chocolate, and citrus with an elimination diet.

❧ Avoid refined sugar (almost always involved in ADHD reactions.)

❧ Use organically grown foods when possible.

❧ The ongoing diet should be high in vegetable proteins and whole grains, with plenty of fresh fruits and vegetables, and no junk or fast foods.

❧ Have a green salad every day.

❧ Include calming tryptophan-rich foods like turkey, fish, wheat germ, yogurt and eggs.

❧ **Effective superfoods:**
❧ **Crystal Star CALCIUM SOURCE™ extract in water as a rapid calmative.**
❧ **Lewis Labs high phos. lecithin.**
❧ Organic Gourmet Nutritional Yeast Extract before bed.

Herbal Therapy

Poor immune response and allergies are factors in all of these disorders.

❧ **Jump start herbal program:**
Crystal Star RELAX CAPS™ or Planetary Formulas CALM CHILD drops or **capsules as needed.** ☺
❧ **EVENING PRIMROSE oil for critical EFAs.**

❧ **Add Crystal Star VALERIAN/WILD LETTUCE extract for extra calming.**
❧ **GINKGO BILOBA extract for inner ear balance problems often present.**
❧ **GINSENG/LICORICE ELIXIR™.**

❧ **Effective fatty acid sources:** (GLA sources to improve body "electrical connections.")
❧ Black currant oil
❧ Borage oil
❧ Source Naturals GLA 240
❧ **High omega-3 flax oil.**

❧ **Effective teas:**
❧ **Catnip** ☺
❧ Hops/lobelia
❧ Rosemary as a natural antioxidant.

❧ **Effective extracts:**
❧ **HAWTHORN leaf, berry & flower**
❧ **BLACK WALNUT as an anti-fungal**
❧ **Gotu Kola for nerve stress.**

Supplements

Avoid aspirin and amphetamines of all kinds if your child has these disorders.

❧ Stress B Complex with extra pantothenic acid 100mg and B_6 100mg. to activate serotonin in the brain. Add Natren HEALTHY TRINITY for proper synthesis of B vitamins.

with

Vitamin C with bioflavonoids, up to 2000mg daily. Best in powder form, 1/4 teasp. every 2 hours in juice.

❧ Twin Lab GABA plus or Country Life RELAXER CAPS as needed.

❧ **Effective homeopathic remedies:**
❧ **Hylands CALMS and CALMS FORTE**
❧ *Argenticum nit.*
❧ *Arsenicum*
❧ Nature's Way RESTLESS CHILD

❧ Taurine 500mg daily. ☺

❧ **Choline/inositol for brain balance.** ♂
with
Premier LITHIUM .5mg as directed, and magnesium 400mg.

❧ Glycine powder in liquid with passion flower extract drops.

Lifestyle Support Therapy

❧ Relaxation techniques such as massage therapy and biofeedback have shown some success.
❧ **Also baking soda and sea salt baths.**

❧ Prescriptions for Ritalin, Cylertor, and Atarax, short-term sedative drugs for hyperactive disorders, often make the condition worse with long use. They have side effects of nervousness, insomnia, unhealthy weight loss, stunted growth, stomach aches, skin rashes, headaches and hallucinations. Avoid them if you can. Try diet improvement first.

❧ **Read food labels carefully. Avoid all food products with preservatives, (BHT, MSG, BHA, etc.) additives and colors.**
❧ **Eliminate red meats (nitrates) and canned or frozen foods (too much salt).**
❧ **Reduce carbonated drinks (Excess phosphorus).**

❧ **Reflexology points:**

adrenals
diaphragm
pituitary
brain

Common Symptoms: *Behavior symptoms include extreme emotional instability, compulsive, aggressive, destructive behavior, short attention span, can't sit still; self-mutilation, chronic liar, doesn't follow directions or listen, impatient and defiant. Motor coordination symptoms include poor muscle harmony, speech problems; dyslexia; accident proneness. Cognitive/perceptual problems include slow learning and reasoning, unusual chronic thirst, chronic cold symptoms with sneezing and coughing.*

Common Causes: *Mineral and EFA deficiencies from too many refined and junk foods; food intolerances to preservatives and additives; prostaglandin imbalance; hypoglycemia; heavy metal (esp. lead) poisoning causing excess ammonia waste in the brain; prescription drugs that make the condition worse by blocking EFA conversion in the brain.*

See HYPOGLYCEMIA AND EPILEPSY DIETS in this book, or OPTIMAL EATING FOR CHILDREN DIET in COOKING FOR HEALTHY HEALING by Linda Rector Page, for more information.

Back Pain

Lumbago ❋ Herniated Disc ❋ Scoliosis

The spine is the major seat of human nerve structure, and as such manifests many of the body's emotional, psychological and physical stresses. 80% of Americans suffer back pain at some point in their lives and almost 40% wind up with crippling back pain. Back pain is second only to childbirth as a reason for hospitalization, and it can last for months. Major back surgery, like removing discs may do more harm than good. In addition to diet improvement and supplementation, a good chiropractor or massage therapist who treats more than just the physical problem, is often the best answer.

Diet & Superfood Therapy

❧ **It is critical to drink at least 6 glasses of water daily. Much back and rheumatoid pain is due to chronic dehydration. You need to keep acid particles flushed to keep kidneys functioning well.**

❧ Uric acid aggravates back pain. Avoid red meats, pasteurized dairy and caffeine.

❧ The diet should be high in minerals and vegetable proteins. Vegetarians have stronger bone density.

❧ **Reduce the fat in your diet. The greater the deposits of fatty plaque, the greater the degeneration of spinal discs.** ❧

❧ Effective superfoods:
—**Crystal Star ENERGY GREEN™ drink** or SYSTEMS STRENGTH™ for absorbable minerals and chlorophyll strength.
—A protein drink, like Nappi THE PERFECT MEAL, or Solgar WHEY TO GO.
—Take a potassium broth (pg. 167) once a week for kidney cleansing.
—AloeLife ALOE GOLD concentrate, 2 TBS. in water as an anti-inflammatory.

Herbal Therapy

☙ **Jump start herbal program:**
—**Crystal Star STRESSED OUT™ extract to help immediate pain.**
—**ANTI-FLAM™ caps or extract for pain control.**
—**SILICA SOURCE™ complex extract for collagen growth.**

☙ Crystal Star RELAX CAPS™ or ANTI-SPZ™ capsules for spasm control.
—BACK TO RELIEF™ caps, an analgesic.
—BLDR-K TEA™ if kidneys are inflamed. ♀
and

☙ Alta Health SIL-X silica extract for strength and collagen building.

☙ **Effective herbal compresses:**
—Hops or comfrey w. lobelia
—Home Health CASTOR OIL PACKS
—**Cayenne/ginger heat packs** ♂

☙ **Massage into back:**
—B&T *TRIFLORA GEL*.
—Chinese WHITE FLOWER oil. ♀
—**PRN PAIN FREE lotion.** ♂
—DMSO with ALOE GEL. ♂
—New Chapter Arnica/Ginger gel.
—Aromatherapy lavender or chamomile essential oils.

Supplements

⚘ **Quercetin with Bromelain, 2 daily to reduce swelling/inflammation.**
—**Enzymatic Therapy GS COMPLEX or AR-MAX as directed, or Bovine tracheal cartilage as directed, or**
—**Twin Lab CSA 250mg 1 daily, with L-Carnitine 500mg for muscle strength.**

⚘ **Take homeopathic *Horse Chestnut* ·** results in about 3 to 6 days.

⚘ Stress B Complex with extra B_6 100mg daily and B_{12} SL 2000mcg.
or

⚘ Nature's Bounty internasal B_{12} for spine cell development;
—COQ$_{10}$ 30mg 3x daily. with Nature's Life BROMELAIN/PAPAIN.

⚘ DLPA as needed for chronic pain. ♀
or
⚘ Country Life LIGATEND capsules. ♂

⚘ **Vitamin C 3-5000mg with bioflavonoids, and a high magnesium CAL/MAG CITRATE formula, with Boron 3mg daily for better uptake.**

Lifestyle Support Therapy

If you have fallen or bruised the spine or tailbone, and have persistent pain after 5 days, see a qualified massage therapist or chiropractor.

🐾 Regular, non-jarring exercise is the most important key in treating and preventing back pain. Exercises, such as swimming, cycling, walking, rowing and cross-country skiing build back strength.

🐾 **Upper back pain:** sleep on your side with your knees bent and a fat pillow under your head; or on your back with a thin pillow under your head and a big pillow under your knees. Avoid sleeping on your stomach if possible.

🐾 Apply Centipede Kitty's OXY-GEL to affected areas every 24 hours. Or take an energy/oxygen bath (pg. 176).

🐾 New research shows that more than 2 days bed rest with a bad back weakens muscles. Always sleep on a firm mattress.

🐾 **Reflexology points:**

spine & kidney

Common symptoms: Spinal stress and pain; inability to do even small bending or pushing actions; sometimes inability to move at all.
Common Causes: Poor posture; improper lifting, sitting or standing; arthritis; deep-seated emotional stress; kidney malfunction, usually from dehydration; high heels; overweight; protein, calcium and other nutrient deficiency; green vegetable deficiency; osteoporosis or osteoarthritis; sleeping on a mattress that is too soft; congenitally poor spinal alignment. Causes for back conditions can be as wide-ranging as a herniated disc and family financial problems. Scoliosis curvature is thought to be inherited.

Bad Breath & Body Odor

Halitosis ❧ Bromidrosis

Both of these conditions are manifestations of the same problem - poor diet, poor food digestion, causing rotting food and bacteria formation that the body throws off through the skin and breath. There are many very effective natural mouth fresheners and deodorizers. Make sure you don't have a more serious problem than just poor food assimilation. Rule out cavities, gum disease and sinus infections for bad breath first.

Diet & Superfood Therapy

Diet change and cleansing your internal environment is the single most beneficial thing you can do to get rid of bad breath and body odor.

🌿 Start with a short 24 hour liquid diet (pg. 158) with apple juice and 1 TB. psyllium husks, or Crystal Star CHO-LO FIBER TONE™ to cleanse the bowel.

🍃For one week, add liquid chlorophyll to apple or carrot juice to neutralize stomach acids and cleanse the digestive tract.

🌿 Then make sure your diet has crunchy, cleansing, fiber-rich foods like fresh fruits and green vegetables. Eat high chlorophyll foods like parsley and sprouts.

🍃Eat plenty of cultured foods such as yogurt or kefir for intestinal flora activity.

🍃Drink 6-8 glasses of water daily to keep the body flushed and clear.

🌿 Eat light, less concentrated foods - especially reduce or avoid red meats and heavy animal protein, caffeine, fried foods, and heavy sweets.

Eat smaller, meals, and chew well for best enzyme activity.

🌿 **Effective superfoods:**
🍃**Crystal Star ENERGY GREEN™ drink.**
🍃**Nutricology PROGREENS.**
🍃**GreenFoods BETA-CARROT.**
🍃Solaray ALFAJUICE capsules.

Herbal Therapy

🌿 **Jump start herbal program:** Crystal Star PRE-MEAL ENZ™ extract before meals, or AFTER MEAL ENZ™ extract at or after meals.
🍃**BITTERS & LEMON CLEANSE™** extract, or GREEN TEA CLEANSER™ every morning to boost liver and digestion.

🌿 Breath & body freshening teas:
🍃Peppermint
🍃Fenugreek/sage
🍃Rosemary
🍃Alfalfa/mint
🍃Natureworks HERBAL BITTERS

🌿 Put pinches of cloves, ginger, cinnamon, nutmeg or anise in a cup of water and drink as a natural antacid; or chew a few aromatic seeds like anise, cardamom or fennel for breath freshening.
🍃BioForce GOLDENROD extract as directed, or DENTAFORCE BREATH SPRAY.

🌿 **Keep colon and bowel clean with a gentle laxative such as HERBAL TONE, or a laxative tea such as Crystal Star LAXA-TEA™, or AloeLife FIBER-MATE.**♀

🌿 Control low-grade mouth infections with propolis lozenges or odorless garlic caps daily, or tea tree oil rubbed on gums to control lowgrade infections.

Supplements

🌀 **Think zinc for body odor. Take 15-50mg daily.**♂

🌀 **Effective digestive aids:**
🍃**Acidophilus 4-6 x daily.**
🍃**Betaine HCl with papain before each meal (especially before meat protein), or Schiff ENZYMALL tabs with ox bile.**♀
🍃Liquid chlorophyll, 1 teasp. in water after meals.

🌀 Daily vitamin aids: vitamin C 1000mg with 500mg bioflavonoids 3x, and B Complex 100mg.

🌀 High Omega-3 fish or flax oils to improve circulation and blood fat release.

🌀 **For morning breath:** Just before bedtime, floss between all teeth, then brush with baking soda rather than toothpaste. Brush your tongue but do not use mouthwash. Morning breath should be eliminated or greatly reduced.

🌀 **Effective mouth deodorizers:**
🍃Del's BREATH DROPS
🍃TIBS essential oil breath drops.
🍃Breath Assure caps.
🍃Desert Essence tea tree mouthwash.
🍃Peri-dent herbal gum mouthwash.

Lifestyle Support Therapy

Give your body a chance to digest your food. Don't eat for 2 hours before bed.

☞ **Exercise to cleanse metabolic wastes being improperly expelled through skin and lungs.**
🍃Take a mineral salts bath such as Para Labs BATH THERAPY, or an herbal bath like Olbas HERBAL BATH once a week.♀

☞ Clean teeth with myrrh gum powder, or Toms toothpaste with myrrh. Brush teeth and tongue after every meal.

☞ **Effective body deodorants:**
🍃Dab underarms/feet with vinegar.
🍃Natural salt crystal deodorant.
🍃Tom's deodorants (all kinds).
🍃Apply aloe vera gel under arms.♀

☞ Use a dry skin brush, or a "bath beauty cloth" all over the body daily to remove toxins coming out through the skin. Then shower with an oatmeal/honey scrub soap.

☞ Wear natural fiber clothing so the skin can breathe. Wear sandals when possible.

☞ **Reflexology point:**

food assimilation♂

Common Symptoms: *Bad taste in the mouth and mouth odor; foul smelling perspiration.*

Common Causes: *Poor diet with a green vegetable deficiency; poor digestion; enzyme deficiency; inadequate protein digestion, leading to indigestion; poor mouth or body hygiene; sluggish intestinal system and chronic constipation; stress and anxiety; gum disease and tooth decay; food intolerances; HCl deficiency; low grade chronic throat infection; smoking; liver malfunction; post-nasal drip from a chronic sinus infection; candida yeast infection.*

Bedwetting
Child & Adult Enuresis

Bedwetting, after the normal age of 3 to 7 years old, affects about 5 million children, mostly male. It also affects over 150,000 adults. Most experts agree that barring any physical/mechanical obstruction or infection, bedwetting is probably psychologically based. However, nutritional therapies have had such notable success in this area that we cannot help but believe that nutritional deficiencies are also a part of the problem.

Diet & Superfood Therapy

❧ Avoid oxalic acid-forming foods, such as cooked spinach, sodas, rhubarb, caffeine, cocoa, chocolate, etc.

❧ No junk foods. Avoid refined sugars, salty or extra spicy foods as irritants. ⚘

❧ Avoid food colorings, preservatives and pasteurized cow's milk as possible allergens.

❧ Take a small glass of cranberry/apple juice each morning to clean the kidneys.

❧ No liquids before bed. Eat a little celery instead to balance organic salts. ⚘

❧ A spoonful of honey before bed. ⊛

Herbal Therapy

❧ **Jump start herbal program:**
  ✻**Crystal Star BLDR-CONTROL™ extract in water before dinner. Use half strength for children.** ⊛
  ✻**CALCIUM SOURCE™ capsules or extract drops in water.**

❧ Crystal Star RELAX CAPS™ or VALERIAN/WILD LETTUCE extract in water for stress-related bedwetting. ⊛

❧ Give the child cinnamon sticks to chew on before bed. ⊛

❧ Effective teas: Use as extract drops in water if possible.
  ✻Thyme ⊛
  ✻Scullcap
  ✻Cinnamon bark ⊛
  ✻Horsetail at dinner
  ✻Cornsilk
  ✻Plantain

❧ **Effective tea combinations:**
  ✻Parsley/oatstraw/juniper/uva ursi.

❧ GINKGO BILOBA extract in water, mixed with a little honey before bed.

Supplements

✒ **Homeopathic remedies:**
  ✻**Hylands *BEDWETTING* tablets before bed.** ⊛
  ✻BSI *Equisetum.*
  ✻Standard *Enuraid* (adults).

✒ Minerals strengthen tissues:
  ✻Twin Lab LIQUID K PLUS.
  ✻Mezotrace SEA MINERAL COMPLEX chewable. ⊛
  ✻Country Life CAL SNACK, milk-free chewable calcium. ⊛

✒ Twin Lab CSA 250mg 1 daily.

✒ **Floradix LIQUID MULTI-VITA-MIN daily.** ⊛

✒ Magnesium 100mg daily.

Lifestyle Support Therapy

☞ See a good chiropractor or massage therapist if a compressed nerve or an obstruction is the suspected cause.

☞ Muscle testing (applied kinesiology) is effective here in determining what allergies may be the cause.

☞ Good circulation is a key. Good daily exercise is an answer; especially bicycle riding.

☞ **Effective TLC:** ⊛
  ✱Leave a night light on so the child will feel free to get up at night.
  ✱Give a relaxing massage before bed to ease muscles and fears. Try lavender oil.
  ✱Decrease your child's stress about bedwetting by giving encouragement rather than punishment. Praise him for not wetting the bed.
  ✱Make sure home emotional environment is supportive.
  ✱Make sure bedtime is regular and stress-free. Consider a happy bedtime story.

☞ Guided imagery techniques have had some success. Within the first few hours of sleep, give the child reassuring messages without waking him.

See also CHILDHOOD DISEASES pages in this book for more information.

Common Symptoms: Involuntary urination during the night beyond toilet training age.
Common Causes: Unusually deep sleep patterns with decreased REM sleep; inherited organ weakness; allergies - especially food allergies; excess sugar, salt, spices or dairy in the diet; food allergies; stress, emotional anxiety and behavioral disturbances; bad dreams; hypoglycemia or diabetes; compressed nerve or congenital obstruction in the bladder area...

Bladder Infections

Bacterial Cystitis ❀ Incontinence

Recurrent bladder infections are common in women; less common in men (theirs are mostly as a result of prostate problems). Bladder infections are the most frequent reason a woman seeks medical attention; pain can be all-consuming during the acute stage. Over 75% of American women have at least one urinary tract infection in a ten year period, almost 30% have one once a year. About 15% of menopausal women experience them, usually in the first years of menopause when body chemistry is changing. Staph and strep infections and diabetes may also affect the kidneys, making the problem more serious - an alarming number of cases result in kidney failure.

Diet & Superfood Therapy

Changing body pH is important. Diet is the biggest factor for doing this.

❧ Avoid acid-forming foods - caffeine, black tea, tomatoes, cooked spinach, chocolate.
➻**Avoid sugary foods, carbonated drinks, concentrated starches, fried, salty and fatty foods, sugars, pasteurized dairy and refined foods.** Reduce meat protein.
➻Add plenty of alkalizing foods: celery, watermelon juice, ume plum balls, green drinks, potassium broth (pg. 167).
➻A yeast-free diet is best, with no baked breads during healing.

❧ **During acute stage:** take 2 TBS. cider vinegar and honey in water each a.m., yogurt at noon, a glass of white wine at night.
➻**Dilute cranberry juice (unsweetened), 8 glasses daily, and carrot/beet/cucumber juice every other day to reduce infection.**
➻**Increase urine flow: Drink a minimum of 10 glasses of distilled water, diluted, unsweetened fruit juices and herbal teas daily to keep acid wastes flushed.**

❧ **Effective superfoods:**
➻Green Foods GREEN MAGMA drink daily during healing.
➻Crystal Star BIOFLAV. FIBER & C SUPPORT™ with cranberry.
➻Klamath BLUE-GREEN SUPREME.

Herbal Therapy

If infections develop regularly after intercourse, rinse the vagina and labia with golden seal/echinacea tea.

❧ **Jump start herbal program:**
➻**At the first hint of a bladder infection, take Crystal Star BLDR-K™ caps, 2 every 3 hours, and/or BLDR-K™ tea. ♀♂ or PROX FOR MEN™ caps. ♂**
➻**with two ANTI-BIO™ capsules each time if problem is severe.**
or
➻Goldenseal/echinacea extract, Solaray CORNSILK BLEND caps, or uva ursi caps, daily for 10 days, then Crystal Star BLDR-K™ extract.

❧ **Effective aromatherapy sitz bath oil:**
➻3 drops tea tree oil, 2 drops bergamot oil, 2 drops cypress oil, 2 drops thyme oil, 1 drop eucalyptus oil. Take a sitz bath 2x daily for ½ hour.

❧ **Aromatherapy abdomen massage:**
➻1-oz. almond oil, 3 drops sandalwood oil, 2 drops cedarwood oil, 2 drops cypress oil, 1 drop benzoin resin, 1 drop frankincense oil.

❧ **For incontinence:**
➻**Crystal Star BLDR-K CONTROL™.**
➻Standard Homeopathics *Enuraid*.

Supplements

The active chemical in many spermicidal creams and foams, nonoxynol-9, causes recurring cystitis and yeast infections. Also look to your oral contraceptives.

❧ **As soon as you feel any symptoms, take NUTRIBIOTIC GRAPEFRUIT EXTRACT caps as directed, and a glass of water with 1 teasp. baking soda in it.**
and
➻**Take 1000mg ascorbate or Ester C with bioflavonoids, bromelain 500mg, mycelized A & E, and Lysine 1000mg every 2 hours during the day.**

❧ Dr. DOPHILUS 2 caps 3x daily to replace friendly flora, especially if taking antibiotics. May also use 1 TB. acidophilus powder in warm water as a douche. ♀
with
➻Garlic caps 6 daily, zinc 30mg B₆ 500mg daily and high Omega 3 flax oil.

❧ Take Future Biotics VITAL K and uva ursi caps for 14 days to disinfect. On the tenth day, take Solaray CRAN-ACTIN caps, 2 daily.

❧ **Homeopathic remedies are effective for both infections and incontinence.** Check with a knowledgeable professional for the remedy that fits your symptoms.

Lifestyle Support Therapy

Acupuncture can sometimes relieve pain almost immediately.

❧ Apply wet heat, or hot comfrey compresses across lower back and kidneys to relieve pain and ease urination.
➻Take extended hot sitz baths.

❧ For accompanying hemorrhage, take 1 oz. marshmallow rt., steep in 1 pt. hot milk. Take every ½ hr. to staunch bleeding.

❧ **Take a mild catnip or chlorophyll enema to clear acid wastes.**

❧ **Urinate as soon as possible after sexual intercourse. Do not use a diaphragm if you are prone to bladder infections.** ♀
➻Do not use colored toilet paper. ♀

❧ **Reflexology point:**

bladder

❧ **For incontinence:**
➻Biofeedback and acupuncture have been successful for incontinence in both women and men, regardless of cause.
➻Do toning Kegel exercises.

See also INTERSTITIAL CYSTITIS page in this book for more information.

Common Symptoms: Frequent, urgent, burning, painful urination, especially at night; pain in lower back and abdomen below the navel; often chills and fever as the body tries to throw off infection; strong, turbid, foul-smelling urine; cloudy or bloody urine. If you have pain above the waist, it may be a kidney infection or kidney stones instead of a bladder infection.

Common Causes: The result of a cold infection, then aggravated by overuse of antibiotics; venereal disease; fecal bacteria, usually E.coli that migrate up the urethra; stress; spermicide and contraceptives; kidney malfunction; food allergens; aluminum cookware, deodorants, etc.; lack of adequate fluids to keep the body flushed; poor elimination; tampons or diaphragms pinching the neck of the bladder, hampering waste elimination.

Bladder Infections

Interstitial Cystitis ⁜ Chronic Urethritis

Chronic UTIs may not be due to infection. Interstitial cystitis, a non-bacterial form affecting one in 20 women with bladder infections, has been called "migraine of the bladder," because many of the same things that either trigger or benefit migraine headaches affect interstitial cystitis the same way. It seems to be an auto-immune disease, resulting from low immune strength. Attend to healing immediately, because of the great pain, and because the bladder can shrink to a size where it will only hold 1 or 2 ounces. A natural approach is best; antibiotics do not help and may aggravate this type of cystitis - actually attacking the bladder lining when there is no infection to attack.

Diet & Superfood Therapy

Cranberry juice is not beneficial for interstitial cystitis.

Avoid trigger foods:

Aged protein foods such as yogurt, pickled herring, preserved or smoked meats, cheeses, yeasted breads, sauerkraut, citrus fruits, citrus juices and red wine until condition normalizes.

Avoid all caffeine-containing foods, spicy foods, soy sauce, and foods with additives like NutraSweet.

Begin drinking water immediately when you feel an infection coming.

Increase leafy greens and fiber foods.

Take veggie drinks (pg. 168) and carrot juice during acute stages, and as a preventive.

Cleanse the kidneys with watermelon juice, or watermelon seed tea. Strengthen them with well-cooked beans and sea vegetables.

Effective superfoods:

Nutricology PRO-GREENS.

Solaray ALFAJUICE as a potent antioxidant and green source.

Sun CHLORELLA 1 pkt. daily for 1 month.

AloeLife ALOE GOLD juice before meals.

Herbal Therapy

Jump start herbal program:

Crystal Star BLDR-K™ extract and/ or BLDR-K™ tea, or cat's claw tea 3 cups daily.

A full course of ECHINACEA extract or PAU D' ARCO/ECHINACEA extract.

ANTI-FLAM™ caps inflammation.

ANTI-SPZ caps for pain.

6 extra goldenseal capsules, or ANTI-BIO™ caps a day during acute periods if needed.

and then

Solaray CENTELLA ASIATICA extract caps.

Omega 3 flax oil caps 3 x daily.

Effective teas:
- **Cornsilk**
- **Dandelion/nettles**
- **Uva ursi** or buchu tea
- Astragalus
- Watermelon seed

Effective extracts:

GINKGO BILOBA extract

BILBERRY extract as an anti-inflammatory.

Nutribiotic GRAPEFRUIT SEED EXTRACT drops in water as directed for 1 month.

Supplements

The active chemical in many spermicidal creams and foams, nonoxynol-9, increases the risk of all types of cystitis.

At the first signs of an impending infection, take a teasp. of baking soda in a glass of water to alkalize the urine before it reaches the bladder.

Then a calcium carbonate capsule every 12 hours for a time-release effect.

CoQ_{10} 30mg 3x daily.

with

Mycelized A & E to help reduce interstitial cystitis scarring.

and

Zinc 30mg daily to combat infection.

Vitamin C therapy: ascorbate or Ester C powder, $^1/_4$ teasp. every hour during acute stages to help restore normal immunity.

and

Lysine 1000mg with bromelain 500mg 6x daily.

Enzymatic Therapy ACID-A-CAL capsules 4-6 daily.

Nature's Plus vitamin E 800IU daily.

Lifestyle Support Therapy

Do not wear tampons if you have recurring cystitis.

Acupuncture works well for symptom relief.

Reflexology point:

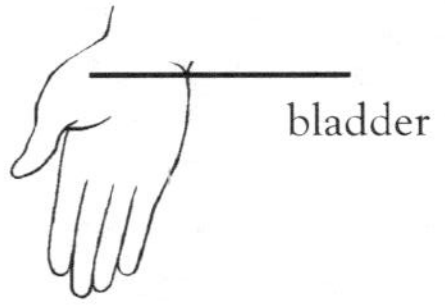

Press alternating hot and cold compresses against the pubic bone and clitoris. Press hard.

Hot sitz baths during an infection help bring cleansing circulation to the infected area. See aromatherapy sitz baths on the previous page.

Position of bladder/urethra:

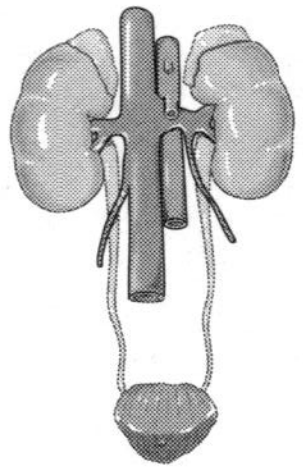

Common Symptoms: *Scarred, tough, atrophied bladder, so that normal urination is impossible; pain goes away during urination, then immediately returns; breakdown of bladder tissue, even when infection is not present; cloudy urine with foul odor; systemic fever and aching.*

Common Causes: *Sometimes accompanies endometriosis; environmental and food allergies; lowered immunity; dietary "triggers" causing acidity in the system; pelvic congestion from chronic constipation, lowered libido, or heavy, painful menstrual periods; dehydration.*

See also BACTERIAL CYSTITIS *page in this book for more information.*

Bone Health

Healing Bone Breaks ✤ Preventing Brittle Bones ✤ Cartilage Regrowth

Continuing research is showing that several common medications put bone health at risk: L-thyroxine - a thyroid stimulant; cortico-steroid drugs such as hydrocortisone, cortisone and prednisone - prescribed for rheumatic conditions and respiratory diseases; phenytoin and phenobarbital - anti-seizure drugs; heparin - a blood thinner; and furosemide - a diuretic; Ibuprofen - a pain killer; over use of aspirin and NSAIDS drugs like naproxen; No-DOZ - a stimulant.

Diet & Superfood Therapy

Vegetarians have denser, better formed bones, and stronger immune systems.

❧ Maintain a mineral-rich vegetable protein diet. Love your liver. It is vital to bone marrow formation. Keep it healthy.
    —Avoid red meats, refined foods, and acid-forming foods like fried and fast foods, and cola drinks.
    —Sugar inhibits calcium absorption.
    —Caffeine causes a loss of calcium.
    —Excess salt decreases bone density.

❧ **If you have prematurely gray hair, it may be a sign you have decreased mineral bone mass:**
    —for calcium and silicon: green vegetables, fish and seafood, sea vegetables, whole grains, tofu, yogurt.
    —for boron: dried fruits, nuts and seeds, honey, a little wine.
    —for vitamin C: papayas, kiwi, strawberries, bell peppers, broccoli, cantaloupe. ❧

❧ **Effective superfoods:**
    —**Crystal Star SYSTEMS STRENGTH™.**
    —Organic Gourmet NUTRITIONAL YEAST extract or MISO broth before bed.
    —Green Foods BETA CARROT.
    —Solaray ALFAJUICE for active Vit. K.
    —AloeLife ALOE GOLD for HCL.

Herbal Therapy

Absorbable minerals are key factors in bone building. Herbs are one of the best ways to get them.

❧ **Jump start herbal program:**
    —Crystal Star PRO-EST OSTEO PLUS™ roll-on, and/or CALCIUM SOURCE™ caps or extract for balanced calcium. with
    —Crystal Star SILICA SOURCE™ extract or Flora VEGE-SIL for collagen formation.

❧ *Phyto-hormone-containing herbs can be an important part of continuing bone health and formation. Effective estrogen/progesterone balancing herbs:*
    —**Crystal Star FEM-SUPPORT™** ♀♂
    —Black cohosh/sarsaparilla caps
    —Dong quai/damiana extract ♂
    —**Royal jelly/ginseng** ♂

❧ **Effective herbal bone healers:**
    —Nettles ♀
    —Horsetail extract

❧ **For cartilage regrowth:**
    —Enzymatic Therapy MYO-TONE.
    —**Crystal Star BIOFLAVS. FIBER & C SUPPORT™ drink daily,** or Enzymatic Therapy HERBAL FLAVONOIDS.
    —**BILBERRY extract (bioflavonoids also have estrogen-like activity).**

Supplements

There is much more to strong bones than just calcium. Without the proper amounts of other minerals as well as vitamin D - you won't absorb the calcium.

❧ **For general bone health:**
    —Calcium ascorbate C 3000mg.
    —Vitamin B$_6$ 250mg daily.
    —A & D 25, 000IU/1000IU daily.
    —**Mezotrace SEA MINERAL COMPLEX**
    —Vitamin E 400IU.
    —CoQ$_{10}$ 60mg 2x daily.

❧ **For bone density:**
    —Transitions PROGEST CREAM.
    —Enzymatic Therapy OSTEO PRIME.
    —Flora VEGE-SIL or Body Essentials SILICA GEL.
    —Jarrow HYDROXYAPATITE.

❧ **Bone knitters/healers:**
    —**Twin Lab CSA capsules.**
    —Ethical Nutrients BONE BUILDER.
    —Nature's Bounty vitamin B$_{12}$ every 3 days.

❧ **For bone breaks:**
    —Take homeopathic *Arnica Montana.*
    —Apply *Arnica* gel for swelling.
    —Apply a green clay or turmeric paste poultice and cover with gauze.

Lifestyle Support Therapy

❧ Aerobic exercise and light weight training are some of the best ways to build and elasticize bones.
    —Get some sunlight on the body every day possible for natural vitamin D.

❧ NO SMOKING. It increases bone brittleness and inhibits bone growth.

❧ Swim or walk in the ocean when possible; or take daily kelp or dulse tablets.

❧ Avoid aluminum pots and pans, deodorants and fluorescent lighting. Both leach calcium from the body.

See also OSTEOPOROSIS page in this book for more information.

Common Symptoms: Brittle bones with easy bone breaks; poor bone healing; prematurely gray hair (before 40), is sometimes a sign of decreased bone mineral mass.
Common Causes: Mineral deficiency or poor assimilation; poor diet with too many refined foods, and too much meat protein, causing phosphorus imbalance; enzyme deficiency; heavy metal or drug toxicity; steroids or too many cortico-steroid drugs; stress; too much alcohol and/or tobacco.

Brain Health

Better Memory & More Mental Activity ✻ Less Mental Exhaustion & Burn-Out

The brain controls the entire body. It is our primary health maintenance organ and the seat of energy production. Although it makes up only 2¹/₂% of our body weight, it uses almost 25% of our available oxygen, more than 25% of available glucose and 20% of our blood supply! When it is functioning well, total body health is improved. The brain is an incredibly sensitive organ, responding quickly but only temporarily to drugs and short term stimulants. The best way to get good, long term, brain enhancement is to feed it and use it. Brain nutrients have a rapidly noticeable effect on increased brain performance. Good, consistent brain nourishment can straighten out even grave mental, emotional and coordination problems.

Diet & Superfood Therapy

The brain needs constant, rich sources of vitamins, minerals, amino acids and antioxidants from your diet to function optimally. Unrefined, fresh foods offer the most nutrients.

❧ **Include frequently in the diet:**
Sea vegetables, fish, esp. tuna, and sea foods, (cold water fish are excellent as brain food because they are primarily fat and water), sprouts, fertile eggs, wheat germ, unsaturated oils, brown rice, tofu, apples, oranges, grapefruit, wheat germ and beans.

❧ Drink plenty of pure water every day.

❧ Make a brain food: mix 2TBS. each: lecithin for phosphatides and memory lapses., brewer's yeast for myelin formation. Take 1-2TBS. daily.

❧

❧ **Effective superfoods:**
✻Nutricology PRO-GREENS w. EFAs
✻Solgar EARTH SOURCE GREENS & MORE w. EFAs.
✻Crystal Star SYSTEMS STRENGTH for brain minerals.
✻Nappi THE PERFECT MEAL.
✻Klamath BLUE-GREEN SUPREME.
✻BeWell VEGETABLE JUICES.
✻Future Biotics VITAL K drink.

Herbal Therapy

Many mineral-rich herbs provide key bio-chemical ingredients for effective neurotransmission.

❧ **Jump start herbal program:**
Crystal Star MENTAL CLARITY™ capsules, CREATIVI-TEA™, or MEDITATION™ tea.
and
✻GINKGO BILOBA extract 3x daily for enhanced blood flow to the brain.

❧ *Half the weight of the brain is EFAs.*
✻EVENING PRIMROSE oil 2-4 daily for good brain electrical connections. ♀

❧ **Herbal neurotransmitter stimulants:**
✻Cayenne
✻Dandelion/gotu kola caps
✻Aromatherapy thyme oil

❧ **Ginsengs are key brain nutrients:**
-Crystal Star SUPER GINSENG 6™.
-Crystal Star MENTAL INNER ENERGY™ extract.
✻Ginseng/Gotu Kola capsules. ♂
✻Ginseng/Damiana capsules. ♂

❧ **Herbal brain foods:**
✻Rosemary
✻Royal jelly
✻Fo-Ti root
✻Parsley/sage tea

Supplements

Alcohol, tobacco and drugs depress brain function - increasing the need for neurotransmitter replenishment through brain foods nutrients.

❧ **Anti-oxidants are the brain key:**
✻Pycnogenol 50mg 3x daily ♀
✻CoQ₁₀ 60mg 2x daily.
✻Nature's Bounty. B₁₂ internasal gel
✻Premier GERMANIUM with DMG daily, esp. if there is brain cancer.
✻Carnitine 500mg daily. ♀

❧ Glutamine pwdr. ¹/₄ teasp. with Glycine pwdr. ¹/₄ teasp. ♀

❧ **Phosphatidyl Serine (PS)** 1000mg or Choline 600mg, or Phos. Chol. daily.

❧ **B Complex** 150mg. w/ extra niacin 500mg, and B₆.

❧ **Other good brain nutrients:**
✻Klamath POWER 3 caps
✻Source Naturals MENTAL EDGE
✻Chromium picolinate 200mcg ♂
✻Omega-3 fish/flax oils
✻Magnesium 800mg with GINKGO BILOBA extract ♂
✻Tyrosine 500mg
✻Zinc Picolinate 30mg daily ♂
✻Dr. Diamond DIAMOND MIND caps
✻Super Nut. EINSTEIN'S FORMULA ♂

Lifestyle Support Therapy

More oxygen and increased circulation are the bodywork goals for better brain function. Build more brain circuits by reading and playing mental games. (Do a Sunday crossword puzzle.)

☞ Get some mild aerobic exercise, such as a daily 20 minute walk. Practice deep brain breathing. (See Bragg's booklet on this subject.)

☞ Cheerfulness, optimism and relaxation assure better brain function. (Listening to music is especially good.)

☞ Tobacco, alcohol, marijuana inhibit brain release of vasopressin, impairing memory, attention and concentration.

☞ **Reflexology point:**

squeeze all around fingers and hand

☞ Position of the brain in the body:

See also MENTAL HEALTH page in this book for more information.

Common Symptoms: Spaciness and lack of concentration; inability to remember well or for a reasonable length of time.
Common Causes: Lack of protein, potassium or other minerals that causes mental burnout; overwork with no rejuvenating "down time"; stress; sometimes viral activity; poor diet.

Bronchitis
Acute & Chronic

Chronic bronchitis is an infectious condition in which excessive mucous is secreted in the bronchi. The typical victim is forty or older, with lowered immunity from prolonged stress, fatigue or smoking. The disease usually develops slowly over a course of years, but will not go away on its own. Bronchial walls thicken and the number of mucous glands increases. The person becomes increasingly susceptible to respiratory infections. The recent type of viral bronchitis, which affects women, is very hard to treat, and lasts from 3 weeks to 5 months. Chronic bronchitis can be incapacitating, and lead to serious, even potentially fatal lung disease. Acute bronchitis, inflammation of the bronchial tree, is generally self-limiting, like a bad chest cold, with eventual complete healing.

Diet & Superfood Therapy

ᕫ Go on a short mucous cleansing liquid diet (pg. 162) to clear the body of mucous. Then follow a largely vegetarian, cleansing diet for 3 weeks. Reduce fats, dairy, salt and clogging heavy foods.

☞Take cleansing soups broths, hot tonics, high vitamin C juices, vegetable juices and green drinks. (pg. 168).

☞Take lemon juice in water each morning and flax seed tea each night during acute stages to alkalize the blood and cleanse the colon.

☞Avoid sugars, dairy, starchy, and fatty foods during healing to reduce congestion. Keep the bowels clean so that the system can eliminate excess mucous.

ᕫ **Make an onion/honey syrup:** Put 5 to 6 chopped onions and ¹/₂ cup honey in a pot and cook over very low heat for two hours. Strain and take 1TB. every two hours; or use the onion garlic broth on page 171.

☙

ᕫ **Effective superfoods:**
☞**Crystal Star SYSTEMS STRENGTH™ drink mix daily for 1 month.**
☞AloeLife ALOE GOLD 2 TBS. daily.
☞Liquid chlorophyll 1 tsp. in water before each meal.

Herbal Therapy

ᕫ **Jump start herbal program:**
Crystal Star BRNX™ extract with ANTI-BIO™ capsules or extract 6x daily, with
☞**FIRST AID™ caps, 4 to 6 daily, a powerful anti-oxidant to relieve acute conditions, and X-PECT TEA™ expectorant, or GINSENG/LICORICE™, a tonic expectorant or GINSENG/REISHI extract.**

☞Follow with cayenne/ginger capsules to cleanse the inner system of tissue mucous. May also apply cayenne/ginger compresses to the chest.

ᕫ **Cardiotonic herbs:** 3 to 4 x daily:
☞Mullein
☞Cayenne/Garlic

ᕫ Han HONEY LOQUAT syrup. ☺

ᕫ **Expectorant herbs:**
☞Bayberry
☞Lobelia
☞USNEA extract ♂
☞Licorice root. ♂
☞Hyssop/horehound

ᕫ **Bronchitis tea formula:**
Steep in a pot with 4 cups water for 25 minutes - licorice rt., horehound, lemon grass, osha, coltsfoot, lobelia, pleurisy rt., mullein. ☺

Supplements

Avoid cough suppressants. Coughing helps get rid of mucous.

ᕫ Ester C or ascorbate vitamin C crystals with bioflavonoids 1000mg in water, 5-10,000mg or to bowel tolerance at first, then reducing to 3-5000mg daily. Take with magnesium 400mg 2x daily.

ᕫ Zinc lozenges as needed every two hours, with Cysteine 500mg for chest congestion and Flora VEGE-SIL to relieve inflammation. ♀

ᕫ **Matrix Health GENESIS H₂O₂ OXY-SPRAY on the chest.**

ᕫ **Bromelain 1500mg - as an anti-inflammatory daily.** ♀

ᕫ **Effective anti-oxidants:**
☞Twin Lab LYCOPENE for the lungs.
☞**Beta carotene 100,000IU with garlic caps 6 daily and bee pollen 1000mg.**
☞CoQ₁₀ 100mg 2x daily.
☞Country Life DMG SL tabs.

ᕫ Enzymatic Therapy THYMU-PLEX caps.

ᕫ Homeopathic remedies:
☞Hylands *HYLAVIR tabs.* ☺
☞B&T *Bronchitis/Asthma Aid.*

Lifestyle Support Therapy

Air pollutants are probably responsible for more chronic bronchitis than any other one cause. Avoid smoking, secondary smoke and smog-plagued areas. Get fresh air and sunshine every day.

ᕫ Take a hot sauna; follow with a brisk rubdown, and chest/back percussion with a cupped hand to loosen mucous.

☞Apply alternating hot and cold witch hazel compresses to the chest. Use eucalyptus oil in a vaporizer.

☞Deep breathing exercises daily, morning & before bed to clear lungs.

☞Avoid inhaling cold air. Cover mouth and nose with a scarf or mask so that infectious micro-organisms are not sucked into the lungs.

ᕫ Rub tea tree oil on the chest. ☺

ᕫ **Reflexology point:**

lungs

ᕫ Bronchi:

Common Symptoms: *Acute Bronchitis:* symptoms like a deep chest cold; slight fever; inflammation; headache, nausea, lung and body aches; hacking, mucous-producing cough. **Chronic Bronchitis:** bronchial tissue becomes inflamed, and mucous becomes thicker and more profuse; difficult breathing and shortness of breath from clogged airways; repeated attacks of acute bronchitis; chest congestion; mucous-producing cough and wheezing that lasts for 3 months or more; fatigue; weakness and weight loss; low grade lung infection.
Common Causes: High mucous and acid-forming diet; suppressive "cold preparations;" lack of exercise and poor circulation; smoking and smog; low immunity, stress and fatigue.

See "COOKING FOR HEALTHY HEALING" by Linda Rector-Page for a complete non-mucous forming diet.

Bruises, Cuts & Abrasions

Easy Bruising ✲ Hard To Heal Wounds

If there is continued, excessive and frequent bruising see a physician for a clotting time blood test.

Diet & Superfood Therapy

❧ The diet should be light, low fat, and mineral-rich to lay a solid foundation for strong capillaries and skin.
* Eat plenty of fresh greens every day.
* Eat vitamin K rich foods, such as alfalfa sprouts, sea vegetables, green peppers, citrus fruits and green vegetables.
* Avoid pasteurized dairy foods during healing. They are too clogging.

❧ For a cut or abrasion:
* Apply wheat germ oil directly.
* Apply honey.
* Squeeze a fresh lemon on the area to clean and disinfect.
* Apply an onion compress.

❧ For bruises:
* Apply wheat germ oil directly
* Take Solaray TURMERIC capsules
* Apply pineapple slices directly to a bruise; orange to a black eye ☘

❧ Effective superfoods:
Take a veggie drink once a week, especially for hard-to-heal wounds (page168).
* Crystal Star ENERGY GREEN™ drink.
* Crystal Star BIOFLAVONOID, FIBER & C SUPPORT™ drink.
* Sun CHLORELLA.
* **Solaray ALFAJUICE.**
* **Aloe Life ALOE GOLD drink.**
* Y. S. ROYAL JELLY/GINSENG drink.

Herbal Therapy

❧ **Jump start herbs for cuts & wounds:**
Apply Crystal Star ANTI-BIO™ gel with una da gato, or GINSENG SKIN CARE™ gel with germanium and vitamin C.
* **Take Crystal Star ANTI-BIO™ capsules or extract to prevent infection.**
* Apply aloe vera gel as needed.

❧ Take internally for cuts & wounds:
* **EVENING PRIMROSE OIL for hard to heal wounds with BILBERRY extract.**
* Propolis lozenges; take and apply propolis extract directly.
* **Deva FIRST AID drops, or Bach Flower RESCUE REMEDY drops.** ♀

❧ **Effective topicals for cuts & wounds:**
* Cayenne tincture to stop bleeding; take drops internally as needed for shock.
* PAU D' ARCO/ECHINACEA extract. ☺
* GOLDEN SEAL/MYRRH salve.
* Nature's Pharmacy MYR-E-CAL.
* St. John's wort oil.

❧ **Jump start herbs for bruises:**
* **Crystal Star SILICA SOURCE™ or bilberry extract for capillary strength and collagen formation and apply VARIVEIN™ roll-on, with Solaray CENTELLA-VEIN caps.**
* Golden seal solution
* Tea tree oil ☺
* **Body Essentials SILICA GEL.**

Supplements

❧ **For cuts & wounds:**
* Nutribiotic grapefruit seed extract SKIN SPRAY to counteract infection.
* Apply vitamin E oil. Take 400IU daily.

❧ Ester C w/ bioflavs. and rutin, 5 grams daily. Apply weak solution directly to cut.
* Take w. panto. acid 500mg for collagen formation; zinc picolinate 50mg 2x daily.
* Vit. K 100mcg 3x daily for clotting.
* Cal/mag/zinc tabs for faster healing.
* **Nutricology GERMANIUM150mg for a month if wound is slow healing.** ♂
* Enzymatic Therapy DERMA-ZYME ointment, especially for slow healing cuts. ♀

❧ **For bruises:**
* **Quercetin with bromelain 500mg. Take for 48 hrs. until bruising subsides.**
* Ascorbate vitamin C with bioflavs and rutin 1000mg every 2 hrs. during healing.
* Vitamin K, 100mcg 4 daily.

❧ **Apply to bruises:**
* Enzymatic Therapy CEL-U-VAR cream.
* Prick open/apply a vitamin A&D cap.
* Make a paste of bromelain/papain powders - apply directly; enzyme therapy.

❧ **Homeopathic remedies:**
* Arnica Montana and arnica cream
* Ledum for severe bruises ♀

Lifestyle Support Therapy

Do not take aspirin if you bruise easily.

☞ **For a cut or abrasion:**
* Place ice packs on the area immediately to stop bleeding and reduce trauma.
* Apply alternating hot and cold witch hazel compresses, or clean with H_2O_2 and apply tea tree oil drops every 2 to 3 hours.
* Apply B & T *CALIFLORA*, or a good calendula gel. Then apply homeopathic *Hypericum* tincture. Note: For a deep cut do not apply calendula gel right away. It heals so fast that the outside closes up before the inside is healed. Apply after the inside begins to heal.
* Yarrow compresses for clotting.
* Essential thyme oil - white blood cells.

☞ **For bruising:**
* Apply ice often; squeeze bruise to release blood congestion; rub vigorously.
* Matrix Health Genesis OXY-SPRAY. ♀
* Apply B & T *ARNIFLORA* gel.
* **Make strong rosemary/thyme tea. Strain; add to a hot bath. Soak 25 min.**
* Rosemary essential oil after a bruise.

☞ **Effective compresses for bruises:**
* Comfrey rt. and comfrey cream.
* Aloelife ALOE VERA SKIN GEL.
* DMSO a.m. and p.m. for 3 days. ♀

Common Symptoms: *For bruises: Black and blue skin discoloration; sometimes vein damage.*
Common Causes: Bruises: *Vit. K deficiency; thin capillary and vein walls; poor collagen formation; mineral-poor diet. Easy bruising is usually found in people who are overweight, or who take anti-clotting drugs.*
Unusual easy bruising is also an early warning sign of cancer. Hard to heal wounds: occur because bioflavonoids are deficient.

Burns

1st, 2nd & 3rd Degree ✤ Sunstroke / Heatstroke

Get medical help fast for anything other than a first degree or small second degree burn. Don't use over-the-counter-burn medications over large body areas or for serious burns. They are for minor burns only. If there is severe itching, redness or swelling, or if fever, chills or great fatigue appear, get to a medical clinic.

Diet & Superfood Therapy

✥ Apply ice water immediately, then vinegar soaked compresses.

✥ Drink plenty of fluids, especially potassium broth (pg. 167) and veggie drinks (pg. 168). Get plenty of proteins and mineral-rich foods for fast tissue repair.

✥ **For immediate relief with no blistering or irritation, dip cotton balls in strong fresh ginger juice or strong black tea and apply.**

✥ Effective compresses:
—Honey ☺
—Cold black tea
—Egg whites or raw potato for scalds.
—Use baking soda or cider vinegar in warm water for acid/chemical burns.

✥ Electrolyte replacement foods for heatstroke/suntroke:
—**Alacer EMERGEN-C, 2 pkts. in water.**
—Lemonade, limeade, mineral water.

✥ Effective superfoods:
—Nutribiotic PRO GREENS.
—Crystal Star ENERGY GREEN™ drink.
—Crystal Star BIOFLAVONOID, FIBER & C SUPPORT™ drink.
—Future Biotics VITAL K several times daily for fluid loss.
—Sun CHLORELLA 1 pkt. daily.

Herbal Therapy

✍ **Jump start herbal program:**
—Apply Aloe Life ALOE SKIN GEL to stop burning; then Crystal Star ANTI-BIO™ GEL, or St. John's wort oil.
—**Use ANTI-FLAM™ caps or extract to take down swelling.**
—Bach Flower RESCUE REMEDY, especially if there is the threat of shock.
—Apply Calendula gel or Pau d' Arco gel frequently as needed.

✍ Effective herbal compresses:
—Comfrey root/wheat germ oil/honey
—Tea tree oil ☺
—Thyme oil
—White oak bark
—Flax oil and mullein ☺
—Chamomile
—Fresh plantain herb leaves

✍ Make a strong tea, strain and apply:
#1 Elder blossoms, red clover, yarrow and golden seal. Strain and apply.
#2 Comfrey, nettles, marshmallow, scullcap, red clover and apply.

✍ Flora VEGE-SIL caps, Crystal Star SILICA SOURCE™ extract or horsetail tea for healing and new collagen formation.

✍ **Green tea or gotu kola tea, 2 cups daily for nerve and tissue healing.**

Supplements

✦ **Nutribiotic grapefruit seed extract SKIN SPRAY to counter infections.**

✦ **Effective antioxidants:**
—Nutricology GERMANIUM 150mg.
—Ascorbate vitamin C 3-5000mg daily. Make a solution of **ascorbate** crystals in water and apply.
—Apply natural vitamin E oil every 3-4 hours. Take vitamin E w. selenium.

✦ American Biologics SUB-ADRENE for cortex formation 3 drops, 3x daily.

✦ **Homeopathic burn remedies:** *Arnica* for severe burns, followed by:
—*Hypericum* tincture
—*Apis* for a stinging burn
—*Phosphorus* for electrical burns
—*Urtica Urens* for 2nd degree burns that itch and sting.

✦ For fluid loss:
—B Complex 100mg.
—Solaray CAL/MAG with D and potassium for fluid/potassium loss.

✦ Proteolytic enzymes for healing, especially bromelain 500mg and papain.

Lifestyle Support Therapy

☞ Flush with cold water; then apply ice packs until pain is relieved.
—Apply Matrix Genesis OXY-SPRAY.
—AloeLife ALOE SKIN GEL.

☞ **Effective, soothing applications:**
—Colloidal silver to combat infection.
—Body Essentials SILICA GEL frequently.
—Cold green clay poultices.
—New Chapter ARNICA GINGER GEL.

☞ **If the burn is 3rd degree, treat for shock until help arrives.**
—Cayenne: 1/4 teasp. tincture, or 2 opened capsules in 1 tsp. warm water for shock.
—Cut away loose clothing that has not adhered to the skin.
—Apply ice water if skin is not charred. If charred, apply cloths dipped in aloe vera gel or juice, or a fresh comfrey leaf poultice.

☞ **For sunstroke/heatstroke:**
—Apply ice packs and wrap the person in a cold wet sheet. Get medical help for shock immediately. See SHOCK THERAPY, page 401.
—Give the person an electrolyte drink or a little salty water. No alcoholic drinks- they dehydrate.

Common Symptoms: *1st degree - sunburn or heat exposure, minor blistering and pain.*
2nd degree - blistering, scarring, gland structure damage; hair follicles burned off.
3rd degree - extensive tissue damage; oozing, charring, severe loss of body fluids; electrolyte loss and shock.

Heat and sunstroke are an over-reaction to heat and sun exposure, characterized by rapid pulse, and a "shocky" condition which can even lead to brain damage.

See also SUNBURN/SKIN DAMAGE for more information.

Bursitis

Acute & Chronic Tendonitis ✤ Tennis Elbow

Inflammatory conditions in the tendons or bursa, the sac-like membrane that contains joint protecting fluids. Both conditions can develop calcified deposits in the shoulder, elbow, hip or knee. Both can result from strain, a blow to the affected body part, or in the case of bursitis, as a secondary symptom of arthritis or rheumatism.

Diet & Superfood Therapy

See the ARTHRITIS DIET in this book for more information.

❧ Relieve pain from acidosis by avoiding acid-forming foods, such as caffeine, salts, refined foods, red meats, and nightshade plants like tomatoes and eggplant.

❦Keep the body vegetarian and alkaline with foods like celery, avocados, potatoes, wheat germ, sweet fruits, sprouts, greens, brewer's yeast, oats and sea vegetables.

❦Keep the kidneys flushed with carrot/beet/cucumber juice.

❧ For organic calcium uptake:
❦Salmon and sea foods
❦Dark leafy greens
❦Cultured foods
❦Broccoli and cauliflower

❧ Take high Omega-3 flax oil 1 tsp. 3x daily. Improvement usually in 2- 6 weeks.

❧ Effective superfoods:
❦Crystal Star BIOFLAVONOID, FIBER & C SUPPORT™ drink as needed.
❦Solaray ALFAJUICE. ♀
❦Aloe Falls ALOE/GINGER JUICE.

Herbal Therapy

❧ Jump start herbal program:
❦ADR-ACTIVE™ capsules for essential cortex formation, and RELAX™ capsules for stress relief.
❦Apply Body Essentials SILICA GEL to joints. Take internally as directed.
with
❦Nutricology GERMANIUM 150mg and PRN PAIN-FREE gel.

❧ Alive Energy MAXIMUM MOBILITY.

❧ Apply B&T *TRI-FLORA* analgesic gel, or hot comfrey/olive oil compresses.
with
Solaray TURMERIC capsules as an anti-inflammatory.

❧ Apply a lobelia/mullein poultice.

❧ Change body pH:
❦ Crystal Star ALKALIZING/ENZYME BODY WRAP™ (almost immediate).
❦Cornsilk tea to flush kidneys
❦Crystal Star CLEANSING & PURIFYING TEA™.
❦ Alta Health CANGEST caps or Natren BIFIDO FACTORS. ♀

Supplements

❧ Enzyme therapy:
❦Biotec EXTRA ENERGY ENZYMES with SOD 6-10 daily.
❦Quercetin Plus 3 daily with extra bromelain 500mg.
❦Prevail MOBIL-EASE.

❧ For inflammation:
❦Enzymatic Therapy ACID-A-CAL capsules to dissolve sediment.
❦American Biologics INFLAZYME FORTE as directed.

❧ Country Life LIGA-TEND as needed, or 4 daily.

❧ Take DLPA 500-750mg as needed.

❧ Nature's Bounty B₁₂ nasal gel.

❧ Ascorbate vitamin C or Ester C with bioflavonoids and rutin 3000mg daily for collagen formation.

❧ Solaray BIO-ZINC or zinc picolinate daily.

❧ American Biologic A & E EMULSION FORTE with SUB-ADRENE extract.
and
❦Niacinamide 500mg 2x daily for 1 week, then once daily with DMG 125mg.

Lifestyle Support Therapy

Smoking and tobacco are acid-producing habits.

☙ Take a mineral or epsom salts bath once a week. Apply hot castor oil packs to affected areas.
❦Use affected area gently. Intense athletic activity is inadvisable until trauma is relieved.
❦Acupuncture is effective for bursitis.

☙ Apply ice packs to inflamed area during acute stages. Apply wet warm compresses in later stages for fast healing.
❦ Matrix Health GENESIS OXY-SPRAY to affected areas every 24 hours.
❦DMSO roll-on as needed.
❦Biochemics PAIN RELEAF.

☙ Regular mild aerobic and stretching exercises keep joint system free.

☙ Reflexology point:

shoulder
shoulder

Common Symptoms: *Both tendonitis and bursitis involve inflammation and tenderness where tendons affix to bones, causing limited motion in the affected body part. The pains are usually severe and shooting with swelling and redness, especially in the morning and in damp weather. Intense pain when lifting or backward rotating the arm.*
Common Causes: *Poor diet causing metabolic imbalance; stress; toxemia; a direct blow or repetitive pressure to a bursa area.*

See also ARTHRITIS pages in this book for more information.

Cancer

Whole Body Recommendations

By the turn of the century, cancer is expected to be the number one cause of death in America. Cancer used to be extremely rare. Is our late twentieth century lifestyle really that bad? The dramatic increase is only minimally due to new diagnostic tests or to new technology instead of nature. Over 200 different diseases are now classified as cancer. Chasing every cancer classification with a drug for the different requirements and ramifications of each one is futile. I feel the only chance for success is to use every part of our lifestyle to normalize cells that are out of control.

Diet & Superfood Therapy

Make your vegetable juices fresh in a juicer to help stop cancer pain.

❧ Follow the macrobiotic diet on the next page to begin healing.

➻Have miso, shiitake mushrooms, sea veggies and brewer's yeast every day.

➻Take a carrot/beet/cucumber juice once a week to clean liver and kidneys.

➻Reduce meat proteins and fat.

❧ **The best cancer-fighting foods:**

➻**carotene-rich foods:** carrots, yams, all red, orange and yellow fruits, green vegetables, tomatoes, red grapefruit.

➻**antioxidant-rich foods:** garlic, onions, broccoli, wheat germ, sea vegetables and leafy vegetables.

➻**steamed cruciferous vegetables:** broccoli, cabbage, cauliflower, kale.

➻**protease inhibitors:** beans (esp. soy), rice, potatoes, corn.

➻**high fiber foods:** whole grains, especially brown rice, fruits and vegetables.

➻**lignan foods:** fish, flax oil, walnuts.

❧ **Effective superfoods:**

➻AloeLife ALOE GOLD juice.
➻Green Foods GREEN ESSENCE drink
➻BeWell juices, tomato and fruit.
➻Y.S. ROYAL JELLY/GINSENG drink. ♂
➻Sun CHLORELLA 2 pkts. daily.
➻Klamath BLUE-GREEN SUPREME.

Herbal Therapy

❧ **Jump start herbal program:**

➻**Ginseng therapy shows outstanding results. Crystal Star CAN-SSIAC™ extract tea and GINSENG/REISHI extract.**

➻**Especially with iodine therapy: J.R.E. IOSOL extract or Crystal Star SYSTEMS STRENGTH™ drink daily.** ♀

or

❧ Crystal Star DETOX™ capsules and PAU D' ARCO/ECHINACEA extract as directed, and GREEN TEA CLEANSER™ every morning. ♂

with

➻**Maitake mushroom extract daily, and turmeric (curcumin) extract daily.**

❧ **Cancer-fighting herbs:**

➻Siberian ginseng extract or capsules
➻**Una da gato - especially if liver fluke parasites are involved (most cancers)**
➻GINSENG/LICORICE ELIXIR™.
➻Pau d'arco tea, 4 cups daily.
➻Garlic - an anti-oxidant, 6-10 daily.
➻GINKGO BILOBA to enhance immunity.
➻Health Aid America SIBERGEN.

❧ **Herbs to reduce the effects of chemotherapy and radiation:**

➻Reishi mushroom
➻Astragalus
➻Echinacea/goldenseal root caps
➻High Omega-3 flax oil, 3x daily.

Supplements

Too much iron may increase the risk of cancer. We recommend iron-rich herbs instead of supplements if you need iron.

☞ Nutricology MODIFIED CITRUS PECTIN as directed, with
➻Enzymatic Therapy THYMUPLEX.

☞ **Enzyme therapy:**
➻**Quercetin Plus w/Bromelain 3x daily.**
➻Rainbow Light ADVANCED ENZYME SYSTEM.
➻Enzymatic Ther. QUERCEZYME PLUS.
➻Prevail VITASE.
➻Natren TRINITY, for liver support.

☞ **Cartilage is a key:**
➻Lane Labs BENE-FIN caps.
➻Nutricology CAR-T-CELL emulsion.
➻VitaCarte BOVINE TRACHEAL cartilage.

☞ **Anti-oxidants are anti-carcinogenic:**
➻Nutricology GERMANIUM 150mg
➻CoQ₁₀ 200mg 3x daily
➻Beta carotene 100,000IU 2x daily
➻PCOs 100mg 3x daily
➻Ester C with bioflavonoids 6 daily
➻Orange Peel Ent. PRO-N-50 PLUS ♂
➻Biotec CELL GUARD w. SOD ♀

☞ Experimental ANTI-NEOPLASTIN THERAPY. Ask your alternative health care provider.

Lifestyle Support Therapy

☞ Get aerobic exercise regularly. It is an antioxidant nutrient in itself. No healing program will make it without some exercise.
➻Get some sunlight on the body every day possible (esp. for organ cancers).

☞ Avoid tobacco in all forms, synthetic hormones, particularly estrogen, X-Rays, excessive alcohol and caffeine.

☞ **Take a coffee enema once a week for a month (1 cup strong brewed in a qt. of water) or chlorella implants.**
➻**Wheat grass retention enema.**

☞ Poultices for external growths:
➻AloeLife ALOE SKIN GEL
➻Garlic/onion poultice
➻Comfrey leaf poultice
➻Green clay poultice
➻**Crystal Star GINSENG SKIN REPAIR™ GEL or ANTI-BIO™ gel with una da gato.**

☞ Apply Matrix Health GENESIS OXYGEL to affected areas, or rub on soles of feet every 24 hours; and/or take a frequent energy/oxygen bath (pg. 176).

☞ Apply kukui nut oil for chemotherapy or radiation burning. ♀

Common Causes: Cancer in not a single entity with a single cause, but a complex, multi-dimensional disease involving many factors. Ninety percent of all cancer is a result of diet and lifestyle habits or environmental pollutants and chemicals. At least 20,000 of the 70,000 chemicals people come in contact with regularly are toxic. Hereditary factors account for 5% of cancer cases, but even these are largely influenced by diet and environment. Lifestyle causes mean that we can positively affect many cancer source factors ourselves - both to prevent cancer from occurring and helping ourselves when it has.

See the following pages for signs, early symptoms and recommendations for specific cancer sites.

Intensive Building & Balancing Macrobiotic Diet

A macrobiotic diet is very effective against cancer, helping to rebuild healthy blood and cells, and preventing diseased tissue from continued growth. This way of eating is non-mucous forming, low in fat foods that can alter body chemistry and enhance cancer potential in the cells, and high in vegetable fiber and protein. It is stimulating to the heart and circulatory system through its emphasis on oriental foods such as miso, bancha green tea, and shiitake mushrooms. It is alkalizing with umeboshi plums, sea vegetables and soy food. It is high in potassium, natural iodine and other minerals. Its greatest benefit is that it is cleansing and strengthening at the same time, and offers a truly balanced way of eating that is easily individualized for one's environment, the seasons, and the constitution of the person using it. The strict form recommended here for an intensive healing program should be followed for three to six months.

Before each meal, and before bed, take 2 to 4 TBS. aloe juice concentrate in water (detoxifies and eases nausea if you are undergoing chemotherapy or radiation).
On rising: take a potassium broth or essence (page 167), or carrot/beet/cucumber juice, or cranberry concentrate (2 teasp. in water) or red grape juice; and a vitamin/mineral drink such as Nutritech ALL 1, or Crystal Star SYSTEMS STRENGTH™, or a vegetable superfood drink like Green Foods BETA CARROT.

Breakfast: a mix of 2 TBS. each: brewer's yeast, wheat germ, lecithin, bee pollen granules. Sprinkle some on a whole grain cereal, granola or muesli; or mix with yogurt and dried fruit; use on fresh fruit, such as strawberries or apples with kefir or kefir cheese; add a whole grain breakfast pilaf such as Kashi, bulgur or millet, with apple juice or kefir cheese topping.

Mid-morning: take a veggie drink (pg. 168), Sun CHLORELLA, Green Foods GREEN MAGMA, Crystal Star ENERGY GREEN™ or fresh wheat grass juice. Add 1 teasp. Bragg's LIQUID AMINOS; and/or an herb tea, such as pau d'arco, Essiac tea, or Crystal Star CAN-SSIAC™ drops in water as a tea, or MEDITATION™ tea; or a glass of fresh carrot juice, or a cup of miso soup, such as Organic Gourmet MISO BROTH & GINGER, with sea vegetables snipped on top. (Have 2 TBS. dry sea vegetables daily.)

Lunch: have some steamed broccoli or cauliflower with brown rice, tofu and a little soy cheese; or an oriental stir fry with brown rice and miso sauce; or a fresh green salad with whole grain pitas; or a black bean, onion or lentil soup, or a 3 bean salad; or falafels in pita bread with some raw or steamed veggies and tamari dressing; or a cabbage slaw with oriental sesame dressing.

Mid-afternoon: a cup of green tea, Crystal Star GREEN TEA CLEANSER™, and some whole grain crackers with kefir cheese or a soy spread; or raw veggies dipped in gomashio.

Dinner: have a brown rice, millet, bulgur, or kasha casserole with tofu, or tempeh and some steamed vegetables, or a hearty dinner salad with some sea veggies, nuts and seeds, and whole grain bread or chapatis, or baked, broiled or steamed fish or seafood with rice and peas or other veggies, or a baked veggie casserole with mushroom/yogurt or kefir cheese sauce; or stuffed cabbage rolls with rice, and baked carrots with tamari and a little honey.

Before bed: have a cup of Organic Gourmet savory mushroom or ginger broth, or a relaxing herb tea, such as alfalfa/mint or red clover tea, or a glass of organic apple juice.

NOTE: IN ORDER FOR THE MACROBIOTIC BALANCE TO BE SET UP AND WORK CORRECTLY WITH THE BODY, SEVERAL FOODS AND FOOD TYPES MUST BE AVOIDED:
• Red meat, poultry, preserved, smoked or cured meats of all kinds, and dairy products
• Coffee, black teas and carbonated drinks
• Nightshade plants, such as tomatoes, potatoes, peppers and eggplant
• Sugars, corn syrup and artificial sweeteners; and tropical and sweet fruits
• All refined, frozen, canned and processed foods; hot spices, white vinegar, and table salt

SUPPLEMENTS AND HERBAL AIDS FOR THE INTENSIVE MACROBIOTIC DIET:
• Maitake mushroom extract or tea several times daily; wheat germ oil or germanium 150mg to add tissue oxygen.
• Ascorbate vitamin C crystals in water 3 to 5000mg daily, with GINKGO BILOBA EXTRACT drops.
• Mega-potency acidophilus and Green Foods GREEN MAGMA or chlorella or Crystal Star SYSTEMS STRENGTH™ drink to combat the effects of chemotherapy.
• Crystal Star CAN-SSIAC™ extract with panax ginseng, IODINE/POTASSIUM SOURCE™ capsules, and high omega-3 FLAX OIL to inhibit tumor growth.

BODYWORK FOR THE INTENSIVE MACROBIOTIC DIET:
• Get morning sunlight and mild exercise every day possible to accelerate the passage of toxins.
• Overheating therapy is effective for degenerative disease. See page 178 for the proper technique at home.

See COOKING FOR HEALTHY HEALING by Linda Rector Page for an initial cleansing and complete diet program for cancer control.

An Objective Look At Cancer

The natural healing world regards cancer as an unhealthy body whose defenses can no longer destroy abnormal cells - a view that has engendered remarkable healing success.

Here is a new look at cancer facts you can use to make healing choices.

• Cancer cells are normal cells that have been altered by a chemical or other insult that allows the cell to survive, but without the controls of normal cells. Cancer cells can no longer do their assigned job for the body. Cancer cells have only one job....to survive.

• Cancers are opportunistic, attacking when immune defenses and bloodstream health are low. Promote an environment where cancer and degenerative disease can't live - where inherent immunity can remain effective. These diseases do not seem to grow or take hold where oxygen and minerals (particularly potassium) are high in the vital fluids.

• Most cancers are a result of poor diet and nutrition. Many cancers respond well to diet improvement. Nutritional deficiencies accumulate over a long period of time - too much refined food, fats and red meats; too little fiber and fresh foods; natural vitamin and mineral imbalances. These deficiencies eventually change body chemistry. The immune system cannot defend properly when biochemistry is altered. It can't tell its own cells from invading toxic cells, and sometimes attacks everything or nothing in confusion.

• Cancerous cells seem to crave dead de-mineralized foods. If you like junk foods, starving them out isn't easy, but as healthy cells rebuild, the cravings subside.

• Cancers seem to live and grow in the unreleased waste and mucous deposits in the body. Avoid red meats, pork, fried foods, refined carbohydrates, sugars, caffeine, preserved or artificially colored foods, heavy pesticides and sprayed foods. All of these clog the system so that the vital organs cannot clean out enough of the waste to maintain health.

• Enzyme therapy is effective against cancer. It improves immune response, it chemically alters tumor by-products to lessen cancer's side effects, and it changes the tumor's surface to make it vulnerable to immune system response. Avoid antacids. They interfere with enzyme production, and the body's ability to carry off heavy metal toxins.

• **Love your liver!** It is a powerful chemical plant that keeps the immune system going. **Love your thymus!** It is the seat of the immune system.

• Anti-angiogenesis is effective against cancer to prevent new blood supply for cancer cell division and growth. Shark cartilage and bovine tracheal cartilage interrupt angiogenesis.

• Overheating therapy has been effective against cancer. See page 178 for an in-home method.

• Glutamine deprivation therapy is effective against cancer. Glutamine is needed for cancer cell division. A product called Tributyrate interrupts cancer cells from storing glutamine.

• Guided imagery has been effective in helping the immune system to work better, and the hormone system to stop producing abnormal cells.

• Regular exercise is almost a "cancer defense" in itself. Exercise acts as an antioxidant to enhance body oxygen use; it also accelerates passage of waste out of the body. Exercise alters body chemistry to control fat retention, a key involvement with cancer.

• The best chance for cancer isn't drugs or surgery - it's diet and lifestyle choices you can make yourself. Fresh foods, superfoods and herbs (and the phyto-chemicals they contain), are very powerful cancer fighters. You may have to return to a juice and raw foods diet several times, but the deep body healing power is there.

• To treat cancer successfully, you must enhance immune response first.

Cutting Your Risk

How can we take more control of our health and our lives to prevent cancer? It seems like we're assaulted from all sides by cancer activators that we can't control. It's easy to get the idea that anything and everything can cause cancer. Yet, most cancer is preventable. You can go a long way toward protecting yourself and your family from cancer-causing factors.

Here are 6 watchwords for cutting your risk:

1 Improve your diet in 3 ways: **#1)** Reduce your intake of fat. Environmental toxins become lodged in the fatty tissue of the animals in our food chain, and in tissue of humans who are exposed to them. Fat from cancer tissue regularly tests almost double the safe amount of chlorinated pesticides. **#2)** Reduce your intake of red meats. Cancer onset is closely related to the protein and fat in red meats, fast foods and fried foods. **#3)** Eat vegetables every day. The more fruits and vegetables you eat, the less your cancer risk, regardless of the type of cancer. People who eat plenty of fruits and vegetables have half the risk of people who eat few fruits and vegetables. Even small to moderate amounts of fruits and vegetables make a big difference. Two fruits and three vegetable servings a day have shown amazing anti-cancer results. Eating fruit twice a day, instead of twice a week, can cut the risk of lung cancer by 75%, even in smokers. Avoid tobacco in any and all forms.

3 Keep your immune system strong. U.S. industries alone generate 88 billion pounds of toxic waste per year. The EPA estimates 90% of them are improperly disposed of. Environmental toxins can damage cell DNA, which leads to cell mutation and tumor development.

4 Use enzyme therapy in 2 ways: **#1) Have a fresh green salad every day as a source of hydrolytic enzymes to stimulate immune response. #2)** Take CoQ$_{10}$ 30mg daily to give the immune system a boost.

5 Detoxify and cleanse your body at least twice a year. Certain superfoods and juices accelerate natural body detox activity and prevent the genetic ruin of cells, a prelude to cancer.

2 Exercise at least 3 times a week. While one out of three Americans falls victim to cancer, only one out of seven **active** Americans does.

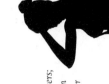
Breast Self Exam

Recommendations For Specific Cancer Sites

Cancer is not one disease, but many. There are four types of cancerous growths: 1) **carcinomas**, which affect the skin, glands, organs and mucous membranes; 2) **leukemias**, which are blood cancers; 3) **sarcomas** which affect connective tissue, bones and muscles; 4) **lymphomas**, which affect the lymph system. There can be more than one type of cancer in a particular location. The link between all cancers is that certain cells have been de-sensitized to normal growth constraints. The damaged cells grow uncontrolled and may move (metastasize) to other sites in the body. Obviously, cancer is complex. There is no simple solution. Vigorous treatment is necessary on all fronts. But, more people are overcoming this devastating disease every day.

Use the specific site recommendations along with the general cancer healing recommendations on page 254.

Breast Cancer

Over 185,000 women fall victim to breast cancer **every year. Over 50,000 die of it annually.** Post-menopausal, overweight women have the highest risk, with 75% of all cases occurring in women over 40. Being more than 25% above your recommended weight increases risk, because fat cells store environmental estrogens, pesticides, organo-chlorine residues and other chemical toxins, proven cancer causes. Weight gain around age 30 increases the long-term risk of breast cancer, too. A 10-pound increase raises the risk by 23%, a 15-pound increase by 37%, and a 20-pound increase by 52%. Also at risk are women who have overly high, or imbalanced estrogen secretions, e.g., those who had their first period before age 12, those who did not go through menopause until after age 55, those who did not have a child before age 30, and those who did not carry a pregnancy full-term. Women who have a diet high in meats and dairy products have a higher risk. Many food animals are injected with hormones that add to the environmental estrogens circulating in a woman's body. Women who eat soy foods have lower levels of circulating estrogen. Vegetarians have fewer instances of breast cancer because they process estrogen differently...and they are less exposed to hormone-injected animals like beef and pork. Long term synthetic estrogen and/or oral contraceptive use, and estrogen-containing pesticides are also a risk factor for breast cancer. Indeed, there is a veritable assault on female hormone balance from man-made estrogens. Regular exercise is a key to fighting breast cancer, because it favorably alters body chemistry to control fat retention which stores excess estrogen, and to increase fat metabolism, which helps flush out excess and environmental estrogens. Try to limit your exposure to environmental estrogens.

The largest breast cancer increase is in women who were born in the baby boom after World War II, an era that ushered massive amounts of chemicals and new drugs, such as super-strong antibiotics, hormone therapy, and processed foods into American life. Most were developed during the press of wartime, without the normal years of testing for long term health effects. After the war, a great many of these substances got incorporated into agriculture and household products. Most pesticides, household chemicals and common plastics - the major estrogen imitators, did not exist before World War II. Man-made estrogens, also called environmental or xenestrogens, can stack the deck against women by increasing their estrogen levels hundreds of times. Only in the last five years has anyone realized how common environmental estrogens are in today's world. Smoking and long secondary smoke exposure increase risk, women with low melatonin levels are more at risk, women who work around electromagnetic fields have a 38% greater risk. Breast or prostate cancer in a woman's father's family doubles her risk. Chemotherapy does **not** seem to improve a woman's chances for survival, especially if the cancer has spread to the lymph nodes.

About mammograms: Radiation from X-Rays can severely harm breast tissue and cell balance, especially those from older mammography machines. Although mammograms have improved in the last 20 years both in clarity and amount of dosage, we still hear enough horror stories about swift fibroid onset to recommend that mammograms should not be done routinely or without suspected cause. Because a younger women's breasts are so dense, a mammogram screening her breasts only detects dangerous lesions about 50% of the time. No study has shown that death rates from breast cancer are reduced by mammogram screening in women under 50. Since even low-dose radiation can cause breast fibroids, mammograms in this age group should only be necessary if there are abnormal findings such as lumps or nipple infections. Even in women over fifty, where the effect of radiation is less, if there is no family breast cancer history or suspected reason for alarm, mammograms should be undertaken with care. Check out your chosen facility thoroughly. By the time a tumor has reached the size that can be detected, it has probably been growing for 10 years or more and has likely spread to other body areas. While early detection can mean less radical medical intervention, early detection is not prevention. A healthy lifestyle should be the primary goal.

Symptoms include discharge from the nipple, breast lumps or thickening, scaly skin patches around the nipples; change in breast texture or color, persistent enlargement of lymph nodes in the armpit, breast changes that are not related to regular menstrual cycle, chronic swelling and sores around the mouth, gums or jaw, hypothyroidism, especially if linked to iodine deficiency.

Therapy: Reduce the fat in your diet to 15% or less of calorie intake. Especially avoid fats from sugary foods, dairy products and high sugar alcohol. Increase your fiber and anti-oxidants from fruits, vegetables, whole grains and beans. Especially add vegetables like broccoli, cabbage, and cauliflower, because these vegetables contain elements with estrogen-reducing effects. Reduce or eliminate all meats in your diet, even chicken and turkey, unless you can find an organic supply that has no hormone injections. Fish is fine. Salmon is especially beneficial. Add sea vegetables to your diet. Certain minerals, such as copper, zinc, chromium, manganese and magnesium are critical to detoxification pathways in the body. They protect us from the cancer-promoting effects of chemical overload. Sea vegetables are a highly absorbable source of plant minerals. Hypothyroidism is regularly involved in breast cancer. Sea vegetables are a naturally-occurring iodine source that balances thyroid activity. Two TBS. daily of dried sea vegetables are a therapeutic dose; or take Crystal Star POTASSIUM/IODINE caps. Add selenium for extra antioxidant protection 200mcg. daily.

Take Crystal Star EST-AID™ extract or PRO-EST WOMEN'S DEFENSE™ roll-on - lab-tested, proven cancer inhibiting formulas. Take REISHI/GINSENG extract, 2 times daily for 6 months. Take royal jelly, ¼ teasp. daily in panax ginseng tea to boost adrenal activity. Take EVENING PRIMROSE OIL, 2000mg daily. Use fresh rosemary in your cooking; drink rosemary tea frequently.

Add vitamin C, up to 10,000mg with bioflavonoids, (or quercitin 1000mg), and Co-Q₁₀, up to 300mg daily. Add shark or bovine tracheal cartilage (or Nutricology CAR-T-CELL), to inhibit the formation of new blood vessels that feed tumor growth. Both cartilage substances have shown remarkable activity, even when standard therapy failed. Take PCO's, 100mg 3x daily (from white pine bark or grape seeds). They are some of the most potent antioxidants and free radical scavengers known.... 50% more potent than vitamins E or C. Consider Nutricology LACTOFERRIN - one of the newest natural therapies to show promise for breast cancer. Low body levels of the antioxidant hormone melatonin may raise breast cancer risk. Consider a small melatonin supplement of .1 to .3mg at night.

Prostate Cancer

Prostate cancer is the most common cancer in males in the U.S., striking one in nine men over age seventy. Today, striking at an ever earlier age, over 200,000 new cases of prostate cancer are detected every year, with the annual death rate approaching 50,000 men. Prostate cancer is clearly associated with the conversion of normal testosterone to di-hydro-testosterone by the enzyme 5-alpha reductase, which is itself a consequence of a high fat, high sugar, low fiber diet. and high cholesterol foods like red meats. A low-fat, vegetarian diet is a proven weapon against this kind of cancer, because high fiber, low-fat foods excrete hormones linked to prostate cancer. Since sperm counts have dropped by 50% and prostate cancer has doubled in the last 50 years, new studies are focusing on environmental estrogens and other pollutants as they affect male hormones, and put men (as well as women) at risk. A monthly self-exam should be a part of your prevention plan, especially if you are over fifty. Consider with caution, supplemental melatonin .1 to .3mg, at night as a prostate cancer deterrent.

About the PSA test: The medical world has gotten better at diagnosing prostate cancer, largely because of super-sensitive blood tests like the Prostate Specific Antigen (PSA) test. In fact, the PSA test is producing an epidemic of prostate radiation and surgery, the treatment of choice for prostate cancer in America. Radiation and surgery procedures are escalating even though they can be as devastating as the disease, and studies indicate that surgery only extends life a few months at best. Almost 2% of men die within 90 days of prostate cancer surgery, and 8% experience severe heart and lung complications. Both treatments regularly cause incontinence and impotence, because surgery and radiation damage nerves that lead to the penis and rectum. Over 10% of men become impotent after surgery for prostate cancer, and more than 12% become incontinent. Radiation treatments also frequently initiate a free radical cascade that reduces immune response. Always get a second opinion if you are diagnosed with prostate cancer. While most elderly men have some prostate cancer cells, most do not die of prostate cancer. It is such a localized, non-invasive form of cancer, that life expectancy with surgery and radiation is practically the same as with no treatment. The European way of "watchful waiting" would seem to be a better choice for avoiding the enormous pain and disability if surgery is not absolutely necessary. There is, however, growing concern worldwide about invasive prostate cancer, which rapidly engulfs the organ and spreads throughout the body. The incidence of this deadly form of prostate cancer is noticeably increasing among men in their 40's and 50's in all industrialized countries.

Symptoms include lumps in prostate and/or testicles, thickening and fluid retention in the scrotum, and persistent, unexplained back pain. There is frequency of urination, difficulty in starting and stopping urination, feelings of urgency or straining, and other symptoms similar to prostatitis. As the cancer outgrows the small prostate gland, it often eats its way into the bladder or rectum, or even the pelvis and back, causing severe damage.

Therapy: Improve your diet immediately: Reduce dietary fats to 15% or less of calorie intake. Include carotene-rich, antioxidant, lycopene-rich foods like tomatoes, and/or beta-carotene 100,000IU daily. Add soy foods to your diet. The soybean has at least five proven anti-cancer agents, with anti-estrogenic activity that can retard the development of hormone related cancers such as prostate cancer. Add 4 to 6 grams of fiber to your daily diet from complex carbohydrates such as those in whole grains, vegetables and fresh or dried fruits. Have a fresh green salad every day. Especially add cancer-fighting, cruciferous vegetables like broccoli and cauliflower, and other green and orange vegetables.

Ginseng/royal jelly therapy has been successful. Take Y.S. or Beehive Botanical products with these two ingredients daily. Take una da gato and GINSENG/LICORICE ELIXIR™. Both the ginsenosides of panax ginseng and the triterpenoids of licorice root have been tested for their ability to stifle quick-growing cancer cells and in some cases, cause pre-cancerous cells to return to normal. Add a phyto-hormone-rich herbal compound to balance hormone levels. Crystal Star PROX™ and PRO-EST PROX™ roll-on with saw palmetto, pygeum, and potency wood have been lab tested for inhibiting the DHT form of testosterone. Take EVENING PRIMROSE oil as an EFA, 4 daily to suppress the growth of prostate cancer cells, and zinc 50mg daily. Valuable supplements include a glycine, alanine, glutamic acid amino acid combination to normalize sugar use in the body, antioxidants like CoQ$_{10}$, 300mg daily, shark or bovine tracheal cartilage capsules (or Nutricology CAR-T-CELL), and garlic capsules 8 daily to retard cancerous cell growth. Take vitamin C 10,000mg daily (best as an ascorbic acid flush - page 445), glutathione 50mg 2x daily and cysteine 500mg daily. Add PCOs from grapeseed or white pine, 100mg 2x daily, especially for invasive prostate cancer. Exercise is a must for men dealing with prostate cancer, as well as early morning sunlight on the body for vitamin D, at least 15 minutes every day possible. (African American men have a 40% higher rate of prostate cancer than white men because they synthesize less vitamin D. Black men should consider supplementing with 400IU vitamin D daily.)

✂

Cervical, Uterine (Endometrial) Cancer

Overweight women are particularly likely to develop cancer of the cervix and/or uterine lining. Post menopausal women, between the ages of 55 and 75, especially those who have never been pregnant, (or conversely, have had more than five births), are vulnerable. Women who take "estrogen only" replacement therapy (ERT) for menopausal symptoms are especially at risk (symptoms are clearly aggravated by excess estrogen). Women with high blood pressure, and those who have used oral contraceptives for 5 or more years at a time, those who have a history of sexually transmitted diseases, especially cervical dysplasia, and those who have benign uterine fibroids, have all recently been linked to cervical and uterine cancer. If localized cervical cancer is not treated, it usually spreads to underlying connective tissue, nearby lymph glands, the uterus, and the genito-urinary tract. Serious vaginal infections such as trichomonas, and exposure to carcinogenic substances, such as heavy metals, asbestos, herbicides and nicotine, should be warning signs. The drug tamoxifen can also increase the risk of endometrial cancer.

Early symptoms include unusual bleeding or discharge between menstrual periods, painful, heavy periods, vaginal discharge or bleeding during intercourse indicating the presence of polyps.

Therapy: Reduce fatty meats, red meats, eggs and butter in your diet immediately. The correlation between these foods and uterine cancer is undeniable. Fresh fruits and vegetables (especially cruciferous vegetables, carrots and artichokes) are protective for their fiber and anti-carcinogen nutrients. Include soy foods in your diet 3 times a week for protein and genistein. Avoid tobacco - it secretes toxins into cervical mucous, significantly increasing the risk of cervical and endometrial cancer. Take calcium to prevent pre-cancerous lesions from becoming cancerous. Take EVENING PRIMROSE OIL, or high Omega-3 flax oil daily. Take high potency royal jelly 2 teasp. daily, oceanic-carotene 100,000IU daily Ester C 5 to 10,000mg daily, vitamin E 800IU daily with selenium 200mcg. Take green superfoods such as Green Foods GREEN MAGMA, or Crystal Star ENERGY GREEN™ drink. Use Transitions PROGEST CREAM™ for natural progesterone protection.

Note: the American Cancer Society has quietly dropped its recommendation that women have a PAP test every year - advocating it only if the woman is at high risk. If you have a Type II PAP smear, take green drinks daily, use Crystal Star WOMAN'S BEST FRIEND™ capsules for 3 to 6 months, Lane Labs BENE-FIN shark cartilage 6 daily, and folic acid 800mcg daily.

✂

Colon & Colo-rectal Cancer

Because America's diet is still loaded with fat and low in fiber, colon cancer has become the number two cause of cancer death in the United States, 150,000 people die every year from colon cancer. Overweight men are particularly at risk. A low fat, high fiber diet can dramatically reduce the development of benign polyps that usually lead to colon cancer. **Experts estimate that 90% of colon cancer is avoidable through diet improvement!** Other risk factors include a family history of colon cancer (mostly from family diet habits), severe ulcerative colitis or Crohn's disease. Smoking is linked to colon cancer. There may be pain and gas in the lower right abdomen. Colon cancer begins as polyps on the colon walls. For precancerous polyps, take vitamin C with bioflavonoids 5000mg daily and Green Foods GREEN MAGMA drink. You can test for colon cancer yourself. See self test on page 448.

Symptoms include persistent diarrhea, changing to persistent constipation for no apparent reason, blood in the bowel movement, and a change in shape of the stool to a thin, flattened appearance. There is also unusual weight loss and fatigue.

Therapy: high fiber and low fat are still the dietary key for colon cancer. Add whole grain cereals, (particularly wheat bran) fresh vegetables, especially cruciferous vegetables, soy foods as protease inhibitors and for genistein estrogen balance, legumes and other high fiber (but low roughage) foods, like dried fruits, to the diet. Include carotene-rich, antioxidant foods like tomatoes, fresh greens and cruciferous vegetables. Have a green salad every day. Add calcium rich foods like dark greens and broccoli. Numerous studies show that daily exercise and sunshine lower the risk of colon cancer. Drink a cup of green tea or Crystal Star GREEN TEA CLEANSER™ daily.

Inhibitory antioxidant vitamins include vitamin C 5000mg daily with bioflavonoids, beta carotene 100,000IU, vitamin E 800IU with selenium 200mcg Omega-3 rich flax oil (effective in reversing precancerous changes in the rectum) and folic acid 800mcg daily. Drink green tea, or Crystal Star GREEN TEA CLEANSER™ daily as a preventive; flax seed tea for fiber and cleansing. Take Nutricology MODIFIED CITRUS PECTIN as directed. Take CoQ$_{10}$, 60mg 5x times daily, L-Carnitine 500mg daily and acidophilus 3x daily with meals to normalize the colon environment.

Garlic is a proven colon cancer inhibitor; 6 to 10 capsules daily, may reduce tumors by 75%. Turmeric extract (curcumin) reduces tumor development. Take shark cartilage, to inhibit tumors from forming new blood vessels. Tumors even shrink from lack of nutrients as the blood vessels shrivel. Shark cartilage is also rich in calcium, a specific preventive for colon cancer. Bovine tracheal cartilage helps the immune system resist abnormal growth of cancer cells, by activating lymphocytes that slow down cell multiplication. Take a GLA source such as EVENING PRIMROSE oil, 6 daily or flax seed oil. Ginseng-based adaptogen combinations are proving to speed healing and normalize cell structure. Ginseng enhances antibody response, strengthens the immune properties of the cellular connective substance, lowers or raises red and white blood cells according to need, normalizes cell structure and has a distinct activity against radiation. GINSENG/REISHI extract has shown clinical results against colon cancer cells. People who have had polyps surgically removed recover faster and build more healthy new cells when they drink a ginseng tea such as Crystal Star GINSENG 6 SUPER TEA™ during healing. GINKGO BILOBA and astragalus extracts nourish the body's defense system against tumor development. Shiitake mushrooms contain the much studied polysaccharide, lentinan, an anti-cancer agent and immune cell stimulant.

Note: The herbal formula ESSIAC appears to be effective for colon cancer. But in our own experience, it does not go far enough toward immune enhancement, nor is it complex enough to address cancer as it exists today. Crystal Star CAN-SSIAC™ formula with pau d'arco for immune response, and panax ginseng for reverse transformation activity on malignant cells may be more effective.

Ovarian Cancer

Women at risk seem to be those who have never had children, who are past menopause and overweight from a high fat diet, and have a family history of cancer. Long term estrogen replacement therapy increases ovarian cancer risk. NutraSweet is implicated in ovarian cancer. Avoid it, especially in hot drinks. Check product dates that contain NutraSweet. Old NutraSweet breaks down into DKP, a tumor-causing product. Talcum powder is linked to ovarian cancer. The mineral particles get trapped in the ovarian (and fallopian) tissue. Use a talc-free condom during intercourse, and do not dust your perineum with talcum. Asbestos exposure is also implicated, as well as certain anti-inflammatory drugs (salicylates, non-steroidals, and cortico-steroids).

Symptoms: In early stages, ovarian cancer is asymptomatic, except for some bloating and abdominal discomfort. There are often no symptoms until the cancer has metastasized.

Therapy: Add omega-3 rich flax oil to your diet, or take EVENING PRIMROSE OIL 1000mg daily. Enrich your diet with fresh fruits and vegetables, especially cruciferous vegetables. Keep fats low, and include soy foods for protein instead of meats or dairy products. Add sea vegetables as a source of iodine therapy, especially if a thyroid disorder is involved. Avoid fried foods and eggs.

Take shark cartilage or bovine tracheal cartilage as directed to arrest angiogenesis growth of tumors. Take high potency royal jelly 2 teasp. daily with ginseng. Take Crystal Star GINSENG/LICORICE ELIXIR™. Add anti-oxidant supplements - beta-carotene 100,000IU daily, especially from marine sources; Ester C, up to 10,000mg with bioflavonoids daily, vitamin E 800IU daily with selenium 200mcg. Take garlic 8 - 10 capsules daily. Take green superfoods such as Green Foods GREEN MAGMA, or Crystal Star ENERGY GREEN™ drink. Use Transitions PRO-GEST CREAM for natural progesterone protection. Early morning sunlight protects the ovaries with vitamin D. Get 15 minutes of sunlight on the body daily.

Bladder / Kidney Cancer (Renal Cell Carcinoma)

Bladder and kidney cancers are rising in America, (more than 50,000 new cases every year) especially in women who started smoking in the decades of 1960 to 1980. Smoking has been implicated as the main cause in both bladder and kidney cancers. A history of cystitis and polycystic kidney disease add to the risk.

Signs and Symptoms include blood in the urine, urinary difficulty, sometimes side or loin pain. (These can also be signs of problems other than cancer.)

Therapy: Increase your intake of fresh vegetables, especially carrots, or Green Foods BETA CARROT. Have fruit in the morning and at night before retiring. Have cold water fish twice a week. Studies show that probiotics, like high potency lactobacillus help prevent bladder cancer recurrence. Take Nutricology MODIFIED CITRUS PECTIN (MCP). Increase your anti-oxidant intake with beta-carotene 100,000IU, vitamin E 800IU, vitamin C 5000mg, 200mg B$_6$, folic acid 800mcg, and zinc 50mg daily. Add sea vegetables to your diet for further antioxidants and iodine therapy.

Lung Cancer

Smoking and second-hand smoke exposure hurts everybody and puts everyone more at risk for cancer, even unborn fetuses. Even with all the media and medical attention on the hazards of smoking, lung cancer is still rising in the U.S. - at the astounding rate of **153,000 deaths per year, and 175,000 new cases annually.** Eighty-five percent of lung cancer cases are attributable to cigarette smoke, (including the new, potentized marijuana strains, which are 100 times more likely to cause lung cancer than cigarettes). The remaining 15% is attributed to heavy metal, toxic chemicals (pesticides and herbicides), radioactive exposure, chronic bronchitis and T.B.

Symptoms include a persistent cough and chest pain, hoarseness, a sore throat, and increasingly, blood in the sputum. The cough changes and worsens, and chest pain increases as the cancer grows. There is unusual sweating, feverishness and unhealthy weight loss as the disease progresses.

Therapy: Primary therapy is fresh fruits and vegetables, especially lycopene-rich foods like tomatoes. I recommend at least 3 servings of fresh vegetables 3 times a day. Lung cancer has been reduced by 75% with this nutritional therapy! Concentrate on high carotene foods and dark orange and green vegetables. Regard broccoli as a healing gift for lung cancer. Reduce all dairy foods in your diet. Your increased vegetable intake can supply more absorbable calcium sources. Add sulphur-rich garlic and onions to your **daily** diet, and soy foods 3 times a week. Reduce fat calories to no more than 20% of your diet. Drink green tea daily or take Crystal Star GREEN TEA CLEANSER™. Take beta-carotene, 100,000IU particularly from marine sources. Take Crystal Star MINERAL SPECTRUM™ capsules, rich in watercress, a proven lung cancer deterrent. Take vitamin E 1000IU with selenium 200mcg, B complex 150mg, Vitamin B₁₂ w/ folic acid, Nutricology GERMANIUM 200mg, and Nutricology LACTOFERRIN as directed; garlic 6 - 10 daily, royal jelly with Siberian ginseng extract 4x daily, and reishi mushroom tea or capsules for interferon. Apply Matrix Health GENESIS OXY-GEL to the chest regularly.

Stomach & Esophageal Cancer

A high fat, low fiber diet is always linked to stomach cancer and stomach polyps. The elderly are particularly at risk, because of decreasing HCL production and lack of dietary fiber. Stomach cancer takes a long time to develop, sometimes as much as fifteen years. Smoking is a high risk factor. Dietary habits contribute to onset - a high intake of meat proteins and nitrates, and low intake of fresh fruits, vegetables and olive oil (and the vitamins C and E in them).

Major Symptoms: Pernicious anemia; chronic indigestion and gastritis; pain after eating.

Therapy: A diet with plenty of fresh vegetables is the key, especially cruciferous vegetables, like broccoli and cabbage. I recommend at least 3 servings per meal for antioxidants and vitamin C. Add soy foods to your diet, at least three times a week for protease inhibitors. Add whole wheat and wheat bran. Eat garlic and onions in some form every day, and add garlic 8 caps daily or Enzymatic Therapy GARLINASE. Add glutathione-rich foods like avocados, asparagus, grapefruit, oranges and tomatoes, or take glutathione 50mg 2x daily. Limit alcohol to a small drink a day. Limit salt to less than 2500mg a day. Limit cured meats and smoked foods like bacon, ham or hot dogs, and eat them with a source of vitamin C like broccoli or green peppers. Reduce caffeine intake. Drink green tea, or Crystal Star GREEN TEA CLEANSER™ as therapy and a preventive. Take green superfoods, like Green Foods GREEN MAGMA or Crystal Star ENERGY GREEN. Take CoQ₁₀ 60mg 3x daily. Take proteolytic enzymes, such as Enzymatic Therapy PROTA-ZYME, or Solaray HCL with PEPSIN, and pancreatin for protein digestion. Take Crystal Star GINSENG/LICORICE ELIXIR™ daily. Eat small frequent meals - no large meals. Inhibitory vitamins are beta-carotene, C and E 800IU with selenium 200mcg. Take garlic 10 tabs daily. Take shark cartilage caps, 8-14 daily before meals.

Liver & Pancreatic Cancers

Organ cancers are some of the most difficult to deal with, because they are so deep in the body, because their influence on other parts of the system is so widespread, and because they metastasize quickly. Beware of the drug *loratadine*, an antihistamine. It causes liver tumors in animal testing.

Therapy: Guided imagery is successful as a method of reaching liver and pancreatic cancers. Use magnetic therapy, especially to reduce abdominal bloating. Avoid alcohol consumption. Reduce fats and add soy foods to your diet, at least three times a week as a protease inhibitor. A diet with plenty of fresh vegetables is the key, especially cruciferous vegetables, like broccoli and cabbage, and lycopene-rich foods like tomatoes. I recommend at least 3 servings per meal for antioxidants and vitamin C. Green drinks are essential: Crystal Star ENERGY GREEN™, Green Foods GREEN ESSENCE or GREEN MAGMA, or Sun Chlorella WAKASA GOLD. Add high omega-3 flax oil 2 teasp. and Enzymatic Therapy LIQUID LIVER to any drink. Use Nutricology CAR-T-CELL shark emulsion. Herbal medicines have a proven record. Mega-doses are important at first. Include in your therapy: schizandra, MILK THISTLE SEED, garlic, dandelion, GINKGO BILOBA, pau d'arco, ECHINACEA, goldenseal, saw palmetto, Crystal Star GINSENG/LICORICE ELIXIR™ and Solaray ALFAJUICE tablets. **Enzyme therapy is critical in organ cancers (like Nature's Secret REZYME program).** Enzymatic Therapy MEGA-ZYME, pancreatin, and proteolytic enzymes, CoQ₁₀ 300mg daily, L-Carnitine 500mg daily, Chromium picolinate 250mg daily, Glutathione 100mg daily, and vitamin C 10,000mg with bioflavonoids daily.

Brain Cancer

Most brain tumors grow very slowly, for years, but when they become large, progressive problems develop quite rapidly. The use of pesticides in pest strips have been linked to brain cancer, especially in children. Excessive intake of Nutrasweet in sodas and pre-prepared foods has produced a high incidence link with brain tumors. The brain is also often a site for the metastasis of other tumors, usually from the lungs and breast. **Symptoms** include fatigue, skin itchiness, night sweats, unusual weight loss, stomach discomfort (because of a swollen spleen); anemia is usually present.

Therapy: Drink plenty of raw vegetable juices and AloeLife ALOE GOLD juice (use ALOE MASTERS for children). Use superfoods like Green Foods GREEN ESSENCE, or WHEAT GERM extract. Use a fresh grape juice poultice on the nape of the neck. Leave on until dry; continue treatment until tumor regresses. Take Premier GERMANIUM w. DMG 3x daily. Take vitamin E with selenium 200mcg. Take GINKGO BILOBA extract to increase brain circulation. Use Nutricology VITA-CARTE bovine tracheal cartilage for glioblastoma multiform tumors.

Lymphoma

Lymphomas are cancers of the lymphatic system, including Hodgkin's and non-Hodgkin's diseases and lymphatic leukemia. Lymphomas are related to mercury fillings in the mouth. Check them first to see if you should have them removed. Exposure to herbicides, solvents and vinyl chloride petro-chemicals have been implicated in both Hodgkin's and non-Hodgkin's diseases, especially when immunity was already compromised because of long term conditions like hypoglycemia or prescription drug addiction.

Early signs include swollen lymph nodes. If the lymph nodes stay swollen for more than 3 weeks, you should get a medical diagnosis. Frequent and often painful, burning urination; blood in the urine; extreme lethargy.

Therapy: Start with a liver cleansing diet, (See page 163 in this book.) Green superfoods have shown the most promise, especially Sun Chlorella WAKASA GOLD, and AloeLife ALOE GOLD drinks. Use American Biologics DIOXYCHLOR as directed, reishi or maitake mushroom extracts, Nutricology GERMANIUM 200mg daily, high potency royal jelly, ¹/₂ teasp. 4x daily, and Crystal Star ANTI-BIO™ extract 6 daily to clear the lymph nodes of poisons.

❧

Skin Cancer

Skin cancer is an undeclared epidemic of our time. It is the most common (one in every three cancers is skin cancer), and the fastest rising (800,000 new cases each year) of all cancers. Over 90% of skin cancers are caused by over-exposure to the sun's harmful ultra-violet rays, radiation that is increasing in toxicity as the earth's protective ozone layer is steadily depleted. There is also evidence that a genetic predisposition to certain reactions with the sun's UV rays is involved. Exposure to coal tar, creosote, and radium all show up in skin cancers. Age (usually 55 or over), and gender (50% more males gets skin cancer), are factors. Caucasians and people who have received a blistering sun-burn any time in their lives are most at risk.

There are 3 kinds of skin cancer: 1) **squamous cell carcinoma**, fast growing, characterized by a red papule or a psoriasis-looking patch with scaly crusted surface, appearing on sun-exposed areas of the body. Later, it becomes hard and nodular; may become a lesion on the face, lips or ears. Generally curable with appropriate treatment; 2) **basal cell carcinoma**, least dangerous, but most common. They do not metastasize, are characterized by small, shiny, firm nodules, or ulcerated crusted lesions that look like local dermatitis. A shiny, pearly border develops after 3 or 4 months with a central ulcer; **malignant melanoma**, a deeply rooted cancer that arises from the same type of cells found in moles. It is serious, and can be fatal, because it can metastasize to other organs of the body, especially lymph nodes. Early signs of melanoma look just like a freckle or mole. Warning signs include itchiness, tenderness, hardening, or any visible change in size or color in the mole.

Diet Therapy: Reduce the fat in your diet immediately. Stop smoking. Smoking is linked to recurrence of skin cancers. Eliminate alcohol; reduce wine intake to 2 small drinks a day or less. Eat leafy greens every day. Eat green, orange and yellow vegetables at least three times a week. Eat cold water fish like salmon twice a week. Take 1 teasp. each, wheat germ oil and brewer's yeast in AloeLife ALOE GOLD juice 2x daily: Avoid sugars, caffeine and caffeine-containing foods.

General skin cancer therapy: Drink green tea, or take Crystal Star GREEN TEA CLEANSER™ super tea and apply GINSENG SKIN REPAIR GEL™. Take highest potency Beehive Botanicals ROYAL JELLY with propolis and ginseng to normalize skin cells. Alpha hydroxy acids help normalize the epidermis, such as Zia Cosmetics CITRUS NIGHT TIME SMOOTHER. Take CoQ₁₀ 60mg daily, and EVENING PRIMROSE OIL caps 1000mg daily for better cell oxygenation. Take Flora VEGE-SIL for connective tissue growth. Take proteolytic enzymes like Enzymatic Therapy PROTA-ZYME, and/or bromelain 1500mg to reduce swelling. Take turmeric capsules with 2 cups of burdock tea daily. Take Nutricology GERMANIUM 150mg as an immuno-stimulant.

For basal cell carcinomas: Use American Biologics DIOXYCHLOR, or Genesis OXY-GEL, Aloe Life ALOE SKIN GEL, ascorbate or Ester C powder, ¹/₂ teasp. hourly to bowel tolerance during healing, for collagen production and connective tissue growth, and shark cartilage capsules. Also open a shark cartilage capsule and mix with ¹/₄ teasp. vitamin C crystals and DMSO as a skin transporter and apply. Results usually in 3 to 4 weeks.

For squamous cell carcinoma: Take beta carotene 100,000IU (or drink Be Well CAROTENE JUICES), vitamin E 800IU w/ selenium, and apply tea tree oil, BioForce ECHINACEA CREAM, a germanium solution in water, a garlic paste, (also take garlic capsules 6 to 8 daily).

For malignant melanomas: Eat a few apricot kernels every day, take pycnogenol 100mg 3x daily, and apply Matrix Health GENESIS OXY-GEL or American Biologics DIOXYCHLOR, Apply Crystal Star ANTI-BIO™ gel, calendula gel, or a goldenseal/myrrh solution. Apply a vitamin C /garlic paste solution, or open a shark cartilage capsule and mix with ¹/₄ teasp. vitamin C crystals and DMSO as a skin transporter and apply.

Wear protective clothing when out in the sun, Always use sun screen, and avoid tanning salons and sunlamps if you are fair skinned. Get early morning sunlight on the skin every day for 15 minutes. Early sun can help heal ulcerations. Midday sun aggravates them. Skin cancer healing applications include hot comfrey compresses, dry mustard plasters, tea tree oil, propolis tincture, green clay poultices, B & T CALIFLORA gel, or Centipede KITTY'S OXY-GEL on affected area, and on to soles of feet. (Usually a noticeable change in 3 weeks.)

❧

CANCER PREVENTION
is the key

Candida Albicans

Candidiasis ❧ Thrush ❧ Leaky Gut Syndrome

Candidiasis is a state of inner imbalance, not a germ, bug or disease. Candida albicans is a strain of yeasts commonly found in the gastro-intestinal and genito-urinary areas of the body. It is generally harmless, but when resistance and immunity are low, the yeast is able to multiply rapidly, feeding on sugars and carbohydrates in these tracts. It releases toxins into the bloodstream, and causes far-reaching problems. It is a stress-related condition, brought about because the body is severely out of balance and the immune system is seriously compromised. Repeated rounds of antibiotics, birth control pills or cortico-steroids, a nutritionally poor diet high in refined carbohydrates and alcohol, and a lifestyle short on rest encourage candida.

Diet & Superfood Therapy

The food recommendations for the initial diet are critical for controlling candida yeast proliferation to normal levels. Candida yeasts grow on carbohydrates, preserved, processed and refined foods, molds, and gluten breads.

🌿 **Do not eat the following foods for the first month to 6 weeks:** Sugar or sweeteners of any kind, gluten bread and yeasted baked goods, dairy products (except plain kefir or kefir cheese, yogurt or yogurt cheese), smoked, dried, pickled or cured foods, mushrooms, nuts or nut butters (except almonds and almond butter), fruits, fruit juices, dried or candied fruits, coffee, black tea, caffeine, carbonated drinks, (the phosphoric acid binds up calcium and magnesium) alcohol or foods containing vinegar. Avoid drugs, like anti-biotics, steroids, cortico-steroids, and tobacco.

❋*This is a long, restrictive list,* but for the first critical weeks, when the energy-sapping yeasts must be deprived of nutrients and killed off, it is the only way.

🌿 **Acceptable foods during the first stage:** Plenty of fresh and steamed veggies (especially onions, garlic, ginger root, cabbage, and broccoli) poultry, seafoods and sea veggies, olive oil, eggs, mayonnaise, brown rice, amaranth, buckwheat, barley, millet, soy and vegetable pastas, tofu and tempeh, plain yogurt, rice cakes/crackers, some citrus fruit and herb teas. Have a green drink and/or miso soup every day.

❋*This is a short, limited list;* but diet restriction is the most important way to stop yeast overgrowth.

Herbal Therapy

Use herbs to restore body homeostasis.

🌿 **Jump start herbal program:**
To kill the yeasts:
❋Pau d' Arco tea 4 cups daily, or Crystal Star PAU D' ARCO/ECHINACEA extract, CAND-EX™ caps with FEM-SUPPORT™ extract and CRAN-PLUS™ tea.
❋Add BLACK WALNUT EXTRACT and garlic 6-10 capsules daily, and CHOLO FIBER TONE™ 3 times a week.

🌿 **For adrenal and thyroid support:**
❋Crystal Star SYSTEMS STRENGTH™
❋**Crystal Star ADR-ACTIVE™**
❋EVENING PRIMROSE OIL caps
❋Enzymatic Therapy ADRENAL complex

🌿 **For bowel /digestive regulation:**
❋Crystal Star GINSENG/LICORICE ELIXIR.
❋**Crystal Star BWL-TONE IBS™ caps.**
❋AloeLife FIBER-MATE drink.
❋Chamomile tea, 4 cups daily.
❋Planetary Formulas TRIPHALA caps.

🌿 **Build immunity/discourage infection:**
❋Pau d' Arco tea soak for nails.
❋ECHINACEA extract, tonic dose.
❋Astragalus and hawthorn extracts.
❋Crystal Star ANTIOXIDANT CAPS™.

🌿 **For tissue oxygen:**
❋Nutricology GERMANIUM 150mg.
❋Rub Genesis OXY-SPRAY on abdomen.

🌿 **To clean the liver and detoxify:**
❋Crystal Star LIV-ALIVE™ caps.
❋Natren BIFIDO-FACTORS.
❋MILK THISTLE SEED extract.

Supplements

Rotate anti-yeast and antifungal products, so that yeast strains do not build up resistance to any one formula.

🌿 **Bowel flora/probiotic therapy:**
❋**Natren BIFIDO FACTORS.**
❋Prof. Nutr. DR. DOPHILUS as directed. (May also be used as a vaginal application.)

🌿 **Anti-fungals to help kill the yeasts:**
❋Am. Biologics DIOXYCHLOR.
❋Solaray CAPRYL.
❋Shark cartilage as directed.
❋**Natren GY-NA-TREN caps and inserts.**
❋**Nutribiotic GRAPEFRUIT SEED extract.**

🌿 **Use enzyme therapy for allergies:**
❋Bromelain 750mg daily.
❋Enzymatic Therapy PROTA-ZYME and MEGA-ZYME.
❋Pancreatin 1400mg with HCL.

🌿 **For liver and immune support:**
❋**Red marine algae.**
❋**Biotin 1000mcg with Nature's Secret ULTIMATE B complex and taurine.**
❋Zinc picolinate 50mg.
❋Oceanic carotene 100,000IU.
❋Enzymatic Therapy IMMUNO-PLEX and LIVA-TOX formulas.

🌿 **Effective superfoods & protein drinks:**
❋**Crystal Star ENERGY GREEN™ drink.**
❋JRE EGG WHITE PROTEIN.
❋Nutricology PROGREENS.
❋**Future Biotics VITAL K.**
❋Aloe Falls ALOE GINGER juice.
❋AloeLife ALOE GOLD concentrate.

Lifestyle Support Therapy

Exercise and oxygen, and a positive mind and outlook are essential to overcome this body stress. Have a good laugh every day.

🌿 Use applied kinesiology to test for food and product sensitivities.
❋Avoid antibiotics, birth control pills and steroids unless absolutely necessary.

🌿 Get enough sleep. Adequate rest is primary for the body to overcome debilitating, yeast-induced fatigue.

🌿 **Effective vaginal treatment:**
❋**Soak infected areas in tea tree oil solution. Use in water as a vaginal douche.**
❋**Nutribiotic GRAPEFRUIT SEED extract as a vaginal douche or enema.**
❋**Garlic douche or vaginal insertion.**
❋**Acidophilus capsule insertions.**
❋**Make up a garlic, echinacea, myrrh solution in a squirt bottle and wash perineum after defecating to keep from reinfecting.**

🌿 For thrush: use tea tree oil, homeopathic *thuja,* Nature's Pharmacy MYR-E-CAL, and BLACK WALNUT extract. Disinfect toothbrush with 3% H_2O_2 frequently.

🌿 **Reflexology point:**

Liver — Adrenals
Colon

See also NAIL FUNGUS *and* SKIN FUNGAL INFECTIONS.

Do You Have Candidiasis?

Most of the orthodox medical community still chooses not to recognize, diagnose or treat Candidiasis seriously. Thus, the alternative professions of Naturopathy, Homeopathy, Chiropractors and massage therapists have seen and dealt with most cases over the past fifteen years. Their energy and dedication have dramatically advanced the knowledge and understanding of the symptoms and etiology of Candidiasis, to better pin-point symptoms and treatment, to shorten healing time, to lessen overkill, and to understand the large, overriding psychological aspect of the disease.

☞**Ask yourself the following questions as a measure of self-diagnosis. Several "yes" answers should alert you to Candidiasis.**

• Have you recently taken repeated rounds of antibiotic or corticosteroid drugs, such as Symycin, Panmycin, Decadron, Prednisone, etc. or acne drugs for 1 month or longer?
• Have you been troubled by PMS, vaginitis or vaginal yeast infections, endometriosis, abdominal pains, prostatitis, or loss of sexual interest?
• Are you bothered by unexplained frequent headaches, muscle aches and joint pain?
• Do you crave sugar, bread, or alcoholic beverages?
• Are you frequently bothered by chronic fungal infections, such as ringworm, jock itch, nail fungus, athlete's foot? Or hives, psoriasis, eczema or chronic dermatitis?
• Are you over-sensitive to tobacco, perfume, insecticides, or other chemical odors?
• Do you have recurrent digestive problems, gas or bloating? Do you have chronic constipation alternating to diarrhea?
• Are you now taking, or have you previously taken birth control pills for more than 2 years? Have you been pregnant more than twice?
• Are you bothered by chronic fatigue, erratic vision, spots before the eyes, poor memory or continuing nervous tension?
• Do you feel depressed and sick all over, yet the cause cannot be found? Are the symptoms worse on damp, muggy days with joint and muscle pain?

Note: While Candida symptoms appear mostly in women, men and children also get yeast infections. Both sexual partners need to be treated because candida is passed back and forth during intercourse. See "THRUSH" in the Children's Ailments section, and the Fungal Skin Infections page for more information concerning yeast overgrowth in men and children.

☞**Symptoms for candida albicans overgrowth occur in fairly defined stages:**

   1st symptoms: Bowel and bladder problems; heartburn; chronic indigestion with flatulence and bloating; recurring cystitis or vaginitis; chronic fungal skin rashes and nail infections.
   2nd symptoms: Allergy/immune reactions such as asthma, hives, sinusitis, eczema, hayfever, acne; frequent and chronic headaches or migraines; muscle pain and burning; earaches; chronic bronchitis; sensitivity to odors.
   3rd symptoms: Central nervous system reactions, such as extreme irritability; confusion; a "spacey" feeling and night time panic attacks; memory lapses and the inability to concentrate; chronic fatigue and lethargy, often followed by acute depression.
   4th symptoms: Gland and organ dysfunctions such as hypothyroidism, adrenal failure, and hypoglycemia; ovarian problems, frigidity and infertility; male impotence and lack of sex drive.
Note: Candida albicans can mimic the symptoms of over 140 different disorders. For instance, chronic fatigue syndrome, salmonella, intestinal parasite infestation and mononucleosis exhibit similar symptoms, but are treated very differently. Have a test for candida before starting a healing program to save time, expense, and for more rapid improvement.

☞**Golden Rules for controlling candida overgrowth:**
   Candida albicans is an opportunistic yeast strain that takes advantage of lowered immunity to overrun the body. Healthy liver function and a strong immune system are the keys to lasting prevention and control of candida overgrowth. The whole healing/rebuilding process usually takes from 3-6 months or more, and is not easy. The changes in diet, habits and lifestyle are often radical. Some people feel better right away; others go through a rough "healing crisis." (Yeasts are living organisms - a part of the body. Killing them off is traumatic.) But most people with candida are feeling so bad anyway, that the treatment and the knowledge that they are getting better, pulls them through the hard times. Be as gentle with your body as you can. Give yourself all the time you need, at least 3 to 6 months. Of course you want to get better quickly, but multiple therapies all at once can be self-defeating, psychologically upsetting, and too traumatic on the system. Just stick to it and go at your own pace.

☞A COMPREHENSIVE, SUCCESSFUL PROTOCOL FOR OVERCOMING THIS DISEASE INCLUDES THE FOLLOWING STAGES:
   Stage 1: Kill the yeasts through diet change and supplement therapy. Avoid antibiotics, cortico-steroid drugs and birth control pills, unless there is absolute medical need.
   Stage 2: Cleanse the dead yeasts and waste cells from the body with a soluble fiber cleanser or bentonite. Colonic irrigation and herbal implants are effective here.
   Stage 3: Strengthen the digestive system by enhancing its ability to assimilate nutrients. Strengthen the afflicted organs and glands, especially the liver. Restore normal metabolism, and promote friendly bacteria in the gastro-intestinal tract.
   Stage 4: Rebuild the immune system. Stimulating immune well-being throughout the healing process supports faster results.

☞

Candida Cleansing Diet For The First Two Months Of Healing

Diet change is the most effective way to rebuild strength and immunity from candida overgrowth. The initial cleansing diet on this page concentrates on releasing dead and diseased yeast cells from the body. This phase usually requires 2-3 months for complete cleansing. It may also be used as the basis for a "rotation diet," in which you slowly add back individual foods during healing that caused an allergic reaction to candida. As you start to see improvement, and symptoms decrease (usually after three months), start to add back some whole grains, fruits, juices, a little white wine, some fresh cheeses, nuts and beans. Go slowly, add gradually. Test for a food sensitivity all along the way until it is gone. Don't forget that sugars and refined foods will allow candida to grow again.

Note: We have been working successfully with candidiasis since 1984 and have found repeatedly that a too-rigid diet does not work over the long term, because the sufferer cannot stick to it (except in a very restricted, isolated environment), and the body becomes imbalanced in other ways. In addition, we are learning that the disease itself, and the immune response to it are changing. The recommended diets in "HEALTHY HEALING" and "COOKING FOR HEALTHY HEALING" are real people diets, used by people suffering from candida who have shared their experience with us. They are being continually modified to meet changing needs and to take advantage of an ever-widening network of information.

***Make sure you are eating beta-carotene-rich foods, and iodine and potassium-rich foods. They are most effective food nutrients against candida.*

On rising: take 2 tsp. cranberry concentrate, or 2 tsp. lemon juice in water, or a fiber cleanser like AloeLife FIBERMATE or Crystal Star FIBER & HERBS COLON CLEANSE™ to clean the kidneys; or a cup of Crystal Star GREEN TEA CLEANSER™, or 1 teasp. raw unfiltered apple cider vinegar with 1 teasp. honey, if there is flatulence.

Breakfast: take NutriTech ALL 1 vitamin/mineral drink in water; then take 1 or 2 poached or hard boiled eggs on rice cakes with a little butter or flax oil;
or almond butter on rice cakes or wheat free bread; or oatmeal with 1 TB. Bragg's LIQUID AMINOS; or amaranth or buckwheat pancakes with a little butter and vanilla.

Mid-morning: take a vegetable drink (page 168) or Sun CHLORELLA or Green Foods GREEN MAGMA, or Crystal Star SYSTEMS STRENGTH™ in water;
or a cup of miso soup with sea veggies snipped on top;
or a cup of pau d' arco tea, or chamomile, barberry, or ECHINACEA EXTRACT drops in a cup of water; or a small bottle of mineral water.

Lunch: have a fresh green salad with lemon/olive, flax oil dressing, or Rohe pumpkin seed oil.
or open face rice cake or wheat free bread sandwiches, with a little mayonnaise or butter, some veggies, seafood, chicken or turkey;
or a vegetable or miso soup with sea veggies snipped on top with butter and cornbread;
or steamed veggies with tofu, sea veggies and brown rice;
or chicken, tuna or wheat-free pasta salad, with mayonnaise or lemon/ oil dressing.

Mid-afternoon: have some rice crackers, or baked corn chips, with a little kefir cheese or butter;
or some raw veggies dipped in lemon/oil dressing or spiced mayonnaise;
or a small mineral water and hard boiled or deviled egg with sesame salt or sea vegetable seasoning.

Dinner: baked, broiled or poached fish or chicken with steamed brown rice or millet with flax oil and veggies;
or a baked potato with Bragg's LIQUID AMINOS, or a little kefir cheese, or lemon oil dressing;
or an oriental stir fry with brown rice, sea veggies and a miso or light broth soup;
or a tofu and veggie casserole with sea veggies; or a small omelet with veggie filling;
or a vegetarian pizza with snipped sea veggies on top, on a chapati or pita crust; or a hot or cold wheat-free, vegetable pasta salad.

Before bed: have a cup of herb tea such as chamomile, peppermint, or Crystal Star AFTER MEAL ENZ™ extract drops in water, or a cup of miso soup.

Note: Brewer's yeast does not cause or aggravate candida albicans yeast overgrowth. It is still one of the best immune-enhancing foods available.

Supplementation should be included in the cleansing diet phase to boost body energy in the yeast reduction and killing process. See the vitamin/mineral and herbal suggestions on the preceding page. For best results choose supplements to help kill the yeasts, to balance and restore intestinal flora, to help clean the liver, for bowel regulation, glandular rebalance, and allergic reactions. See "COOKING FOR HEALTHY HEALING," by Linda Rector Page for a complete control diet for Candida Albicans - to enhance liver function for detoxification, improve digestion, create an environment for better nutrient assimilation, and build immunity to prevent recurrence.

Carpal Tunnel Syndrome
Repetitive Strain Wrist Injury

While carpal tunnel syndrome has long been a problem for knitters and needleworkers, and those doing repetitive task jobs, such as carpenters, musicians and assembly-line workers, it is becoming a common ailment of the computer age, affecting more than one out of ten Americans who work on computer terminals. Standard medical treatment is usually cortisone shots to control swelling, or in severe cases, surgery to enlarge the carpal tunnel opening. Natural therapies can both relieve pain and act as a preventive to the development of CTS.

Diet & Superfood Therapy

❧ B₆ deficiency, because of toxins in the environment, may be a cause of CTS. Make sure your diet is rich in vitamin B₆ foods, such as whole grains, liver, green leafy vegetables, beans and legumes.

❧ Eat plenty of fresh foods with at least one green salad every day. Add celery for good cell salt activity, and sea vegetables or miso soup to alkalize.

❧ Avoid caffeine, hard liquor and soft drinks. They bind magnesium.
—Avoid other oxalic acid-forming foods, such as cooked spinach, rhubarb and chocolate.

❧ Take a glass of lemon juice and water each morning. Make a mix with 2 teasp. each: lecithin granules, brewer's yeast, molasses, toasted wheat germ; add 1TB. to the daily diet.
☙

❧ **Effective superfoods:**
—Green drinks (pg. 168).
—Fresh carrot juice or Green Foods BETA CARROT drink.
—Crystal Star BIOFLAV., FIBER & C SUPPORT DRINK™ for collagen support and tissue integrity.

Herbal Therapy

❧ Jump start herbal program:
—**Crystal Star RELAX CAPS™ for nerve restoration.**
with
—**ANTI-FLAM™**, or Solaray TURMERIC capsules for inflammation to **reduce inflammation and SILICA SOURCE™ extract for rebuilding collagen and connective tissue.**
and
—CALCIUM SOURCE™ for tissue strength.

❧ EVENING PRIMROSE OIL caps 500mg, 4 daily for prostaglandin balance. ☿

❧ GINKGO BILOBA extract 2-3x daily for increased circulation.

❧ **Effective nerve relaxers:**
—Scullcap
—Passion flower
—Lobelia

❧ Flora VEGE-SIL caps 2-3x daily.

❧ Homeopathic:: Hylands *NERVE TONIC* or *Arsenicum* as needed ☿

❧ Massage affected areas frequently.
—Apply cajeput oil or Chinese WHITE FLOWER oil.

Supplements

❧ **Vitamin B₆ 250mg daily, with B Complex 100mg for 3 months.**
and
—**Bromelain 750mg to reduce inflammation, and niacin (flush-free if desired) 500mg 2x daily to increase circulation.**
and
—**Ascorbate vitamin C with bioflavonoids 3-5000mg daily for connective tissue formation.**

❧ Enzymatic Therapy LIQUID LIVER with SIBERIAN GINSENG. ♂

❧ **Solaray QBC-PLEX, or Quercetin 2 daily with bromelain 750mg.**
and
—Vitamin E 400IU 2x daily.

❧ Nutrapathic CALCIUM/COLLAGEN capsules.

❧ **Effective natural pain control:**
—**Country Life LIGATEND** ♂
—GABA with Taurine
—DLPA 500mg as needed ♀
—Twin Lab CSA as needed

Lifestyle Support Therapy

❧ **Self Test for CTS:** Hold out your right hand, bend your left index finger and tap the middle of your right wrist where wrist joins your hand. If you get a tingling sensation or shooting pains down your fingers, you probably have carpal tunnel problems.

❧ Both chiropractic and hypnosis are effective for a variety of repetitive strain injuries. Surgery is usually unnecessary.

❧ **Reflexology point:**

nerves
lungs

❧ Massage area with Matrix Health GENESIS OXY-SPRAY.

❧ **Affected area:**

Common Symptoms: Poor grip; intense numbness, tingling, pain and swelling in the wrist and hand, often involving shoulder nerves as well; chronic muscular weakness and atrophy; nerve inflammation.
Common Causes: Continued stress on the wrist, hand and arm nerves from repetitive tasks; vitamin B₆ deficiency; and/or birth control pills creating a B₆ deficiency, leading to the disorder; underactive thyroid; too much protein; lack of magnesium; glandular imbalance during pregnancy; body electrical system "shorts" from prostaglandin imbalance.

Cataracts & Macular Degeneration
Lens Opacity

Cataracts are the leading cause of impaired vision in America, affecting over 4 million people. Cataract surgery is the most common operation for people over 65 - performed over 1 million times a year. Most operations have to be repeated in 2 to 5 years. Natural therapies can arrest and reverse early cataracts. Age-related macular degeneration (AMD), a disease of the central part of the retina (the part of the eye responsible for fine vision), affects 9 million Americans and is the leading cause of blindness in the elderly. AMD can be greatly aided or reversed with nutritional therapy.

Diet & Superfood Therapy

Keys to eye health: preventive diet and lifestyle.

♌ Reduce intake of fats, cholesterol foods, and salt. Add food sources of magnesium, such as seafoods, whole grains, green vegetables, molasses, nuts and eggs.
☛Avoid refined carbohydrate, all sugars, red meats, and caffeine. Avoid rancid foods - sources of harmful free radicals.

♌ "See" foods to prevent cataracts:
Blood sugar stability is a key factor. Include green leafy veggies, sea vegetables, seafood, celery, citrus fruits, brewer's yeast, sprouts, apples and apple juice. Add legumes for sulphur-containing amino acids.
☛For three months, a daily carrot juice.

♌ "See" foods for macular degeneration:
☛Eat lutein-rich foods, especially kale, collard greens and spinach.
☛Eat natural zinc-rich foods: fish and seafoods, sea vegetables, whole grains, beans and pumpkin seeds.

♌ Effective superfoods:
☛Crystal Star BIOFLAV., FIBER & C SUPPORT™ drink. with rutin.
☛Aloe vera juice (without ascorbic acid); take internally, use as eyedrops 2x daily.
☛Green Foods BETA CARROT.
☛Klamath BLUE GREEN SUPREME for macular degeneration.

Herbal Therapy

♌ Jump start herbal program:
☛Use Crystal Star EYEBRIGHT HERBS™ tea as an eyewash.
☛Take BILBERRY extract for PCO activity as soon as cataracts or macular degeneration become known, to decrease sorbitol accumulation, and help remove chemicals from the eyes.
and
☛GINKGO BILOBA extract.
☛SUGAR STRATEGY HIGH™ capsules for sugar regulation.♂

♌ High potency royal jelly 2 teasp. daily, with spirulina tabs 4-8 daily.♀

♌ PCOs 100mg daily from grapeseed or white pine.

♌ Homeopathic *SILICEA* tabs.

♌ Herbs for cataracts:
☛Eyebright eyewash
☛Rosehips eyewash
☛Ginkgo biloba extract caps 4 daily
☛Shark cartilage

♌ Herbs for macular degeneration:
☛BILBERRY
☛Aloe vera juice ♂
☛GINKGO BILOBA extract
☛Chamomile

Supplements

♌ Anti-oxidants are key nutrients for both problems, especially in the de-activation of heavy metals and pollutants:
☛Enzymatic Therapy ORAL NUTRIENT CHELATES as directed. ♂
☛Nutricology germanium150mg. ♂
☛Ascorbate Vitamin C with bioflavonoids 5000mg daily.
☛Glutathione 50mg 2x daily.
☛Vitamin E 400IU 2x daily.
☛Beta carotene 150,000IU daily.
☛Cysteine 1000mg 2x daily.
☛Zinc 50mg daily.

♌ Country Life MAX FOR MEN AND MAXINE FOR WOMEN as preventives.
☛Enzymatic Therapy ACID-A-CAL caps, with chromium picolinate 200mcg.

♌ Other important nutrients:
☛Riboflavin 10mg 2x daily.
☛Taurine 500mg 2x daily.
☛Solaray VIZION capsules.
☛Nature's Life I-SIGHT.

♌ For cataracts:
☛Quercetin plus with bromelain.
☛Copper 3mg with manganese 5mg.

♌ For macular degeneration:
☛Nutricology OCUDYNE with Lutein.
☛HCL tabs for best food assimilation.

Lifestyle Support Therapy

❧ Do long slow neck rolls and other good eye exercises (see Bates Method book).

❧ Avoid long exposure to the sun. Get your exercise early in the day. Wear wraparound sunglasses for protection.
☛Stop smoking and avoid secondary smoke. Smokers are 63% more likely to develop cataracts.

❧ Avoid aspirin, commercial antihistamines and cortisone as detrimental to eye health.

❧ Wear amber or blue-blocking sunglasses, especially when driving.

❧ Reflexology point:

eyes

squeeze and press
all around eye fingers

cataract and AMD area

Common Symptoms: Cataracts: appear as cloudy or opaque areas on the crystalline lens of the eye which focuses light, (they block light entering the eye). Macular degeneration: blurry, distorted vision; decreased reading ability, even with large type; faded colors. Glasses do not help. Driving is very difficult because of blind spots.
Common Causes: Cataracts: Free radical damage from heavy metal/environmental pollutants or UV rays; too much dietary fat, sugar, salt and cholesterol; linked to diabetes, poor circulation and constipation; liver malfunction; protein deficiency with poor enzyme activity. Macular degeneration: poor digestion; linked to UV sunlight. People with light colored eyes are more at risk.

Also see DIET FOR DIABETES CONTROL in this book for more information.

Cellulite

Fatty Deposits Under The Skin

Cellulite is actually a combination of fat, water and trapped wastes beneath the skin - usually on otherwise thin women. When the body's circulation and elimination process become impaired, connective tissue loses its strength. Unmetabolized fats and wastes become trapped in the vulnerable cells just beneath the skin and form the puckering skin effect we know as cellulite. Because it is unattached material, dieting and exercise alone can't dislodge cellulite. An effective program for cellulite release should be in four parts: 1) Stimulate elimination functions. 2) Increase circulation and metabolism. 3) Control excess fluid retention. 4) Re-establish connective tissue elasticity.

Diet & Superfood Therapy

See "COOKING FOR HEALTHY HEALING" by Linda Rector-Page for a complete cellulite diet.

A low fat diet is the key:
- Have a fresh salad every day. Have 1 or 2 fresh or steamed vegetables at every meal. Have brown rice once a day.
- Eat fruits and juices in the morning.
- Use small amounts of unsaturated oils.
- Have Omega-rich fish and seafood twice a week. Have 2 TBS. sea vegetables 3 or 4 times a week in a soup or salad.
- Graze - eat smaller, more frequent meals, instead of 2 to 3 large ones.
- Drink 6 to 8 glasses of water or healthy liquids every day.

The cellulite blacklist:
- All fried and fatty foods.
- Heavy caffeine use, carbonated drinks, and hard liquor.
- Red meats.
- Full-fat, pasteurized dairy foods.
- Salty foods - use herbal seasoning.

Effective superfoods:
- Crystal Star antioxidant SYSTEMS STRENGTH™ drink or capsules.
- Crystal Star BIOFLAV.FIBER & C SUPPORT for collagen support.
- Carrot/beet/cucumber juice, to clean the liver so it can metabolize fats better.

Herbal Therapy

Jump start herbal program: Crystal Star THERMO-CEL-LEAN™ roll-on gel with CEL-LEAN™ caps or CEL-LEAN™ tea, before meals.

and

- META-TABS capsules to stimulate thyroid function and tone tissue.
- HOT SEAWEED BATH™ to stimulate circulation and potentiate lipolysis.
- EVENING PRIMROSE oil 1000mg 2 daily for EFAs and prostaglandin balance.
- THERMO-CITRIN GINSENG™ caps for extra fat and calorie burning help.
- GINSENG/LICORICE ELIXIR™ for system and sugar level balance.

Crystal Star AMINO-ZYME™ capsules with LIV-ALIVE™ tea to energize cells and metabolize fats.

Other effective herbals:
- MILK THISTLE SEED extract for liver support in metabolizing fats.
- Crystal Star SILICA SOURCE™ extract for connective tissue/collagen support.
- HAWTHORN extract to reduce blood fat levels and stabilize heart rate.

Rub-on cellulite-fighting oils:
- Antioxidants rosemary and thyme.
- Peppermint to increase metabolism.
- Juniper to stimulate circulation.

Supplements

Don't smoke. It impedes both circulation and metabolism.

Silica tightens connective tissue:
- Natureworks SILICA GEL
- Body Essentials SILICA GEL internally, 1 TB. in 3-oz. liquid, and externally on problem areas.

Solaray CENTELLA ASIATICA or CENTELLA VEIN caps.

Enzymatic Therapy CELL-U-VAR cream and capsules as directed.

Carnitine 500mg daily.

with

- Biotec AGELESS BEAUTY tabs to dissolve and flush rancid fats and waste material.

Effective liver aids to help metabolize fats:
- Educated Beauty SLEEK & CHIC cellulite contouring cream.
- High Omega-3 flax or fish oils.
- Rainbow Light TRIM-ZYME.
- Source Naturals SUPER AMINO NIGHT caps.

Apply Matrix Health GENESIS H_2O_2 OXY-SPRAY to fatty areas. (In some cases the fat globules release by coming out through the skin in little white bumps.)

Lifestyle Support Therapy

The four bodywork steps:
- **Kneading massage** - from periphery toward the heart. Use a dry skin brush, loofa or ayate cloth to stimulate lymph glands.
- **Regular aerobic exercise** - to tone tissue, increase circulation and maintain underlying tissue integrity. An arm-swinging walk every day, especially after a large meal is the best choice for cellulite. *It helps maintain a slim subcutaneous fat layer by keeping the body slender and toned.*
- **Body wraps:** Crystal Star TIGHTENING & TONING BODY WRAP™, a rapid inch-loss treatment.
- **Seaweed baths:** to release trapped toxins in the cells.

Do thigh creams work? Some of them do. Natural products don't have the risky side affects. Choose one with AHAs, herbal antioxidants and theophyllisilane.
- **Jason THIGH THERAPY NIGHTTIME, and THIGH Rx DAYTIME gel and body spray.**
- **Chae BODY THERAPY.**

Reflexology point:

thyroid gland

liver

Common Symptoms: Lumpy, rippled skin around thighs, hips and love handles; trapped waste and fluid in pockets beneath the skin. When regular fat is squeezed the skin appears smooth - cellulitic skin will ripple like an orange peel, or have the texture of cottage cheese. Tightness, heaviness in the legs; soreness and tenderness when tissue is massaged.

Common Causes: Sometimes a family trait, but usually poor nutrition resulting in liver exhaustion and reduced fat metabolism. (Fats are often thrown off as lumpy "chicken fat.") Inadequate exercise; poor elimination and sluggish circulation; insufficient water intake; stress; imbalanced estrogen activity; environmental pollutants; crash dieting with rapid regain of weight.

See also WEIGHT LOSS & CONTROL pages in this book for more information.

Cerebral Palsy
Muscle / Nerve Dysfunction

Cerebral palsy is the most common crippling childhood disorder. Cerebral palsy is a broad term for brain-centered motor disorders which usually occur before or during birth, or in the first few months after birth. Damage to the cerebrum causes a paralysis (palsy) in one or more parts of the body. The damage is sustained throughout adulthood. Premature infants with very low birth weight (less than $3^{1}/_{2}$ pounds) are at high risk for developing cerebral palsy, especially if the mother has been addicted to drugs.

Diet & Superfood Therapy

Absorbable minerals are key factors in bone building. Herbs are one of the best ways to get them.

☙ A modified macrobiotic diet is effective. See pg. 211 in this book, and "COOKING FOR HEALTHY HEALING" by Linda Rector-Page for a complete daily diet.

☙ Eat organically grown foods as much as possible. Include plenty of leafy greens in the diet with a fresh salad every day.

☙ Go on a cleansing juice fast one day a week until symptoms improve (usually 3-4 months). Take a potassium broth (pg. 167) every other day during the cleanse.

☙ Avoid all refined foods, saturated fats, red meats, fried or fatty foods, caffeine and canned foods.

☙ Make a mix with 2TBS. each: brewer's yeast, lecithin, toasted wheat germ. Take some daily over cereal or in juice.

☙ **Effective superfoods:**
♣Crystal Star SYSTEMS STRENGTH™.
♣Organic Gourmet NUTRITIONAL YEAST or MISO extract in water before bed.
♣Beehive Botanicals ROYAL JELLY with SIBERIAN GINSENG drink or capsules.

Herbal Therapy

☙ **Jump start herbal program:**
Crystal Star RELAX CAPS™ 2-4 daily as needed for tension, with EVENING PRIMROSE OIL caps 6 daily.
and/or
♣ANTI-SPZ™ capsules or CRAMP BARK COMPLEX™ extract.
♣BLDR-K CONTROL™ for urinary incontinence.
♣HAWTHORN extract 4x daily for circulation and a feeling of well-being.
♣MINERAL SPECTRUM™ caps for stability and alkalinity.

☙ **Effective herbal anti-oxidants:**
♣Rosemary
♣GINKGO BILOBA extract for brain and nerve stability.

☙ Matrix Health GENESIS H_2O_2 OXY-SPRAY applied to affected muscle areas.

☙ An effective nerve tea:
One part each of gotu kola, bilberry, ginger, butcher's broom and scullcap.

Supplements

☙ Magnesium 800mg daily for better muscle/nerve coordination.
♣Pregnant women at risk for premature births and toxemia, especially from drugs, should take magnesium 400mg during prenatal months to reduce risk of brain injury associated with birth asphyxia.
♣Twin Lab CSA for spinal/nerve pain and tension.
♣**Tyrosine 500mg daily for L-Dopa formation.**

☙ **Country Life RELAXER caps (GABA with Taurine).** ♀

☙ B Complex 150mg. daily, with
♣Am. Biologics SUB-ADRENE. ♀
♣ITC SUPER SUNSHINE B powder for muscle atrophy. ♂

☙ **Choline therapy:**
♣Twin Lab CHOLINE/INOSITOL caps.
♣Phosphatidyl choline. ♂
♣Egg Yolk Lecithin 6 daily.

☙ **Effective anti-oxidants:**
♣Octacosonal 1000mg 4 daily.
♣Natural vitamin E 400IU 3x daily.
♣CoQ_{10} **60mg daily.**

Lifestyle Support Therapy

☙ Stay away from all pesticides, agricultural sprays. Many affect the nervous system if an individual is very sensitive.

☙ Use hot and cold hydrotherapy to stimulate circulation.

☙ Continuing massage of the muscles is a key deterrent to atrophy.

☙ **Reflexology point:**

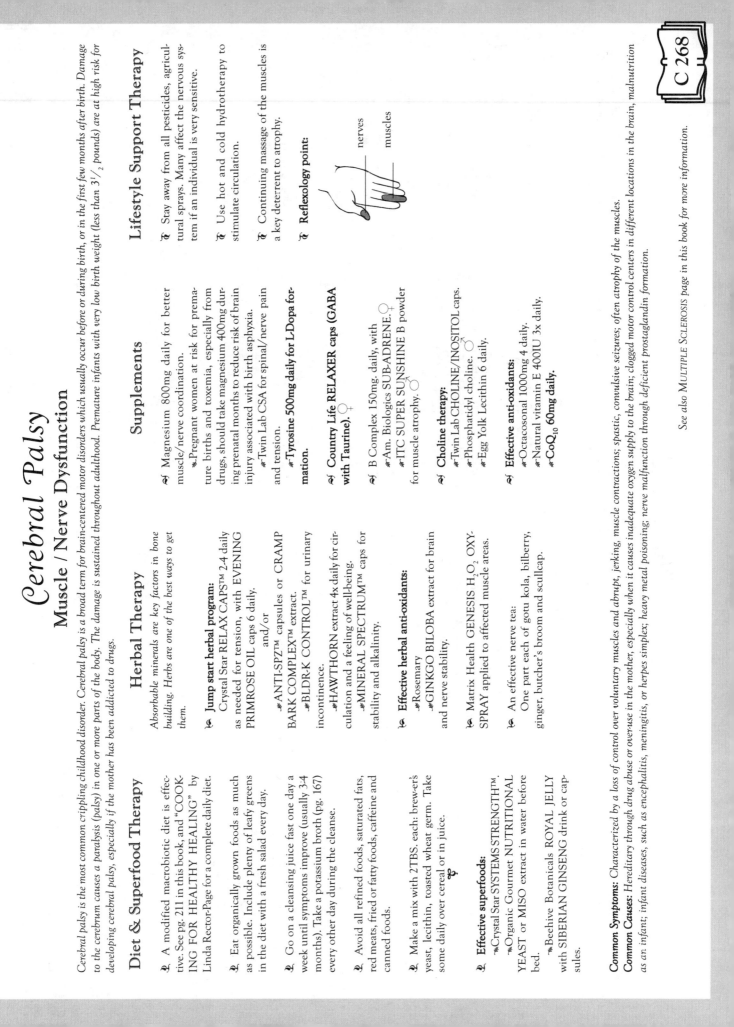

nerves

muscles

Common Symptoms: *Characterized by a loss of control over voluntary muscles and abrupt, jerking, muscle contractions; spastic, convulsive seizures; often atrophy of the muscles.*
Common Causes: *Hereditary through drug abuse or overuse in the mother, especially when it causes inadequate oxygen supply to the brain; clogged motor control centers in different locations in the brain, malnutrition as an infant; infant diseases, such as encephalitis, meningitis, or herpes simplex; heavy metal poisoning; nerve malfunction through deficient prostaglandin formation.*

See also MULTIPLE SCLEROSIS *page in this book for more information.*

Chicken Pox
Varicella-Zoster Virus

Chicken pox is a herpes-type virus disease, usually a childhood ailment, lasting from seven to ten days. One bout of chicken pox provides immunity against recurrence for the rest of your life. Adults are vulnerable if they did not have chicken pox as children. It can be life-threatening if the child has a compromised immune system (such as a cancer patient undergoing chemotherapy treatment). Complications commonly include ear infections and secondary skin infections.

Diet & Superfood Therapy

✿ Take 2 lemons in water with a little honey every 4 hours to flush the system of toxins and clean the kidneys.

✿ Stay on a liquid diet for the first 3 days of infection, with plenty of fruit and vegetable juices. Then have a raw foods diet, some apples, bananas, yogurt, avocados and a fresh salad daily for the rest of the week.

✿ Avoid all dairy products except a little yogurt or kefir cheese. ⊛

✿ Dab honey or wheat germ oil on scabs to heal and prevent infection. ⊛

🌿 **Effective superfoods:**
⟡Crystal Star SYSTEMS STRENGTH **for minerals and body balance.**
⟡Beehive Botanicals fresh royal jelly in honey. Take internally and apply.
⟡Klamath POWER 3 caps or **BLUE GREEN SUPREME drink.**
⟡**BeWell VEGETABLE JUICE.**

Herbal Therapy

Many mineral-rich herbs provide key biochemical ingredients for effective neurotransmission.

✿ **Jump start herbal program:**
Crystal Star ANTI-HST™ **caps to reduce itching, and** ANTI-FLAM™ **to reduce inflammation, and** WILD LETTUCE/ VALERIAN **extract in water to help calm and relax the child.** ⊛
and
⟡Crystal Star THERA-DERM™ tea and wash. Take internally, and apply with cotton balls to lesions.
⟡**Apply** LYSINE/LICORICE GEL **to sores.** Crystal Star ANTI-BIO™ gel frequently if sores become infected.
⟡Take cayenne/lobelia caps every 3 to 4 hours.

🌿 **Effective topical applications:**
⟡Make a rosemary/calendula wash: 1 handful dried herb each to 1 qt. water. Dab on sores every 2 to 3 hours.
⟡Comfrey salve, or fresh comfrey leaf compresses.
⟡Aloe vera gel, or AloeLife SKIN GEL.
⟡**St. John's** wort oil or salve.
⟡Apply a golden seal/myrrh solution.
⟡A strong tea of yellow dock, burdock and golden seal every 4 hours.

Supplements

✿ **Extra vitamin C is essential. Begin taking vitamin C as soon as diagnosis is made:**
⟡**Ascorbate vitamin C or Ester C crystals,** ¼ **teasp. every 2-3 hours to bowel tolerance, to flush the tissues, relieve itching, and neutralize the viral activity.** ⊛
⟡Beta carotene 25,000IU.
⟡Natural vitamin E 400IU daily. Apply E oil to scabs as well.
⟡**Zinc 30mg 2x daily for a month after disease has run its course to re-establish immunity.**

✿ Raw thymus glandular to encourage the production of T-lymphocytes.

✿ **Effective homeopathic remedies:**
⟡Apply B & T CALIFLORA gel.
⟡*Rhus Tox*
⟡*Pulsatilla*

✿ Use Nutribiotic GRAPEFRUIT SEED SKIN SPRAY to control infection and heal sores.

✿ Apply Matrix Health GENESIS OXY-SPRAY to affected areas to reduce scarring. ⟡Apply Home Health SCAR-GO to heal scars.

Lifestyle Support Therapy

✿ Do not give aspirin. It has been linked to Reye's syndrome, a rare but deadly disease that can afflict children after bouts of chicken pox or some types of flu. It also tends to aggravate sores.

✿ Use a catnip enema twice during acute stage to clean out toxins. ⊛

✿ Effective baths for skin itching and healing:
⟡Peppermint/ginger
⟡**Cider vinegar/sea salt**
⟡**Oatmeal**
⟡Ginger root
Note: Wet compresses of any of the above may be applied often to control itching.

✿ **Effective applications:**
⟡Thursday Plantation ANTISEPTIC CREAM
⟡AloeLife ALOE SKIN GEL
⟡Lemon Balm cream

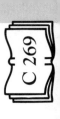

Common Symptoms: Mild fever and headache, with small, flat, pink, blister-type lesions all over the body that erupt, crust and leave a small scar. The blisters and scabs are highly infective and extremely itchy. Keep the child isolated from other children, frail elderly people, or those who have never had chicken pox.

Common Causes: An airborne viral infection, usually allowed to become virulent by reduced immunity from a poor diet - too many sugars, sweets, refined carbohydrates, and mucous-forming foods; lack of green vegetables.

See also CHILDHOOD DISEASE pages (pg. 114ff) in this book for more information.

Cholesterol

Hyperlipidemias ✻ High Serum LDL or VLDL ✻ High Triglycerides

Cholesterol is a fat-related substance in the body that is needed for many processes related to nerve and hormone functions. Poor metabolism and over-indulgence in high cholesterol foods lead to serious deposits in arterial linings, and to gallstones. There are two kinds of cholesterol. HDL (high density lipo-protein, or good) cholesterol, LDL/VLDL (low density and very low density lipo-proteins, or bad) cholesterol. Triglycerides are a sugar-related blood fat that travels with cholesterol as lipo-proteins. High triglycerides can cause blood cells to stick together, impairing circulation and leading to heart attack. High cholesterol levels do not increase heart disease risk in people 70 and older, and some cholesterol-lowering drugs are actually harmful. Ask about yours.

Diet & Superfood Therapy

See "COOKING FOR HEALTHY HEALING" by Linda Rector-Page for a complete daily diet.

❧ Cholesterol in foods such as eggs is not the culprit. (Eggs are a whole food, with phosphatides to balance the cholesterol.) The big contributor to high blood cholesterol levels is saturated fat and over-eating.

✱Vegetarians who occasionally eat eggs and small amounts of low fat dairy are at the lowest risk for arterial or heart disease.

❧ A low fat, high fiber diet is the key to reducing cholesterol. Reducing sugar is the key to lowering triglycerides.

✱Foods that lower cholesterol: soy foods, olive oil, whole grains like oats, high fiber foods like fresh fruits and vegetables, yogurt and cultured foods and yams.

✱Substantially reduce or avoid animal fats, red meats, fried foods, fatty dairy foods, salty/sugary foods, refined foods.

✱Eat smaller meals, especially at night.
✱A little wine with dinner reduces stress and raises HDLs.

❧ Effective superfoods:
✱ Crystal Star CHO-LO FIBER TONE™ drink daily for 1 to 2 months.
✱Lewis Labs BREWER'S YEAST.
✱Y.S. ROYAL JELLY/GINSENG drink.
✱Green Foods WHEAT GERM extract.
✱Klamath BLUE GREEN SUPREME.

Herbal Therapy

✺ Jump start herbal program:
✱Crystal Star CHOLEX™ caps, 3 daily for 2 months with GINSENG/REISHI extract.
and/or
✱Crystal Star HEARTSEASE/CIRCU-CLEANSE™ tea, and HAWTHORN extract 2 to 3x daily.
✱GREEN TEA CLEANSER™ each morning.

✺ Take PCOs from pine or grapeseed to inhibit and prevent LDL oxidation, 100mg daily.

✺ Source Naturals MEGA-GLA or EVENING PRIMROSE OIL 4 daily.♀

✺ Herbs that help raise HDL's:
✱Solaray ALFA JUICE caps.
✱Suma root
✱Panax ginseng (also protects the liver)

✺ Herbs to lower LDL/triglyceride levels:
✱Grifon MAITAKE mushroom caplets
✱Cayenne/Ginger capsules 2 daily
✱Una da gato
✱Fenugreek seed tabs
✱Garlic 6 tabs daily (decreases 9%) ♂
✱Solaray TURMERIC extract tabs.

✺ Help the liver lower cholesterol:
✱Dandelion root
✱MILK THISTLE SEED extract
✱Goldenseal/Myrrh extract

Supplements

✑ If dietary means have not been successful, use niacin therapy to reduce all blood fats and benefit nerves. (Do not use if glucose intolerant, have liver disease or a peptic ulcer.) Flush free niacin is OK.
✱1500mg daily ♀
✱1000mg daily ♂
✱Bio-Resource LO-NIACIN with glycine 500mg if sugar sensitive.
✱Solaray CHROMIACIN or CHROME-MATE to regulate sugar use.

✑ Golden Pride FLORMULA ONE oral chelation w/ EDTA A.M./P.M.
✱NAC to lower blood fats over all.

✑ Enzymatic Therapy GUGGUL-PLUS guggulipids 3x daily to reduce both LDL, VLDL, and triglyceride levels.

✑ Lipotropics to enhance the liver:
✱Solaray LIPOTROPIC 1000.♀
✱Vitamin E 400IU, 2x daily with B₆.
✱ITC SUPER SUNSHINE B powder.♂
✱Omega-3 rich flax oil capsules daily.

✑ Antioxidants to help raise HDLs:
✱Carnitine 1000mg. daily.
✱CoQ₁₀ 60mg daily (especially if taking cholesterol-lowering drugs).
✱Ester C with bioflavs. 2000mg daily.
✱Beta carotene 100,000IU daily.

Lifestyle Support Therapy

Accurate lipoprotein and cholesterol fractions testing is available, and is worthwhile as a means of monitoring your progress.

☞ Ideal cholesterol levels should be from 140 to 165 mg/dl, with LDL cholesterol from 30 to 50 mg/dl, and HDL cholesterol from 80 to 90 mg/dl. (Over 244 is an ideal heart attack victim; 210 is the average American level.)
✱Ideal triglyceride levels should be around 200 to 240 mg/dl. Every 1% increase in blood cholesterol translates into a 2% increase in heart disease risk.

☞ Reduce your body weight. Most overweight people have abnormal metabolism.
✱If you are 10 pounds overweight, your body produces an extra 100mg. of cholesterol every day.

☞ Take a brisk daily walk or other regular aerobic exercise of your choice to enhance circulation and boost HDL.
✱Eliminate tobacco use of all kinds. Nicotine raises cholesterol levels.

☞ Practice a favorite stress reduction technique at least once a day. There is a correlation between high cholesterol and aggression. Men especially who are the most emotionally repressive have the highest cholesterol levels.

Common Symptoms: *Plaque formation on the artery walls; poor circulation; leg cramps and pain; high blood pressure; difficult breathing; cold hands and feet; dry skin and hair; palpitations; lethargy; dizziness; allergies and kidney trouble.*

Common Causes: *Stress; diet high in saturated fats and sugars; low in soluble fiber; EFA deficiency. Oxidized LDL-cholesterol poses a particular health hazard to the heart, as it significantly contributes to the accumulation of arterial plaque. An English study shows that not only is this progression inhibited, but the process may be prevented from even occurring by taking PCOs.*

See also HEART DISEASE pages in this book for more information.

Chronic Fatigue Syndrome
Epstein Barr Virus ✤ Hypoadrenalism ✤ Hypotension

Chronic fatigue syndrome (CFS) is sometimes referred to as a condition without a cause. In reality, the opposite is true. There are a wealth of causative factors. Although pinpointing an exact virus cause is inconclusive, it is widely accepted that a virus or group of viruses are involved. Epstein-Barr virus (EBV), herpes simplex viruses (genital and oral), and cytomegalovirus (CMV) are clearly implicated. Candida albicans yeast and parasite infestations are also highly suspect. Incredibly, new research shows that the polio virus, long considered conquered, may be resurfacing 20 to 30 years after childhood vaccinations against it, as Post-Polio Syndrome, now seen as Chronic Fatigue.

Diet & Superfood Therapy

People who suffer from chronic fatigue need supernutrition.

❧ Keep the diet at least 50% fresh foods during intensive healing time. Emphasize foods that build immunity. Include often:
❋defense foods: cruciferous vegetables;
❋antibody forming foods: onions and garlic;
❋oxygenating foods: wheat germ;
❋high mineral, B Complex foods: sea vegetables and brown rice;
❋high fiber foods: prunes and bran;
❋cultured foods: yogurt and miso;
❋protein foods: sea foods and whole grains.

❧ CFS association with hypoglycemia is well-known. Also see *Diet for Hypoglycemia* on page 338 in this book.

❧ Avoid allergen-prone, body-stressing foods; junk and fast foods; foods that contain caffeine, refined sugars, alcohol, dairy, gluten and chemical agents.

❧ Effective superfoods: Immune defense cells are created in bone marrow. Keep new cell development strong with protein. Take a protein drink every morning:
❋Solgar WHEY TO GO (lactose-free)
❋Crystal Star SYSTEMS STRENGTH™ (also combats hypothyroidism), and GREEN TEA CLEANSER™ to detox.
❋Nutricology PRO-GREENS, or Klamath BLUE GREEN SUPREME, or Nature's Life SUPER GREEN PRO-96.
❋Beehive Botanicals Royal Jelly, Pollen, Propolis and Siberian Ginseng drink.

Herbal Therapy

❧ Jump start herbal program:
❋Crystal Star FEM-SUPPORT™ extract with ashwagandha; ard GINKGO BILOBA extract as needed.
❋Crystal Star ADRN-ACTIVE™ caps or extract, with BODY REBUILDER™, and EVENING PRIMROSE oil 4 daily.
❋PRO-EST BALANCE™ roll-on, with maitake mushroom caplets for the first 3 months of healing.
❋Crystal Star GINSENG/LICORICE ELIXIR™ with POTASSIUM/IODINE™ caps as needed.

❧ Effective body balancers: (take 15 to 30 drops in water for best results.)
❋Suma
❋GINSENG/REISHI extract
❋HAWTHORN extract
❋Siberian ginseng extract, or Rainbow Light ADAPTO-GEM ♀

❧ Effective liver detoxifiers:
❋Nutricology ALIVE & WELL caps
❋MILK THISTLE SEED extract
❋Crystal Star LIV-ALIVE™ caps

❧ Immune builders: (take as teas)
❋Astragalus
❋Chamomile/Angelica blend
❋GINSENG/CHLORELLA™ extract
❋Pau d'arco

❧ Anti-viral herbs:
❋St. John's wort (also an antidepressant)
❋Crystal Star ANTI-VI™ tea or extract
❋Garlic capsules 5 daily

Supplements

❧ Effective anti-oxidants:
❋Nutricology GERMANIUM 150mg.
❋Carnitine 500mg daily.
❋Vit. E 400IU with selenium 200mcg.
❋PCOs - pine or grapeseed, 50mg 3x daily
❋Vitamin C or Ester C crystals with bioflavonoids, $1/4$ teasp. every half hour to bowel tolerance - to flush the tissues and act as an anti-viral agent, for 10 days. Then reduce to 3 - 5000mg daily.
❋Marine carotene 100,000IU daily.

❧ Non-depleting energizers:
❋Food Science DMG sublingual tabs
❋Source Naturals DIBENCOZIDE B_{12} and B Complex 100mg daily.
❋Magnesium 1000mg daily

❧ For immune stimulation: Health Aid Amer. SIBERGEN with Enzymatic Therapy THYMUPLEX tablets, biotin 1000mcg, and Tyrosine 500mg daily. ♀
❋CoQ₁₀ 100mg 3x daily.
❋Magnesium 500mg daily.

❧ For detoxification:
❋Biotec CELL GUARD tablets.
❋American Biologics DIOXYCHLOR with taurine tablets.
❋Nutribiotic GRAPEFRUIT SEED EXTRACT capsules.

❧ Enzyme therapy:
❋Bromelain 500mg daily
❋Future Biotics VITAL K
❋Natren BIFIDO FACTORS probiotics
❋Pancreatin with HCL

Lifestyle Support Therapy

Note: High doses of aspirin, NSAIDS and cortisone for arthritic pain can hamper your body's ability to maintain bone strength.

☞ Take a daily deep-breathing walk for tissue oxygen uptake. Walk at least twenty minutes to stimulate lymphatic system and cerebral circulation.
☞Get some early morning sunlight on the body every day possible for vitamin D.

☞ Apply Matrix Health GENESIS OXY-SPRAY onto soles of the feet for body oxygen. Alternate use, one week on and one week off. Too much reactivates symptoms. A little is great; a lot is not.

☞ Relax. An optimistic mental attitude and frame of mind play a major role in releasing body stress, a big factor in lowered immunity. Remember that immune stimulation itself has an anti-viral effect.

☞ Stretching exercises and massage will cleanse the lymph system and enhance oxygenation. Use hot and cold alternating hydrotherapy to stimulate circulation.
☞ Take a wheat grass enema, once a week, to help detoxification.

☞ Avoid tobacco in all forms. Nicotine destroys immunity. It takes 3 months to rebuild immune response even after you quit.

☞ Overheating therapy is effective in controlling and overcoming Epstein-Barr Virus. See page 178 for at-home technique.

Call the CFS Hotline (800) 442-3437, and see MONONUCLEOSIS in this book for more information.

Do You Have Chronic Fatigue Syndrome?

Most researchers believe CFS is a result of mixed infections, with several pathogens involved. Environmental pollutants and contaminants also contribute to CFS by reducing immune response and allowing CFS a path to develop. In addition, growing evidence points to exhausted adrenal glands from high stress life-styles and an imbalance in the hypothalamic-pituitary-adrenal (HPA) axis. *CFS is a response (or lack of immune response) to the ever-increasing mental, emotional and physical stresses in our environment. Susceptibility to chronic viral infections has become more and more prevalent in the last decades. As our immunity drops lower and lower, almost anything can be the final trigger for CFS. Onset is abrupt in almost 90% of cases.*

Natural healers and therapists have now been working with fatigue syndromes and EBV since the early eighties. These problems represent a degenerative imbalance in the endocrine/metabolic systems of the entire body, so are quite difficult to diagnose and treat. **Over 85% of CFS victims are women, usually between 30 and 50, who are outgoing, productive, independent, active, overachievers.** It affects close to 2 million people in America today. The number of people suffering from medically incurable viral conditions is increasing at an alarming rate. No conventional medical treatment or drug on the market today can help fatigue syndromes; most hinder immune response and recovery.

Knowledge is part of the cure for CFS. Here are some things to recognize:

1) CFS develops from EBV or other opportunistic retro-viruses that attack a weakened immune system. But it is maintained through other agents: a history of mononucleosis and/or yeast related problems, emotional stress, environmental pollutants that cause chemical sensitivities, smoking, widespread use of antibiotic or cortico-steroid drugs, a low nutrition diet, or low levels of cortisol (an immune-stimulating hormone that is secreted in response to stress). I suggest a test for candida albicans yeast, mononucleosis, herpes virus or other conditions with similar symptoms, so they can be ruled out first.

2) Chronic fatigue syndromes act like recurring systemic viral infection, viruses that often go undetected because their symptoms mimic simple illnesses like colds, flu, or acute, but less debilitating, mononucleosis. Following the acute stages these retro-viruses penetrate the nuclei of immune system T-cells where they are able to survive and replicate indefinitely. Multiplication of the virus and recurring symptoms appear with a rupturing of the organism and its release into the bloodstream. This can occur at any time, but almost always arises when the person is under stress or has reduced immune response due to a simpler illness such as a cold or cough.

3) Chronic Fatigue and EBV take longer to overcome than Candida or Herpes. The symptoms are similar, but viral activity is more virulent and debilitating to the immune system, and entrenchment in the glands (especially the adrenals), organs (especially the liver) and circulatory system (hypotensive) is more deep-seated. It takes two to four weeks to notice consistent improvement, and six months or longer to feel energetic and normal. However, most people do respond to natural therapies in three to six months. Many achieve near normal functioning in two years even though the virus may persist in the body.

4) CFS symptoms are greatly reduced by aerobic exercise. Even light stretching, shiatzu exercises, or short walks are noticeably effective when they are done regularly every day.

5) Good diet and lifestyle habits are paramount in keeping the body clear of toxic wastes and balancing the lymphatic system. Drink plenty of fresh liquids, and clear the bowels daily.

6) Mind and attitude play a critical role in the status of the immune system and energy levels for overcoming CFS. Be gentle with yourself. Don't get so wound up in the strictness of your program that it further depresses you and takes over your life. The people who learn to identify and manage mental, emotional and physical stress in their lives recover fastest. Laughter is still the best medicine.

Symptomology For Chronic Fatigue Syndrome - A CFS Profile

The outward symptoms for chronic fatigue conditions are similar to mononucleosis, HIV infection, candidiasis, cytomegalovirus, M.S., lupus and fibrocystic myalgia. There are many AIDS-like reactions, but CFS does not kill, is not sexually transmitted as once thought, and tends to go into remission. Get tested for viral titers that measure your body's reaction to the virus, or elevated levels of EBV anti-bodies so that your treatment will be correct.

• **First symptoms** include persistent, debilitating fatigue where there has been no previous history of fatigue, that does not resolve with bed rest, and that is severe enough to reduce average daily activity below 50% percent of normal for that person for at least 6 months. The person experiences classic flu or mononucleosis symptoms - chronic low grade fever, throat infections without pus, unexplained muscle weakness, lethargy, gastro-intestinal disturbance, and sore lymph nodes in the armpit and neck.

• **Second symptoms** include ringing in the ears, exhaustion, chronic depression and self-doubt, moodiness and irritability, fogginess, disorientation and muddled thinking, continued low grade infection and fever, worsening allergies, diarrhea, sharper muscle aches and weakness, numbness and tingling in the limbs, and vertigo.

• **Third symptoms** include extreme fatigue, isolation, herpes infections, aching ears and eyes, night sweats, blackouts, extremely low immune response resulting in frequent infections, paranoia, chronic exhaustion, weight loss and loss of appetite, MS-like nerve disorder with heart palpitations.

CFS Support Groups are a good idea. CFS National Society: (800) 234-0037; CFS Infoline: (800) 442-3437; CFS Hotline (800) 597-4237.

Circulation Problems

Sluggish Blood Flow ✤ Claudication ✤ Raynaud's Disease

Sluggish circulation can stem from many body conditions. It transports heat from the inner body to the skin. It carries antibodies to areas of infection. It helps move waste products to channels of elimination. Sluggish circulation is one of the first signs of serious disorders. High blood pressure, arteriosclerosis, varicose veins, phlebitis, and heart disease are all connected with circulatory system health. Investigate further if your condition does not improve. Raynaud's disease is characterized by numbness and cold hands and feet even in warm weather.

Diet & Superfood Therapy

See the High Blood Pressure pages and Healthy Heart Diet in this book.

❧ Keep the colon clear and your cholesterol down with a high fiber diet; at least 60% fresh foods.

➛Eat citrus fruits, juices and dried fruits; they have good bioflavonoid content to strengthen vein and tissue walls.

➛Avoid red meats, fried and fatty foods, excess caffeine, salts, refined foods, sugar.

➛Drink plenty of healthy fluids, especially for Raynaud's disease.

➛Eat smaller meals more often. Avoid large or heavy meals.

❧ **Circulation drink:** take some daily for almost immediate improvement: Mix $^1/_2$ cup tomato juice, $^1/_2$ cup lemon juice, 6 teasp. wheat germ oil, 1 teasp. brewer's yeast.

❧ **Effective superfoods:**
➛Crystal Star BIOFLAV. FIBER & C SUPPORT™ drink, and on alternating days, CHO-LO-FIBER TONE™ drink.
➛Rainbow Light GARLIC & GREENS.
➛Green tea daily or Crystal Star GREEN TEA CLEANSER™.
➛**New Moon GINSENG GINGER WONDER syrup as desired.**

Herbal Therapy

❧ **Jump start herbal program:**
Crystal Star HEARTSEASE/HAW-THORN™ capsules with HAWTHORN or GINKGO BILOBA extract;♂ orHEARTSEASE/CIRCU-CLEANSE™ tea daily.♀
➛**Cayenne/ginger caps 4 daily, or as needed, especially for cold hands and feet.**

❧ **Effective circulation tonics:**
➛BILBERRY extract 2-3x daily
➛SIBERIAN GINSENG extract ♂
➛Ginger extract daily
➛Solaray CENTELLA ASIATICA caps
➛Crystal Star CHINESE ROYAL MU™ tea.

❧ Herbal antioxidants:
➛Rosemary
➛Panax ginseng
➛GINSENG/CHLORELLA extract.

❧ Butcher's broom caps or tea as a natural blood thinner. (Use only temporarily.) ♂

❧ **Ginseng Company CYCLONE CIDER.**

❧ **For claudication:** rub **CAPSAICIN cream on legs.** ♂
➛GINKGO BILOBA extract
➛Hot sea salt compresses

Supplements

❧ **Effective antioxidants:**
➛**Carnitine 500mg 2x daily.**
➛**Quercetin with bromelain 500mg.**
➛OPCs from pine or grapeseed.
➛Nutricology GERMANIUM 150mg.
➛CoQ$_{10}$ 30mg 2x daily.
➛Solaray TRI O$_2$ capsules.
➛**Vit. E w/ selenium 400IU daily.**
➛**Ester C with bioflavonoids 500mg 2 tabs 3x daily.**

❧ Nature's Bounty B$_{12}$ internasal gel every 3 days; and
➛**Enzymatic Therapy ORAL NUTRIENT CHELATES as directed.** ♂

❧ **Niacin therapy:** 250mg 3 - 4x daily, with PABA 500mg 2x daily. ♂
➛Solaray CHROMIACIN capsules. ♂

❧ High Omega-3 flax oil 3x daily. ♀

❧ **For Raynaud's syndrome (cold hands and feet):** follow a hypoglycemic diet, take IODINE/POTASSIUM SOURCE™ caps, New Moon GINGER WONDER syrup and magnesium 400mg 2x daily.

❧ **For claudication:** Solaray CENTELLA VEIN caps, and enzyme therapy with aspergillus oryzae - a protease enzyme.

Lifestyle Support Therapy

❧ Biofeedback has been notably successful for cold hands and feet.
➛Avoid things that restrict blood flow, like smoking and alcohol.

❧ Apply alternating hot and cold cayenne/ginger compresses to areas in need of stimulation. Or wrap feet in towels soaked in cayenne/ginger solution.
➛Use a dry skin brush over the body before your daily shower.

❧ **See a chiropractor or massage therapist for a structure work-out to clear any obstructions and open energy pathways.**

❧ **Take a brisk aerobic walk every day to get your blood moving.**

❧ **Effective aromatherapy:**
➛Juniper oil
➛Rosemary oil
➛Sage oil

❧ Apply Crystal Star THERMO-CEL-LEAN™ gel as directed.

❧ **For claudication:** sit with legs elevated when possible. Don't wear knee high hosiery. Massage your legs each morning; or
➛Take a daily morning walk.

Common Symptoms: Cold hands and feet; poor memory; migraine headaches; numbness; ringing in the ears and hearing loss; dizziness when standing quickly; shortness of breath; high triglyceride and cholesterol levels; varicose veins. In Raynaud's disease fingers turn white due to lack of blood, because small arteries contract and cut off blood flow.

Common Causes: Cholesterol plaque on artery walls; low fiber diet and constipation; lack of exercise; toxic or obstructed system; poorly managed stress. Raynaud's disease is usually the result of an underlying circulatory cause like atherosclerosis or using a jackhammer or chain saw on the job over many years.

See COOKING FOR HEALTHY HEALING by Linda Rector-Page for a complete diet for circulatory improvement. diet.

Colds
Upper Respiratory Infections

The common cold is quite common. Within any two week period during high risk seasons, about a third of America suffers from a cold. A cold is usually an attempt by the body to cleanse itself of wastes, toxins and bacterial overgrowth that have built up to the point where natural immunity cannot handle or overcome them. The glands are always affected, and as the endocrine system is on a 6 day cycle, a normal cold usually runs for about a week as the body works through all its detoxification processes. Natural remedies are effective in speeding recovery and reducing discomfort.

Diet & Superfood Therapy

To prevent a cold: keep immune response strong with optimum nutrition. During high risk seasons, get plenty of rest and regular exercise.

♣ When you have a cold:

Go on a liquid diet during **acute stage,** with green or potassium drinks (pg.167) to clean out infection and mucous.

✸Then eat light meals when fever and acute stage has passed - fresh and steamed vegetables, fresh fruits and juices, and cultured foods for friendly intestinal flora.

✸Avoid dairy products of all kinds, red meats, sugars and fried or fatty foods.

✸Chicken soup increases mucous release.

✸Drink six to eight glasses of liquids daily, especially green tea.

✸ Take 2 TBS. cider vinegar, and 2 teasp. honey in water, or garlic/ginger tea each morning, and garlic/miso soup each night.

✸Or 2 TBS. each lemon juice and honey, and 1 teasp. fresh grated ginger at night.

♣ To release quantities of mucous all at once, take fresh grated horseradish in a spoon with lemon juice, and hang over the sink; or use onion/garlic syrup (page 253) for gentler mucous release, especially for a streaming cold.

♣ Effective superfoods:

✸Crystal Star BIOFLAV., FIBER & C SUPPORT™ drink for nasal congestion - clears in 15 to 20 minutes; GREEN TEA CLEANSER™ to combat infection.

✸Balance your intestinal structure with Solgar WHEY TO GO protein drink.

Herbal Therapy

♣ Jump start herbal program:
During acute phase:

✸Crystal Star FIRST AID CAPS™ every hour during acute stages to promote sweating and eliminate toxins. (Use as a preventive in initial stage.)

✸Zand HERBAL LOZENGES, or

✸Beehive Botanical PROPOLIS THROAT SPRAY every 2 hours. ⊛

then

✸ **ANTI-BIO™ capsules or extract to flush the lymph glands for 6 days.**
✸Throat coats: COFEX™ TEA

-Elderberry/mint/yarrow tea

✸Crystal Star ZINC SOURCE™ extract and hot ginger compresses to the chest.

♣ Make a "cold" cocktail: Mix in a glass with aloe vera juice - ¼ teasp. vitamin C crystals, 2 teasp. SAMBUCOL elderberry syrup, ½ teasp. turmeric powder (or 1 opened capsule curcumin), 1 opened capsule echinacea, ½ teasp. propolis extract. Works great!

♣ During recovery phase:

✸USNEA extract for both viral and bacterial infections. ♂

✸Crystal Star HERBAL DEFENSE TEAM™.

♣ Effective system cleansers:

✸Cayenne/ginger capsules
✸Echinacea/golden seal capsules
✸Cayenne/garlic capsules
✸Zand DECONGEST extract
✸Crystal Star X-PECT-T™ ⊛

♣ Stimulate immunity:

✸Crystal Star COLD SEASON DEFENSE™
✸Zand ASTRAGALUS extract. ♀

Supplements

✸ Ester C or vitamin C crystals, ¼ teasp. every half hour to bowel tolerance to flush the body and neutralize toxins. Use also as a preventive to decrease the length and severity of colds and to boost immunity.

✸ Nutribiotic GRAPEFRUIT SEED extract spray, or gargle (3 drops in 5-oz. water) to release mucous and phlegm.

✸H_2O_2 nasal spray: (make with several drops of 3% solution in 5-oz. water) to reduce congestion and clear sinuses. ♂ ♀
✸Nutribiotic NASAL SPRAY & EAR DROPS.

✸ For coughs: Planetary formulas OLD INDIAN COUGH SYRUP and Olbas COUGH SYRUP and pastilles.
✸Zinc lozenges to kill throat bacteria.

✸ Stimulate immunity:
✸CoQ_{10} 30mg 3x daily.
✸Nutricology LACTOFERRIN caps.

✸ High risk season preventives:
✸Beta carotene 25,000IU 4x daily.
✸Zinc 30mg daily. ♂
✸Garlic caps 6 daily.
✸Acidophilus liquid 3 tsp. daily. ⊛

✸ Effective homeopathic remedies:
✸Boiron OSCILLOCOCCINUM
✸B&T ALPHA CF tabs
✸Eupatorium Perfoliatum ⊛
✸Hylands C PLUS ⊛

✸ Enzyme therapy:
✸Prevail DEFENSE FORMULA

Lifestyle Support Therapy

Avoid drug store cold remedies. They halt the body cleansing/balancing processes, and generally make the cold last longer.

☞ Open all channels of elimination with hot baths or showers, hot broths and tonics, (pg. 170) brandy and lemon, and catnip enemas.

✸To prevent colds, start taking alternating hot and cold showers at the beginning of cold season every day to stimulate immune response. Repeat any time you feel the first signs of discomfort.

☞ Aromatherapy steams, with or without a vaporizer are effective:

✸Eucalyptus opens sinus passages.
✸Wintergreen relieves nasal congestion.
✸Mint or chamomile relieve headache.
✸Tea tree oil combats infection.

☞ Rest is important. Adequate sleep is necessary. Light exercise is better than vigorous exercise during a cold.

☞ A massage therapy treatment can open up blocked body meridians.

☞ Acupressure press points:

✸For a scratchy, hoarse throat: press between the nail and the first joint of the thumb, just behind the nail, on the outside.

✸To unclog a stuffy nose: press on the cheek, at the flare of the nostrils where they join the cheek.

See FLU page for what to do for flu.

What If You Have Chronic Colds?

Even though rhino-viruses are involved in the misery we know as a cold, we are constantly exposed to these organisms without them causing a cold. Reduced immune system health is the deciding factor in whether you "catch" a cold or not. There seem to be almost as many drugstore cold remedies as there are colds, most of them symptom-suppressing with side effects. Since a cold is usually a cleansing condition, I feel it is often just better to let it happen so your body can start fresh, with a stronger immune system. Yet, without a doubt, it is hard to work, sleep, and be around other people with miserable cold symptoms. Traditional wisdom is effective for minimizing misery while your body gets on with its job of cleaning house.

1) Take a daily walk to rev up your immune system, and give your body some fresh air. A walk puts cleansing oxygen into your lungs, and stops you from feeling sorry for yourself. It works wonders!
2) Take ascorbate vitamin C or Ester C, 1000mg every hour, preferably in powder form with juice, throughout the day. Take zinc lozenges as needed, or propolis throat spray.
3) No smoking or alcohol (other than a little brandy and lemon). They suppress immunity. Avoid refined foods, sugar, and dairy foods. They increase production of thick mucous.
4) Eat lightly but with good nutrition. Nutrient absorption is less efficient during a cold. A vegetarian diet is best at this time so the body won't have to work so hard at digestion.
5) Drink plenty of liquids; 6-8 glasses daily of fresh fruit and vegetable juices, herb teas, and water. These will help flush toxins through and out of the system.
6) Keep warm. Don't worry about a fever unless it is prolonged or very high. (See fevers as cleansers and healers) Take a long hot bath, spa or sauna. Lots of toxins can pass out though the skin. Increase room humidity so the mucous membranes will remain active against the virus or bacteria.
7) Stay relaxed. Let the body concentrate its energy on cleansing the infection. Go to bed early, and get plenty of sleep. Most regeneration of virus-damaged cells occurs between midnight and 4 a.m.
8) Think positively about becoming well. Optimism is often a self-fulfilling prophecy.

Do You Have A Cold Or The Flu? Here's How To Tell.

Colds and flu are distinct and separate upper respiratory infections, triggered by different viruses. (Outdoor environment - drafts, wetness, temperature changes, etc. do not cause either of these illnesses.) The flu is more serious, because it can spread to the lungs, and cause severe bronchitis or pneumonia. In the beginning stages, the symptoms of colds and flu can be similar. Both conditions begin when viruses (that, unlike bacteria, cannot reproduce outside the cells), penetrate the body's protective barriers. Nose, eyes and mouth are usually the sites of invasion from cold viruses. The most likely target for the flu virus is the respiratory tract. Colds and flu respond to different treatments. The following symptomatic chart can help identify your particular condition and allow you to deal with it better.

A Cold Profile Looks Like This:
• Slow onset. No prostration.
• Body aches - largely due to the release of interferon (an immune stimulator)
• Rarely accompanied by fever and headache.
• Localized symptoms such as sore throat, sinus congestion, listlessness, runny nose and sneezing.
• Mild fatigue and weakness as a result of body cleansing.
• Mild to moderate chest discomfort, usually with a hacking cough.
• Sore or burning throat common.

A Flu Profile Looks Like This:
• Swift and severe onset.
• Early and prominent prostration with flushed, hot, moist skin.
• Usually accompanied by high (102° -104°) fever, headache and sore eyes.
• General symptoms like chills, depression and body aches.
• Extreme fatigue, sometimes lasting 2-3 weeks.
• Acute chest discomfort, with severe hacking cough.
• Sore throat occasionally.

Cold Sores & Fever Blisters
Canker Sores * Mouth Herpes (Simplex 1)

These mouth sores are quite common and indicate recurrent body chemistry imbalance, sometimes coupled with a hypothyroid condition and usually triggered by a food allergy. They can occur on the lips, tongue, inside the cheeks or on the gums. They are generally the result of a herpes simplex virus 1 infection, occurring after a fever, illness, body stress, and resulting reduced immunity. They can also be caused by nutrient deficiencies, or hormone imbalance, such as before menses. Mouth sores occur most often in women, generally because of hormone imbalances during the menstrual cycle. They are more prevalent in winter than warm months, unless the lips get sunburned.

Diet & Superfood Therapy

☙ Body acid/alkaline balance is important: Add more cultured foods to your diet for prevention: yogurt, kefir, sauerkraut, etc.

☙ Avoid high arginine foods, such as coffee, peanut butter, nuts, seeds, corn, etc. Avoid red meats, caffeine, refined and fried foods, sugars and sweet fruits.

☙ Eat a mineral-rich diet: plenty of salads, lots of raw and cooked vegetables, whole grains. Baked potatoes and steamed broccoli are especially good.
☙Drink a fresh carrot juice once a week.

☙ Tannins and bioflavonoids help. Apply:
⚘ Red wine residues
⚘ Green tea cold tea bags
⚘ Grape juice

☙ Effective superfoods:
⚘ Crystal Star SYSTEMS STRENGTH™ drink to alkalize the body. Take BIOFLAV., FIBER & C SUPPORT drink for concentrated food flavonoids.
⚘ Lewis Labs BREWERS YEAST, take **2 TBS. daily.**

☙ Take aloe vera juice internally. Apply aloe vera skin gel frequently.

Herbal Therapy

☙ Jump start herbal program:
⚘Crystal Star HRPS™ capsules 4-6 daily, to alkalize and heal; ANTI-FLAM™ to reduce pain and inflammation.
⚘Apply LYSINE/LICORICE GEL™
⚘Source Naturals RED ALGAE.

☙ Crystal Star RELAX CAPS™ as needed to calm the tension often causing sores; or
⚘Burdock tea 2 cups daily to balance hormones.♀

☙ Licorice extract, or GINSENG/LICO-RICE extract, or a mouthwash made from deglycyrrhizinated licorice chewable tablets - apply directly, take internally.

☙ Apply St. John's wort salve. Take St. John's wort capsules or Crystal Star ANTI-VIT™ extract as anti-virals.

☙ Effective herbal mouthwashes: swish around in mouth several times daily.
⚘White oak extract, an astringent ♂
⚘Camomile flowers ♀
⚘Lemon balm tea or extract
⚘Red sage

☙ Propolis lozenges - apply propolis extract directly, and take under the tongue to boost immune response, or use Beehive Botanicals PROPOLIS THROAT SPRAY.

Supplements

☙ Ester C or ascorbate vitamin C crystals with bioflavonoids: Take ¼ teasp. every 2-3 hours in juice. Make a strong solution in water and apply directly to sores every half hour until they subside.
with
⚘B Complex 100mg. daily with extra B₆ 250mg, and pantothenic acid 100mg for adrenal support, 3x daily.
⚘Use zinc lozenges several times daily.

☙ Dr. Diamond HERPANACINE capsules as directed 2x daily.
⚘Enzymatic Therapy HERPILYN cream.

☙ Take Lysine 1000mg daily. Apply SUPER LYSINE PLUS cream on blisters.

☙ Source Naturals ACTIVATED QUERCETIN with Bromelain 500mg 2x daily.

☙ Prof. Nutrition DR. DOPHILUS, or Natren LIFE BIFIDO-FACTORS, ¼ teasp. 4x daily in ⊛ water or dissolve opened capsules in water and rinse mouth 3x daily.

☙ Effective homeopathic remedies:
⚘Hylands *Hylavir* ⊛
⚘Natrum *Muriaticum*

☙ For leukoplakia (pre-cancerous mouth sores), use selenium 200mcg daily.

Lifestyle Support Therapy

☙ **During the acute stage:**
Apply Nutribiotic GRAPEFRUIT SEED SKIN SPRAY to sore as needed.

☙ **Effective rinses to alter mouth pH:**
⚘Golden seal solution, or goldenseal/myrrh solution. Swish in mouth every half hour.
⚘Echinacea solution in water.

☙ **Effective topical applications:**
⚘Matrix GENESIS OXY-SPRAY
⚘Calendula ointment
⚘BLACK WALNUT tincture
⚘Tea tree oil
⚘Comfrey/aloe salve
⚘Red raspberry tincture
⚘B & T homeopathic *SSSTING STOP*

☙ Apply ice packs frequently. Follow with vitamin E oil.

☙ Check your toothpaste. It should be sodium-lauryl-sulfate free.

☙ Relax more. Get plenty of sleep and rest.
⚘Use sunblock more often.

Common Symptoms: *Contagious herpes simplex virus sores on the face and mouth. (Don't kiss if you have a cold sore.) They begin with a small, sore bump, and turning into a very sore, often pussy blister. Lips and inside of the mouth are usually also sore.*

Common Causes: *Herpes simplex virus 1; B Complex, iron or folic acid deficiency; high arginine foods diet; reduced immunity; Sodium-lauryl-sulfate toothpaste; premenstrual tension and consequent hormone imbalance; Crohn's disease; gluten sensitivity; over-acid diet; recurring virus infection; emotional stress.*

See IMMUNITY page in this book for extra help.

Colitis & Irritable Bowel Syndrome (IBS)

Ulcerative Colitis ❖ Spastic Colon ❖ Ileitis

A chronically inflamed colon is often a result of food allergies, usually a gluten reaction to wheat, or cheese, corn or eggs or other sensitivity. Colon membranes become irritated, and the body forms pouchy pockets in reaction. In severe cases ulcerous lesions line the sides of the colon. Natural therapies are effective and reduce the need for drugs. Many sufferers see dramatic results.

Diet & Superfood Therapy

Diet changes are a must. Healing herbs will not work without diet changes.

❧ **During the acute stage:** Go on a mono diet for 2 days with apples and apple juice.
➽ Then eat a low fat diet with plenty of fiber, but low roughage. Foods should be lightly cooked, never fried, with few salts.
➽ Include fresh fruits, fruit fiber from prunes, apples and raisins, green salads with olive oil and lemon dressing, whole grain cereals, such as oatmeal and brown rice, and steamed vegetables.
➽ Have a glass of mixed vegetable juice (page 168) daily for the first two weeks.
➽ Eat cultured foods, such as yogurt and kefir for friendly intestinal flora.
➽ Have fresh carrot juice 3x a week.
➽ Keep the body well-hydrated.
➽ Eat smaller, more frequent meals. No large meals.

❧ **Avoid coffee and caffeine-containing foods:** nuts, seeds, dairy and citrus fruits while healing. Spicy foods are an irritant.

❧ **Effective superfoods:**
➽ Crystal Star CHO-LO FIBER TONE™ drink at bedtime for 2 weeks.◯↗
➽**Wakunaga KYO-GREEN.**
➽**AloeLife ALOE GOLD drink.**

Herbal Therapy

❧ **Jump start herbal program:**
➽Take Planetary Formulas TRIPHALA caps and Crystal Star BWL-TONE IBS™.
➽Add una da gato capsules (cat's claw), BITTERS & LEMON CLEANSE™ drops, or MILK THISTLE SEED drops in water each morning if desired.

or

➽ Crystal Star GREEN TEA CLEANSER™ 2 cups daily with 2 to 3 peppermint oil drops added, 2x daily.

❧ **Effective anti-spasmodics:**
➽Crystal Star RELAX CAPS™, ANTI-SPZ caps or CRAMP BARK COMPLEX™ extract ◯+
➽Chamomile tea
➽VALERIAN/WILD LETTUCE extract

❧ **Soothing teas for irritation:**
➽Slippery elm
➽Pau d' arco
➽Rosemary

❧ **Immune system support is crucial:**
➽Royal Jelly with ginseng 2 teasp. daily.
➽Alfalfa tablets 6-10 daily, or Solaray ALFA-JUICE caps.
➽Bee pollen 2 teasp. daily.

❧ Apply warm ginger compresses to spine and stomach and drink peppermint tea.

Supplements

Liquid and chewable supplements are best for colitis irritation.

❧ **Probiotics - enzyme therapy is important:**
➽Country Life BROMELAIN with 2000gdu activity. ◯↗
➽Chewable papaya enzymes
➽Alta Health CANGEST powder
➽Solaray SUPER DIGESTAWAY
➽Enzymatic Therapy chewable DGL tabs before meals, PEPPERMINT PLUS (enteric-coated peppermint oil) between meals and GUGGULPLUS each morning
➽An electrolyte replacement drink if there is diarrhea. ◯
➽Chlorophyll liquid 3 teasp. daily in water before meals.
➽Pancreatin enzymes - full strength
➽Natren TRINITY as directed in water to rebalance bowel flora. ◯

❧ Source Naturals NAG capsules; or
➽American Biologics SHARKILAGE capsules as directed.

❧ High Omega-3 flax oil 3 teasp. daily as an anti-inflammatory.

❧ Nature's Secret ULTIMATE MULTI PLUS 2x daily for 2 months.

❧ **Homeopathy:** *SILICEA* or *NUX VOMICA* tablets.

Lifestyle Support Therapy

Many elimination channel problems mimic IBS. A physical exam can help pinpoint the problem. If there is appendicitis-like sharp pain, seek medical help immediately.

❧ Effective gentle enemas to rid the colon of fermenting wastes and relieve pain:
➽Peppermint tea
➽White oak bark
➽Slippery elm
➽Chamomile
➽Lobelia

❧ Biofeedback is especially helpful for IBS as a stress reduction technique.

❧ **Acupressure help:**
➽Stroke abdomen up, across and down.

❧ **Watchwords:**
➽Do not take aspirin. Use an herbal analgesic, or non-aspirin pain killer.
➽Avoid antacids. They often do more harm than good by neutralizing body HCl.
➽Consciously practice relaxation techniques like meditation to reduce stress.

See also CROHN'S DISEASE for more information.

Common Symptoms: First symptoms include weakness, lethargy and fatigue; then abdominal cramps and pain; recurrent constipation, usually alternating with bloody diarrhea; rectal hemorrhoids, fistulas and abscesses; mucous in the stool; urgency to defecate; dehydration and mineral loss; unhealthy weight loss with abdominal distention.
Common Causes: Excess refined foods and sweets; lack of dietary fiber; food allergies; yeast disease like candida albicans; heavy smoking and/or caffeine use; vitamin K deficiency; anemia and electrolyte imbalance; emotional stress, depression and anxiety; too many antibiotics, causing reduced immunity; a small number of cases are genetically prone.

Constipation & Waste Management
Colon & Bowel Health

The colon and bowel are the depository for all waste material after food nutrients have been extracted and processed to the bloodstream. It is hardly any wonder that up to 90% of all diseases generate from an unclean colon. Decaying food ferments, forms gases, as well as 2nd and 3rd generation toxins, and the colon becomes a breeding ground for putrefactive bacteria, viruses, parasites, yeasts, molds, etc. Ideally, one should eliminate after each meal. Bowel transit time should be approx. 12 hours. To promote healthy bowel function, include plenty of fiber and liquids in your diet, exercise regularly and establish a regular daily time for elimination.

Diet & Superfood Therapy

Diet awareness is the key to colon health.

❧ Start with a short colon cleansing juice diet (pg. 157) to rid the bowel of wastes.

✻Then, follow a low fat, largely vegetarian diet, with plenty of fruits, whole grains, salad greens, and cultured foods like yogurt to establish good intestinal flora.

✻Make fiber the key; it doesn't get digested; it simply moves through your system, helping other foods to move along with it.

✻Drink 6-8 glasses of healthy liquids every day; avoid milk and dairy drinks.

✻Avoid all high fat, sugary, processed and fried foods and dairy foods; they don't allow your body to get rid of waste easily.

✻Chew food well, and eat smaller meals. No large heavy meals.

❧ **An easy make-it-yourself fiber drink:** mix equal parts of flax seed and oat bran in water. Let sit overnight. Take 2 TBS. in the morning in juice.

❧ **Effective superfoods:**
✻Crystal Star BIOFLAV., FIBER & C SUPPORT™ drink for 3 gms. fiber per serving, or CHO-LO-FIBER TONE™ drink.
✻Aloe Falls ALOE JUICE with GINGER
✻**Nutricology PRO GREENS with flax.**
✻Solgar WHEY TO GO protein drink.
✻Or. Peel Enterprises GREENS PLUS.

Herbal Therapy

❧ **Jump start herbal program:**
✻**Crystal Star FIBER & HERBS COLON CLEANSE™ capsules 2, 3x daily. and/or**
✻LAXA-TEA™ to flush wastes gently and quickly the first few days.

❧ Planetary Formulas TRIPHALA to promote a firm, healthy odor-free stool.

❧ MILK THISTLE SEED, or dandelion extract to enhance bile output and soften stool.

❧ **Herbal laxatives and regulators:**
✻Senna leaf and pods (use sparingly - a little goes a long way.)
✻Cascara sagrada to increase peristalsis and normalize evacuation.
✻AloeLife FIBER-MATE drink. ♂
✻Bee pollen 2 teasp. to regulate intestinal function.
✻HERBALTONE caps. ♀
✻Solaray TETRA CLEANSE.
✻Omega-3 flax seed oil capsules to prevent constipation.
✻Fennel/ginger caps 4 at a time (also freshens breath.)
✻Garlic capsules, 4 daily.

Supplements

Avoid drugstore antibiotics, antacids and milk of magnesia. They kill friendly intestinal flora.

✌ **Quick fix for occasional constipation: Take 3000 to 5000mg vitamin C with bioflavonoids over a two hour period. Voila!**

✌ **Probiotics to prevent constipation:**
✻Professional Nutrition Dr. DOPHILUS
✻Solaray MULTI-DOPHILUS
✻Natren TRINITY
✻Alta Health CANGEST powder (also helps liver function)
✻Prevail INNER ECOLOGY
✻**Prevail FIBER-ZYME 2x daily.**

✌ **Colon cleansing aids:**
✻**Nature's Secret A.M./P.M. ULTIMATE CLEANSE.**
✻**TRIM MAX by Body Breakthrough**
✻**Zand QUICK CLEANSE**
✻**Earth's Bounty OXY-CLEANSE**

✌ Take a *food source* multi-vitamin to control initial gas and stomach rumbling as the additional dietary fiber combines with the minerals in the G.I. tract.

✌ Apple pectin or HCL tablets at meals.♂

Lifestyle Support Therapy

The protective level of fiber in the diet can be easily measured:
1) the stool should be light enough to float.
2) bowel movements should be regular, daily and effortless.
3) the stool should be almost odorless, signalling decreased transit time in the bowel.
4) there should be no gas or flatulence.

☙ Take a colonic irrigation to start your program. **A grapefruit seed extract colonic is extremely effective, especially if there is colon toxicity along with constipation.** (Dilute to 15 to 20 drops per gallon of water.)

☙ Take a catnip enema once a week to keep cleansing well. (See page 446)
✻Note: Enemas may be given to children. Use small amounts according to size and age. Allow water to enter very slowly; allow them to expel when they wish.

☙ Take a brisk daily walk to stimulate regularity.

☙ Stroke and press each of the reflexology points for 3-5 minutes:

colon points

See DIVERTICULITIS page in this book for more information.

Common Symptoms: Infrequent bowel movements; flatulence and gas; fatigue, nausea and depression; nervous irritability; coated tongue; headaches; bad breath and body odor; mental dullness; sallow skin.
Common Causes: Poor diet with too little fiber, and too much fast, fried, sugary, low-residue foods; especially cheese and cow's milk; drugs, travel and stress all affect bowel regularity; too much red meat, pasteurized dairy, caffeine and alcohol; overeating and eating late at night; overuse of drugs and laxatives; hypothyroidism; lack of exercise.

Step-By-Step Diet Change For Colon Health

Most poor health conditions extend from poor elimination in one way or another. Elements causing constipation and colon toxicity come from three basic areas:

1) Chemical-laced foods, and pollutants in the environment, ranging from relatively harmless to very dangerous. The body can tolerate a certain level of contamination. When that individual level is reached, and immune defenses are low, toxic overload causes illness. A strong system can metabolize and excrete many of these toxins, but when the body is weak or constipated, they are stored as unusable substances. As more and different chemicals enter and build up in the body they tend to interreact with those that are already there, forming mutant, second generation chemicals far more harmful than the originals. Evidence in recent years has shown that most bowel cancer is caused by environmental agents.

2) Over-accumulation of body wastes and metabolic byproducts that are not excreted properly. These wastes can also become a breeding ground for parasite infestation. A nationwide survey reveals that one in every six people studied had one or more parasites living somewhere in their bodies! An astounding figure.

3) Slowed elimination time, allowing waste materials to ferment, become rancid, and then recirculate through the body tissues as toxic substances. These and other factors result in sluggish organ and glandular functions, poor digestion and assimilation, lowered immunity, faulty circulation, and tissue degeneration.

The key to avoiding bowel problems is almost always nutritional. A high fiber, low fat diet, with lots of fresh foods is important to both cure and prevent waste elimination problems. Diet improvement can also correct the diseases waste elimination problems cause. Even a gentle and gradual improvement from low fiber, low residue foods helps almost immediately. In fact, graduated change is often better than a sudden, drastic about-face, especially when the colon, bowel or bladder are painful and inflamed. Constipation is normally a chronic problem, and while body cleansing progress can be felt fairly quickly with a diet change, it takes from three to six months to rebuild bowel and colon elasticity with good systolic/diastolic action. There is no easy route, but the rewards of a regular, energetic life are worth it. See also *THE BODY SMART SYSTEM* by Helene Silver for more information.

After the initial cleansing juice diet, (see page 157), the second part of a good colon health program is rebuilding healthy tissue and body energy. This stage may be used for 1 to 2 months. It emphasizes high fiber through fresh vegetables and fruits, cultured foods for increased assimilation and enzyme production, and alkalizing foods to prevent irritation while healing. During this diet avoid refined foods, saturated fats or oils, fried foods, meats, caffeine or other acid or mucous forming foods, such as pasteurized dairy products.

On rising: take a glass of AloeLife ALOE VERA JUICE, with 1 teasp. liquid acidophilus added; or Crystal Star CHO-LO FIBER TONE™ capsules, or drink mix in apple or orange juice.

Breakfast: Soak a mix of dried prunes, figs and raisins the night before; take 2 to 4 TBS. with 1 TB. blackstrap molasses, or mix with yogurt; or make a mix of oat bran, raisins, and pumpkin seeds, and mix with yogurt or apple juice, or a light veggie broth. Add 2 teasp. brewer's yeast or Lewis Labs FIBER YEAST; and have some oatmeal or a whole grain cereal, granola or muesli with yogurt or apple juice; or have a bowl of mixed fresh fruits with apple juice or yogurt.

Mid-morning: take a veggie drink (page 168), Sun CHLORELLA, Green Foods GREEN ESSENCE, or Crystal Star ENERGY GREEN™ drink; or pau d'arco, green tea or Crystal Star GREEN TEA CLEANSER™ to alkalize the system. or a fresh carrot juice;

Lunch: have a fresh green salad every day with lemon/olive oil dressing, or yogurt cheese or kefir cheese; or steamed veggies and a baked potato with soy or kefir cheese; or a fresh fruit salad with a little yogurt or raw cottage cheese topping.

Mid-afternoon: have another fresh carrot juice, or Crystal Star SYSTEMS STRENGTH™ drink; and/or green tea or slippery elm tea. and/or some raw crunchy veggies with a vegetable or kefir cheese dip, or soy spread.

Dinner: have a large dinner salad with black bean or lentil soup; or an oriental stir fry and miso soup with sea vegetables snipped on top; or a steamed or baked vegetable casserole with a yogurt or soy cheese sauce; or a vegetable or whole grain pasta with a light lemon or yogurt sauce.

Before bed: have some apple or papaya juice; or another glass of aloe vera juice with herbs; or Crystal Star CHO-LO FIBER TONE™ drink or capsules, or BIOFLAV, FIBER & C SUPPORT™ drink.

Cough

Chronic Cough ❧ Dry, Hacking Cough ❧ Smokers Cough

A continuing cough, one that lasts more than 2 or 3 weeks, is not the result of infection per se, but evidence of continuing throat irritation from smoking, environmental pollens, or chemical pollutants. It should be regarded as a sign of reduced immunity, and treated both topically, and as part of an immune-stimulating program.

Diet & Superfood Therapy

🌿 Start with a short colon cleansing juice diet (pg. 159) to rid the bowel of current wastes.

➤ Take 2TBS. honey and 2TBS. lemon juice in water or cider vinegar to stop the tickle.

➤ Drink cleansing fruit juices. Eat high vitamin C foods, such as sprouts, green peppers, broccoli, citrus and cherries.

➤ Take a cup of hot black tea with the juice of 1 lemon and 1 teasp. honey.

➤ Take a cup of hot water with 2TBS. brandy and 2TBS. lemon juice.

🌿 Avoid pasteurized dairy products during acute stages.

🌿 Make your own honey/onion cough syrup: Slice a large onion into rings and place in a bowl. Cover with honey and let stand 24 hours. Strain off liquid mixture and you have an anti-microbial cough elixir.

🌿 **Effective superfoods:**
➤ **Crystal Star BIOFLAV, FIBER & C SUPPORT™ drink.**
➤ AloeLife ALOE JUICE.
➤ Y.S. ROYAL JELLY with ginseng drink.

Herbal Therapy

🍃 **Jump start herbal program:** **Crystal Star COFEX TEA™, especially at night. Usually works within 24 hours.**
➤ **X-PECT™ TEA as an expectorant.**
➤ **ANTI-SPZ™ capsules, 4 at a time as needed for spasmodic coughing, or** Nature's Way ANTSP tincture.
➤ **GINSENG/LICORICE ELIXIR™** drops directly on the throat.

🍃 **Use propolis extract under the tongue or lozenges as desired, or Beehive Botanicals PROPOLIS THROAT SPRAY.**

🍃 **Other effective topicals: use directly on the throat:**
➤ Horehound, licorice, and wild cherry drops, or syrups.
➤ **Slippery Elm lozenges. ♂**
➤ Zand HERBAL lozenges. ♀

🍃 **Effective teas or steams:**
➤ Wild cherry to suppress a cough
➤ Coltsfoot for a cough with mucous (small amounts only)
➤ **Sage or rose hips tea with lemon juice, honey, and fresh ginger root.**
➤ Clove tea for spasmodic coughing.
➤ Marshmallow for a dry cough.

🍃 Garlic capsules 4 to 6 daily.

Supplements

✥ **Strengthen immune response:**
➤ Ascorbate vitamin C or Ester C powder: ¼ teasp. every half hour to bowel tolerance.

with

➤ Beta-carotene 25,000IU 2x daily.

✥ **Effective lozenges:**
➤ **Zinc gluconate lozenges as needed.**
➤ Ricola lozenges/pearls.
➤ Olbas Cough Syrup and pastilles.

✥ **Effective homeopathic remedies:**
➤ BioForce *Biotussin* drops and tablets.
➤ Hylands *Cough Syrup.*
➤ B&T *Cough Syrup.*
➤ Standard Homeopath *Hylavir* tablets.
➤ Bioforce Santasapina cough drops.

Lifestyle Support Therapy

🌿 Eliminate smoking and secondary smoke from your environment.

🌿 **Effective gargles:**
➤ Tea tree oil drops in water
➤ Slippery elm tea
➤ Aloe vera juice
➤ Echinacea/goldenseal solution

🌿 Steam eucalyptus, peppermint or tincture of benzoin in a vaporizer at night.

🌿 Avoid commercial cough syrups, and drugstore over-the-counter medicines. They often make the problem worse by suppression, which forces the infection deeper into the tissues.

See SORE THROAT, COLDS & FLU pages in this book for more information.

Common Symptoms: Hacking, dry or chronic coughing with no phlegm or mucous eliminated; a reflex reaction to an obstruction of the airways; chronic, rough smoker's-throat cough from constant irritation.
Common Causes: Low grade chronic infection of throat and sinuses (often the hanging-on result of a cold or flu); mucous-forming diet; allergies; environmental irritants; cigarette smoking or secondary smoking irritation.

Crohn's Disease
Regional Enteritis

Crohn's disease, chronic inflammation of the digestive tract, affects about 2 million Americans today. It is characterized by painful ulcers that form in one or more sections, or all along the length of the gastrointestinal lining. When the ulcers heal they leave thick scar tissue that narrows and hardens the tract and adversely affects elimination. Poor assimilation of nutrients is always involved; accompanying ulcerous bleeding often causes anemia. A strictly followed, highly nutritious, mild foods diet has proven to be an effective, non-toxic alternative to cortico-steroid drugs.

Diet & Superfood Therapy

❧ **Diet improvement is the key:**

1) Start with an alkalizing liquid diet for 3 days: carrot and apple juice, grape juice, pineapple and green vegetable drinks.

2) Then add mild fruits and vegetables for a week: carrots, potatoes, yams, apples, papayas, bananas, etc.

3) Add steamed and raw vegetables, brans, cultured foods for 2 weeks: yogurt, kefir, miso, etc., and especially fresh salads.

4) Add rice, whole grains, wheat germ, tofu, fish and seafood for healing protein.

5) The continuing diet should be high in complex carbohydrates, fiber and fresh vegetables, and low in fats. **(Avoid too much fiber during flare-ups.)**

❧ Avoid nuts, seeds, and citrus while healing. Eliminate red and fatty meats, saturated fats (especially from dairy foods), and fried foods.

➥ Drink only bottled water. Over treated tap water can wreak havoc on an inflamed bowel.

☙

❧ **Effective superfoods:**
➻Crystal Star ENERGY GREEN™
➻Green Foods GREEN MAGMA
➻Solgar WHEY TO GO protein drink
➻AloeLife ALOE GOLD JUICE
➻Y.S. ROYAL JELLY with ginseng
➻Lewis Labs FIBER YEAST each A.M. ♀♂

Herbal Therapy

Crohn's disease sufferers can react to almost anything, no matter how mild or soothing. Start slowly, noting your reactions carefully.

❧ **Jump start herbal program:**
➻**Crystal Star BWL TONE™ caps and/or GREEN TEA CLEANSER™, or CAN-SSIAC™ extract for 3 months.**

with

➻ANTI-FLAM™ extract in water to ease pain without aspirin salicylates, and ALOE VERA JUICE 4 glasses daily.

❧ **EVENING PRIMROSE OIL caps 500mg 2x daily.** ♀

❧ Flora ESSENCE drink 2-oz daily. Use in Wisdom of the Ancients YERBA-MATE or fenugreek tea for best results.

❧ **Mix 1 teasp. bee pollen in a cup of chamomile tea. Take 2x daily.**

❧ Effective herbal anti-oxidants to scavenge free radicals involved in Crohn's.
➻Garlic capsules 4-6 daily.
➻Una da gato caps
➻Pau d' Arco

❧ Effective herbal flavonoids:
➻HAWTHORN extract
➻BILBERRY extract
➻Rose hips

Supplements

Use liquid or powdered supplements whenever possible for the least irritation.

❧ **Strengthen immune response:**
➻Ascorbate vitamin C with bioflavonoids powder, ¹⁄₄ teasp. 4 to 6x daily.
➻Glutamine 500mg - as effective as prednisone in controlling Crohn's and GI integrity.
➻OPCs from grapeseed, 50mg 3x daily.
➻Am. Biologics DIOXYCHLOR.

✓ **Take daily for enzyme therapy:**
➻Quercetin with bromelain 750mg, or Solaray QBC complex.
➻Dr. DOPHILUS, or Natren TRINITY powder ¹⁄₄ teasp. 3x daily, before meals.
➻Chewable bromelain 40mg or papaya enzymes after meals. ♂

✓ Enzymatic Therapy IBS capsules, LIQUID LIVER w. Siberian ginseng, with chewable DGL tablets as needed.

and

➥**Omega-3 flax oil capsules daily to reduce inflammation.**♀

❧ **Replace depleted nutrients:**
➻Zinc picolinate 15-30mg daily. ♂
➻Magnesium 200mg3x daily.
➻B Complex liquid with extra B₂, B₆, and pantothenic acid.
➻Nature's Bounty internasal B₁₂ gel.
➻Vitamin E 400IU daily 2x daily.

Lifestyle Support Therapy

Avoid commercial antacids. They eventually make the inflammation worse by causing the stomach to produce more acids.

➻ Consciously work to reduce stress in your life. Acupuncture, yoga and meditation have all been successful with Crohn's.

➻ Eat smaller meals, more frequently.

➻ Use peppermint tea enemas once a week for the first month of healing.

➻ Apply hot, wet ginger compresses to stomach and lower back.

➻ **Reflexology points:**

stomach & colon

➻ Crohn's disease region:

Common Symptoms: Inflammation and soreness along the entire G.I. tract; bouts of diarrhea with a low grade fever; raised white blood cell counts; abdominal distention, tenderness and pain from food residue and gas; abnormal weight loss and depression; anemia.

Common Causes: A diet with low fiber, excess refined sugar and acid-forming foods, leading to a severely inflamed colon which forms deep ulcers along the entire length of the digestive tract from rectum to mouth. Malnutrition is common in Crohn's disease. Multiple food intolerances, particularly to wheat and dairy; emotional stress; zinc deficiency.

See DIVERTICULITIS and COLITIS pages in this book for more information.

Cysts & Polyps
Benign Tumors * Lipomas * Wens

Benign growths of varying size - found both internally on the intestinal, urethral, genital passage linings, and externally anywhere on the skin. They often arise from an excessive growth of fat cells. They are responsive to the body's growth-regulating mechanisms and quite receptive to natural therapies. They can be annoying, unsightly, and in some cases lead to cancer.

Diet & Superfood Therapy

❧ Go on a short 1 to 3 day liquid diet (page 157) to set up a healing environment, stimulate the liver and clean the blood. Then follow with a fresh foods diet for the rest of the week.

❧ Avoid red meats, caffeine, pasteurized dairy products and acid-forming foods.

❧ Eliminate saturated fats (mostly animal fats), fried foods, chocolate, margarine, shortening and other refined fats.

❧ Add more fish, seafoods, sea vegetables and unsaturated oils, such as flax and sunflower oil to the diet.

❧ **Effective superfoods:**
 ✺Crystal Star SYSTEMS STRENGTH™ drink.
 ✺Sun CHLORELLA 1 packet daily.
 ✺AloeLife ALOE JUICE each morning.
 ✺**Add 1 TB. wheat bran to any can of BE WELL JUICE daily for 3 months to prevent colon polyps. Take in the morning.**

Herbal Therapy

❧ **Jump start herbal program: Crystal Star has a successful program.**
 ✺**Use PAU D' ARCO/ECHINACEA or MILK THISTLE SEED extracts 4x daily to clear lymph nodes and regulate liver function.**
 ✺**Crystal Star ANTI-BIO™ extract as an anti-infective, and apply ANTI-BIO™ gel directly.**
         and
 ✺**EVENING PRIMROSE OIL 500mg 6 daily to balance fat metabolism.**

❧ **Apply Nutribiotic GRAPEFRUIT SEED EXTRACT directly, 2x daily, especially if the growth is increasing in size.**
 ✺Add Solaray CENTELLA ASIATICA caps 4 daily for cytotoxic effects.

❧ Apply tea tree oil for 4 to 6 weeks. ☺

❧ Apply AloeLife SKIN GEL.

❧ Take pau d' arco tea 4 cups daily for a month. Rub on Crystal Star PAU D' ARCO/ECHINACEA extract. ♀+
 ✺Add garlic caps 8 daily or cayenne garlic caps 4 daily, for a month.

❧ Take turmeric caps 6 daily, (Curcumin) extract 4x daily for 1-2 months. ♂

Supplements

❧ **Strengthen immune response:**
 ✺Beta carotene 25,000IU every 4 hours for a month.
 ✺Ascorbate vitamin C crystals with bioflavonoids ¹⁄₄ teasp. 4x daily for a month.
 ✺**CoQ₁₀ 60mg 2x daily.**
 ✺**Vitamin E 800IU daily, with selenium 200mcg daily.**
 ✺Propolis lozenges - apply propolis extract directly, and take under the tongue. Zinc picolinate 50mg 2x daily for a month. Then a maintenance dose of 30mg daily. ♂

❧ **For lipomas and wens:** Lane Labs BENE-FIN shark cartilage caps, 9 daily.
 ✺Carnitine 500mg 2x daily.
         with
 ✺High omega 3 flax oil 3x daily to control fat metabolism.

❧ **For colon polyps:** 1500mg daily calcium with Nature's Secret ULTIMATE A.M./ P.M. CLEANSE.

❧ Nutricology GERMANIUM 150mg daily.

❧ **Folic acid 400mcg to correct formation.** ♀+

❧ Vit. B₆ 250mg 2x daily until condition clears. ♂+

Lifestyle Support Therapy

❧ Homeopathic remedies work to reduce cysts and polyps. See a good homeopath who can recommend the correct treatment for your type of growth.

❧ Apply Crystal Star GINSENG SKIN REPAIR GEL™ with germanium and vitamin C for several weeks.
 ✺Apply liquid garlic directly with a cotton swab.
 ✺Apply Martin PYCNOGENOL GEL.
 ✺Apply fresh comfrey compresses.

❧ Don't smoke. Nicotine aggravates gland imbalances that allow deposits to form.

❧ **Massage into affected area daily, Matrix Health GENESIS OXY-SPRAY for 3 weeks, for noticeable reduction without pain.**

❧ Scrub skin with a loofah or dry skin brush regularly to keep sebaceous glands

See FIBROID AND TUMOR pages in this book for more information.

Common Symptoms: *A lump or bulge seen or felt under the skin (usually movable); in the case of vaginal cysts, there is often bleeding during intercourse; where there are colon, bladder or cervical polyps there is often rectal, urinal or vaginal bleeding; wens usually form over nerve ganglia.*
Common Causes: *Internal toxicity and infection; diet contains excess acid or mucous forming foods; poor assimilation/digestion of fats; for sebaceous cysts, gland outflow blocked with sebum deposits; accumulation of dead skin cells, local cosmetic irritants.*

Dandruff
Seborrheic Dermatitis & Pityriasis

Pityriasis (simple dandruff) is a dry skin problem, and can usually be controlled with a better diet, cleansing and brushing. Seborrheic dandruff appears as dry, flaky particles of skin in the hair. While it looks like a dry skin condition, it is actually the opposite - too much oil is being produced, clogging the highly active sebaceous glands. It can result from a variety of conditions, both physical and emotional, appearing when skin cells turn over at a faster rate than normal and break away in large flakes into the hair. It tends to occur more in the winter and fall months. Diet improvement is the key to long term dandruff control for either kind of dandruff.

Diet & Superfood Therapy

♀ Eat vegetable proteins like soy, brewer's yeast and wheat germ, with plenty of fresh fruits and vegetables to keep your metabolically active scalp cells working right.

➶Reduce sugars, starchy foods and animal fats. Sugar depletes the body of B vitamins.

➶Eliminate fried foods. They clog the body so it can't eliminate wastes properly.

➶Avoid allergenic foods like dairy products, refined flours, chocolate, nuts and shellfish. These are sometimes involved with dandruff.

➶Add sulphur-rich foods: Lettuce, oats, green pepper, onions, cucumber, eggs, fish, cabbage, wheat germ.

➶Eat cultured products like yogurt and kefir to encourage healthy intestinal flora and better digestion. ✂

♀ Effective superfoods:
➶Crystal Star SYSTEMS STRENGTH™ for absorbable minerals.
➶Nature's Life SUPER GREEN PRO-96 for extra vegetable protein. ♀♂
➶YS ROYAL JELLY 3-4 teasp. daily.

Herbal Therapy

➷ Jump start herbal program:
Crystal Star ANTI-BIO™ extract or capsules with MINERAL SPECTRUM™ capsules, and EVENING PRIMROSE OIL capsules for EFAs.
➶GREEN TEA CLEANSER™ to keep the system metabolically active.
and
➶SILICA SOURCE™ extract, or Flora VEGE-SIL for healthy hair growth. ♀♂

➷ Effective herbal scalp treatments:
➶Mix the juice from fresh grated ginger with an equal amount of sesame oil. Rub on scalp at night. Rinse in the morning. Use for 1 week.
➶Steep bay leaves in olive oil until fragrant. Rub on scalp before shampoo. Leave on 30 minutes and shampoo out.
➶Massage jojoba or rosemary oil into scalp. Leave on 1 hour. Shampoo out.

➷ Effective mineral hair rinses:
➶Rosemary/yarrow
➶Nettles
➶Chaparral
➶Steep cider vinegar and peppermint oil drops in 1 cup water. Rinse hair. ♂

Supplements

➷ Vit. E with selenium 400IU daily. ♀
with
➶Biotin 600mcg daily.
➶Zinc picolinate 50mg 2x daily. ♂

➷ Omega-3 flax oils 3x daily.

➷ B Vitamins are important for skin and scalp hair health:
➶B Complex 100mg daily with extra B₆ 100mg, folic acid 400mcg, PABA 1000mg and niacin 500mg for increased circulation.

➷ Lubricate and balance with oil-based vitamins:
➶Schiff EMULSIFIED A & D.
➶Lecithin caps or choline/inositol caps, 2 daily.
➶Rainbow Light MULTI-CAROTENE COMPLEX.
➶Nature's Secret ULTIMATE OIL. ♀

Lifestyle Support Therapy

Avoid over-the-counter commercial ointments that often do more harm than good by clogging sebaceous glands.

➷ Add a few drops Nutribiotic GRAPE-FRUIT SEED EXTRACT to shampoo, and use daily.

➷ Use jojoba, aloe vera, or biotin based shampoos.
➶Add drops of tea tree oil to hair rinse, and use daily. Or use tea tree oil shampoo.
➶Rinse the hair with cider vinegar and water after every wash to keep sebum deposits from clogging pores. Or use a natural shampoo specifically designed to remove build-up.

➷ Get some regular circulation-stimulating exercise daily.

➷ Massage head with both hands and all the fingers at once, for 5 minutes every day to stimulate scalp circulation and slough dead skin cells.

See also ECZEMA/PSORIASIS page in this book for more information.

Common Symptoms: *Scaling flakes on scalp, eyebrows and sometimes the face; redness, weeping and itching, burning scalp; sometimes a crust formation.*
Common Causes: *Sebaceous gland malfunction; an allergic reaction to a hair care product; too much alcohol, saturated fat, sugar and starch in the diet; essential fatty acid deficiency; lack of green vegetables; excessively strong or harsh hair dyes.*

Depression

Paranoia ✳ Mood Affective Disorder ✳ Manic-Depressive Disorder

Depression is the most common adult psychiatric disorder, and it's on the rise worldwide. Mood disorders currently affect almost 16 million people. Depression is both a mental and emotional state that stems from a wide range of causes, and affects women more than men. In general, there seem to be five underlying origins for depression. 1) Great loss, as of a spouse or child, and the inability to mourn or express grief; 2) Bottled-up anger and aggression turned inward; 3) Negative emotional behavior, often learned as a child, that controls relationships; 4) Biochemical imbalance characterized by amino acid and other nutrient deficiencies; 5) Drug-induced depression. Many prescription drugs create nutrient deficiencies.

Diet & Superfood Therapy

If you are taking MAO inhibitor drugs, you must control your diet with care: avoid alcohol, cheese, red meat, yeast extract and broad beans - foods rich in tyrosine.

♋ Food and nutrition are key factors in the brain's behavior and well-being.
↘Make vegetable protein about 15% of total calorie intake to minimize depression. Include fish, sea foods and legumes.
↘Make sure you are getting good vegetable and whole grain fiber daily.
↘Eat foods rich in calcium, magnesium and B vitamins.
↘Have a glass of carrot juice 2 to 3x a week with a pinch of sage and 1 teasp. Bragg's LIQUID AMINOS for adrenal stress.
↘Drink bottled water. Treated water can cause neurotransmitter imbalances.
↘Make a mix of lecithin granules, brewer's yeast, wheat germ, pumpkin seeds; take 2 TBS. daily.
↘Eliminate all preserved, refined and junk foods. Avoid sugary foods, alcohol and caffeine because they wreak havoc on blood sugar levels.

🏵

♋ Effective superfoods:
↘Crystal Star SYSTEMS STRENGTH™.
↘GreenFoods WHEAT GERM extract. ♂
↘Nutrex HAWAIIAN SPIRULINA. ♂
↘Beehive Botanicals ROYAL JELLY with GINSENG and bee pollen. ♀

Herbal Therapy

Be aware that the two major classes of antidepressant drugs seem to block the effect of herbal nervines. St. John's wort is contra-indicated if you are taking PROZAC.

♋ Jump start herbal program:
Crystal Star RELAX™ caps for nerve repair, DEPRESS-EX™ extract or capsules for mental calm, with St John's Wort.
↘GINKGO BILOBA extract.
↘Kava-Kava or Enzymatic Therapy KAVA TONE as directed. ♀

♋ Liver support:
↘Crystal Star GREEN TEA CLEAN-SER™.
↘MILK THISTLE SEED extract

♋ Nervine tonics and relaxants:
↘Crystal Star INCREDIBLE DREAMS™ tea before retiring, or make an anti-depression pillow with **fresh-dried** mugwort leaves, rosemary, California poppies, lemon balm and mint. Stuff a pillow for sweet sleep.

♋ Adaptogens to normalize:
↘**High potency panax ginseng, or Crystal Star MENTAL INNER ENERGY™ formula with kava kava.** ♂
↘**Bach Flower RESCUE REMEDY.**
↘Black cohosh if hormone related.
↘**Gotu kola for nerve support.**
↘Siberian ginseng extract or Rainbow Light ADAPTOGEM caps. ♀

Supplements

Prolonged depression increases risk of osteoporosis.

✔ **Flora NERVE GUARD with Nature's Bounty B$_{12}$ internasal gel every other day for 1 to 2 months.**

✔ **5-HTP 50-100mg daily for 2 months.**

✔ **Country Life Maxi-B with taurine daily, and MOOD FACTORS capsules as needed.** ♂

✔ Depression relievers:
↘Magnesium 500mg 2x daily.
↘**DLPA 750-1000mg as needed.**
↘Tyrosine 500mg, with extra B$_6$ 100mg 2x daily.

✔ **Quercetin with bromelain daily.**
↘Melatonin 3mg at bedtime for 3 mo. ♂
↘Country Life RELAXER caps. ♀
↘Natrol SAF caps. ♀
↘GABA caps.

✔ Brain oxygenators:
↘Germanium with suma
↘**CoQ$_{10}$ 30mg 3x daily**
↘Glutamine 1000mg daily

✔ **Vitamin C with bioflavonoids is a natural tranquilizer and helps withdrawal from drugs and chemical dependencies.**

Lifestyle Support Therapy

In general, avoid the amino acid phenylalanine, as in NutraSweet and some amino acid formulas. Many depressed people react allergically to phenylalanine.

🌿 **Before you try PROZAC, (it has had more side effect complaints than any other drug) ask your doctor about hypnotherapy, biofeedback or acupuncture. All three of these relaxation techniques have had good success in overcoming chronic depression.**

🌿 **Exercise worry and anxiety away. Give yourself plenty of body oxygen. Exercise is an anti-depressant nutrient in itself.**
↘Sunlight therapy - get some on the body every day possible for Vit. D.

🌿 Do brain breathing exercises. (See Bragg's BRAIN BREATHING book).

🌿 Yoga stretches or a shiatsu massage can clear the mind and refresh the body.

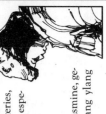

🌿 Stop smoking. It contracts capillaries and arteries, and slows circulation, especially to the brain.

🌿 **Aromatherapy:**
↘Essential oils of jasmine, geranium, rosemary, ylang ylang and basil.

Common Symptoms: *Manic episodes alternating with deep depression; excessive self-reproach and guilt; fatigue; unusual drowsiness; inability to think and disorientation; memory loss; wired feeling; paranoia attacks; headaches; sweating, palpitations; loss of interest in pleasure; poor food absorption and significant weight loss even if meals are good; recurrent thoughts of death or suicide.*

Common Causes: *Hypoglycemia or other sugar imbalance; sugar or alcohol dependency; chemical or food allergies; glandular imbalance with high copper levels; drug abuse; hypothyroidism; prescription drug addiction or intolerance; negative emotions discharging hormonal secretions into the bloodstream; the inability to cope with prolonged and intense stress.*

See also ANXIETY AND CHRONIC FATIGUE SYNDROME pages for more information.

Diabetes

High Blood Sugar * Type 1 (Juvenile Diabetes) * Type 2 (Adult-Onset Diabetes)

Type 2, adult-onset diabetes mellitus, ought to be an auto-immune disorder, is a chronic degenerative disease in which the body's ability to use carbohydrates is impaired by disturbances in normal insulin mechanisms. It afflicts more than 12 million Americans. With its complications, it is the third leading cause of death in the U.S. Type 2 diabetics produce insulin, the hormone that helps convert food into energy, but it isn't used properly (insulin resistance), causing glucose to build up in the bloodstream, and depriving cells of the nutrients they need. Type 1 diabetes is a juvenile-onset condition, is more severe, and is almost entirely dependent on insulin injections to sustain life. Both types benefit from diet improvement, exercise and certain natural supplements. Diet improvement is absolutely necessary to overcoming diabetes. High blood sugar is also an indication of high triglycerides.

Diet & Superfood Therapy

Avoid cow's milk especially and all fatty dairy foods.

☘ Eliminate sugars, alcohol, fried, fatty, **refined and high cholesterol foods.**
*Complex carbohydrate, like whole grains and vegetables, **are a key** to reducing insulin requirements.
*High fiber foods are a key, and in some mild cases can lead to discontinuation of insulin therapy. Fiber improves control of glycemia and glucose metabolism, lowers cholesterol and triglyceride levels, and promotes weight loss.
*Chromium-rich foods are a key: whole grains, brewer's yeast, string beans, eggs, cucumbers, soy foods, liver and organ meats, onions and garlic, fruits, shiitake mushrooms, wheat germ, etc.
*Have a daily green salad with Omega-3 flax oil dressing. Eat salmon twice a week.
*The continuing diet should be low in fats and total calories, largely vegetarian, with alkalizing foods, olive oil and most proteins from vegetable sources. ☘

☘ Effective superfoods:
*AloeLife ALOE CONCENTRATE, 1 teasp. in water.
*Sun CHLORELLA 15-20 tabs daily.
*Lewis Labs BREWER'S YEAST.
*Klamath BLUE GREEN SUPREME.

Herbal Therapy

☘ Jump start herbal program:
Crystal Star SUGAR STRATEGY HIGH™ capsules and turmeric capsules to encourage insulin balance; GINSENG 6 SUPER TEA™ to lower blood sugar levels.
*EVENING PRIMROSE OIL capsules 1000mg daily for needed EFAs.
*BODY REBUILDER™ - stable energy.
*ADR-ACTIVE™ caps or ADRN™ extract for cortex support. ♂♀

☘ Grifon MAITAKE MUSHROOM caplets.

☘ Sugar-balancing teas:
*Dandelion/licorice
*Fenugreek seed
*Siberian ginseng ♂
*Rosemary

☘ Insulin forming herbs:
*Pau d' arco
*Garlic oil capsules
*BILBERRY extract
*Burdock tea, 2 cups daily for 3 mo.
*Astragalus

☘ Use stevia herb instead of sugar for sweetening. It does not have sugar's insulin requirements.
*Take gymnema sylvestre extract before meals to help repair the pancreas, and damage to cells in the liver and kidneys.

Supplements

✦ GTF Chromium or chromium picolinate 200mcg 2x daily,

✦ High dose biotin treatments - 1000mcg 6x daily, to lower blood sugar levels.

✦ Magnesium/potassium/bromelain 3 daily to control blood pressure.

✦ To normalize pancreatic activity:
*Alta Health CANGEST caps.
*Twin Labs CSA caps
*Futurebiotics VITAL K.
*Glutamine 500mg with carnitine 500mg. ♂
*Raw pancreas glandular.

✦ American Biologics VANADIUM 20mcg 3-4x daily.

✦ Solaray B₁₂ 2000mcg and B Complex 100mg, with pantothenic acid 500mg daily to encourage adrenal activity, niacin 250mg to stimulate circulation, and zinc 30mg for more immune strength.

✦ Ester C 3000mg daily to increase insulin tolerance/normalize pancreatic activity.

✦ DHEA to increase cells sensitivity to insulin. ♂♀

✦ Health Aid America SIBERGIN to stabilize blood sugar. ♂

Lifestyle Support Therapy

☘ Exercise regularly to increase metabolic processes and reduce need for insulin. ♂

☘ A regular deep therapy massage is effective in regulating sugar use.

☘ Don't smoke. Nicotine increases sugar desire.

☘ Avoid phenylalanine. No Nutra-Sweet, etc. (Check labels on colas, diet drinks, etc.)

☘ If overweight, loose the excess. Poor biochemistry often results from being overweight. A fiber weight loss drink, such as:
*Crystal Star CHO-LO FIBER TONE™ or AloeLife FIBER-MATE are effective.

☘ Alternating hot and cold hydrotherapy to stimulate circulation.

☘ **Reflexology points:**

pancreas
adrenals

Common Symptoms: *High blood sugar; constant hunger with rapid weight change; dry, itching skin; excessive thirst; lack of energy; kidney malfunction leading to bladder and prostate problems, and excessive urination with high sugar in the urine; obesity; hypertension; accelerated aging.*

Common Causes: *Poor diet with too many refined foods, fats and carbohydrates; insulin, chromium, HCL deficiencies; possibly a virus; glucose and fat metabolism malfunction leading to obesity; pancreas and liver malfunction from excess caffeine, alcohol and stress overloads; inherited proneness usually accompanied by several allergies; hypothyroidism.*

See the Diabetes Control Diet on the following page.

Blood Sugar Balancing Diet For Diabetes Control

Although many Type 2 diabetics must take insulin to regulate blood sugar levels, others can balance their blood sugar without drugs by following a controlled diet and getting regular exercise.

Diabetes makes a person want to eat more, so it can be brought on by eating too much fat, too many sugary foods and excess refined carbohydrates. Pancreatic activity and other vital organs become damaged, the body loses the ability to produce or use insulin correctly, and high blood sugar results. As less and less simple carbohydrates and sugars are metabolized, they keep accumulating in the body and are stored as fat. Excess body fat and lack of exercise bring on insulin resistance, and energy is prevented from moving into the cells. The following diet, in addition to reducing insulin requirements and balancing sugar function in the bloodstream, has the nice "side effect" of healthy weight loss.

The key to this diet is in supplying slow-burning complex carbohydrate fuels, primarily from vegetables, that do not need much insulin for metabolism. Slow-release nutrients, such as legumes prevent rapid blood sugar spikes. Good diabetic meals are small, frequent, largely vegetarian, and low in fats of all kinds. Proteins come from soy foods and whole grains that are rich in lecithin and chromium. Fifty to sixty percent of the diet consists of fresh and simply cooked vegetables for low calories and high digestibility.

All sugars, refined, fried and fatty foods are excluded.

On rising: take the juice of two lemons in a glass of water with 2 teasp. CHLORELLA granules.

Breakfast: take a heaping teaspoon of Crystal Star CHOL-LO FIBER TONE™ or other natural high fiber drink mix, in apple juice or water, to regulate and balance the sugar curve; and/or make a mix of 2 TBS. each: brewer's yeast, wheat germ, lecithin granules and rice or oat bran. Sprinkle some daily on your choice of breakfast foods, or simply mix into yogurt with fresh fruit and some grated almonds on top;
have 1) poached egg on whole grain toast, 2) muesli, whole grain or granola cereal with apple juice or vanilla soy milk, 3) buckwheat or whole grain pancakes with apple juice or molasses.

Mid-morning: have a green drink such as Crystal Star ENERGY GREEN™ or Green Foods GREEN ESSENCE;
and some whole grain crackers or muffins with a little soy spread or kefir cheese;
and a refreshing, sugar balancing herb tea, such as licorice, dandelion, or pau d'arco tea.

Lunch: have a green salad, with celery, sprouts, green pepper, marinated tofu, and mushroom soup;
or baked tofu, tofu burgers or turkey with some steamed veggies and rice or cornbread;
or a baked potato with a little yogurt or kefir cheese, or soy cheese and some miso soup with sea vegetables;
or a whole grain sandwich, with avocado, low fat or soy cheese, a low fat sandwich spread and watercress leaves.

Mid-afternoon: have a glass of carrot juice, diluted with water;
and/or fruit juice sweetened cookies or muffins with a bottle of mineral water or herb tea;
or some watercress/cucumber sandwiches with kefir cheese sandwich spread;
or a hard boiled egg with sesame salt, or a veggie dip, and a bottle of mineral water.

Dinner: Keep it light - have a baked or broiled seafood dish with brown rice and peas;
• or a Chinese stir-fry with rice, veggies and miso soup;
• or a Spanish beans and rice dish with onions and peppers;
• or a light northern Italian polenta with a hearty vegetable soup, or whole grain or veggie pasta salad;
• or a mushroom quiche with whole grain crust and yogurt/wine sauce, and a small green salad.
• A little white wine is fine with dinner for relaxation and has surprisingly high chromium content. Beware of overconsumption of alcohol, because it can cause blood sugar to soar.

Before bed: take another heaping teasp. CHOL-LO FIBER TONE™ mix in apple juice;
and/or Organic Gourmet NUTRITIONAL YEAST or MISO, 1 teasp. in warm water.

• Avoid caffeine and caffeine-containing foods, hard liquor, food coloring and sodas. (Even "diet" sodas have phenylalanine in the form of NutraSweet, and will affect blood sugar levels).

• Avoid tobacco in any form. Nicotine increases the desire for sugar and sugary foods.
• Never stop or reduce insulin without monitoring by your physician.

Controlling Other Problems Associated With Diabetes

Diabetes frequently leads to other health problems. Use the recommendations as needed for specific diabetic complications along with your diabetes healing program.

CATARACTS, GLAUCOMA, DIABETIC RETINOPATHY (DAMAGED RETINA), RETINITIS AND IMPAIRED VISION: Ginkgo biloba extract 3x daily; PCOs from grapeseed or white pine bark, 100mg 3 to 4 times daily to reduce vascular fragility; Quercetin Plus with bromelain, **Lane Labs BENE-FIN shark cartilage caps** as directed for blood vessel and capillary support; magnesium 400mg 3x daily; Ascorbate vitamin C or Ester C powder with bioflavonoids, $1/4$ teasp. at a time, 4 to 6 x daily; vitamin E 400IU 3 x daily, especially for retinitis; BILBERRY extract, Solaray VIZION capsules, or Solaray CENTELLA ASIATICA; B Complex 100mg daily

CARDIOVASCULAR COMPLICATIONS- HEART DISEASE/HIGH BLOOD PRESSURE (PEOPLE WITH DIABETES ARE 250 TIMES MORE LIKELY TO SUFFER FROM STROKE): Ginkgo biloba 3x daily; PCOs from grapeseed or white pine bark, 100mg 3 to 4 times daily; gymnema sylvestre extract to lower blood lipids; taurine to reverse blood clotting; vitamin E as an anti-oxidant to increase blood flow and to decrease platelet aggregation. To help keep arteries and circulatory system free of fats: Omega-3 flax oil 3x daily, with B_{12} sublingual or internasal gel, with carnitine 500mg and BILBERRY extract. To help lower cholesterol: niacinamide 500mg 2x daily, and chromium picolinate 200mcg daily, or Solaray CHROMIACIN.

CHRONIC DIABETIC OBESITY: You must lower your sugary, fatty foods intake. Get help with this from stevia herb, or gymnema sylvestre herb before each meal for pancreatic normalization and increase in insulin output; Lewis Labs FIBER YEAST daily in the morning, and/or Lewis Labs WEIGH DOWN DIET DRINK with chromium picolinate; chromium picolinate 400mcg daily; L-carnitine 500mg daily. A weekly dry sauna helps regulate sugar use and control cravings

NEPHROPATHY, KIDNEY DISEASE RESULTING FROM DIABETIC SMALL BLOOD VESSEL MALFUNCTION: avoid red meats - eat fish or chicken instead - especially salmon; take **gymnema sylvestre** water soluble extract before meals; Lane Labs BENE-FIN shark cartilage capsules for blood vessel and capillary support.

DIABETIC CIRCULATORY PROBLEMS AND ULCERS: consider chelation therapy. Today, it is an easy clinic procedure... and it works. Try Health Papers CETA CLEANSE as directed. Take American Biologics emulsified vitamin A & D 25,000/1,000IU. (beta-carotene is not effective for diabetics, who cannot convert it to A in the liver). Drink aloe vera juice every morning. Take zinc/methionine 30mg 2x daily to improve zinc status without affecting copper levels. Clean diabetic ulcers of necrotic tissue and apply a comfrey poultice, B & T CALIFLORA gel, AloeLife SKIN GEL, tea tree oil/olive oil compresses, or Country Comfort GOLDENSEAL/MYRRH salve.

FOOD ALLERGIES: when being tested for glucose tolerance, be sure to take food tolerance tests to determine food allergies. There is a definite link between cow's milk and Type 1 Childhood Diabetes. Aspartame (especially in sweeteners like NutraSweet, Sweet 'N' Low and Equal) deplete insulin reserves. Effective supplements include HCL with meals, digestive enzymes after meals, such as Solaray DIGEST-AWAY and Alta Health CANGEST, or Prevail DAIRY ENZYME FORMULA for lactose intolerance. Keep the diet high in fresh raw fruits and vegetables, with lots of soluble vegetable and grain fiber. Avoid acid-forming foods like red meats and hard cheeses, refined carbohydrates, and preserved foods.

ACCELERATED AGING (ESPECIALLY ARTERIOSCLEROSIS): anti-oxidants are the key: chromium picolinate 200mcg 3x daily. Caution note: Diabetics progressively lose the ability to heal from cuts and wounds as they age. It is recommended that they cut toenails straight across or have a professional do it.

NEUROPATHY, DAMAGE TO THE NERVOUS SYSTEM CHARACTERIZED BY NUMBNESS, TINGLING, PAIN AND CRAMPING IN THE EXTREMITIES: Follow a vegetarian diet; take Quercetin with Bromelain 2x daily (or Solaray QBC COMPLEX); PCOs from grapeseed or white pine bark, 100mg 3x daily to reduce vascular fragility; gotu kola capsules 2, 3x daily for nerve support; GINKGO BILOBA or BILBERRY extract 2, 3x daily; EVENING PRIMROSE OIL capsules 1000mg 4 daily; biotin 1000mcg 6x daily; Capsaicin cream applied to affected areas; vitamin B_{12} internasal gel every other day for a month; vitamin C 3000mg daily; magnesium 400mg 2x daily; L-carnitine 500mg daily; Choline/inositol for nerve damage.

Diarrhea

Chronic Diarrhea ❀ Traveler's Diarrhea ❀ Lack Of Nutrient Absorption

Uncomfortably frequent, fluid and excessive bowel movements. Diarrhea is one of the body's best methods of rapidly throwing off toxins. Unless diarrhea is chronic, or continues for more than two to three days, it is best to let it run its cleansing course. Note: No drugstore remedy I have found is as effective as diet correction with herbs or natural supplements.

Diet & Superfood Therapy

♌ **For chronic diarrhea:**
➛Go on a short juice fast for 24 hours (pg. 158) to clean out harmful bacteria.
➛Then take daily for 3 days: Miso soup with sea vegetables, papaya juice, bananas, a green salad, toast, and brown rice with steamed vegetables.

♌ **For travel diarrhea and irregularity:**
➛Eat high fiber foods as much as possible during your trip, especially brown rice, salads and vegetables.
➛Add yogurt to your travel diet.
➛Take black orange pekoe tea with a lemon and a pinch of cloves.
➛Eat only very ripe bananas for 24 hours - esp. if in a 3rd world country.
➛**Have a glass of wine with meals. It is 6 times more effective in killing bacteria than *Pepto Bismol.***

♌ Add fiber to your continuing diet with whole grain brans, brown rice and fresh vegetables. Add yogurt, kefir and cultured foods for friendly flora.
➛Avoid dairy products, fatty and fried foods during healing.
➛Drink plenty of liquids to keep from getting dehydrated and losing minerals.
➛Eat only small meals during healing. Chew food well.

Herbal Therapy

🍃 **Jump start herbal program:**
➛**For traveler's diarrhea:** Crystal Star TRAVELERS COMFORT™ (with ginger), followed by ANTI-BIO™ caps or extract to counter gastro-intestinal infections.
➛**For chronic diarrhea: BWL TONE-IBS™ capsules for gentle bowel rebalance. ♦New Moon GINGER WONDER syrup as needed. Take SILICA SOURCE™ extract for rebuilding strong bowel tissue.**

🍃 **All-in-one diarrhea aid:** Crystal Star GREEN TEA CLEANSER™ with 1/4 teasp. ginger powder, 15 drops myrrh extract and 1 teasp. Bragg's LIQUID AMINOS added. ♀

🍃 For traveler's diarrhea:
➛Bee pollen, 2 teasp. 2x daily, or Beehive Botanical POLLEN PLUS caps, and kelp tabs 6 daily.

🍃 **Effective balancing teas:**
➛Raspberry, rich in needed minerals
➛**Peppermint/Slippery elm**
➛Horsetail
➛Bayberry/barberry ♂
➛Blackberry/elderberry/cinnamon ⊛
➛Catnip or thyme tea ♂
➛White oak bark ♂

🍃 Chlorophyll liquid 1 teasp. in water 3x daily before meals. ♂

Supplements

⚘ **Bowel balancing:**
➛**Prof. Nutrition DR. DOPHILUS, or Natren TRINITY, or Alta Health CANGEST powder 1/2 teasp. 3x daily in water or juice.**
➛Garlic capsules 6 daily.
➛Pancreatin enzymes.
➛Activated charcoal tabs on a temporary basis with Cal/Mag/Zinc caps at night. ♂
➛Quercetin with bromelain, esp. if the cause is food allergies. ⊛
➛Vitamin A 10,000IU. ⊛

⚘ **Homeopathic remedies:**
➛Nux Vomica
➛Hylands *Diarrex.* ⊛
➛*Chamomilla*

⚘ **For chronic diarrhea:**
➛American Biologics DIOXYCHLOR.
➛Nutribiotics GRAPEFRUIT SEED extract
➛Niacin therapy 250mg 3x daily. ♀

⚘ **Effective superfoods:**
➛Crystal Star SYSTEMS STRENGTH™ to replace lost electrolytes - stimulate enzyme activity.
➛Salute ALOE VERA JUICE with HERBS morning and evening.
➛Sun CHLORELLA 15-20 tabs daily.
➛BeWell juices for body balance.
➛Future Biotics VITAL K.
➛Lewis Labs FIBER YEAST daily for B vitamins and fiber, or brewer's yeast tablets.

Lifestyle Support Therapy

☙ Mix 1 TB. **each:** psyllium husk, flax seed, chia seed, and slippery elm in water. Let soak for 30 minutes. Take 2 TBS. at night for 2 days before bed.

☙ If no inflammation is present, use mild catnip enemas to rid the body of toxic matter. ♂
➛Take fenugreek seed tea enemas to soothe inflamed tissues.

☙ Apply ice packs to the middle and lower back to stimulate nerve force.

☙ **To curb symptoms:**
➛Two teasp. roasted carob powder in water with 1 teasp. of cinnamon 2x daily.
➛Two TBS. cider vinegar in hot water with honey 2 to 3x daily.
➛BLACK WALNUT HULLS extract.
➛Alacer MIRACLE WATER.
➛Apple pectin capsules 3 daily. ♂
➛**For babies:** give finely grated apples followed by oatmeal. ⊛
➛For older children, give oat flakes; let them chew and wet them with saliva; don't give any other food for at least 2 hours. ⊛

Common Symptoms: *Loose, watery, frequent stools, often with abdominal pain and dehydration; sometimes vomiting and fever; general fatigue.*

Common Causes: *Poor food absorption, and lack of fiber in the diet; enzyme and chronic vitamin A deficiency; intestinal parasites; colitis; food poisoning; reaction to rancid or unripe foods; food allergy - particularly lactose intolerance; food allergies and reactions to chemicals in foods; reaction to water and/ or foods in foreign countries; too many antibiotics, or a reaction to other drugs; viral/bacterial infection. Note: hemorrhoids are linked to diarrhea and obesity conditions - not constipation as one might think.*

See also PARASITE INFECTIONS page for more information.

Diverticulosis

Diverticulitis ✴ Inflamed Bowel Disease

Diverticular disease is common today, affecting almost 40% of Americans over 50. It mimics many of the symptoms of Irritable Bowel Syndrome. Bowel mucous membranes become inflamed from fermented, uneliminated food residues. The constipated colon forms protruding pouch-like hernias in its walls in an effort to trap toxic waste and protect the body from main-canal infection. However, if constipation continues, and the diet is not improved, the pouches (diverticula) themselves become painfully infected, and may perforate leading to contamination in the abdominal area.

Diet & Superfood Therapy

Diet improvement is the main solution.

♉ Start with a short juice diet for 3 days (pg. 157). Use carrot, apple, grape or carrot/spinach juice.

➥Add oat or rice bran and take 2 TBS. molasses with a banana and plain yogurt daily. Eat prunes for occasional constipation.

➥Then add mild fruits and vegetables, such as carrots, bananas, potatoes, yams, papayas, broccoli, etc.

➥Finally, as inflammation subsides and healing begins, add brown rice, millet, cous cous, tofu, baked fish or seafood as lean protein sources.

➥Eat plenty of cultured foods for healthy G.I. flora; yogurt, kefir, miso, etc.

➥Eliminate dairy products, fatty and sugary foods, red meats and fried foods during healing. Reduce wheat and dense grains, nuts and seeds during healing.

♉ Drink 6 to 8 glasses of water and healthy liquids (see below) ❧

♉ **Effective superfoods:**
➥**Crystal Star CHO-LO-FIBER TONE™.** ♂
➥**Green Foods GREEN MAGMA.**
➥**AloeLife ALOE GOLD juice drink** to soothe pain and gently aid bowel action.
➥**Solgar WHEY TO GO protein drink.**
➥Green Foods GREEN MAGMA.

Herbal Therapy

Absorbable minerals are key factors in bone building. Herbs are one of the best ways to get them.

♉ **Jump start herbal program:**
➥**Crystal Star BWL TONE IBS™ capsules 2-3x daily for 3 months to heal and tone bowel tissue.**
➥**Add EVENING PRIMROSE OIL for EFAs to normalize bowel function.**
and
➥**Pau d' arco tea 3 cups daily or una da gato capsules.**

❧ Use Crystal Star ANTI-BIO™ drops in water, or other echinacea/goldenseal combination, or garlic extract if there is infection, several times daily.
➥Use ANTI-FLAM™ drops in water or other white willow combination if there is inflammation.
➥Use Crystal Star ANTI-SPZ™ capsules **with wild yam**, or other cramp bark combination for spasmodic pain and cramping.

❧ **Bowel soothing teas:**
➥Slippery elm
➥Comfrey/fenugreek
➥Alfalfa/mint

Supplements

Liquid and chewable supplements are preferable for ease and gentleness.

♉ B complex vitamins, such as Nature's Secret ULTIMATE B, Source Naturals Co-ENZYMATE B, or Twin lab B Complex Liquid with Iron, to curb stomach gas and rumbling as fiber combines with minerals.

♉ **Enzyme therapy is very important:**
➥Dr. DOPHILUS or Natren TRINITY powder $\frac{1}{2}$ teasp. 3x daily with meals.
➥Nature's Plus chewable BROMELAIN 40mg or chewable PAPAYA ENZYMES at each meal.
➥Enzymatic Therapy DGL chewables.
➥Chlorophyll liquid before meals.
➥Whey complex powder after meals for bowel rebalance. ♀
➥Rainbow Light ADVANCED ENZYME SYSTEM capsules. ♀

♉ Solaray ALFAJUICE caps.

♉ Enzymatic Therapy THYMU-PLEX to help immune response.

Lifestyle Support Therapy

Avoid drugstore antacids. They eventually make the problems worse by causing the stomach to produce more acids.

❧ Take peppermint, fenugreek, or catnip enemas once or twice a week for bowel cleansing and rebalancing.

❧ Massage therapy treatments often help. ♀

❧ Active people are less prone to diverticular disease. Take a brisk walk every day possible. Walk outdoors to get a vitamin D boost.

❧ Apply wet hot compresses to abdomen and lower back to stimulate systolic/diastolic action.

❧ **Diverticulitis area:**

Sigmoid

Common Symptoms: Inflammation and soreness in the colon mucous membranes from unpassed food residues and gas; chronic constipation; abdominal pain, cramping and distention; alternating constipation and diarrhea; sometimes severe bleeding, especially from long-standing problems in the elderly.

Common Causes: Fiber deficiency from too many refined foods, leading to weakening of the colon wall, and formation of pockets that look like worn out tire bulges; chronic constipation; thyroid deficiency; emotional stress causing colon spasms; obesity; causing compressed or prolapsed colon structure.

See also COLITIS/IBS and the CONSTIPATION CLEANSING DIET pages for more information.

Down's Syndrome

Genetic Mental Retardation ✦ Mongolism

Down's syndrome, a genetic condition caused by an extra 21st chromosome, is characterized by both physical and mental retardation. Untreatable by conventional medicine, vanguard work is being done for nutritional therapies. Studies show that some retarded dysfunction and behavior is learned, not inherited, and that Down's syndrome victims have immune deficiencies, particularly greatly accelerated free-radical damage that are thought to be largely responsible for the accelerated aging progress of the condition. Because of this, most Down's victims do not live very long lives. Those that do almost always fall prey to Alzheimer's disease.

Diet & Superfood Therapy

Better nutrition can improve IQ and physical health in Down's syndrome, which represents both a glycogen storage and protein metabolism problem.

➋ Eat only fresh foods for 3-4 days to clear the body of toxic waste, and provide a clean working ground for nutritional therapy.
—Then, insist on a highly nutritious diet of fresh and whole foods, rich in vegetable proteins and magnesium foods.
—Eliminate all refined foods, sugars, pasteurized dairy and alcohol. Reduce high gluten foods.
—Take Alacer MIRACLE WATER for brain potassium.

➋ Make a mix of brewer's yeast, lecithin and wheat germ; take 2 TBS. daily: ✿

➋ **Down's Syndrome is thought to be a metabolism disease today rather than an inherited disease. Enzyme therapy from superfoods is critical:**
—Nutricology PRO-GREENS with flax seed oil EFAs.
—Crystal Star SYSTEMS STRENGTH™.
—Klamath BLUE GREEN SUPREME.
—Nappi THE PERFECT MEAL.
—Long Life IMPERIAL TONIC w. EPO.
—BeWell VEGETABLE JUICES.

Herbal Therapy

➋ **Jump start herbal program:**
Thyroid balance is a key: Crystal Star IODINE/POTASSIUM caps, or 4 kelp tablets daily, or 2 TBS. of sea veggies daily sprinkled on soup or a salad.
—**CHLORELLA/GINSENG extract drops in water daily for immune strength.**
and
—**GINKGO BILOBA extract 3x daily.**

➋ **Herbal antioxidants:**
—EVENING PRIMROSE OIL caps 4-6 daily for 3-4 months for prostaglandin balance.
—YS high potency royal jelly, ginseng and honey tea, 1 cup daily, or use the royal jelly paste 2 teasp. daily.
—Crystal Star GINSENG/REISHI extract for immune stimulation.
—Garlic caps 4 daily.
—Siberian ginseng extract
—Crystal Star CREATIVI-TEA™.

➋ Other effective herbs: take for 3-4 months to see noticeable improvement.
—**Gotu kola for nerve strength.**
—Crystal Star SILICA SOURCE™ drops to help collagen production.
—Chamomile to relax spasms.
—Crystal Star TINKLE TEA™ to help gently reduce fluid retention.

Supplements

➌ **Abundant anti-oxidants are the Down's Syndrome key to counteract the excess production of internal H_2O_2:**
—DMG sublingual 1 daily or Premier germanium with DMG (half dose for children).
—Vitamin E 400IU with selenium 200mcg.
—CoQ_{10}, 30mg 3x daily.
—Ester C 550mg with bioflavonoids 4 to 6 daily with **Flora VEGE-SIL caps to help the body produce collagen.**
—Marine carotene 25,000 3x daily.
—Solaray 2000mcg B_{12} every other day.

➌ **Solaray pancreatin 1300mg with Enzymatic Therapy THYMUPLEX for immune strength.**

➌ Country Life MAXI-B with taurine, and extra B_6 100mg for nerve strength, or Country Life RELAXER capsules with Taurine 500mg for stress symptoms.

or

—**Choline 600mg 4 daily, or phosphatidyl choline (PC 55), or phosphatidyl serine (PS) as directed.**

or

—ACETYL-CARNITINE - 20mg for every 20lbs, of body weight. ☺

Lifestyle Support Therapy

More oxygen and increased circulation are the bodywork goals for better brain function. Build more brain circuits by reading and playing mental games.

➼ Play soothing classical or new age music in the home. It works wonders.

➼ Expose the body to early morning sunshine daily if possible for vitamin D.

➼ Avoid pesticides, heavy metals, (cadmium, lead and mercury), and aluminum.

➼ Massage therapy helps circulation and tissue strength.
➼ Do deep breathing exercises every morning to oxygenate the brain.
➼ Stay interactive with other people and especially animals.

➼ Reflexology brain points:
—Pinch the end of each toe. Hold for 5 seconds.
—Squeeze all around the hand and fingers.

See the HYPOGLYCEMIA DIET and ALZHEIMER'S DISEASE pages in this book for more information.

Common Symptoms: *Slow reactions and motor dysfunction; poor collagen and connective tissue causing weakness, poor muscle tone and joints; learning disability; withdrawal from, and poor behavior with people; thyroid disease; gland and hormone deficiencies giving the person a "retarded," mongoloid appearance.*

Common Causes: *Drugs, either given to the child or taken by the mother when pregnant; immune system dysfunction from free radical damage from excessive SOD production; excess water fluoridation; too much sugar and refined foods; heavy metal poisoning altering brain chemistry; hypoglycemia and glycogen storage deficiency; allergies; birth trauma.*

Earaches

Excessive Earwax ❋ Otitis Media ❋ Otitis Externa (Swimmers Ear)

The most common type of infection in adults is swimmer's ear - inflammation of the outer ear canal. Middle ear infections are common in children (a third of all childhood doctor visits) whose eustachian tubes have not fully formed. Frequent use of antibiotics for these types of ear infections are almost never justified, because common use often results in thrush in children and candidiasis in adults. A ruptured eardrum can result from diving, a hard slap on the ear, a loud explosion or a serious middle ear infection.

Diet & Superfood Therapy

Breast feed your baby; breast fed kids have far less ear infections as they grow up. Nursing mothers should avoid dairy products if their babies are prone to ear infections.

⚘ **If earaches are chronic,** keep the diet low in fats and reduce mucous-forming foods like dairy products.

☙During healing, eliminate all milk and dairy products, sugars and protein-concentrated foods, such as peanut butter. Do not take sweet fruit juices in full strength. The high natural sugars may feed bacteria.

☙Reduce all sugary and refined foods.

☙Many ear infections are the result of food reactions. Eliminate MSG, and check for food additives and preservatives, the biggest offenders.

⚘ Drink lots of water and diluted liquids like pineapple juice to keep mucous secretions thinned.

☙Use ice packs instead of heat on the ear to relieve pain. ♂

⚘ Press out and strain onion juice onto a small cotton plug. Place in the ear for fast, effective relief and infection fighting. ⚥

⚘ **Effective superfoods:**
☙Crystal Star BIOFLAVONOID, FIBER & C SUPPORT™ drink as needed.
☙Liquid chlorophyll in water 3x daily.

Herbal Therapy

Enhancing immune defenses is a primary factor in controlling chronic earaches in both adults and children.

⚘ **Jump start herbal program:**
Crystal Star ANTI-BIO™ capsules 4 to 6 daily, or extract 4x daily to clear infection. (Extract may also be used as ear drops morning and evening.)
☙**ANTI-HST™ capsules - a decongestant to take down swelling and shrink swollen membranes. Also use before an airplane flight to relieve ear congestion.**
☙**ASPIR-SOURCE™ capsules 4 at a time for pain.** ⊛ **or ANTI-FLAM™ for inflammation in adults.**

⚘ **Effective herbal ear oil drops:**
☙Mullein oil
☙Turtle Island warm EAR OIL drops.
☙Warm garlic oil ear drops; take garlic tabs 4x daily for immune response.
☙Warm lobelia extract in the ear. ⊛
☙Castor oil drops. ⊛
☙Calendula oil.

⚘ Effective soothing teas:
☙Chamomile for pain. ♀
☙Yarrow
☙Angelica root

⚘ Use ECHINACEA extract in water as a gargle and internally. ♂

Supplements

Beware of having medical drainage tubes placed in children's ears. They may damage hearing.

⚘ Mix together white vinegar and 70% isopropyl alcohol; drop in the ear for 30 seconds. Rinse out. Three times daily.
or
☙**Use a small dropper and flush ear gently with a food grade dilute solution of 3% H_2O_2 to cleanse infection.**

⚘ **Effective homeopathic remedies:**
☙NatraBio *EARACHE.* ⊛
☙*Pulsatilla* and *Kali Mur.* ⊛
☙*Chamomilla* for irritability. ⊛
☙*Belladonna* for throbbing pain.

⚘ Acidophilus powder - $\frac{1}{4}$ teasp. in juice 4x daily, with ascorbate or Ester vitamin C 3-5000mg daily with bioflavs.

⚘ **Beta carotene 25,000IU 4x daily, with**
☙**Zinc lozenges 30mg under the tongue until dissolved.**
☙ Enzymatic Therapy LYMPHO-CLEAR to flush lymph glands.
and
☙**Nutribiotic GRAPEFRUIT SEED extract to clear infection.**

⚘ Mix warm vegetable glycerine and witch hazel. Soak a piece of cotton and insert in the ear to draw out infection.

Lifestyle Support Therapy

While most childhood earaches can successfully be treated at home, there are illness signs that indicate medical treatment:
- if acute pain and loss of hearing does not respond within 48 hours.
- if fever does not abate within 3 days.
- if there is dizziness, bloody discharge, or redness around the ear.
- if there is difficult breathing or vomiting.

☙ Massage ear, neck and temples. Pull ear lobe 10 times on each ear. Fold ear shell over and back repeatedly until blood suffuses area. Big yawn several times.

☙ Use ear candles as directed.

☙ **For excess earwax:** Have the ear flushed for infection by a doctor.
☙Then press firmly but gently behind, then in front of the ear. Pull lobe up and down to work wax out. Fold ear shell in half. Open and fold repeatedly for circulation.
☙Put 3 drops of warm olive oil in each ear to soften wax; flush with warm water.

☙ **Reflexology point:**

ear
ear

Common Symptoms: Acute, stabbing pain in the mastoid, eustachian and ear area; swelling, inflammation, thickness and temporary loss of hearing in the ear; slight fever and general fussiness in a child - nausea and vomiting in a baby; bleeding or pusy discharge from the ear; extreme tenderness when the earlobe is pulled; sometimes temporary hearing loss because of congestion.

Common Causes: Residue of a cold, flu or bronchial infection settling in the ear; viral infection; too many mucous-forming foods such as dairy products; food allergies; high altitude, cold and decompression in air travel; in children, often the inner ear structure is not fully developed and canals and eustachian tubes become easy breeding areas for bacterial infection.

See also COLD AND FLU pages in this book for more information.

Eating Disorders

Anorexia Nervosa ❖ Bulimia

For over thirty-five percent of American women, and over seventy-five percent of American teen-age girls, looking good means being bone thin. Fashion models are presented as both the aesthetic standard and the health standard. Striving to meet this abnormal standard translates to thinness at any cost - specifically to eating disorders that are extremely hard to overcome, and which eventually result in other disabling health problems. Within 20 years of diagnosis, there is a mortality rate of almost 40%! Men are not completely exempt. Bodybuilders, male models, etc. have competition from ever-thinner rivals, and can suffer reduced testicular function from starving.

Diet & Superfood Therapy

Emphasis must be on optimal nutrient foods for body regeneration. See The Forever Diet in "COOKING FOR HEALTHY HEALING" by Linda Rector Page.

☙ Eat a high vegetable protein, high complex carbohydrate diet. Eat breakfast - with whole grain cereals, fruit, yogurt, etc.
☞NO junk foods, heavy starches or sugars. They disrupt normalization of body chemistry.
☞Eat slowly; chew well; have small meals often for best absorption.
☞Make a mix of brewer's yeast, or Bio-Strath YEAST EXTRACT, wheat germ, blackstrap molasses; take 2 TBS. daily:

☙ Superfoods can be lifesavers:
☞Crystal Star SYSTEMS STRENGTH™.
☞Future Biotics VITAL K liquid daily.
☞Protein drinks: Nappi THE PERFECT MEAL, or Solgar WHEY TO GO.
☞Green drinks for blood-building: (pg. 168) or Crystal Star ENERGY GREEN™, or Nutrex HAWAIIAN ENERGIZER.
☞Carrot juice (page 168) or Green Foods BETA CARROT.
☞Y.S. ROYAL JELLY 3-4 teasp. daily.
☞Crystal Star nutrient-rich LIGHT WEIGHT™ meal replacement drink is well-accepted by people struggling with eating disorders - satisfying nutrition requirements without excess calories or any fats.

Herbal Therapy

☙ **Jump start herbal program:**
Crystal Star ZINC SOURCE™ extract or capsules with POTASSIUM/IODINE SOURCE™ caps; and
☞BODY REBUILDER™ capsules with ADR-ACTIVE™ caps, 2 each daily.
☞FEEL GREAT™ capsules 2x daily for a feeling of well-being and strength.

☙ BIOFLAV., FIBER & C SUPPORT™ drink, 1 daily for 1 month to help change body chemistry, and normalize body functions.
with
☞RELAX CAPS™ 2 daily to rebuild and normalize nerve structure.
☞Flora VEGE-SIL caps, or Crystal Star SILICA SOURCE™ extract for new collagen/tissue growth. ♀✝

☙ Ginseng can be a key for energy and balance without calories:
☞Root To Health POWER PIECES (panax ginseng in honey). ♀✝
☞Beehive Botanical GINSENG/ROYAL JELLY caps.
☞Crystal Star GINSENG SUPER 6™.

☙ **To stimulate appetite and digestion:**
☞Ginseng/Gotu Kola caps
☞Acidophilus complex powder $1/4$ teasp. 3x daily in water, with Enzymatic Therapy PARAZYME for absorption.

Supplements

Girls don't realize that the very minerals they are losing through vomiting are the ones that help them control their weight - potassium and iodine stimulate the thyroid to keep metabolism, and therefore calorie-burning, strong.

☙ **Mineral therapy is effective.** Many minerals are lost from vomiting and laxatives. (Minerals also help to regain normal menstrual periods.)
☞Zinc is a key. Severely zinc-deficient individuals can't manufacture a key protein that allows them to taste. Chewable zinc lozenges or 30mg. capsules 3x daily. (Add extra tyrosine 500mg if needed.)
☞Mezotrace SEA MINERAL COMPLEX.

☙ Nature's Bounty vitamin B_{12} internasal gel, sublingual B_{12} or folic acid with B_{12} for healthy cell growth and energy.

☙ **Enzyme therapy for nutrient assimilation.**
☞Enzymatic Therapy MEGA-ZYME.
☞Rainbow Light ADVANCED ENZYME SYSTEM.

☙ A good food source multiple daily, such as Country Life MAXINE, or Nature's Secret ULTIMATE MULTI PLUS. ♀

☙ A GABA compound for stress relief and nerve building - Natrol SAF or Country Life RELAXER.

Lifestyle Support Therapy

Since there is a high correlation between sexual abuse and eating disorders, psychological counseling is often helpful. It can help in understanding the almost universal problem of low self-esteem that triggers this type of harmful behavior, and in beginning to deal with it. Therapy during healing reinforces the idea that destructive thinking and behavior can change, and self-confidence of the patient reestablished.
☞*See Eating Disorder Self-Test on page 444 in this book.*

☞ Improve self-esteem; cultivate relationships with positive people. Keep company with those in whose company you feel good about yourself.
☞Get some mild exercise every day for lung, heart and muscle rebuilding.
☞Get regular massage therapy treatments.

☞ **Reflexology point:**

food assimilation

Common Symptoms: Extreme malnutrition from vomiting/laxatives (bulimia) that discharges most nutrients; or refusing to eat (anorexia); belligerent, impolite, aggressive behavior; low blood pressure, slow heartbeat; hard fecal stools; fluid retention; reduced metabolism; cold hands and feet; dry skin, brittle, dull hair; tooth decay and yellow teeth; cessation of menses. Bulimia sufferers have a swollen rack and eroded tooth enamel from excessive vomiting, broken blood vessels on the face, low pulse rate and blood pressure and extreme weakness.

Common Causes: Eating disorders are usually caused by complex cultural or emotional problems that end up turning into a form of compulsive psychosis.

Hotlines with good information: ANAD: (708) 831-3438; Am. Anorexia/Bulimia Assoc. (212) 501-8351.

Eczema & Psoriasis
Atopic Dermatitis

Eczema is an itchy, inflammatory skin disease found on the tender areas of elbows, knees, wrists and neck. *Psoriasis* is a common adult skin disorder, marked by plaques and silvery scales on the skin, caused by a too-rapid replication and pile up of skin cells. It usually affects the scalp, and the outsides of the elbows, wrists, knees, etc. Drugs can produce dramatic short-term results, but the problem reappears after they are discontinued. Natural therapies have had notable achievement in both skin conditions because they get to the root of the problem. Natural methods take several months to produce consistent improvement, but they offer lasting results. *Afflicted individuals have trouble converting linoleic acid to gamma-linolenic acid. It is most common in infants and children.*

Diet & Superfood Therapy

A healthy, low fat diet is a key factor. Most severe psoriasis sufferers are overweight.

⚕ A high fiber, high mineral diet with lots of vegetable protein is the key to clearing and preventing eczema.

⚕ Go on a short 3 day cleansing diet (pg. 157) to release acid wastes.
  ☀Take 1 TB. psyllium husk, Sonne bentonite or Crystal Star CHOL-LO-FIBER TONE™ in water morning and evening.
  ☀Take a green drink daily (see below)
  ☀Take 3 cranberry or apple juices daily.
  ☀Eliminate refined fatty or fried foods, alcohol and red meats.
  ☀Then follow a sugar-free, milk-free, low-fat and alkalizing diet with 60-70% fresh foods, whole grains, seafood and sea vegetables for iodine therapy.
  ☀Make a skin health mix of lecithin granules, brewer's yeast, and unsulphured molasses and take 2 TBS. daily. ☞

⚕ Effective superfoods:
  ☀Crystal Star BIOFLAV., FIBER & C SUPPORT™ to help tissue integrity.
  ☀Nutricology PROGREENS.
  ☀AloeLife ALOE SKIN GEL; apply and drink aloe juice every morning.
  ☀Green Foods GREEN MAGMA.
  ☀Crystal Star ENERGY GREEN™.

Herbal Therapy

☙ Jump start herbal program:
  Crystal Star THERADERM™ caps, or BEAUTIFUL SKIN™ caps with ECHINACEA extract for 3 months.
  ☀Take BEAUTIFUL SKIN™ tea internally 2 cups daily, and apply to lesions with soaked cotton balls.
  ☀Apply ZINC SOURE™ spray topically.
  ☀Turmeric therapy: take the equivalent of 1-oz. (or about twelve "00" capsules) turmeric daily for six weeks. Often dramatic results in fresh new skin without recurrence.

☙ Crystal Star ADRN™ extract drops help form adrenal cortex, RELAX CAPS™ ease stress, and MILK THISTLE SEED drops 2x daily enhance liver function. ♀

☙ Effective topical/internal solutions:
  ☀Myrrh/goldenseal root extract
  ☀Licorice root extract tea
  ☀Abkit CAMO-CARE cream.
  ☀Nettles extract.
  ☀Crystal Star ANTI-BIO™ gel with una da gato.
  ☀Propolis extract.

☙ Effective GLA sources: Use for at least 3 to 6 months in decreasing doses.
  ☀EVENING PRIMROSE OIL 4-6 daily
  ☀Borage or black currant seed oil
  ☀Nature's Secret ULTIMATE OIL

Supplements

Support healthy liver function. It is a key to normalizing skin balance.

❧ Dr. Diamond HERPANACINE capsules as directed. ♀

❧ Lane Labs BENE-FIN shark cartilage capsules 2 daily for 3 months. ♂

❧ Melatonin .1 to .3mg at bedtime for 2 to 3 months.

❧ Flora VEGE-SIL tabs 3 daily, with

❧ EVENING PRIMROSE OIL with natural vitamin E 5x daily for 3 months. ♀
  or
  ☀High omega-3 flaxseed oil 3 daily.

❧ Ester C w/ bioflavonoids 3000mg daily for tissue/collagen regrowth and to to decrease histamine skin reactions.
  and
  ☀Beta carotene 100,000IU daily.

❧ Zinc picolinate 50mg 2x daily, with germanium 150mg daily, and vitamin E 400IU with selenium 200mcg (or mix zinc oxide with vitamin E oil from capsules and apply to sores). ♀

❧ B Complex 100mg with extra pantothenic acid 500mg & PABA 1000mg.

Lifestyle Support Therapy

Give your body a chance to digest your food. Don't eat for 2 hours before bed.

☘ Exercise is important to keep circulation healthy and body wastes released.
  ☀Expose affected areas to early morning sunlight daily for healing Vitamin D. A gradual suntan is ideal.
  ☀Swim or wade in the ocean, or take kelp foot baths for iodine therapy.
  ☀Take a catnip or chlorophyll enema once a week to release acid toxins.

☘ Effective local applications:
  ☀Zia PAPAYA ENZYME PEEL ♀
  ☀Tea tree oil or Witch hazel
  ☀Jojoba oil (for scalp psoriasis) ♂
  ☀Matrix Health GENESIS OXY-SPRAY
  ☀Advanced Research PAU d' ARCO gel
  ☀Hot ginger, goldenseal or fresh comfrey leaf compresses

☘ Stress management is a key. Depression and emotional stress can cause and aggravate psoriasis flare-ups.
  ☀Acupuncture is successful for eczema.
  ☀Overheating therapy (pg. 178) is effective for psoriasis.

☘ For childhood eczema rash: bathe areas with strong chamomile tea, then apply an oatmeal paste and let dry. Repeat for 3 or 4 days until clear. ☺

Common Symptoms: Chronic silvery red, scaly, skin rash or patches on knees, elbows, buttocks, scalp or chest that flare up irregularly; skin is continually dry and thickened even when not in the weeping, blistered stages; "oil drop" stippling of the nails; sometimes accompanying arthritis.
Common Causes: Overuse of drugs/antibiotics; chronic stress or depression; eczema is associated with diabetes, asthma, candida allergies, psoriasis with arthritis; hypothyroidism; EFA deficiency; liver malfunction; thin bowel walls allowing wastes elimination through the skin; excess fatty, animal foods in the diet and poor protein digestion; heavy smoking.

See also Skin Healing pages in this book for more information.

Emphysema
Smoker's Pulmonary Disease

Emphysema is a wasting pulmonary disease that affects smokers almost exclusively. It is characterized by loss of elasticity and dilation ability, and scarring/thickening of delicate lung tissue. Breathing becomes ever more difficult as the lungs progressively scar. The lung exchange of oxygen and carbon-dioxide is seriously affected to the point of extreme breathlessness and the inability to take a deep breath at all. The person feels asphyxiated. If an emphysema sufferer continues to smoke, emphysema is usually fatal. See the STOP SMOKING page in this book.

Diet & Superfood Therapy

Eliminate food and inhalant allergens to improve emphysema symptoms.

✿ Go on a short mucous cleansing juice diet for 3-5 days (pg. 157).

✿ Then, eat a largely fresh foods diet with increased vegetable protein, from whole grains, tofu, nuts, seeds and sprouts. Have a green salad every day, and add vitamin B rich foods such as brown rice and eggs frequently.

✿ Add extra protein to the diet in the form of sea foods and sea vegetables for additional B_{12}.

✿ Have a glass of fresh carrot juice every day for a month (pg. 168), then every other day for a month.

✿ Eliminate mucous-forming foods such as pasteurized dairy, red meats, and caffeine.

✿ **Effective superfoods:**
✿ Wakunaga KYO-GREEN drink.
✿ Crystal Star SYSTEMS STRENGTH™.
✿ Solgar EARTH SOURCE GREEN & MORE drink.
✿ Beehive Botanical ROYAL JELLY with Siberian ginseng 2 teasp. daily, ♀ or Long Life IMPERIAL TONIC with royal jelly and EPO. ♂
✿ AloeLife ALOE GOLD juice 2x daily.

Herbal Therapy

✿ **Jump start herbal program:**
Crystal Star RSPR™ CAPS and TEA 2x daily for tissue oxygen uptake.
✿ GINSENG/LICORICE ELIXIR™ for adrenal support and to reduce lung inflammation.
✿ Crystal Star ANTI-BIO™ capsules 2x daily to counteract infection, and X-PECT™ tea to expel mucous congestion.

✿ **Effective lung healers:**
✿ Comfrey/fenugreek tea
✿ Mullein/lobelia extract
✿ Pleurisy root tea

✿ **Herbal antioxidants to improve lung tissue oxygen:**
✿ PCOs from grapeseed or white pine, 100mg 3x daily.
✿ Rainbow Light GARLIC & GREENS caps, 6 daily with 1 tsp. olive oil in juice - to dissolve mucous, and detoxify. ♀
✿ Sun CHLORELLA 3x daily.

✿ Crystal Star HEAVY METAL™ if chemical pollutants are the cause. Use WITHDRAWAL SUPPORT™ capsules if heavy marijuana smoking is the cause.

✿ Take 5 drops anise oil in 1 teasp. brown sugar 3x daily before meals.

Supplements

✿ **Anti-oxidants are key factors:**
✿ Co Q_{10} 100mg 2x daily. ♂
✿ Nutricology germanium 150mg.
✿ Vit. E 1000IU with selenium.
✿ Premier GERMANIUM w. DMG. ♀
✿ Beta or marine carotene 100,000IU with copper caps to improve elasticity of lung tissue.
✿ **Vitamin C crystals with bioflavonoids $1/4$ teasp. every hour to bowel tolerance daily for at least a month. (an ascorbic acid flush to neutralize lung poisons and encourage tissue elasticity.)**

✿ High B Complex 150mg daily with pantothenic acid 500mg, with extra folic acid 800mcg. ♀

✿ Enzymatic Therapy LUNG COMPLEX and ADRENAL COMPLEX; and LIQUID LIVER w. Siberian ginseng caps.
✿ Twin Labs LYCOPENE - an anti-oxidant specific for the lungs.

✿ Propolis extract 3x daily or Crystal Star BIO-VI™ extract with propolis.

✿ BioForce ASTHMASAN homeopathic.

Lifestyle Support Therapy

☞ Avoid smoking and secondary smoke, including smog and other air pollution. (Use Enzymatic Therapy NICO-STOP formula to help stop smoking.)

☞ Do deep breathing exercises for 3 minutes every morning when rising to clean out the lungs.
☞ Take a brisk deep breathing daily walk to increase oxygen.

☞ Get some early sunlight on the body every day possible.

☞ **Steam head and nasal passages with eucalyptus and wintergreen herbs.**

☞ Use 1 teasp. food grade 3% solution H_2O_2 in 8-oz. water in a vaporizer at night.

☞ **Reflexology point:**

lung

See the MUCOUS CLEANSING DIET in the ASTHMA section for more information.

Common Symptoms: *Chronic bronchitis with shortness of breath, continuing post-nasal drip and congestion; frequent colds; coated tongue; bad breath; frequent hacking cough, especially during exhalation and speaking; lack of energy and general vitality because of lack of oxygen.*
Common Causes: *Smoking and secondary smoke; air and environmental pollution; excess refined foods and dairy products; allergies; heavy metal pollution from industry; poor circulation and elimination of poisons by the lungs.*

Endometriosis
Pelvic Inflammatory Disease (PID)

Endometriosis is a condition caused by mislocation and overgrowth of uterine endometrial tissue, and attachment of this tissue to other organs. It is normal tissue growing in abnormal places. Menstrual flow is heavy and painful, and much of the waste blood flows back through the fallopian tubes instead of through the vagina normally. Endometriosis increases risk for uterine and breast fibroids, and is often followed by CFS or Fibromyalgia. An immune-enhancing program that addresses liver therapy, improves emotional stress, body trauma, and relieves pain is the most effective.

Diet & Superfood Therapy

See the Hypoglycemia Diet in this book, or "COOKING FOR HEALTHY HEALING" by Linda Rector Page for more information.

❧ **Eat an immune power diet:**
—Go on a short 24 hour juice diet (pg. 158) to clear out acid wastes. (This helps you to work on the integrity of the liver and digestive system first. Repeat 24 hour diet before menses.)
—Lower fat intake to reduce body fat and excess circulating estrogen.
—Then follow a vegan diet with the addition of cold water fish. Eat cultured foods, fresh fruits and green salads, whole grains and cereals until condition clears.

◆ **Especially add soy foods.**
—Eliminate all forms of caffeine from the diet permanently. Restrict refined sugars, alcohol, salt, red meats and dairy products during healing. Keep all animal fats and high cholesterol foods low, to prevent excess estrogen production, a clear cause of endometriosis. Particularly avoid chocolate, tropical oils, fried and fast food of all kinds.
✿

❧ **Effective superfoods:**
—Green Foods GREEN MAGMA, or Crystal Star ENERGY GREEN™ drinks.
—Crystal Star SYSTEMS STRENGTH™ for iodine and potassium therapy.
—Nutricology PRO-GREENS w. flax oil.

Herbal Therapy

Note: Bitters herbs can be excellent cleansers of pelvic congestion, but should be avoided during painful flare-ups.

❧ **Jump start herbal program:**
Crystal Star WOMAN'S BEST FRIEND™ caps 6 daily, and bur-dock tea 2 cups daily **for 3 months,**
—PRO-EST BALANCE™ roll-on, for progesterone stimulation and to control pain, and WOMEN'S STRENGTH ENDO™ tea **as a body-balancing adaptogen.**
—**EFA therapy:** EVENING PRIMROSE OIL caps 1000mg 4 daily.

❧ Black cohosh extract to dissolve adhesions of abnormally placed tissue.
—Dandelion leaf to help metabolize excess estrogen.

❧ **Adjunctive herbal therapy:**
—Crystal Star ANTI-FLAM™ to relieve inflammation; ADRN™ extract for adrenal cortex balance; RELAX CAPS™ for stress reduction - 2 at a time as needed.
—VITEX extract for pituitary support.

❧ **Energy-building liver therapy:**
—ECHINACEA and MILK THISTLE SEED extracts.
—NatureWorks SWEDISH BITTERS or Crystal Star BITTERS & LEMON CLEANSE™.

Supplements

Avoid cortico-steroid drugs commonly given for endometriosis - esp. prednisone.

❧ **Gland therapy for pain relief:**
—Enzymatic Therapy OVARY-UTERUS COMPLEX and LYMPHO-CLEAR 3x daily.
—NUCLEO-PRO F for pain relief. Chew tablets for faster results.
—American Biologics SHARKILAGE 750mg as an anti-infective.
—**Transitions PRO-GEST CREAM or OIL rubbed on the abdomen.**

❧ **Nature's Secret ULTIMATE B, and extra folic acid 400mcg, B₆ 100mg and Floradix herbal iron 3x daily.**

❧ **Immune enhancement:**
—CoQ₁₀ 60mg 3x daily.
—Marine carotene 100,000IU daily
—Ester C with bioflavonoids 3000mg.
—Future Biotics VITAL K liquid potassium 3 teasp. daily
—Vitamin E 400-800IU 2 daily
—Ascorbic acid flush: ascorbate vitamin C powder with bioflavonoids - ¼ teasp. in juice every hour until stool turns soupy.

❧ **EFA and liver therapy:**
—Omega-rich flax or fish oil.
—Solaray LIPOTROPIC PLUS complex.
—**Nature's Secret ULTIMATE OIL.**
—Choline 1000mg with inositol 500mg.

Lifestyle Support Therapy

Before you jump into surgery or any drastic treatment decision, endometriosis fibroids often go away when glands and hormones rebalance, such as after pregnancy and birth, or menopause.

☙ Use stress reduction techniques like, massage therapy and acupuncture.

☙ Avoid all chloro-fluorocarbon products and any other known toxic chemical or environmental pollutants.
—Avoid all IUDs. They are a major contributor to endometriosis.

☙ Get mild exercise and early morning sunlight on the body every day.

☙ **Effective douches:**
—Garlic
—Mineral water

☙ **Reflexology point:**
—Press both sides of the foot just below the ankle bone, 2x daily for 10 seconds each.

☙ Boluses and vaginal packs are effective in drawing out internal infection. Use castor oil packs or see the formula in HOME PROTOCOLS in this book. Make sure there are long rest times between pack or bolus use - 1 week of use to 3 weeks rest.

Common Symptoms: *Severe cramping and abdominal/rectal pain, swelling and bleeding during menses, ovulation and sex; fluid retention; enlarged ovaries; irritable bowel and gas; pinched nerve-type pain; unusual insomnia; excessive menstruation and prolonged cycles; irregular bowel movements; possible infertility; endometrial tissue on cervix, vaginal walls, vulva and rectum.*

Common Causes: *Excess levels of estrogen, deficient progesterone, hormone imbalance that causes abnormal biochemical processes in the endometrium; sexually transmitted chlamydia, cervical dysplasia or vaginal warts; magnesium deficiency; hypoglycemia; EFA deficiency and prostaglandin imbalance; X-Ray consequences; high fat diet with too much caffeine and alcohol.*

Call the ENDOMETRIOSIS hotline 1-800-992-ENDO: for updated information.

Energy

There's no doubt about it - stress and fatigue are becoming more a part of our lives - putting our energy resources in jeopardy. Some of us feel tired most of the time. Almost all of us feel the need of a pick-me-up during a long day. Yet, turning to drugs or controlled substances for stimulation is asking for trouble. The overuse of stimulants is dependency, irritability and lethargy, further reducing energy in a downward spiral. Even traditional food energizers like caffeine, sodas or sugar can end up making us feel more nervous and restless. Natural energizers have great advantages over chemically processed stimulants. They don't exhaust the body, and are supporting rather than depleting. They can be strong or gentle as needed.

Increasing Stamina & Endurance ✦ Overcoming Fatigue, Nerve Exhaustion & Mental Burn-Out

Diet & Superfood Therapy

☙ A balanced, high energy diet should consist of 65-70% complex carbohydrates, fresh fruits, vegetables, whole grains and legumes; 20-25% protein, from nuts, seeds, whole grains, legumes, soy, yogurt and kefir, sea foods and poultry; 10-15% fats from sources such as unrefined vegetable, nut and seed oils, eggs and low-fat dairy.

✻Foods that fight fatigue include potassium and magnesium-rich foods, complex carbohydrates, high vitamin B and C foods, and iron-rich foods.

✻Reduce sugar, caffeine, (it drains adrenals) and dairy foods.

✻Take a high protein drink every morning (pg. 175, or see below). Add spirulina or bee pollen granules if desired.

✻Drink plenty of healthy liquids daily.

✻Have a little white wine at dinner for mental relaxation and good digestion.

❧

☙ Effective superfoods:
✻Alacer EMERGEN-C granules in water
✻Nutri-Tech ALL 1 vit./mineral drink
✻Crystal Star ENERGY GREEN™.
✻Nappi THE PERFECT MEAL drink
✻Aloe vera juice in the morning
✻Nature's Life SUPER-PRO 96 drink
✻Beehive Botanicals ginseng/royal jelly
✻Nutrex HAWAIIAN SPIRULINA ◯
✻Future Biotics VITAL K drink
✻Bragg's LIQUID AMINOS

Herbal Therapy

☙ Energizers for men:
✻Crystal Star HIGH PERFORMANCE™, SUPER MAN'S ENERGY™, MALE GINSIAC™, and ADRN™ extracts.
✻SARSAPARILLA extract
✻Chinese red ginseng
✻Bioforce GINSAVENA
✻Dragon Eggs SAGES GINSENG

☙ Energizers for women:
✻Crystal Star BODY REBUILDER™ with ADR-ACTIVE™ capsules; FEM-SUPPORT™ extract with ashwagandha, EVENING PRIMROSE oil, especially for recovery from fatigue; HIGH ENERGY™ tea, RAINFOREST ENERGY™ tea and caps, FEEL GREAT tea.
✻HAWTHORN extract for well-being.

☙ Ginseng is a highly recommended natural energizer for both sexes:
✻Crystal Star ACTIVE PHYSICAL ENERGY, FEEL GREAT™, GINSENG SUPER 6 ENERGY™ capsules and tea.
✻Ginseng Co. CYCLONE CIDER
✻Siberian ginseng extract ♂
✻Rainbow Light ADAPTO-GEM.
✻Crystal Star GINSENG/LICORICE ELIXIR™.

☙ Mental energizers:
✻Crystal Star MENTAL INNER ENERGY™.
✻GINKGO BILOBA extract

Supplements

☙ Fatigue and a poor diet deplete chromium, magnesium and B vitamins:
✻B Complex 100mg with extra pantothenic acid 500mg 2x daily. ♀
✻Nature's Bounty B₁₂ internasal gel or dibencozide every three days. Take with tyrosine 500mg for best results. ♂
✻Chromium picolinate 200mcg daily.
✻Country Life TARGET MINS - potassium/magnesium aspartate, or Solaray magnesium/potassium asporotate with bromelain.

☙ Effective anti-oxidants/energizers:
✻Country Life B₁₅ DMG SL tabs ♂
✻Unipro LIQUID DMG
✻CoQ₁₀ 30mg, 2x daily
✻Vitamin C with bioflavs, 3000mg daily
✻Glutamine 1000mg. daily ♀
✻Zinc picolinate 50-75mg
✻Earth's Bounty OXY-CAPS as directed
✻Full spectrum, pre-digested amino acid compound, 1000mg. daily, **or** Phenylalanine 500mg. 1 to 2x daily.

☙ Gland and organ energizers:
✻Enzymatic Therapy BIO-VITAL ONE, and THYROID & TYROSINE COMPLEX. ♀
✻Raw Pituitary
✻Raw Brain
✻Raw Liver

☙ Rainbow Light ULTRA ENERGY PLUS. ♀

Lifestyle Support Therapy

If symptoms are chronic for more than 6 months, get a test for EBV, chronic fatigue syndrome, or Candida albicans.

☜ Take a brisk walk or other aerobic exercise every day for tissue oxygen. Aerobic exercise stimulates endorphins and replenishes oxygen in the entire body.
✻Stretch out for 5 minutes both morning and before bed to release energy blocks.
✻Get some early morning sunlight on the body every day day possible.
✻Have a full spinal massage for increased nerve force.
✻Take alternating hot and cold hydrotherapy showers to increase circulation.

☜ Get good sleep. Feeling rested has everything to do with the amount of energy you have.

☜ **Acupressure energizer:** squeeze point between eyes where brows come together.

☜ Energy drainers:
✻Smoking and second-hand smoke.
✻Excess alcohol is both a depressant and dehydrator.
✻Drugs of all kinds, taken to excess, can result in lethargy and dependency.

See also BRAIN HEALTH page in this book for more information.

Common Symptoms: *Lack of energy for even everyday tasks; mental depression; lethargy.*

Common Causes: *Poor eating habits - lack of proper nutrition; protein deficiency caused by extreme "new age" eating beliefs; too much sugar; emotional stress; low thyroid, liver and adrenal activity; anemia; stress; allergies, diabetes, chronic fatigue syndrome, mononucleosis, anemia or Candida albicans conditions; abuse of tobacco, caffeine, drugs or alcohol; pessimistic outlook on life.*

Epilepsy
Petit Mal ✻ Partial Seizures

Epilepsy is a neurological disorder that involves recurrent electrical disturbances in the brain, causing seizures. 1) Petit mal - a short seizure with a blank stare; most common in children; 2) Grand mal - a long seizure with falling, muscle twitching, incontinence, gasping, and ashen skin. 3) Partial seizures - muscle jerking, sensing things that do not exist. Most people have no memory of an attack. Many commonly used anti-convulsant drugs today are so strong and so habit forming that even non-epileptic people have bad reactions and seizures when cut off suddenly. Nutritional medicines can make drugs unnecessary. If you decide to use natural therapies, or try methods other than drugs, taper off gradually. If seizures recur, return to the anti-convulsants briefly to let the body adjust.

Diet & Superfood Therapy

There must be a diet and lifestyle change for there to be permanent control and improvement. Consider a rotation diet to check for food allergy reactions.

2. Start with a 3 day liquid diet (pg. 157) to release mucous from the system.
   *✻Then follow a diet with at least 70% fresh foods. Have a green salad every day.
   *✻Add cultured foods such as yogurt and kefir, tofu, brown rice and other whole grains.
   *✻After a month, add eggs, small amounts of low fat dairy, legumes and seafoods.
   *✻Eat organically grown foods whenever possible to avoid seizure triggers in pesticides.
   *✻Eliminate foods with preservatives or colorings; refined foods, sugars, fried and canned foods, red meats, pork, alcohol, caffeine, and pasteurized dairy products.

2. **Superfoods are very important:**
   *✻Crystal Star SYSTEMS STRENGTH™ for iodine, potassium and broad spectrum nutrient support. ☺
   *✻Organic Gourmet NUTRITIONAL YEAST or MISO extract before bed.
   *✻Amazake RICE DRINKS.
   *✻AloeLife ALOE GOLD drink.

Herbal Therapy

2. Jump start herbal program:
   Crystal Star RELAX CAPS™ and ANTI-SPZ™ caps as needed, and EVENING PRIMROSE OIL caps 4-6 daily for 2 months, then 3-4 daily for 1 month to balance body electrical activity.
   with
   *✻LIV-ALIVE™ caps and MILK THISTLE SEED extract to support the liver, especially if you are taking Dilantin and Depakote drugs.
   *✻HEARTSEASE/ANEMI-GIZE™ capsules to strengthen spleen for tissue oxygen and red blood cell formation.

2. **Calming teas:**
   *✻Catnip ☺
   *✻Scullcap, 3 cups daily - with vitamin E 400IU and C 500mg for best results.
   *✻Siberian ginseng or Rainbow Light ADAPTO-GEM caps.
   *✻Hyssop

2. Transitions PROGEST as directed. ♀

2. Minerals help stabilize:
   *✻Nature's Life TRACE MINERAL COMPLEX caps. ☺
   *✻Mezotrace SEA MINERAL caps
   *✻American Biologics MANGANESE FORTE.
   *✻(Also consider Health Papers oral chelation CETA CLEANSE with EDTA.)

Supplements

2. Country Life MAXI-B w/taurine and B$_6$ as an anti-convulsant.
   and a good calcium 1000mg/magnesium 500mg supplement daily to reduce excitability of the nerves.
   *✻Nature's Bounty B$_{12}$ SL or internasal.
   *✻Alta Health SL MANGANESE with B$_{12}$.
   *✻Natren TRINITY for probiotic aid.

2. Country Life RELAXER caps with GABA and taurine 500mg 2x daily.
   *✻Glutamine 500mg daily or DMG sublingual, 1 daily.

2. Choline/inositol or phosphatidyl choline for brain balance. ☺
   with
   *✻Atrium LITHIUM 5mg as directed, and magnesium 400mg. ♂

2. **For childhood epilepsy:**
   *✻Floradix liquid multiple vit./min. complex for body balance. ☺
   *✻Nature's Way ANTSP tincture, or lobelia tincture under the tongue as emergency measures. ♂
   *✻Carnitine 250mg with folic acid 400mcg esp. if taking Dilantin.

Lifestyle Support Therapy

2. Take lemon juice or catnip enemas once a month to keep the body pH balanced and toxin-free.

2. Get some outdoor exercise every day for healthy circulation.

2. Epileptic seizures are usually short, with immediate recovery of consciousness.
   *✻Do not attempt to restrain the person. Catch him if he falls. Loosen any constricting clothing clothing.
   *✻Let the person lie down and get plenty of fresh air. Clear away sharp or hard objects. Cushion the head.
   *✻Squeeze the little finger very firmly during a seizure.
   *✻Do not put anything in the person's mouth or throw water on the face. Turn head to let excess saliva drain out.
   *✻Deep sleep usually follows a seizure.

2. Biofeedback has been successful in shortening and limiting seizure attacks.

Common Symptoms: *Brief seizures, often with motor disability; loss of memory, and often loss of consciousness; sometimes there is falling down and jerking with foam at the mouth.*
Common Causes: *Inability of the body to eliminate wastes properly with a resultant overload on the nervous system; heavy metal toxicity; allergies; EFA, magnesium and other mineral deficiency; hypoglycemia; sometimes drugs or alcohol; deficient metabolic function and prostaglandin formation.*

See also the HYPOGLYCEMIA DIET in this book, or COOKING FOR HEALTHY HEALING by Linda Rector Page.

Eyesight

Weak Eyes ✲ Blurred Vision ✲ Swollen, Bloodshot, Burning Eyes ✲ Itchy, Watery Eyes

Ninety percent of what we learn during our lives we learn through sight. The eyes are not only the windows of the soul, but windows to body health as well. Eyes often reflect imbalances elsewhere in the system. No other sense is so prone to poor health conditions. Your lifestyle profoundly affects your "eyesight." As with so many other body systems, the liver is the key to healthy eyes. The most stressful eyesight situations are reading, using a computer for most of your workday, and a sedentary lifestyle. Take good care of your eyes!

Diet & Superfood Therapy

Liver malfunction is a common cause of eye problems. Keep it clean and well-functioning.

❦ Keep plenty of protein in the diet from sea and soy foods, whole grains, low fat dairy foods, eggs, sprouts and seeds.
~Increase vitamin A and high mineral foods, such as leafy greens, endive, carrots, broccoli, sea vegetables and parsley.
~Include vision foods like broccoli, sunflower and sesame seeds; leeks, onions, cabbage and cauliflower; barley, blueberries and watercress.
~Take a vision drink twice a week: Mix 1 cup carrot juice, ½ cup eyebright tea, 1 egg, 1 TB. wheat germ, 1 tsp. rosehips powder, 1 tsp. honey, 1 tsp. sesame seeds, 1 tsp. brewer's yeast, 1 tsp. kelp.
~Reduce sugar intake. Avoid refined foods, esp. margarine/shortening, pasteurized dairy, and red meats. These foods cause the body to metabolize slowly, use sugars poorly, and form crystallized clogs. ❧

❦ Effective superfoods:
~Green Foods BETA CARROT.
~Solgar EARTH SOURCE GREENS & MORE w. EFAs.
~Crystal Star SYSTEMS STRENGTH™.
~ALOE VERA JUICE, internally and as a eyewash.
~BeWell VEGETABLE JUICE.

Herbal Therapy

Seeing sparks of light or color with your eyes closed indicates stress.

❧ Jump start herbal program:
Crystal Star EYEBRIGHT HERBAL™ capsules 4-6 daily, with BILBERRY extract and LIV-ALIVE™ capsules 4-6 daily.

❧ Soothing, clarifying eyewashes:
~Crystal Star EYEBRIGHT HERBAL™ tea
~Sea vegetables tea for blurry vision.
~Aloe vera juice. ♂
~Raspberry tea or green tea especially for bloodshot eyes.
~For clarity and brightness: bathe eyes in a rosemary solution. (Better than Visine)
~Borage seed tea wash for sore eyes.
~Goldenseal tea, esp. for infected eyelids.
~Calendula tea for scleroderma.

❧ For eye health: Parsley root capsules 4 daily or eyebright tea with kelp tabs 6 daily. ♀

❧ Liver support for eye health:
~MILK THISTLE SEED extract.
~Dandelion root tea. ♂

❧ For strain and eye fatigue:
~GINKGO BILOBA extract to support healthy circulation to the eye area.
~Passionflower extract.
~PCOs from grapeseed 50mg 2x daily.

Supplements

Most eye-improving supplements need 2 to 3 months for effectiveness.

❧ For eye health and to lessen risk of disease:
~Zinc 30-50mg daily
~Taurine 500mg daily
~Beta carotene, up to 150,000IU daily
~Vit. E 400IU with selenium 200mcg.

❧ Bioflavonoids to strengthen eye vessels:
~Quercetin Plus with bromelain daily.
~PCOs from grape seed or white pine. 100mg with Vitamin D 400IU.
~Enzymatic Therapy I-TONE. ♂

❧ Chromium picolinate 200mcg to regulate sugar use, and Vit. B₂ 100mg daily.

❧ Nature's Life I-SIGHT with zeaxanthine.

❧ For tired, itchy red or painful eyes:
~B Complex 100mg with extra B₂ ♀
~Boiron OPTIQUE (allergic reactions).
~Ascorbate vitamin C 500mg 3x daily

❧ For color blindness: Solgar oceanic carotene 25,000IU (from Dunaliella Salina).

❧ For "computer" eyes:
~Press points under eyebrows; press points in inner corners of eyes; squeeze eyebrows; look up, down, right and left every half hour. Clean your screen.

Lifestyle Support Therapy

Relaxation techniques for the eyes are the key to better vision, especially if they are under strain. All it takes is a minute or two out of every hour. Eye exercises help both myopia and presbyopia. (See the Bates Method book for more information.)

❧ Eye relaxation techniques:
~Blink regularly to cleanse, lubricate and de-stress the eyes.
~Change your focus every 3 to 5 minutes, esp. driving or using a computer.
~Massage temples; pinch skin between the brows.
~Bathe eyes in a cool saline solution, witch hazel, or chamomile tea; or bathe eyes in ice water - then squeeze them shut for a few seconds to increase blood flow to the area.
~Palm your eyes to rest them; 3x daily for 10 seconds per time.

❧ Bad substances for eyes: cocaine, excessive use of chemical diuretics, sulfa drugs or tetracycline, aspirin, nicotine, phenylalanine, hard liquor, hydrocortisone.

❧ Reflexology point:

eye points - squeeze all around on fingers

See the following pages for information on other vision problems.

Common Symptoms: *Poor, often degenerating vision; easily strained eyes, blurring more as the day goes on; frequent headaches over the eyes; spots and floaters before the eyes.*
Common Causes: *Liver malfunction; environmental pollutants; allergies; poor diet deficient in usable proteins and minerals, excessive in sugars and refined foods; thyroid problems; allergies; serious illness; prescription and other drug abuse.*

Therapy For Other Vision Problems

THE MIND/BODY CONNECTION PLAYS A BIG ROLE IN GOOD VISION. EMOTIONAL HARMONY HAS AN IMPACT ON THE WILLINGNESS TO SEE.

❧•**CATARACTS** - See page 266.

❧•**CONJUNCTIVITIS INFECTION** - an inflammation of the lining of the eyelid is often caused by a viral infection, and can be extremely contagious. Therapy: 1 drop castor oil in the eyes 3x daily, and zinc 50mg 2x daily; teas and/or washes, such as BILBERRY, tansy tea, aloe vera juice, chamomile, or chickweed. Palm eyes to release infection and stimulate circulation. Apply yogurt, grated potato or apple to inflammation; **use homeopathic *Belladonna* or Boiron *OPTIQUE* remedy.** Take PCOs from grapeseed or white pine to help new tissue grow back healthy, 100mg 2x daily.

❧•**DRY EYES, (Sjögren's syndrome)** - a sudden onset problem, characterized by dryness of eyes, mouth, skin and all mucous membranes, and the inability to tear, often accompanies rheumatoid arthritis, scleroderma and systemic lupus. It is caused by a vitamin A deficiency, and by lowered immune response, and affects 9 times more women than men. Eliminate common food allergens and processed foods, such as milk and other pasteurized dairy products, corn, wheat, and nightshade plants (including tobacco and the drug Motrin which is nightshade-based.) Increase green vegetable, whole grain and fiber intake. Reduce all refined sugars, red meats and saturated fats. Increase cold water fish, sea foods and calcium foods like broccoli in your diet. Increase water and healthy fluid intake. Bathe the eyes daily with aloe vera juice. Take high omega-3 flax or EVENING PRIMROSE OIL capsules, 4 daily. Take 3000mg ascorbate vitamin C daily; emulsified vitamin A and E 25,000IU/400IU, to clear and support tear pathways; taurine 500mg 2x daily; butcher's broom tea or Crystal Star HEARTSEASE/CIRCU-CLEANSE™ tea to clear circulation, BILBERRY and GINKGO BILOBA extracts act as natural antihistamines; B complex 100mg with extra B$_2$, and zinc 30-50mg daily. Take Crystal Star CALCIUM SOURCE™ capsules for extra absorbable calcium.

❧•**DARK CIRCLES UNDER THE EYES** - usually caused by iron deficiency, but also an indication of liver or kidney malfunction or chronic allergies. Take Floradix liquid iron; use chamomile or green tea teabags over the eyes for 15 minutes.

❧•**DYSLEXIA** - color therapy eyewear has had some success. Pick whatever color glasses make your ability to read easier. Wear for 30 minutes at a time.

❧•**FLOATERS AND SPOTS BEFORE THE EYES** - these may be Bitot's spots, hard, elevated white spots on the whites of the eyes, bits of debris that cast shadows over the retina, or scotoma, blind spots in the vision field because of retina trouble. Take bioflavonoids 520mg. daily; Vit. K 100mcg 2x daily; Choline/Inositol; vitamin A & D, 25,000IU/400IU, or emulsified A & E 25,000IU/400IU to help remove lens particles, 4x daily; pantothenic acid 500mg with B$_6$ 250mg; Ascorbate vitamin C or Ester C; rub Matrix Health GENESIS OXY-SPRAY on the feet at night for several months; dandelion root tea and eyewash.

❧•**GLAUCOMA** - caused by a build-up of pressure in the front compartment of the eye. See page 314.

❧•**MACULAR DEGENERATION** - the leading cause of blindness in people over 60, oxidation to the macular blood vessels causes the tissues to break down. It may also be brought on by long-term exposure to ultraviolet and blue light from the sun. People with light-colored eyes seem to be more at risk. Symptoms of developing macular degeneration include blurry or distorted vision, decreased reading ability, even of large lettering. Colors are less bright; there are blind spots when looking straight ahead, even though peripheral vision is good. Driving becomes difficult and vertical lines are wavy. Glasses cannot help. Macular degeneration is often reversible with nutritional therapy. ***See page 266 for therapy information.***

❧•**MYOPIA (NEAR SIGHTEDNESS)** - only 2% of second grade children are nearsighted; by the end of high school, the figure is 40%; by the end of college, more than 60% of students are nearsighted! In addition to the general recommendations for better eyesight on the previous page, use ascorbate C powder 5000mg daily; Vitamin D 1000IU; Solaray VIZION; BILBERRY extract or caps; Enzymatic Therapy VISION ESSENTIALS capsules.

❦ **NIGHT BLINDNESS** - Take BILBERRY or GINKGO BILOBA extract capsules or liquid; PCOs from grapeseed or white pine 100mg 3x daily; CoQ$_{10}$ 60mg 3x daily; use amber glasses when doing daytime driving. Carotenoids such as beta or marine carotene up to 100,000IU daily are key. Take Enzymatic Therapy HERBAL FLAVONOIDS 4 daily.

❦

❦ **OVER-SENSITIVITY TO LIGHT (photophobia)** - Ascorbate vitamin C, American Biologics A & E EMULSION as directed; BILBERRY extract. Natural sunlight nourishes eyes. Face the sun **with the eyes closed** for 5 seconds. Then cover eyes with palms for 5 seconds. Repeat 10 times to relax eyes and reduce light sensitivity.

❦

❦ **PRESBYOPIA (middle age far-sightedness)** - If you have to wear glasses, use an **under-corrected prescription** to encourage your eyes to work with the glasses, not passively depend on them. Add B complex vitamins like Nature's Secret ULTIMATE B daily.

❦

❦ **PROTRUDING/BULGING EYES** - generally denotes a thyroid problem. Iodine therapy has had some success in these cases. See page 313.

❦

❦ **RETINITUS PIGMENTOSA** - the progressive degeneration of the rods and cones of the retina. Common symptoms are night blindness and a narrow vision field. Take BILBERRY or GINKGO BILOBA extract capsules or liquid. Take CoQ$_{10}$ 60mg 4x daily (especially effective if the case is not severe); PCOs from grapeseed or white pine 100mg 3x daily, taurine 500mg daily, zinc picolinate 50mg daily. Omega-3 lipids such as flax or fish oils. Take vitamin E 400IU 2x daily if retinitis is hemorrhagic.

❦

❦ **RETINAL DETERIORATION** - occurs when the retinal epithelium, the thin layer of cells located behind the receptor cells does not function properly in providing nutrients to or removing wastes from the crucial light receptor cells. The photo-receptors die and vision loss is irreversible. GINKGO BILOBA and BILBERRY extracts and PCOs have proven effective.

❦

❦ **SHINGLES NEAR THE EYES (herpes zoster)** - high dose vitamin C crystals $^{1}/_{4}$ teasp. in water every hour until the stool turns soupy - about 8000-10,000mg daily; vitamin E 400IU with selenium 200mcg daily, Nature's Bounty vitamin B$_{12}$ sub-lingual. (See also HERPES page in this book.)

❦

❦ **STYES & EYE INFLAMMATION** - painful, pimple-like infections of the eyelids. Natural therapies work well when treatment is early. Origins stem from allergic, viral, herpes-type infections. In these cases, use buffered vitamin C eye drops (must be sterile solution), vitamin A, and zinc. If the cause is a bacterial infection, do not squeeze, use Crystal Star ANTI-BIO™ extract drops in water (may also be used to bathe the affected area); or bathe eyes in aloe vera juice, chamomile tea, raspberry leaf tea, eyebright tea, yellow dock tea or goldenseal root tea. Apply hot, strained calendula tea compresses. Mix one drop aged garlic extract in 4 drops distilled water and drop into infected eye. Take vitamin A and D capsules 25,000IU/400IU, and omega 3 flax oil. Take Crystal Star ANTI-FLAM™ or ANTI-BIO™ caps or extract to help reduce inflammation. Use Boiron *OPTIQUE* homeopathic eye irritation remedy. Alternating hot and cold compresses on the affected areas to relieve discomfort. Eye inflammation compress: 1 TB. eyebright herb, $^{1}/_{2}$ TB. powdered comfrey or parsley root, $^{1}/_{2}$ TB. powdered goldenseal root, 1 pint boiling water. Add herbs and steep for 30 minutes, covered. Apply to cotton balls and then to affected areas. May use hot and alternate with cold compresses to stimulate drainage of infection. Or simply use the white of an egg and spread it on a cloth or bandage; then apply to affected area.

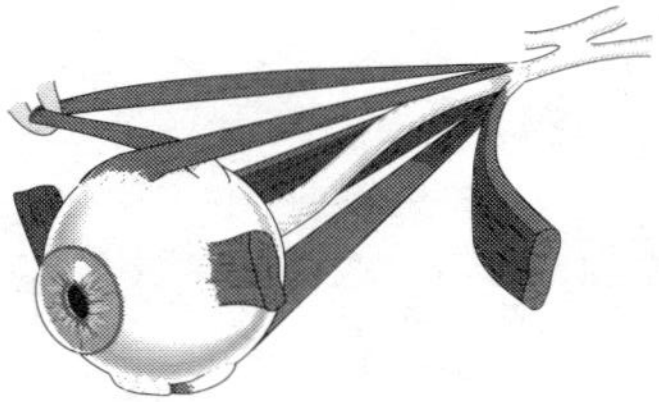

Fevers

Nature's Cleansers & Healers

A slight fever is often the body's own way of clearing up an infection or toxic overload quickly. Body temperature is naturally raised to literally "burn out" harmful poisons, to throw them off through heat and then through sweating. The heat from a fever can also de-activate virus replication, so unless a fever is exceptionally high (over 103° for kids and 102° for adults) or long lasting (more than two full days), it is sometimes a wise choice to let it run its natural course, even with children. Often they will get better faster.

Administer plenty of liquids during a fever - juices, water, broths. Bathe morning and night during a feverish illness. Infection and wastes from the illness are largely thrown off through the skin. If not regularly washed off, these substances just lay on the skin and become partially reabsorbed into the body. As there is usually substantial body odor during a cleansing fever as toxins are being eliminated, frequent baths and showers help you feel better, too. A cup of hot bayberry or elderflower tea, or cayenne and ginger capsules, will speed up the cleansing process by encouraging sweating and by stimulating circulation.

Watchwords for fevers and kids: It's probably ok unless: 1) you have an infant with a temperature over 100°; 2) the fever has not abated after three days, and is accompanied by vomiting, a cough and trouble breathing; 3) your child displays extreme lethargy and looks severely ill; 4) your child is making strange, twitching movements.
Remember: Fevers are a result of the problem and a part of the cure.

Diet & Superfood Therapy

❧ Stay on a liquid diet during a fever to maximize the cleansing process: bottled water, fruit juices, broths and herb teas.

❧ Carrot/beet/cucumber juice is a specific to clean the kidneys and help bring a fever down.

❧ Sip on lemon juice with honey all during the morning; grapefruit juice during the evening.
↬Add plenty of healthy liquids to the daily diet all during the illness.

❧ After a fever breaks, take hot tonic drinks (pg. 170).

❧ **Effective superfoods:**
↬Crystal Star SYSTEMS STRENGTH™.
↬Solgar WHEY TO GO - lactose-free with probiotics.

Herbal Therapy

Do not give aspirin to children to reduce a fever. Give herb teas instead, like peppermint or catnip.

❧ **Jump start herbal program:** Crystal Star ANTI-BIO™ caps or drops as an anti-infective.
↬Lobelia tincture drops in water every few hours and Crystal Star FIRST AID TEA FOR KIDS™.

❧ Use a fever to fight a cold or flu. Take Crystal Star FIRST AID CAPS™ until sweating occurs, usually within 24 hours.
↬Then, COLD SEASON DEFENSE™ to help rebuild immune strength.

❧ **Fever teas:**
↬Catnip/peppermint/ginger
↬Elderflower/sage
↬Boneset/white willow ♀
↬Yarrow ♀
↬Thyme
↬Fenugreek or sassafras tea with lemon and honey.

Supplements

✺ Vitamin A 10,000IU or beta carotene 25,000IU ♀♀ every 6 hours as an anti-infective.

✺ Vitamin C crystals ¼ teasp. every ½ hour in juice or water to bowel tolerance as an ascorbic acid flush.
↬Add garlic capsules 3x daily.

✺ Effective homeopathic remedies:
↬Bioforce *Fiebresan* drops
↬Natra-Bio *Fever* tincture
↬Hylands *Hylavir* flu or cold tablets
↬Homeopathic remedies for sudden fever onset: *Arsenicum album, Belladonna, Aconite.*

Lifestyle Support Therapy

☙ Take catnip enemas to cleanse the elimination channels.

☙ Use cool water sponges, or alcohol rub-downs to reduce a fever.
↬Apply peppermint tea cooling compresses to the head.

☙ Take ECHINACEA extract to encourage the lymph glands to throw off toxins.
↬Then sponge off with cool water, and follow with a brisk towel rub.

☙ Take a sauna to sweat toxins out.

Common Symptoms: Hot, dry, flushed skin; lethargy.
Common Causes: Bacterial or viral infection in the system that the body is trying to throw off; sometimes a sign of more serious problems, such as mononucleosis, Epstein-Barr virus, or diabetes.

See also INFECTIONS & INFLAMMATION page for more information.

Fibroids

Breast (Cystic Mastitis) ✦ Uterine (Myomas or Fibromas)

One out of 1500 American women between 35 and 49 have fibroid breast growths. Uterine fibroids are more common than blue eyes! Hormone imbalances, primarily too much estrogen and an under-active thyroid are the normal cause for both breast and uterine fibroids. Fibroids are not cancer, and have little chance of becoming cancerous before menopause. Natural therapies have been consistently successful in helping a woman avoid fibroid surgery. Care for your liver to prevent fibroids. The liver metabolizes and regulates body hormones (particularly estrogens).

Diet & Superfood Therapy

Painful breast swelling and excessive uterine bleeding have disappeared within a matter of weeks with the change to a low fat, vegetarian diet.

1. Follow a low fat, fresh foods vegetarian diet (50-60% fresh foods) to rebalance gland functions and relieve symptoms. High fats mean imbalanced estrogen levels - a clear cause of fibroids. Obesity from a high fat diet also increases risk.

➝Avoid caffeine and caffeine-containing foods, such as chocolate. Avoid cooked spinach, rhubarb and carbonated sodas.

➝Avoid hormone-laden red meats, hard alcohol and refined sugars that can cause iodine deficiency.

➝Avoid concentrated starches, full fat dairy products, and hard liquor. Avoid fried, sugary and salty foods, especially smoked or preserved meats during menses.

➝Get adequate high quality protein daily (about 60-70 grams) from largely vegetable sources to avoid saturated fats: whole grains, sprouts, tofu and soy foods, sea foods, low fat dairy and poultry, etc.

➝Increase intake of B vitamin-rich foods, such as brown rice, wheat germ and wheat germ oil (4 teasp. daily) and brewer's yeast.

➝Add miso, sea vegetables, and leafy greens to neutralize toxins. Eat diuretic foods -cucumber and watermelon to flush them out.

➝Have fresh apple or carrot juice every day during healing.

Herbal Therapy

Ϙ **Jump start herbal programs:**

For breast fibroids: Crystal Star WOMEN'S BALANCE FIBRO™ caps for 3 mos. with EVENING PRIMROSE oil and saw palmetto, 2-4 caps daily.

➝Then Crystal Star FEMALE HARMONY™ caps or VITEX extract 2x daily.

➝BITTERS & LEMON CLEANSE™ extract to help metabolize/regulate estrogens.

➝Crystal Star PRO-EST BALANCE™ roll-on directly to fibrous areas.

➝Use an echinacea/goldenseal formula to flush lymph glands.

For uterine fibroids: Crystal Star WOMAN'S BEST FRIEND™ 4-6 daily for 3 months, with EVENING PRIMROSE OIL caps 6 daily, and LIV-ALIVE™ caps, or MILK THISTLE SEED extract for liver function.

➝Beware of straight dong quai extract if you have uterine fibroids - it may increase bleeding. **Use centella asiatica instead.**

➝Crystal Star ANTI-SPZ™ caps, 4 at a time, or CRAMP BARK extract for pain.

➝**Consider: Crystal Star BLDR-K™ to prevent bladder problems: PRO-EST BALANCE™ roll-on for progesterone levels.**

Ϙ **Iodine therapy** is often effective in 3-4 months: J.R.E. IOSOL drops, or Crystal Star IODINE SOURCE™ extract, 2-3x daily. Take with vitamin E for best results.

➝Apply a comfrey leaf poultice to nodules.

Supplements

Homeopathic treatment of fibroids has been notably successful for fibroids.

❧ **Nutricology germanium** 150mg daily or CoQ_{10} 60mg 4-6x daily as healing anti-oxidants.

❧ **Vitamin E** 800IU daily with folic acid 800mcg daily during healing.
and/or

➝**High omega-3 oils, and/or shark cartilage as anti-infectives 3x daily.**

❧ **J.R.E. IOSOL drops as directed.**

❧ Ascorbate Vitamin C or Ester C powder with bioflavonoids 5000mg daily in divided doses.

❧ Matrix Health GENESIS OXY-SPRAY rubbed directly on the fibroids. Noticeable reduction in 3-6 weeks.

❧ Enzymatic Therapy RAW MAMMARY caps with MEGA-ZYME capsules.

❧ Alta Health SIL-X silica for collagen regrowth.
℞

❧ **Superfood supplements:**

➝Crystal Star ENERGY GREEN™ drink and SYSTEMS STRENGTH™ drink.
➝Klamath BLUE GREEN SUPREME drink with spirulina.

Lifestyle Support Therapy

The medical answer for fibroids is early detection, surgical biopsies and then removal. But, the tests are often inaccurate (15% false negatives and 30% false positives), and the attendant invasive medical procedures cause anxiety, pain and expense. We have found that there is a very real risk in receiving regular doses of radiation through mammograms, even low dose radiation. Breast tissue is so sensitive that the time between a mammogram and fibroid growth is sometimes as little as three months.

➝Do not take synthetic estrogen compounds of any kind. They keep fibroids growing even after menopause.

☙ Try to avoid mammograms and chest X-rays. (See above.) X-rays also contribute to iodine deficiency.

☙ Get some outdoor exercise every day for tissue oxygen.

➝No smoking. Avoid secondary smoke.

☙ **External poultices:** green clay and castor oil packs, applied directly.

☙ **Reflexology point:**

R & L breast points

uterus

Common Symptoms: Breast fibroids: moveable, rubbery nodules near the surface of the breasts, causing painful breast swelling, **Uterine fibroids:** benign growths (between the size of a walnut and an orange) that appear on the uterine walls cause excessive menstrual bleeding; back and abdominal pain, and bladder infections; painful intercourse; infertility or the inability to sustain pregnancy.
Common Causes: Too much caffeine and too much fat in the diet; EFA deficiency; hormone imbalance with an abnormal response to estrogen and progesterone and an underactive thyroid; obesity; genetic factors; high-dose birth control pills; X-rays. Benign growths usually cease after menopause; **new growths after menopause** may mean breast or uterine cancer.

Fibromyalgia
Immune-deficient Muscle Disease

Fibromyalgia is a debilitating, often painful muscle disease, involving neuro-hormonal imbalances and impaired deep sleep. Generally considered a stress-related immune disorder, many symptoms mimic those of Chronic Fatigue Syndrome (CFS) and arthritis. Researchers now estimate that up to ten million Americans (mostly mid-life women) suffer from fibromyalgia. Although labeled untreatable and incurable, it may be vastly helped by natural therapies. See also Chronic Fatigue Syndrome for more information.

Diet & Superfood Therapy

The HYPOGLYCEMIA diet in this book is a good place to start diet improvement.

❧ Go on a short 3 to 5 day cleansing and detoxification liquid diet (page 157).
➳A largely vegetarian diet can have very beneficial influence on blood toxins and fibrinogen that affects coagulation.
➳Make your diet rich in whole foods, low in processed foods, sugars, and saturated fats.
➳**Avoid red meats and caffeine.**
➳**Eliminate common food allergens.**

❧ Keep the diet at least 50% fresh foods during intensive healing time. Emphasize foods that build immunity. Include often:
➳oxygenating foods: wheat germ.
➳high mineral, B Complex foods: sea vegetables and brown rice.
➳high fiber foods: prunes and bran.
➳cultured foods: yogurt and miso.

❧ Superfoods are important:
➳Crystal Star CHO-LO FIBER TONE™ drink or GREEN TEA CLEANSER™ as on-going body cleansers.
➳Sun CHLORELLA packets or tabs.
➳Be Well juices.
➳**Klamath BLUE GREEN SUPREME.**
➳**Aloe Life ALOE GOLD drink.**
➳Solgar EARTH SOURCE GREENS & MORE.
➳**Y.S. ROYAL JELLY/GINSENG.**

Herbal Therapy

❧ Jump start herbal program:
Crystal Star PRO-EST BALANCE™ to address neurohormonal imbalance; **ADRN-ACTIVE™** capsules for adrenal deficiency.
➳**ANTI-FLAM™** capsules or extract to help with headaches and inflammation.
➳**AR-EASE™** caps as a joint rebuilder and collagen tonic; very relieving.
➳**GINKGO BILOBA** for circulation.
➳**RELAX CAPS™** for nerve support.
➳**NIGHT CAPS™** for REM sleep.
➳**MENTAL INNER ENERGY™** with kava kava and ginseng for energy.

❧ Drink 2 cups of burdock tea daily as a hormone balancer and blood cleanser for the musculo-skeletal system. Take with Crystal Star FEM SUPPORT™ extract and una da gato caps for best results.

❧ Effective herbal anti-depressants:
➳Gotu kola helps neurotransmission
➳**St. John's wort extract for REM sleep patterns.**
➳Enzymatic Therapy **KAVA-TONE.**

❧ Effective herbal pain management:
➳Black cohosh extract, an anti-inflam.
➳**PRN PAIN-FREE** gel with cayenne.
➳Rosemary tea to increase corculation.
➳Wood betony - a tonic for headaches.
➳Solaray **TURMERIC (curcumin) as a prime anti-inflammatory.**

Supplements

❧ **Antioxidants are a key:**
➳PCOs from grapeseed or white pine bark 100mg 3x daily.
➳Vitamin C up to 5000mg daily with extra bioflavonoids 500mg.
➳Vitamin E 400IU with selenium.
➳American Biologics SUB-ADRENE.
➳Solaray QBC, quercetin with bromelain to take down inflammation.
➳Beta-carotene 50,000IU 2 x daily.
➳**L-Carnitine 1000mg daily.**

❧ **NAG (glucosamine sulfate) - a cartilage nutrient - 500mg 6 daily.**

❧ **Magnesium/malic acid, or Ethical Nutrients MALIC/MAGNESIUM** to alleviate tender points and improve circulation.
➳Also effective, Enzymatic Therapy KREBS CYCLE CHELATES.

❧ **Melatonin .1-.3mg** at retiring to help normalize sleep patterns.

❧ Enzyme therapy:
➳Bromelain 1500mg daily.
➳Pancreatin 1300mg before meals.

Lifestyle Support Therapy

❧ Those with fibromyalgia are generally not physically fit. Build up a slow, low-impact aerobic exercise program - 20 minutes a day for body oxygen and muscle tone.
➳Add weight bearing exercise for 10 minutes a day to start.

❧ **Relaxation techniques are crucial:**
➳Choose from meditation, guided imagery, yoga, biofeedback, and progressive muscle relaxation - all of which have had success with fibromyalgia in developing a positive mind/body stance to work with the disease.
➳Regular, monthly massage therapy treatments have had notable success.

❧ Local, gentle heat applications are effective, **especially with a gentle massage.**

Common Symptoms: Painful, tender, recurrent points aching all over the body; persistent, diffuse musculo-skeletal pain; fatigue, weakness, headaches, confusion, migraine headaches, chronic diarrhea and irritable bowel, poor sleep patterns and nervous symptoms like depression, and hypoglycemia - symptoms of mild cortisol deficiency; stomach and digestive problems; shortness of breath with high uric acid. Other symptoms include cardiovascular problems, allergies, stiffness and anxiety.

Common Causes: Vitamin and mineral deficiencies. It is associated with mitral valve prolapse. Being overweight and a smoker compounds fibromyalgia.

Access the FIBROMYALGIA/ CHRONIC FATIGUE SYNDROME Network for more information. 1- (800) 853-2929.

Flu

Viral Respiratory Infection

Flu infections are longer-lasting and stronger than colds. Flu treatment programs work best in a series of stages. The ACUTE, or infective stage, includes aches, chills, prostration, fever, sore throat, etc., and usually lasts for 2 to 4 days. The RECUPERATION, or healing stage, replenishes the body's natural resistance. This phase should be followed for one to two weeks. The IMMUNE SUPPORT stage should be followed for two to three weeks, especially in high risk seasons. Recovery from flu is often slow, with a good deal of weakness.

Diet & Superfood Therapy

During the acute stage: take only liquid nutrients - plenty of hot, steamy chicken soup, hot tonics and broths to stimulate mucous release (pg. 170). Vegetable juices and green drinks (pg. 168) to rebuild the blood and immune system.
✻Have ginger/garlic broth every day.

During the recuperation stage: follow a vegetarian, light "green" diet.
✻Have a salad every day, cultured foods like yogurt and kefir for friendly flora replacement, and steamed vegetables with brown rice for strength.

For immune support and all stages:
✻Avoid refined foods, sugars, and pasteurized dairy foods; they increase mucous clogging and allow a place for the virus to live. Avoid alcohol and tobacco; they are immune suppressors.
✻Avoid caffeine foods; they inhibit iron and zinc absorption.

If you just can't seem to "get over it," make up 1 gallon of Crystal Star CLEANSING & FASTING™ tea, and take 5 to 6 cups daily with 12 - 15 FIBER & HERBS COLON CLEANSE™ capsules daily until the virus is removed.

Effective superfoods:
✻Crystal Star SYSTEMS STRENGTH™ drink to alkalize, return body vitality and rebuild healthy blood.
✻Wakunaga KYO-GREEN
✻Green Foods GREEN MAGMA

Herbal Therapy

Jump start herbal program:
During the acute stage: **Crystal Star ANTI-VI™ extract as needed several times daily, or ANTI-BIO™ extract or capsules every 2 hours until improvement is noticed.**
or
FIRST AID CAPS™ to raise body temperature and reduce virus multiplication, and CLEANSING & PURIFYING TEA™ or GREEN TEA CLEANSER™ sipped all during the day.

Effective anti-viral herbs:
✻ECHINACEA ANGUSTIFOLIA
✻USNEA EXTRACT, 🖐 or Crystal Star BIO-VI™ extract with propolis.
✻St. John's Wort
✻Lomatium
✻Osha root tea
✻SAMBUCOL - elderberry syrup
✻Scullcap root

Boneset tea to inhibit flu virus, relieve pain and induce sweating.

Effective recovery herbs:
✻Calendula tea 4 cups daily.
✻Astragalus capsules or extract
✻Cayenne/bayberry capsules - to normalize gland activity.
✻Wisdom of the Ancients SYMFRE tea.

Adaptogen immune strength herbs:
✻Sun CHLORELLA tabs or granules.

✻Ginseng Co. CYCLONE CIDER for achy, sore throat and increase circulation. ♂

Supplements

During acute stage: Ester C or ascorbic acid crystals: $1/4$ teasp. every half hour to bowel tolerance to flush the body and neutralize toxins.
and
✻Zinc lozenges to deactivate virus activity in the throat, or Nutribiotic GRAPEFRUIT SEED SKIN SPRAY.

Effective anti-infective/antioxidants:
✻Nutricology germanium 150mg.
✻Beta-carotene 100,000IU
✻Matrix Health H_2O_2 OXY-CAPS.
✻OPCs from white pine or grapeseed, 100mg 3x daily.

Effective immune support:
✻Raw thymus to build cell immunity, or Enzymatic Therapy THYMUPLEX.
✻Prof. Nutrition DR. DOPHILUS in papaya juice. 🖐
✻CoQ₁₀, 60mg 3x daily.
✻Pantothenic acid for adrenal support.

Homeopathic remedies against flu:
✻Boiron OSCILLOCOCCINUM
✻B&T Alpha CF
✻BioForce FLU RELIEF
✻Hylands remedies specific to individual symptoms of the flu. 🖐

Lifestyle Support Therapy

Flu shots can affect immune response. Beware.

☞ **During the acute stage:**
Sweating is effective at the first sign of infection. Heat de-activates viruses.
1) Take 1 cayenne cap and 1 ginger cap.
2) Take a hot bath with tea tree oil.
3) Go to bed for a long sleep, so the body can concentrate on healing.
✻During the next several days, take a hot sauna, spa, or bath to raise body temperature and increase circulation.

☞ Gargle with a few drops of tea tree oil or ginger root tea in water for sore throat; or use New Moon GINGER WONDER SYRUP. 🖐

☞ Take a catnip enema to cleanse out flu virus from the intestinal tract.

☞ To begin the immune support phase: Get a complete massage therapy treatment to cleanse remaining pockets of toxins, and clear body meridians. Plus it makes you feel so good again!

See COMMON COLD pages for diagnosis information. See COLDS & IMMUNITY pages in this book for extra help.

Foot Problems

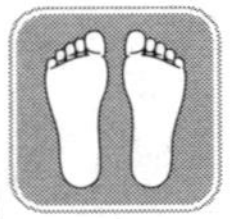

Bone Spurs ✤ Plantar Warts ✤ Callouses ✤ Corns ✤ Bunions

Bunions *- thickened layers of skin on the sides of the big toe.* ***Callouses*** *- thickening of the skin formed on the site of continual pressure - usually on the hands or feet.* ***Corns*** *- thickening of the skin, hard or soft, on the feet.* ***Plantar warts*** *- painful, sometimes ingrowing, warts on the sole of the foot.* ***Bone spurs*** *- a horny out growth, usually on the heel, often the result of acid/alkaline imbalance in the body. May accompany rheumatoid arthritis, because individuals with this disease are deficient in stomach acid and normal enzyme production.*

Diet & Superfood Therapy

Go on a 24 hour (pg. 158) vegetable juice liquid diet to clear out acid wastes. Then eat lots of fresh raw foods for a month.
- Have a green salad every day.
- **Drink black cherry juice daily.** Take a green drink or carrot/beet/cucumber juice every 3 days to flush the kidneys and rebalance the acid/alkalinity.

Avoid fats, fried foods, sugars and alcohol. Avoid red meats, caffeine, chocolate, sodas, and other oxalic acid-forming foods.
- Eat a low salt diet.
- Eat 2-3 apples a day.

Make sure your diet is rich in whole foods, vegetables and fiber, low in sugars, meat and saturated fats.
- Eliminate hard liquor and fried food.

Effective enzyme balancing foods:
- Miso soup, lecithin 2 tsp. daily, fresh vegetables, brewer's yeast, cranberry juice.

Effective superfoods:
- Crystal Star ENERGY GREEN™ drink.
- Sun CHLORELLA packets or tabs.
- **Kyolic KYO-GREEN.**
- **Aloe Life ALOE GOLD drink.**
- Solaray ALFA-JUICE.

Herbal Therapy

Jump start herbal program:
Crystal Star AR-EASE™ capsules to dissolve crystalline deposits, with BITTERS & LEMON CLEANSE™ extract each morning and ECHINACEA extract during the day.
- **Take ANTI-FLAM™ caps to take down inflammation.**

and

- **Flora VEGE-SIL, or apply Body Essentials SILICA GEL.** ♀

Effective topical herbal applications:
- Propolis tincture.
- Echinacea extract drops.
- BioForce ECHINACEA cream.
- **Tea tree oil 2-3x daily.**
- A weak golden seal root solution.
- Dandelion stem juice 3x daily. Let dry each time.
- A mixture of wintergreen oil, witch hazel, and black walnut extract.
- NatureWorks SWEDISH BITTERS.

Effective herbal poultices:
- Mix green clay and liquid chlorophyll.
- Flaxseed/garlic powder paste. ♂

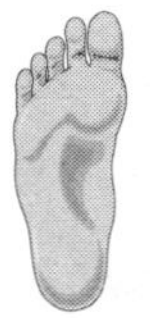

For heel pain (usually a thyroid-related problem): take EFAs from EVENING PRIMROSE oil, Crystal Star SILICA SOURCE™ and ANTI-FLAM™ caps, Omega-3 flax oil, or Nature's Secret ULTIMATE OIL w. vit. E.

Supplements

Enzymatic Therapy ACID-A-CAL. ♀
and/or
- **CHERRY FRUIT extract.** ♂

Country Life LIGA-TEND for at least 1 month, with Magnesium/Potassium/Bromelain capsules for enzymes. ♂

or

Betaine HCl, or Prevail VITASE with meals for proteolytic enzymes. ♀

and

Quercetin Plus w/ Bromelain to take down inflammation.

Effective topical applications:
- **Nutribiotic GRAPEFRUIT SEED SKIN SPRAY or ointment full strength, and take the capsules 2x daily.**
- **Mix vitamin C crystals with water to a paste. Apply and take vitamin C up to 5000mg daily with extra bioflavonoids 500mg.**
- Vitamin E 400IU daily. Apply E oil.

Cal/mag/zinc 4 daily with B Complex 100mg 4 daily.

Beta-carotene or oceanic carotene, 50,000IU 2 x daily.

Lifestyle Support Therapy

For best results, soak feet in warm water before using topical applications.

Crystal Star ALKALIZING ENZYME WRAP™ to rebalance body chemistry.

Effective foot soaks:
- Make a footbath with 2 handfuls of comfrey root to 1 gallon warm water. Soak feet 15 minutes daily.
- Epsom salts soak.

For corns, callouses, bunions:
- Biochemics PAIN RELEAF.
- Rub on green papaya skins. ♀
- Apply Body Essentials SILICA GEL directly or as a compress.
- Apply olive oil compresses to corns.
- Apply raw garlic poultices to bunions.
- Miracle of Aloe FOOT REPAIR.

For plantar warts and bone spurs:
- Soak feet in the hottest water you can stand for as long as you can.
- Matrix Health OXY-SPRAY directly on a wart or bone spur twice daily. Removal takes about 2 months.
- Apply DMSO for pain and to help dissolve crystalline deposits. ♂
- Home Health CASTOR OIL PACKS.
- Mix vitamin C crystals and water to a paste. Apply to spur, and secure with tape. Leave on all day for several weeks.

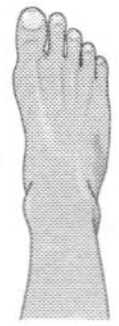

Common Symptoms: *Staph or strep type infection; pain and inflammation of nodules and growths on the feet.*
Common Causes: *Toxemia; kidney malfunction causing acid/alkaline imbalance; too many sweets, caffeine and saturated fats; excess sebaceous gland output causing poor skin elimination of wastes; poor calcium elimination. Low acid diet aggravating liver congestion and poor or irregular kidney function; insufficient stomach acid; constipation and toxemia from excess fats and refined carbohydrates; too little vegetable protein.*

See additional diet suggestions on ARTHRITIS AND GOUT pages in this book.

Frostbite

Chillblains ✣ Possibility Of Gangrene

If untreated, severe frostbite of the extremities can turn into a gangrenous condition, in which blood flow stops, and tissue becomes numb, oxygen-deprived and dies. If treated right away, this type of dry, non-infected gangrene, responds successfully to natural self-therapy. Wet gangrene is the result of an infected wound, which prevents drainage and deprives the affected tissues of cleansing blood supply and immune-stimulating oxygen. See an emergency clinic if you have wet gangrene.

Diet & Superfood Therapy

❧ For frostbite: paint on, but do not rub in, warm olive oil. Massage in for gangrene.

➥Or paint on honey to arrest infective bacteria development and stabilize the skin balance.

➥Give the person warm drinks or green drinks, but no alcohol. It constricts blood flow.

➥Eat a high protein diet for the two weeks after exposure, with plenty of whole grains to speed recovery.

❧ **Effective superfoods:**
➥Crystal Star ENERGY GREEN™ drink and capsules.
➥**Nature's Life PRO GREENS 96.**
➥Beehive Botanicals ROYAL JELLY/ GINSENG and bee pollen drink.
➥Sun CHLORELLA tabs 20 daily.
➥FutureBiotics ViTAL K 3 teasp daily.

Herbal Therapy

❧ **Jump start herbal program:**
Crystal Star GREEN TEA CLEANSER™ or HEARTSEASE/CIRCU-CLEANSE™ tea.
➥GINKGO BILOBA extract.
➥FIRST AID CAPS™, or Ginseng Co. CYCLONE CIDER to help raise body temperature. ♂

❧ Effective herbal compresses mixed with olive oil:
➥Marshmallow root
➥Slippery elm
➥Comfrey/plantain
➥**Ginger/cayenne powder**

❧ Effective extracts:
➥**BLACK WALNUT HULLS** as an anti-microbial
➥Myrrh gum as an anti-infective
➥Witch hazel as an anti-septic

❧ **Circulation stimulants:**
➥Butcher's broom extract - apply locally mixed in water and take internally (temporarily only).
➥Crystal Star HEARTS-EASE/HAW-THORN™ caps 4 daily, with sage tea 2 cups daily.

❧ Apply AloeLife ALOE SKIN GEL often to affected areas - several times daily.

Supplements

✐ Bach Flowers **RESCUE REMEDY every 5 minutes under the tongue as needed for shock.**

✐ Vitamin C powder with bioflavs. and rutin, 1/4 teasp. every half hour for 6 days for collagen and tissue rebuilding.

✐ Vitamin E 400IU. Take internally and prick a capsule - apply oil to affected areas.

✐ Matrix GENESIS OXY-SPRAY or Centipede KITTY'S OXY-GEL. Rub on affected area several times daily until healing begins.

✐ **Effective anti-oxidants:**
➥CoQ$_{10}$, 60mg 3x daily.
➥PCOs from grapeseed or pine, 100mg 3x daily.
➥Nutricology GERMANIUM for wound healing, 150mg for 2 months.

✐ Enzymatic Therapy ORAL NUTRIENT CHELATES. Then follow with a full-spectrum multi-vitamin complex for 1 month to help redevelop tissue.

Lifestyle Support Therapy

☞ Get the person to a heated room immediately.
➥Gently stroke the kidneys toward the middle of the back.
➥Cover warmly, so frostbitten areas will warm up gradually.
➥If case is severe, wrap in gauze so blisters don't break. Elevate legs. Do not rub blisters.
➥Use alternating warm and cool hydrotherapy to stimulate circulation. No hot water bottles, hair dryers, or heating pads. Slow warming is the key.
➥If case is very severe, immerse areas in warm water and massage very gently under water for 5-10 minutes.

☞ Apply Body Essentials SILICA GEL.
➥CAPSICIN creme
➥or calendula/comfrey salve.

☞ **Effective applied oils:**
➥Cajeput oil
➥Mullein oil
➥**Olive oil**
➥Tea tree oil, which sloughs off old and infected tissue, and leaves healthy tissue intact.
➥Biochemics PAIN RELEAF.

See also SHOCK THERAPY *page for more information.*

Common Symptoms: *Frostbite is the freezing of cold-exposed extremities, and its effects of redness, swelling, blistering, numbness, etc. Circulation slows, causing skin to become hard, blue-white and numb. Dry gangrene symptoms include dull, aching pain and coldness in the area. Pain and skin pallor are early signs of dry gangrene. As the flesh dies, pain can be intense; once it is dead, the flesh becomes numb and turns dark.*
Common Causes: *Prolonged exposure of the feet and hands to severe cold; poor circulation; arteriosclerosis; an infected wound; a diabetic condition.*

Fungal Skin Infections
Athlete's Foot ✣ Ringworm ✣ Impetigo

Fungal infections are characterized by moist, weepy, red patches on the body. Though opportunities for risk seem to be everywhere, fungal infections do not take hold when there is healthy immune response. Stimulating and rebuilding immunity is the key to controlling recurring infections. Athlete's foot (ringworm of the feet) and other fungal infections thrive in dampness and warmth. Make sure that any concurrently occurring fungal infections (such as athlete's foot and "jock itch") are treated simultaneously, so that infection is not continually passed from one area to another.

Diet & Superfood Therapy

Maintaining healthy bowel flora is crucial to overcoming fungal conditions.

♌ Avoid foods such as red meats, cola drinks, caffeine, sugary foods and fried foods as prime culprits for fungal imbalance conditions.

♌ Diet watchwords:
✽Eat plenty of cultured foods like yogurt, tofu and kefir to keep the body alkaline and nutrients fully absorbed.
✽Add lots of fresh fruits and vegetables to the diet during healing.
✽Keep dietary protein high for fastest healing: from sea foods and sea vegetables, sprouts, eggs, soy foods, poultry and vegetables.
✽Drink 6-8 glasses of water daily to keep elimination system free and flowing.

♌ Foods to avoid:
✽Eliminate pasteurized dairy products.
Keep the diet low in sugary carbohydrates and carbos from pasta, whole grains and nuts. (Vegetable carbohydrates are fine).
✽Omit red meats, fried and fatty foods during healing.

♌ Effective superfoods:
✽Apply AloeLife SKIN GEL; drink aloe vera juice daily.
✽Balance your intestinal structure with Solgar WHEY TO GO protein drink.

Herbal Therapy

Note: Griseofulvin™ tabs for toenail fungus can affect liver function.

✍ Jump start herbal program:
Apply Crystal Star FUNGEX™ gel or ANTI-BIO™ gel with una da gato.
✽Apply tea tree oil as needed.

✍ Take EVENING PRIMROSE OIL caps 4 daily for 2 weeks for fungal peeling; apply **Miracle of Aloe FOOT REPAIR for athlete's foot fungus;**
and take
✽Garlic extract or **turmeric extract capsules** daily to destroy fungal bacteria.

✍ **Topical herbals for skin funguses:**
✽Open a capsule of Crystal Star antifungal WHITES OUT #2™. Make a solution with water. Dab twice daily onto affected areas; or open a WHITES OUT™ #2 capsule and apply directly to toes.
✽Apply lomatium extract to area, or Crystal Star ANTI-VI™ extract.♂
✽**Make an anti-fungal footbath with tea tree oil, marshmallow root and black walnut hulls extract. Soak feet for 20 minutes daily.**♀

✍ For ringworm:
✽Basil tea skin wash.
✽Myrrh extract - internally and applied.♀
✽*Thuja* - externally and internally for both thrush and ringworm.☺

Supplements

Avoid drug overuse, particularly long courses of antibiotics and cortisones.

✍ Apply Nutribiotic GRAPEFRUIT SEED SKIN SPRAY to any fungal condition.

✍ Stimulating immune response is the key to preventing recurring infection:
✽**Beta carotene 50,000IU**♂
✽Zinc 50mg 2x daily.♀
✽Lysine 1000mg daily.

✍ Effective anti-fungals:
✽Amer. Biologics DIOXYCHLOR liquid.
✽Matrix Health GENESIS OXY-SPRAY
✽Solaray CAPRYL caps♀
✽American Biologics SHARKILAGE

✍ Effective enzyme therapy:
✽Schiff ENZYMALL
✽Alta Health CANGEST
✽Acidophilus caps before meals.
Nature's Plus JR. DOPHILUS ☺
Natren TRINITY
Prof. Nutrition Dr. DOPHILUS
✽Dissolve acidophilus in water and apply to area directly.

✍ Crush or open and mix together in a bowl: B₂ 500mg, niacin 1000mg, pantothenic acid 500mg. Add 2 tsp. sesame oil and 2 tsp. brewer's yeast. Apply at night. Put on a sock to cover - leave on overnight.

Lifestyle Support Therapy

Get early morning sunlight on the body every day possible for healing vitamin D.

♋ For athlete's foot and toenail fungus:
✽Keep feet well aired and dry. Keep shoes well-aired and change socks daily. Go barefoot as much as possible where appropriate. Expose feet to natural sunlight every day to inhibit fungal growth.
✽Dab cider vinegar between toes daily.
✽Apply opened garlic capsules between the toes every morning and night.
✽Apply a honey/garlic poultice to area.
✽Apply tea tree oil; use tea tree oil soap.
✽Apply baking soda daily and soak your feet in warm epsom salts water for 10 minutes; dry carefully; then apply witch hazel freely before you go to bed.

♋ For ringworm and impetigo:
✽Take garlic oil capsules 6 daily. Apply a garlic poultice and cover for 3 days.
✽Apply Matrix Genesis OXY SPRAY.
✽Pat on cider vinegar, or garlic vinegar, or rub papaya skins to affected areas.
✽Apply a goldenseal/myrrh solution.
✽Take Epsom salts baths for 20 minutes.

♋ For thrush: rinse mouth with a dilute tea tree oil solution for thrush. Keep bathroom cups/toothbrushes clean to prevent re-infection. Soak toothbrush in grapefruit seed extract solution.☺

Common Symptoms: Patchy, itching skin infection; area will be dry, scaly, cracked, bleeding and tender, with bacterial odor. Or, moist, weepy skin patches that do not dry out, such as ringworm, foot and toenail fungus, a non-healing cut, mouth or nail infections; excessive belching from gas; unexplained allergies; persistent headaches; acne; diaper rash in babies.
Common Causes: Broad spectrum antibiotic and prescription drug use that kills friendly digestive flora and lowers immune defenses; synthetic steroid use; birth control pills; poor hygiene. For athlete's foot or toenail fungus, tight or non-porous shoes, so that perspiration cannot evaporate; infection from fungus micro-organisms; yeast overgrowth.

Gallbladder Disease
Gallstones ❖ Cholecystitis

The gallbladder helps digest fats through production of bile. About 20 million Americans have gallstones, which are formed from bile components (cholesterol, bile pigments and salts) that do not dissolve and crystallize as stones. As the stones enlarge, the gallbladder becomes inflamed, causing severe pain that feels like a heart attack, and in some cases can be life threatening if left untreated. Stones can also block the bile passage, causing pain and digestive incapacity. High risk factors include poor diet with high cholesterol and low bile acids, obesity, certain drugs, age, and the presence of Crohn's disease. More men than women suffer from gallbladder problems, especially cholecystitis, (acute gallbladder inflammation). Gallstones are far easier to prevent than to reverse.

Diet & Superfood Therapy

The primary factor in both prevention and control is diet improvement, especially the elimination of red meats and fatty foods. A vegetarian, high fiber diet is the best protection.

☙ **Go on a short juice and gallbladder flush fast for 3 days. (See next page). In the acute pain stage, all food should be avoided. Only pure water should be taken until pain subsides.**

☙ After your gallbladder flush, take a glass of cider vinegar and honey in water each morning for prevention and oxygen uptake.
  ✷One TB. lecithin grains before each meal.
  ✷One TB. brewer's yeast and 1 TB. olive oil daily.

  ✷Avoid all dairy products except cultured dairy, such as yogurt. Add artichokes, pears and apples to the diet.

  ✷Eat small meals more frequently. No large meals. Drink 6 glasses of water daily for bile maintenance. ❧

☙ **Effective superfoods:** Note: A predisposing factor for gallstones is excessive sugar consumption. Do not take highly sweetened protein powder drinks.
  ✷**Crystal Star CHO-LO FIBER TONE™ morning and evening.**
  ✷AloeLife FIBER MATE powder.

Herbal Therapy

Increasing bile solubility is the goal.

☙ **Jump start herbal program:
Herbal cholagogues to effect bile flow:**
  ✷**NatureWorks SWEDISH BITTERS** —Crystal Star BITTERS & LEMON CLEANSE™ extract to help dissolve bile solids.
  ✷**ALOE VERA JUICE with HERBS daily, with MILK THISTLE SEED extract drops added to each glass.**

☙ **Crystal Star STN-EX™ capsules with lemon juice and water or LIV-ALIVE™ tea.**

☙ Turmeric extract (curcumin) 2x daily as an anti-inflammatory.

☙ **For gallstones:**
  ✷Chamomile or gravel root tea, 5-7 cups daily for a month to dissolve stones.
  ✷Peppermint tea
  ✷Solaray ALFAJUICE caps.
  ✷Gynemna sylvestre capsules before meals to reduce dietary sugar which helps form stones.

☙ Apply cold milk compresses to the abdomen area.

☙ Effective gallbladder teas:
  ✷Wild yam root ♀
  ✷Catnip
  ✷Dandelion leaf and root ♂

Supplements

☙ **Lipotropics are a key:**
  ✷Choline/Inositol 2 daily with Vit. E 400IU and Biotin 600mcg.♀
  ✷High Omega-3 flax seed oil 3x daily.
  ✷Vitamin A 25,000IU & D 1000IU.
  ✷Methionine before meals.
  ✷Solaray LIPOTROPIC 1000.
  ✷Phosphatidyl choline 500mg.

☙ Taurine 1000mg. daily to increase bile formation.

☙ **Enzyme therapy:**
  ✷Full-spectrum digestive enzymes with meals to stimulate bile, such as Alta Health CANGEST, Rainbow Light ADVANCED ENZYME SYSTEM or Prevail DIGEST.
  ✷Two acidophilus complex caps before meals, and 1 HCL tablet after meals.

☙ Ascorbate vitamin C or Ester C 550mg with bioflavonoids 6 daily. ♂

☙ **For sugar balance:**
  ✷Glycine caps for sugar regulation, with taurine to keep bile thinned.
  ✷Chromium picolinate 200mcg.
  ✷Spirulina caps in between meals with vitamin B complex 100mg to help stabilize blood sugar.

Lifestyle Support Therapy

☙ Take coffee, garlic or catnip enemas every 3 days until relief.

☙ Take olive oil flushes for 2-3 weeks until stones pass. (See next page.)
  ✷Apply castor packs to the abdomen.

☙ A sedentary lifestyle is a major high risk factor. Get mild regular exercise and reduce body fat to keep the system free and flowing.

☙ Acupuncture and acupressure have been successful for gallbladder disease.

☙ **Reflexology point:** right foot only

liver & gallbladder

☙ Gallbladder area:

Common Symptoms: Recurrent abdominal pain bloating and gas; intense pain in the upper right abdomen during an attack, sometimes accompanied by fever and nausea if there are gallstones; belching, pain, and bloating after a heavy meal; headache and bad temper; sluggishness, nervousness.
Common Causes: Too many fatty and fried foods, and lack of ability to digest them; chronic indigestion and gas from too much dairy and refined sugars; food allergies (eliminate the offending food to stop attacks); parasite infections can lead to calcium composition stones; high cholesterol sediment (coagulated serum fats that do not pass); birth control pills; lack of regular exercise.

See also Liver Healing pages for more information.

Therapeutic Gallstone Flushes & Healing Diets

Gallbladder cleansing flushes have been very effective in passing and dissolving gallstones. Depending on the size of the stones and the length of time they have been forming, the flushing programs may last from 3 days to a month. Have a sonogram before embarking on a flush to determine the size of the stones. If they are too large to pass through the bile and urethral ducts, they must be dissolved first, using the STN-EX™ herbal program for 1 month, or other surgical methods must be used. Note: If olive oil is hard for you to take straight, sip it through a straw. See previous page and COOKING FOR HEALTHY HEALING by Linda Rector Page for a complete diet program to prevent gallstones.

NINE DAY GALLSTONE FAST & FLUSH. This program has often been successful in passing gallstones without surgery. After stones have been passed, the next diet phase should concentrate on healing the liver/gallbladder area, and preventing further stone formation.

1) Repeat this mild 3 DAY OLIVE OIL & LEMON LIQUID DIET below for 3 days:

On rising: take 2 TBS. olive oil and the juice of 1 lemon in water;
Breakfast: take a glass of carrot/beet/cucumber juice; or a potassium juice or broth. (pg. 167)
Mid-morning: have 1 to 2 cups of chamomile tea.
Lunch: take another glass of lemon juice in water with 2 TBS. olive oil; and a glass of black cherry juice, carrot juice or organic apple juice.
Mid-afternoon: have 1 to 2 cups of chamomile tea.
Dinner: have another glass of organic apple, carrot or black cherry juice.
Before bed: take another cup of chamomile tea.

2) Follow with a FIVE DAY ALKALIZING DIET. Drink 6-8 glasses of bottled water each day:

On rising: take 2 TBS. cider vinegar in water with 1 teasp. honey; or 2 TBS. lemon juice in water, or a glass of fresh grapefruit juice.
Breakfast: take glass of carrot/beet/cucumber juice, or a potassium broth or juice.
Mid-morning: have 1 to 2 cups of chamomile tea, and a glass of organic apple juice.
Lunch: take a green drink like Green Foods GREEN MAGMA, or Crystal Star ENERGY GREEN™ and a fresh green salad with lemon/oil dressing. Have a cup of dandelion tea after lunch.
Mid-afternoon: have 1 to 2 cups of chamomile tea, and another glass of grapefruit juice or apple juice.
Dinner: have a small green salad with lemon/oil dressing; or some steamed veggies with brown rice or millet; and another glass of organic apple juice.
Before bed: have another cup of chamomile or dandelion tea.

3) Finish with a ONE DAY INTENSIVE OLIVE OIL FLUSH:

Starting around 7 P.M. on the evening of the 5th day of the alkalizing diet: make a mix of 1 pint of pure olive oil and 9-10 juiced lemons; take ¼ cup of this mix every 15 minutes until it is gone, (about 3-4 hours). Lie on the right side for better assimilation if desired.

✂

FOUR DAY INTENSIVE OLIVE OIL FLUSH. Take 6-8 glasses of bottled water throughout each day:

1) Repeat the stronger cleansing diet below for 4 days

On rising, and every 2 hours throughout the day for three days: take a glass of apple or pear juice. Take a coffee, catnip or garlic enema each day.
Before bed on the 3rd day: take ½ cup olive oil mixed with ½ cup lemon juice. Sip slowly. Sleep on your right side with a hip pillow to concentrate the remedy in the gallbladder area.
On the morning of the 4th day: take a garlic enema. The stones will often pass during the day.

2) Follow with a TWO DAY ALKALIZING DIET: To rebalance the system and build a preventive environment against gallstones. Repeat for 2 days. Drink 6-8 glasses of bottled water each day.

On rising: take 2 TBS. cider vinegar or lemon juice in water, or a glass of fresh grapefruit juice.
Breakfast: take a potassium juice or essence (pg. 167).
Mid-morning: take a cup of chamomile tea and a glass of pear or apple juice.
Lunch: have a green drink (pg. 168) or Sun CHLORELLA or Green Foods GREEN MAGMA granules in water; and a small fresh green salad with lemon/oil dressing.
Midafternoon: take a cup of dandelion root tea, and a glass of apple, pear or black cherry juice.
Dinner: have a small green salad, and some steamed vegetables with brown rice or millet and a glass of apple juice.
Before bed: have a cup of chamomile or dandelion tea.

✂

Gastric Diseases

Chronic Gastritis ❖ Gastroenteritis ❖ Gastric Ulcers

Gastric diseases refer to ulcerative disorders of the upper gastro-intestinal tract. Stomach acids and some enzymes can damage the lining of the G.I. tract if natural protective factors are not functioning normally. Current medical treatment for these problems focuses on reducing stomach acidity - a symptom - rather than addressing the long term cause of the problem. Many of these treatments are extensive, with definite side effects, and a tendency to alter the normal structure of the digestive tract walls. The alternative approach focuses on rebuilding the integrity of the stomach lining and normalizing G.I. tract pH and function.

Diet & Superfood Therapy

❧ Emphasis should be on alkalizing foods. Include plenty of soluble fiber foods, whole grains, brown rice, fresh fruits and vegetables, etc. Eat cultured foods for friendly G.I. flora. Have a green salad daily.

❧ **Juices for stomach acid balance:**
  ❀Carrot
  ❀Carrot/cabbage, a stomach healer
  ❀Pineapple/papaya
  ❀Have a glass of non-carbonated mineral water every evening.

❧ Avoid alcohol, except a little wine at dinner. Eliminate caffeine, tobacco, aspirin and all fried foods.
  ❀Avoid dairy products, except cultured foods; they contribute to stomach acidity.
  ❀Eat small meals more frequently. No large meals. Chew everything well.
  ☿

❧ **Effective superfoods:**
  ❀**Crystal Star SYSTEMS STRENGTH™**
  ❀**Solgar WHEY TO GO protein drink.**
  ❀**Lewis Labs BREWER'S YEAST.**
  ❀**Crystal Star ENERGY GREEN™.**
  ❀**AloeLife ALOE GOLD JUICE.**
  ❀**Green Foods BETA CARROT.**
  ❀YS royal jelly 3-4 teasp. daily.
  ❀New Moon GINGER WONDER or GINSENG GINGER syrup.

Herbal Therapy

❧ **Jump start herbal program:**
  Crystal Star BITTERS & LEMON™ extract to balance gastrointestinal region; RELAX CAPS™ for nerve stress as needed, MINERAL SPECTRUM™ caps 4 daily.
  ❀**Holistic PROPOLIS LOZENGES.**
  ❀**GINKGO BILOBA extract 2-3x daily.**
  ❀**PAU D'ARCO/GINSENG extract.**
  ❀Una da Gato capsules or tea.

❧ **Herbal anti-inflammatories:**
  ❀Chamomile
  ❀Turmeric (curcumin)
  ❀**Ginger to tone intestinal walls.**

❧ **Herbal wound healers:**
  ❀Calendula tea
  ❀**Aloe vera juice**
  ❀Goldenseal/myrrh extract 3x daily

❧ **Herbal astringents to lessen bleeding:**
  ❀Red raspberry tea
  ❀Plantain tea
  ❀**Turmeric capsules** ♂

❧ **Gastric soothing teas:**
  ❀Pau d'arco/**Peppermint tea**
  ❀Marshmallow
  ❀Slippery elm
  ❀**Hops/Valerian/Scullcap tea to relax esophagus.** ♀
  ❀Celandine extract tablets in water

Supplements

Tagamet and Zantac, drugs prescribed regularly (one billion dollars in sales yearly) for ulcers and other gastric problems, can be addictive. They also inhibit bone formation and proper liver function. DGL normalizes these functions after drugs.

❧ **Enzyme therapy and natural digestive aids:**
  ❀Prevail ACID-EASE tablets
  ❀HCL for stomach acid
  ❀Activated charcoal to release gas
  ❀Liquid chlorophyll 1 tsp. before meals
  ❀**Enzymatic Therapy BROMELAIN before meals,** ♂ **or DGL after meals.** ♀
  ❀Pancreatin for fat digestion
  ❀Raw pancreas for enzymes
  ❀Schiff ENZYMALL with ox bile

❧ **Probiotics rebalance digestion:**
  ❀**Prof. Nutrition DR. DOPHILUS complex before meals.** ♂
  ❀Natren TRINITY powder in water.

❧ Magnesium to soothe membranes, or Country Life magnesium/potassium/bromelain capsules 2 before meals. ♂

❧ **Oral Gamma Oryzonal 300mg daily.**

❧ Jarrow BIOSIL, 6 drops in warm water, or Flora VEGE-SIL caps. ♀

Lifestyle Support Therapy

Avoid cortico-steroid drugs. They often result in ulcers. Antacids offer minor symptomatic, or no relief. Excess use of aspirin increases gastric problem risk.

☞ Relaxation techniques like biofeedback are successful for many gastric problems.
  ❀Take a "constitutional" walk after meals. Don't eat when upset, angry or anxious.

☞ **Acupressure points:**
  Pull middle toe on each foot for 1 minute.

☞ **Reflexology point:**

diaphragm,
solar plexus
stomach

☞ Upper gastro-intestinal region:

Common Symptoms: Chronic poor digestion, with sharp abdominal and chest pains; heartburn and tenderness; nausea and acid bile reflux in the throat; asthma-like symptoms, often irritable bowel symptoms; hoarseness and chronic cough.

Common Causes: Poor diet with too many fried, fatty foods, sugars, and refined foods; poor food combining, and drinking with meals; overeating - esp. excessively spiced foods: eating too fast, too much and too often; acidosis; intestinal parasites; food allergies or candida yeast overgrowth; too much caffeine and alcohol; steroid use; stress.

See also HIATAL HERNIA, DIVERTICULITIS, COLITIS AND CROHN'S DISEASE pages for more

Glandular Health
Deep Body Balance

Glands are organs that secrete fluids. There are two types of glands in the body - exocrine (glands regulated by the hypothalamus, that secrete their fluids through ducts, like the salivary and mammary glands; and endocrine (glands that emit their secretions directly as hormones into the bloodstream). Because they work at such a deep body level, our endocrine glands are involved with almost every body function. The health of the endocrine system interacts directly with our foundation genetics, determining genetic potential. Proper gland function gives us a basis for living life to the fullest.

Diet & Superfood Therapy

❧ For best results in a gland balance program, start with a 24 hr. detox diet - watermelon only - to rapidly flush and cleanse.

☛Then eat a high vegetable protein diet for at least a month: whole grains, brown rice, nuts, seeds and sprouts.

☛Include "good gland foods:" sea foods and sea veggies, fresh figs and raisins, pumpkin and sesame seeds, green leafy vegetables, broccoli, avocados, yams, and dark fruits.

☛Drink 6 glasses of bottled water daily. The glands are affected first by dehydration. **Avoid red meats, caffeine, preserved and all refined foods.**

❧ Make a mix of brewer's yeast, wheat germ, and sesame seeds, take 2 TBS. daily in juice or on a salad:
🜛

❧ Superfoods: *Glands need greens!*
☛Crystal Star ENERGY GREEN™
☛Solgar EARTH SOURCE GREENS & MORE
☛Nutricology PRO GREENS w. flax
☛Crystal Star SYSTEMS STRENGTH™
☛AloeLife ALOE GOLD JUICE.
•YS royal jelly w. ginseng 4 teasp. daily

Herbal Therapy

Herbs work through the glands, at the deepest levels of the body processes. The complex, holistic nature of herbal activity make them ideal support for endocrine health.

❧ **Jump start herbal program:**
Crystal Star MINERAL SPECTRUM™ caps twice daily.
☛FEEL GREAT™ caps or tea with ADRN™ extract for gland homeostasis.
☛HEAVY METAL CLEANSE™ capsules if you are regularly exposed to toxic pollutants. The glands are very sensitive to pollutants.

❧ **Pre-digested raw glandulars:**
Solaray MALE CAPS with raw orchic and PROSTATE CAPS with raw prostate.
☛Enzymatic Therapy glandulars are highly recommended, especially THYMUPLEX, PARA-CAL, NUCLEO-PRO M, and PRO-50 prostate tissue for men, and NUCLEO-PRO F and RAW MAMMARY for women.

❧ Sea vegetables are gland nourishers:
☛Kelp tabs 6 daily
☛2 TBS. mixed sea veggies sprinkled on a soup or salad.

❧ Gland energizers:
☛Siberian ginserg ♂
☛Mullein ♀

❧ Gland oxygenating teas:
☛Yellow dock/sage tea ♂
☛Burdock tea ♀
☛Barberry tea

❧ High potency YS ROYAL JELLY 2 teasp. ♂♀
☛Y.S. ROYAL JELLY/GINSENG daily. ♀

Supplements

Raw glandular extracts offer biochemical nutritional support for stress and fatigue affecting glands. They can improve gland health dramatically by delivering cell-specific and gland specific factors.

❧ B Complex 100mg with extra pantothenic acid 500mg, and digestive enzymes like Rainbow Light DOUBLE-STRENGTH ALL-ZYME.

❧ **Effective mineral complexes:**
☛Mezotrace SEA MINERAL COMPLEX tabs 2-4 daily.
☛Future Biotics VITAL K LIQUID.

❧ J.R.E. IOSOL drops, with Vitamin E 400IU 2 daily for iodine therapy. ♀

Lifestyle Support Therapy

❧ Avoid air and environmental pollutants as much as possible. Your glands are the first to feel their damaging effects.

❧ Take a regular 20 minute "gland health" walk every day.

❧ **Acupressure points:** stroke the top of the foot on both feet for 5 minutes each to stimulate endocrine and hormone secretions.

❧ **Reflexology points:**

all gland health

☛Thump the thymus point briskly each morning 6 times to stimulate immune response.

Common Symptoms: *Poor assimilation of nutrients; adrenal and pancreas exhaustion; constant tiredness; hypoglycemia.*
Common Causes: *Mineral deficiency; stress; hypothyroidism; environmental pollutants; too much sugar, alcohol, caffeine, tobacco and drugs.*

See COOKING FOR HEALTHY HEALING by Linda Rector Page, for gland and organ target diets. See following page for information on specific glands.

Recommendations For Maintaining The Health Of Specific Glands

❧ **ADRENALS** - the adrenals lie just atop the kidneys, and are composed of two distinct parts - the adrenal medulla and the adrenal cortex. The medulla secretes the hormones epinephrine (adrenaline) and norepinephrin in the "fight or flight" response. These hormones also maintain involuntary functions like heart rate, breathing and digestion. The adrenal cortex secretes corticosteroid hormones, formed from cholesterol. Corticosteroids perform functions from the metabolism of glucose, suppression of allergies, to mineral retention, and sex hormones, including DHEA, thought to have anti-aging effects, as well as therapeutic benefits for diabetes, obesity and asthma. An herbal formula to stimulate some of these corticosteroid hormone effects might include **licorice root, wild yam root, panax ginseng, bupleurum, Siberian ginseng and turmeric.** See page 220 for a complete discussion of adrenal health.

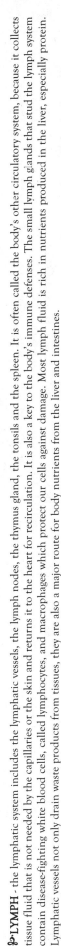

❧ **LYMPH** - the lymphatic system includes the lymphatic vessels, the lymph nodes, the thymus gland, the tonsils and the spleen. It is often called the body's other circulatory system, because it collects tissue fluid that is not needed by the capillaries or the skin and returns it to the heart for recirculation. It is also a key to the body's immune defenses. The small lymph glands that stud the lymph system contain disease-fighting white blood cells, called lymphocytes, and macrophages which protect our cells against damage. Most lymph fluid is rich in nutrients produced in the liver, especially protein. Lymphatic vessels not only drain waste products from tissues, they are also a major route for body nutrients from the liver and intestines.

To revitalize the lymph system with diet: Take a glass of lemon juice and water regularly in the morning, and a glass of papaya juice in the evening. Include plenty of potassium-rich foods regularly, such as sea vegetables, broccoli, bananas and seafood. Avoid caffeine, sugar and alcohol during healing.

To stimulate lymph flow: 1) activate muscles with regular exercise and stretching. Start every exercise period with deep, diaphragmatic breathing. 2) elevate feet and legs for 5 minutes every day, massaging lymph node areas. 3) take a hot and cold hydrotherapy treatment at the end of your daily shower. Mini-trampoline exercise clears clogged lymph nodes. Both acupuncture and acupressure have been successful. Eliminate aluminum cookware, food additives, and alum-containing foods and deodorants.

Herbal recommendations : Crystal Star ANTI-BIO™ caps or extract for white blood cell formation, REISHI/GINSENG™ extract to enhance immune health. A good lymph tea blend might include white sage, astragalus, echinacea root, oregon grape root and dandelion root.

Supplement recommendations: Enzymatic Therapy LYMPHO-CLEAR, Lane Labs BENE-FIN shark cartilage for leukocyte production, EVENING PRIMROSE OIL caps, and Flora VEGE-SIL.

❧ **PANCREAS** - the pancreas is located just behind the stomach. It functions as both an exocrine and an endocrine gland, secreting hormones directly into the bloodstream as well as digestive enzymes into the small intestine to activate the body's enzyme processes. Its hormone, glucogon, controls blood sugar levels and digestive enzymes. Today, pancreas glandular therapy is used for digestive disorders, and as an antimicrobial and anti-inflammatory. Alcoholism, excessive use of prescription drugs and poor nutrition can mean pancreatitis, a painful condition related to gallbladder problems, that can become critical. Sugary foods should be avoided if you have a weak pancreas. Nutrients to help maintain pancreatic health include chromium picolinate 200mcg daily, phosphatidyl choline to aid in fat digestion, and pancreatin, a digestive enzyme.

❧ **OVARIES** - the ovaries on either side of the pelvic cavity, produce the female eggs for reproduction, and two hormones, estrogen and progesterone, responsible for maintaining secondary sexual characteristics, and preparing the uterus and breasts for the reproductive cycle. *See Hormone Health & Balance pages for more.*

❧ **PITUITARY** - the pituitary is called the master gland, regulating all glandular activity. The major symptoms of pituitary deficiency involve the nervous system, mental processes (especially mental burn-out brought on by stress), healing, blood sugar levels and body fluid balance. The **Pineal Gland** lies just under the pituitary gland, behind the eyes, is highly responsive to light waves; it is the body's light meter. Many health problems result from our modern day indoor lifestyle, in which we receive distorted light waves from sunglasses, eyeglasses, window glass, fluorescent lights and contact lenses. Both pineal and pituitary benefit from 20 minutes a day in early morning sunlight. The pineal helps balance the endocrine system, regulating our body rhythms, sleep patterns, fertility and the development of consciousness.

Dietary recommendations: include plenty of green leafy vegetables. Have a veggie drink (pg. 168) or Future Biotics VITAL K drink, or Crystal Star ENERGY GREEN™ drink once a week. Eat complex carbohydrates like broccoli, potatoes, sprouts, peas, dried fruits, whole grains and brown rice. Take fresh fruit juices each morning. Drink 6 glasses of bottled water daily. Avoid beer, sweet wines, refined foods, sugar, heavy pastries, and canned foods. Avoid all MSG-containing foods and preserved foods.

Supplement recommendations : include a multi-mineral complex, vitamin C or Ester C with bioflavonoids and rutin, Nature's Bounty B$_{12}$ internasal gel every other day, Glutamine 500mg 4x daily for growth hormone, B Complex 100mg daily, with extra B$_6$ 250mg and PABA 1000mg daily, Flora VEGESIL caps and Enzymatic Therapy RAW PITUITARY caps.

Herbal recommendations for pituitary/pineal health: Crystal Star GINSENG 6 SUPER™ TEA or GINSENG/LICORICE ELIXIR™ twice daily; IODINE/POTASSIUM™ caps, or Solaray ALFA-JUICE caps; Beehive Botanicals royal jelly and honey drink mix daily and gotu kola/damiana caps. Sea vegetables of all kinds work synergistically with the pituitary in glandular formulas.

Acupressure points: press for 10 seconds, 3x each, over the left eyebrow for pituitary stimulation; on the forehead where the eyebrows meet for pineal stimulation.

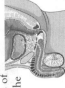

PROSTATE - the prostate is a large male gland that lies just below the neck of the bladder, and around the top of the urinary tract. The primary function of the prostate is to help the semen move through the urethra during ejaculation. It also produces an alkaline fluid which carries the sperm from the testes into the vagina. This fluid greatly enhances the chances of fertilization because it balances the acid environment of the uterus for the sperm. The prostate enlarges during sexual arousal. If there is prolonged arousal without ejaculation, the pressure from the prostate on the testicles becomes very uncomfortable. *See BENIGN PROSTATIC HYPERPLASIA on page 390 for more information.*

SPLEEN - the spleen is the largest mass of lymphatic tissue in the body. It produces lymphocytes, destroys worn-out blood cells, and serves as a blood reservoir. During times of great stress or hemorrhage, the spleen can release its stored blood to prevent shock. Depletion symptoms include anemia, pallor, extreme slimness, poor memory and sluggishness.

Dietary recommendations for spleen health: Take a carrot/beet/cucumber juice every day for 1 week, then every other day for another week to "spring clean" these glands of stored toxins. Then, build up red blood cells with a potassium broth (pg. 167, a veggie drink (pg. 168), Green Foods GREEN ESSENCE drink, or Crystal Star ENERGY GREEN™ drink, and a leafy green salad every day. Include brown rice and alfalfa sprouts frequently.

Herbal recommendations for spleen health: Crystal Star HEARTSEASE/ANEMI-GIZE™ caps with HAWTHORN extract for blood building and tone, GINSENG 6 SUPER™ tea or red root tea for continued enhancement. Spleen enhancing tea: 4-oz. hawthorn, 1-oz. cardamom, 1-oz. safflowers, 1-oz. lemon balm, 1-oz. red sage; take 2 cups daily.

Supplement recommendations for spleen health: include: Enzymatic Therapy LIQUID LIVER w. GINSENG, LYMPH/SPLEEN COMPLEX, or GOLDEN SPLEEN 500, Vitamin E 400IU daily for red blood enhancement, marine carotene 50-100,000IU daily, liquid chlorophyll 3 teasp. daily with meals, zinc picolinate 30mg daily and Natren TRINITY, $^1/_2$ teasp. in water 2x daily.

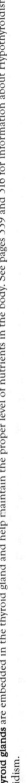

TESTES - the male gonads, are located in the scrotum. The testicles are the workhorses of the male reproductive system, producing the sperm and the male hormone testosterone. Testosterone causes the development of male secondary characteristics - face and body hair (and the male pattern receding hairline), body odor, voice change, enhanced muscles, male sexual organs and the increased oiliness and coarseness of a man's skin (a factor that means men's skin ages about ten years behind the skin of women). Testosterone also establishes the male sex drive, but has nothing to do with male erection. Some men do experience a decrease in testosterone production as they age, especially if his diet and lifestyle are not conducive to healthy gland function. The symptoms of this endocrine imbalance are similar to a woman's menopause and are called andropause.

THYMUS - the thymus lies between the thyroid gland and the heart. Known as the "master gland" of the immune system, the thymus gland is vital to the production of T-lymphocyte cells and thymic hormones, vital to cell-mediated immunity. The thymus is easily damaged by oxidation and free-radicals. Therapeutic uses of thymus glandulars include help against chronic infections, food allergies, auto-immune disorders and cancer therapy.

Anti-oxidants are critical to thymus health: vitamin E with selenium and beta-carotene can help protect the thymus. Zinc, vitamin B$_6$ and vitamin C help produce thymic hormones. Enzymatic Therapy THYMUPLEX capsules,

Herbal recommendations for thymus health: Echinacea and echinacea/goldenseal/myrrh combinations are prime herbals for increasing the activity of white blood cells and stimulating the production of interferon. Panax ginseng is also an effective adaptogen. Crystal Star GINSENG/LICORICE ELIXIR™ acts synergistically for the thymus.

THYROID - the thyroid gland folds around the front and sides of the windpipe at the base of the neck. It is responsible for metabolism which provides vital energy resources for every body activity. It secretes the high iodine hormone thyroxin. The two most common thyroid disorders are hypothyroidism, where the thyroid is not producing enough thyroxin (a problem that is increasing in our heavily polluted, nutrient-poor environment), and hyperthyroidism, caused by the secretion of too much thyroxin (as in Grave's Disease). Signs of an underactive thyroid include depression, unusual fatigue, hair loss (especially in women), obesity, breast fibroids and poor immune response. Iodine and potassium rich sea vegetables and herbs are some of the best nutrients to take for thyroid health.

The **parathyroid glands** are embedded in the thyroid gland and help maintain the proper level of nutrients in the body. See pages 339 and 316 for information about Hypothyroidism and Hyperthyroidism.

See RAW GLANDULARS, page 86 in this book for more information on supplementing the glands. See HORMONE HEALTH & BALANCE pages for more on glands and hormones.

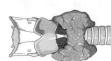

Glaucoma
Eyeball Fluid Pressure & Hardening

While glaucoma affects over 2 million people in America, it is often undetected. Chronic glaucoma, frequently asymptomatic in the early stages, is characterized by a build up of pressure in the eyeball. If the pressure is not relieved, the eyeball may harden, harm the retina and damage the optic nerve. Collagen, as the most abundant and necessary protein in the eye, is responsible for eye tissue strength and integrity. Improved collagen metabolism by the body can be a key to the relief of pressure on the eye. Glaucoma is also often the result of, and accompanied by, liver malfunction.

Diet & Superfood Therapy

Avoid food and environmental allergens.

✿ Go on a fresh foods diet for 2 weeks to clear the system of inorganic crystalline deposits. Take one of the following every day during these 2 weeks:
　✿Carrot/beet/cucumber/parsley juice
　✿Fresh carrot juice
　✿Potassium broth (pg. 167)

✿ Avoid all refined sugars, caffeine and foods containing caffeine.

✿ **Vitamin A-rich foods for eyes:** endive and leafy greens, carrots, sea foods and sea vegetables, broccoli.

✿ **Vitamin C sources for eyes:** Citrus juice, green peppers, cucumbers, carrot juice, beets. ☿

✿ **Effective superfoods: the eyes require a great deal of nourishment.**
　✿**Klamath BLUE GREEN SUPREME.**
　✿**Crystal Star ENERGY GREEN™ and BIOFLAV, FIBER & C SUPPORT™.**
　✿**Solgar EARTH SOURCE GREENS & MORE drink.**
　✿**Beehive Botanical ROYAL JELLY with Siberian ginseng 2 teasp. daily.**
　✿**AloeLife ALOE GOLD JUICE 2x daily, also dilute and use as an eyewash.**

Herbal Therapy

The liver must be cleansed for there to be real advancement against the problem.

✿ **Jump start herbal program:** Crystal Star EYEBRIGHT COMPLEX™ capsules 4 daily to strengthen eyes, with RELAX CAPS™ to ease tension.
　✿GINKGO BILOBA extract or cayenne capsules to normalize circulation to the optical system.
　✿IODINE/POTASSIUM SOURCE™ caps for iodine imbalance. ☿
　✿Crystal Star BITTERS & LEMON CLEANSE™ as a liver cleanser.

✿ **Effective eye washes:**
　✿Crystal Star EYEBRIGHT™ tea
　✿Weak goldenseal solution
　✿Ayurvedic coleus forskohlii
　✿Chamomile tea
　✿Fennel seed compresses.

✿ Effective herbal "greens:" spirulina tabs 6 daily; Solaray ALFAJUICE capsules.

✿ For formation of collagen and tissue integrity:
　✿BILBERRY extract
　✿**Solaray VIZION caps with bilberry**
　✿Gotu kola/ginseng ☿♀

Supplements

↪ **Vitamin C therapy is critical to reduce intracellular pressure:**
　✿**Ascorbate Vit. C with bioflavonoids and rutin, 10,000mg. or more daily. Take 1/4 teasp. at a time in water every hour as an ascorbic acid flush.**
　and
　✿**Bathe eyes daily with a weak ascorbate C/bioflavonoid solution in water.**
　and
　✿**Quercetin with bromelain 6 daily.**

↪ Lane Labs BENE-FIN shark cartilage.

↪ Nutricology OCUDYNE II with lutein.

↪ OPCs from grapeseed or white pine, 100mg 3x daily;
　✿**with Glutathione 50mg 2x daily.** ♂

↪ Enzymatic Therapy ORAL NUTRIENT CHELATES to help relieve pressure and crystallized particles in eye arteries. ♀

↪ Beta carotene 150,000IU daily.

↪ Nature's Life I-SIGHT 2x daily.

↪ **Vitamin E 400IU daily to help remove lens particles.** ♂
　✿add magnesium 800mg daily. ♀

Lifestyle Support Therapy

✿ Relax more. Strive for a less stressful lifestyle.
　✿Stop smoking. It constricts eye blood vessels and increases pressure.

✿ Get a good spinal chiropractic adjustment or massage therapy treatment.

✿ Avoid cortico-steroid drugs, tranquilizers, epinephrine-like or atropine drugs, aspirin and over-the-counter antihistamines. These drugs tend to inhibit or destroy collagen structures in the eye.

✿ Reflexology point: Important in breaking up crystalline deposits:

eyes

✿ Eyeball and interior:

Common Symptoms: Colored halos around lights; eye inflammation with reddened eyes; great eye area pain and headaches; tunnel vision - loss of peripheral vision; blurred vision; inability to tear; fixed and dilated pupils. Acute closed-angle glaucoma is extremely serious, an eye emergency with severe, throbbing eye pain, and loss of vision if pressure is not relieved within 36 hours.
Common Causes: Chronic glaucoma is more prevalent than acute glaucoma. Overuse of steroid and other drugs - see list above; diabetes; food allergies; poor collagen metabolism; too much dietary caffeine and sugar; prolonged emotional stress; allergies; adrenal exhaustion; liver malfunction; watching TV too long in the dark; thyroid imbalance; arteriosclerosis.

See LIVER CLEANSING AND EYESIGHT pages for more information.

Gout

Arthritis Of The Toe & Peripheral Joints

Gout is a common type of arthritis, suffered primarily (90%) by overweight, middle-aged males. It occurs when there is too much uric acid in the blood, tissues and urine. Joints, tendons and kidneys are normal gout sites. The natural healing approach is simple and successful. Improving gout involves diet change to eliminate high purine foods and heavy alcohol that causes sedimentary precipitates. It reduces dietary fat for weight loss and cholesterol reduction. It advocates cleansing of the kidneys to normalize uric acid levels in the blood and tissues.

Diet & Superfood Therapy

Gout is clearly caused by dietary factors. Lowering fats, meat proteins, and white flour grains are the diet key.

♦ Go on a bladder/kidney liquid cleansing diet (pg. 161) to rid the body of acid wastes.

—Follow with a diet of 75% fresh foods for a month to balance uric acid formation.

—Drink 4 glasses of black cherry juice and 6 glasses of water daily to flush and neutralize uric acid. Eat plenty of dark fruits.

—Eat high potassium foods: fresh cherries, bananas, strawberries, celery, broccoli, potatoes, and greens to put acid crystals in solution so they can be eliminated.

—Avoid high purine foods, including red meats, rich gravies, broths and bouillon, sweetbreads, organ meats, mushrooms, asparagus, dry peas, cooked spinach and rhubarb, sardines, anchovies, crab.

—Eliminate alcohol during healing; it inhibits uric acid secretion from the kidneys.

—Avoid high levels of fructose in any food or drink. Reduce caffeine, fried foods, and all saturated fats.

♦ **Effective superfoods:**

—Potassium broth (page 167), or **Crystal Star ENERGY GREEN™ drink.**

—Crystal Star SYSTEMS STRENGTH™ for iodine and potassium therapy.

—Nutricology PRO-GREENS with flax.

—**Aloe vera juice each morning.**

Herbal Therapy

Herbal support can take down inflammation and enrich body flavonoids.

♦ **Jump start herbal program: Crystal Star AR EASE™ or ANTI-FLAM™ capsules, with ADRN™ extract 2x daily.** ○

—**Herbal diuretics are effective in reducing swelling without potassium loss: BLDR-K COMFORT™ caps or BLDR-K™ tea.**

♦ Hypothyroidism is usually involved in gout. Take sea vegetables or Crystal Star IODINE/POTASSIUM caps to normalize thyroid activity.

♦ Many herbs are rich in anthocyanosides and flavonoids - a key to overcoming gout.

—HAWTHORN extract 4x daily
—BILBERRY extract 4x daily
—**Crystal Star BIOFLAV, FIBER & C SUPPORT™ drink daily.**
—**PCOs from grapeseed and white pine bark, 100mg 3x daily.**

♦ Solaray ALFAJUICE tabs, and Enzymatic Therapy CHERRY JUICE extract.

♦ Buchu tea to help dissolve and flush inorganic crystal sediment.

♦ BioForce *DEVILS CLAW* extract to reduce uric acid and cholesterol levels.

Supplements

✒ **Quercetin 1000mg with bromelain 1500mg 3x daily until relief to reduce inflammation. (For both acute and preventive benefits.)**

✒ Ascorbate vitamin C powder with bioflavonoids and rutin, ¼ teasp. every 4 hours daily for a month.

✒ **Enzymatic Therapy ACID-A-CAL capsules as needed; ORAL NUTRIENT CHELATES to help dissolve heavy metal, inorganic calcium and cholesterol build-up.**

✒ **Nutricology GERMANIUM 150mg to reduce pain and swelling.**

✒ **B Complex 100mg with extra B₆ 250mg and folic acid 800mcg 3x daily.**

✒ Biotech CELL-GUARD with SOD, 6 daily.

✒ Future Biotics VITAL K 3 teasp. daily for potassium, with vitamin E 400IU and niacin 500mg. to increase circulation.

✒ Glycine 500mg daily. with chromium picolinate 200mcg to regulate sugar levels.

Lifestyle Support Therapy

❧ Weight reduction is a key factor to ease pressure on feet and legs. But lose it slowly. Rapid weight loss shocks your metabolism and can trigger a gout attack.

❧ Apply plantain, ginger, or fresh comfrey compresses to inflamed area.

❧ Check your high blood pressure medicine. Several of them cause formation of inorganic crystal sediments.
*Avoid aspirin. It can raise uric acid levels.

❧ Use Crystal Star ALKALIZING ENZYME HERBAL BODY WRAP™ to neutralize acids and balance body pH right away.

❧ Apply topical DMSO with aloe vera to painful area to help dissolve crystalline deposits.

See ARTHRITIS pages in this book for more information

Common Symptoms: Extremely painful joints in the foot and big toe; tenderness, redness, swelling - sometimes chills and fever; gradual joint destruction with longer and longer attacks.
Common Causes: Tiny, needle-like crystals of uric acid in blood and body fluids caused by overeating, too much red meat, refined food, alcohol, sugar, caffeine, etc. that an over-loaded kidney does not excrete properly; overuse of drugs, such as thiazide diuretics causing potassium deficiency; lead toxicity; obesity; hypoglycemia.

Grave's Disease
Hyperthyroidism

Grave's disease is an auto-immune disease involving thyroid imbalance (increased thyroid secretion), and characterized by an overactive metabolism. Every body process seems to speed up - digestion, nervous energy, impatience, perspiration, the onset of tiredness (but the inability to rest adequately), hair loss, unhealthy weight loss, rapid heartbeat, climate sensitivity, even aging. Grave's disease affects women far more than men. Overactive thyroid conditions respond well to diet improvement and herbal supplements. Many drugs for these conditions have dangerous side effects.

Diet & Superfood Therapy

❧ For the first month of healing, follow a diet of about 75% fresh foods. Include plenty of vegetable proteins from sprouts, sea vegetables, soy foods and whole grains.

➥Add B vitamins and complex carbohydrates from brown rice and vegetables for stabilizing energy.

➥Have a potassium or green drink frequently (pg. 167, 168) and see below.

➥Eat plenty of cultured foods for friendly G.I. flora.

➥Make a mix of brewer's yeast, wheat germ, lecithin; take 2 TBS. daily.

➥Drink 8 glasses of water daily, and carrot juice 3x a week; take papaya juice for adrenal support. Avoid stimulant foods such as caffeine and carbonated drinks.

❧ Thyroid-balancing foods include: raw cruciferous vegetables, like cabbage, cauliflower, broccoli, kale and brussels sprouts, beets, and spinach. **(Cooking inactivates much of the thyroid lowering ability.)**

❧ **Effective superfoods:**
➥Crystal Star SYSTEMS STRENGTH™ drink for absorbable iodine and potassium
➥Nutri-Tech ALL 1 vit./mineral drink
➥Crystal Star ENERGY GREEN™
➥Nature's Life SUPER-PRO 96 drink
➥Beehive Botanicals ginseng/royal jelly
➥Future Biotic VITAL K, 2 teasp. daily

Herbal Therapy

☙ **Jump start herbal program:**
Crystal Star HEAVY METAL™ caps with bugleweed to reduce the thyroid hormone T4, and IODINE/POTASSIUM™ capsules 2-4 daily as thyroid balancers,
with
➥**LIV-ALIVE™ tea or MILK THISTLE SEED extract for 2 months for liver support.**

and

➥EVENING PRIMROSE OIL or borage oil caps 500mg 4 to 6 daily. ♀

☙ **Herbal thyroid balancers:**
➥GINKGO BILOBA extract
➥ECHINACEA extract
➥Mullein/lobelia
➥**HAWTHORN leaf, berry and flower**
➥Astragalus capsules 4 daily.

Supplements

✔ Enzymatic Therapy THYROID/TYROSINE COMPLEX 4 daily.
➥Rainbow Light MASTER NUTRIENT SYSTEM food-source multiple daily.

✔ **Immune enhancers:**
➥**CoQ$_{10}$, 60 mg 3x daily.**
➥Marine carotene, such as Solgar OCEANIC CAROTENE 100,000IU daily.
➥Ester C with bioflavs. 550mg 6 daily.
➥Zinc picolinate 50-75mg daily.

✔ Enzymatic Therapy LIQUID LIVER with Siberian ginseng, or Siberian ginseng extract capsules 2000mg.

✔ Stress B Complex with extra B$_2$ 100mg, and B$_6$ 100mg. ♀

✔ **American Biologics SUB-ADRENE.**

✔ **Rainbow Light ADAPTOGEM caps.**

✔ Twin Lab LIQUID K, 2 teasp. daily.

✔ **To calm thyroid storms:**
➥Calcium citrate 4 daily
➥Lecithin 1900gr daily
➥Vitamin E 800IU daily

Lifestyle Support Therapy

❧ Exercise daily to the point of breathlessness and mild sweating.

❧ Get some early morning sun on the body every day possible. Wade and swim in the ocean frequently to access naturally-occurring thyroid minerals.

❧ Acupressure points: press points on both sides of the spinal column at the base of the neck, 3 times for 10 seconds each.

❧ **Reflexology point:**

thyroid/thymus

❧ Eliminate over-the-counter diet pills. Their ingredients can both bring on and aggravate a thyroid imbalance problem.

thyroid region

LARYNX
PARATHYROID
GLAND
THYROID GLAND
CAROTID ARTERY
TRACHEA

See also GLAND HEALTH *page in this book for more information.*

Common Symptoms: *Bulging eyes and blurred vision; fatigue; restlessness and irritability; insomnia; nervous tension; sweating and tremors; unhealthy weight loss; systolic hypertension, mood swings, and sometimes mental psychosis during a "thyroid storm."*

Common Causes: *Autoimmune traits are thought to be partially caused by inheritance; stress; overuse of diet pills; mental burnout and fatigue; zinc deficiency; anorexia syndrome.*

Gum Disease

Periodontal Disease ✴ Pyorrhea ✴ Gingivitis

Periodontal (literally surrounding the teeth) disease is a progressive disorder affecting not only the gums but the bone structure around the teeth. Almost half the U.S. population over 35 years of age has some form of periodontal disease. But gum problems can occur at any age. Today, many children show signs of gingivitis. Gum disease is an outward sign of an internal imbalance of body chemistry. In most cases, holistic therapies are successful alternatives to surgery, involving body chemistry change through diet improvement, supplements and irrigation techniques.

Diet & Superfood Therapy

Alert: New findings are showing that risk of gum and mouth cancers are related to highly fluoridated water.

♉ Avoid acid-forming foods, such as tomatoes, sugars, refined foods, colas and carbonated drinks.

➼Eat raw, crunchy, fiber foods to stimulate the gums; apples, celery, Grape Nuts cereal, seeds, whole, chewy grains. Have a green salad every day.

➼Eat high vitamin C foods, such as broccoli, green peppers, papaya, cantaloupe, and citrus fruits.

➼ Eat vitamin A and carotene-rich foods, such as dark green leafy vegetables, yellow and orange vegetables and fruits, fish and sea vegetables.

➼Avoid caffeine.

➼Rub gums with halved fresh strawberries, baking soda, honey, or lemon juice.

➼Eat cultured foods for friendly digestive bacteria.

➼Chew your food thoroughly. ✍

♉ **Superfoods are very important:**
➼Crystal Star BIOFLAV, FIBER & C SUPPORT™ drink (no sugars).
➼Sun Chlorella drink - 1 pkt. daily.
➼AloeLife ALOE GOLD drink.

Herbal Therapy

♌ **Jump start herbal program:**
➼Open up a Crystal Star ANTI-BIO™ capsule or use ANTI-BIO™ extract, and rub directly on gums to counter infection.
➼Crystal Star ANTI-FLAM™ caps for gingivitis and abscesses.
➼GINKGO BILOBA extract for gum disease.
➼**Gotu Kola extract for gum healing.**
➼MINERAL SPECTRUM™ capsules to strengthen gums (takes about 3 weeks).
➼EVENING PRIMROSE OIL caps as an effective EFA source, 4 daily.

♌ **Effective herbal applications to stop bleeding and counter infection:**
➼Goldenseal/myrrh powder - make into a poultice and place directly on gums.
➼**Tea tree oil; an anti-infective** ☺
➼Witch hazel
➼LICORICE ROOT extract ♂
➼Cayenne extract to relieve pain
➼Calendula extract
➼Aloe vera juice/myrrh
➼St. John's wort dilute tea solution to promote healing.
➼Chlorophyll liquid 3 teasp. daily before meals. Also make into a solution with water and apply directly to gums daily.

♌ Siberian ginseng or ECHINACEA extract drops 2-3x daily. ♂

Supplements

♋ **Ascorbate vitamin C powder with rutin and bioflavonoids, 5000mg daily.** Also make into a solution with water. Rub directly onto gums, and take 1 teasp. daily.
➼**Quercetin with bromelain for inflammation, with Lysine 500mg 2x daily.**
➼CoQ$_{10}$ 60mg. 2x daily for almost immediate relief. Continue for prevention.

♋ American Biologics DIOXYCHLOR gel. Rub directly on gums.
➼**Body Essentials SILICA GEL 1 TB. in 3 oz. water 3x daily.** Also rub directly on gums as an anti-inflammatory.

or

➼**Vitamin E caps 400IU.** Take internally; prick caps to rub oil directly on gums.
➼Or vitamin A & E emulsion, 25000IU 4x daily.

♋ Quantum GUM THERAPY, or Enzymatic Therapy ORA BASICS with WILLOCIN caps for pain.

♋ **Effective homeopathic remedies:**
➼Arsenicum Album
➼Ferrum Phos.
➼Hypericum

♋ Nature's Life LIQUID CALCIUM PHOS. FREE with vitamin D. ♀ or Cal/Mag/Zinc to reduce alveolar bone loss. ♂

Lifestyle Support Therapy

Don't smoke - smoking sabotages gum health.

ॐ Chew propolis lozenges. Use propolis toothpaste. Rub on propolis tincture.
➼Folic acid solution mouthwash.♀♂
➼Beehive Botanical toothpaste, or Thursday Plantation TEA TREE toothpaste for gum disease.

ॐ Effective gum massages to control pain and soothe inflammation:
➼**Clove oil - dilute**
➼Eucalyptus oil - dilute
➼Lobelia extract

ॐ **Put 4-5 drops tea tree oil, or Nutribiotic GRAPEFRUIT SEED extract or Rainbow Light HERBA-DENT extract in a water pik and use daily for recurring gum infections.**

ॐ **Daily watchwords for gum health:**
➼Brush teeth well twice a day.
➼Floss well once a day.
➼Eat sugarless, low fat snacks.
➼Rinse your mouth immediately after eating. Rinse with a salt water solution whenever you feel the first signs of gum infection.

ॐ **Reflexology point:**

teeth & gums

Common Symptoms: red, swollen, tender gums that bleed when you brush, chronic bad breath that no amount of mouthwash will help, loose or shifting teeth, pus between the teeth and gums, receding gums that leave the root surface of teeth exposed, the loss of even cavity-free teeth; changes in the bite; hot and cold sensitivity in the mouth.

Common Causes: plaque formation on the gums that hardens into tartar, forming deep pockets between gums and teeth roots leading to loosened teeth and eventual bone damage; nutritional deficiencies, especially vitamins A, C, D and calcium; allergies; lack of fresh foods; too much red meat, refined foods, sugar, alcohol and soft drinks; poor tooth brushing; diabetes.

See also the HYPOGLYCEMIA DIET in this book, or COOKING FOR HEALTHY HEALING by Linda Rector-Page.

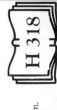

Hair Growth

Healthy Hair ❦ Graying Hair

Healthy hair is a mirror of both good nutrition and common-sense, daily care. Natural hair care products are being enthusiastically rediscovered all over America. Hair consists of protein layers called keratin. In healthy hair, the cell walls of the hair cuticle lie flat like shingles, leaving hair soft and shiny. In damaged or dry hair, the cuticle shingles are broken and create gaps that make hair porous and dull. Hair problems are never isolated conditions. They are the result of more basic body imbalances. In fact, changes in hair are often the first indication of nutritional deficiencies.

Diet & Superfood Therapy
Nutrition is the real secret to healthy hair.

❧ Feed your hair a high vegetable protein diet. Make a mix of the following hair foods and take 3 TBS. daily: wheat germ (oil or flakes), blackstrap molasses, brewer's yeast and sesame seeds.

❧ **Healthy hair foods:**
⁂Carrots, green peppers, lettuces, bananas, strawberries, apples, peas, onions, green peppers, cucumbers and sprouts, green tea. Have aloe vera juice in the morning.

⁂Avoid saturated fats, sugars and processed, refined foods.

⁂**Poor liver function is often the cause of unhealthy hair. Too much alcohol, caffeine and drugs put a heavy load on the liver and rob the body of B vitamins.**

❧ Kitchen cosmetics for hair: Wet hair, blot, and apply 4 TBS. mayonnaise. Wrap in a towel for 30 minutes. Rinse/shampoo.
⁂Mix yogurt and an egg. Apply to hair. Wrap in a towel for 30 minutes. Rinse and shampoo.

❧ **Effective superfoods:**
⁂**Crystal Star SYSTEMS STRENGTH™.**
⁂A low fat protein drink every morning can have a dramatic effect on dry hair texture: Nappi THE PERFECT MEAL, or Solgar WHEY TO GO.

Herbal Therapy
Minerals are critical to hair health. Herbs are good, absorbable sources.

❧ **Jump start herbal program:**
Natural silica is a source of hair strength: **Crystal Star SILICA SOURCE™ extract daily**; Alta Health SIL-X, or Flora VEGE-SIL capsules.
⁂**HEALTHY HAIR & NAILS™ tea as a rinse and shine.**
⁂**ADR-ACTIVE™ caps and ADRN™** extract to prevent graying.
⁂Rosemary sprigs steeped in wine for enhanced uptake of minerals.
⁂**Sea vegetables are excellent for hair health: IODINE/POTASSIUM SOURCE™ 2 capsules, or 6 kelp tablets daily.**
⁂**EFAs are imperative to hair health: EVENING PRIMROSE oil capsules 6 daily.**

❧ **Herbal hair enhancers to blend through hair and scalp:**
⁂Camocare concentrate for dazzle.♀♂
⁂Jojoba oil for sebum deposits.♀♂

❧ **Herbal hair nourishers:**
⁂Strength: horsetail, oatstraw
⁂Scalp irritation: chamomile, comfrey
⁂Hair body: sage, calendula ♀♂
⁂Luster: nettles, rosemary
⁂Dry hair: burdock, nettles
⁂Oily hair: witch hazel, lemon balm
⁂Graying hair: fo-ti root

Supplements

❧ **For color/growth, take together daily:**
⁂**PABA 1000mg, molasses 2 TBS, pantothenic acid 1000mg, folic acid 800mg.**

❧ **B Complex 100mg daily with extra B₆ 100mg and folic acid 800mcg.** with extra
⁂**Nature's Bounty B₁₂ internasal gel every 3 days. New hair starts in about 3 weeks; especially effective after illness or radiation treatments.**

❧ **Amino acid therapy:**
⁂Cysteine 500mg 2 daily, vitamin C with bioflavonoids 6 daily.
⁂Tyrosine 500mg 2x daily.

❧ Mezotrace SEA MINERAL COMPLEX 3 daily with boron 3 mg for mineral uptake.

❧ Homeopathic *Silicea.*

❧ **Biotin 600mcg daily with choline/inositol capsules.**♂

❧ **Effective shampoos:**
⁂Home Health olive oil and aloe vera
⁂Jojoba for damaged, brittle and over-processed hair.♂
⁂Shampoo with wheat germ oil.♀

Lifestyle Support Therapy

☞ Massage the scalp every morning for 3 minutes to waken the brain and stimulate hair growth.
⁂Sunlight helps hair grow, but too much sun dries and damages. Be careful.

☞ Use alcohol-free gels as style holders, not hair sprays that damage hair and pollute the atmosphere.
⁂Wash hair in warm, not hot water. Rinse in cool water for scalp circulation. Condition regularly.

☞ What about henna? Is it a good choice for hair coloring? Henna is a natural non-carcinogenic plant used for centuries for body coloring. It offers body while it colors - often dramatically. Henna works best on thin, light, porous hair.

☞ **Effective hair rinses:**
⁂Nettles/sage/rosemary to darken.
⁂Rosemary/sage to shine dark hair.
⁂Kelp or sea water for body.
⁂Cider vinegar for pH balance.
⁂Chamomile/lemon to blonde.
⁂Rosemary/nettles for dry hair.
⁂Mix 1 egg yolk with the second shampooing for bounce/protein.
⁂Mix olive oil with drops of essential lavender and rosemary oil and use as a hot oil treatment.

See next page and LIVER HEALTH pages in this book for more information.

Common Symptoms: *Too dry or too oily hair; lots of falling hair; flaky deposits on the scalp; brittle hair with split ends; lack of bounce and elasticity.*
Common Causes: *Poor diet with several mineral deficiencies; lack of usable protein; poor circulation; recent illness and drug residues; liver malfunction resulting in loss of hair.*

Hair Loss
Alopecia ✤ Male Pattern Baldness

Over 30 million men and 20 million women have thinning or falling hair. Although androgenic alopecia is hereditary and not easily reversible, there are other factors, both internal and external, involved in most hair loss that can indeed result in hair improvement, thickness and regrowth. Hair health depends on blood supply, circulation and nutrition. Your therapy choice must be vigorously followed. Occasional therapy will have little or no effect. Two months is usually the minimum for really noticeable growth.

Diet & Superfood Therapy

❧ Diet is very important. Eat foods rich in silica and sulphur, such as onions, garlic, sprouts, horseradish, green leafy veggies, carrots, bell peppers, eggs, apricots, cucumbers, rice, and seeds.
　Eat foods rich in iodine and potassium, such as sea vegetables and sea foods for growth and thickness.
　Add soy foods to your diet, for phyto-hormones, plant protein and vitamin E.
　Drink 6 glasses of water daily.
　Reduce salt, sugar and caffeine - avoid fat, refined and preserved foods.
　Especially eliminate animal fat from your diet.

❧ Make a mix of wheat germ flakes, brewer's yeast flakes, pumpkin seeds, chopped dulse; take 2 TBS. daily in food: ♀

❧ Effective superfoods:
　Crystal Star SYSTEMS STRENGTH™ drink for absorbable minerals.
　NutriTech ALL 1 vitamin/mineral drink.
　AMAZAKE rice drinks for B vitamins.
　Beehive Botanicals ROYAL JELLY, POLLEN and SIBERIAN GINSENG drink.

Herbal Therapy

❧ Jump start herbal program:
Natural silica is a source of hair strength: Crystal Star SILICA SOURCE™ extract, horsetail tea, or Flora VEGE-SIL capsules.
　GINSENG/REISHI extract internally.
　IODINE/POTASSIUM SOURCE™ capsules, or 6 kelp tablets daily.
　GINKGO BILOBA extract for regrowth.
　EFAs are imperative to hair growth: EVENING PRIMROSE oil or borage oil caps.

❧ Herbal hair stimulants:
　Ginger tea rub; leave on 15 min.
　Cayenne extract rub: use directly on scalp before shampooing. Leave on for 30 minutes.
　Rosemary/dulse hair rinse.
　White sage for thinning hair.

❧ Male pattern baldness is a condition emanating from testosterone production; treat your prostate to treat your hair loss: herbal prostate remedies include saw palmetto, potency wood, panax ginseng and pygeum africanum, or Crystal Star PROX FOR MEN™ or Ethical Nu: MAXI-PROS PLUS.

❧ Phyto-estrogen and hormone balancing herbs can help hair loss in women:
　Crystal Star GINSENG/LICORICE ELIXIR™, use internally and rub on scalp.
　Black cohosh, dong quai, burdock combination, or Crystal Star EST-AID™ caps.

Supplements

❧ Take daily: 2 TBS. or more blackstrap molasses, PABA 1000mg, pantothenic acid 1000mg, and zinc 30mg for 2 months. with
　CoQ$_{10}$ 60mg 3x daily to improve circulation.

❧ Biotin 1000mcg daily, with Choline/inositol 1000mg daily and Enzymatic Therapy THYMULUS capsules.

❧ Ageless Products NU HAIR, or SILICEA GEL. ♀♂

❧ Hair nourishers:
　High B Complex daily with extra niacin 500mg daily,
　Ester C with bioflavonoids and rutin 550mg, 4 daily,
　Vitamin E 400IU daily.
　Pancreatin 1300mg at meals.
　Mezotrace SEA MINERAL COMPLEX 2x daily.
　High Omega -3 flax oils 3 daily. ♀
　Nature's Plus ULTRA HAIR tabs.

❧ Cysteine 500mg daily with zinc 75mg daily, especially if hair loss is related to low thyroid with zinc deficiency. ♂

Lifestyle Support Therapy

☞ External factors that cause hair loss are tight hairstyles and curlers, hot rollers, and chemicals for perming or straightening.
　Discontinue commercial hair coloring and hair dryers.

☞ Head circulation is a key:
　Finger massage scalp vigorously for 3 minutes every morning.
　Brush dry hair well for 5 minutes daily.
　Rinse for several minutes with alternating hot and cold shower water.
　Use a slant board once a week for 15 minutes.

☞ Effective scalp conditioners:
　Biotin treatments and shampoos
　Jojoba oil and shampoo to relieve sebum build-up, like HOBE ENERGIZER TREATMENT shampoo.
　Aloe vera oil and shampoo. ♂

☞ Get some outdoor exercise every day possible for body oxygen.

☞ Rinse hair with sea water or apple cider vinegar for thickness.

☞ Aromatherapy oils for falling hair: sage, cedarwood, rosemary, thyme. ♀♂

Common Symptoms: Thinning or complete loss of hair by either men or women (both male and female pattern baldness occur).
Common Causes: Poor circulation; poor diet with excess salt and sugar and too little protein; dandruff or seborrhea; plugs of sebum, high cholesterol; heredity; gland imbalance (especially the thyroid) in women from postpartum changes or discontinuance of birth control pills and overproduction of male sex hormones - (hair loss above the temples in women can mean a possible ovarian or adrenal tumor); chemotherapy and high blood pressure drugs; B vitamin deficiency; prolonged emotional stress or anxiety; surgery; severe illness or anemia; mineral deficiencies; hypothyroidism.

See previous page and LIVER HEALTH & CLEANSING pages for more information.

Headaches

Migraines ❧ Cluster Headaches (Vascular Headaches)

Cluster headaches are two or more sudden, extremely painful headaches a day, localized over the eyes or a spot on the forehead, usually coming in cycles for several days, with long periods of remission, recurring every few months. They stem from an imbalance in the frontal part of the brain, and affect the nerves in the face. There are no advance warning symptoms. Vasodilation is a key factor. Migraines affect 15% of American men and 30% of American women. A migraine usually indicates vascular instability potentiated by chronic stress, cranial artery constriction and inadequate blood supply to the brain. Inflammation, vasodilation, serotonin release and histamine reactions can be successfully addressed by natural healing methods. Indeed, sometimes these work when nothing else does.

Diet & Superfood Therapy

❧ Food sensitivities accompanying these types of headache are often from a favorite food that one craves. Watch out for "trigger foods" and avoid them.

➛Avoid pickled fish and shellfish, aged and smoked meats and other nitrate-containing foods, aged cheeses, red wines, avocados, caffeine, chocolate, cultured foods like yogurt and refined sweeteners.

❧ At the first signs of migraine type headache: take 1-2 cups of strong coffee to prevent blood vessel dilation, or a glass of carrot/celery juice.

❧ Eat high magnesium foods to reduce throbbing and contractions: dark leafy greens, fresh sea foods and sea vegetables, nuts, whole grains, molasses.
➛Eat vitamin C rich foods: broccoli, hot and bell peppers, sprouts, cherries, citrus.
➛Avoid red meats and dairy products, excess caffeine (withdrawal can be a precipitator), soft drinks (phosphorus binds up magnesium), MSG, and hard liquor.
➛**Drink green tea or Crystal Star GREEN TEA CLEANSER™ as a preventive.**
❧

❧ **Effective superfoods:**
➛Crystal Star SYSTEMS STRENGTH™.
➛BeWell juices.

Herbal Therapy

A colon cleanse is very effective in stopping vascular-type headaches.

❧ **Jump start herbal program:**
➛**For migraines:** Crystal Star MIGR-EASE™ caps or MIGR™ extract and RELAX CAPS™ as needed for pain and prevention.

➛**For cluster headaches:** Crystal Star CLUSTER CAPS™ and STRESSED OUT™, extract, with ASPIR-SOURCE™ caps for frontal lobe pain. Rub on CAPSAICIN cream.

or

➛Feverfew extract capsules or liquid or MIGR™ extract with feverfew, or Quantum MIGRELIEF™ extract.♀

❧ Capsicum/ginger capsules, 2 daily, or Crystal Star MENTAL INNER ENERGY™ caps with kava kava;♀ or
➛Take 1 ginger capsule dissolved in water at first sign of visual disturbance. ♂☙

❧ EVENING PRIMROSE OIL, 4 daily for **prostaglandin balance, with royal jelly.**

❧ **Effective for vascular type headaches:**
➛**Crystal Star FEM-SUPPORT™ or DEPRESS-EX™ for hormone-related headaches.**
➛**Enzymatic Therapy KAVA-TONE**♀ +
➛**GINKGO BILOBA extract.**
➛Rainbow Light GARLIC & GREENS
➛Scullcap/Rosemary/sage tea
➛**Lavender essence, aromatherapy**

Supplements

Niacin is helpful for some types of headaches, but not recommended for cluster headaches.

❧ **DLPA 1000mg for pain control and for natural endorphin formation.**♀ and/or Twin Lab GABA PLUS, or Country Life RELAXER capsules for brain stress control.♂
➛**Transitions PROGEST oil - apply to temples every ½ hour.**♀

❧ Niacin therapy for migraines: up to 500mg daily to normalize circulation. Take with Stress B Complex and extra B$_6$.
and
➛**Nature's Bounty internasal B$_{12}$ gel every other day as a preventive.**

❧ Nature's Plus QUERCETIN PLUS 500mg 2x daily with magnesium 500mg 2x daily, to prevent nerve twitching.

❧ **Anti-oxidants are a key:**
➛**Nutricology GERMANIUM 150mg.**♂
➛Twin Lab CSA caps .
➛Solgar 5-HTP 50-100mg as needed.
➛Omega-3 fish or flax oils 3x daily.
➛Melatonin, an antioxidant hormone - esp. for cluster headaches, 3mg at night, one week on one week off.

❧ Glutamine 500mg 2x daily, with Nature's Life CAL/MAG preacidified liquid 3 teasp. daily.

Lifestyle Support Therapy

Avoid smoking and secondary smoke. It constricts blood vessels.

☞ Put an ice pack on the back of the neck to reduce swelling, or put your feet in cold water to draw blood from the head.

☞ **Almost immediate results:** a coffee enema to stimulate liver and normalize bile activity; a bowel movement may relieve vomiting.

☞ Effective physical therapies to decrease intensity of attacks:
➛Chiropractic manipulation
➛Acupuncture and acupressure
➛Massage therapy
➛Biofeedback/relaxation training
➛Deep breathing exercises
➛Fresh air and exercise
➛Magnetic therapy

☞ **Reflexology point:** press and/or apply ice.

☞ **Reflexology therapy:** Apply pressure to inside base of the big toe 3 times for 10 seconds each time. Massage temples for 5 minutes. Breathe deeply. Do 10 neck rolls. Pull ear lobes for 5 seconds. Rub back and all around ear shell.

See the HYPOGLYCEMIA DIET in this book to help blood sugar regulation.

Common Symptoms: *Nutritional awareness is a must for preventing all migraine-type headaches. Cluster headaches mean severe, localized pain; dilated blood vessels with irritated adjacent nerves; localized nasal histamine reactions; sensitivity to light; restlessness. Migraines mean many symptoms, including constriction/dilation of brain, scalp and face blood vessels, lasting anywhere from 4 hours to two days; recurrent several times a month; a preceding aura, light sensitivity, visual problems and halos appearing around lights; nausea and vomiting, made worse by light and movement; intense, long-lasting pain, usually on one side of the head; water retention.*

Common Causes: *Vascular instability from chronic stress; too much caffeine, fat and sugar; pituitary/hormone serotonin imbalance; platelet aggregation; over-acid system stripping away protective nerve sheath; food allergies/sensitivities; lack of friendly intestinal flora; liver blockage; overuse of drugs; magnesium deficiency.*

Headaches

Stress & Tension Headaches ✦ Sinus Headaches

Tension headaches: muscle contractions of the scalp and back of the head, usually caused by stress or fatigue. They may last for hours or days. *Sinus headaches:* congestion and inflammation of the nasal sinuses.

Diet & Superfood Therapy

See LIVER CLEANSING and HYPOGLYCEMIA diet suggestions in this book for more.

♫ Go on a short 24 hour juice fast (pg. 158) to remove congestion. Drink lots of water and lemon, and veggie drinks (pg. 168) or potassium broth. (pg. 167).

❁Follow the next day with a very alkaline diet: apples and apple juice, cranberry juice, sprouts, salads and some brown rice.

❁Make a mix of brewer's yeast, lecithin granules, cider vinegar and honey; take 2 TBS. daily to restore body balance.

♫ Avoid for headache trigger foods:
❁Additive and chemical-laced foods
❁Salty, sugary or wheat-based foods
❁Caffeine-containing foods
❁Dairy foods, especially cheese
❁Condiments, sulfites, MSG
❁Too much alcohol, beer, wine

♫ Apply cold black tea bags to the eyes for 15 minutes. ♀ ♂

♫ Effective superfoods:
❁Nutricology PRO-GREENS w. EFAs.
❁Solgar EARTH SOURCE GREENS & MORE with EFAs.
❁Crystal Star SYSTEMS STRENGTH™ for minerals.

Herbal Therapy

Mineral-rich herbs provide key bio-chemical ingredients for neuro-transmission.

♫ Jump start herbal program: **Crystal Star RELAX™ caps 2 as needed to help rebuild nerve sheathing. ❁ANTI-FLAM™ for inflammation.**
❁ASPIR-SOURCE™ for frontal pain.
❁STRESSED OUT™ ext. for tension. ♂
❁FEM-SUPPORT™ for hormone-related stress headaches. ♀
❁ANTI-HST™ for sinus headaches.

♫ EVENING PRIMROSE OIL 500mg, and Enzymatic Therapy KAVA-TONE. ♂

♫ Soothing extracts:
❁VALERIAN/WILD LETTUCE ⊛
❁Scullcap
❁GINKGO BILOBA

♫ Soothing teas:
❁Wisdom of Ancients Yerba Mate
❁St. John's wort
❁White willow bark ♂
❁Chamomile ○
❁Catnip/sage

♫ **Rosemary as an antioxidant.** Drink rosemary tea, or mix the essential oil in hot water and inhale as an effective steam; or take the extract under the tongue.

Supplements

❀ **Bromelain 500mg as needed. Acts like aspirin without the stomach upset.**

❀ Magnesium citrate 800mg daily with taurine.
❁Country Life MAXI-B with taurine.

❀ Niacin therapy 100mg or more as needed daily to keep blood vessels and circulation open.

❀ **Effective antioxidants:**
❁**DLPA 1000mg or a GABA compound such as Country Life RELAXER caps for brain relief.**
❁Nutricology GERMANIUM 150mg. ♂
❁Natrol Ester C 550mg with bioflavonoids and rutin 3 - 4 daily.

❀ **Homeopathic remedies:**
❁**Hylands Calms Forte.** ♀
❁*Kali Phos, Bryonia, or Mag. Phos.* for frontal headaches.
❁*Kali Sulph., Kali Mur or Ferr. Phos* for headaches in the back of the head.
❁Hylands *Hylavir.* ⊛
❁*Nux Vomica* for hangover headaches.

Lifestyle Support Therapy

☞ Take a brisk walk. Breathe deeply for oxygen. The more brain oxygen, the fewer headaches.

☞ Rest. Lie down with the head higher than the body.

☞ Apply an ice massage on the back of the neck and upper back. It will dramatically reduce pain.
❁Apply onion or horseradish poultices to the nape of the neck **or soles of the feet** to relieve inflammation.

☞ Have a chiropractic adjustment, shiatsu massage, or massage therapy treatment if headaches are chronic. Take CSA 250mg daily, if spinal misalignment is the cause.

☞ **Aromatherapy:**
❁Apply lavender oil on temples. ♂
❁Peppermint oil on temples. ♂
❁Eucalyptus for sinus headaches.

☞ **Reflexology point:**

Apply an ice cube on the hand point for fast relief.

See also STRESS page in this book for more information.

Common Symptoms: Pain over the eyes, a dull ache in the forehead and temples; inability to sleep; irritability.

Common Causes: Emotional stress; food allergies or sensitivities; eyestrain; muscle tension; pinched nerve; constipation; too much caffeine, salt, sugar or MSG intake; hypoglycemia; artificial sweeteners like Aspartame (NUTRASWEET, EQUAL); water retention; PMS; poor circulation; poor posture; sluggish liver; jawbone misalignment (TMJ); arthritis; Candida albicans; drug toxicity; arteritis (inflammation of the artery).

Hearing Loss

Tinnitus ✳ Ringing in the Ears

Hearing loss is the third most common health problem for people over 65. In 1992, more than 25 million Americans suffered hearing loss. Hearing problems are the consequence of a wide spectrum of causes (see below). The ones addressed here are the result of externally or nutritionally-based causes - as opposed to internal bone fusions that need surgical attention. Lose excess weight. Fat clogs the head, too. See Hypoglycemia Diet pages in this book for additional diet suggestions.

Diet & Superfood Therapy

❧ Reduce dietary fats, cholesterol and mucous-forming foods. Avoid refined sugars, heavy starches and concentrated foods.

➥Eat light to hear better - plenty of vegetable proteins, sprouts, whole grains, fruits, and cultured foods.

➥Take fresh grated horseradish in a spoon with lemon juice. Hang over a sink to release excess mucous and clear head passages.

❧ **For ringing in the ears:**
➥Go on a short 3 day mucous cleansing diet (pg. 157). Then eat fresh foods for the rest of the week. Have plenty of salads and citrus fruits.

➥Then, for a month, eat a mildly cleansing diet. Avoid all clogging, saturated fat foods. Reduce dairy products. Add plenty of vegetable fiber foods.

➥Have a glass of lemon juice and water each morning.

➥Keep the diet very low in sugars, salt, and dairy foods.

➥Drink only bottled water.
☙

❧ **Effective superfoods:**
➥Sun CHLORELLA drink daily.
➥New Moon GINGER WONDER syrup.
➥Crystal Star CHOLO-FIBER TONE™.

Herbal Therapy

❧ **Jump start herbal program:**
Crystal Star ANTI-HST™ caps to relieve pressure in ears and sinus canals.
➥**GINKGO BILOBA extract 3x daily for ringing in the ears and circulation.**
➥Put 6 drops garlic oil and 3 drops goldenseal extract in the ear. Hold in with cotton. Repeat daily for a week. Flush out with vinegar and water.

❧ **Silica helps elasticize vascular walls:**
➥Crystal Star SILICA SOURCE™.
➥Flora VEGE-SIL.
➥Body Essentials SILICA GEL 1 TB. in 3-oz. liquid 3x daily.

❧ ECHINACEA extract liquid with SIBERIAN GINSENG extract caps 4 daily. ♂

❧ Effective ear extracts: (Dilute in water to use as drops).
➥Lobelia
➥Angelica root ♀
➥Peppermint
➥Mullein oil drops to relieve pain.

❧ **For ringing in the ears:**
➥Licorice rt. extract
➥Summer savory and rose water tea. Use internally; also as drops in the ear.
➥**Cayenne/ginger caps for circulation.**

Supplements

One of the common high-dose aspirin side effects for arthritic sufferers is ringing in the ears.

➥ Take a good hearing mix - one of each:
➥Emulsified A 25,000IU
➥Ester C with bioflavonoids
➥Mezotrace MULTIMINERAL
➥Magnesium 400mg
➥Glutamine 500mg

➥ Mega C therapy: Use ascorbate or Ester C crystals $1/4$ teasp. every half hour to bowel tolerance for 1 week.

➥ Nutricology GERMANIUM150mg daily. ♂

➥ Enzymatic Therapy ORAL NUTRIENT CHELATES, two packs daily to open clogged arteries and stimulate blood. ♀
➥B Complex for regrowth of damaged microscopic hairs in the ear canal.

➥ **For ringing in the ears:**
➥**Alta Health manganese and B₁₂.**
➥**PCOs from grapeseed or white pine 100mg 3x daily.**
➥Beta carotene 150,000IU daily ♂
➥Niacin therapy: 500mg daily. ♀
➥Vitamin C with bioflavonoids, 3000-5000mg daily for 3 months. ♀

Lifestyle Support Therapy

❧ Massage neck, ear and temples. Pull earlobes - top front and back to clear passages of excess wax or mucous.
➥Use diluted 3% H₂O₂ to gently clean out excess ear wax or obstructions.
➥Smoking limits blood flow to the inner ear.

❧ Avoid continuous loud noise. (Listening to loud rock music through headphones on a regular basis results in major ear problems.)

❧ **Acupressure point:**
Squeeze the joints of the ring finger and the 4th toe, covering all sides for several minutes each day.

❧ **For ringing in the ears:**
➥Avoid high doses of aspirin.
➥Massage the ear as above.
➥Acupressure: stroke gently downward from the top of the temple to the bottom of the cheek with the nails for 30 seconds on each side.

❧ **Reflexology point:**
ears

Common Symptoms: *Degenerative hearing loss; feeling of fullness and clogging in the ear; obstructed ear passages; no pain, but an extremely annoying ringing sound in the head.*
Common Causes: *Arteriosclerosis; allergies; thickening of ear passages or fluid congestion in the middle ear reducing vibration; excess ear wax; mucous clog; infection or inflammation; swelling and congestion; chronic bronchial mastoid and sinus inflammation; hypoglycemia (raised blood insulin causes poor carbohydrate metabolism); a diet with too many mucous-forming foods; poor digestion (low HCL); poor circulation; high blood pressure; imbalance in the inner ear; low immune defenses; raised copper levels; metabolic imbalance.*

See HEALTHY HEART DIET and EAR INFECTIONS page for more information.

Heart Disease

Arrhythmias ✳ Palpitations ✳ Tachycardia ✳ Atrial Fibrillation

Arrhythmias: Electrical disruptions that affect the natural rhythm of the heart. **Palpitations:** the heart beating out of sequence. **Atrial fibrillation:** episodic heart flutter, shortness of breath and the uncomfortable awareness of the racing of the heart, sometimes accompanied by dizziness or fainting; may predispose a person to having a stroke. **Atrial tachycardia:** too rapid contractions of the heart coming on in sudden attacks; usually associated with coronary artery disease. May increase the risk of congestive heart failure.

Diet & Superfood Therapy

❧ Keep your diet low in fats, salt and calories. Have a fresh green salad and some whole grain protein every day.

☛ Add sunflower and sesame seeds, miso soup, rice and oat bran, green leafy vegetables frequently to the diet.

☛ Drink a bottle of mineral water every day.

☛ Make a mix of lecithin granules, toasted wheat germ, brewer's yeast, chopped sea vegetables; sprinkle 2 TBS. daily on a salad, soup or protein drink.

☛ Take a green drink once a week esp. during initial healing. (See page 168, or below.)

❧ Arrhythmias can be aggravated by coffee, tea, alcohol, or nicotine. Reduce these stimulants if you are prone to arrhythmias. ☙

❧ **Effective superfoods:**
☛ Crystal Star SYSTEMS STRENGTH™ drink or capsules for daily potassium.
☛ Solgar WHEY TO GO protein drink.
☛ Sun CHLORELLA.
☛ New Wonder GINSENG/GINGER WONDER syrup.
☛ NutriBiotic PRO-GREENS.
☛ Klamath BLUE GREEN SUPREME with spirulina and SOD.
☛ Beehive Botanicals ROYAL JELLY/ GINSENG drink.

Herbal Therapy

❧ **Jump start herbs for palpitations:** Crystal Star HEARTSEASE/HAW-THORN™ caps as a preventive measure.
☛ HAWTHORN leaf, berry and flower extract as needed to regulate.
☛ GINKGO BILOBA extract helps prevent ischemia-caused fibrillation.
☛ EVENING PRIMROSE OIL for EFAs, 4 daily, or Omega-3 flax oils 3 daily.
☛ IODINE/POTASSIUM caps™ 2 daily. ♂♀

❧ Berberine-containing herbs - goldenseal, Oregon grape, or barberry help arrhythmias caused by fatty deposits on the arteries.

❧ Cayenne/ginger caps or Solaray COOL CAYENNE 2 daily, or Heartfoods cayenne products (increase strength gradually). ♂

❧ **Heart regulating herbs:** usually work within 1 minute for simple palpitations.
☛ Cayenne extract drops.
☛ Ginseng Co. CYCLONE CIDER. ♀
☛ HAWTHORN extract drops.
☛ Siberian ginseng 2 daily.
☛ Valerian extract for tachycardia.

❧ **Circulation teas:**
☛ Butcher's broom
☛ Rosemary tea (or rosemary wine sips)
☛ Ginger capsules
☛ Peppermint/sage

Supplements

DIGOXIN, often given for arrhythmias, has side effects that include G.I. irritation, hearing and visual disturbances, headaches and dizziness. Lifestyle and diet change are better ways to avoid arrhythmias.

❧ **Antioxidants are key preventives:** OPCs from white pine or grapeseed.
☛ Future Biotics VITAL K daily.
☛ Liquid chlorophyll 1 teasp. daily in water before each meal. ♂
☛ CoQ₁₀ 60mg 3x daily.
☛ Carnitine 500mg 2x daily. ♀
☛ Vitamin E 400IU w. selenium 200mcg.

❧ Take taurine 500mg 2x daily with Ester C 550mg 2x daily for stability. **and** Solaray CHROMIACIN 3x daily to normalize circulation. (Do not take high doses of isolated niacin.)

❧ Country Life RELAXER capsules and CALCIUM/MAGNESIUM/POTASSIUM capsules, or CAL/MAG/BROMELAIN caps.

❧ Stress B Complex 150mg w. extra B₆ 100mg.

❧ Magnesium 800mg daily, especially if you have had heart surgery. ♂
☛ Rainbow Light CALCIUM PLUS with high magnesium, 4 daily. ♀♂

Lifestyle Support Therapy

See How To Take Your Own Pulse in the on pg. 445. If your pulse is over 80 and remains that way, you should make some diet improvements and get a further heart diagnosis.

☛ Plunge the face into cold water when arrhythmia occurs to stop palpitations.

☛ Avoid soft drinks. The phosphorus binds up magnesium and makes it unavailable for heart regularity.

☛ **Reflexology point:**

heart points

☛ **Heart/artery action area:**

Common Symptoms: *Irregular and/or rapid heartbeat; uncomfortable awareness of your heartbeat; skipped heartbeats and shortness of breath; a feeling that you cannot breathe; light-headedness; often chest discomfort.*

Common Causes: *Poor diet with too much refined sugar and saturated fat; lack of exercise/aerobic strength; obesity; smoking; stressful lifestyle; high blood pressure; diabetes.*

See the following HEALTHY HEART pages for more information.

Heart Disease

Cardiovascular Disease ✤ Angina ✤ Coronary ✤ Heart Attack ✤ Stroke

Almost unknown before the turn of this century, today, two-thirds of America suffers from some kind of cardiovascular disease -heart attack, coronary , hypertension, atherosclerosis, stroke, rheumatic heart and more. A million of us die because of heart problems each year. Nutritional and natural therapies are proving to reduce mortality better than aggressive medical intervention or the most advanced drug treatment. Heart problems in women are different than those of men, because they are hormone-dependent. Hormone balance is an important protective factor.

Diet & Superfood Therapy

Food plays a major part in preventing of heart disease.

A healthy heart diet has plenty of magnesium and potassium rich foods: fresh greens, sea vegetables, flavonoids from pitted fruits, green tea and wine, sea foods, tofu, brown rice and whole grains, garlic and onions.

- Reduce fat to no more than 10% of total daily calorie intake. Especially limit fats from animal sources and hydrogenated oils.
- 70% of daily calories from complex carbohydrates like vegetables and grains; 20% of calories from low fat protein sources.
- Eat less than 100mg per day of diet cholesterol. Keep cholesterol below 160.
- Add 8 glasses of bottled water daily to your diet. It is the best diuretic for a healthy heart. (Chlorinated/fluoridated water destroys vitamin E in the body).
- A glass or two of wine with dinner can relieve stress and raise HDLs.
- Make a hearty morning mix of lecithin granules, toasted wheat germ, brewer's yeast, chopped dry sea vegetables, molasses; take 2 TBS. daily over cereal.
- Pay conscious attention to eliminating red meats, caffeine and caffeine-containing foods, refined sugars, fatty, salty and fried foods, prepared meats and soft drinks. The rewards are worth the effort.

Effective superfoods:

- Crystal Star SYSTEMS STRENGTH™ drink or IODINE/POTASSIUM caps.
- ALOE VERA juice with herbs.
- Beehive Botanicals ROYAL JELLY, POLLEN, SIBERIAN GINSENG drink.
- New Moon GINGER WONDER syrup.

Herbal Therapy

Jump start herbal program:

In an emergency; 1 tsp. cayenne powder, or drops of cayenne tincture in water will often bring a person out of a heart attack or coronary.

- **Take 1/2 dropperful HAWTHORN extract every 1/2 hour. Take 1/2 dropperful daily as preventive support.**
- **EVENING PRIMROSE oil for EFAs and prostaglandin balance, 4 daily. Prostaglandins regulate arterial muscle tone.**
- **GINSENG/REISHI or GINKGO BILOBA extracts to improve blood flow to the heart, 2-3x daily.**
- Crystal Star HEARTSEASE/HAWTHORN caps, or HEARTSEASE/CIRCU-CLEANSE™ tea to strengthen cardiovascular system and keep it clean and clear.

Effective heart tonics:

- Cayenne/ginger capsules, or Heart Foods HEART FOOD CAYENNE caps.
- Spirulina, liquid chlorophyll, or Klamath BLUE GREEN SUPREME drink.
- Ginseng Co. CYCLONE CIDER ♀
- Garlic oil capsules
- Wheat germ oil caps
- Gotu kola caps
- **Siberian ginseng extract caps 2000mg or tea 2 cups daily.** ♂

Effective phyto-estrogen heart protective herbs for post-menopausal women:

- **Crystal Star FEMALE HARMONY™ capsules and tea, or FEM-SUPPORT™ extract.** ♀
- **DONG QUAI/DAMIANA extract**
- **VITEX extract**
- **Licorice root extract, caps, tea, or GINSENG/LICORICE ELIXIR™ extract**

Supplements

Beware of calcium channel blockers. They block many body functions and are being implicated in aggravated cardiovascular problems. Actively explore the alternatives with your physician, such as magnesium 800mg daily.

Golden Pride FORMULA ONE oral chelation w/ EDTA as directed.

Cardio-tonic antioxidants:

- **CoQ_{10}, 60mg. 3x daily.**
- Nutricology GERMANIUM 150mg.
- ITC Super Sunshine B INOSITOL.
- Carnitine 500mg daily.
- Grapeseed PCOs 100mg 3x daily.
- Biogenetics BIO-GUARD enzymes.
- Ascorbate or Ester C with bioflavonoids, up to 5000mg daily for interstitial tissue elasticity, arterial integrity and prevent little strokes. Take with vitamin E with selenium 200mcg for synergistic activity.
- Country Life DMG B_{15} 125mg SL. ♂
- B_1 50mg esp. if taking diuretics; B_6 to help unclog arteries, 50-100mg.

Heart disease preventives:

- Chromium picolinate or Solaray CHROMIACIN and HAWTHORN BLEND for arterial plaque and insulin resistance.
- Omega-3 fish and flax oils 3x daily.
- Bromelain 1550mg regularly to prevent a heart attack by increasing fibrinolysis and inhibiting platelet aggregation.
- Folic acid to keep homocysteine levels down, with B_6 100mg and Nature's Bounty B_{12} for synergistic results.
- Magnesium 800mg, or Country Life CALCIUM/MAGNESIUM/BROMELAIN.

Lifestyle Support Therapy

Bite down on the tip of the little finger to help stop a heart attack.

- **Apply hot compresses and massage chest of the victim to ease a heart attack.**

When administered immediately following symptoms of a heart attack, aspirin has been shown to reduce mortality through its ability to reduce arterial blockage.

Take alternate hot and cold showers frequently to increase circulation.

Stop smoking. Tobacco constricts circulation.

Take some mild regular daily exercise. Do deep breathing exercises every morning for body oxygen, and to stimulate brain activity.

Consciously add relaxation and a good daily laugh to your life. A positive mental outlook does wonders for stress.

Reflexology points:

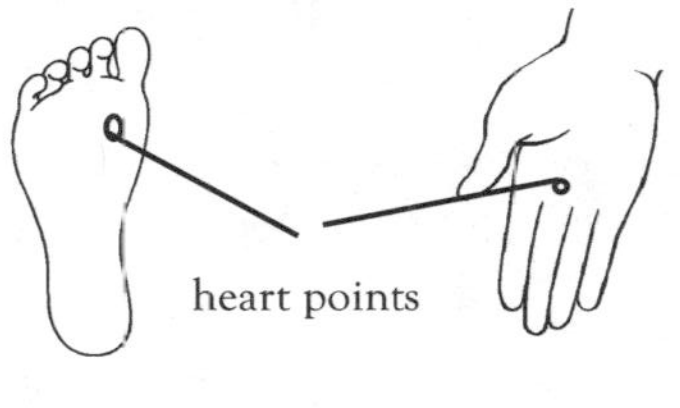

See the HEALTHY HEART DIET on the following pages for more information.

Diagnosing Your Cardiovascular Problem

Signs that you are suffering a heart attack or stroke: 1) sudden weakness or numbness of the face, arm and leg, usually on one side of the body; 2) trouble talking or understanding speech; 3) fluctuating state of consciousness, with tingling sensations; 4) dimness or loss of vision, particularly in one eye; 5) sudden severe headache and dizziness, leading to unsteadiness or a sudden fall. A heart attack or stroke does most of its damage in the first six hours. *CALL AN EMERGENCY ROOM IMMEDIATELY IF YOU FEEL YOU ARE HAVING A HEART ATTACK OF ANY KIND.*

ANGINA: A warning sign of a heart attack. There will be recurring, sudden, intense chest pains, lasting 30 seconds to 1 minute, with a vise-like grip of pressure across the chest. People usually feel the first angina attacks during physical exertion because one or more arteries are partially clogged. With the blood supply to the heart reduced, it functions inefficiently and painfully. Do not ignore this type of sign as "just indigestion." May also be brought on by emotional stress, exposure to cold, or overexertion.
•**Therapy for angina:** Go on a vegetarian, very low fat diet (see page 327 in this book). Take 1000mg carnitine 2x daily and CoQ_{10} 60mg 4 daily; cayenne/ginger capsules, 2 daily; HAWTHORN extract as needed; high Omega-3 flax or fish oil 3x daily; vitamin C 3-5000mg daily with bioflavonoids and L-lysine 1000mg daily to scour arteries and eliminate angina pain; vitamin E 400IU 2x daily; Use **Golden Pride FORMULA ONE, oral chelation w/ EDTA 2 packs morning and evening.**

ATHEROSCLEROSIS: Almost all heart attacks develop from long standing atherosclerosis, clogging of the arteries resulting from degeneration of the artery walls which are narrowed by fat and cholesterol plaque lesions. There can be an embolism when these break loose into the bloodstream. **Arteriosclerosis** means both clogging and loss of elasticity of the arteries, resulting in the most common cardiovascular ailment - **HIGH BLOOD PRESSURE, page 332. (See also HIGH CHOLESTEROL LEVELS, page 270.)**
•**Therapy for atherosclerosis:** vitamin B_6, 100-200mg daily; vitamin C 3000mg daily with bioflavonoids; Enzymatic Therapy GUGUL PLUS; **Golden Pride FORMULA ONE,** oral chelation w/ EDTA 2 packs A.M./P.M.; ginger capsules 2x daily to inhibit platelet aggregation.

MYOCARDIAL INFARCTION, (a CORONARY or CORONARY THROMBOSIS): This is the epidemic heart attack, with permanent damage to the heart muscle, or death. If the build-up of plaque in the coronary arteries continues, eventually one will become narrowed to the point of total obstruction. Instantly the part of the heart served from that artery is without blood supply. In five minutes it will suffer damage or even death from the cut off of oxygen. The heart stops beating; the blood supply to the brain is cut off. There is excruciating pain, starting in the lower chest and spreading throughout the upper half of the body, and a weak, rapid pulse with perspiring, pale skin. Blood pressure drops dangerously, there is dizziness and then unconsciousness. Fever usually follows this kind of attack.
•**Therapy for a coronary:** Liquid carnitine for myocardial infarction during an attack. NAC inhibits heart damage from free radicals after an infarction and CoQ_{10} 60mg 4 daily. Use magnesium to help prevent a coronary, 400mg 2x daily; folic acid to keep homocysteine levels down, with B_6 100mg and Nature's Bounty B_{12} for synergistic results; Fo-Ti to increase heart vigor. Antioxidants are a key (see previous page), especially those with high bioflavonoids and carotenes, and garlic 6 capsules daily. Women might use a DHEA supplement as a preventive after menopause; HAWTHORN extract as needed, especially after a heart attack to normalize heart rate. Take regular proteolytic enzymes to prevent inflammation, such as Country Life CALCIUM/MAGNESIUM/BROMELAIN tablets, and vitamin E 400IU daily.

STROKE: A stroke occurs when there is a blockage of the blood supply to the brain, similar to that of a coronary, the difference being cell death in the brain. Even a partial loss can kill tissue; oxygen-deprived brain tissue dies within minutes. The effects of a stroke can range from temporary loss of speech or vision, disordered behavior, thought patterns and memory, to paralysis, coma and death. See the top of this page for signs you may be having a stroke. Ask for a stethoscope neck check (for a *bruit* sound) if you think you are at risk.
•**Therapy after a stroke:** Unknown to most people, 80% of strokes are preventable. Take1000mg carnitine 2x daily and HAWTHORN extract as needed. Use **Golden Pride FORMULA ONE, oral chelation w/ EDTA 2 packs a.m./p.m..** Take a cup of Japanese green tea, or Crystal Star GREEN TEA CLEANSER™ each morning. Eat cold water fish twice a week - salmon and halibut are two of the best. Add more fruits and vegetables (and less caffeine and alcohol) to your diet. Have a green salad every day. Reduce salty **and sugary** foods. Add fiber. Snip dry sea vegetables over your salad, or take Crystal Star IODINE/POTASSIUM caps. (See Healthy Heart Diet page 327.) Vitamin C 300mg daily with bioflavonoids 500mg; Future Biotics VITAL K PLUS drink for potassium. Take a B Complex vitamin with extra folic acid 800mcg; add vitamin E as an antioxidant; magnesium to normalize heart muscle action. Meditation and acupuncture both show success as relaxation techniques against stroke.

ISCHEMIA: Reduction of blood flow to the heart and cell oxygen starvation, caused by atherosclerosis, the fatty deposits along the coronary artery walls. Ischemia leads to angina, coronary or congestive heart failure. Signs of ischemia are high blood pressure; poor circulation; aching feet, legs and muscles, or numbness and weakness in the legs; gradual mental deterioration, weakness and unsteadiness; diagonal earlobe crease. **Transient ischemia** (small, short heart attacks) signs include sudden onset of weakness, tingling and numbness on one side, speech difficulty, double vision and vertigo.
•**Therapy for ischemia:** CoQ_{10} 60mg 4 daily; BILBERRY extract to protect integrity of the microvessel walls; garlic capsules 6 daily, ginger capsules to normalize circulation; Citrin 50mg. 3x daily.

CONGESTIVE HEART FAILURE: A damaged heart weakened by arteriosclerosis or other disease such as hypothyroidism, ceases to pump effectively. Circulation is inefficient; organs and tissues become clogged with blood. Early symptoms include abnormal fatigue, and shortness of breath after exertion. Ankles and feet usually swell, and there is nausea and gas. Later symptoms are greater heart exhaustion and fluid in the lungs. High iron stores after menopause may put a woman at increased CHF risk. Exercise helps the body get rid of excess iron.
•**Therapy for congestive heart failure:** Magnesium, 800mg daily; CoQ_{10} 60mg 4 daily; CSA (chondroitan sulfate A); taurine 500mg daily; DHEA supplement for post-menopausal women; magnesium to help the heart muscle work better, 800mg daily. (Country Life CALCIUM/MAGNESIUM/BROMELAIN for even better activity.) GINSENG/REISHI extract - immune-strengthening preventive; HAW-THORN extract as needed; Crystal Star ANTI-FLAM™ caps to reduce inflammation; vitamin C 3000mg daily with bioflavonoids; BILBERRY extract daily; Ayurvedic Coleus Forskohlii.

MITRAL VALVE PROLAPSE (MVP): the mitral valve is one of several gates within the heart that regulates oxygen-rich blood flow. A prolapse of the gate valve is a common abnormality of the heart. It sometimes causes palpitations or rapid heart rate, anxiety attacks or night time panic attacks, shortness of breath, and usually physical weakness. While benign arrhythmias are fairly common, the uneven flow of blood increases the likelihood of clot formation in people under 45, who also have a higher rate of stroke during their younger years. MVP is often inherited as a result of conditions that affect the collagen structures throughout the body. Small, thin women are more likely to have a mitral valve prolapse.
• **Therapy for mitral valve prolapse:** 1000mg L-carnitine 3x a day to relieve symptoms; HAWTHORN extract as needed during the day or at night; Crystal Star HEARTSEASE/HAWTHORN capsules or Solaray HAWTHORN BLEND; GINKGO BILOBA to normalize circulation; an herbal combination, such as Crystal Star FEMALE HARMONY™, with phyto-estrogen herbs and small amounts of vasodilators have been used as protectives for women. Relaxation techniques like meditation, shiatzu and biofeedback are a good idea, along with daily mild exercise, such as leisurely swimming or a brisk walk.

CARDIOMYOPATHY: an insidious type of heart failure with a deadly weakening of an enlarged heart muscle and only a fraction of the blood the body needs being pumped.
• **Therapy for cardiomyopathy:** Use CoQ₁₀ 100mg. 3 daily; HAWTHORN extract as needed; GINKGO BILOBA or ginger capsules daily to normalize circulation; CAL/MAG/BROMELAIN 1500mg.

TACHYCARDIA: a heartbeat so rapid that the heart cannot deliver blood efficiently. It can be fatal. **PALPITATIONS:** the heart beating irregularly. **FIBRILLATION:** more serious than tachycardia, there is a weak, irregular quiver to the heartbeat. See page 323.

HYPERTENSION: See HIGH BLOOD PRESSURE, page 332.

PERIPHERAL VASCULAR DISEASE: reduction of blood to the smaller blood vessels. See **Varicose Veins,** page 422.

Note: Modern medicine is now suggesting regular intake of aspirin to prevent life-threatening strokes and heart attacks. The justification is that aspirin inhibits a specific enzyme, making the blood less prone to dangerous clotting. Ginger not only inhibits the same enzyme, it does so without side effects.

Quick Heart Rehabilitation Check Program

This program is designed especially for those of you who have survived a heart attack or major heart surgery. Coming back is tough. Beginning and sticking to a new lifestyle that changes almost everything about the way you eat, exercise, handle stress, and even the smallest details of your life, is a challenge. The following mini-rehabilitation program is a blueprint that you can use with confidence. It addresses the main preventive needs - keeping your arteries clear and your blood slippery - goals that clearly can be achieved through a good diet and exercise. This program has proven successful against heart disease recurrence.

• Reduce fats to at least 15% of your diet; less if possible. Limit polyunsaturates (margarine, oils) to 10%. Add mono-unsaturates (olive oil, avocados, nuts, seeds)
• Eat potassium-rich foods for cardiotonic activity: fresh spinach and chard, broccoli, bananas, sea vegetables, molasses, cantaloupe, apricots, papayas, mushrooms, tomatoes, yams, or take a high potassium drink regularly, such as potassium broth (pg. 167), Crystal Star SYSTEMS STRENGTH™ drink, or Future Biotics VITAL K. (a serving of high potassium fruits or vegetables offers about 400mg of potassium); a serving of the above drinks offers approx. 1000-1250mg of potassium)
• Eat plenty of complex carbohydrates, such as broccoli, peas, whole grain breads, vegetable pastas, potatoes, sprouts, tofu and brown rice.
• **Have a fresh green salad every day.**
• Have several servings of cold water fish or seafood every week for high omega 3 oils.
• Have a glass of white wine before dinner for relaxation and better digestion. Add miso and oat or rice bran to your diet regularly.
• Eat magnesium-rich foods for heart regulation: tofu, wheat germ, bran, broccoli, potatoes, lima beans, spinach, chard.
• Eat copper-rich foods for clear arteries: oysters, clams, crab, fish, brewer's yeast, fresh fruit and vegetables, nuts, seeds.
• Eat high fiber foods for a clean system and alkalinity: whole grains, fruits and vegetables, legumes and herbs.

CHOOSE SEVERAL OF THE FOLLOWING SUPPLEMENTS AS YOUR INDIVIDUAL DAILY MICRO-NUTRIENTS:
• **Heart regulation and stability:** Sun CHLORELLA tabs 15 daily; magnesium 400mg; carnitine 500mg; evening primrose oil 4 daily; gotu kola herb.
• **Clear arteries:** Solaray CHROMIACIN; selenium; omega 3 flax or fish oils 3x daily; **Health Papers CETA CLEANSE oral chelation w/ EDTA 2 packs A.M./P.M.**
• **Antioxidants:** Wheat germ oil raises oxygen level 30%; chlorophyll; vitamin E 400IU with selenium; pycnogenol; CoQ₁₀ 30mg; GINKGO BILOBA extract, rosemary, or chaparral.
• **Cardiac tonics:** HAWTHORN extract; cayenne, or cayenne/ginger capsules; garlic; SIBERIAN GINSENG extract; gotu kola.
• **Anti-cholesterol/blood thinning:** Ginger; butcher's broom; taurine 500mg; **Golden Pride FORMULA ONE, oral chelation w/ EDTA 2 packs morning and evening**
• **Healthy blood chemistry:** Chromium picolinate; Ester C 500mg with bioflavonoid, especially if you have had by-pass surgery.

Diet is the single most influential key to heart health. In general, refined, high fat, high calorie foods create cardiovascular problems, and natural foods relieve them. Americans get over half their calories from processed foods that are high in calories and low in nutrients. Fried foods, salty and sugary foods, low fiber foods, pasteurized dairy products, red meats and processed meats, tobacco, hard liquor and caffeine all contribute to clogged and reduced arteries, LDL cholesterol, high blood pressure and heart attacks. Almost all cardiovascular disease can be treated and prevented with improvement in diet and nutrition. You can carve out health with your own knife and fork. The following diet is for long-term heart and circulatory health. It's easy to live with, and has all the necessary elements to keep arteries clean, and heart action regular and strong. It emphasizes fresh and whole foods, high mineral foods with lots of potassium and magnesium, oxygen-rich foods from green vegetables, sprouts and wheat germ (wheat germ oil can raise the oxygen level of the heart as much as 30%), and vegetable-source proteins. It all adds up to today's definition of living well. Pleasure is derived from improved health and vitality instead of rich food and drink. The rewards are high, a longer, healthier life, and control over your life.

On rising: take a high protein or high vitamin/mineral drink such as NutriTech ALL 1 or Nature's Plus SPIRUTEIN in orange or grapefruit juice, or a cup of Japanese green tea.

Breakfast: Make a mix of 2 TBS. each; lecithin granules, wheat germ, brewer's yeast, honey, and sesame seed. Sprinkle 2 teasp. every morning on fresh fruits, such as apricots, peaches, apples or nectarines, or mix with yogurt;
and/or have a poached or baked egg with bran muffins or whole grain toast and kefir cheese; or some whole grain cereal or pancakes with a little maple syrup.

Mid-morning: have a veggie drink (pg. 168), or Green Foods GREEN ESSENCE drink, a potassium drink (pg. 167), Crystal Star SYSTEMS STRENGTH™ drink, or all natural V8 juice (pg. 168) or a cup of rosemary or peppermint tea; and/or some crunchy raw veggies with a kefir cheese or yogurt dip; and/or a cup of miso soup with sea veggies snipped on top.

Lunch: have a cup of fenugreek tea with additions: 1 teasp. honey, 1 teasp. wheat germ oil, 1 teasp. lecithin granules or liquid;
then have a tofu and spinach salad with some sprouts and bran muffins;
or a high protein salad or sandwich with nuts & seeds and a black bean or lentil soup;
or an avocado, low fat cheese or soy cheese sandwich on whole grain bread;
or a seafood and whole grain pasta salad with a light tomato sauce;
or a light veggie omelet and small green salad;
or some grilled or braised vegetables with an olive oil dressing and brown rice.

Mid-afternoon: have a cup of peppermint tea, or Crystal Star Chinese ROYAL MU™ tonic tea;
and/or a cup of miso soup with a hard boiled egg, or whole grain crackers; or a glass of carrot juice, or Personal V-8 (pg. 168).

Dinner: have a broccoli quiche with a whole grain or chapati crust; and a cup of onion soup;
or a baked seafood dish with brown rice and peas;
or a whole grain, steamed vegetables and tofu casserole;
or an oriental stir fry with light soup and rice;
or grilled fish or seafood and a small green salad and baked potato;
or a salmon or veggie souffle with a light sauce and salad.
Note: A little white wine before dinner is fine for relaxation, digestion and tension relief. Wine has an enzyme that breaks up blood clots. Avoid commercial antacids that neutralize natural stomach acid and invite the body to produce even more acid, thus aggravating stress and tension.

Before bed: have another cup of miso soup, or a cup of Organic Gourmet SAVORY SPREAD paste broth in hot water, apple or pear juice, or chamomile tea.

Daily heart disease prevention supplementation should include: vitamin E 400IU, Solaray CHROMIACIN, or niacin 250mg daily; CoQ₁₀, 60mg, and flax oil 3x daily; Siberian ginseng extract caps, 2000mg or extract, ½ dropperful daily; Vitamin C 3000mg daily with bioflavonoids, or Crystal Star BIOFLAV, FIBER & C SUPPORT™ drink; EVENING PRIMROSE OIL caps, 2 to 4 daily; HAWTHORN extract, 1 dropperful daily as a heart tonic.

Preventive bodywork should include: research demonstrates over and over again that people who exert themselves for either recreation or work are strikingly free of circulatory diseases.
• Get regular daily exercise. To be effective for heart, circulation and artery health, the heart rate and respiration must rise to the point of mild breathlessness for 5 minutes each day. A regular daily walk, or other aerobic exercise, such as dancing, swimming or jogging strengthens the whole cardiovascular system. It also reduces stress, the underlying cause of all disease.

See COOKING FOR HEALTHY HEALING by Linda Rector Page for a complete heart diet and healing program.

Hemorrhage

Internal Bleeding ✣ Excessive Bleeding ✣ Blood Clotting Difficulty

The suggestions on this page refer to first aid for minor or non-life threatening problems. Obviously, you should get to an emergency room or call an ambulance if there is an emergency situation. Nosebleeds, bleeding gums and urinary tract bleeding are types of bleeding that can be addressed with these remedies. Once the bleeding has been arrested, the idea with natural remedies is, as always, to address the underlying causes (such as weak membranes or capillary structure) that allow the bleeding to be excessive.

Diet & Superfood Therapy

ℛ **Make a variety of sprouts a regular part of your diet for natural Vitamin K to help clotting.**
➻Other high vitamin K foods: kale, spinach and all dark green veggies, broccoli, cauliflower, and eggs.

ℛ Have a glass of carrot/spinach juice frequently.
➻Take a green vegetable drink (pg. 168) once a week.

ℛ Eat plenty of papayas. Use citrus peel directly on the bleeding area.
❦

ℛ **Effective superfoods:**
➻**Crystal Star BIOFLAV, FIBER & C SUPPORT™ drink** with extra bioflavonoids to increase tissue integrity.
➻**Crystal Star ENERGY GREEN™** drink at least once a week to build healthier blood balance.
➻Liquid chlorophyll 3 teasp. daily.
➻Beehive Botanical ROYAL JELLY/ POLLEN/SIBERIAN GINSENG drink for stronger blood.

Herbal Therapy

ℛ **Jump start herbal program:**
Capsicum, take 1 teasp. in a cup of hot water to stop bleeding. **(Take with an eyedropper on the back of the tongue if it is too hot to swallow.)**
➻**Clotting tea combo:** Licorice root, comfrey root, shepherd's purse, goldenseal root, cranesbill.

ℛ **Hemostatic clotting herbs:**
➻Plantain and water paste
➻Witch hazel
➻Cayenne powder, or take 2 capsules cayenne and 2 caps BILBERRY extract
➻Calendula salve or poultice
➻AloeLife SKIN GEL

ℛ Internal bleeding control:
➻Pau d' arco tea
➻Turmeric capsules
➻Comfrey root
➻Shepherd's purse

ℛ Herbal astringents/flavonoids to tighten and strengthen veins and capillaries. All may be used both externally and internally to check bleeding:
➻White oak bark ♂
➻Myrrh extract
➻Bilberry
➻**Solaray CRANESBILL blend** ♀
➻Goldenseal extract

Supplements

ℛ **OPCs from grapeseed or white pine** 100mg 3x daily.

ℛ **Solaray CALCIUM CITRATE caps 4 daily.** ♀

ℛ Vitamin C therapy for collagen and interstitial tissue formation: use Ester C or ascorbic acid crystals with bioflav-onoids and rutin. Take up to 5000mg daily.
and/or
➻Quercetin with bromelain 4 daily.

ℛ Vitamin K 100mcg 3x daily to maintain micro-flora integrity.

ℛ **Propolis tincture; apply directly, and take internally 4x daily.** ♂

ℛ Vitamin E 400IU and selenium 200mcg for blood building.

ℛ **Effective homeopathic remedies:** especially for clotting difficulties from dental or cosmetic surgery:
➻*Ferrum Phos.* for bright red bleeding.
➻*Arnica* for bleeding accompanied by bruising, or nosebleeds
➻*Phosphorus* for persistent bleeding.

Lifestyle Support Therapy

☞ **Acupressure point:**
Press the insides of the thighs with the fingers just above the knees, for 10 seconds at a time.

☞ **Body pressure points:**
➻Hold arm in the air on the side of the bleeding to decrease pressure.
➻Pull knuckle of the middle finger on either hand until it pops, to lower blood pressure and tension.

☞ Apply direct pressure to a vein or artery. Get to a doctor and treat for shock.
➻Use cold cloths or ice packs.

☞ Don't use aspirin or other blood-thinning drugs such as Heparin if you are at risk for internal hemorrhaging.

☞ Sprinkle alum powder on the wound - Ayurvedic remedy.

Common Symptoms: *Inability to clot even small wounds; internal pain as with a rupture or ulcer; easy bruising and ulcerations; broken blood vessels; black stools when there are stomach ulcers.*
Common Causes: *Broken blood vessels; weak vein and vessel walls; internal wounds from a blow or accident; lack of vitamin K in the body, from heredity, or sometimes from eating irradiated foods which deplete vitamin K in the system; over-use of aspirin or other blood thinning drugs.*

See also SHOCK TREATMENT page in this book for more information.

Hemorrhoids
Piles ❀ Anal Fissure

Swollen, inflamed veins and capillaries around the anus that often protrude out of the rectum. There is usually constipation and thus, because of straining, rectal bleeding. New research also shows a link with diarrhea and hemorrhoids. The pain and discomfort of hemorrhoidal itch and swelling are well known. A change in diet composition and natural therapies can help you avoid drugs and surgery.

Diet & Superfood Therapy

Diet improvement is the key to permanently reducing hemorrhoids.

❧ Take 1 TB. olive oil or flax seed oil before each meal. Include plenty of fiber foods in your diet, particularly lots of vegetable cellulose, such as stewed and dried fruits, brans, vegetables.
—Include sprouts and dark greens for vitamin K to inhibit bleeding.
—Take 2 TBS. cider vinegar mixed with honey each morning.
—Drink plenty of healthy liquids throughout the day, like juices and mineral water and Wisdom of the Ancients YERBA MATÉ tea.
—Avoid refined, low fiber foods, and acid forming foods, such as caffeine and sugar.
—Keep meals small, so the bowel and sphincter area won't have to work so hard.

❧ Apply papaya skins or lemon juice directly to inflamed area to relieve itching. ❧

❧ Effective superfoods:
—Crystal Star BIOFLAV, FIBER & C SUPPORT™ drink with bioflavonoids to increase tissue integrity.
—YSK WAKASA CHLORELLA GOLD.
—AloeLife ALOE GOLD drink and apply ALOE SKIN GEL to hemorrhoids.
—Liquid chlorophyll 3 teasp. daily.

Herbal Therapy

❧ Jump start herbal program:
—**Crystal Star HEMR-EASE™ capsules for 2 weeks to relieve inflammation and encourage healing. (May also be used as a suppository).**
—**Crystal Star HEMR-EASE GEL™ with VITAMIN C or ANTI-BIO™ gel with una da gato.**
—Add GINKGO BILOBA extract, or Solaray CENTELLA caps for vascular tone.
—Add LIV-ALIVE™ tea to clear sluggishness, and BWL-TONE IBS™ caps or butcher's broom tea for gentle healing.

❧ Healing suppositories: use cocoa butter as the delivery medium.
—Goldenseal/myrrh
—Slippery elm
—Garlic/comfrey
—Cranesbill/yarrow ♀
—White oak bark/yarrow ♂

❧ Apply calendula ointment. Take stone root tea, 3 cups daily for a month.

❧ **Hemorrhoid tea:** mix equal parts comfrey root, wild yam, and cranesbill. Take internally and apply directly.

❧ **For anal fissure:** take internally and apply Crystal Star ANTI-BIO™ caps; apply ANTI-BIO™ gel with una da gato.

Supplements

❧ Vitamin C therapy for collagen and interstitial tissue formation: use Ester C or ascorbic acid crystals with bioflavs. and rutin. Take up to 5000mg. daily; make a solution in water to apply directly.
—Add Source Naturals activated quercetin with bromelain 4 daily, or PCOs from grapeseed or white pine, 2 daily.
—Bromelain 1500mg caps with lecithin caps 1900gr daily.

❧ Vitamin K 100mcg 2x daily with Vitamin B_6 250mg daily.

❧ NatureAde SOFT-EX tablets to soften stool short term. ♂

❧ Enzymatic Therapy HEMTONE capsules to stop rectal bleeding with THYMU-PLEX tabs 3x daily. ♀

❧ Vitamin E 400IU daily. Also apply to inflamed area for healing.

❧ BioForce *Hemorrhoid Relief* homeopathic remedy.

❧ Use a bee pollen 1000mg tablet as a suppository. Insert 1 daily.

❧ EVENING PRIMROSE oil caps 4 daily. ♀

Lifestyle Support Therapy

☞ Effective rectal applications:
—Ice packs
—Witch hazel - apply as needed.
—Hylands HEMMOREX.
—MotherLove RHOID BALM or SITZ BATH.

☞ Effective enemas: ♀
—Nettles ♀
—Chlorella or spirulina
—Cayenne/garlic
—Nutribiotic GRAPEFRUIT SEED extract - 20 drops per gallon of water.

☞ Effective compresses:
Alternating hot and cool water to stimulate circulation, or cold water compresses every morning.
—Horsetail tea - frequently
—Elderberry
—Butcher's broom ♂

☞ Take a good half hour walk every day.
—Put feet on a stool when sitting on the toilet to ease strain.

☞ Reflexology points:

colon and rectum points

See also COLON HEALTH & CONSTIPATION pages for more information.

Common Symptoms: *Pain, itching and rectal bleeding with bowel movements; inflamed anal fissure; protruding swellings.*
Common Causes: *Junk food diet with too many refined, fried, fatty, low residue foods and not enough healthy hydrating liquids; constipation with habitual straining; pregnancy; overeating; lack of exercise, too much sitting; Vit. B_6 deficiency; acid/alkaline imbalance, especially from drugs such as anti-depressants and pain killers, or antacids and laxative abuse; liver exhaustion; allergies; obesity; diarrhea.*

Hepatitis

Severe Viral Liver Infection ✣ Jaundice

*There are several types of viral hepatitis. **Type A:** a viral infection passed through blood and feces; **Type B:** a sexually transmitted viral infection carried through blood, semen, saliva and dirty needles; sometimes develops into chronic hepatitis; **Type C:** a post-transfusion form. **Type D:** caused by Epstein-Barr virus and cytomegalovirus; **Non-A, non-B:** higher mortality viruses passed through transfusion blood products, which frequently develop into chronic hepatitis. Severity of hepatitis ranges from chronic fatigue to serious liver damage, and even to death from liver failure or liver cancer. Natural therapies have had outstanding success in hepatitis cases, both in arresting viral replication, and in regeneration of the liver and its functions.*

Diet & Superfood Therapy

❧ **Hepatitis Healing Diet:**

✻**For 2 weeks:** Eat only fresh foods: salads, fruits, juices, bottled water. Take a glass of carrot/beet/cucumber juice every other day. Take a glass of lemon juice and water every morning. Take Sun CHLORELLA granules daily.

✻**Then for 1 to 2 months:** Take carrot/beet/cucumber juice every 3 days, and papaya juice with 2 teasp. spirulina each morning. Eat a high vegetable protein diet, with steamed vegetables, brown rice, tofu, eggs, whole grains and yogurt. Avoid meat protein.

✻**Then for 1 more month:** Take 2 glasses of tomato juice/wheat germ oil/brewer's yeast/lemon juice every day. Take a daily glass of apple/alfalfa sprout juice. Continue with vegetable proteins, cultured foods, fresh salads and complex carbs for strength.

❧ Avoid refined, fried, fatty foods, sugars, heavy spices, alcohol and caffeine during healing. ♀

❧ **Superfoods: green drinks are critical**
✻Nutricology PRO-GREENS with Flax.
✻Crystal Star SYSTEMS STRENGTH™ for 1 month as a drink, or for 3 months as caps.
✻Klamath BLUE GREEN SUPREME.
✻Sun CHLORELLA drink.
✻AloeLife ALOE GOLD drink with spirulina tabs 6 daily.
✻Green Foods WHEAT GERM EXTRACT.

Herbal Therapy

❧ **Jump start herbal program:**
Crystal Star LIV-ALIVE™ capsules 46 daily, with LIV ALIVE™ tea 2 cups daily for 1 month. Reduce dose to half the 2nd month.
✻Add HEARTSEASE/ANEMIGIZE™ caps to build blood, and ANTI-HST™ caps as needed to control histamine reactions for 1 month. Reduce dose to half 2nd month.
✻Add GINSENG/LICORICE ELIXIR™ to rebuild normalize liver function. ♂
✻Nutribiotic GRAPEFRUIT SEED extract 10 drops 3x daily for 1 month in juice. Also apply to lesions, or apply Crystal Star ANTI-BIO™ gel™ to lesions.
✻For long term liver support: use MILK THISTLE SEED extract BITTERS & LEMON CLEANSE™ each morning for 3 months.
✻Echinacea/St. John's wort therapy for lymphatic support: alternate 4 days of ECHINACEA extract and 4 days of St. John's wort extract. ♀

❧ **Liver detoxifying teas:**
✻Oregon grape/red clover
✻Gotu kola/licorice root
✻Pau d'arco/calendula

❧ **Effective liver tonics:**
✻Dandelion root extract.
✻Astragalus extract under the tongue.
✻Lobelia extract in water.
✻Reishi mushroom or GINSENG/REISHI extract. ♀

Supplements

✷ Beta carotene 150,000IU daily, with B Complex 150mg, and Nature's Bounty internasal B₁₂ gel daily for 1 month and extra folic acid 800mcg. Then reduce beta carotene to 50,000IU, and B Complex to 100mg daily.
✷Take Ascorbate Vitamin C crystals, up to 10,000mg daily in water, to bowel tolerance for 1 month.
✷Add a strong multiple vitamin/mineral such as Solaray MULTI-VITA MEGA-MINERAL.
✷Rainbow Light LIVA-GEN extract as directed, with ADVANCED ENZYME SYSTEM.

✷ Alta Health CANGEST if detection is early: Take 1 teasp. powder in water 2-3x daily for 7 days; then 1 teasp. 4x daily at meals and bedtime for 7 days.

or

✷ Natren BIFIDO FACTORS daily for 1 month, with CoQ10 60 mg 2x daily as an immune stimulant.

✷ Solaray LIPOTROPIC PLUS caps with TURMERIC extract 300mg, 1 daily. ♂
and/or
✷ Enzymatic Therapy LIVA-TOX, with THYMU-PLEX caps for thymus strength as directed with THISTLE-PLEX. ♀

✷ Nutricology GERMANIUM 150mg daily.

Lifestyle Support Therapy

Count on 2 weeks for emergency detox measures; 1-3 months for healing the liver and rebuilding blood and body strength.

☞ Get plenty of bed rest, especially during the acute infectious stages.

☞ Overheating therapy has been effective for Hepatitis. See page 178 in this book.

☞ **Use chlorophyll implants twice weekly for the first two critical weeks of healing to detoxify.**

☞ Avoid all alcohol, amphetamines, cocaine, barbiturates, or tobacco of any kind.

☞ Use hot castor oil packs over the liver area.

☞ **Reflexology point:**

liver

Common Symptoms: *All forms of hepatitis are characterized by great fatigue, flu-like symptoms of exhaustion and diarrhea; enlarged, tender, congested, sluggish liver; loss of appetite to the point of anorexia, nausea; dark urine, gray stools; sometimes vomiting; skin pallor and histamine itching; depression; skin jaundice; cirrhosis of the liver.*
Common Causes: *Infectious hepatitis is primarily a lifestyle disease - with almost 90% of intravenous drug users, and 85% of homosexuals infected. Others at risk include dental and medical workers, and over 25% of people receiving blood transfusions. Hepatitis can lead to liver cancer, cirrhosis and is sometimes itself fatal.*

See LIVER CLEANSING DIET and SEXUALLY TRANSMITTED DISEASES for more information.

Hiatal Hernia
Esophageal Reflux Disease (GERD)

A **hiatal hernia** occurs when a part of the stomach protrudes through the diaphragm wall, causing difficulty swallowing, acid burning and reflux in the throat, and great nervous anxiety. Today's American diet habits mean that a hiatal condition is common. **Esophageal reflux disease** is due to leaking of stomach acid back into the lower esophagus and acid coming up into the throat. This can also occur in severe cases of osteoporosis, when the rib cage and upper body have collapsed to the point where normal food transit is impeded.

Diet & Superfood Therapy

❧ Eat only raw or lightly steamed vegetable-source fiber foods during healing.
  ☛Drink 2 glasses of fresh carrot or apple juice every day.
  ☛Take 2 glasses of mineral water or aloe vera juice daily.
  ☛When digestion has normalized, follow a **low fat, low salt, high fiber diet**.
  ☛Eat smaller meals more frequently. No large meals. No liquids with meals. Eat slowly so that you are less likely to swallow air and belch.

❧ Foods that aggravate a hiatal hernia are coffee, chocolate, red meats, hard alcohol drinks, and carbonated drinks.
  ☛Eliminate fried and spicy foods because they slow the rate at which your stomach empties, allowing food to travel backwards to the esophagus. Avoid nuts, seeds, acidic juices and gas-producing foods during healing. ❧

❧ **Effective superfoods:**
  ☛AloeLife or Salutè ALOE VERA juice with herbs every morning.
  ☛Crystal Star CHO-LO FIBER TONE™ drink for gentle cleansing fiber.♂
  ☛Sun CHLORELLA 15-20 tabs daily for 1 month, or liquid chlorophyll 3 teasp. daily at meals.
  ☛Transitions EASY GREENS.

Herbal Therapy

ᴥ **Jump start herbal program:**
  ☛Crystal Star ANTI-FLAM™ caps 4 daily, and ANTI-SPZ™ caps 2 with each meal, or CRAMP BARK COMBO™ extract ½ dropperful at a time as needed for pain and spasms.
  ☛**Combine with a "bitters" formula to stimulate the liver, bile formation, fat digestion** - BITTERS & LEMON CLEANSE™ extract in the morning, or MILK THISTLE SEED extract for 1 to 3 months.
  ☛Propolis extract ½ dropperful every 4 hours during an attack.

ᴥ **Soothing, effective teas:**
  ☛Pau d' arco tea.
  ☛Chamomile tea ♀+
  ☛Licorice root
  ☛Slippery elm or marshmallow tea as needed to soothe inflamed tissue.

Supplements

ᴥ **Enzyme therapy is a key:**
  ☛Pancreatin 1400mg with meals.
  ☛Prevail DIGEST formula
  ☛Natren TRINITY.
  ☛Enzymatic Therapy CHEWABLE DGL as needed.
  ☛Bromelain 750mg as needed.
  ☛Alta Health CANGEST caps or powder 3x daily. ♀
  ☛National Enzyme Co. FORMULA #1 for proteolytic enzymes.

ᴥ Source Naturals ACTIVATED QUERCETIN or Quercetin 3 daily to reduce inflammation, **with bromelain and vitamin C for best results.**
  ☛**Enzymatic Therapy GASTRO-SOOTHE as directed.**

ᴥ Schiff EMULSIFIED A 25,000IU 2x daily.

ᴥ Zinc gluconate lozenges under the tongue as needed. ♂

Lifestyle Support Therapy

Commercial antacids often do more harm than good; they can upset stomach pH causing it to produce even more harmful acids.

☞ No smoking. Avoid all tobacco.

☞ Lose weight. Tone the abdomen with exercise. Watch posture to avoid slouching. Wear loose, comfortable, non-binding clothing.

☞ Apply a green clay pack to the area.

☞ **Reflexology point:**

— stomach and diaphragm

☞ Yellow color therapy eyewear - wear until hernia is gone, esp. during meals.

☞ Have a chiropractic adjustment to the area.

☞ To prevent night time reflux, elevate head of bed on 6 to 8" blocks. Don't eat within two hours of your bedtime.
  ☛Don't lie down after eating.

Common Symptoms: Chest pains and proneness to heartburn after eating; belching, excess gas and bloating; difficulty swallowing and a full feeling at the base of the throat; hiccups and regurgitation; pressure behind the breast-bone; raised blood pressure; diarrhea; inflammation and gastro-intestinal bleeding, usually with a stomach ulcer; mental confusion and nerves.

Common Causes: Food allergies; short esophagus; overeating; obesity; food allergies; enzyme deficiency; constipation from a low residue diet and too many refined and acid-forming foods; osteoporosis and bone collapse of upper body structure; tobacco; too tight jeans or underclothing.

See also INDIGESTION/HEARTBURN page for more information.

High Blood Pressure
Hypertension

High blood pressure is a major problem in today's fast-paced, high-stress world. It causes 60,000 deaths a year and directly relates to more than 250,000 deaths from stroke. It is a silent condition that steals health and is a precursor to serious cardiovascular disease that can steal life. Most cases of high blood pressure are caused by arteriosclerosis and atherosclerosis - factors that can be brought under control by diet and lifestyle improvement. In fact, recent clinical studies show that people with hypertension who make good life changes fare much better than those on anti-hypertensive prescription drugs.

Diet & Superfood Therapy

Keep body weight down. One of the biggest risk factors is increased fat storage.

❧ Go on a liquid juice diet for 1 day every week for 2 months to improve body chemistry and reduce excess blood fats:
—Have citrus juices or a potassium essence drink (pg. 167) in the morning. Make a mix of wheat germ, omega-3 flax oil, brewer's yeast; take 2 TBS. daily.
—Have a veggie green drink (pg. 168), V-8 juice, or carrot juice at mid-day;
—Apple, pear or papaya juice before dinne.
—Have chamomile tea or Organic Gourmet SAVORY SPREAD broth at bedtime.
—Then follow the High Blood Pressure Diet on the next page: include lots of vitamin C, magnesium and potassium-rich foods, like broccoli, bananas, dried fruits, potatoes, seafood, bell peppers, avocados, cauliflower, brown rice and leafy greens.
—Avoid refined foods, caffeine, salty, sugary, fried, fatty foods, prepared meats, heavy pastries and soft drinks. All cause potassium depletion and allow arterial plaque build-up.
❧

❧ **Effective superfoods:**
—**Sun CHLORELLA drink daily to lower blood fats, with 1TB. Body Essentials SILICA GEL mixed in the drink.**
—Salute ALOE VERA juice with herbs.
—Future Biotics VITAL K drink daily.

Herbal Therapy

❧ **Jump start herbal program:**
—**Crystal Star HEARTSEASE H.B.P.™ caps or tea daily, with POTASSIUM/IODINE SOURCE™ caps and HAWTHORN extract daily for tonic support and palpitations.**
—TINKLE™ caps for edema; ADR-ACTIVE™ for fatigue, GINKGO BILOBA for circulation, GREEN TEA CLEANSER™ for stroke risk.
—**RELAX CAPS™ or GINSENG/REISHI extract for anti-hypertension activity.**
—EVENING PRIMROSE oil for EFAs.♀♁

❧ **Effective circulation tonics:**
—**Garlic oil, or onion/garlic caps 6 daily.**
—Cayenne/ginger 4 daily, or New Moon GINGER WONDER syrup before meals.
—Suma caps 6 daily
—BILBERRY for herbal flavonoids
—Siberian ginseng extract caps.♁

❧ **Effective tension reducing herbs:**
—Hyland's *CALMS FORTE* tabs ♀♁
—Solaray EUROCALM caps.
—Ayurvedic coleus forskohlii - Enzymatic Therapy has COLEUS FORSOHLII extract.

❧ **Effective diuretic herbs:**
—Uva ursi extract
—Dandelion extract

❧ **Aromatherapy:** Lavender, marjoram, ylang ylang oils.

Supplements

Most high blood pressure medicines cause potassium and magnesium deficiency. If you are taking diuretics, supplement with vitamin C, potassium and B Complex.

❧ **Vitamin E therapy: Take 1 100IU capsule daily for 1 week, then 4 capsules daily for 1 week, then 2 400IU capsules daily for 2 weeks.**
—**Add 1 selenium 100mcg, and 1 Ester C with bioflavs each time. for hypertension caused by toxic heavy metals.**
—Add tyrosine to inhibit hypertension
—PCOs from grapeseed as antioxidants.♂

or

❧ Nature's Secret ULTIMATE B daily with extra B_6 100mg, niacin 100mg 3x daily.
—Add omega-3 fish or flax oils 3 daily, with bromelain 500mg. to digest fats, and chromium picolinate 200mcg. daily to combat insulin resistance.♁

❧ Vitamin C 3000mg daily with bioflavonoids and rutin for venous integrity.

❧ CoQ_{10} 60mg 2x daily, and Country Life RELAXER capsules with GABA, and melatonin 3mg at bedtime for 3 months.

❧ Rainbow Light CALCIUM PLUS capsules with high magnesium, 6 daily.♀

❧ **Golden Pride FORMULA ONE oral chelation a.m. and p.m. with EDTA, with gugulipids to lower cholesterol.**♂

Lifestyle Support Therapy

You have high blood pressure if you have a repeated reading over 150/90mmHg.
If you have a high blood pressure problem, monitor your progress often with a home or free drugstore electronic machine reading.

❧ Avoid tobacco in all forms to dramatically lower blood pressure. Smoking also aggravates high blood sugar levels. Eliminate caffeine and hard liquor. (A little wine at night with dinner is fine, and can actually lower stress and hypertension.)

❧ Exercise is important. Take a brisk 30 minute walk every day, with plenty of deep lung breathing.
—Relaxation techniques are very important. Massage and meditation are two of the best for hypertension.

❧ Use a dry skin brush all over the body frequently to stimulate circulation.

❧ **Reflexology point:**
—Pull middle finger on each hand 3x for 20 seconds each time, daily.

❧ Avoid phenylalanine (especially as found in Nutra-Sweet) and over-the-counter antihistamines.

Common Symptoms: *Headaches; irritability; dizziness and ringing in the ears; flushed complexion; red streaks in the eyes; fatigue and sleeplessness; edema; frequent urination; depression; heart arrhythmia; chronic respiratory problems.*

Common Causes: *Clogging arterial fats and increased fat storage; calcium/fiber deficiency; thickened blood from excess mucous and waste; insulin resistance and poor sugar metabolism; thyroid imbalance; obesity; lack of aerobic exercise; too much salt and red meat, causing raised copper levels; kidney malfunction; auto-toxemia from constipation; prostaglandin imbalance.*

See the HEALTHY HEART pages in this book for more information.

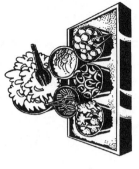

High Blood Pressure Prevention Diet

Eighty-five percent of high blood pressure is both treatable and preventable without drugs. The most beneficial thing you can do to reduce high blood pressure is a diet change. Reduce and control salt use. (See About Low Salt Diets, pg. 209). Eat smaller meals more frequently; consciously undereat. It is worth noting that vegetarians have less hypertension and fewer blood pressure problems. Lifestyle change must be made for there to be permanent control of high blood pressure. Pay conscious attention at first to eliminating foods that aggravate high blood pressure - red meats, caffeine, fried and fatty foods, soft drinks, refined pastry, salty foods and prepared meats, but the rewards are high - a longer, healthier life - and control of your life.

On rising: Have a glass of lemon water and honey, and/or a high vitamin/mineral drink such as Nutri-Tech ALL 1 or Crystal Star SYSTEMS STRENGTH™ drink.

Breakfast: Make a mix of 2 TBS. each: lecithin granules, wheat germ, brewer's yeast, honey, and sesame seeds. Sprinkle some on fresh fruit or mix with yogurt; and/or have a poached or baked egg with bran muffins or whole grain toast, and kefir cheese or unsalted butter; or some whole grain cereal or pancakes with a little maple syrup.

Mid-morning: Have a veggie drink (pg. 168) or Sun CHLORELLA or Crystal Star ENERGY GREEN™ drink, or Green Foods GREEN ESSENCE, or natural V-8 juice or mint tea: and/or a cup of miso soup with sea veggies snipped on top, or low-sodium ramen noodle soup; and/or some crunchy raw veggies with a kefir cheese or yogurt dip.

Lunch: Have one cup daily of fenugreek tea with 1 teasp. honey, and 1 teasp. wheat germ oil;
then have a tofu and spinach salad with some sprouts and bran muffins;
or a large fresh green salad with a lemon oil dressing. Add plenty of sprouts, tofu, raisins, cottage cheese, nuts, and seeds as desired;
or have a baked potato with yogurt or kefir cheese topping, and a light veggie omelet;
or a seafood and vegetable pasta salad;
or some grilled or braised vegetables with an olive oil dressing and brown rice;
or a high protein whole grain sandwich, with avocados and low fat or soy cheese.

Mid-afternoon: Have a bottle of mineral water, a cup of peppermint tea, or a tea made from Crystal Star GINSENG/LICORICE ELIXIR™ extract, or ROYAL MU™ tonic tea. and/or a cup of miso soup with a hard boiled egg, or whole grain crackers; or some dried fruits, and an apple or cranberry juice.

Dinner: Have a baked vegetable casserole with tofu and brown rice, and a small dinner salad;
or a baked fish or seafood dish with rice and peas, or a baked potato;
or a vegetable quiche (such as broccoli, artichoke, or asparagus), and a light oriental soup;
or some roast turkey and cornbread dressing, with a small salad or mashed potatoes with a little butter;
or an oriental vegetable and seafood or chicken stirfry, with a light, clear soup and brown rice;
  • A little white wine is fine with dinner for relaxation, digestion and tension relief.

Before bed: Have a cup of miso soup, or Organic Gourmet NUTRITIONAL YEAST OR MISO broth, apple juice, or some chamomile tea.

Note #1: Particular foods to eliminate if you have high blood pressure: canned and frozen foods, cured, smoked and canned meats and fish, commercial peanut butter, soy sauce, bouillon cubes and condiments, fried chips and snacks, canned and dry soups.
Note #2: Avoid commercial antacids that neutralize natural stomach acid and invite the body to produce even more acid, thus aggravating stress and tension.

SUGGESTED SUPPLEMENTS FOR THE HIGH BLOOD PRESSURE PREVENTION DIET:
• Siberian ginseng extract caps, 2000mg, or extract, ¹/₂ dropperful daily.
• Vitamin C 3000mg daily with bioflavonoids, or Crystal Star BIOFLAVONOID, FIBER & C SUPPORT™ drink.
• EVENING PRIMROSE OIL caps, 2 to 4 daily with vitamin. E and selenium 400IU daily, or Omega-3 oils, from flax or cold water fish, 1000mg daily.
• Sun CHLORELLA, 1 packet granules, or 15 tabs daily, or Klamath POWER 3 caps.
• Aloe vera juice with herbs for digestion.

☞ Regular exercise is a key factor in circulatory health. Take a brisk walk every day.

Hormone Imbalance Problems

Rebalancing For Men ✳ Rebalancing For Women

Hormones help regulate everything from energy flow; to inflammation; to a woman's monthly cycle; to a man's hair growth. Using lifestyle therapy to rebalance hormone ratios gently harmonizes your body, rather than regulating hormone levels by injection; especially after trauma, stress or serious illness, such as prostate or testicular problems for men, and after a hysterectomy, childbirth, a D & C, or an abortion for a woman. This allows the body to achieve its own hormone levels and bring itself to its own balance at its deepest levels.

Diet & Superfood Therapy

♋ Start with a modified macrobiotic diet for 2 weeks (pg. 211) with seasonal fresh foods, whole grains, brown rice and vegetable protein.

✹Make a hormone balance mix of wheat germ oil, lecithin granules, brewers yeast and flax oil: add 1 TB. to a fruit smoothie each morning.

✹Add soy foods (tofu, tempeh, soy milk, etc.) to your diet for hormone normalizing isoflavones.

✹Add complex carbohydrate-rich, building foods to your diet: broccoli, peas, cauliflower, yams, wheat germ, nuts and seeds, and whole grains

✹Drink 6 glasses of bottled water daily.

✹Avoid sugary foods, refined foods and canned foods.

ॐ

♋ **Effective superfoods:**
✹Nutricology PRO-GREENS.
✹Solgar WHEY TO GO protein drink.
✹Nappi THE PERFECT MEAL.
✹Crystal Star ENERGY GREEN™.
✹Transitions EASY GREENS.
✹Green Foods GREEN MAGMA daily.
✹Beehive Botanical ROYAL JELLY/ GINSENG drink.
✹AloeLife aloe juice 2-4 TBS. daily.

Herbal Therapy

✍ **Jump start herbal program:**
For male hormone balance: Crystal Star MALE PERFORMANCE™ capsules for 3 months.

✹SIBERIAN GINSENG extract daily.
✹GINSENG/LICORICE ELIXIR™.

✍ Effective hormone combinations:
✹Panax ginseng/Damiana
✹Panax ginseng/Sarsaparilla
✹Licorice root/Dandelion root

✍ Smilax extract 10-15 drops daily with Beehive Botanical ROYAL JELLY/GINSENG/POLLEN caps.

✍ **For female hormone balance:** Crystal Star FEM-SUPPORT™ extract, or FEMALE HARMONY™ caps or tea, with EVENING PRIMROSE OIL 1000mg 2 daily, or VITEX extract.
✹PRO-EST BALANCE™ roll-on.

✍ Y.S. ROYAL JELLY/GINSENG drink with VITEX or dong quai/damiana extract.

✍ **For both sexes:** Crystal Star ADR-ACTIVE™ capsules or extract with FEEL GREAT™ caps or tea.

✹Y.S. GINSENG/HONEY tea.
✹Rainbow Light ADAPTO-GEM caps.

Supplements

If you are taking synthetic estrogen or progesterone for glandular problems, it can destroy vitamin E in the body, allowing greater risk for heart, cancer and other diseases. Supplementation is advisable to counteract this.

◐ **For male hormone balance:**
✹Cal/mag/zinc 4 daily, or zinc 75mg.
✹Carnitine helps sperm cells "swim" to their destination. Men with low sperm motility have low carnitine.
✹Raw glandular therapy includes: raw pancreas, raw orchic, and raw pituitary.

◐ L-Glutamine 500mg 4x daily to stimulate the pituitary to produce rejuvenating growth hormone.

◐ **For female balance:**
✹Optimal Nutrients DHEA or Body Ammo FOUNTAIN of YOUTH creme.
✹B Complex 100mg daily with extra pantothenic acid 1000mg.

◐ **For both sexes:**
✹Long Life IMPERIAL TONIC with royal jelly and evening primrose oil.

◐ **Effective GLA sources for EFAs:**
✹Evening primrose oil 2-4 daily.
✹Twin Lab MAX-EPA
✹Nature's Secret ULTIMATE OIL.

Lifestyle Support Therapy

Note: Muscle Testing (Applied Kinesiology), is useful for determining which hormonal herbs or supplements are specific to an individual problem. Once the simple technique is learned, (see a nutritional consultant, a holistic chiropractor, or a massage therapist, or page 445 in this book), it can easily be done at home to determine which supplements are right for your condition.

☞ Relaxation techniques for hormone balance:
✹Chiropractic adjustment. ♂
✹**Massage therapy treatment, to reestablish unblocked meridians of energy and increase circulation.**
✹**Abdominal breathing.**
✹Yoga stretches every morning.

☞ Take a good brisk exercise walk every day.

☞ Get morning sunlight on the body every day possible, on the genitalia for men, on the arms for women.

Common Symptoms: For Women: *painful, difficult menstruation, or absence of menstruation; spotting between periods; depression; mood swings and irritability; water retention.*
For Men: *Prostate pain and inflammation; lack of abdominal tone; poor urinary and sexual function.*
Common Causes: *Birth control pills or vasectomy; adrenal exhaustion due to stress; severe dieting or body building; surgery or long illness; protein or iodine deficiency; calcium deficiency; B Complex or EFA deficiencies; hysterectomy; synthetic steroid use.*

See the following pages and the Gland Health pages for more information.

Hormones Are Incredibly Important To Our Health

Hormones are incredibly minute glandular secretions, produced from chemical substances called steroids. Steroids affect the part of the brain that influences sexual behavior. In men, the prostate and testes release the essential male hormone testosterone. In women, the ovaries secrete the sex hormones estrogen and progesterone. But, estrogens, female hormones, and androgens, male hormones, occur in both sexes, just in different ratios and amounts.

Women with hysterectomies are only beginning to see the harm that removing delicate glands, or treating fragile hormones with drugs can do.

Science has long debated whether a vasectomy, the contraceptive procedure which severs or seals off the vessel that carries sperm from the testes, increases the risk of prostate cancer in men. New studies on two large groups of men, show that vasectomies do increase risk of prostate cancer. In one study of 73,000 men, 300 of the men developed prostate cancer between 1986 and 1990. The men with vasectomies had a 66% greater risk of prostate cancer than did the men without vasectomies. In a separate study, vasectomies increased the risk of prostate cancer by 56%. As sperm builds up in the sealed-off vas deferens after a vasectomy, the body re-absorbs the cells. This confuses the immune system, making it less alert to tumor cells. Sometimes the body's immune defenses try to mount a response against its own tissue. In addition, a vasectomy affects hormone secretions in the testes, and lowers prostatic fluid. When the natural movement of sperm and hormones is artificially prevented, a host of male health problems result.

What About Environmental Hormones?

Pesticides, plastics, herbicides and a wealth of other new chemicals contain man-made estrogens. People are assaulted today by hormones in meats, dairy products, and drugs such as hormone replacement therapies for both sexes. Only in the last five years has anyone realized how common environmental estrogens are in today's world. Science is just beginning to accept, although naturopaths have known for some time, that man-made estrogens, also called environmental or xenoestrogens, can stack the deck against women by increasing their estrogen levels hundreds of times.

There is a link between pesticides and breast cancer. Pesticides, like other pollutants, are stored in body fat areas like breast tissue. Some pesticides including PCB's and DDT compromise immune function, overwork the liver and affect the glands and hormones the way too much estrogen does. One study shows 50 to 60% more dichloro-diphenyl-ethylene (DDE) and polychlorinated bi-phenols, (PCB's) in women who have breast cancer than in those who dont. The quantity of DDT in body tissues is also higher. In fact, some researchers suggest that the reason older women are experiencing a higher rate of breast cancer may be that these women had greater exposure to DDT before it was banned. The dramatic rise in breast cancer is consistent with the accumulation of organo-chlorine residues in the environment. Israel's recent history offers a case study. Until about 20 years ago, both breast cancer rates and contamination levels of organo-chlorine pesticides in Israel were among the highest in the world. An aggressive phase-out of these pesticides has led to a sharp reduction in contamination levels, followed by a dramatic drop in breast cancer death rates.

Women aren't the only ones endangered by the estroger-imitating effects of chemicals and pesticides. Although controversial, there is substantial evidence that supports the role played by man-made estrogens in hormone imbalances that threaten male health and fertility, too. The most alarming statistics relate to sperm count and hormone driven cancers. The dramatic rise in prostate cancer deaths over the last 40 years is another wake-up call to change our environment for health.

While the rate of prostate cancer has doubled since World War II, male sperm counts have declined by half - a trend that has led to speculation that environmental, dietary, and lifestyle changes in recent decades are interfering with a man's ability to manufacture sperm. Semen analysis tests of both sperm count and quality over the last few decades show us undeniably that total sperm count as well as sperm quality of the general male population has been deteriorating. In 1940, the average sperm count was 113 million per ml. In 1993 that value had dropped to 65 million. Total amount of semen has also fallen dramatically, from 3.5ml in 1940 to 2.74ml in 1993. These changes mean that men have only about 39% of the sperm counts they had in 1940.

The greatest threat comes from industrial chemicals, like poly-chlorinated bi-phenols,(PCBs), as well as dioxin, and pesticides used for agriculture. I recommend that men especially avoid hormone-injected meats and dairy products, and herbicide-sprays to avoid the exogenous estrogen factor.

There is grim news about estrogenic chemicals and developing fetuses, too. Male and female hormones must remain in balance in an embryo for sexual organs to develop normally. In early stages, a fetus is capable of developing either set. Hormone balance determines whether the child will be male or female. Exogenous estrogens can upset this balance, resulting in children with stunted male sex organs or with both sets of sex organs.

What About Plant or Phyto-Hormones?

Plant or phyto-hormones are remarkably similar to human hormones. They can be accepted by hormone receptor sites in our bodies, and, at $1/_{400th}$ to $1/_{50,000th}$ the strength of human hormones, they are extremely gentle and safe, exerting a tonic, nourishing effect rather than drug-like activity. Although used for centuries by both men and women, we are just beginning to understand their power and properties for modern needs. Recent studies on soy foods and herbs such as ginseng, black cohosh and wild yam clearly show hormone-normalizing effects. See MENOPAUSE pages for more complete information about both synthetic and phyto-hormones.

Controlling Specific Problems Involved With Hormone Imbalance

Deficient hormone secretions can be caused by, or lead to, other conditions, like hot flashes, night sweats, contraceptive and synthetic hormone side effects, frigidity, low libido and prostaglandin imbalance.

❧**FOR HOT FLASHES & NIGHT SWEATS:** Crystal Star EST-AID™ capsules and/or FEM-SUPPORT™ extract; Body Ammo DHEA cream (from soy) with VITEX extract; vitamin E 800IU; EVENING PRIMROSE OIL caps 500mg 4 daily; Nature's Secret ULTIMATE B daily with Ester C 1000 to 3000mg daily.

❧**TO OVERCOME SIDE EFFECTS FROM SYNTHETIC HORMONES OR BIRTH CONTROL PILLS:** Nature's Plus vitamin E 800IU, Country Life MAXINE capsules daily, B Complex 100mg daily, with extra B$_6$ 250mg, sub-lingual B$_{12}$ and folic acid 800mg daily; emulsified A & D 25,000IU/1,000IU; Ester C 550mg with bioflavonoids, 6 daily; Solaray CALCIUM CITRATE SUPREME capsules, 4-6 daily; Crystal Star FEM-SUPPORT™ extract 2-3x daily.

❧**FOR FRIGIDITY, PAINFUL INTERCOURSE, OR DRY VAGINA:** (*See MENOPAUSE page in this book for more information.*) High potency YS or Premier 1 royal jelly 2 teasp. daily, and/or YS GINSENG TEA with honey, 1 cup daily; vitamin E 800IU, EVENING PRIMROSE OIL, 4 daily for EFAs, with extra B$_6$ 250mg, Transitions PRO-GEST cream, rubbed on the abdomen regularly, Country Life MAXINE capsules, 2-3 daily, Crystal Star WOMEN'S DRYNESS™ extract as needed, LOVE CAPS FEMALE™, FEM-SUPPORT™ extract and CUPID'S FLAME™ tea, Country Life ADRENAL with TYROSINE, or Enzymatic Therapy THYROID with TYROSINE capsules, 4 daily.

❧**TO REBALANCE PROSTAGLANDIN FORMATION:** (Prostaglandin imbalance can lead to breast and uterine fibroids, arthritis, eczema, menstrual difficulties, high blood pressure and cholesterol, and a tendency to gain weight.) Avoid saturated fats, especially from red meats and pasteurized, full fat dairy products. Take high Omega-3 oils from cold water fish or flax seed oil 3x daily. Or use EVENING PRIMROSE or Nature's Secret ULTIMATE OIL capsules 4-6 daily for 3 months.

✂

What About Male Impotence and Infertility?

Many men are concerned about their ability to achieve or maintain an erection, premature ejaculation, the frequency with which they are able to have intercourse and the recovery period in between. Male infertility is also reaching alarming proportions today for a wide variety of lifestyle and environmental reasons. For most men, these are problems of the dinner table, not the bedroom. Stress reduction techniques like hypnotherapy, and natural therapies for reversing infertility have been notably successful for men, because poor nutrition and emotional stress are so clearly implicated as causes. Hypoglycemia, depression, marijuana and/or other pleasure drug use, arteriosclerosis, environmental or heavy metal poisoning, too much alcohol and tobacco and protein deficiency also contribute to impotence.

The first step is to lose weight if you are overweight. Many men can correct their weight simply by improving their diet. Junk, chemical-laced, and processed foods are undeniably a factor in male weight control problems **and** impotence. Eat a high vegetable protein diet, with plenty of whole grains and soy foods. Take a high protein drink every morning, such as Solgar WHEY TO GO. Include a green leafy salad every day. Add plenty of potassium and selenium-rich foods. Avoid red meats (they may contain exogenous estrogens), and prepared meats, such as luncheon or sandwich meats, that contain nitrates. Reduce dietary salt and sugar.

Make and take a "potent-C" drink every morning for 3 months: For 4 drinks, blender blend: 1 cup sliced strawberries, 1 banana, 1 cup papaya chunks, 1 cup pineapple/coconut juice, 1 cup amazake rice drink, 2 TBS. honey, 2 TBS. toasted wheat germ, 2 TBS. pumpkin seeds, 2 TBS. lecithin, 2 TB. brewer's yeast, 1 egg, 1 TB. sesame seeds, 2 teasp. vanilla.

Herbs to consider for hormonal energy and libido include: Crystal Star LOVING MOOD FOR MEN™ extract, SUPER MAN'S ENERGY TONIC™ or LOVE CAPS MALE™ caps, and Strength Systems YOHIMBE with tyrosine 500mg. daily (use with caution), or Unipro LIQUID DMG daily for fastaction. Crystal Star MALE PERFORMANCE™ caps and MALE GINSIAC™ extract for long term hormone building. To increase sperm count, take licorice/damiana caps, highest potency royal jelly 2 teasp. daily. or Crystal Star GINSENG/ LICORICE ELIXIR™ 2x daily, for several months. Avoid clothing and tiny bicycle seats that holds the testes too close to the body. (Body heat hampers sperm production.) Also avoid electric blankets, hot tubs and saunas because of too much heat. For sperm agglutination, take vitamin C 3-5000mg daily.

Ginseng formulas are clearly helpful. Ginseng is a regenerative herb (the only herb that tests positively for plant testosterone). It does not make the normal male body into a superman. Good examples include: ginseng/royal jelly ampules, Siberian ginseng extract, Chinese red ginseng caps, ginseng/sarsaparilla caps, ginseng/damiana caps, ginseng/cayenne capsules, ginseng/gotu kola caps, Ho-Shou-Wu, BioForce GINSAVENA extract, PEP COBRA tabs as desired.

Supplements for male potency include: Crystal Star PRO-EST PROX™ roll-on; Heart Foods KEEP IT UP to help erection; EVENING PRIMROSE or Nature's Secret ULTIMATE OIL capsules, 4 daily; Country Life MAX caps daily with zinc 50mg daily, niacin 50mg daily (not niacinimide), up to 3000mg daily for circulation, Alta Health magnesium chloride 6 daily on a full stomach, for 1 week, then 3 daily for 3 weeks. Raw glandular therapy for male impotence includes Solaray MALE CAPS with orchic extract, raw pituitary, Country Life MAX caps with orchic, adrenal and prostate. (Take glandulars with tyrosine and carnitine 500mg **each,** and vitamin E 400IU for best results.

Lifestyle is a key factor in impotency - stop smoking, using hard liquor and recreational drugs. Get regular exercise; breath deeply as you do it. Get early morning sunlight on the body and genitals when possible. Take alternating hot and cool showers for circulation. Squeeze testicles daily to stimulate them, one squeeze for each year of your life.

✂

Hypoglycemia
Low Blood Sugar

Hypoglycemia, often called a "sugar epidemic" today, is a condition in which the pancreas regularly overreacts to repeated high sugar intake by producing too much insulin. Excess insulin results in lowering blood sugar too much as the body strives to achieve proper glucose/insulin balance. This is particularly harmful to the brain, the most sensitive organ to blood sugar levels, which requires glucose as an energy source to think clearly. Hypoglycemia causes a change in the way the brain functions. Small fluctuations disturb one's feeling of well-being. Large fluctuations cause feelings of depression, anxiety, mood swings, fatigue and even aggressive behavior. Sugar balance is also needed for muscle contractions, the digestive system and nerve health.

Diet & Superfood Therapy

Nutrient deficiencies always accompany hypoglycemia. A healthy diet is critical.

🌿 Go on a 24 hour liquid diet (pg. 158) if low blood sugar symptoms appear regularly. Add a high nutrient, sugar-free protein powder (see below). A feeling of well-being will return rapidly.

—Sugar and refined carbohydrates must be avoided. Omit natural sugars, too, such as honey, molasses, maple syrup, and alcohol until sugar balance is achieved.

—Include some vegetable protein at every meal. Include high fiber foods to help stabilize blood sugar swings.

—Add whole grains, fresh fruits and vegetables, low fat dairy products, seafoods, sea vegetables, soy foods and brown rice frequently. Eat plenty of cultured foods such as yogurt and kefir for G.I. flora.

—Reduce full fat dairy, fried, fatty foods, fast foods, pastries, red and prepared meats.

—Eliminate alcohol (the worst for hypoglycemics), refined foods, caffeine, preserved foods and red meats permanently.

🌿 Effective superfoods: protein drinks help build a "floor" under a sugar drop.
—Nature's Life SUPER GREEN PRO.
—Nappi THE PERFECT MEAL
—Crystal Star ENERGY GREEN™ drink
—Lewis Labs BREWER'S YEAST.
—BE WELL juices during a sugar drop.

Herbal Therapy

🌿 Jump start herbal program:
Crystal Star SUGAR STRATEGY LOW™ capsules and tea, with ADR-ACTIVE™ caps or ADRN™ extract to nourish exhausted adrenals.
—GINSENG 6 SUPER TEA™ to help remove sugar from the blood.
—CHO-LO FIBER TONE™ or other good fiber cleanse morning and evening to absorb unnecessary carbohydrates and balance sugar curve.

🌿 Tonics for adrenal support:
—Beehive Botanical or Y.S. ROYAL JELLY WITH GINSENG caps or drink.
—EVENING PRIMROSE OIL caps.
—Gotu kola caps.

🌿 To help stabilize blood sugar swings:
—Crystal Star GINSENG/LICORICE ELIXIR™ as needed.
—1 teasp. each: spirulina granules, and bee pollen granules in a fruit juice, or Nutrex HAWAIIAN SPIRULINA, between meals.
—AloeLife ALOE GOLD concentrate 1 teasp. 3x daily before meals.

Supplements

Glucose homeostasis depends on a wide range of micro-nutrients - many of which are in short supply in the American diet.

❧ Effective chromium therapy choices:
—GTF Chromium 200mcg.
—Solaray CHROMIACIN.
—Chromium picolinate 200mcg daily.
—DMG B_{15} 125mg SL
—American Biologics VANADIUM.

❧ Enzyme therapy is important:
—Pancreatin with meals
—Prevail GLUCOSE FORMULA
—Alta Health CANGEST

❧ B Complex 100mg 2x daily with extra PABA 100mg, and pantothenic acid 500mg.
and
—Vitamin C 3000mg w. bioflavonoids. (Take vitamin C immediately during an attack).

❧ CoQ10 60mg 3x daily for 3-6 weeks,

❧ American Biologics MANGANESE.

❧ Country Life GLYCEMIC FACTORS and MOOD FACTORS capsules as needed.

❧ Glutamine 500mg daily. ♂

❧ Enzymatic Therapy HYPO-ADE caps, with RAW ADRENAL.

Lifestyle Support Therapy

Hypoglycemia and diabetes stem from the same causes. Hypoglycemia is regularly a way station on the road to serious diabetes. Lifestyle changes for hypoglycemia pay off handsomely for total health, too.

🌿 Eat 6 to 8 mini-meals throughout the day to keep blood sugar levels up. Large meals throw sugar balance way off, especially at night.

🌿 Eat relaxed, never under stress.
—Relaxation techniques that are successful for hypoglycemia include regular massage therapy treatments

🌿 Get some exercise everyday to work off unmetabolized acid wastes.

🌿 Some oral contraceptives can cause glucose intolerance and poor sugar metabolism. Ask your doctor.

🌿 Reflexology point:

pancreas

Common Symptoms: Manic/depressive psychological states; irritability, often violence; restlessness and insomnia; anxiety, depression and a feeling of going crazy; dizziness, general shakiness and trembling; ravenous hunger and craving for sweets; heart problems; lethargy or hyperactivity; nausea; blurry vision; frequent headaches or migraines; great fatigue.

Common Causes: Poor diet or excess dietary sugar causing abnormally low levels of glucose in the blood; poor pancreas function; drinking alcohol on an empty stomach; prolonged fasting or dieting for weight loss; food allergies; too much alcohol, caffeine or nicotine; stress; exhausted adrenals, kidney failure or liver damage; hypothyroidism; too large meals.

See next page and Low Blood Sugar Test on page 450 for more information.

Diet For Hypoglycemia Control

The two key factors in hypoglycemia are stress and poor diet. Both are a result of too much sugar and refined carbohydrates. These foods quickly raise glucose levels, causing the pancreas to over-compensate and produce too much insulin, which then lowers body glucose levels too far and too fast. The following diet supplies the body with high fiber, complex carbohydrates and proteins - slow even-burning fuel, that prevents these sudden sugar elevations and drops. Small frequent meals should be eaten, with plenty of fresh foods to keep sugar levels in balance. I recommend a diet like this for 2 to 3 months until blood sugar levels are regularly stable. Other watchwords: 1) Eat potassium-rich foods, such as oranges, broccoli, bananas, and tomatoes. 2) Eat chromium-rich foods, such as brewer's yeast, mushrooms, whole wheat, sea foods, beans and peas. 3) Eat some high quality vegetable protein at every meal.

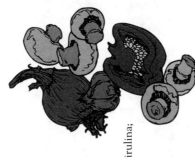

On rising: take a "hypoglycemia cocktail," 1 teasp. each in apple or orange juice to control morning sugar drop: glycine powder, powdered milk, protein powder, and brewer's yeast;
or a protein/amino drink, such as Nature's Life SUPER GREEN PRO or Crystal Star SYSTEMS STRENGTH™.

Breakfast: a very important meal for hypoglycemia, should include ¹⁄₃ of daily nutrients; have some oatmeal with yogurt and fresh fruit;
or poached or baked eggs on whole grain toast with a little butter or kefir cheese;
or a whole grain cereal or granola with apple juice, soy milk or fruit, yogurt and nuts;
or some whole grain pancakes with an apple or fruit sauce;
or some tofu scrambled "eggs" with bran muffins, whole grain toast and a little butter.

Mid-morning: have a veggie drink (page 168), Green Foods GREEN MAGMA with 1 teasp. Bragg's LIQUID AMINOS, or Crystal Star ENERGY GREEN™ drink as a liver nutrient;
and/or a balancing herb tea, such as licorice, dandelion, or Crystal Star SUGAR STRATEGY LOW™ tea;
and some crisp, crunchy vegetables with kefir or yogurt cheese;
or cornbread or whole grain crackers, or bran muffins with butter or kefir cheese.

Lunch: have a fresh salad, with a little cottage cheese or soy cheese, nut, noodle or seed toppings, and lemon oil dressing;
and/or a high protein sandwich on whole grain bread, with avocados, low fat cheese, and mayonnaise;
or a bean or lentil soup with a tofu or shrimp salad or sandwich;
or a seafood and whole grain pasta salad;
or a vegetarian pizza on a chapati crust with low fat or soy mozzarrella cheese.

Mid-afternoon: have a hard boiled egg with sesame salt, and whole grain crackers with yogurt dip;
and/or a licorice herb tea, such as Crystal Star GINSENG/LICORICE ELIXIR™ in water, another green drink, such as Klamath BLUE GREEN SUPREME with spirulina;
or yogurt with nuts and seeds.

Dinner: have some steamed veggies with tofu, or baked or broiled fish and brown rice;
or an oriental stir fry with seafood and vegetables, and miso soup with sea vegetables;
or a whole grain or vegetable Italian pasta dish with a verde sauce and hearty soup; add green beans for good pancreatic support.
or a Spanish beans and rice dish, or paella with seafood and rice;
or a veggie quiche on whole grain crust and a small mushroom and spinach salad;
or roast turkey with cornbread stuffing and a light soup.
  * Before bed: have a cup of Organic Gourmet NUTRITIONAL YEAST or MISO broth; or papaya juice with a little yogurt.

♪Suggested supplements for the Hypoglycemia Control Diet:
•To support adrenal glands depleted by stress and hypoglycemic reactions, take B complex 100mg, and vitamin C 3000-5000mg daily, (or immediately during a sugar drop attack).
    or Crystal Star ADR-ACTIVE™ caps or ADRN™ extract, or Enzymatic Therapy RAW ADRENAL extract; and/or add 2 teasp. daily of YS ROYAL JELLY to a protein or green drink.
•To balance sugar use in the bloodstream, take GTF chromium or chromium picolinate 200mcg, or Solaray CHROMIACIN daily, with DMG B₁₅ sublingually.
•To improve carbohydrate digestion, take Alta Health CANGEST, with spirulina or bee pollen granules, morning and evening.
•To increase oxygen uptake and add minerals, take CoQ10 60mg and Mezotrace SEA MINERAL COMPLEX daily or Nature's Path TRACE-LYTE liquid minerals in juice.

Hypothyroidism

Sluggish Thyroid Syndrome ✤ Parathyroid Disease ✤ Goiter

Sluggish Thyroid Syndrome is the most commonly occurring hormonal disturbance in America today. Hypothyroidism, low thyroid function, is a condition where the thyroid is not producing enough thyroxin hormone. The brain is sensitive to low thyroid levels; the primary signs of the disease are slowed brain functions. Eight times more women than men are hypothyroid. To determine your thyroid condition: Take your basal temperature for 10 minutes on rising in the morning. Do not move while taking temperature. It should be between 97.8 and 98.2 for health. Below this, a sluggish thyroid exists. Temperature will return to normal as treatment begins to work. If menstruating, take temperature on the 2nd, 3rd and 4th day of menses.

Diet & Superfood Therapy

☽ Follow a 75% fresh foods diet for a month to rebalance metabolism. Have a fresh green salad every day.

⚕Eat plenty of iodine-rich foods, such as sea vegetables, sea foods, fish, mushrooms, garlic, onions and watercress.

⚕Eat vitamin A-rich foods such as yellow vegetables, eggs, carrots, dark green vegetables, raw dairy.

⚕Take a veggie drink (pg. 168) or a potassium broth (pg. 167) several times weekly. (Also see superfoods below.)

⚕Use an herb salt instead of table salt.

⚕Avoid refined foods, saturated fats, sugars, white flour and red meats.

⚕Avoid "goitrogens," foods that prevent the use of iodine: cabbage, turnips, peanuts, mustard, pine nuts, millet and soy products. (Cooking these foods inactivates the goitrogens.)

⚕Cancer of the thyroid has been linked to highly fluoridated water.

☙

☽ **Effective superfoods:**
⚕Crystal Star SYSTEMS STRENGTH™ drink or capsules daily for 2 to 3 months.
⚕Klamath BLUE GREEN SUPREME.
⚕Nature's Life SUPER GREEN PRO-96.
⚕Green Foods WHEAT GERM extracrt.
⚕Sun CHLORELLA drink or tabs daily.
⚕Transitions EASY GREENS drink.

Herbal Therapy

The thyroid needs body iodine to produce its hormones. An imbalanced thyroid invariably causes over-production of estrogen with numerous attendant problems for women. Herbal iodine sources are effective without side effects.

☙ **Jump start herbal program:**
⚕Crystal Star IODINE SOURCE™ extract or IODINE/POTASSIUM SOURCE™ caps 2x daily, or META-TABS 2 daily, with ADRN-ACTIVE™ extract 2x daily and EVENING PRIMROSE oil, 4 daily.

☙ Other iodine balancing herbal sources:
⚕J.R.E. IOSOL drops.
⚕Kelp tabs 8 daily, with cayenne 3 daily.
⚕Enzymatic Therapy ENZODINE.
⚕Solaray ALFA JUICE caps.

☙ **For goiter:** apply BLACK WALNUT extract as a throat paint, and take ½ dropperful 2x daily; apply calendula compresses twice a day for a month.

☙ GINSENG/PAU d' ARCO extract or Siberian ginseng extract 2x daily.

☙ Effective daily teas:
⚕Sarsaparilla extract tea
⚕Gotu kola
⚕Dandelion

Supplements

Do not take iron supplements along with thyroid hormone medication. It binds up the thyroxine, rendering it insoluble.

⚘ **Raw glandular therapy:**
⚘Raw Thyroid complex
⚘Raw Pituitary
⚘Raw Adrenal glandular, or Country Life ADRENAL COMPLEX w. tyrosine. ♂
⚘**Enzymatic Therapy THYROID/TYROSINE COMPLEX.** ♀
⚘ Nutri-PAK thyroxin-free double strength thyroid.

⚘ **CoQ$_{10}$ 60mg daily with B$_{12}$ SL.**

⚘ Emulsified A 25,000IU 3x daily, or beta carotene 100,000IU daily, with Vitamin E 400IU daily.
⚘Ascorbate vitamin C with bioflavonoids 3000mg daily.

⚘ Magnesium/potassium/bromelain caps 2 daily, and zinc 75mg daily.♀
⚘Cal/mag/potassium caps 2 daily, with zinc 50mg daily.♂

⚘ Tyrosine 500mg with L-lysine 500mg 2x daily, or Taurine 500mg with L-lysine 500mg 2x daily.

⚘ B Complex 100mg with extra B$_2$ 100mg, B$_1$ 500mg and B$_6$ 200mg.

Lifestyle Support Therapy

Do you gain weight easily? Are you constantly fatigued? Ringing in the ears? Thin, falling hair? Generally constipated? Sensitive to cold? No enthusiasm? Extra dry skin?

☞ Take a brisk half hour walk daily; exercise increases metabolism and stimulates circulation.
⚕Sun bathe in the morning. Sea bathe and wade whenever possible.

☞ **Acupressure point:**
Press hollow at base of the throat to stimulate thyroid, 3x for 10 seconds each.

☞ Avoid fluorescent lights and fluoride toothpaste. They deplete vitamin A in the body.

☞ **Reflexology point:**

thyroid/thymus

☞ Color therapy: for hypothyroid - wear orange glasses 20-30 min; switch to blue for 5 minutes. Reverse for hyperthyroid.

☞ The drug levothyroxine, frequently given for hypothyroidism, can cause significant bone loss. Ask your doctor. Avoid antihistamines and sulfa drugs.

Common Symptoms: Mental depression, and emotional instability; muscle weakness and fatigue; poor memory; lethargy; headaches; deep, slow speech; hoarseness; coarse hair and loss of hair; swollen, cold hands and feet; constipation; pale, sallow, thick, dry skin; swelling of the face, tongue and eyelids; excessive and painful menstruation; nervousness and heart palpitations; unexplained weight gain. In children, hypothyroidism may result in retarded growth and mental development. Goiter symptoms include enlargement of the thyroid gland, usually a woman's problem.
Common Causes: Iodine depletion, often from X-rays or low dose radiation, such as mammograms; environmental pollutants that deplete vitamin A in the body; overuse of diet pills and other drugs; vitamin A, E and zinc deficiency; PMS.

See GLAND BALANCE pages and NUTRIENT DEFICIENCY TEST FOR SLUGGISH THYROID (page 438) for more information.

Immunity

Building Stronger Immune Response

The immune system is responsible for both pro-active and protective activities against substances encountered in the environment. The main elements of the immune system are the thymus gland, bone marrow, the spleen, the complement system of enzymatic proteins, and the lymphatic system with white blood cells and lymphocytes, the backbone of immune defenses. The immune system is ever-vigilant, constantly searching for proteins, called antigens, that don't belong in our bodies. It can deal with a wide range of pathogens - viruses, funguses, bacteria and parasites. It can even recognize potential antigens, such as drugs, pollens, insect venoms and chemicals in foods, and malignant cells and foreign tissue, such as transplanted organs or transfused blood.

Diet & Superfood Therapy

Immunity is the body system most sensitive to nutritional deficiency.

ᐛ The U.S. diet of processed foods, 20% sugars, and 37% fat, suppresses immunity. Saturated fats, such as those in pastries, fried foods, and red meats are the worst culprits. Refined foods offer little nutrition. Avoid junk and processed foods. Reduce dairy and sugary foods.

—Take a balanced protein drink every morning for strength. (pg. 175, or below.)

—Eat a generally cleansing/building, low fat diet, with plenty of fresh foods, fiber foods, whole grains, sea foods, eggs and cultured dairy foods, such as yogurt and kefir for friendly G.I. flora.

—Food enzymes are basic to immune response. Include fresh fruits and vegetables and a green salad in your diet every day. Especially include enzyme-rich garlic, papaya and sea vegetables.

ᐓ

ᐛ **Immune-enhancing superfoods:**
—Crystal Star BIOFLAV, FIBER & C SUPPORT™ drink, SYSTEM STRENGTH™ drink and GREEN TEA CLEANSER™.
—AloeLife ALOE GOLD JUICE. ♂♀
—Solgar EARTH SOURCE GREENS.
—Y.S. or Beehive Botanical ROYAL JELLY/SIBERIAN GINSENG and POLLEN drink.
—Sun CHLORELLA 1 packet daily.
—Nappi THE PERFECT MEAL protein.
—BioStrath YEAST ELIXIR w. HERBS.

Herbal Therapy

ᐘ **Jump start herbal program:**
Crystal Star HERBAL DEFENSE TEAM™ caps, extract or tea, for 2 months.
—GINSENG 6 SUPER TEA™.
—EVENING PRIMROSE oil for EFAs.
—GINSENG/CHLORELLA extract. ♂
—ANTIOXIDANT HERBS™ caps.
—FEEL GREAT™ tea and caps to rebuild strength and a feeling of well-being. ♀

ᐘ **Enzyme therapy herbs:**
—MILK THISTLE SEED extract
—Green tea
—Goldenseal and Oregon grape
—Licorice root

ᐘ **Immuno-modulating tonic herbs:**
—Siberian ginseng
—Propolis and royal jelly
—ECHINACEA root
—Panax ginseng or Suma root
—Zand HERBAL INSURE extract

ᐘ **Immune-enhancing antioxidant herbs:**
—White willow
—Astragalus
—Hawthorn extract
—Pau d'arco or PAU d'ARCO/GINSENG.

ᐘ **Mushrooms for interferon production:**
—Planetary Formulas REISHI SUPREME.
—Reishi amd maitake mushrooms.

Supplements

Our environment is so polluted. I feel almost everyone needs to supplement.

ᐕ **Solgar SOD 2000 units for 6 weeks, with B Complex 100mg, Nature's Bounty internasal B$_{12}$, and Mezotrace SEA MINERALS.**
—Vitamin C/Ester C with bioflavonoids 3000mg with zinc 50mg daily.

ᐕ **Effective immune stimulant products:**
—Source Naturals WELLNESS
—Enzymatic Therapy THYMU-PLEX
—American Biologics OXY-FORTE 5000
—Country Life WELL-MAX with PCOs
—Rainbow Light DEEP DEFENSE
—Future Biotics VITAL K

ᐕ **Antioxidants prevent thymus shrinkage:**
—PCOs from grapeseed/white pine 100mg 2 daily.
—Nutricology GERMANIUM 150mg.
—Beta or marine carotene 25,000IU
—Nutricology Laktoferrin 100mg daily.
—Solaray QBC COMPLEX
—CoQ$_{10}$ 60mg 2x daily. ♂

ᐕ **Thymus enhancement:** Enzymatic Therapy THYMULUS or THYMUPLEX, or Nutricology organic thymus. Tap the thymus with the knuckles every morning to stimulate activity.

ᐕ **Enzyme therapy:** Prevail DEFENSE FORMULA, or Natren TRINITY daily.

Lifestyle Support Therapy

℞ Tobacco/nicotine in any form is an immune depressant. The cadmium content causes zinc deficiency. It takes 3 months to get immune response even after you quit.

℞ Get quality rest - immune power builds the most during sleep.

—Get regular daily exercise to keep system oxygen high. Disease does not readily attack in a high oxygen, high potassium environment.

—Stop and smell the roses occasionally. A conscious, free-flowing emotional life is fundamental for inner harmony.

—Have a good laugh every day. It's the best immune booster.

—Aromatherapy is effective: lavender or rosemary oil.

℞ Relaxation techniques are immune-enhancers. A positive mental attitude makes a big difference in how the body fights disease. Use creative visualization to establish belief and optimism, and biofeedback or massage therapy to reduce stress.

℞ Environmental pollutants, particularly pesticides, lower immunity. Eat organically grown foods whenever possible.

℞ Eliminate recreational drugs. Reduce prescription drugs, especially antibiotics and cortico-steroids that depress immunity.

See next page for more information.

Common Symptoms: Chronic and continuing infections, colds, respiratory problems; Candida yeast overgrowth; chronic fatigue; chronic allergies.
Common Causes: Glandular malfunction, usually because of poor diet and nutrition; staph infection; prolonged use of antibiotics and/or cortico-steroids, (long-term use of these drugs can depress the immune system to the point where even minor illness can become life-threatening.); some immunization shots; Candida albicans yeast overgrowth; great emotional stress; food and other allergies; environmental and heavy metal pollutants; radiation.

What Does The Immune System Really Do?

We hear so much about immune system breakdown today. Yet, most of us don't know very much about it, or how it works. It's really an amazing part of our bodies. The immune system is the body's most complex and delicately balanced infrastructure. While the workings of other body systems have been well known for some time, the complex nature and dynamics of the immune system have been largely a mystery. One of the problems in comprehending immune response is its highly individual nature. It's a personal defense system that comes charging to the rescue at the first sign of an alien force, such as a harmful virus or pathogenic bacteria. Personal immune response shows us that there is so much more to our healing than the latest wonder drug. It shows us that we are the ultimate healer of ourselves.

The immune system is not responsive to drugs for healing. Even doctors admit that most drugs really just stabilize the body, or arrest a harmful organism, to allow the immune system to gather its forces and take over. The character of immune response varies widely between people, making it almost impossible to form a drug that will stimulate immunity for everyone. But natural nutritive forces, like healing foods and herbal medicines **can and do** support the immune system. They enhance its activity, strengthen it, and provide an environment through cleansing and detoxification for it to work at its best.

Immune defense is autonomic, using its own subconscious memory to establish antigens against harmful pathogens. It's a system that works on its own to fend off or neutralize disease toxins, and set up a healing environment for the body. It is this quality of being a part of us, yet not under our conscious control, that is the great power of immune response. It is also the dilemma of medical scientists as they struggle to get control of a system that is all pervasive and yet, in the end, impossible to completely understand. It is as if God shows us his face in this incredibly complex part of us, where we are allowed to glimpse the ultimate mind-body connection.

Maintaining strong immune defenses in today's world is not easy. Daily exposure to environmental pollutants, the emotional and excessive stresses of modern lifestyles, chemicalized foods, and new virus mutations are all a challenge to our immune systems. Devastating, immune-deficient diseases are rising all over the world. Reduced immunity is the main factor in opportunistic diseases, like candida albicans, chronic fatigue syndrome, lupus, HIV, hepatitis, mononucleosis, herpes II, sexually transmitted diseases and cancer. These diseases have become the epidemic of our time, and most of us don't have very much to fight with. An overload of antibiotics, antacids, immunizations, cortico-steroid drugs, and environmental pollutants eventually affect immune system balance to the point where it cannot distinguish harmful cells from healthy cells.

I see traditional medicine as "heroic" medicine. Largely developed in wartime, its greatest strengths are emergency measures - the ability to arrest a crisis, destroy or incapacitate pathogenic organisms, reset and re-attach broken body parts, and stabilize the body so it can gather its healing forces. Because drugs work in an attempt to directly kill harmful organisms, it is easy to see that their value would be for emergency measures, and for short term use.

But, three unwanted things often happen with **prolonged** drug use: 1) Our bodies can build up a tolerance to the drug so that it requires more of it to get the same effect. 2) The drug slowly overwhelms immune response so the body becomes dependent upon it, using it as a crutch instead of doing its own work. 3) The drug misleads the body's defense system to the point that it doesn't know what to assault, and attacks everything in confusion. This type of over-reaction often happens during an allergy attack, where the immune system may respond to substances that are not really harmful. Most of the time, if we use drugs wisely to stimulate rather than over kill, if we "get out of the way" by keeping our bodies clean and well nourished, the immune system will spend its energies rebuilding instead of fighting, and strengthen us instead of constantly gathering resources to conduct a "rear guard" defense.

The very nature of immune strength means that it must be built from the inside out. The immune system is the body system most sensitive to nutritional deficiencies. Giving your body generous, high quality, natural remedies at the first sign of infection improves your chances of overcoming disease before it takes serious hold. Powerful, immune-enhancing superfoods and herbs can be directed at "early warning" problems to build strength for immune response. Building good immune defenses takes time and commitment, but it is worth it. The inherited immunity and health of you, your children and your grandchildren is laid down by you.

Here Are The Immune System Checkpoints To Keep You Healthy:

✔ Take high potency green, "superfoods," several times a week, such as Sun CHLORELLA, Green Foods GREEN MAGMA, Solaray ALFAJUICE, Klamath POWER 3, wheat grass, spirulina, or Crystal Star ENERGY GREEN™ drink. The composition of chlorophyll is very similar to that of human plasma, so these foods provide a "mini-transfusion" to detoxify your bloodstream.

✔ Include sea vegetables, such as kelp, hijiki, dulse, kombu, wakame, and nori in your daily diet for their therapeutic iodine, high potassium, and sodium alginate content; or take Crystal Star SYSTEMS STRENGTH™ drink, or POTASSIUM/IODINE SOURCE™ sea plant complex.

✔ Take a high potency lactobacillus or acidophilus complex, such as Natren TRINITY, Dr. DOPHILUS, or Solaray MULTI-DOPHILUS for friendly G.I. flora, and good food assimilation.

✔ Enzymes are basic to immune response. Have fresh fruits and vegetables every day for plant enzymes; take supplements like Biotec CELL GUARD w. SOD, or Solgar SOD INDUCERS.

✔ Include anti-oxidant supplements, like PCOs from grapeseed and white pine, vitamin E with selenium, beta carotene, zinc, CoQ$_{10}$, germanium and vitamin C. Herbs with anti-oxidant qualities include echinacea, panax ginseng, reishi and maitake mushrooms, goldenseal, Siberian ginseng, rosemary, licorice root, astragalus, suma, burdock, and pau d' arco.

✔ Nourish the thymus gland (your immune-stimulating gland) with a raw thymus glandular supplement, such as Enzymatic Therapy THYMULUS or THYMU-PLEX.

✔ Regular aerobic exercise keeps system oxygen high, and circulation flowing. Disease does not readily overrun a body where oxygen and organic minerals are high in the vital fluids.

✔ The immune system is stimulated by a few minutes of early morning sunlight every day. But avoid excessive sun. Sun *burns* immunity.

✔ Laughter lifts more than your spirits. It also boosts the immune system. Laughter decreases cortisol, an immune suppressor, allowing immune response to function better.

See COOKING FOR HEALTHY HEALING by Linda Rector-Page for a complete diet to build and maintain strong immunity.

Indigestion & Heartburn

Gas * Bloating * Flatulence

Good food digestion and assimilation is at the "heart" of health. When digestion is not optimum, problems go beyond the usual symptoms of gas and bloating. Energy is reduced, constipation results from metabolic byproducts that are not eliminated, allergic reactions, diarrhea and fatigue can all ensue. In cases of chronic indigestion, the immune system suffers drastically, allowing viral and other infections, such as candidiasis and chronic fatigue to take hold. Good digestion is important!

Diet & Superfood Therapy

See page 452 for a Food Combining Chart.

✿ Eat an alkalizing diet, with plenty of cultured foods such as yogurt, kefir and miso soup, high fiber foods like whole grains, fresh vegetables and fruits, enzyme-rich foods like papaya and pineapple.

✿ Avoid fatty, spicy, sugary and acid-forming foods. Omit fried foods, red meats, fatty dairy products, dried fruits, sodas and caffeine. Eat smaller meals. Chew food very well. No smoking or fluids with meals. A glass of white wine is OK for better absorption.

✿ To cleanse the digestive system and establish good enzyme production:
Start with a cleansing, pectin mono diet of apples and apple juice for 2 days.
Then for 4 days use a diet of 70% fresh foods and steamed brown rice for B vitamins to rebalance digestion.
Take 1 tsp. cider vinegar in water, (If it makes your heartburn go away, you need more stomach acid - HCL).
Add fresh vegetables and high fiber foods gradually.

✿ Effective superfoods:
➤Crystal Star ENERGY GREEN™ drink.
➤Solgar WHEY TO GO protein drink.
➤Sun CHLORELLA
➤Salute ALOE JUICE W. HERBS.

Herbal Therapy

✿ Jump start herbal program:
Crystal Star AFTER MEAL ENZ™ extract in water as needed; PRE-MEAL ENZ™ before meals; BITTERS & LEMON CLEANSE™ extract each morning as a preventive.
➤CRAMP BARK COMBO™ as needed.
➤GINSENG/LICORICE ELIXIR™ for heartburn.
➤SYSTEMS STRENGTH™ drink for long term enzyme activity and alkalizing.

✿ To relieve gas quick: pinches of cinnamon, nutmeg, ginger, cloves in water - drink down.
➤Umeboshi plum paste

✿ Good digestion teas: 🖐
➤Catnip/fennel 🖐
➤Slippery elm
➤NatureWorks SWEDISH BITTERS.
➤Peppermint/spearmint
➤Wild yam ♀♂
➤Chamomile
➤Alfalfa/mint
➤Thyme 🖐

✿ Effective herbal digestive caps:
➤Turmeric extract (curcumin)
➤Garlic/parsley
➤Ginger capsules.

✿ Solaray ALFAJUICE caps.

Supplements

✿ Effective enzyme therapy:
➤ Bromelain 500-750mg daily, or Nature's Plus chewable bromelain 40mg.
➤Enzymatic Therapy MEGA-ZYME
➤Am. Health PAPAYA CHEWABLES
➤Pancreatin capsules 1400mg
➤Prevail ACID EASE, or BEAN/VEGI ♂
➤FutureBiotics VEGETARIAN ENZYMES.
➤Betaine HCL capsules after meals

✿ Probiotics for friendly flora:
➤Solaray SUPER DIGEST AWAY ♀
➤Prof. Nutrit. DR. DOPHILUS caps
➤Nutrition Now Children's PB 8 ⊛
➤Natren TRINITY.

✿ For belching and burping:
➤AkPharma BEANO drops
➤Hylands *Indigestion* after meals
➤Country Life DIGESTIVE FORMULA

✿ For gas and bloating:
➤Activated charcoal - short term
➤BioForce *Indigestion Relief*

✿ For diarrhea:
➤Activated charcoal tabs - short term
➤Apple pectin tabs ♀

✿ For acute indigestion:
➤Enzymatic Therapy DGL tabs
➤Raw pancreas glandular ♀

Lifestyle Support Therapy

Commercial antacids neutralize stomach acid, inviting the stomach to produce even more acid, often making the condition worse in the long run. New tests are even showing that chronic use of aluminum-containing antacids causes bone loss. Avoid over using anti-biotics. They destroy friendly flora in the digestive tract, too.

✿ Apply ginger compresses to abdominal area. Take 2 ginger capsules as needed to break up gas.
➤Take peppermint oil drops in a cup of water. (Also helpful if there is irritable bowel syndrome).
➤**For flatulence: take a catnip or slippery elm enema for immediate relief.**

✿ Lie on your back and draw knees up to chest to relieve abdomen pressure.

✿ Try to eat when relaxed. Meals eaten in a hurry or under stress contribute to poor digestion. Life isnt going to slow down on its own. You need to make a conscious effort to lessen digestive stress. Try a short walk before eating.

✿ **Reflexology point:**

food assimilation —

See page 30 for a complete discussion of enzyme therapy.

Common symptoms: *Gnawing, burning pain and tenderness occurring directly after food consumption; excess gas and abdominal distention; passing foul gas; poor food assimilation.*

Common Causes: *Poor food combining; eating too much food, and too many refined, fatty and spicy foods; allergies to sugar, wheat or dairy; enzyme deficiency; overeating; candida yeast overgrowth; food allergies; too much caffeine, sodas and acid-forming foods; chronic constipation from lack of fiber; diverticulitis; vegetable protein deficiency; HCl deficiency.*

Infections & Inflammation

Staph Infection ❦ Bacterial Infections ❦ Viral Infections

*A **staph infection** involves a staphylococcus micro-organism, is usually virulent, and is often food-borne. Antibiotic measures are effective. A **bacterial infection** involves pathogenic microbial bacteria. Antibiotic agents are normally effective. A **viral infection** involves virus organisms that infiltrate the deepest regions of the body and live off the body's cell enzymes. Virus infections are virulent, deep-reaching and tenacious. Antibiotics are not effective. Antiviral treatment must be vigorous, since viruses can both mutate and move to escape being overcome. All infections regularly cause painful inflammation as the body reacts to overcome them. Chronic recurring infections can indicate low thyroid function.*

Diet & Superfood Therapy

❧ For any infection:

★A quick, enzyme therapy detox and cleanse: use 3 parts water to 1 part fresh pineapple juice; drink 8 glasses in 24 hours.

★Then take 6 glasses of vegetable juices (pg. 168), or potassium broth (pg. 167) in the next 24 hours.

★Then eat only fresh foods and brown rice for three days to keep the body alkaline and free flowing.

★Take a glass of lemon juice and water each morning to stimulate kidney filtering.

★Include vegetable source proteins for faster healing; sea vegetables and sea foods, whole grains, sprouts, and soy foods.

★Avoid all sugars, refined foods, caffeine, colas, tobacco and alcohol (except for a little wine) during healing. ❦

❧ **Effective superfoods:**

★Crystal Star SYSTEMS STRENGTH™, daily during healing; then ENERGY GREEN™ for strength and body chemistry balance.

•Nutricology PROGREENS. ♂

•Future Biotics VITAL K drink. ♀

•**Aloe vera juice, such as AloeLife ALOE VERA GOLD, morning and evening.**

★Green Foods GREEN MAGMA.

★Sun CHLORELLA.

★Klamath BLUE GREEN SUPREME.

Herbal Therapy

Herbs are well suited to management of infective conditions that are resistent to medical treatment.

❧ **Jump start herbal program:**

★**Viral infection:** Destroy the active virus. Crystal Star ANTI-VI™ or ANTI-BIO™, or garlic, goldenseal, myrrh, astragalus, propolis or St. John's wort extracts; or Lane Labs BENE-FIN shark cartilage capsules.

★**Limit bacterial harm** with echinacea, myrrh, garlic, Siberian ginseng, una da gato caps, or Crystal Star ANTI-FLAM™.

★**Raise immunity** with reishi or maitake mushroom, calendula tea, and ECHINACEA.

★**Restore homeostasis** with Crystal Star GINSENG 6 SUPER caps or tea. ♀

❧ **Staph infection:**

★ECHINACEA extract, and see above. ♂

★Propolis extract for thymus activity. ♂

★**Use una da gato or turmeric caps to take down inflammation.**

❧ **Bacterial infection:**

★**Destroy the active microbe.** Crystal Star ANTI-BIO™ extract or capsules. (FIRST AID CAPS™ in acute stages.) Turmeric (curcumin) as an anti-inflammatory.

★**Raise immunity** w. propolis, garlic echinacea or GINSENG/REISHI mushroom extracts.

★**Flush out released lymphatic toxins** with senna tea or BLDR-K™ extract. ♀

Supplements

Don't take iron supplements during an infection. Tends to make the bacteria grow faster.

❧ **Viral infection:**

★Lane Labs BENE-FIN shark cartilage to take down inflammation.

★Vitamin C crystals with bioflavs., ½ teasp. in water every hour during acute stages, reducing to 5000mg daily.

★Amer. Biologics INFLAZYME FORTE. ☜

★Hylands *Hylavir* tablets ☜

★Prof. Nutr. DR. DOPHILUS or Natren BIFIDO FACTORS, 2 caps with meals.

★PCOs from grapeseed or white pine.

❧ **Staph infection:**

★Nutribiotic GRAPEFRUIT SEED extract

★**Vitamin C crystals with bioflavs., ½ teasp. in water every hour during acute stages, reducing to 5000mg daily.**

★Bromelain 1500mg daily.

★Raw thymus 3x daily for immune defenses. ♀

❧ **Bacterial infection:**

★Nutribiotic GRAPEFRUIT SEED extract

★Dr. DOPHILUS or Natren BIFIDO FACTORS, 2 caps 3x daily with meals.

★Beta carotene 100,000IU daily, or quercetin with bromelain (Solaray QBC complex), as an anti-inflammatory.

★Source Nat. ACTIVATED QUERCETIN.

★PCOs from grapeseed or white pine.

★Vitamin C crystals with bioflavonoids.

Lifestyle Support Therapy

❧ Topical anti-infective applications:

★Crystal Star ANTI-BIO™ gel.

★Garlic poultice for inflammation.

★Matrix GENESIS 1000 H_2O_2 OXYSPRAY, especially for staph infections.

★Tea tree oil as an antiseptic.

★Nutribiotic GRAPEFRUIT SKIN SPRAY.

★Green clay packs for swelling.

★Honey - antiseptic, antibiotic and antimicrobial properties.

★**AloeLife ALOE SKIN GEL.**

❧ Overheating therapy is extremely effective in controlling virus replication. Even slight temperature increases can lead to considerable reduction of infection. See page 178 for the technique.

★Or raise blood temperature by taking a hot sauna, and by hot ginger/cayenne compresses applied to the affected area.

★Use alternating hot and cold hydrotherapy, pg. 177, to stimulate circulation.

★Activate kidney cleansing with a chamomile or chlorophyll enema.

★Get some early morning sunlight on the body every day possible.

★Get plenty of rest. Healing is at its peak during sleep.

❧ For children: use osha root tea.

★Aromatherapy essential oils for infants: 1 drop tea tree oil, 1 drop essential oil of lavender, 1 drop calendula oil in juice. ☜

Common Symptoms: *Inflammation, boils, sores, and abscesses; breakdown of tissue into waste matter and pus; sore throat, cough, and headache; high temperature and fever; reduced vitality; chronic fatigue and lethargy.*

Common Causes: *Lowered immunity; overuse of antibiotics; chronically low nutrition diet with too many refined foods and too few green vegetables; food or environmental allergies.*

See also FUNGAL AND PARASITIC INFECTIONS in this book for more information.

Infertility

Conception Difficulty For Both Men & Women

One in six married couples has trouble conceiving and completing a successful pregnancy in America today. About 40 percent of the time the problem lies with the man....not enough sperm, weak or malformed sperm, a sexually transmitted infection, or a reproductive system obstruction; hindrances are zinc deficiency, too much alcohol, and tobacco. About 40 percent of the time the problem lies with the woman.... hormonal difficulties, irregular release of eggs, scar tissue from a sexually transmitted disease, or endometriosis; prime inhibitors are anxiety, emotional stress, severe anemia, and hormonal imbalance. In the remaining 20 percent of the cases, the inability to conceive is related to problems with both the man and woman...reduced immunity.

Diet & Superfood Therapy

Diet is an all-important key. The body does not readily allow conception without adequate nutrition. Consciously follow a healthy diet and lifestyle for at least six months before trying to conceive. See "COOKING FOR HEALTHY HEALING" by Linda Rector-Page for a complete diet for infertility.

For both sexes:

—Eat plenty of whole grains, cultured foods such as yogurt, sea foods and sea vegetables, fresh fruits and vegetables.

—Take a daily morning protein drink, such as one from page 175 or see below.

—Reduce dairy products, esp. women, fried and fatty foods, sugary and junk foods.

—Avoid tobacco, alcohol, except moderate wine, caffeine (esp. women), red meats (they may have synthetic hormones), and chemical-laced foods.

For men: Make a mix of brewer's yeast, bee pollen granules, wheat germ, pumpkin seeds; blend 2 teasp. into each drink below.

—Eat zinc foods: oysters, wheat germ, onions, sunflower and pumpkin seeds.

Effective superfoods:

—Crystal Star BIOFLAV, FIBER & C SUPPORT.

—Green Foods WHEAT GERM extract.

—Beehive Botanical ROYAL JELLY w. pollen and Siberian ginseng 2 teasp. daily.

—New Moon GINGER WONDER.

Herbal Therapy

For women:

—**Crystal Star FEMALE HARMONY™ or FEM-SUPPORT™ extract, with EVENING PRIMROSE OIL for EFAs, 4-6 daily.**

or

PRO-EST BALANCE™ roll-on wild yam cream for 1 month with high potency royal jelly 2 tsp. daily and VITEX extract.

—Histidine 500mg - more sexual enjoyment.
—B₆ to increase progesterone.
—Siberian ginseng extract.
—Red raspberry tea.
—Licorice extract or GINSENG/LICORICE ELIXIR™.

—Cayenne/ginger caps.
—**DONG QUAI/DAMIANA - discontinue after pregnancy is achieved.**

For men:

—Effective ginseng combinations: Crystal Star MALE GINSIAC™ extract, MALE PERFORMANCE™ caps, ginseng/damiana caps,

—Damiana/licorice
—Siberian ginseng extract
—Propolis tabs 2 daily
—Crystal Star ADRN™ extract daily with highest potency YS royal jelly 2 teasp. daily.
—**Smilax 8x extract 2-3x daily.**
—Saw palmetto extract caps or Crystal Star PROX™ for men caps with saw palmetto and pygeum africanum.

—HAWTHORN extract 3-4x daily.

Supplements

For women:

—Enzymatic Therapy NUCLEO-PRO F, or STEREO-PLEX MF, with RAW OVARIAN extract and RAW FEMALE glandular.

—Vitamin E 400IU 2x daily, with C 1000mg daily and A & D 25,000IU daily.

—B Complex such as Nature's Secret ULTIMATE B with extra B₆ 100mg, PABA 1000mg and folic acid 800mcg daily.

—Nature's Bounty B₁₂ gel.

—Rainbow Light CALCIUM 1200mg with high magnesium 1200mg.

For men:

—Enzymatic Therapy NUCLEO-PRO M caps or STEREO-PLEX MF; Solaray MALE CAPS with orchic extract, raw pituitary, or Country Life MAX with orchic.

—Source Naturals DIBENCOZIDE 10,000mcg.

—Carnitine 500mg daily with chromium picolinate 200mcg daily, and L-arginine 500mg for increased sperm count/motility (except if you have herpes).

—Vitamin E 800IU w. selenium 200mcg.

—Vitamin C 3000mg daily and niacin 500mg for low sperm counts/sperm clumping.

—Zinc 75mg daily.

—Vitamin D 1000IU daily with beta-carotene 50,000IU daily.

—Calcium/magnesium 1000/500mg for testosterone balance.

Lifestyle Support Therapy

For both parents: Do not smoke; avoid secondary smoke. Avoid areas with smog and pollutants as much as possible.

—Get regular mild exercise every day.

Reflexology points:

penis,
coccyx,
prostate,
uterus

For women: anxiety and infertility are linked. Consciously relax more. Acupuncture treatments have been successful for women as relaxation techniques.

—For vaginal pH balance douche right before intercourse: use baking soda/honey for over-acid condition, vinegar/water for overalkaline.

—Alternate hot and cold sitz baths to stimulate circulation.

—Use aromatherapy rose oil.

—Avoid NSAIDS drugs.

For men: avoid bikini underwear, hot electric blankets, and hot water beds.

—Sun bathe in the early morning, nude if possible for 15 minutes.

—Stress and abnormal sperm production are linked. Relax.

Common Symptoms: Difficulty in both conceiving and bearing a child, a condition of both man and woman.

Common Causes: Female: Nutrient deficiency and hypoglycemia from too many refined foods; emotional stress; chlamydia or pelvic inflammatory disease; obstruction in the fallopian tubes; toxicity from drugs or environmental pollutants; birth control pills causing hormone imbalance; vaginal pH imbalance and allergic reaction to partner's sperm. Male: False estrogens lowering sperm production; prolonged marijuana or other drug use; radiation/toxic chemical poisoning; steroid use; poor nutrition/lack of protein; hypoglycemia; ductal obstruction; gland malfunction; chlamydia.

See HORMONE IMBALANCE PAGE, OR HAVING A HEALTHY BABY section, page 106 for more information.

Insect Bites & Stings
Bees ✴ Wasps ✴ Mosquitos ✴ Non-Poisonous Spiders

Insect bites can be annoying, painful, even dangerous, because of the diseases transmitted through them. Natural therapies provide time-proven defense against insect bites and stings. Chemical repellents have racked up many reports of toxic side effects in the last few years. The following are recommendations for persons mildly affected by insect poisons. If you are violently allergic, with chest tightness, wheezing, hives or intense pain and severe swelling, get emergency medical treatment immediately.

Diet & Superfood Therapy

❧ Household products help to take down swelling:
- raw onion slices
- raw potato slices
- lemon juice and vinegar
- wet mud packs
- tobacco and water paste
- toothpaste
- cologne or rubbing alcohol
- honey mixed w.1 drop peppermint oil
- baking soda or sea salt
- ice packs
- charcoal tabs or burnt toast
- wheat germ oil
- chlorophyll liquid
- green clay packs

❧ Avoid consuming sugar and alcohol for 24 hours before you are going to be in mosquito territory.
- ✴Avoid bananas and nuts and other serotonin-rich foods that attract insects.
- ✴Avoid meats and sweets for faster healing.
- ✴Avoid alcohol - it causes the skin to swell and flush, aggravating bites and stings.

❧ **Effective superfoods:**
- ✴Sun CHLORELLA to reestablish body balance.
- ✴AloeLife ALOE SKIN GEL - apply.

Herbal Therapy

☙ **Jump start herbal program:**
Crystal Star ANTI-HST™ and ANTI-FLAM™ caps to take down rash or swelling.
- ✴Add Bach Flower RESCUE REMEDY.
- ✴Apply neem oil.
- ✴ECHINACEA to flush lymph glands.

☙ Mix the following oils and apply to exposed areas for prevention: citronella, pennyroyal, eucalyptus, in a base of safflower oil.

☙ For prevention: rub fresh elder leaves or elder/chamomile tea on area regularly.
- ✴HEART FOODS TICKWEED PLUS with neem oil for prevention.

☙ **Effective local herbal applications:**
- ✴B&T SSSTING STOP gel. ⊛
- —Comfrey leaf poultice.
- —Turmeric powder
- —Witch hazel
- —Pau d'arco gel
- —Tea tree oil

☙ **Effective herbal compresses:**
- ✴Hot parsley leaf
- ✴Black cohosh
- —Chamomile

☙ Take a few drops of cayenne extract in warm water every ¹/₂ hour to stimulate the circulatory defense mechanism.

Supplements

✎ **Vitamin C therapy: Use calcium ascorbate powder. Take ¹/₄ teasp. every 15 minutes right after the bite, then ¹/₄ teasp. every few hours until pain and swelling are gone. Also mix some powder to a paste with water and apply directly.**
- ✴Pantothenic acid 1000mg as an antihistamine for swelling.

✎ For prevention, take vitamin B₁ like Source Naturals CO-ENZYMATE B for a month during high risk seasons - 100mg for children, ⊛ 500mg for adults.

✎ Quercetin Plus with bromelain or Source Naturals ACTIVATED QUERCITIN. Take every 4 hours for inflammation.

✎ **Effective applications:**
- ✴American Biologics DIOXYCHLOR on a piece of cotton as needed.
- ✴Dissolve PABA tablets in water and apply.
- ✴Body Essentials SILICA GEL.

✎ **Homeopathic remedies:**
- ✴*Ledum* tincture to relieve swelling and stinging.
- ✴*Apis* ointment for puffiness.
- ✴*Cantharis* for inflammation.

Lifestyle Support Therapy

🕭 **Environmental preventives:**
- ✴Sprinkle garlic or eucalyptus powder around the house.
- ✴Sprinkle sassafras tea or dried tomato leaves around the house.
- ✴Sprinkle vanilla water around the house.
- ✴Wear light colors - remain cool and dry. Cover up in the early morning and evening.

🕭 To lessen the effect of the bite, keep quiet, and keep the affected area below the level of the heart. Pull out a bee stinger with tweezers.
- ✴Apply cold or ice pack compresses, and see shock page in this book if reaction is severe.

🕭 Avoid flowery scents and perfume to escape bees. They think you are a source of pollen!

🕭 Natural repellents: Re-apply often - repellency is based on aroma. Don't use on fine fabrics.
- ✴Citronella for mosquitoes and flies.
- ✴Cedarwood for fleas and ticks.
- ✴Eucalyptus for most flying insects.
- ✴Lemon grass for broad range of insects.
- ✴Pennyroyal for fleas (do not use if pregnant).
- ✴Peppermint, rosemary, thyme, geranium and lavender for flies and fleas.

See BRUISES, CUTS & ABRASIONS pages for more information.

Common Symptoms: *Pain, swelling, itching, and redness around the bite area; more severe reactions include nausea, dizziness, headache, chills, fever, allergic and histamine side-effects.*

Insomnia

Sleep Disorders ✢ Sleep Apnea ✢ Snoring

Millions suffer from insomnia, twisting, turning, agonizing through the night, battling anxiety and rumpled bedding. Americans consume over a million and a half pounds of tranquilizers annually! Insomnia itself seems to be due largely to psychological, rather than physical factors. Maintaining sleep involves nighttime blood glucose levels. A blood sugar drop promotes awakening by sugar-regulatory hormones. Avoid commercial sleeping pills. They interfere with the ability to dream, and interrupt natural sleeping patterns. They interact adversely with alcohol and tranquilizers because the nervous system never really relaxes. Eventually they lose their sleep promoting effectiveness in as little as 3-5 days of use. Natural therapies are conservative, non-addictive and effective.

Diet & Superfood Therapy

Don't worry about "making up" lost sleep One good night's sleep repairs fatigue.

✍ Eat only a light meal at night. Good late-night "sleepytime" snacks about an hour before bedtime: bananas, celery and celery juice, wheat germ and wheat germ oil, brown rice, a little warm milk, lemon water and honey, brewer's yeast, Organic Gourmet NUTRITIONAL YEAST broth, with 1 TB. Bragg's LIQUID AMINOS in water.
↝Have a glass of wine at dinner for minerals, digestion and relaxation.
↝Have a small glass of bottled mineral water at bedtime.
↝Don't take caffeine drinks except in the morning.
↝Avoid a heavy meal in the evening, especially if under a great deal of stress.
↝Avoid salty and sugary foods before bed. Dont eat too late.
✿

✿ **Effective superfoods:**
↝B&T *Alfalco*, homeopathic Alfalfa tonic drink before bed.
↝Beehive Botanicals SIBERIAN GINSENG/ROYAL JELLY drink.

Herbal Therapy

It takes several days of common-sense therapy to establish good sleep patterns.

✍ **Herbal Jump start program:**
Crystal Star RELAX CAPS™ or NIGHT CAPS™ ♀ NIGHT *ZZZ*™ extract, ♂ or GOODNIGHT™ tea. ♀ 🜨
↝VALERIAN/WILD LETTUCE extract.
↝REISHI/GINSENG extract.
↝For quality sleep and dream recall: INCREDIBLE DREAMS™ tea.

✍ Passion flower capsules or extract, if weaning away from sleeping pills.

✍ **Aromatherapy for insomnia:** chamomile or lavender oils on temples, pillow, bottoms of feet. ♀ Make a hops/rosemary sleep pillow. Sprinkle with a little alcohol to enhance aromatherapy.

✍ **Effective night time teas:**
↝Chamomile for relaxation or snoring
↝Catnip/lemon balm 🜨
↝**St. John's wort**

✍ Enzymatic Therapy KAVA TONE especially if under a great deal of stress. ♀ ♂

¶ Effective drops in water:
↝**Floradix HERBAL REST liquid**
↝**Crystal Star CALCIUM SOURCE™** ♀ ♂
↝Scullcap extract

Supplements

A lack of balanced calcium and magnesium in the blood can cause one to wake up at night and not be able to return to sleep.

✍ Rainbow Light CALCIUM PLUS with high magnesium, with B Complex 100mg, ♀ ♂ or Enzymatic Therapy RELAX-O-ZYME. ♀

✍ **Homeopathic remedies:**
↝Hyland's *CALMS FORTE* ♀
↝*Chamomilla* 🜨
↝*Nux vomica* for over-indulgence. ♂
↝Boiron *QUIETUDE.*

✍ Melatonin, 3mg for sleep disorders (if your melatonin is low) on a temporary basis, to reset you biological clock, esp. if over 45.
↝**5-Hydroxy tryptophan, 50-100mg.**

✍ One each for sleep when there is pain: ♀ DLPA 500mg, Calcium/magnesium capsule.

✍ GABA 500mg and glycine capsules before bed, especially if hypoglycemic. ♂

✍ **For nightmares:**
↝B₁ 500mg at night for 1 to 2 months
↝Niacinimide 500mg.
↝**Bach Flower Remedies.**

✍ Restless legs/nocturnal myoclonus:
↝Vitamin E 400IU before bed.
↝Folic acid 800mcg daily. ♀

Lifestyle Support Therapy

☞ Snoring - which causes insomnia for your mate, has two causes: 1) an obstruction or narrowing of the airway; 2) sleep apnea - the snorer actually ceases to breathe because the tongue blocks the throat.
↝Get off your back. Elevate your head. Lose some weight. Cut back on alcohol at night. Clear your nose before bed. Avoid tranquilizers and CNS depressants at night.
↝Go to bed earlier to control snoring.
↝BREATHE RIGHT nasal strips.

☞ **Stress reduction techniques:**
↝Biofeedback, yoga, hypnotherapy, and regular massage therapy treatments.
↝Gaze at a lighted candle for 3 minutes before retiring.
↝Before bed breathing stretch: take 10 deep breaths; wait 5 minutes; take 10 more.
↝Use a "white noise" machine.
↝Take an epsom salts bath before bed.

☞ **Sleep stealers:**
↝Alcohol interrupts sleep patterns.
↝Nicotine - a long-lasting stimulant.
↝Coffee and caffeine.
↝Too much long term stress.

☞ Exercise in the morning, outdoors if possible; a "sunlight break" promotes sleep 12 hours later, and keeps circadian rhythm regular. Take a "constitutional walk" before bed.

Common Symptoms: Chronic inability to sleep; prematurely ended or interrupted sleep; difficulty falling asleep; snoring and sleep apnea can be a serious disorder, linked to high blood pressure, irregular heartbeat, headaches and excessive fatigue.

Common Causes: Chronic stress, tension, depression and anxiety; the inability to "turn your mind off;" too much caffeine; pain; hypoglycemia; overeating; too much salt and sugar; B Complex deficiency; nicotine or other drugs; asthma; indigestion and toxic liver overload; too high copper levels. Snoring can be caused by poor food digestion.

See also STRESS & TENSION page for more information.

Kidney Disease

Nephritis * Kidney Stones * Bright's Disease

Kidney infections are usually severe, serious, and should be attended to immediately. Nephritis *involves chronic inflammation of the kidney tissues. In* Bright's disease *(usually connected with diabetes) the blood becomes toxic from an overload of unfiltered wastes. Inflammation develops with blood in the urine, high blood pressure and water retention.* Kidney stones *form when minerals that normally free float in the kidney fluids, combine into crystals. When there is an overload of inorganic mineral waste and too little fluid, the molecules can't dissolve properly and form sharp-edged stones. It takes from 5 to 15 hours of vigorous and urgent treatment to dissolve and pass small stones. Ten percent of all men and 5% of all women have a kidney stone by the time they're seventy.*

Diet & Superfood Therapy

Prevention through improved diet and exercise is the best medicine.

❧ **A short 3 day kidney cleanse to remove toxic infection and help dissolve stones:**
—Each morning take 2 TBS. cider vinegar or lemon juice in water. Take one each of the following juices daily: carrot/beet/ cucumber, cranberry, potassium broth (pg. 167), and a green veggie drink (pg. 168).
—**Take 2 cups watermelon seed tea daily if there are kidney stones.**
—**Take aloe vera juice before bed.**
—**Take 8 glasses of water each day.**
—Take 2TBS. olive oil through a straw every 4 hours to help dissolve stones.
—**Then,** a simple low salt, low protein, vegetarian diet with 75% fresh foods for a week.
—Avoid all refined, fried, fatty foods, and cola drinks during healing. Avoid salts, sugars, and caffeine-containing foods. Eliminate dairy products. Reduce all animal protein.
—Continue for 2 to 3 weeks with the diet on the following page.

❧ **Effective superfoods:**
—**Crystal Star ENERGY GREEN™.**
—Transitions EASY GREENs.
—**Klamath BLUE GREEN SUPREME.**
—Future Biotics VITAL K drink daily.
—Aloe Falls ALOE JUICE with ginger.
—**Sun CHLORELLA 2 pkts. daily.**

Herbal Therapy

❧ **Jump start herbal program:**
Crystal Star ANTI-BIO™ capsules 4 daily til infection clears; then STN-EX™ capsules for a month to help dissolve stones.
—**Then, GREEN TEA CLEANSER™** every morning for another month.
—**BLDR-K™ caps or tea with GINKGO BILOBA extract as needed for prevention.**
Other options:
—AFTER MEAL ENZ™ extract.
—HAWTHORN or BILBERRY extract. ♀+
—EVENING PRIMROSE oil 4 daily.

❧ **Kidney balancing herbs:**
—Parsley/cornsilk tea. ♀+
—St. John's wort if incontinent.
—Solaray ALFAJUICE daily.

❧ **Kidney detoxifiers:**
—Burdock root tea, ECHINACEA extract 4x daily, garlic/cayenne caps 6-8 daily.
—**Dandelion extract esp. for nephritis.**

❧ **For kidney stones:** drink a quart daily of any of these teas to help dissolve:
—Chamomile, rosemary or rosehips, ♀+
or dandelion/nettles. ♀+

❧ **Kidney flushing teas: (Crystal Star IODINE/POTASSIUM daily if taking diuretics.**
—Watercress, cleavers or couch grass ♀+
—Uva Ursi/juniper

Supplements

Eliminate iron supplements during healing. Avoid L-cystin - aggravates crystallization in the kidneys.

❧ **For kidney inflammation:**
—**B Complex 100mg; extra B$_6$ 100mg daily and magnesium 800mg daily.**
—Natren TRINITY or Prof. Nutrition Dr. DOPHILUS $1/2$ teasp. 3-4x daily.
—**American Biologics A & E EMULSION,** or beta-carotene 100,000IU.
—High omega-3 flax oil daily or Choline/ Inositol caps 4x daily.
—**Country Life CAL/MAG/POTASS.**
—Enzymatic Therapy LIQUID LIVER with GINSENG, and RENATONE 2x daily.♂
—Zinc 50mg 2x daily. ♂

❧ **For kidney stones:**
—Flora VEGE-SIL caps 2 daily for kidney stone prevention.
—Enzymatic Therapy ACID-A-CAL caps 2-4 daily to help dissolve sediment.♂
—**Ascorbate or Ester C powder in water; $1/4$ teasp. every hour to bowel tolerance until stones pass - about 5000mg.**
—Solaray LIPOTROPIC PLUS daily.
—Solaray CALCIUM CITRATE 4 daily, with QBC for inflammation. ♂
—**B complex 100mg with extra B$_6$ 100mg and magnesium 400mg 2x daily, and vitamin K 100mcg.**
—Golden Pride FORMULA ONE oral chelation with EDTA. ♂

Lifestyle Support Therapy

Kidney stones are extremely painful, but very preventable.

❧ Take a daily brisk walk to keep kidney function flowing.
—Avoid commercial antacids during healing. Avoid NSAIDS drugs. They have been implicated in kidney failure cases.
—Avoid smoking and secondary smoke.

❧ Apply moist heat packs, comfrey compresses, and/or alternating hot and cold compresses on the kidney area.
—Apply white flower oil or tiger balm to kidney area 2-3x daily.
—**Apply compresses to kidney area,** like hot ginger/oatstraw, cayenne/ginger, mullein/lobelia.

❧ **Use capsicum, spirulina or catnip enemas 2-3x weekly to stimulate better kidney function.**

❧ **Reflexology points:**

kidney points

—In addition, press on the back, on the tops of both hip bones, 3x for 10 seconds.

See following page for a KIDNEY CLEANSING DIET.

Common Symptoms: *Kidney disease means painful, frequent urination; chronic lower back pain and fatigue; chills and fever; fluid retention.* **For kidney stones,** *there may be no apparent symptoms except a dull ache in the lower back, until the stone blocks the urinary tract, which results in excruciating, radiating pain. Then there is very painful urination; nausea, fever and vomiting.*
Common Causes: *Excess sugar, red meat, carbonated drinks, sugars and caffeine in the diet; diabetes; allergies; heavy metal poisoning; excess aluminum; EFA deficiency; overuse of prescription or pleasure drugs; B vitamin and magnesium deficiency; overuse of aspirin, salt and chemical diuretics.*

Kidney Cleansing & Rebuilding Diet For Kidney Stones

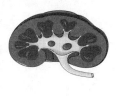
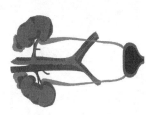

This diet is recommended to normalize kidney activity after the 3 day liquid cleanse on the preceding page. Intense pain should have ceased. Follow for 2 to 3 weeks after acute stage has passed. (Use for 2 to 3 months for chronic problems.) Keep salt and protein low for at least 3 weeks. The diet is vegetarian, emphasizing fresh and cultured foods to alkalize the system. It is low in proteins, starches and carbohydrates, allowing the body to spend more energy on healing than on dealing with heavier foods. It is high in fiber, which results in lowering urinary calcium waste. It eliminates acid-forming foods, such as caffeine and caffeine-containing foods, salty, sugary and fried foods, soft drinks, alcohol, and tomatoes. They all inhibit kidney filtering. It also avoids mucous-forming foods, like pasteurized dairy products, heavy grains, starches and fats, in order to relieve irritation and sediment formation, to continue cleansing activity, and to normalize kidney function. Kidney stones plague people who eat a rich, high fat diet. A vegetarian diet is best. An ongoing kidney health diet should always be low in cholesterol and saturated fats to prevent further kidney stone formation.

Note #1: Drink at least 8 glasses of bottled water every day if you are prone to kidney problems, so that waste and excess minerals are continuously flushed through the body.
Note #2: OLIVE OIL FLUSHES under the Liver Cleansing Diet in this book may also be used successfully for kidney stones.
Note #3: Do not use TUMS for indigestion. They have a history of increasing risk for stone formation.
Note #4: Avoid oxalic acid-forming foods, like spinach, rhubarb, chard, chocolate, black tea, grapes and celery.

On rising: take a glass of lemon juice in water with 1 teasp. honey; or 2 TBS. apple cider vinegar in water with 1 teasp. honey; or 2 TBS. cranberry juice concentrate in water with $\frac{1}{4}$ teasp. ascorbate vitamin C crystals added; or Crystal Star GREEN TEA CLEANSER™.

Breakfast: a glass of papaya or apple juice, or fresh watermelon juice, or a bowl of watermelon chunks; then fresh tropical fruits, such as papaya, mango, or banana.

Mid-morning: have a green drink such as Sun CHLORELLA or Green Foods GREEN MAGMA, or Crystal Star ENERGY GREEN™ drink; or a glass of apple juice; or dandelion, watermelon seed, or parsley tea, or Crystal Star BLDR-K™ tea.

Lunch: have a green salad with lots of cucumbers, spinach, watercress and celery, with lemon/oil or yogurt dressing; and/or baked or marinated tofu; with sesame seeds and wheat germ; or a Chinese vegetable salad with bok choy, daikon, pea pods, and other Chinese greens, with a cup of miso or ramen noodle soup with sea veggies.

Mid-afternoon: have a cup of alkalizing, sediment-dissolving herb tea, such as cornsilk, plantain, dandelion leaf or oatstraw, or another cup of Crystal Star BLDR-K™ tea; or some asparagus stalks and carrot sticks with kefir or yogurt cheese; or fresh apples and pears with kefir or yogurt dip.

Dinner: have some brown rice with tofu and steamed veggies; or steamed asparagus with miso soup and snipped, dry sea veggies on top; or a baked potato with kefir cheese or 1 teasp. butter, and a spinach salad; or baked or broiled salmon with millet and baked onions.
Note: A glass of white wine is fine at dinner for alkalizing and relaxation.

Before bed: have another apple or papaya/mango juice; or miso soup with sea vegetables snipped on top; or Organic Gourmet NUTRITIONAL YEAST or MISO/GINGER broth in hot water.

☜SUGGESTED SUPPLEMENTS FOR THE KIDNEY CLEANSING & REBUILDING DIET
•Continue with 3-5000mg ascorbate vitamin C daily in juice or water, $\frac{1}{2}$ teasp. every 4 hours, and beta carotene, or emulsified A 25,000IU 4x daily.
•Take a concentrated green food supplement, such as Green Foods GREEN MAGMA, Klamath POWER 3 caps, or Crystal Star ENERGY GREEN™ drink before meals.
•Take Enzymatic Therapy ACID-A-CAL caps to dissolve sedimentary waste, with bromelain 500mg daily.
•Take a milk-free acidophilus powder in juice or water, as needed 2-3 times daily, with garlic caps, or flax oil capsules.

☜BODYWORK FOR THE KIDNEY CLEANSING/REBUILDING DIET
•Continue with wet, hot compresses and lower back massage when there is inflammation flare up, especially lobelia or ginger fomentations.
•Take hot saunas when possible to release toxins and excess fluids, and to flush acids out through the skin. A swim after a sauna is wonderful for body tone.
•Take 3 to 5000mg ascorbate vitamin C with bioflavonoids for a month to acidify urine and prevent further stones.
•Take hot and cold, or Epsom salts sitz baths to stimulate circulation.

See COOKING FOR HEALTHY HEALING by Linda Rector Page for a complete diet for kidney health.

Leukemia
Blood & Bone Marrow Cancer

Leukemias are cancers which originate in the tissues of the bone marrow, spleen and lymph nodes. They are characterized by excessive production of white blood cells and seem to result from a failure of the bone marrow to function adequately. The spleen and liver are infiltrated and damaged by the excess leukocytes. Lymph nodes and nerves are also affected. Thirty-thousand Americans are diagnosed each year with leukemias - 20,000 die as a result of it. Natural treatments, especially in conjunction with cytotoxic drugs have improved the remission rate of this type of cancer to over 50%.

Diet & Superfood Therapy

Food healing value is lost very quickly in this disease. Make sure the diet is very nutritious to make up for this.

❧ **Start with a cleansing/detoxification program (pg. 164) for 2 months.** Follow with a macrobiotic diet program, using organically grown foods (pg. 211) for 3 to 4 months with no animal protein and lots of alkalizing foods.

❋High vegetable proteins are the key after initial detoxification. Eat lots of green leafy vegetables on a continuing basis for red blood cell formation. Include plenty of potassium-rich foods.

❋To clean vital organs, take a glass of carrot/beet/cucumber juice every day for the first month of healing; every other day for the second month; once a week the third month. Add a potassium broth every other day (pg. 167).

❋Take 2 glasses of cranberry juice daily.

❋Avoid alcohol, junk and chemicalized foods, refined sugars and red meats.

❧ **Effective superfoods:**
❋Green Foods BETA CARROT and GREEN MAGMA drinks.
❋Wakasa GOLD, liquid CHLORELLA.
❋Beehive Botanicals Royal Jelly with Siberian Ginseng and Propolis 4x daily.
❋AloeLife ALOE VERA GOLD daily.
❋Nutrex HAWAIIAN SPIRULINA.

Herbal Therapy

❧ **Jump start herbal program:**
Crystal Star DETOX™ caps with GREEN TEA CLEANSER™ 2x daily, or 2 cups of burdock tea daily to detoxify the blood.

❋Crystal Star CAN-SSIAC™ or Flora FLOR-ESSENCE Essiac liquid for 2 months.

❋Turmeric capsules (curcumin) to take down organ swelling.

❋LIV-ALIVE™ capsules with MILK THISTLE SEED extract for 2 months to revitalize liver function.

❋Then add HEARTSEASE/ANEMI-GIZE™ caps to rebuild marrow.

❧ **Herbal red blood cell builders:** 🌀
❋Liquid chlorophyll 🌀
❋Floradix LIQUID IRON
❋Crystal Star GINSENG 6 SUPER TEA™.
❋Crystal Star IRON SOURCE™ extract.
❋Yellow dock tea ♀
❋Siberian ginseng extract
❋Health Aid America SIBERGEN.
❋Garlic/cayenne caps 8 daily.

❧ **Herbal cell normalizers:**
❋Crystal Star GINSENG/REISHI extract, or GINSENG/CHLORELLA extract.
❋HAWTHORN extract. ♀
❋PAU d'ARCO/ECHINACEA extract to normalize the lymphatic system.
❋Mezotrace SEA MINERAL COMPLEX 4 daily for needed minerals. 🌀

Supplements

✍ **Beta or marine carotene 150,000IU daily for at least 6 weeks.** and
❋Nutricology CAR-T-CELL with Enzymatic Therapy THYMUPLEX tablets. and

❋Ascorbate vit. C or Ester C powder, up to 10,000mg daily with bioflavonoids and rutin for several months.

❋Nature's Bounty internasal B$_{12}$ every other day for body balance/strength.
or

✍ American Biologics DIOXYCHLOR as directed for detoxification with Vita Carte BOVINE CARTILAGE or Nutricology MODIFIED CITRUS PECTIN as directed.

✍ **Anticancer agents:**
❋Nutricology GERMANIUM 150mg.
❋Am. Biologics colloidal silver.
❋Enzymatic Therapy LIQUID LIVER with SIBERIAN GINSENG 4 daily. ♀
❋Glutathione 50mg 2x daily.
❋Matrix Health GENESIS OXY-CAPS.

✍ Niacin therapy: 250mg 4x daily all during healing. ♀

✍ **B Complex 100mg, 4x daily, with extra folic acid, and B$_6$ 250mg.** ♀

✍ Vitamin E 800IU with selenium 200mcg and zinc 50mg.

Lifestyle Support Therapy

☙ Cortico-steroid drugs given to relieve symptoms of leukemia, over a long period of time greatly weaken immunity and bone strength.

☙ **Overheating therapy is effective for leukemia. See page 178 in this book.**
❋Use with a wheat grass enema or implant for best results.

☙ Avoid pesticides, X-rays, microwaves, electromagnetic fields from power lines and radiation of all kinds if possible. There seems to be a clear link between these and leukemia, especially in children.
❋Chemotherapy treatment for other cancers has sometimes been implicated in the development of leukemia.
❋Smoking is linked to leukemia.

☙ Relaxation techniques, such as meditation, imagery, acupuncture and reflexology are effective for leukemias.

☙ **Lymph-Flow Bath:** Put $^1/_2$ **pound each baking soda and sea salt in the tub. Soak for 20 minutes. Dunk head 5 times. Drip dry; stay warm; then shower.**

Common Symptoms: Increase in white blood cells, with no red blood cell production; extreme tiredness and anemia with symptoms similar to pernicious anemia - pallor, easy bruising, bone pain, thinness and weight loss; chronic infections - especially in children; spleen malfunction or loss; swelling of the spleen, liver and lymph nodes.

Common Causes: Indiscriminate use of X-rays and some drugs, especially in children and pregnant women; severe malnutrition with too many refined carbohydrates (especially in children); overfluoridation of the water; thyroid malfunction; deficiencies of vitamin D, iron, B$_{12}$ and folic acid; chronic viral infections; hereditary proneness. See Cancer causes in this book.

See the CANCER DIET in this book, or COOKING FOR HEALTHY HEALING by Linda Rector-Page for a complete healing diet.

Liver Health
Renewal & Revitalization

The health and vitality of all body systems depend to a large extent on the health and vitality of the liver. It is the body's most complex and useful organ - a powerful chemical plant that converts everything we eat, breathe and absorb through the skin into life-sustaining substances. The liver is a major blood reservoir, filtering out toxins at a rate of over a quart of blood per minute. It manufactures bile to digest fats and prevent constipation. It metabolizes proteins and carbohydrates, and secretes hormones and enzymes. Fortunately, since we live in an increasingly toxic world, the liver has amazing regenerative powers. Be good to your liver!

Diet & Superfood Therapy

Keeping fat low in your diet is crucial for liver vitality and regeneration. Optimum nutrition is the best liver protection.

Follow an alkalizing, rebuilding diet for a month with high quality vegetable protein. (A brief version is on page 352.)

➤Take daily during healing: 1 TB. each lecithin granules and brewer's yeast, 2-3 glasses cranberry or apple juice and 6-8 glasses of bottled water.

➤Avoid red meats and other acid-forming foods such as caffeine, alcohol, refined starches and dairy products during all healing phases. Reduce sugars, saturated fats and fried foods permanently.

Liver health and support foods include:
➤Vegetable fiber foods that absorb excess bile and increase regularity.
➤Potassium-rich foods: sea foods, dried fruits.
➤Chlorophyll-rich foods: leafy greens and sea vegetables.
➤Enzyme-rich foods: yogurt and kefir.
➤Sulphur-rich foods: garlic and onions.

Effective superfoods:
➤Green Foods BETA CARROT.
➤Beehive Botanicals ROYAL JELLY, GINSENG, POLLEN drink.
➤Crystal Star SYSTEMS STRENGTH™.
➤George's ALOE VERA JUICE.
➤CHLORELLA 1 pkt. daily/1 month.

Herbal Therapy

Jump start herbal program:
Crystal Star LIV-ALIVE™ caps and tea, with BITTERS & LEMON CLEANSE™ extract for intense cleansing.
➤MILK THISTLE SEED extract in aloe vera juice for protective benefits.
➤GREEN TEA CLEANSER™ to normalize liver function.
➤GINSENG/LICORICE ELIXIR™ as an ongoing liver tonic.
➤HEARTSEASE/ANEMIGIZE™ caps to rebuild liver and spleen activity or IRON SOURCE™ extract.

"Bitters" herbs for the liver:
➤Solaray TURMERIC extract caps (curcumin) to stimulate bile flow.
➤NatureWorks SWEDISH BITTERS.
➤Roast dandelion and burdock root.

A complete liver renewal program can take from three months to a year. **Liver vitality herbs:** Pau d'Arco tea or Crystal Star PAU d' ARCO/GINSENG extract in water.
Reishi mushroom extract, or Crystal Star GINSENG/REISHI extract.
➤Royal jelly 2 teasp. daily.

Liver rebuilding herbal tonic: Mix 4-oz. hawthorn berries, 2-oz. red sage, 1-oz. cardamom. Steep 24 hours in 2 qts. of water. Add honey. Take 2 cups daily.

Supplements

The liver is a vast storehouse for vitamins, minerals, and enzymes. It secretes them as needed to build and maintain healthy cells.

A "spring cleaning" inositol cocktail: ITC SUPER SUNSHINE B, or Source Naturals CO-ENZYMATE B daily with a good lipotropic, such as Solaray LIPOTROPIC PLUS - esp. if taking contraceptives. or

High omega-3 flax seed oil 3x daily with liquid chlorophyll 3 teasp. daily, and AloeLife FIBERMATE.

Natren TRINITY, or Dr. DOPHILUS, or Alta Health CANGEST, ¼ teasp. 3x daily, or take Prevail LIVER FORMULA caps.

Liver antioxidants:
➤Ascorbate vitamin C 500mg every hour during cleansing stage, then 3000mg daily.
➤Nutricology GERMANIUM 150mg.
RBeta Carotene 100,000IU
➤Carnitine 500mg.
➤CoQ₁₀ 60mg 3x daily.
➤PCOs from grapeseed or white pine 100mg daily.

Enzymatic Therapy LIVA-TOX or Liquid Liver with Siberian Ginseng. Then add THYMU-PLEX to rebuild immunity,

Lifestyle Support Therapy

The liver is dependent on the amount and quality of oxygen coming into the lungs. Exercise, air filters, time spent in the forest and at the ocean, and drinking pure water are important.

Overheating by raising blood temperature is effective. See pg. 178 in this book.

Good liver lifestyle practices:
➤Eat smaller meals, minimize eating late at night.
➤Get adequate, regular sleep.
➤Exercise every day, with a good brisk aerobic walk.
➤Avoid taking saccharin-containing foods and acetaminophen drugs over a long period of time.

Take one coffee enema during your detoxification cleanse; (1 cup coffee to 1 qt. distilled water.)
➤Wheatgrass implants are also effective.

Take several saunas if possible during a liver cleanse for faster, easier detoxification.

Reflexology point:

liver

Common Symptoms: Sluggish system; general depression and melancholy; unexplained weight gain and great tiredness; poor digestion; food and chemical sensitivities; PMS; constipation and congestion; nausea and shakes; dizziness; dry tongue and mouth; jaundiced skin and/or liver spots; skin itching.

Common Causes: Too much alcohol and/or drugs; too much sugar, refined, low nutrition foods, and preservatives; overeating - esp. too much animal protein; low fiber; low vegetable diet; exposure to toxic environmental chemicals and pollutants; stress; hepatitis virus; long-term use of prescription drugs (especially antibiotics and tranquilizers).

See COOKING FOR HEALTHY HEALING by Linda Rector Page and the following pages for more information.

Liver Disease
Cirrhosis ❀ Jaundice

Cirrhosis, or scarring, of the liver tissue is a serious, degenerative condition, preventing the liver from its proper function. It is the second biggest killer of people between 45 and 65 in America today. Usually a consequence of alcohol abuse, it is also almost always a part of other severe liver infections, such as hepatitis, EBV, and AIDS related syndromes. If your diet is nutrient poor, the liver becomes exhausted, and even more serious debilitation results.

Diet & Superfood Therapy

A continuing optimum nutrition diet is the key to liver regeneration.

❧ If condition is acute, go on a 3 day liquid detoxification diet (see next page) to clean out toxic waste.

➤Take a carrot/beet/cucumber juice daily for 1 week, then every other day for a week, then every 2 days, then every 3 days, etc. for a month.

➤Then take a glass of lemon juice and water each morning.

➤Include two glasses of carrot juice daily for a month during healing.

➤Eat plenty of fresh fruits and vegetables. Particularly eat vegetable protein such as sprouts, whole grains, tofu, wheat germ, and brewer's yeast.

➤Avoid all alcohol, fried, salty or fatty foods, caffeine, sugar and tobacco.

❧ Make a mix of lecithin, brewer's yeast and wheat germ oil; add 2 tsp. to the daily diet.
❦

❧ **Superfoods are very important:**
➤Crystal Star ENERGY GREEN™.
➤Wakunaga KYO-GREEN.
➤AloeLife **ALOE GOLD drink.**
➤Green Foods GREEN ESSENCE.
➤Sun **CHLORELLA 1 pkt. daily.**
➤Solgar WHEY TO GO protein drink.

Herbal Therapy

❧ **Jump start herbal program:**
Crystal Star LIV-ALIVE™ caps, or extract 3x daily, and/or LIV-ALIVE™ tea (3 cups daily for 3 weeks, then 1 cup daily for a month.)
➤GREEN TEA CLEANSER™ daily for 3 to 6 months. ♂
➤**MILK THISTLE SEED extract 3x daily especially against alcohol damage.**
➤**GINSENG 6 SUPER TEA™ to help heal internal scarring.**

❧ **Herbal liver antioxidants:**
➤Solaray **CENTELLA ASIATICA:**
➤Oregon grape root
➤Dandelion root
➤Garlic capsules 4 daily.
➤Solaray ALFAJUICE caps.

❧ Make the following tea mix. Take 1 cup daily: bilberry, ginkgo biloba lf., ginger rt.

❧ Barberry tea for jaundice until clear.

Supplements

➣ **Carnitine 500mg 2x daily.** ♀

➣ **Effective lipotropics, to prevent fat accumulation in the liver:**
➤Choline 600mg
➤Phosphatidyl choline
➤Solaray LIPOTROPIC PLUS caps
➤Methionine 2x daily
➤Lecithin capsules 2 daily

➣ For severe liver dysfunction, see HEPATITIS in this book and use the following:
➤Enzymatic Therapy LIVA-TOX caps.
➤Choline/inositol 100mg.
➤L-Glutamine 500mg 2x daily.
➤Beta-carotene 100,000IU daily.
➤**Natren BIFIDO FACTORS 3x daily to cleanse and restore liver tissue.**
➤**Klamath POWER 3 caps as directed.**
➤**Enzymatic Therapy SUPER MILK THISTLE COMPLEX with artichoke.**
➤Enzymatic Therapy GARLINASE.

➣ **Effective liver anti-oxidants:**
➤Vitamin E 400IU with selenium 100mcg 2x daily.
➤**Ascorbate vitamin C crystals 5000mg daily or to bowel tolerance.**
➤Country Life DMG B$_{15}$ SL, 1 daily.
➤Nutricology GERMANIUM 150mg.
➤CoQ10 60mg 3x daily.

Lifestyle Support Therapy

☞ Take a coffee enema once a week for a month to flush out and stimulate liver activity. (1 cup strong brewed in a quart of water), or chlorella or spirulina implants.

☞ Smoking is bad for liver health. Try even harder to quit all forms of tobacco.

☞ Drink 6-8 glasses of pure water daily. Take an early morning sunbath whenever possible.

☞ **Reflexology point:**

liver

☞ **Liver area:**

See next page for a LIVER DETOX DIET.

Common Symptoms: *Sluggish, reduced energy; constipation alternating to diarrhea; often jaundice; skin itching/irritation; bags under the eyes. Severe symptoms include anemia and large bruise patches. As cirrhosis progresses, there is increasing weakness, jaundice and abdominal distention.*
Common Causes: *Liver toxicity from excess alcohol and/or drugs; environmental pollutants; excess refined foods and sugars; long term malnutrition.*

left lobe
ligamentum teres
right lobe

Liver Detoxification Diet

Since any toxic substance can harm the liver, and since most of us are continually assailed by toxins in our food, water and air, it is generally realized that none of us has a truly healthy liver. The good news is that the liver has amazing rejuvenating powers, and can continue to function even when as many as 80% of its cells are damaged. A clean, functioning liver produces natural antihistamines to keep immunity high, neutralizes and destroys poisons in the body, cleanses the blood and discharges waste into the bile, metabolizes and helps excrete fat and cholesterol, helps form and store red blood cells and iron, aids digestion, maintains hormone balance, and remarkably enough, regenerates its own damaged tissue. A liver cleanse and detoxification twice a year in the spring and fall is highly recommended to maximize its activity, using the extra vitamin D from the sun to help.

On rising: take a glass of 2TBS. lemon juice or cider vinegar in water with 1 teasp. honey, and 1 teasp. royal jelly; or Crystal Star BITTERS & LEMON CLEANSE™ extract in water .
If an olive oil flush or coffee enema are to be included in the cleanse, now is the time to take them.
Breakfast: take a glass of carrot/beet/cucumber juice, or a potassium broth (pg. 167); or a glass of organic apple juice. Add ¹/₂ teasp. dairy free acidophilus powder.
Mid-morning: have an apple or cranberry juice; or a cup of Crystal Star LIV-ALIVE™ tea; or a vegetable green drink (page 168), or Sun CHLORELLA, or Crystal Star ENERGY GREEN™ drink.
Lunch: have a glass of fresh carrot juice, or another glass of organic apple juice.
Mid-afternoon: have a cup of peppermint, pau d' arco, or roasted dandelion root tea; or another vegetable green drink, or Crystal Star GREEN TEA CLEANSER™, or LIV-ALIVE™ tea.
Dinner: have another glass of organic apple juice; and/or a Crystal Star SYSTEMS STRENGTH™ drink or another potassium broth.
Before bed: take another glass of lemon juice or cider vinegar in water. Add 15 drops of MILK THISTLE SEED extract.

☙ **Suggested supplements for the Liver Detoxification Diet:**
•Add one teasp. royal jelly, or ascorbate vitamin C crystals, ¹/₄ teasp. at a time, or 15 drops MILK THISTLE SEED extract to any above liquids.
•Drink six to eight glasses of bottled water every day to encourage maximum flushing of liver tissues.
☙ **Bodywork for the Liver Detoxification Cleanse:**
•Only mild exercise should be undertaken during the fast. Get plenty of early morning sunlight every day possible. Get adequate rest during the cleanse.
•Take a hot sauna each day of this cleanse for optimum results. Take an spirulina implant once a week followed by 1¹/₂ teasp. acidophilus in water.

Liver Rebuilding Diet

This diet is high in alkalizing fresh foods (60%), and vegetable proteins, dairy free, and low in fats. All alcohol, caffeine and caffeine-containing foods, saturated fats, and red meats should be avoided while on this diet. It may be used for 1 month, after the Liver Detox Diet above to rebuild healthy liver function, or by itself for a week or more, as a mild "spring cleaning" for the organs at any time. A continuing diet for liver health should be lacto-vegetarian, low fat, and rich in vegetable proteins and vitamin C foods for good iron absorption. Note: Take small meals more frequently all during the day, rather than any large meals.

On rising: take a glass of lemon juice and water with 1 teasp. honey.
Breakfast: Make a mix of 2 TBS. each: brewer's yeast, lecithin, and high omega 3 flax oil. Take 2 teasp. each morning in prune, organic apple or cranberry juice; and have some fresh fruit, like grapefruit or pineapple; and/or a whole grain cereal or muesli with apple juice or fruit yogurt on top.
Mid-morning: have a veggie green drink (pg. 168), Sun CHLORELLA or Green Foods GREEN MAGMA; and/or a cup of miso soup with 2 TBS. sea veggies snipped on top; or a cup of Crystal Star GREEN TEA CLEANSER™, or SYSTEM STRENGTH™ drink.
Lunch: have a large fresh green salad with lemon/olive oil dressing; and a glass of fresh carrot juice and some whole grain crackers with a yogurt, kefir or soy spread; or marinated, baked tofu with brown rice or millet, and a small spinach/sprout salad with a light olive oil dressing.
Mid-afternoon: have a cup of miso soup, or an alkalizing herb tea, such as chamomile, dandelion root, or pau d' arco; and/or a hard boiled egg and a cup of plain or goat's milk yogurt.
Dinner: have a baked potato with kefir cheese or soy cheese dressing, and a large dinner salad with low-fat mayonnaise; or a light vegetable steam/stir fry with vegetables, seafood or tofu; or some steamed veggies with a light Italian or tofu dressing, and brown rice, millet or bulgur wheat; or a vegetable souffle or casserole with a light noodle broth.
Before bed: have an herb tea, like dandelion root, chamomile or Crystal Star ROYAL MU TEA™, or a glass of apple juice or prune juice, or a cup of Organic Gourmet NUTRITIONAL YEAST broth.

☙ **Suggested supplements for the Liver Rebuilding Diet:**
•Add 1 teasp. royal jelly, ascorbate vitamin C crystals, ¹/₄ teasp. at a time, or 15 drops MILK THISTLE SEED extract to any of the above liquids.
•Take a veggie green drink (pg. 168), Sun CHLORELLA, Crystal Star ENERGY GREEN™ drink, or Green Foods GREEN MAGMA frequently for red blood cell formation.
☙ **Bodywork For The Liver Rebuilding Diet:**
•Take a brisk walk every day to cleanse the lungs, increase circulation, and oxygenate the blood. Stretching exercises are particularly helpful to tone liver tissue.

See COOKING FOR HEALTHY HEALING by Linda Rector Page for a complete Liver Healing Diet.

Low Blood Pressure

Hypotension

Even though we hear much less about it, chronically low blood pressure is also a threat to good health. LBP is abnormal blood pressure due to a variety of causes, from a reaction to drug medication, an electrolyte-loss response to a disease, or an endocrine or nerve disorder. LBP is also a sign that arterial system walls and tissue are weak; blood and fluid can leak and abnormally distend them, and prevent good circulation. Natural treatment works well when there are symptoms such as dizziness or light-headedness upon standing up, or faintness, indicating a reduction of cerebral flow.

Diet & Superfood Therapy

✿ Follow a fresh foods diet for a week, with veggie drinks (pg. 168), potassium broth (pg. 167), brewer's yeast, and green salads. Take a lemon and water drink every morning with 1 teasp. honey.

Then, follow a modified macrobiotic diet for 1-2 months, stressing vegetable proteins, green salads with celery, miso, onions, garlic and other alkalizing foods, and dried or fresh fruits.

➤Include strengthening complex carbohydrates, such as peas, broccoli, potatoes and whole grains.

➤Avoid canned and refined foods, animal fats, red meats, and caffeine. Reduce all high cholesterol, starchy foods.

✿ Bioflavonoids are the key for stronger blood vessels:
➟Citrus juices, esp. pineapple juice
➟Juice of *whole grapes*
➟Japanese green tea
➟Knudsen RECHARGE electrolyte drink, or Alacer MIRACLE WATER

✿ Effective superfoods:
➟Crystal Star SYSTEMS STRENGTH™ drink or caps for absorbable minerals.
➟Protein drinks: Nappi THE PERFECT MEAL, or Solgar WHEY TO GO.
➟Future Biotics VITAL K, 6 teasp. daily.

Herbal Therapy

♔ Jump start herbal program:
Crystal Star HEARTSEASE/HAWTHORN™ capsules 2-4 daily for a month, with 8 garlic caps or 4 cayenne/ginger caps daily.
➤Then, ADR-ACTIVE™ capsules 2x daily for a month with extra GINKGO BILOBA or HAWTHORN extract.
➤BITTERS & LEMON CLEANSE™ extract for metabolism support.

♔ Crystal Star HEARTSEASE/CIRCU-CLEANSE™ tea for prevention.
➤Crystal Star GREEN TEA CLEANSER™ during entire healing period. ♀

♔ Flavonoid-rich herbs for tissue tone:
➟HAWTHORN extract 2-3x daily
➟BILBERRY extract
➟Gotu kola extract
➟Lemon peel tea
➟Hibiscus tea
➟Rosehips tea

♔ Blood pressure normalizing herbs:
➟Siberian ginseng 4-6 daily
➟Cayenne/ginger 4 daily
➟Garlic 6-8 daily
➟**Kelp 8-10 daily**
➟Dandelion root caps 4 daily ♀
➟Rosemary for nerve balance ♀

Supplements

Avoid the amino acids phenylalanine and tyrosine.

✧ Magnesium 400mg 4x daily, or Solaray CAL/MAG CITRATE, 1000mg calcium and 1000mg magnesium, or Rainbow Light CALCIUM PLUS with high magnesium; with extra zinc 30mg 2x daily. ♀

✧ Vitamin E therapy for 8 weeks: work up from 100IU daily the first week, to 800IU daily, adding 100mg. daily each week. ♂

✧ B Complex 100mg daily with extra B$_1$ 100mg and pantothenic acid 500mg.

✧ Antioxidants are important:
➤PCOs from grapeseed and white pine for extra high flavonoids.
➤Germanium 150mg 2x daily.
➤Vitamin C with bioflavonoids and rutin 3000mg daily.

✧ Enzymatic Therapy LIQUID LIVER with SIBERIAN GINSENG.

✧ Vitamin K 100mcg 2 daily for capillary strength.

✧ Floradix LIQUID IRON.

Lifestyle Support Therapy

Sometimes tiredness and lack of energy are a sign of low blood pressure. Check out your symptoms.

❧ Acupressure, chiropractic spinal manipulation and shiatsu therapy are all effective in normalizing circulatory function.
➤Alternating hot and cold hydrotherapy (pg. 177) revs up circulation.

❧ Avoid tobacco and secondary smoke.

❧ Consciously try to relax the whole body once a day with short meditation, yoga exercises and rest.

❧ Do deep breathing exercises (See Bragg's book) to stimulate circulation and oxygenate the system.
➤Stand up slowly to allow blood pressure to normalize.

Common Symptoms: Malfunction of the circulatory system's systole/diastol action; thinning of the blood; great fatigue and easy loss of energy; low immunity and susceptibility to allergies and infections - particularly opportunistic disease like candida yeast overgrowth.

Common Causes: Poor diet with vitamin C and bioflavonoid deficiency causing a "run-down" condition; kidney malfunction causing system toxemia; emotional problems; anemia; overuse of drugs that lower immunity.

See CHRONIC FATIGUE SYNDROME pages in this book for more information.

Lung Disease

Sarcoidosis ❖ Tuberculosis ❖ Cystic Fibrosis

Chronic pulmonary diseases have increased dramatically in the last decade. Three that have been part of this unusual rise are discussed here. Sarcoidosis is a systemic viral infection with widespread, grainy lesions on tissue or organs. The lungs and liver are both usually affected, with a chronic cough and difficulty breathing. Tuberculosis is a highly contagious, bacterial infection that's on the rise in America. It is characterized by bloody sputum, a chronic cough, shortness of breath and fatigue, night sweats, serious weight loss and chest pain. Cystic fibrosis is an inherited childhood disease characterized by recurring lung infections and severe malnutrition from lack of nutrient absorption.

Diet & Superfood Therapy

High quality protein is needed to heal lung diseases.

♇ Go on a short mucous cleansing liquid diet (pg. 162). Then, use the following lung cleansing diet for two weeks:
  ❧Lemon or grapefruit juice and water each morning with 1 tsp. honey; or water-diluted pineapple juice as a natural expectorant.
  ❧Fresh carrot juice or potassium broth (pg. 167) daily.
  ❧Take two fresh green salads daily.
  ❧Steamed vegetables with brown rice and tofu or seafood for dinner.
  ❧Cranberry or celery juice before bed.

♇ A continuing diet for lung health should be high in vegetable proteins and whole grains, low in sugars and starches.
  ❧Include cultured foods such as yogurt and kefir for friendly G.I. flora.
  ❧Include pitted fruits- apricots, peaches, plums are lung specifics.
  ❧Include brewer's yeast 2 teasp. daily.
  ❧Take a protein drink each morning.

♇ **Effective superfoods:**
  ❧Salute ALOE VERA JUICE with herbs, 1 glass daily.
  ❧Crystal Star SYSTEMS STRENGTH™.
  ❧**Nappi THE PERFECT MEAL protein.**
  ❧Green Foods **BETA CARROT.**
  ❧Nature's Life SUPER GREEN-PRO.

Herbal Therapy

☙ **Jump start herbal program:**
Crystal Star ANTI-BIO™ 4x daily for 1 week; then 2x daily with RESPR™ caps 4 daily for 2 months.
  ❧Add RESPR™ tea or DEEP BREATHING™ tea 2 cups daily for increased results.
  ❧Add HEAVY METAL™ caps if lungs are subject to lots of environmental pollution.
  ❧PAU D'ARCO / ECHINACEA extract or pau d'arco tea 3 cups daily as lung healers.
  ❧EVENING PRIMROSE OIL capsules 4-6 daily especially if there is lung pain.

☙ **For Tuberculosis:**
  ❧High potency royal jelly 2 teasp. daily.
  ❧Calendula ointment chest rubs. ♀
  ❧Body Essentials SILICA GEL on the chest. ♀

☙ **For sarcoidosis:**
  ❧Planetary TRIPHALA caps as directed.
  ❧**Melatonin 3mg at night to reduce nodules.**
  ❧Klamath POWER 3 caps.
  ❧**Garlic caps 6-8 daily.**

☙ **For cystic fibrosis:** ⊗
  ❧Echinacea/goldenseal capsules or Crystal Star ANTI-BIO™ extract in water.
  ❧High Omega-3 flax oil, 2 teasp. daily.
  ❧GINSENG/LICORICE ELIXIR™ a body-strengthening expectorant, dilute in water.
  ❧Expectorant herbs, like licorice, marshmallow root, pleurisy root, thyme or coltsfoot.

Supplements

❧ **Effective anti-oxidants are a key:** (They may be given to children in reduced dose as protection from future lung diseases.)
  ❧**Beta-carotene 100,000-150,000IU daily, with B Complex 100mg, extra B₆ 100mg, and B₁₂ 2000mcg.**
  ❧Vitamin C 5000mg w. bioflavonoids.
  ❧American Biologics OXY-5000.
  ❧**Nutricology GERMANIUM 150mg.**
  ❧PCOs 100mg 3x daily.
  ❧**Twin Labs LYCOPENE 5-10mg.**

❧ **H₂O₂ therapy:** Matrix Health OXY-CLEANSE caps, or American Biologics DIOXYCHLOR for 1 month. Rest for a month; resume if needed. There will be intense and prolonged coughing, as accumulated waste is released. H₂O₂ works to destroy chronic infection in the lungs and provide nascent oxygen to the tissues. ♂

❧ **For T.B. - on the rise in America:**
  ❧Beta-carotene 150,000IU.
  ❧CoQ₁₀ 100mg 3x daily. ♀
  ❧Quercetin with Bromelain daily. ♂
  ❧Vitamin C to bowel tolerance daily.

❧ **For cystic fibrosis:** ⊗
  ❧Enzymatic Therapy LUNG COMPLEX and THYMULUS complex.
  ❧RAW PANCREAS to help absorption.
  ❧Natren LIFE START daily.

Lifestyle Support Therapy

☙ Avoid all CFCs. They are as harmful to your lungs as they are to the atmosphere.
  ❧Avoid tobacco and secondary smoke.
  ❧Get plenty of fresh air and sunshine, away from air pollution.

☙ Scratch the arm lightly, for 5 minutes daily, along the meridian line from the shoulder to the outside of the thumb to clear and heal lungs.
  ❧For cystic fibrosis, use gentle percussion on the chest to keep mucous from clogged airways. ⊗
  ❧Take a catnip or chlorophyll enema once a week to clear body toxins out faster.

☙ **Reflexology points:**

lung points

☙ **Lung area:**

Common Symptoms: Constant coughing, inflammation and pain; bloody expectoration; difficulty breathing; difficulty performing even simple activities without shortness of breath. Cystic fibrosis symptoms include very salty sweat from dysfunctional sweat glands.

Common Causes: Environmental and heavy metal pollutants, such as chlorofluorocarbons and smoking; malnutrition, and vitamin A deficiency; suppressive over-the-counter cold and congestion remedies that don't allow the lungs to eliminate harmful wastes properly. Cystic fibrosis is genetically inherited.

See the ASTHMA DIET in this book or "Cooking For Healthy Healing" by Linda Rector-Page for a complete lung healing diet.

Lupus

Systemic Lupus Erythematosus

Lupus is a multi-system, auto-immune, inflammatory, viral disease affecting over half a million Americans, more than 80% of them black and Hispanic women. The immune system becomes disoriented and develops antibodies that attack its own connective tissue. Joints and blood vessels are affected producing arthritis-like symptoms. Kidneys and lymph nodes become inflamed; in severe cases there is heart, brain and central nervous system degeneration. Orthodox treatment has not been very successful for lupus. Natural therapies help rebuild a stable immune system. Our experience shows that you feel worse for 1 or 2 months until toxins are neutralized. Then, suddenly, as a rule, you feel much better. A natural program works, but requires many months of healing.

Diet & Superfood Therapy

♨ Diet therapy reduces the symptoms of lupus. Follow the ARTHRITIS CLEANSING DIET in this book for three months:

✺The diet should be 60-75% fresh foods during this time. Avoid nightshade plants like eggplant, tomatoes, tobacco.

✺Take potassium broth (pg. 167) every day for 1 month, then every other day for 1 month, then once a week the 3rd month.

✺Then follow a modified macrobiotic diet (pg. 211) until blood tests clear, (sometimes 2-3 years, but healing success rate is good). Take aloe vera juice 1-2 glasses daily.

✺Make sure your diet is very low in fat. A vegetarian diet is strongly recommended to increase fatty acids and decrease fats.

✺Avoid red meats, sugars, starchy foods.

♨ See "COOKING FOR HEALTHY HEALING" by Linda Rector-Page for a complete, effective healing diet.

♨ **Effective superfoods:**
✺Wakunaga KYO-GREEN drink.
✺**Crystal Star SYSTEMS STRENGTH™ drink** to re-establish tissue integrity.
✺**Nutricology PRO-GREENS with flax.**
✺Beehive Botanical ROYAL JELLY with Siberian ginseng 2 teasp. daily.
✺AloeLife ALOE GOLD JUICE 2x daily, FIBERMATE 2x daily.
✺Sun CHLORELLA 15 tabs daily.

Herbal Therapy

♨ **Jump start herbal program:**
Crystal Star LIV-ALIVE™ caps and tea daily for 1 month, with EVENING PRIMROSE oil 6 daily for EFAs, and bupleurum extract 2x daily.

✺**ANTI-BIO™ w. AR-EASE™ or ANTI-FLAM™ caps as needed for inflammation.**

✺**BODY REBUILDER™, GINSENG 6 SUPER TEA™, and ADR-ACTIVE™ capsules to rebuild energy.**

✺**GREEN TEA CLEANSER™ to re-establish homeostasis.**

✺Pau d' arco tea 3-4 cups daily or PAU d'ARCO/ECHINACEA extract in water as an anti-infective.

✺Apply ANTI-BIO™ gel with una da gato - apply to roughened skin patches.

✺Gotu Kola capsules 4 daily as a central nervous stimulant.

✺Solaray TURMERIC extract as an anti-inflammatory.

♨ **Effective immune stimulants:**
✺High potency royal jelly, 40,000mg or more, 2 teasp. daily ♀♂
✺Crystal Star GINSENG/REISHI extract
✺Zand IMMUNE HERBAL extract

♨ **Hormone balancing aids:**
✺Sarsaparilla extract
✺Crystal Star GINSENG/LICORICE ELIXIR™

Supplements

❧ Body Ammo DHEA with Cat's Claw and Glucosamine 50mg 3x daily.♀

❧ **For the liver:**
✺Twin Lab EGG YOLK LECITHIN.
✺Enzymatic Therapy LIQUID LIVER with SIBERIAN GINSENG.
✺Nature's Secret ULTIMATE B with extra B_6 200mg daily, for effective EFAs.
✺Nature's Bounty B_{12}, and CoQ_{10} 100mg 3x daily to block toxicity from drugs and rebuild cell structure.
✺Future Biotics VITAL K 4 teasp. daily.

❧ **American Biologics SUB-ADRENE 3-5 drops 3 to 4 times daily.**♀

❧ Ascorbate vit. C 5000mg daily with bioflavonoids and rutin, or Quercetin with bromelain 3x daily as an anti-inflammatory.

❧ **Omega-3 flax oil caps for inflammation.** ♂

❧ **Immune building supplements:**
✺Nutricology GERMANIUM 150mg
✺Enzymatic Therapy THYMU-PLEX
✺Health Aid SIBERGIN as directed
✺Nutricology CAR-T-CELL as directed

❧ Probiotics normalize the internal system: Natren BIFIDO FACTORS and Alta Health CANGEST for pancreatic enzymes.

Lifestyle Support Therapy

☞ Over-medication for lupus, especially by cortico-steroid drugs is dangerous; they weaken the bones, cause excess weight gain and eventually suppress immune response.

☞ Avoid birth control pills, penicillin, allergenic cosmetics, and phototoxins from UV rays. Any of these can result in a flare-up of lupus.

☞ Get plenty of rest and quality sleep.

☞ Take a walk every day for exercise and stress reduction.
✺Other effective stress reduction techniques include meditation, yoga and acupuncture.

See Arthritis and Immunity sections in this book for more information.

Common Symptoms: *Great fatigue and depression; rough, red skin patches; chronic nail fungus - red at cuticle base; skin pallor; photosensitivity to light; inability to tear; low grade chronic fever; rheumatoid arthritis symptoms; kidney problems; anemia and low leukocyte count; pleurisy; inflammation, esp. around the mouth, cheeks and nose; seizures, amnesia and psychosis; low immunity.*
Common Causes: *Viral infection; degeneration of the body, often caused by too many antibiotics or prescription drugs from Hydrazine derivatives; alcoholism; food allergies; emotional stress; reaction to certain chemicals; latent diabetes; overgrowth of Candida albicans yeasts; chronic fatigue syndrome; triggered by UV sunlight.*

Lyme Disease
Lyme Arthritis

Lyme disease is caused by a micro-organism that is transmitted to humans by the deer tick, a pest no bigger than a freckle. It is a serious, steadily debilitating, degenerative disease, with symptoms much like those of arthritis. It is difficult to guard against. Antibiotics are the current medical treatment of choice, and seem to work in the initial phases, symptoms usually recur after the drugs are withdrawn, and they do not work in the later stages at all. Natural therapies that address the disease as if it were a virus have had the best success. Strong immune enhancement is the best defense.

Diet & Superfood Therapy

See the Hypoglycemia Diet in this book, or COOK-ING FOR HEALTHY HEALING by Linda Rector Page for more information.

❧ A modified macrobiotic diet (pg. 211) is recommended for 2-3 months to strengthen the body while cleaning out and overcoming the disease.
➠Potassium broth (pg. 167) 2x a week.
➠**Have a veggie drink (pg. 168) or a fresh green salad every day.**
➠Take 1 teasp. each daily: wheat germ oil for body oxygen, EGG YOLK LECITHIN, royal jelly 40,000mg or more.
➠Avoid alcohol, tobacco, all refined and caffeine-containing foods, and sugars. Omit red meat, high gluten and starchy foods.

❧ **Effective superfoods:**
➠Green Foods GREEN MAGMA drink.
➠Crystal Star ENERGY GREEN™ drink and ZINC SOURCE™ drops.
➠Sun CHLORELLA, 2 pkts. daily.
➠Nutricology PRO-GREENS w. flax oil.
➠Solgar WHEY TO GO protein drink.

Herbal Therapy

Symptoms show up 3 weeks after tick bite. Use natural therapy after a course of antibiotics.

☙ **Jump start herbal program:**
➠Clean the tick bite with: **tea tree oil, calendula extract, echinacea/goldenseal extract,** or **St. John's wort extract 2-3x daily.**
➠**Then take ANTI-VI™ extract in water 2x daily, one week on and one week off to overcome the virus.**
➠**Use ANTI-FLAM™ caps or extract, or turmeric (curcumin) for inflammation.**
➠Boost immune response with: Crystal Star ANTI-BIO™ caps or extract to cleanse lymph glands; LIV-ALIVE™ caps or extract to enhance liver activity for a month.
➠Then the GINSENG/REISHI™ extract to rebuild immune response, or GINSENG 6 SUPER TEA™ or capsules with suma, to reestablish homeostasis.

☙ **Other effective herbs:**
➠Use myrrh or pennyroyal oil **topically** to both repel and kill lyme ticks.
➠Crystal Star RELAX CAPS™ to re-build nerve structure
-➠Astragalus extract
-➠Garlic capsules 6 daily, or Enzymatic Therapy GARLINASE 4000.

Supplements

Deer ticks also transmit the even more serious pathogen, Ehrlichia, that causes HGE, that can be fatal. Rigorously check for tiny deer ticks if you live in an infested area.

☙ **Anti-infectives:**
➠**Nutricology germanium 150mg daily.**
➠**Matrix GENESIS OXY-SPRAY H$_2$O$_2$ gel** or Centipede KITTY'S OXYGEL to the bite.
➠**Colloidal silver as directed.**
➠**Nutribiotic GRAPEFRUIT SEED extract, 10 drops 3x daily in water.**
➠**Lane Labs BENE-FIN shark cartilage to enhance leukocytes with Enzymatic Therapy THYMULUS complex to help restore immunity.**

☙ **Antioxidants:**
➠Beta or oceanic carotene 100-150,000IU daily with quercitin with bromelain as an anti-inflammatory.
➠Cysteine (or NAC) 500mg 2x daily.
➠Vitamin C or Ester C powder, $^1/_4$ teasp. every hour to daily bowel tolerance as an antioxidant and toxin neutralizer, especially during acute attacks and recurrences.

☙ **Probiotics for homeostasis:**
➠Natren LIFE STAR ⊛ or TRINITY for digestive damage from long courses of antibiotics and to restore nutrient assimilation.
➠Solaray pancreatin 1300mg. 4x daily on an empty stomach.

Lifestyle Support Therapy

☙ Take a hot bath or spa to discourage organism replication, and to relieve pain.

☙ **Environmental preventive measures:**
➠Keep lawns cut short and shrubbery to a minimum where children play.
➠When walking through tall grass or brush, wear long-sleeve shirts and pants, and tape pant legs into socks. Use natural tick repellents on exposed body areas. DEET chemical repellent, while effective, can be fatal if ingested and can cause adverse reactions in children. Put suspicious clothing in the dryer to kill ticks by dehydration. Just washing clothes is not effective.
➠Do a meticulous, daily body inspection if you have been in the woods or live in an infested area. Have a partner inspect for best results. Look for louse-sized arachnids or dark freckle-sized nymphs behind knees, in scalp and pubic hair, in armpits and under waistbands. Apply heat to tick so it will back out. Remove the tick with tweezers as close to the head as possible. Pull straight up. **Do not squeeze or twist it.** (Gut contents will empty into you.) Never touch the tick with your hands. Apply alcohol to bite area. Time is critical. The longer the tick is attached the greater are the risks of serious disease.
➠Check outdoor pets for ticks regularly.

Common Symptoms: *A large red "bulls-eye" rash with a light center, near the site of the bite that becomes as large as 10 to 20 inches; initial flu-like symptoms of chills and aches; unusual fatigue and malaise, head aches and joint pain, especially in children; later symptoms of heart arrythmia, muscle spasms with racking pain, meningitis (brain inflammation), chronic bladder problems, arthritis, facial paralysis and other numbing nerve dysfunctions, and extreme fatigue. Note: Lyme disease symptoms mimic several other disease conditions. Have a simple test done by a health care clinic if you feel that you are at risk.*

Use LymeNet for the latest information (908-390-0005). Treat Lyme Disease early.

Measles
Rubella

Measles is a highly contagious viral infection that attacks a lowered immune system. The first symptoms appear as an upper respiratory cold or flu, followed by a red rash. While usually thought of as a childhood disease, measles also affects adults whose immunity to the virus has not been established. Measles is most communicable in the early stages. Rubella (German measles) is a more severe, and even more contagious form of viral measles, infecting a wider area of the body. Measles effects can be permanent in adults. Keep immunity high for the best defense. Take great care if you are pregnant. Measles can cause birth defects.

Diet & Superfood Therapy

♌ Start with a liquid foods diet for at least 24 hours to increase fluid intake as much as possible. Use fresh fruit and vegetable juices, miso soup, bottled water and herb teas such as catnip, chamomile or rosemary, that will mildly induce sweating and clean out toxins faster.

  *Then follow with a simple, basic diet featuring vitamin A and C-rich fresh foods.

  *Give 1 teasp. acidophilus liquid in citrus juice each morning.

  *Offer fresh fruits all through the morning, with yogurt if desired.

  *Have a fresh green salad each day.

  *Have a cup of miso or clear soup with 1 teasp. brewer's yeast and snipped sea veggies daily.

  *Have a cup of miso (or Ramen) soup each day, and a cup of Organic Gourmet NUTRITIONAL YEAST extract broth before bed.

      ℬ

♌ **Superfoods are very important:**
  *Crystal Star BIOFLAV, FIBER & C SUPPORT™ drink 2x daily.
  *BioStrath original LIQUID YEAST.
  *New Moon GINGER WONDER syrup to soothe a sore throat and provide healing benefits.

Herbal Therapy

♌ Jump start herbal program:
  Crystal Star ANTI-VI™ tea to curb infection, twice daily, and ANTI-FLAM™ extract drops in water to reduce inflammation.
  *FIRST AID CAPS™ 2 daily for 2 days to break out the fever and rash, and start the healing process.

  *Use EYEBRIGHT HERBS™ tea as an eyewash to soothe photosensitivity discomfort. (Keep the room darkened.)

  *ZINC SOURCE™ herbal drops for almost immediate sore throat relief.

  *Use catnip, yarrow or chamomile teas, 3-4 cups daily, as diaphoretics to break out the rash; raspberry, gotu kola or lobelia tea to heal measles skin sores.

♌ **For rubella: use licorice tea or GINSENG/LICORICE ELIXIR™ drops as an expectorant.**

  *St. John's wort extract or capsules, or mullein/lobelia tincture acute stage.

  *Use marjoram tea internally to sweat out rash; externally to soothe skin.

♌ Effective herbal body washes to soothe and heal:
  *Elder flower ☺
  *Peppermint
  *Chickweed
  *Pleurisy root
  *Ginger root

Supplements

☞ **Vitamin A therapy is a key:**
  *Emulsified vitamin A & D 10,000IU/400IU for children as soon as the rash appears. ☺
  *Stronger dosage should be used for rubella - up to 100,000IU in divided doses.

☞ Zinc gluconate lozenges, esp. Zand HERBAL ZINC lozenges for kids. ☺

☞ **Vitamin C therapy is important:**
  *Alacer effervescent EMERGEN-C, 2 to 4x daily in juice, or ascorbate vitamin C 1/4 teasp. 3-4x daily in juice or water.

☞ **Probiotics:** Natren LIFE START or Solaray ACIDOPHILUS FOR CHILDREN 3-4x daily, to replace friendly G.I. flora and rebuild immunity. ♂

☞ Enzymatic Therapy VIRAPLEX or ThYMU-PLEX complex caps.

Lifestyle Support Therapy

Measles vaccinations have a number of side effects for children - be wary.

☞ Use hydrotherapy baths with comfrey or calendula flowers to induce sweating, and neutralize body acids.
  *Apply calendula gel to sores.

☞ Take tepid oatmeal baths to relieve skin itch and rash. ☺

☞ Apply ginger/cayenne compresses to the rash areas.

☞ Frequent hot baths will often release poisons through the rash.
  *Pat aloe vera gel on sores, and also put aloe vera juice in bathwater for skin healing.

☞ **Take garlic or catnip enemas 1-2 times during acute stages to lower fever and clean out infection fast (person should be 8 years or older).**

Common Symptoms: Cold and flu-like symptoms of sneezing, runny nose, red eyes, headache, cough and fever; lymph nodes are usually swollen; fever is followed by a red rash on the face and upper body which sloughs off when the fever drops. With rubella, there is heavy coughing, the rash covers the body; light hurts the eyes; white spots appear in the mouth and throat; there is usually a middle ear infection, and sometimes hearing is affected permanently.

Common Causes: Low immunity from a poor diet, or too many immune-depressing antibiotics or corticosteroid drugs.

See also the CHILDHOOD DISEASES section in this book for more information.

Meningitis
Encephalitis

Meningitis is an infectious, viral disease that causes inflammation of nerves, spine, and brain tissue. It is characterized by deficient blood supply to these areas and therefore deficient oxygen to the brain. Children are especially at risk for permanent brain damage and/or paralysis. Coma or death may ensue if prompt treatment is not undertaken. Medical treatment has been successful with meningitis, but only if received early. Nutritional therapies increase the healing rate substantially. *Encephalitis* is a rarer form of this type of viral infection, with many of the same symptoms. Adults experience severe mental disturbance, disorientation and coma.

Diet & Superfood Therapy

There must be diet and lifestyle change for there to be permanent improvement.

✷ A 24 hour liquid diet (pg. 158) should be used one day each week to keep the body flushed and alkaline.

✷The diet should be 50-75% fresh foods and vegetable juices, with fresh carrot juice and a potassium broth (pg. 167 or veggie drink (pg. 168) 2 to 3x a week.

✷Add cultured foods, such as yogurt and kefir, for friendly G.I. flora establishment.

✷Drink only healthy liquids, 8 glasses daily; take 1 to 2 electrolyte drinks daily.

✷Reduce mucous-forming foods, such as dairy products, red meats, caffeine-containing and refined foods.

✷No sugar, fried, or junk foods at all.

✷ Effective superfoods:
✷Green Foods BETA CARROT drink.
✷Crystal Star SYSTEMS STRENGTH™ and ZINC SOURCE™ drops.
✷AloeLife ALOE GOLD drink.
✷Sun CHLORELLA to reduce inflammation and for healthy tissue growth.
✷Nutricology PRO-GREENS w. flax oil.
✷Orange Peel GREENS PLUS
✷Be Well VEGETABLE JUICES.
✷Knudsen's ELECTROLYTE DRINKS.

Herbal Therapy

✷ Jump start herbal program:
ECHINACEA EXTRACT to helps flush lymph glands as well as fight infection.
✷Crystal Star ANTI-VI™ extract one week on, one week off, alternating with ANTI-BIO™ extract to control infection.
✷Garlic 6 to 8 capsules daily.
✷EVENING PRIMROSE oil or Nature's Secret ULTIMATE OIL caps 4-6 daily.

✷For encephalitis, add homeopathic *Belladonna 200c*, and Alacer EMERGEN-C electrolyte replacement.

✷ Enzymatic Therapy THYMU-PLEX with VIRAPLEX 4 daily to help overcome the virus and boost immunity.

✷ Effective anti-inflammatory herbs:
✷Crystal Star ANTI-FLAM™ caps.
✷Fresh comfrey leaf tea 5 cups daily.
✷Turmeric (Curcumin) caps.

✷ Kelp tabs 6-8 daily.

✷ For nerve support:
✷Scullcap tea
✷Gotu Kola caps 4 daily.
✷Long Life IMPERIAL TONIC (ROYAL JELLY/EPO).♀
✷High omega 3 flax oil 3 teasp. daily.
✷Lobelia extract drops in water.

Supplements

⋙ Anti-oxidants are a key both in supporting treatment and for prevention:
✷Germanium 150mg, in divided doses.
✷PCOs from grapeseed or white pine 50mg 3x daily.
✷Solgar OCEANIC carotene 50,000IU.
✷Quercetin with bromelain with meals to control inflammation.♂
✷Twin Lab CSA for degeneration.♀

⋙ Golden Pride FORMULA ONE oral chelation with EDTA to increase blood flow to the brain.♂

⋙ Niacin therapy: 100-500mg daily. (If a child, use no flush niacin; if adult, use a baby aspirin first to avoid niacin flush).

⋙ Vitamin A therapy is a key:
✷Emulsified vitamin A & D 10,000IU/ 400IU for children as soon as the rash appears.

⋙ B Complex 50mg, with extra B₆ 100mg, and Solaray B₁₂ 2000mcg daily.

⋙ Phosphatidyl choline (Twin Lab PC 55), to nourish brain tissue.♂

⋙ Ascorbate vitamin C or Ester C powder with bioflavonoids, ¼ teasp. every hour during acute phase. Reduce by ½ for maintenance until remission.

Lifestyle Support Therapy

Cortico-steroid drugs taken for meningitis over a long period of time weaken both bone structure and immunity.

♋ Immerse back of the head in warm epsom salts solution several times daily to draw out inflammation. ☺
✷Alternate hot and cold packs on the neck and back of the head to stimulate circulation to the area.

♋ Use catnip enemas to reduce fever, during acute phase and to clear body quickly of infection. ☺

♋ Avoid aluminum cookware, deodorants, and other alum containing products.

♋ Get some fresh air and early morning sunshine every day.
✷Get plenty of rest during healing.

Common Symptoms: Early signs include lethargy, slow thought and movement; sore throat, with a stiff neck and fever, a dark red skin rash, chronic colds with chills, light sensitivity, severe headaches and nausea. Emergency symptoms include stupor, coma, (change in temperature and sleep patterns usually precedes a coma), and convulsions, with acute inflammation of the brain and spinal cord.
Common Causes: Infection by a wide array of viruses; nutritional depletion, especially in children; too many mucous-forming foods; heavy metal or chemical poisoning; constipation; cerebro-vascular disease; psychological trauma.

Acute bacterial meningitis can be rapidly fatal, especially for infants or the elderly. Get emergency help right away for acute symptoms.

Menopause
Women's Change Of Life

Menopause is intended by nature to be a gradual reduction of estrogen by the ovaries with few side effects. In a well-nourished, vibrant woman, the adrenals and other glands pick up the job of estrogen secretion to keep her active and attractive after menopause. Unless you are absolutely sure you need synthetic estrogen replacement, choose a natural menopause. Although almost 90% of women experience some menopausal symptoms, most stem from exhausted adrenals and poor liver function where it does not process estrogens correctly. I strongly recommend a natural menopause. "You'll want to keep the change!"

Diet & Superfood Therapy

Maintain a high level of nutrition to reduce unpleasant menopausal symptoms.

➋ Make sure your diet is at least 50% fresh foods. Eat vegetable, proteins, especially soy foods, instead of meat proteins.

✻Balance estrogen levels by increasing intake of boron-containing foods, such as green leafy vegetables, fruits, nuts and legumes. (Boron also helps harden bones.)

✻Eat calcium-rich foods from vegetables like corn, seeds, tofu, broccoli and leafy greens, and from non-fat dairy products.

✻Add soy foods like tofu and miso.

✻A diet to control hypoglycemia is also beneficial in controlling menopause symptoms. Reduce sugary foods and alcohol.

✻Reduce dietary fat, and mucous-forming foods such as red meats and dairy products. Steam and bake foods - never fry.

✻Eat whole grains. Their high fiber helps regulate estrogen levels.

✻Eliminate carbonated drinks that are loaded with phosphates and deplete the body of calcium and other minerals.

✻Avoid refined foods, caffeine, and hard liquor (a little wine with dinner is fine).

✻Drink bottled mineral water instead.

➋ **Effective superfoods:**
✻Crystal Star BIOFLAVONOID, FIBER & C SUPPORT™ drink as needed.
✻Salute ALOE VERA JUICE W. HERBS.
✻YS GINSENG/ROYAL JELLY drink.

Herbal Therapy

Phyto-hormone-rich herbs have effective, hormone balancing properties that make them a first choice for addressing the complex needs of menopause.

➋ **Jump start herbal program:**
Crystal Star EST-AID™ caps 4 daily the first month, 2 daily the 2nd and 3rd month, to control hormone imbalances and bone weakness accompanying estrogen changes.

✻Then take EASY CHANGE™ caps or roll-on for the year or so of the change; RELAX™, ADR-ACTIVE™, or FEMALE HARMONY™ for a feeling of well-being.

✻EVENING PRIMROSE OIL caps 4 daily -for EFAs to handle mood swings.

✻FEM-SUPPORT™ for long-term balance.

✻MILK THISTLE SEED extract for liver support to help normalize estrogen levels.

✻GINSENG 6 SUPER ENERGY™ caps or tea for phyto-hormones and energy.

➋ **Effective menopause herbs:**
-Dong quai
✻WIld yam for natural DHEA
-Licorice root
✻Black cohosh
✻Panax ginseng for energy and vaginal dryness
-Alfalfa or Solaray ALFA JUICE
✻Royal jelly for 6 mos. - hot flashes

➋ Kelp tabs 8 daily, or J.R.E. IOSOL, or Crystal Star IODINE/POTASSIUM SOURCE™ caps for thyroid balance.

Supplements

➸ Stress B Complex 100mg with extra B6 100mg, pantothenic acid 250mg and PABA 500mg, with flax oil 2 caps 3x daily, especially for mood swings and insomnia.

➸ Enzymatic Therapy NUCLEO-PRO F caps, 2 daily. Chew for immediate results.

➸ Transitions PRO-GEST CREAM daily.

➸ Country Life MAXINE MENOPAUSE.

➸ Body Ammo SOY DHEA as directed.

➸ **Prevail MENO-FEM w. Gamma Oryzanol.**

➸ **Effective menopause nutrients:**
✺Enzymatic THYROID/TYROSINE
✺Enzymatic MAMMARY COMPLEX
✺Enzymatic OVARY/UTERUS COMPLEX
✺Country Life ADRENAL w/TYROSINE
✺Calcium/Magnesium 1000/1000mg.
✺Flora VEGE-SIL for tissue integrity.

➸ **Anti-oxidants are important:**
✺PCOs 50mg 2x daily.
✺**Vitamin E 800IU for vaginal dryness**
✺Solaray TRI-O₂ capsules.
✺**CoQ10 60mg 2x daily.**
✺Ester C with bioflavonoids 550mg 4x daily, especially for hot flashes and excessive menstrual bleeding.

Lifestyle Support Therapy

Lifestyle changes for better body balance:

☛ Exercise regularly outdoors to get the additional advantages of natural vitamin D for bone health. Take a daily brisk walk to keep the system free and flowing.

✻Do deep stretches on rising and each evening before bed.

✻Weight training three times a week along with aerobic exercise is a perfect way to keep tissue and skin from sagging. Weight training also helps you keep the muscle while you lose the fat- an advantage of a natural menopause. When estrogen levels drop naturally, so does some body fat and excess fluids.

✻Get a massage therapy treatment once a month for energy restoration, a body tune-up and a feeling of well-being.

✻Smoking contributes to breast cancer, emphysema, osteoporosis, wrinkling and early menopause. If you still smoke, now is the time to quit!

See following page for a discussion of Estrogen Replacement Therapy.

Common Symptoms: *Erratic estrogen and other hormone secretions by the glands causing hot flashes, insomnia and fatigue; low libido, irritability, calcium imbalance, unstable behavior, mood swings, palpitations; calcium metabolism disturbances causing osteoporosis; skin and vaginal dryness and sometimes atrophy; occasional appearance of male characteristics.*

Common Causes: *Deficient nutrition and lack of exercise; thyroid imbalance; exhausted adrenals; poor food absorption; B vitamin deficiency; emotional stress.*

What About Hormone Replacement Therapy?

There is a firestorm of controversy today about synthetic hormone replacement, and man-made estrogens. What are the real issues? There will be 25 million menopausal women in America by the year 2000. Sixteen million women are currently going through menopause, and already synthetic hormones are the most often-prescribed drug in the U.S. The medical community and the drug companies, for whom synthetic hormones are an incredibly profitable business, have continued to justify the risks because of the perceived advantages to osteoporosis and heart disease prevention. Many physicians prescribe Hormone Replacement Therapy as a lifetime drug, believing that it is the most effective way to prevent osteoporosis and heart disease no matter how good you feel. Yet, the newest research indicates that the benefits for these two diseases are not validated over the long term. In reality, synthetic estrogen does not facilitate deposition of calcium in the bone. It only slows down the leaching of calcium from the bone. Progesterone is seen today as the hormone most responsible for strengthening bone. Many doctors, realizing this, prescribe an HRT combination of a conjugated estrogen substance, and synthetic progesterone, to address bone loss. Even this combination has a downside, because most conjugated synthetic estrogens are composed primarily of the estrogens estrone and estradiol, the primary uterine cancer culprits. *(See the Osteoporosis pages in this book for a detailed discussion of progesterone replacement therapy.)*

I don't believe hormone replacement is the right course for most women. New research, not funded by companies that produce synthetic estrogen, shows that there are numerous problems, side effects and unknowns about drugs that tamper with the deep hormone levels of a woman's body. Unless you have specific, extenuating circumstances, (only about 6% of American women do), a natural menopause is the best way. Even women who don't have a symptom-free menopause, say they feel younger and more energetic than ever, when they address their menopausal changes with gentle, natural remedies. If you are in your 40's or 50's, and are about to be confronted with the great Hormone Replacement Therapy choice, consider carefully before you agree. Of the women past menopause today, about half start synthetic hormone replacement, but only half of those stick with it because of the side effects or fear of cancer risk.

Are the cancer risks as bad as we've all heard?

Knowledge about the pros and cons of hormone replacement therapies is becoming increasingly important as we find out about its extensive side effects, and become painfully aware of the frightening risks. Long speculated by naturopaths, increased cancer risk because of synthetic hormones has now been validated by the latest clinical studies. The threat of breast cancer and uterine cancer are both dramatically escalated, with the risk becoming ever greater as a woman ages. Recent studies indicate that a natural menopause may actually be nature's way of decreasing hormone production to protect women from cancer.

Most hormone replacement therapy prescriptions are for Premarin, made from pregnant mare's urine (under incredibly cruel conditions for the horses), or from hormones synthesized in test tubes. The synthetic partial estrogen, "ethynol estradiol" is a completely man-made substance, not found in nature at all. The newest research seems to show a clear link between the pseudo-estrogens, the partial estrogens, and the risk of breast cancer.

Can we put the pros and cons of synthetic hormones in perspective?

Clearly, women would prefer a natural menopause. Synthetic estrogen increases appetite, causes fluid retention, aggravates mood swings and depression, and localizes fat deposits on the hips and thighs. Many women are never told that they don't have to be on estrogen replacement therapy forever. Nor are they told to reduce dosage gradually, to allow the system to adjust, so that menopause symptoms don't return and body elasticity is not lost. In fact, even when hormone replacement is necessary, many women only need it for a year or less.

Hormone replacement therapy can also destroy Vitamin E in the body, making the risk of heart disease greater, and it is not recommended if a woman has high blood pressure, breast fibroids, high cholesterol, chronic migraines, or endometriosis. Synthetic estrogen replacement should also be avoided if there is a history of breast, bone or uterine cancer, thrombosis, gallbladder or liver disease. Some post-menopausal cancers stem from poor liver function that does not process estrogens safely. Women with a family history of these cancers should not be taking HRT as it exists today.

Here in a nutshell are the things you need to consider about hormone replacement therapy:

- **Estrogen Replacement Therapy pros:** it is thought by the medical world to reduce risk of osteoporosis; it diminishes vaginal dryness; it eliminates hot flashes and distressing body temperature changes; it reduces heart disease risk by raising HDL cholesterol levels; it stabilizes energy levels.
- **Estrogen Replacement Therapy drawbacks:** it artificially manipulates the menstrual cycle, often continuing menstruation or spotting; it increases the risk of breast, bone, uterine and endometrial cancer; it increases risk of gallbladder and liver disease; it increases growth of uterine and breast fibroids; it is contra-indicated if there is endometriosis, high blood pressure, chronic migraines or thrombosis; it may be a lifetime drug.
- **Progesterone Replacement Therapy pros:** it decreases risk of uterine cancer; if used with estrogen, it may decrease risk of heart disease; it may help regulate hormonal balance.
- **Progesterone Replacement Therapy cons:** it increases the risk of breast cancer; it may increase risk of heart disease by decreasing "good" HDL levels.

What about the hormone DHEA? It's been called a youth hormone against menopausal symptoms. It is the most abundant hormone in the body, and it's part of an important cascade of activity that ends in the making of estrogen or testosterone. See the ALTERNATIVE HEALTH ARSENAL for information.

See also OSTEOPOROSIS on pages 377-378 for more information.

Do phyto-hormones from plants really work for humans?

Around the world, in every culture throughout history, plant hormones have helped women through the discomforts of menopause. Plants like soybeans and wild yams, and herbs like black cohosh, ginseng, licorice root and dong quai, have a safety record of centuries. They offer a gentle, effective way to stimulate a woman's own body to produce amounts of estrogen and progesterone that are in the right proportion for her needs as menopause progresses. They help control hot flashes, tighten sagging tissue, lubricate a dry vagina, normalize circulation, and keep her system female. Phyto-hormone-rich herbal compounds are effective, yet safe and gentle. At only 1/400th or less of the potency of synthetic or circulating estrogen, phyto-estrogens do not have the unpleasant side effects of increased appetite, fluid retention and cellulite deposits caused by synthetic hormones. Yet they still offer symptom control and deter osteoporosis for a woman who is not producing enough estrogen on her own. Phyto-estrogens work with the system to help stabilize a woman's estrogen levels - stimulating the glands to produce hormones if estrogens are too low; lowering estrogen levels by competing for, and binding to estrogen receptor sites if levels are too high. The naturally-occurring flavonoids in many phyto-hormone rich herbs exert a similar balancing effect on hormone secretions. Much like the body's own estrogen and progesterone hormones, plant flavonoids helps elevate good cholesterol HDL's and keep arterial pathways clear. Phyto-hormone herbs also increase uterine and organ tone by improving circulation, so they become system tonics for women.

How do phyto-hormones protect a woman from breast and other hormone-driven cancers?

Most hormone-driven cancers like breast, bone, and uterine cancer are the result of excess hormones, especially estrogen. Synthetic hormones are only part of the hormone assault on women (and men) from environmental and pseudo-estrogens like those found in pesticides, herbicides and hormone-injected meat or dairy products. Although many scientists believe that there is no significant difference between man-made and natural hormones, we see over and over again, that even when a lab test can't tell the difference, your body can. Our experience has been that none of the man-made hormones work as well as natural, plant-derived hormones from herbal combinations.

Estriol, the kind of estrogen that naturally rises in women during pregnancy and remains in women after menopause, is thought to be a cancer protective factor for women against breast, and other estrogen-driven cancers, like ovarian and uterine cancers. Estriol is also the type of estrogen found in phyto-estrogen containing herbs, and may be anti-carcinogenic because it closely mimics the natural human pattern. Phyto-estrogens can reduce excess blood estrogen by competing for estrogen receptor sites with a women's own circulating estrogen, and with harmful environmental estrogens in her body. Because the estrogen potency of plant estrogens is so small, they have the net effect of lowering the body's estrogen when they bind to the receptor sites, thus reducing the risk of estrogen-driven diseases.

Natural Therapy For Specific Problems Associated With Menopause

The feelings of ill health which sometimes accompany menopause are due to the body's difficulty in adapting to reduced hormone function. Many of the common problems can be positively influenced or avoided with natural, lifestyle therapies. Herbal remedies give you control of your health during your own individual life change.

❧•HOT FLASHES AND NIGHT SWEATS: the body's temperature-regulating mechanism becomes unstable during the shifting hormone balance of menopause. As estrogen levels drop, the pituitary responds by increasing other types of hormones to re-establish hormone homeostasis. Hot flashes generally last 2 to 4 years after menstruation ends, and subside as the body adjusts to lower levels of hormones. Stress, excess caffeine and excess alcohol trigger hot flashes. Natural therapies: Crystal Star EST-AID™ caps or extract, or FEM-SUPPORT™ extract with ashwagandha, or PRO-EST EASY CHANGE™ roll-on gel; Vitamin E 800IU daily; VITEX extract; Body Ammo SOY METABOLITE DHEA cream; GINSENG tea with honey; 2 teasp. royal jelly daily.

❧•SAGGING INTERNAL TISSUE AND ORGANS: Herbal combinations are particularly well-suited to elasticizing tissue and toning prolapsed organs. Natural therapies: Crystal Star WOMANS BEST FRIEND™ or EST-AID™ or VITEX extracts.

❧•DRY VAGINA: Reduced estrogen levels sometimes cause the mucous membranes of the vagina to become dry, resulting in discomfort or pain during intercourse - just at a time of life when you can be more spontaneous, without fear of pregnancy. Natural therapies: Body Ammo DHEA CREAM, Crystal Star WOMENS DRYNESS™ extract with EST-AID™ extract or FEMALE HAR-MONY™ capsules, Vitamin E suppositories, Vitamin B₆ 500mg daily; apply pure aloe gel.

❧•DEPRESSION, IRRITABILITY, INSOMNIA AND FATIGUE: psychological symptoms that are distressing to many normally practical, well-balanced women. Indeed, many women feel that their lack of energy during menopause is the number one disruption in their lives. Natural therapies: Crystal Star MENTAL INNER ENERGY™ caps with kava kava and ginseng, or FEM-SUPPORT™ extract with ashwagandha, vitamin E 800IU, daily, VITEX extract, Nature's Secret ULTIMATE B COMPLEX; reduce caffeine intake (it affects mood more during menopause).

❧•BODY SHAPE CHANGES: If you have never exercised, now is the time - at least 3x weekly to retain muscle and gain body tone. Natural therapies: Weight training along with moderate aerobic exercise and pre-workout stretches three times a week realizes excellent results, along with Beehive Botanicals ROYAL JELLY/GINSENG and honey drink.

❧•FACIAL HAIR GROWTH/HEAD HAIR LOSS: a common problem involving both hormone levels and mineral uptake. Natural Therapies: Crystal Star FEM-SUPPORT™ with CALCIUM SOURCE extract™, a cal/mag/zinc combination with high magnesium; B Complex 100mg with extra B₆ and Nature's Bounty internasal B₁₂ every other day.

❧•POOR CIRCULATION/TINGLING IN THE LIMBS: a common menopausal condition, especially evident when one takes a deep breath. Natural therapies: HAWTHORN extract, GINKGO BILOBA extract, PCOs from grapeseed or white pine 100mg 2x daily; gotu kola caps or cayenne/ginger capsules as needed.

See MENOPAUSE page for specific phyto-hormone product suggestions.

Menstrual Problems

Excessive Flow (Menorrhagia) ✣ Inter-period Spotting

Progesterone is the factor that assures uniform shedding of the uterine lining - low levels of this hormone result in tissue buildup. At the same time, the relatively high level of estrogen stimulates the uterine lining, causing even more endometrial tissue formation. The combination of these two factors leads to abnormally heavy flow during menstruation, and/or spotting between periods as excess tissue is shed. A low progesterone-to-estrogen ratio also causes PMS symptoms of bloating, irritability and depression during the cycle. Mild to moderate hypothyroidism is almost always involved in menorrhagia; response is often dramatic to herbal iodine therapy.

Diet & Superfood Therapy

Consciously work on nutrition improvement, with emphasis on vegetable proteins, mineral-rich foods and high fiber foods.

❧ Eat plenty of leafy greens, seafood and fish to regulate metabolism.
  ➤Increase Omega-3 rich foods: salmon, cold water fish, sea vegetables, flax seed.
  ➤Add sulphur foods like garlic, onions and turmeric spice.

❧ Restrict intake of animal foods, especially cheese and red meats (many are loaded with the hormone DES that has an effect on human blood).
  ➤Reduce fried, saturated fatty foods, sugars, and high cholesterol foods.
  ➤Avoid caffeine and caffeine-containing foods, hard liquor (a little wine is fine).

❧ Make a mix of brewer's yeast flakes, wheat germ flakes, amaranth grain, lecithin granules; add 2 TBS. to the diet daily.

❧ Effective superfoods:
  ➤Crystal Star BIOFLAV., FIBER & C SUPPORT™ drink daily for tissue strength.
  ➤Y.S. or Beehive Botanical ROYAL JELLY/GINSENG drink.
  ➤Sun CHLORELLA or Crystal Star ENERGY GREEN™ for breakthrough bleeding.
  ➤Green Foods WHEAT GERM extract.
  ➤Carrot juice (page 168) or Green Foods BETA CARROT.

Herbal Therapy

❧ Jump start herbal program:
  Crystal Star FEM SUPPORT™ extract 4x daily with Ashwagandha, and SILICA SOURCE™ for connective tissue.
  ➤Nettles extract, 1/4 tsp. 2x daily.
  ➤MILK THISTLE SEED extract as a mild liver cleanse for spotting.
  ➤IRON SOURCE™ for iron deficiency.
  ➤J.R.E. IOSOL, or Crystal Star IODINE THERAPY™ extract for thyroid balance.
  ➤PRO-EST BALANCE™ as a source of balancing progesterone.

or

❧ FEMALE HARMONY™ caps 2 daily with 2 bayberry capsules, for 2 months to normalize hormone production, esp. if pre-menopausal.
  ➤FLOW-XS™ tea for 6 days.
  ➤Then WOMAN'S BEST FRIEND™ caps 3x daily with VITEX extract as a tissue toner.
  ➤EFAs from EVENING PRIMROSE oil or Flax seed oil to lengthen luteal phase.

or

❧ Make an astringent tea - 3 cups, 3x daily, during and before your period: shepherd's purse 3 cups, cranesbill, red raspberry, periwinkle and agrimony, or Crystal Star GREEN TEA CLEANSER™.
  ➤Take with Crystal Star IODINE/POTASSIUM caps for hypothyroidism.
  ➤Bee pollen caps 1000mg 2 daily.

Supplements

❧ Transitions PROGEST CREAM applied to the abdomen as directed.
  ➤Solgar OCEANIC carotene 25,000IU 4x daily for 1 month.
  ➤Enzymatic Therapy THYROID/TYROSINE for hypothyroidism.
  ➤Flora VEGE-SIL for connective tissue strength.
  ➤Floradix LIQUID IRON for iron deficiency.
  ➤Nature's Secret ULTIMATE OIL for EFAs, 2 daily.

❧ Enzymatic Therapy RAW MAMMARY COMPLEX caps 2-3 daily for almost immediate results; FEM-TROL capsules if periods are too frequent .

❧ Nature's Plus Vitamin E 800IU with probiotics such as Natren TRINITY.

❧ Rainbow Light CALCIUM PLUS capsules 4 at a time daily.

❧ Vitamin K 100mcg 2 daily, with Twin Labs CITRUS BIOFLAVONOIDS and rutin 500mg.

❧ Mezotrace SEA MINERAL COMPLEX 4 daily.

Lifestyle Support Therapy

❧ Acupressure: Press on the insides of the legs about 5" above the knees; 5 minutes on each leg to decrease bleeding.

❧ Apply icepacks to the pelvic area.

❧ Get extra sleep during this time.

❧ Get daily regular exercise to keep system and metabolism flowing.

❧ Reflexology point:

vagina, ovaries, bladder

❧ Avoid drugs of all kinds, even aspirin and prescription drugs if possible. Many inhibit Vitamin K formation.

See MENOPAUSE pages for more information.

Common symptoms: Excessive bleeding for 2 or more days, with large dark clots, spotting between periods. An abnormal (but non-cancerous) PAP smear may occur.
Common Causes: Hypothyroidism; nutrition deficient diet with too much caffeine, salt and red meat, causing hormone and glandular imbalance; uterine fibroids, endometrial polyps or hyperplasia; endometriosis; overproduction of estrogen; too much aspirin or other blood-thinning medications; calcium or chronic iron deficiency; underactive, lazy or low thyroid; Vitamin K deficiency.

Menstrual Problems

Suppressed * Delayed * Irregular

Irregular menstrual periods are among the most common disorders women suffer. Most are related to gland health and lifestyle. Intense body building and training for marathon or competition sports affects menstruation (sometimes to the point of cessation) because a woman's body fat is extremely reduced. The body will not slough off tissue when it feels at risk in forming more. In young girls, menses may be delayed because of abnormally low estrogen levels due to low blood calcium levels, or to eating disorders and crash dieting. Irregular menses due to prolonged emotional stress should be addressed with relaxation and exercise techniques.

Diet & Superfood Therapy

♐ Make sure the diet is very nutritious, with plenty of vegetable proteins and complex carbohydrates. (Your body may not menstruate regularly if it is malnourished).
  ☛Eat brown rice and other B Complex-rich foods like sea vegetables every day.
  ☛Increase Omega-3 rich foods: salmon, cold water fish, sea vegetables, flax seed.

♐ Have a green veggie drink (pg. 168), (or see below) several times a week for healthy blood building.
  ☛Make a mix of toasted wheat germ, lecithin granules, and brewer's yeast; take 2 TBS. each daily for adrenal support.
  ☛Drink plenty of pure water daily.
  ☛Avoid caffeine and caffeine-containing foods, such as chocolate and sodas.

♐ **Effective superfoods:**
  ☛ Crystal Star ENERGY GREEN™ drink or capsules.
  ☛Nutricology PROGREENS.
  ☛Transitions EASY GREENS.
  ☛Beehive Botanical ROYAL JELLY/ GINSENG drink for metabolic balance.
  ☛ Nutrex HAWAIIAN SPIRULINA; take with B Complex 100mg for best results.
  ☛Green Foods GREEEN MAGMA.

Herbal Therapy

♌ **Jump start herbal program:**
  Crystal Star FLOW EASE™ tea daily,
  ☛EST-AID™ caps or EST-AID™ extract, *or*
  ☛FEM-SUPPORT™ extract 2x daily. *or*
  ☛FEMALE HARMONY™ caps and tea with burdock tea 2 cups or VITEX extract **2x daily for abnormal cycles.** *with*
  ☛IRON SOURCE™ for healthy blood composition.

♌ Balancing EFA sources:
  ☛**EVENING PRIMROSE oil 4-6 daily.**
  ☛Nature's Secret ULTIMATE OIL.
  ☛Flax seed oil 3 daily.

♌ **For teenage delayed menses:** Dong quai/ damiana caps or extract 2x daily, with an herbal calcium formula such as Crystal Star **CALCIUM SOURCE™.**

♌ Menstrual problem herbal aids:
  ☛**Turmeric (curcumin) extract to move stagnant blood.**
  ☛Black cohosh to promote menstrual discharge.
  ☛Blue cohosh caps as a uterine tonic.
  ☛**GINSENG/LICORICE ELIXIR™ for hormone balance.**
  ☛Una da Gato caps - irregular menses.

Supplements

✍ Transitions PROGEST CREAM as directed.

✍ B Complex 100mg daily, with extra folic acid 400mcg. *and*
  Nature's Bounty internasal B_{12} every other day.

✍ Nature's Plus Vitamin E 800IU.

✍ Enzymatic Therapy NUCLEO-PRO F caps, with THYROID/TYROSINE and RAW MAMMARY COMPLEX glandulars.

✍ **For delayed teenage menses:** take a good calcium/magnesium supplement with zinc 50mg daily and kelp tabs 8 daily for 2 months.

Lifestyle Support Therapy

☞ **Pelvic compresses:**
  ☛Horehound compresses
  ☛**Ginger compresses**

☞ Alternating hot and cold sitz baths to stimulate pelvic circulation.

☞ Regular mild exercise to keep system free and flowing.
  ☛Consciously try for adequate rest and a reasonable schedule until periods normalize.

☞ **Acupuncture, meditation and massage therapy treatments have all been effective for irregular menses.**

☞ Do knee-chest position exercises for retroverted uterus.

Common Symptoms: *Absence of menses; delayed menses in young girls; irregular menses; with a feeling of continual heaviness and bloating.*
Common Causes: *Poor health or nutrition; gland and hormone imbalance; too much caffeine and too many carbonated drinks; poor organ and abdominal tone; lack of exercise or too much exercise (marathoner's syndrome); extreme, or very low protein, weight loss diet foods; anorexia or excess dieting for weight loss; hypoglycemia; low blood calcium levels; IUD-caused cervical lesions or cysts; venereal disease; stress, emotional shock or depression; adrenal exhaustion; previous birth control pill use causing irregularity; pregnancy aftermath.*

See PMS pages in this book for more information and natural cramps therapy.

Miscarriage

Miscarriage Prevention & False Labor

Miscarriage is often Nature's way of dealing with an abnormal embryo that could not have lived a normal life if the pregnancy had been brought to full term. Rarely is miscarriage the fault of the mother's actions (such as stress, a fall or exercise), except when her nutrition is very poor, or she is addicted to drugs or nicotine. Even then, Nature tries hard to avoid conception under dangerous conditions. Spontaneous miscarriage is most likely to occur in the first tri-mester. Aside from the early discomforts of pregnancy, miscarriage is the greatest threat during this time, especially if the mother is over 35 and had difficulty becoming pregnant.

Diet & Superfood Therapy

♋ A good prevention/building diet should include plenty of magnesium and potassium-rich foods; leafy greens, brown rice, green and yellow veggies, tofu, sprouts, molasses, etc.
　➤Add sea vegetables for naturally occurring vitamin B₁₂ and protein.
　➤NO soft drinks; they bind magnesium and make it unavailable.
　➤Avoid alcohol, caffeine, and drugs. Reduce sugars and refined foods of all kinds.

♋ Be sure to get enough good vegetable protein for the baby's growth: whole grains, sprouts and seeds, low fat dairy foods and sea foods.

♋ Make a mix of lecithin, 4 teasp. wheat germ oil, brewer's yeast and molasses; take 2 TBS. daily.

♋ **Effective superfoods:**
　➤Crystal Star BIOFLAV., FIBER & C SUPPORT™ drink daily for tissue strength and integrity.
　➤Nature's Life SUPER GREEN PRO for extra quality protein.
　➤Earthrise NUTRA GREENS.
　➤NutriTech All ONE daily.

Herbal Therapy

☙ **Jump start herbal program:**
For threatened miscarriage: Have the woman lie very still and give a cup of false unicorn tea every ¹/₂ hour. As hemorrhaging decreases, give the tea every hour, then every 2 hours. Add 6 lobelia extract drops as a relaxer to the last cup.
　➤Give comfrey/wild yam/craneshill tea every hour until bleeding is controlled; or give hawthorn extract ¹/₂ dropperful, and bee pollen 2 teasp. every hour until bleeding is controlled.

☙ Take black haw tea in small doses throughout the danger period for habitual spontaneous abortion.

☙ **For false labor:**
　➤Take 2 caps each cayenne and bayberry, or take lobelia and cayenne extracts together, and get to a hospital or call your midwife immediately.
　➤Red raspberry and catnip tea, or Crystal Star MOTHERING TEA™ all through pregnancy 2-3 cups daily, and kelp tabs 6 daily.
　➤Crystal Star ANTI-SPZ™ caps or CRAMP BARK COMBO™ extract to help stop bleeding.
　➤Nettles tea for uterine hemorrhage.
　➤Blue cohosh for afterpain.
　➤Cramp Bark to prepare for parturition.

Supplements

✐ **Take a strengthening prenatal formula such as Rainbow Light PRENATAL all through pregnancy for a healthier baby and to help prevent miscarriage and birth defects.**

✐ Bioflavonoids and C are a key. *Forty-five percent of chronic aborters have low levels of vitamin C complex.*
　➤**Vitamin C with rosehips or Ester C with bioflavs. and rutin to strengthen veins and blood vessels 2-3000mg daily.**
　➤Alacer SUPER GRAM C II or III.
　➤Solaray QBC with bromelain and C.
　➤Twin Lab CITRUS BIOFLAVS. with rutin 500mg.

✐ Vitamin E 400IU daily during pregnancy as protection against miscarriage.

✐ **Rainbow Light CALCIUM PLUS w. high magnesium.**

✐ B Complex 50mg with Kal B₁₂ with folic acid 2x daily.

✐ Apply Transitions PROGEST CREAM, and take emulsified A & D daily.

✐ Solaray ALFAJUICE caps for chlorophyll antioxidants.

Lifestyle Support Therapy

☞ To determine if the fetus is still alive: take body temperature first thing upon waking. Have a thermometer by the bed, already shaken down, move as little as possible, and take temperature before getting up. The fetus is alive if body temperature is 98.6 or above, unless normal body temperature is low due to abnormally low thyroid metabolism).

☞ Don't smoke. Smokers are twice as likely to miscarry and have low birth weight babies as non-smokers.
　➤Avoid X-rays; they can damage the fetus.

See Having A Healthy Baby in this book for more information.

Common Symptoms: *Spotting to profuse bleeding during pregnancy, usually with cramps, lower back pain and severe abdominal pain.*
Common Causes: *Development of extra fetal chromosomes; chronic infections; latent diabetes; deficient uterine muscle tone; weak blood vessels and capillaries; lack of protein and sufficient nutrition for both mother and child; improper fixing of the fetus to the womb walls; allergic reaction to drugs; overload of prescription and/or recreational drugs.*

Mononucleosis, Infectious

Epstein Barr Virus Infection

Caused by a herpes-type virus, mononucleosis is an opportunistic disease that attacks the respiratory and lymphatic systems with severe flu-like infection. Glands, lymph nodes, bronchial tubes, liver, spleen are all affected. The virus is virulent and highly infectious. Immune response is very weak. The whole body feels the symptoms of fever, sore throat, headache, swollen glands, jaundice, muscle aches and general long-term fatigue. Medical antibiotics are not effective for this virus. Liver, lymph and spleen systems are the main organs involved in healing. Concentrate your efforts on revitalizing these areas. At least three months of rebuilding are needed for restoration of strength.

Diet & Superfood Therapy

High quality vegetable proteins are a key to healing and prevention of further infection.

❧ Begin healing with plenty of cleansing/flushing fruit juices and bottled water for 1 week. Do not fast. Strength and nutrition are too low.

☛Particularly use apple/alfalfa sprout, papaya/pineapple, and pineapple/coconut juices for strength and enzyme enhancement.

☛Then, follow with a week of green drinks, potassium broth (pg. 167), and vegetable juices to cleanse, strengthen and rebuild liver function.

☛Then eat a diet high in vegetable proteins; (brown rice, tofu, nuts, seeds, sprouts, etc.), and cultured foods: (yogurt, kefir, etc.) for rebuilding friendly flora.

☛Add vitamin A and vitamin C rich foods, like fruits and vegetables.

☛Drink plenty of pure water and fruit juices daily to relieve fever and sore throat.

❧ **Effective superfoods:**
☛AloeLife ALOE GOLD drink.
☛Sun CHLORELLA WAKASA GOLD.
☛Crystal Star SYSTEMS STRENGTH™.
☛Nutricology PRO-GREENS w. flax seed oil.
☛**YS or Beehive Botanical ROYAL JELLY/GINSENG drink.**
☛Future Biotics VITAL K drink daily.

Herbal Therapy

❧ **Jump start herbal program:**
Crystal Star ANTI-BIO™ caps or extract, 4-6x daily for 2 weeks to flush toxins from the lymph glands, with CLEANSING & PURIFYING™ tea and LIV-ALIVE™ caps.
☛Then, ADR-ACTIVE™ caps with BODY REBUILDER™ caps 2 each daily.
☛Then, GINSENG 6 SUPER TEA™ for body homeostasis.
☛Then, HAWTHORN extract or MILK THISTLE SEED extract 3-4x daily with FEEL GREAT™ tea and GINSENG SUPER 6™ capsules to re-establish strength. This program has had notable success.

❧ **Effective herbal immune enhancers:** ♂
☛Siberian ginseng extract ♂
☛Astragalus extract
☛Reishi mushroom capsules, Crystal Star REISHI/GINSENG extract or Planetary REISHI MUSHROOM SUPREME. ♀
☛Pau d'arco tea or Crystal Star PAU d'ARCO/ECHINACEA extract ♀
☛St. John's wort extract

❧ Echinacea/goldenseal rt. and garlic to clear lymph glands of infection.

Supplements

☛ **Take during entire 3 month healing time:** your choice of superfood drinks (see Diet & Foods Therapy column), or Solaray ALFA-JUICE.
☛Add Natren BIFIDO FACTORS, or Prof. Nutrition DR. DOPHILUS powder ¹/₄ teasp. in water before meals.
☛Proteolytic enzymes.
☛Twin Labs LYCOPENE.
☛Nutricology GERMANIUM 150mg.
☛CoQ₁₀ 60mg 2x daily.
☛Oceanic-carotene 150,000IU daily.
☛Nature's Bounty internasal B₁₂ gel daily for 1 month, then every other day for a month.
☛Vitamin C powder with bioflavonoids, ¹/₄ teasp. every hour in water to bowel tolerance daily for 1 month. (Reduce dosage in both the 2nd and 3rd month, but continue the C program throughout.)
☛Enzymatic Therapy LYMPH/SPLEEN complex.

☛ **Then enhance immunity:**
☛Biotec CELL GUARD 6 daily.
☛Enzymatic Therapy THYMULUS caps and THYROID/TYROSINE capsules for energy and metabolic increase.

☛ H₂O₂ therapy has been effective. Use Matrix Health OXY-CAPS 1 to 2 daily.

Lifestyle Support Therapy

☞ Bed rest during the acute stages, and regular mild exercise during the rebuilding stages are critical to successfully overcoming mono.

☞ Get early morning sunlight on the body every day possible.

☞ Overheating therapy has been effective for mono. See page 178 for correct home technique.
☛Biofeedback has also been successful.

☞ Avoid all pleasure drugs, caffeine and chemical stimulants. These are often the substances that reduce immunity to its infective point.

☞ **Reflexology point:**

liver & spleen

Common Symptoms: *Severe flu/pneumonia/lung symptoms; swollen lymph nodes; fever and sore throat; loss of appetite and extreme fatigue; totally run-down condition; spleen enlargement; pallor; pain on the upper left side of the abdomen; jaundice as the liver throws off body poisons.*

Common Causes: *An opportunistic disease allowed by a weak immune system; overuse and abuse of pleasure drugs and/or alcohol; liver malfunction.*

See LIVER CLEANSING DIET suggestions and CHRONIC FATIGUE SYNDROME for more information.

Motion Sickness

Jet Lag ❀ Inner Ear Imbalance

Inner ear imbalance is usually at the root of motion sickness symptoms. Deaf people do not get motion sickness. Jet lag is the inability of the internal body rhythm to rapidly resynchronize after sudden shifts in sun time. Our internal clocks are set by hypothalamus-controlled hormonal rhythm and by the pineal glands sensitivity to light. Our bodies instinctively try to maintain stability by resisting time change, causing psycho-physiological impairment of wellbeing and performance. Natural remedies are highly successful without the side-effects of standard Dramamine-type drugs.

Diet & Superfood Therapy

❧ **Before departure:**
Take a cup of Organic Gourmet MISO GINGER BROTH with a pinch of cayenne; ☞or a bowl of brown rice mixed with 3 TBS. brewer's yeast;
☞or one egg white mixed w. lemon juice.
☞and/or strong green tea.

❧ **During the trip:**
☞Suck on a lemon or lime during the trip whenever queasiness strikes.
☞Munch soda crackers to soak up excess acids. Take sugar-free, carbonated sodas. Avoid fried, salty, sugary or dairy foods. They can cause digestive imbalance.

❧ **For jet lag:**
☞Drink water, juices and herb teas to combat dehydration on a flight - but avoid alcohol when flying. It can upset the delicate biochemistry of the nervous system.
☞During re-adjustment, eat high vegetable protein meals when you are trying to stay awake; high carbohydrate meals when you are trying to sleep. Eat complex carbohydrates if you are traveling to high altitudes.

❧ **Effective superfoods:**
☞New Moon GINGER WONDER syrup.⊛
☞Crystal Star BIOFLAV, FIBER & C SUPPORT™ drink before departure.

Herbal Therapy

❧ **Jump start herbal program:**
☞**Ginger caps, or ginger/cayenne caps - better than Dramamine.**
☞**Crystal Star TRAVELERS COMFORT™ extract an hour before traveling. May also take as needed during the trip.**
☞GINKGO BILOBA extract before and during traveling for inner ear balance.
☞GREEN TEA CLEANSER™ each morning for a week before a trip, and during a trip for good stomach enzyme balance. ♀
☞MINERAL SPECTRUM COMPLETE™ caps, about a month before a trip.

❧ **Nerve-soothing herbs are effective:**
☞Peppermint or chamomile tea
☞Crystal Star MENTAL INNER ENERGY™ caps with kava kava and ginseng. ♀

❧ **For jet lag:**
☞**Before a time-change flight: 1 echinacea/goldenseal cap, 2 vitamin C with bioflavonoid tablets, 1 beta-carotene capsule.**
☞GINKGO BILOBA for inner ear balance.
☞Calming herb teas, such as chamomile or passion flower. ♀

❧ **Ginseng is effective for body balance:**
☞Siberian ginseng extract before and as needed during a trip. ♀
☞**Crystal Star GINSENG/LICORICE ELIXIR™ as needed.** ♀

Supplements

❧ B Complex 100mg for several weeks prior to travelling, for better "B" balance, and extra folic acid 400mcg, and Solaray vitamin B₁₂ 2000mcg.

❧ Glutamine 500mg before departure. ♂

❧ Activated charcoal tablets 2-3x before departure to soak up acids. ♂

❧ Take vitamin B₁, thiamine, 500mg - like Dramamine before a trip.

❧ Nutribiotic GRAPEFRUIT SEED extract to overcome the effects of bad food and water or a trip.

❧ **For jet lag:**
☞**Melatonin therapy: take 3mg before retiring during your trip and for two to three days after for best results.**
☞American Biologics OXY-5000 FORTE.
☞Tyrosine 500mg 2 to 3 daily a few days before a trip and during the trip as needed.
☞Vitamin C 500mg chewable 6 daily, with B Complex 2 daily while traveling. ♀
☞Enzymatic Therapy KAVA-TONE for nervous system relaxation. ♀
☞Homeopathic Hyland's *Calms Forte.* ⊛

❧ For jet lag irregularity, have a salad two or three times a day.

Lifestyle Support Therapy

☥ **During an attack:**
☞Massage knee caps for 3 minutes.
☞Massage little finger for 10 mins.
☞Massage back of head at base of skull, and behind ears on mastoids.
☞Massage legs and extremities frequently on a long plane flights.
☞Breathe deeply for 1 minute. Get fresh air and oxygen as soon as possible.

☥ **Reflexology point:**

internal ear

☥ **For jet lag:**
☞Start shifting your sleep/wake cycle in advance to the new time. If traveling long distances, schedule a stop-over if you can.
☞Dont smoke. Stay away from secondary smoke in the airport. Inhaling smoke can keep you toxic for hours.
☞Walk about in the plane to promote circulation and prevent blood stagnation.
☞As soon as you arrive at your destination, get out in the sunlight to help reset your biological clock.
☞Use meditative relaxation tapes.

Common Symptoms: For motion sickness: *nausea, upset stomach and/or vomiting during a vehicle trip; unsettled stomach; queasiness; cold sweats; sleepiness; dizziness; poor appetite. For jet lag; fatigue; lethargy; poor performance; dehydration; inability to sleep well.*
Common Causes: For motion sickness: *inner ear imbalance; mineral deficiency; fear or stress about the trip. For jet lag; circadian rhythm upset.*

See also VERTIGO/DIZZINESS *page in this book for more information.*

Multiple Sclerosis

M.S. ✦ A.L.S. (Amyotrophic Lateral Sclerosis)

Multiple sclerosis is a progressive, central nervous system disease thought to be triggered by an auto-immune reaction to allergens or the HTLV-1 virus. Initial onset usually occurs between age 30 and 45. More women than men seem to be affected. The disease itself results from damage to the sheaths of nerve cells in the brain and spinal cord and has been incurable because the immune system fights against itself. M.S. must be treated vigorously. A little therapy does not work, but long lasting remission and cure are possible if you catch it in time. Natural therapies take 6 months to a year. Strong immune defense is essential. A.L.S. (Lou Gehrig's disease) is a disease of the skeletal muscle nerves that results in progressive muscle wasting as the muscles lose their nerve supply. Treat both M.S. and A.L.S. for nerve damage first, then work on restoring muscle function and immune health.

Diet & Superfood Therapy

Malnutrition and stress often precede M.S.

♉ Follow a cleansing diet for 2 months, similar to a diet for Candida albicans (see pg. 362). Then, follow a modified macrobiotic diet (pg. 211) for 3 to 6 months.

☞The diet should be 70-80% fresh foods, with plenty of salads and green drinks; 15-20% fresh fruits; and 5-10% vegetable proteins from sprouts, legumes and seeds. Eat a bowl of brown rice every day for B vitamins. Eat fish at least three times a week.

☞Take a potassium broth (pg. 167) at least twice a week.

☞Crystal Star BIOFLAV, FIBER & C SUPPORT™ drinks to rebuild nerve tissue.

☞Avoid all refined and fried foods, sugars, full-fat dairy foods, and caffeine-containing foods. Eliminate meats except fish. Reduce starchy and high gluten foods. Eliminate pectin-containing candies.

♉ Effective superfoods:
☞**Sun CHLORELLA 2 packets daily.**
☞**Green Foods WHEAT GERM extract.**
☞**Solgar WHEY TO GO protein drink.**
☞**Crystal Star SYSTEMS STRENGTH™.**
☞**Jarrow EGG YOLK LECITHIN.**
☞**Y.S. ROYAL JELLY 2 teasp. daily.**
☞**Wakunaga KYO-GREEN.**

Herbal Therapy

See a homeopathic doctor for new bee sting therapy. Reported very successful.

♉ Jump start herbal program:
☞**Crystal Star RELAX CAPS™ to feed and help rebuild nerve structure.**
☞PRO-EST BALANCE™ as an assimilable source of wild yam for DHEA, or Body AMMO DHEA from soy.♀
☞GINKGO BILOBA extract for tremor control.
☞**Essential fatty acids are a key: EVENING PRIMROSE OIL caps 4-6, Nature's Secret ULTIMATE OIL and Omega-3 rich flax oils 3x daily are effective.**
☞LIV-ALIVE™ caps and LIV-ALIVE™ tea to clean out toxins,
☞Health Aid America SIBERGIN caps to build blood strength.♂

♉ Solaray ALFAJUICE caps with TURMERIC caps as an anti-inflammatory. ♀

♉ Mezotrace SEA MINERAL COMPLEX daily, and/or scullcap capsules for nerves.

♉ American Biologics SUB-ADRENE for deep body strength.

♉ For A.L.S.: Kombucha mushroom drink, along with a detox method - several reported cases of marked improvement.

Supplements

✺ Nature's Bounty B₁₂ every day for 1 month, then every other day for 2 months.
☞Natren BIFIDO FACTORS ½ teasp. 3x daily before meals.
☞**Phosphatidyl choline (PC55) 2-3x daily, or PHOS. SERINE (PS), 1 daily.**
☞**Beta or marine carotene 100,000IU and cold water fish oils 3x daily, especially helpful for M.S.-related eye damage.**
☞Enzymatic Therapy THYMU-PLEX for immune strength.
☞Ascorbate vitamin C powder, ¼ teasp. every hour to bowel tolerance - daily for a month; then reduce to 5000mg daily.

✺ Enzyme therapy is essential: Pancreatin 1300mg daily, or Enzymatic Therapy MEGA-ZYME daily before meals.

✺ Antioxidants are a key:
☞PCOs 100mg 3x daily.
☞**CoQ₁₀, 60mg 3x daily to help regeneration of myelin sheath.**
☞Nutricology GERMANIUM 150mg.♀
☞Country Life AMINO MAX, with B₆.
☞Country Life DMG B₁₅ SL.♂

✺ Twin Lab CSA for degenerative spine improvement and threonine for energy.

✺ Niacin therapy: 500mg 3x daily, with B₆ 500mg for nerves and circulation.♂

Lifestyle Support Therapy

ॐ Overheating therapy is effective for M.S. See page 178 in this book for effective home technique.

ॐ Sunlight and vitamin D influences the remission of M.S. There are far less incidences of the disease in sun-belt regions.

ॐ Take a catnip enema or spirulina implant once a week for several months.

ॐ Avoid emotional stress, poor diet and excessive fatigue. These trigger the onset of M.S. attacks.
☞Avoid smoking and secondary smoke. You need all the oxygen you can retain.

ॐ Mild daily exercise, chiropractic adjustment, massage therapy and mineral baths are useful in controlling M.S. and A.L.S.

ॐ **Reflexology points:**

nerve points

See Nerve Health page in this book for more information.

Common Symptoms: *Numbness, tingling sensations, and often eventual paralysis; great fatigue; visual loss, preceded by blurring, double-vision and eyeball pain; breathing difficulty; slurred speech; mental disturbance; poor motor coordination/staggering gait; tremors; dizziness; bladder and bowel problems; sexual impotence in men; nerve degeneration; many symptoms mimic Lyme disease.*

Common Causes: *Too many refined carbohydrates and saturated fats, causing poor food assimilation and toxemia from constipation and poor bowel health; lead or heavy metal poisoning; hypoglycemia; Vitamin B₆ B₁₂ and B₁ deficiency; food allergies triggering auto-immune reaction; Candida albicans overgrowth; gland imbalance.*

Muscle Cramps & Spasms
Leg Cramps

Muscle spasms, cramps, twitches and tics are usually a result of body vitamin and mineral deficiencies or imbalances. Most cramping occurs at night as minerals move between the blood, muscles and bones. A good diet and natural supplements have been very successful in fortifying and strengthening the body against nutrient shortages. Improvement is noticeable within one to two weeks. Leg cramps are usually the result of poor circulation.

Diet & Superfood Therapy

❧ Eat vitamin C-rich foods; leafy greens, citrus fruits, brown rice, sprouts, broccoli, tomatoes, green peppers, etc.
* Eat potassium-rich foods; bananas, broccoli, sun flower seeds, beans and legumes, whole grains and dried fruits.
* Add sea vegetables to the diet for extra iodine and potassium.
* Eat magnesium-rich foods; lettuce, bell pepper, green leafy vegetables, molasses, nuts and seafoods.
* Take a veggie drink (pg. 168) 2x a week.
* Drink plenty of healthy liquids. Muscles need fluids to contract and relax.
* Take an electrolyte drink often, such as Knudsen's RECHARGE for good mineral salts transport.
* Avoid refined sugars, processed and preserved foods. Food sensitivities to these are often the cause of twitches and spasms.

❧ **Effective superfoods:**
* Crystal Star SYSTEMS STRENGTH™ drink for iodine and potassium.
* Green Foods GREEN MAGMA with barley grass.
* Crystal Star ENERGY GREEN™ drink
* Nature's Life SUPER-PRO 96 drink.
* Sun CHLORELLA with 1 teasp. kelp.
* Future Biotics VITAL K 3 teasp. daily.
* Nutrex HAWAIIAN SPIRULINA.

Herbal Therapy

❧ **Jump start herbal program:**
* Crystal Star ANTI-SPZ™ caps 4 at a time, or CRAMP BARK COMBO™ extract.
* **ANTI-FLAM™ caps daily, 2 at a time as needed to reduce inflammation; also make a turmeric paste with water and apply on a gauze bandage to area.**
* **GINSENG/LICORICE ELIXIR™ for cortisone-like properties without side effects.** ♂
* **RELAX CAPS™ daily as needed to restore nerve health.** ♀♂
* IODINE/POTASSIUM SOURCE™ caps for deficient minerals.
* EVENING PRIMROSE OIL 4 daily for essential fatty acids.

❧ Flora VEGE-SIL silica caps 3-4 daily for collagen and tissue regeneration.

❧ **Muscle support herbs and herbal tonics:**
* Horsetail/oatstraw
* Rosehips
* Passion flower and Scullcap
* Solaray ALFA-JUICE caps. ♀♂
* Lobelia for cramping
* Crystal Star VALERIAN/WILD LETTUCE extract to calm muscle spasms.
* **Floradix HERBAL IRON for leg cramps.**

❧ Aromatherapy: apply rosemary and juniper essential oils.

Supplements

❧ **Take down inflammation:**
* American Biologics INFLAZYME FORTE to reduce muscle inflammation.
* **Quercetin with bromelain.**
* Source Naturals NAG for cartilage.
* Alacer EMERGEN-C drink.

❧ Homeopathic remedies for muscles:
* Hyland's *Mag Phos* to reduce pain.
* *Arnica Montana* for recovery.

❧ **For men:** Country Life LIGATEND as needed, MAXI-B COMPLEX w/ taurine.
* Magnesium/potassium/bromelain 3 daily, with zinc 75mg, and chromium to help rebuild muscle strength. ♂

❧ **For women:** Solaray CAL/MAG CITRATE 4-6 daily, with vitamin D 1000IU.
* CoQ₁₀ 60mg. 3x daily. ♀

❧ **For both men and women:** Vitamin C or Ester C, up to 5000mg daily with bioflavonoids for collagen formation.

❧ **For leg cramps at night:** B Complex 100mg. daily, with extra B₆ 250mg. and pantothenic acid 250mg. for nerve repair. Take extra B₆ before bed at night as needed.
* Calcium/Magnesium 1000/500mg.
* Vitamin E 400IU daily.
* PCOs 50mg 2x daily.

Lifestyle Support Therapy

Note: If you taking high blood pressure medicine and have continuing muscle spasms, ask your doctor to change your prescription. Some have sodium imbalance that upsets mineral salts in the body.

❧ Take vinegar or epsom salts baths, or apply a hot salt pack, made by heating sea salt in pan, funneling it into an old sock and apply directly to affected area.

❧ Topical applications:
* Arnica tincture
* Lobelia extract

❧ Massage the legs; elevate the feet; slap soles and legs with open palm to stimulate circulation.

❧ Use alternating hot and cold hydrotherapy, or hot and cold compresses applied to the area to ease pain, promote circulation and healing.

❧ Shiatsu and massage therapy are effective in re-aligning the body's "electrical" impulses, and relieving muscle cramps.
* Acupressure is also highly successful. Consult a specialist and see Acupressure & Acupuncture page 22 in this book.
* Take brisk walk every day to relieve leg cramps at night.

Common Symptoms: *Uncontrollable spasms and twitches of the legs, facial muscles, etc.; unexplained leg cramps at night.*
Common Causes: *Metabolic insufficiency of calcium, magnesium, potassium, iodine, trace minerals, and vitamins E, D and B₆; lack of sufficient HCL in the stomach; Vitamin C and silicon deficiency causing poor collagen formation; food allergies to preservatives and colorants.*

See also Sports Injuries pages in this book for more information.

Muscular Dystrophy
Spina Bifida

Muscular dystrophy is a severe weakening of the muscles, and nerve growth due to abnormal development. It affects about 40,000 people in the U.S., mostly young children. In children, muscle and nerve degeneration prohibits the ability to support body weight. Spina bifida is a condition where there is a defect in the nerve growth and development of the spinal column. Children born with spina bifida have poor motor ability and coordination, and are essentially paralyzed from the waist down. Sometimes spina bifida is undiagnosed until adulthood. Natural therapies have been successful in increasing nutrient assimilation, in overcoming EFA deficiency, in rebuilding nerve and muscle tissue, and in balancing prostaglandin formation.

Diet & Superfood Therapy

♋ Go on a short 6-10 day cleansing diet to release accumulated toxins (pg. 157).

➥Then follow an intensive macrobiotic diet for degenerative disease for 2 months, and a modified macrobiotic building diet (pg. 211) for 6 months or more.

➥Take a potassium broth (pg. 167) daily for the first 6-8 weeks of healing. Reduce to once a week for the next 6 months. Add one veggie drink (pg. 168) every week.

➥2 TBS. daily of dried, chopped sea vegetables in a soup or salad for rebuilding mineral and enzyme strength.

➥Mix some lecithin granules, brewer's yeast, wheat germ: take 2 TBS. daily:

➥Avoid all refined foods, caffeine-containing foods, and salty foods.

♋ Eat plenty of leafy greens for folic acid to prevent birth defects like spina bifida.

♋ **Effective superfoods:**
➥Crystal Star SYSTEMS STRENGTH™.
➥Future Biotics VITAL K to 6 teasp. daily.
➥Crystal Star ENERGY GREEN™ drink.
➥Aloe Life ALOE GOLD drink.
➥**Green Foods WHEAT GERM extract.**
➥**Nutricology PRO-GREENS w. flax oil.**
➥Predigested liquid amino acids 1-2 teasp. daily for immediately usable protein building blocks.

Herbal Therapy

☙ **Jumpstart herbal program**
➥**Crystal Star RELAX CAPS™ as needed to rebuild nerve sheath damage, (excellent results.)**
➥**Highest potency royal jelly 50-100,000mg 2 teasp. daily.**
➥**GINKGO BILOBA for muscle weakness.**

➥**High omega-3 flax oil 3x daily, and BODY RE-BUILDER™ caps to support muscle atrophy.**

☙ **Essential fatty acids are a key:**
➥EVENING PRIMROSE oil caps 4-6
➥Omega 3 flax oils 3 daily
➥Nature's Secret ULTIMATE OIL

☙ **Circulatory stimulants:**
➥HAWTHORN extract 2-4x or as needed daily for circulatory tone.
➥Cayenne/ginger caps 6 daily.
➥BILBERRY extract for circulatory tone.

☙ Siberian ginseng extract or Health Aid America SIBERGIN.

☙ Scullcap extract as a healing nervine.

Supplements

✒ Phosphatidyl choline (PC55) 4 daily, or EGG YOLK LECITHIN 2x daily to help neuro-transmission.

✒ **Antioxidants are a key:**
➥PCOs 50mg. 3x daily.
➥**CoQ₁₀ 60mg 3x daily to help regeneration of myelin sheath.**
➥**Nutricology GERMANIUM 150mg.**
➥Vitamin E 800IU or octacosanol 1000mg to protect against cell membrane damage.
➥Beta carotene 100,000IU daily.
➥**Ascorbate vitamin C or Ester C powder with bioflavonoids, ¼ teasp. every 3 hours during main healing period. Then reduce to 3 to 5000mg daily.**

✒ **Health Papers CETA CLEANSE oral chelation with EDTA; with extra niacin 500mg for increased circulation.**

✒ Country Life GLYCINE 500mg with CARNITINE 500mg 4-6 daily, and Nature's Bounty internasal B₁₂ every other day.

✒ **Twin Lab CSA for degenerative spine improvement and Country Life L-Threonine 500mg with B₆ as directed.**

✒ **For spina bifida: take folic acid during pregnancy 400-800mcg daily, and give if there is suspected spina bifida in adulthood.**

Lifestyle Support Therapy

☞ Regular massage therapy treatments are notably helpful for both nerve and muscle normalization.

☞ Overheating therapy has been successful in controlling muscular dystrophy. See page 178 in this book.

☞ Avoid tobacco and alcohol. Question high blood pressure drugs containing sodium. Chemical drugs of all kinds, taken to excess, can lead to increased lethargy and dependency.

☞ Use hot and cold hydrotherapy to stimulate circulation (pg. 177).

☞ Use mineral and therapeutic baths for cleansing and muscle support.

☞ Get early morning sunlight on the body every day possible to rebuild muscle strength.

☞ **Reflexology point:**

nerves & muscles

Common Symptoms: *Muscle weakness and atrophy; nerve damage and atrophy; tremor and palsy; degenerating ability to walk, with frequent falling and stumbling; deep tendon reflexes are usually lost early; occasional loss of bladder control. There may be mild mental retardation in some types of muscular dystrophy.*
Common Causes: *Muscular dystrophy is thought to be a result of an inherited defective gene - often because of folic acid deficiency in the mother; poor diet/food assimilation causing deficient minerals during pregnancy; EFA and prostaglandin deficiency. Spina bifida may be congenital or the result of the mother's nutritional status during pregnancy, such as too little folic acid.*

See COOKING FOR HEALTHY HEALING by Linda Rector Page for complete details of this diet.

Myasthenia Gravis

Muscle Wasting Disease ❖ Facial Tics & Twitches (Bell's Palsy)

Myasthenia gravis is a debilitating muscle disease, now thought to be an immune disorder, because immune antibodies that normally fight infection, instead turn against normal tissue. Largely a woman's problem, it is characterized by progressive weakness and rapid fatigue, beginning with the muscles and nerves of the lips, tongue and face. Breathing and swallowing are also affected. Complete exhaustion and paralysis are a final result. Many of the symptoms as well as successful treatments are the same as for muscular dystrophy. Remission has shown marked success from an improved diet. Bell's palsy is a non-progressing facial nerve disorder characterized by facial paralysis, beginning with muscle weakness on one side of the face and the inability to close one eye.

Diet & Superfood Therapy

♌ Avoid nightshade plants: tomatoes, eggplant, white potatoes, green peppers, etc.

♌ Eat potassium and magnesium-rich foods: from whole grains, leafy greens, and green or potassium drinks (pg. 167).

♌ Take 2 teasp. wheat germ oil daily in juice or water.

♌ **Effective superfoods:**
 ✿Crystal Star ENERGY GREEN™ drink with Barley Grass daily during healing.
 ✿Sun CHLORELLA for blood building and oxygen.
 ✿Crystal Star SYSTEMS STRENGTH™.
 ✿Beehive Botanical ROYAL JELLY/GINSENG drink.
 ✿**Green Foods WHEAT GERM EXTRACT.**
 ✿Future Biotics VITAL K 3-4 teasp. daily.

Herbal Therapy

⬥ **Jumpstart herbal program:**
 Crystal Star RELAX CAPS to feed and rebuild nerve strength, with IODINE/POTASSIUM™ caps for thyroid help.♀
 ✿**EVENING PRIMROSE OIL caps 4-6 daily for EFAs and prostaglandin balance.**
 ✿**GINKGO BILOBA extract 2-3x daily if there is muscle tremor.**
 ✿A pre-digested amino acid complex capsule, or Crystal Star AMINO-ZYME capsules.♀

⬥ **Proper elimination is important to release toxins:**
 ✿Crystal Star FIBER & HERBS COLON CLEANSE™ 4-6 daily for 3 weeks. Then rest for 1 week.

⬥ Take cayenne/ginger capsules 2 at a time as needed to increase circulation. Apply cayenne and ginger compresses to affected areas to help prevent atrophy.

⬥ **SIBERIAN GINSENG extract 3-4x daily for circulation increase.**

⬥ **High potency royal jelly 40-50,000mg 2 teasp. daily.**

Supplements

✐ Transitions PROGEST CREAM as directed with thyroid glandular such as Enzymatic Therapy THYROID/TYROSINE complex. Rapid improvement.

✐ Solaray 2000mcg B$_{12}$ ♀ or Source Naturals Dibencozide 10,000mcg. ♂

✐ Glycine 500mg and/or chromium picolinate 200mcg.

✐ **Effective neuro-transmitters:**
 ✿Choline 600mg. ♂
 ✿Choline/inositol. ♀
 ✿Lecithin 3x daily.
 ✿Phosphatidyl choline (PC 55).
 ✿Phosphatidyl Serine (PS).

✐ Effective antioxidants:
 ✿Octacosanol 1000mg.
 ✿**Vitamin E 800mg.**
 ✿Country Life DMG sublingual.

✐ Twin Lab CSA capsules as directed with Twin Lab EGG YOLK LECITHIN 2-3x daily. Excellent results.

✐ Solaray MEGA B STRESS 100mg daily, with extra pantothenic acid 500mg and B$_6$ 250mg daily.

✐ **For eye tics:** CoQ$_{10}$, 60mg daily.

Lifestyle Support Therapy

☞ Avoid smoking, secondary smoke, and oxygen-depleting pollutants as much as possible.

☞ Get some mild outdoor exercise every day for fresh air and aerobic lung and muscle tone.

☞ Relaxation techniques are helpful because stress aggravates myasthenia gravis symptoms.

✿Massage therapy and shiatsu are both effective in increasing oxygen use and strengthening nerves and muscles.

☞ **Reflexology points:**

muscles & nerves

Common Symptoms: *Severe muscle weakness and fatigue, especially in the upper body; facial muscle weakness (drooping eyelids); inability to perform even small tasks because of lack of strength; progressive paralysis and exhaustion; double vision; poor articulation and speech. Emergency symptoms include great difficulty in breathing and swallowing.*
Common Causes: *Immune disorientation; chemistry failure between the nervous system and the muscles; choline and prostaglandin deficiency causing poor neurotransmission; chronic constipation causing poor elimination of toxins; chronic sugar regulation imbalances.*

See MUSCULAR DYSTROPHY suggestions in this book for more information.

Nails

Nail Health ✴ Nail Fungus

Nails can be very useful as an "early warning system" in diagnosing illness and evaluating health. If the eyes are the "windows of the soul," the nails are considered the "windows of the body." They are one of the last body areas to receive the nutrients carried by the blood, and show signs of trouble before other better-nourished tissues do. Healthy nails are pink, smooth and shiny. Changes in their shape, color and texture signal the presence of disease in the body. Disorders of the blood, glands, circulation and organs as well as nutritional deficiencies all show up in nail conditions. Give yourself 3 to 6 months to achieve nail health.

Diet & Superfood Therapy

Good nutrition and a well-balanced diet are the keys for nail health. Give your program at least a month to show improvement. We have found that nothing seems to happen for 3 weeks, and then noticeable changes appear in the 4th week.

☙ Eat plenty of vegetable protein and calcium foods, like whole grains, sprouts, leafy greens, molasses, and seafood.
　✷Eat sulphur-and-silicon-rich foods, like onions, sea vegetables, broccoli and fish.

☙ For color and texture; mix honey, avocado oil, egg yolk, and a pinch of salt. Rub onto nails. Leave on ¹/₂ hour. Rinse off.

☙ For brittle nails: massage castor oil into nails for a month.

☙ For discolored nails; rub fresh lemon juice around the nail base. Take extra chewable papaya enzymes.

☙ For weak nails; soak daily for 5 minutes in warm olive oil or cider vinegar.

☙ For splitting nails; take 2 TBS. brewer's yeast, or 2 teasp. wheat germ oil daily for a month.

☙ **Effective superfoods:**
　✷Crystal Star SYSTEMS STRENGTH™.
　✷Klamath BLUE GREEN SUPREME.

Herbal Therapy

If your nail problem is a mineral deficiency, herb and plant minerals are best choice supplements.

☙ **Jump start herbal programs: Silica is a key: For 2 months, take:**
　-Horsetail tea or extract 3x daily.
　✷Crystal Star SILICA SOURCE™ extract.
　✷**Flora VEGE-SIL caps.**
　✷Alta Health SIL-X caps 2-4 daily.
　✷Body Essentials SILICA GEL - take internally as directed; apply directly daily.

☙ **To strengthen nails: Crystal Star MINERAL SPECTRUM COMPLETE™ caps, and EVENING PRIMROSE OIL caps 4 daily for a month.**♀✚

☙ **Tea soaks for nails: also take internally**
　-Dulse/oatstraw
　-**Pau d'arco**
　✷Kelp tabs (also take 6-8 daily.)
　✷**Mix a mud face mask in water (don't take internally.)**

☙ **For nail fungus:**
　✷Apply tea tree oil 3-4x daily.
　✷Soak nails in a Nurribiotic GRAPEFRUIT SEED EXTRACT solution - 3 to 4 drops in 8-oz. water until fungus clears.
　✷Soak nails in American Biologic DIOXYCHLOR or Centipede KITTY'S OXYGEL.
　✷Apply a garlic/honey paste to nails; take garlic tabs 8 daily.

Supplements

☙ For growth: Mezotrace SEA MINERAL COMPLEX 2 daily, or cal/mag/zinc caps 4 daily with boron for better mineral up-take.
　✷**FutureBiotics HAIR,SKIN & NAILS.**✚
　✷**Nature's Plus ULTRA NAILS with extra biotin 600mcg 2x daily.**♂

☙ Enzymatic Therapy ACID-A-CAL.♂

☙ **Supplements for nail problems:**
　✷Zinc 50-75mg daily for spots/poor growth.
　✷Vitamin E 400IU daily for breaking nails, ingrown or hangnail infections.
　✷Vitamin A & D for poor growth, ridges and crusty skin around nails.
　✷Betaine HCl and vitamin A for brittleness, splitting and white spots.
　✷Raw thyroid extract for spots or chipping.
　✷Use a green clay poultice to draw out a nail infection; use wild alum (cranesbill) paste with water to relieve inflammation from ingrown or hangnails.

☙ **For nail fungus:**
　✷Nature's Pharmacy MYR-E-CAL a topical fungus spray with myrrh/goldenseal.
　✷Miracle of Aloe MIRACLE FOOT REPAIR for toenail fungus.
　✷1 part diluted DMSO solution mixed with ¹/₂ part oregano oil and ¹/₂ part olive oil - clean nails thoroughly, then rub all over and around nail.

Lifestyle Support Therapy

Note: nail enamels and supplies are among the most toxic environmental polluters. Fake nails or tips add weight to the nails and prevent them from thickening naturally. Nail color dyes penetrate the nail to the skin, often causing allergic reactions. A simple manicure without polish - with beeswax spread on the nails and buffed to a shine can leave your nails naturally beautiful.

☙ If you polish your nails, don't keep them constantly polished. Allow them to breathe at least 1 day a week. To tint nails naturally: make a thin paste of red henna powder and water. Paint on and let dry in the sun. Rinse off. Pretty pink nails with no chipping.

☙ Acupressure treatment: Press 3x for 10 seconds on the moon of each nail, to stimulate circulation.

☙ Do a paraffin (found at beauty supply stores) hand or foot dip to restore nail and skin elasticity. When wax hardens, put on old mittens or socks for ten minutes. (Wax does not adhere.) Peel off for satiny hands and feet.

Nail Signs & Causes: White spots - zinc, thyroid or HCl deficiency; white bands on the nails - zinc/protein deficiency; possible heart disease, or liver problems; **Discolored nails** - Vit. B₁₂ deficiency, kidney or liver problems; **Yellow nails** -Vit. E deficiency, poor circulation, lymph congestion, too much polish; **Green nails** - bacterial nail infection; **Too white nails** - liver malfunction, poor circulation, anemia, mineral deficiency; **Blue nails** - lung and heart problems, drug reaction, blood toxicity from too much silver or copper; **Black bands on the nails** - low adrenal function, chemotherapy or radiation reaction; **No half moons or ridged nails** - Vit. A deficiency, kidney disorder, protein deficiency; **Splitting, brittle or peeling nails** - Vitamin A & D deficiency, poor circulation, thyroid problems, iron, calcium or HCl deficiency; **Poor shape** - iron and zinc deficiency; **Thick nails** - poor circulation; **Dark, spoon-shaped nails** - anemia, B₁₂ deficiency; **Pitted, fraying, split nails** - vitamin C and protein deficiency; **"Hammered metal" looking nails** - hair loss; **Down-curving nails** - heart and liver disorders; **White nails with pink tips** - liver cirrhosis.

Narcolepsy
Chronic Sleeping Disorder ❖ Sleeping Sickness

Narcolepsy is a chronic, neurological sleep disorder involving sleep-wake mechanisms in the brain. Victims are unable to control their sleep spells, and suddenly fall asleep. Sleeping attacks are erratic, recurrent, overwhelming, and can happen at any time - day or night, no matter what the person is doing. Sufferers are easily awakened, although they fall asleep again within an hour or two. Narcoleptics may also experience complete loss of muscle control. There may be up to 200,000 people in the U.S. with narcolepsy (men and women equally). There are two types of the disorder - DDD (dopamine dependent depression), and a type a involving a B₆ deficiency of the dopaminergic system and poor use of body oxygen.

Diet & Superfood Therapy

See the Food Allergy pages in this book and the Food Allergy diet in COOKING FOR HEALTHY HEALING by Linda Rector-Page.

❧ Food allergies are thought to be involved with narcolepsy. A rotation/elimination diet may be helpful. See a nutritional health professional, and start by eliminating common allergens like wheat, corn, potatoes, eggs and dairy food.

❧ The diet should be low in fats and clogging foods, such as dairy products and animal proteins; high in light cleansing foods, such as leafy greens and sea vegetables.
➛Eat brewer's yeast and other foods high in B vitamins, such as brown rice, on a regular basis.
➛Eat tyrosine-rich foods, such as wheat germ, poultry, oats and eggs.

❧ **Superfoods are important:**
➛Sun CHLORELLA pkts daily for natural germanium.
➛Nature's Life SUPER GREEN PRO-96 with flax oil.
➛Nutrex Hawaiian SPIRULINA P.
➛**Klamath POWER 3 capsules or BLUE GREEN SUPREME drink.**
➛**Y.S. ROYAL JELLY/GINSENG drink.**

Herbal Therapy

➷ **Jump start herbal program:**
-➛Ginkgo biloba extract as needed. ♀
➛St. John's wort extract as needed. ♀
➛Crystal Star META-TABS™ or IODINE/POTASSIUM SOURCE™ caps with ADR-ACTIVE™ caps for thyroid and adrenal energy, 2 each daily.
➛RAINFOREST ENERGY™ tea and capsules.

➷ Ginseng helps regulate sleep patterns as well as provides energy:
➛Crystal Star GINSENG 6 SUPER™ tea and GINSENG 6 SUPER™ cap are effective ginseng formulas. ♀
➛GINSENG/LICORICE ELIXIR also helps balance sugar use. ♀
➛SIBERIAN GINSENG extract.

➷ **Start with EFAs for body "electrical" alignment:**
➛EVENING PRIMROSE oil 1000mg 4 daily.
➛Omega 3 flax oils 3-4x daily.
➛Nature's Secret ULTIMATE OIL.

Supplements

Note: when treating for DDD with tyrosine, do not use B₆ therapy.

❧ Enzymatic Therapy THYROID/TYROSINE caps. 4 daily as an anti-depressant, with ADRENAL COMPLEX 2 daily.

❧ B Complex 150mg daily, with extra B₆ 200mg daily.
and/or

❧ Country Life AMINO MAX caps with B₆ daily for at least 2 months, or an amino acid complex for additional protein.

❧ **Antioxidants are critical:**
➛Nutricology GERMANIUM 150mg.
➛CoQ₁₀ 60mg 2x daily.
➛Country Life DMG B₁₅ daily as needed.
➛Unipro DMG liquid, under the tongue as needed. ♀
➛PCOs 100mg 4x daily. ♂

❧ Effective neurotransmitters:
➛Octacosanol 1000mg.
➛Choline 600mg.
➛Choline/Inositol.

❧ Chromium picolinate 200mcg daily, and magnesium 800mg daily for sugar regulation.

Lifestyle Support Therapy

☞ Circadian rhythms (day/night) and regular sleep habits are important for a person with narcolepsy.

☞ Take regular daily exercise for circulation and tissue oxygen.

☞ Biofeedback and chiropractic adjustment have both been effective in correcting the "electrical -shorts" involved in brain-to-motor transmission.

☞ Avoid hallucinogenic drugs - they aggravate frightening nightmares and experience of sleep paralysis where the person is unable to move even though awake. Sometimes a dangerous panic reaction sets in.
✳Hallucinations and dreams are so real in narcolepsy that the person often cannot tell fantasy from reality.

Common Symptoms: symptoms usually begin during the teens with uncontrolled, excessive drowsiness, inappropriate, erratic periods of sleep; longer than normal sleep during regular sleep hours; loss of muscle control (cataplexy) when awake, sometimes triggered by strong emotions, and sleep paralysis, where the person is unable to move while awake ; memory loss; dream-like hallucinations;

Common Causes: Irregular work/sleep schedules that throw off the body clock; hypoglycemia; food allergy; vitamin B₆ or tyrosine deficiency; low thyroid function and metabolism; heredity; constant exposure to physical or mental stress; brain infection; depression accompanying poor brain and adrenal function; poor assimilation and use of body oxygen.

See HYPOGLYCEMIA AND THYROID HEALTH pages in this book for more information.

Nausea

Vomiting ❋ Morning Sickness ❋ Upset Stomach ❋ Infant Colic

Nausea can be caused by many factors - motion sickness, vertigo, exposure to toxic chemicals or even psychological shocks. Over 50% of pregnant women experience high frequency morning sickness nausea during the first trimester. While it is quite understandable that the wide variety of sudden hormone and metabolic changes is contributing to morning sickness, there are also many natural treatments that can lessen the severity. Infant colic and other nausea causes that involve allergic reactions, infection or nervous reactions can also be helped with natural, soothing therapies.

Diet & Superfood Therapy

☙ **For morning sickness:** Keep soda crackers or dry toast by the bed; take some before rising to soak up excess acids; eat ice chips to calm spasms; drink a little fresh fruit juice for alkalinity.

❧Cucumbers soaked in water and eaten will relieve stomach congestion fast.

❧For breakfast, have orange juice sweetened with honey; then a little bran or barley cereal. Sip slowly. Or take only yogurt in the morning; friendly flora will settle digestive imbalance.

❧Take 2 TBS. brewer's yeast flakes in juice or on a salad every day for absorbable and non-toxic B vitamins. (Mix $^1/_4$ teasp. baker's yeast in warm water for non-pregnancy nausea.)

❧Get fiber from vegetables and whole grains to keep bowels clean and flowing.

☙ **For colic:** If you are nursing, the baby's digestion is still dependent on yours. Avoid cabbage, brussels sprouts, onions, garlic, yeast breads, fried foods and fast foods. Refrain from red meat, alcohol, refined sugar and caffeine until a colicky child's digestion improves.

❧Don't give cow's milk to a colicky baby. Chronic upset stomach in an infant indicates a dairy allergy. Goat's milk or soy milk are both better alternatives.

❧Give papaya juice or apple juice.

❧Give lemon and maple syrup in water.

Herbal Therapy

❧ **For morning sickness:**

❧**Ginger capsules or extract on rising.**

❧Crystal Star FEMALE HARMONY™ capsules 2 daily, or VITEX extract daily.

❧**MOTHERING™ TEA or red raspberry tea daily a needed. (Helpful all during pregnancy for balance.)**

❧MILK THISTLE SEED for the liver.

❧Catnip tea w. 1 goldenseal cap on rising.

❧Rose hips vitamin C 500mg daily.

❧ **Effective liver decongestants:**

❧Dandelion/yellow dock

❧ **For nausea:** a light fasting diet of mild liquids and herbal teas.

❧New Moon GINGER WONDER syrup does wonders for any kind of stomach upset.

❧Umeboshi plum paste - especially for over-indulgence nausea.

❧Ginger/peppermint tea

❧Sweet basil tea

❧Alfalfa/mint tea

❧ **For infant colic:**

❧Apply warm ginger compresses to the stomach and abdomen.

❧Turmeric powder $^1/_4$ teasp. in juice.

❧Fennel tea or catnip tea, 1 tsp. in water with a little honey.

❧Peppermint or spearmint tea with a pinch of ginger, or catnip/peppermint tea.

Supplements

❧ **For nausea and morning sickness:**

❧Acidophilus powder - $^1/_4$ teasp. 3x daily, or chewable papaya enzymes to settle stomach imbalance.

❧Premier One OR YS ROYAL JELLY, one teasp. each morning on rising.

❧Homeopathic *Nat. Sulph.*, *Nux Vomica*, or *Ipecac* as needed.

❧**Stress B complex 50mg daily, with extra B₆ 50mg, B₂ 200mg and magnesium 400mg. Vitamin B₆ shots are effective for severe morning sickness.**

❧Country Life RELAXER capsules.

❧Cal/mag/zinc 2 at a time as needed.

For nausea:

❧Activated charcoal 500-1000mg.

❧Vitamin B₆ 50-100mg.

❧ **For infant colic:**

❧Natren LIFE START $^1/_4$ teasp. in water or juice 2-3x daily.

❧Solaray BABY LIFE for mineral and B Complex deficiency.

❧Solaray BIFIDO-BACTERIA powder for infants.

❧Hyland's Homeopathic *Colic* tabs.

❧B Complex liquid - dilute doses in water about once a week

❧Homeopathic *Mag. Phos.* tabs.

❧Small doses of papaya enzymes.

Lifestyle Support Therapy

☙ **For morning sickness:**

❧Deep breathing exercises every morning, and a brisk deep breathing walk every day, for body oxygen.

❧Acupressure points: Press the hollow of each elbow 3x for 10 seconds each.

❧Both biofeedback and hypnotherapy have been effective. See a qualified chiropractor or massage therapist, esp. if nerve reactions are part of the cause.

❧Soft classical or new age music in the morning will help calm you and the baby.

☙ **For simple nausea:**

❧Massage the abdomen with aromatherapy oils like peppermint, chamomile or lavender.

☙ **For infant colic:**

❧**Give a catnip enema once a week, or as needed for instant gas release.**

❧Mix pinches from your spice cupboard in a cup of water - nutmeg, ginger, cinnamon, turmeric, basil, mace, etc. Drink straight down.

Common Symptoms: **Morning Sickness:** *nausea and heaving in the morning or night during the first trimester of pregnancy; gland and hormone upset causing digestive imbalance; sensitivity to food substances.* **Colic:** *excess gas and abdominal discomfort; incessant crying; burping; hiccups.*

Common Causes: **Morning Sickness:** *gland and hormone imbalance as the body adjusts to a new biorhythm; congested liver if yellow bile is vomited; low blood sugar.* **Colic:** *poor diet with too many acid-forming foods, or poor food combination; introduction of protein foods too soon (may form lifelong allergies and colic); mother's acidity during breast feeding; mineral deficiency in the milk formula; enzyme deficiency; Candida albicans yeast overgrowth; poor food absorption; chronic constipation.*

See MOTION SICKNESS *page in this book for more information.*

Nerve Health

Nervous Tension ✦ Anxiety

Along with the brain, your nervous system is the chief means of receiving input messages from your body parts and the outside world. It consists of the central nervous system - brain and spinal cord, peripheral nerves that run from your CNS to all other parts of the body and your autonomic nervous system, and the nerves to your blood vessels, organs and glands. Your nervous system is the first to be affected by stress, tension and emotion. Poor nerve health can spawn a host of physical disorders, such as Alzheimer's and Parkinson's disease, inflammatory reactions like meningitis, loss of muscular movement and control, and impaired coordination. The nervous system also affects mental balance - weak nerves result in neuroses, tension or anxiety.

Diet & Superfood Therapy

♉ **Diet improvement is a key factor in controlling nerve health:**
☛Add to the diet regularly: high fiber foods, fresh greens, vegetable proteins, and natural sulfur foods, like onions, garlic, oat bran, lettuce, cucumbers, and celery.
☛B vitamin foods are important; eat brown rice, whole grains and leafy greens.
☛Keep the diet low in salt and saturated fats.

♉ Effective special foods for nerves:
☛Brewer's yeast for calming B vitamins.
☛Sunflower seeds and molasses for thiamine and iron.
☛Carrot/celery juice for nerve restoration.
☛Veggie drinks (pg. 168) for chlorophyll.
☛Wheat germ oil 1 teasp. daily.
☛Garlic capsules 6 daily

♉ Avoid acid forming foods, such as red meats, caffeine, carbonated drinks - the phosphorus binds up magnesium, making it unavailable. Magnesium is a key mineral in nerve health.

♉ Effective superfoods:
☛Crystal Star **SYSTEMS STRENGTH™**.
☛Sun CHLORELLA packets or tabs.
☛**Aloe Life ALOE GOLD drink.**
☛Solaray ALFA-JUICE.
☛Y.S. ROYAL JELLY/GINSENG.

Herbal Therapy

♌ **Herbal nerve relaxers:**
☛**Crystal Star RELAX™ caps and tea as needed.**
☛Deva Flowers ANXIETY drops.♀
☛Catnip tea ☺
☛HEARTSEASE-H.B.P.™ caps 2-4 daily.
☛STRESSED OUT™ tea or extract. ♂

♌ **Herbal nervine tonics:**
☛Chamomile tea.
☛Aromatherapy peppermint or cinnamon oils.
☛Rosemary ♀
☛Scullcap
☛EVENING PRIMROSE oil caps 4 daily.
☛GINKGO BILOBA extract 2x daily.
☛HAWTHORN extract

♌ **Herbal adaptogens to help the body overcome stress:**
☛**Crystal Star MENTAL INNER ENERGY™ extract with ginseng and kava kava** ♂
☛Siberian ginseng extract ♂
☛Reishi mushroom extract
☛Bee pollen, 2 teasp. daily. ♂
☛**Ginseng/gotu kola** ♀+
☛**Gotu kola for nerve support.**

Supplements

❧ Country Life **MAXI B complex w/ taurine daily, and extra B$_1$ 100mg and B$_6$ 100mg daily.**
☛**Nature's Plus MAGNESIUM/POTASSIUM/BROMELAIN caps.**
☛Phosphatidyl choline 1 daily.

❧ Ascorbate or Ester C 3-5000mg daily with bioflavonoids and rutin 500mg each.

❧ Natren TRINITY or Alta Health CANGEST powder, $1/_4$ teasp. before meals.

❧ Twin Lab TYROSINE 500mg 2x daily as needed.

❧ Rainbow Light CALCIUM PLUS with high magnesium, 4 daily. ♀

❧ Mezotrace SEA MINERAL COMPLEX 2-3 daily.

❧ Vitamin E 400IU daily.

❧ High omega 3 flax oil 3x daily.

Lifestyle Support Therapy

♋ Tobacco and obesity both aggravate nerve disorders and tension. Lose weight and stop smoking.

♋ Wear acupressure sandals for a short period every day to clear reflexology meridians.

♋ **Relaxation techniques are effective:**
☛A brisk walk with deep breathing every day for body oxygen.
☛Techniques like yoga, meditation and massage therapy are wonderful for the nerves.
☛Baking soda or sea salt baths.
☛Regular massage therapy treatments.
☛Gardening, crossword puzzles, hobbies, artwork, etc. can all relieve tension and anxiety.
☛Laughter is the best relief of all.

♋ **Reflexology points:**

nerve points

Common Symptoms: Extreme nervousness and irritability, often with high blood pressure; inability to relax; lack of energy; chronic headaches and neck stiffness; dizziness and blurred vision, palpitations and heart disease proneness.

Common Causes: Too many refined foods, especially sugars; smoking; unrelieved mental or emotional stress; hyperthyroidism and metabolic imbalance; prostaglandin deficiency. Bottle fed babies have a 46% higher risk of developing neurologic abnormalities than breast-fed babies.

Neuritis
Trigeminal Neuralgia

Neuritis (peripheral neuropathy) is an inflammation of a nerve or nerves. It is usually a degenerating process, and often part of a degenerating illness, such as diabetes or leukemia. **Trigeminal neuralgia** is sudden, sharp, severe pains shooting along the course of a nerve - often because of pressure on the nerve trunks, or poor nerve nutrition and an over-acid condition.

Diet & Superfood Therapy

❧ Go on a short 24 hour liquid diet (pg. 158) to rebalance body acid/alkaline pH.
❧Then, for the rest of the week eat mostly fresh foods, with plenty of leafy greens, sprouts, celery, sea vegetables, and enzyme foods such as apples and pineapple. Take a glass of lemon juice and water every morning. Have a potassium broth or essence (pg. 167) every other day.
❧Drink 6 glasses of water with a slice of lemon, lime or cucumber daily.
❧Keep salts, saturated fats and sugars low.
❧Avoid caffeine especially, hard liquor and soft drinks, that bind up magnesium.

❧ Make a mix of lecithin granules, sesame seeds, brewer's yeast, wheat germ; take 2 TBS. daily:

❧ **Effective superfoods:**
❧Crystal Star ENERGY GREEN™ drink.
❧Nature's Life SUPERGREEN-PRO 96.
❧Beehive Botanicals ROYAL JELLY, Siberian ginseng and bee pollen drink.
❧Sun CHLORELLA tabs 20 daily.
❧Future Biotics VITAL K 3 tsp. daily.
❧Biostrath original LIQUID YEAST with herbs.

Herbal Therapy

❧ **Jump start herbal program:** Crystal Star RELAX CAPS™ as needed for rebuilding the nerve sheath, 2-4 daily.
❧IODINE/POTASSIUM caps 2 daily for nerve restoration.
❧GINKGO BILOBA, esp. for facial neuralgia.
❧BILBERRY extract for tissue-toning flavonoids.
❧Solaray Curcumin (turmeric extract) or Crystal Star ANTI-FLAM™ caps 4 daily to take down inflammation.
❧BACK TO RELIEF™ or ANTI-SPZ™ caps as needed for spasmodic pain.

❧ Rub in CAPSAICIN cream directly to area.

❧ EVENING PRIMROSE oil 4 daily, with the following tea daily to rebuild nerves:
❧Equal parts: St. John's wort, peppermint, lavender, valerian, lemon balm, blessed thistle.

❧ **Effective nervine tonics:**
❧Lobelia
❧VALERIAN/WILD LETTUCE, a powerful nerve relaxant.
❧Passion flowers
❧Scullcap

Supplements

❧ **Niacin therapy: 500-1500mg daily to stimulate circulation.**

❧ **Bromelain 500mg 2x daily or American Biologics INFLA-ZYME FORTE as an anti-inflammatory.**

❧ **Neural nutrients:**
❧Stress B Complex 100mg with extra B₆ 250mg folic acid 400mcg.
❧Taurine 500mg.
❧Solaray B₁₂ 2000mcg SL daily.
❧DLPA 750mg as needed for pain.
❧Quercetin 750mg with bromelain 3 daily.

❧ Ascorbate or Ester C with bioflavonoids and rutin, 5000mg daily, to rebuild connective tissue.

❧ Effective homeopathic remedies:
❧Hylands Nerve Tonic
❧Hylands Calms or Calms Forte tabs
❧Aranea Diadema - radiating pain
❧Mag. Phos. - spasmodic pain.
❧Hypericum if nerve injury.
❧B&T TRI-FLORA analgesic gel.

❧ Country Life LIGATEND as needed.

Lifestyle Support Therapy

❧ Get some regular mild exercise every day for body oxygen and circulation.

❧ Use hot and cold hydrotherapy to stimulate circulation (pg. 177).

❧ Do 10 neck rolls as needed at a time to relieve nerve trauma.

❧ Stress management techniques should be a part of any healing program:
❧Chiropractic adjustment, shiatsu, and massage therapy are all effective in controlling nerve disorders.

❧ **Reflexology points:**

nerve points

See COOKING FOR HEALTHY HEALING by Linda Rector Page for a complete diet for nerve conditions.

Common Symptoms: Muscle weakness and degeneration; burning, tingling, numbness in the muscles or nerve area; motor and reflex weakness; facial tics; nerve inflammation.
Common Causes: Spinal pinch or lesions; excess alcohol or prescription drugs; prostaglandin and/or B vitamin deficiency; diabetic reaction; herpes; poor circulation; multiple sclerosis-type weakness and numbness; kidney and gallbladder malfunction; arthritis; lupus; migraines; heavy metal poisoning.

Numbness

Nerve Damage ❖ Nerve Paralysis

Wide-spread suspension or permanent loss of function and sensation of the motor neurons. If there has been an accident or body trauma, there is often cerebral damage as well.

Diet & Superfood Therapy

♌ Go on a short 24 hour liquid diet (pg. 158) to lighten the circulatory load and clean out wastes.
 ➝Then, eat only fresh foods for 3-4 days to alkalize and clean the blood.
 ➝Then add lightly cooked foods to your 75% fresh foods diet for the rest of the week.
 ➝Follow with a modified macrobiotic diet (pg. 211) for 3 weeks, emphasizing whole grains and vegetable proteins, until condition clears.

♌ Mix brewer's yeast and unsulphured molasses and take 2 TBS. daily.

♌ Effective superfoods:
 ➝**Green Foods WHEAT GERM** extract.
 ➝**Crystal Star ENERGY GREEN™.**
 ➝Green Foods GREEN MAGMA, 2 packets daily; add 1 teasp. kelp granules to each drink for nerve restoration.
 ➝**Biostrath original LIQUID YEAST.**
 ➝Future Biotics VITAL K drink 2x daily.
 ➝**Crystal Star SYSTEMS STRENGTH™** drink for highly absorbable potassium, carotenes and iodine.
 ➝Beehive Botanical ROYAL JELLY/GINSENG drink.
 ➝Sun CHLORELLA drink with extra kelp added, 1 teasp. daily.

Herbal Therapy

⚘ **Jump start herbal program:**
 Crystal Star **RELAX CAPS™** 24 at a time, to rebuild nerves, with **GREEN TEA CLEANSER™** every morning and evening.
 ➝HEARTSEASE/CIRCU-CLEANSE™ tea daily to clean out circulatory wastes.
 –**GINKGO BILOBA** extract, 2 to 4 daily.
 –**Gotu kola caps 4 daily.**

⚘ **To strengthen circulation:**
 ➝**HAWTHORN** extract **as needed to strengthen circulation.**
 ➝Cayenne/ginger caps 4 daily, or kukicha twig tea, 2 cups daily with cayenne/ginger caps 3 daily for 1-2 months.
 ➝Butcher's broom tea or caps daily, temporarily, to increase circulation.

⚘ **Effective herbal nervine tonics:**
 –**EVENING PRIMROSE** oil.
 ➝St. John's wort extract to help regenerate nerve tissue.
 –Ginger/oatstraw tea
 –Rosemary
 ➝Passionflower or scullcap tea
 ➝**SIBERIAN GINSENG** extract ♂

⚘ **Topical nerve help applications:**
 ➝Rub on CAPSAICIN™ cream.
 ➝Cayenne/ginger compresses.
 ➝St. John's wort oil.

Supplements

✒ **Neurotransmitter nutrition is critical:**
 ➝Country Life RELAXER with GABA 100mg and taurine, or Twin Lab GABA PLUS supplying 500mg GABA.
 ➝B_6 250mg. 6-8x daily, if numbness is from nerve interference or a stroke.
 ➝**Phosphatidyl Choline (PC55).**
 ➝**Niacin therapy: 500mg daily.**
 ➝**Twin Lab CSA caps. as directed with Twin Lab EGG YOLK LECITHIN 3x daily.**
 ➝Rainbow Light CALCIUM PLUS caps with high magnesium, 4 daily. ♂♀
 ➝L-Glutamine 500mg. ♀

✒ **Vitamin C up to 5000mg daily with bioflavonoids and rutin for nerve connective tissue.**

✒ B Complex 100-150mg daily with extra B_6 500mg. if the extremities are periodically numb. ♂♀

✒ Enzymatic Therapy THYROID/TYROSINE caps, 4 daily.

✒ **Golden Pride FORMULA ONE,** oral chelation therapy with EDTA, A.M. and P.M. as directed. ♂

✒ Apply B&T *TRIFLORA* analgesic gel.

Lifestyle Support Therapy

☞ Avoid alcoholic drinks - symptoms seem to worsen.

☞ Use alternating hot and cold hydrotherapy (pg. 177).

☞ **Stress reduction techniques:**
 ➝Biofeedback for neuro-muscular feedback, acupuncture, massage therapy, shiatsu, and chiropractic adjustment have all shown excellent results.

☞ **Reflexology points:**

nerve points

☞ **Nerves:**

Common Symptoms: *Lack of feeling in various parts of the body; hands, legs, fingers and toes "going to sleep" or tingling; sporadic visual disturbances, such as double vision or a blind spot in the visual field; sometimes personality changes; lower back pain.*
Common Causes: *Poor circulation; thyroid deficiency; pinched nerve or spinal lesions; stroke and brain dysfunction; psychic inhibition, such as from hysteria; multiple sclerosis type nerve damage; nerve damage from a blow or an accident; poor diet with too many mucous-forming foods.*

See also PARKINSON'S DISEASE in this book for more information.

Osteoporosis
Osteomalacia

Osteoporosis is a disease that robs bones of their density and strength, making them thinner and more prone to break. Eventually, bone mass decreases below the level required to support the body. Long considered a woman's problem, because of its female hormone involvement, osteoporosis affects approximately 35 to 50% of post-menopausal women. Osteoporosis also affects men, just at a later age and with less ferocity. Over 25 million Americans suffer from osteoporosis today. Osteoporosis involves hormonal, lifestyle, nutrition and environmental factors. Osteomalacia involves only a decrease of calcium in the bone. Nutritional therapy is a good choice for both treatment and prevention because it offers the broadest base of protection against a wide array of factors.

Diet & Superfood Therapy

Vegetarians have lower risk of osteoporosis; they have denser, stronger bones - particularly after menopause, and in later life.

♁ Have a fresh green salad daily. Take a high vegetable-source protein drink 3 times a week.
✽Sea vegetables contain very effective concentrations of bone building minerals.
✽Eat calcium, magnesium and potassium-rich foods - broccoli, fish and seafood, eggs, yogurt, kefir, carrots, dried fruits, sprouts, miso, beans, leafy greens, tofu, bananas, apricots, molasses, etc.
✽Avoid red meats; reduce animal protein. These are high in phosphates that leach calcium. (Contrary to popular belief, pasteurized milk is not a very good source of absorbable calcium, and can actually interfere with mineral assimilation.)
✽Avoid sugar, caffeine-containing foods, hard liquor, tobacco, and nightshade plants that interfere with calcium absorption.
✽High salt intake accelerates bone loss and decreases bone density.

♁ Superfoods are very important:
✽Crystal Star SYSTEMS STRENGTH™ for broad spectrum mineral support.
✽Green Foods GREEN ESSENCE.
✽Y.S. or Beehive Botanicals ROYAL JELLY/POLLEN/GINSENG drink.
✽Nutricology PRO GREENS w. flax oil.

Herbal Therapy

Beware...ovary removal puts you at greater risk for osteoporosis.

❧ Phyto-hormones are a key:
✽Crystal Star PRO-EST OSTEO™ roll-on.
✽GINSENG/LICORICE ELIXIR™ extract.
✽ACTIVE PHYSICAL ENERGY™ ginseng caps.
✽Black cohosh caps.
✽VITEX extract.

❧ Herbal minerals are another key:
✽Crystal Star CALCIUM SOURCE™.
✽IODINE/POTASSIUM caps.
✽SILICA SOURCE™ extract (dietary silica helps collagen and calcium production.)
✽Horsetail/comfrey rt. tea.
✽Solaray ALFA-JUICE caps.

❧ Herbal bioflavonoids are important: vitamin C deficiency is implicated in osteoporosis. Vitamin C with bioflavonoids is one of the best dietary keys for collagen development. Bioflavonoid-rich herbs, especially in extract form, also have important phyto-hormone like activity.
✽HAWTHORN extract
✽BILBERRY extract
✽GINKGO BILOBA extract

❧ Low stomach acid diminishes calcium absorption. Herbal "bitters" encourage the body to produce more stomach acid.

Supplements

❧ Minerals are a key to bone health:
✽Calcium citrate 1500mg magnesium 1000mg. and boron 3mg for absorption. (Taking too much boron alone can actually cause bone loss.)
✽Mezotrace SEA MINERAL COMPLEX, with Betaine HCl for absorption and vitamin K 100mcg.
✽Flora VEGE-SIL for 6 mcs. or Ethical Nutrients BONE BUILDER with silica.

❧ Apply Transitions PROGEST CREAM as directed. Helpful in both preventing and reversing bone loss, with Nutricology germanium 150mg daily.

❧ B vitamins are important:
✽Nature's Bounty internasal B_{12} every other day, or Solaray B_{12} 2000mcg daily.
✽B complex 100mg daily w. extra B_6 250mg.

❧ Enzymatic Therapy OSTEOPRIME.

❧ Vitamin C or Ester C with bioflavs. up to 5000mg daily for connective tissue, with Vit. D 1000IU, marine carotene 50,000IU, and zinc 30mg daily.

❧ TwinLab CSA or DLPA 750mg for bone pain.

❧ EVENING PRIMROSE oil caps 6 daily, or Nature's Secret ULTIMATE OIL for EFAs.

Lifestyle Support Therapy

☙ Cortico-steroid drugs over a long period of time leach potassium from the system and weaken the bones. Overuse of antibiotic drugs, tobacco, and too much alcohol reduces total mineral absorption.

☙ Smoking cigarettes causes bone loss to women. Smoking a pack a day during adulthood results in a 10% loss in bone density, leaving bones more subject to fracture than those of non-smokers. Smoking also appears to interfere with estrogen production.

☙ Exercise is a nutrient in itself. Weight-bearing exercise is a good way to build bone and prevent bone loss. Duration of exercise is more important than intensity.

☙ Get early morning sunlight on the body every day possible for vitamin D.
✽Avoid fluorescent lighting, electric blankets, aluminum cookware, non-filtered computer screens, etc. All tend to leach calcium from the body.

☙ Reflexology point:

spine

Early warning signs: chronic back and leg pain; bone pain in the spine, affecting cranial nerves; unusual dental problems, such as bone loss in the jaw and tooth sockets, (bone tends to draw away from the teeth, causing them to loosen and in some instances, to fall out); bone fractures from trivial injuries; vision defects or facial tics due to obliteration of bone marrow.

Common Causes: menopausal drop in estrogen levels; mineral and collagen deficiency; thyroid malfunction; poor Vitamin C assimilation; prostaglandin/EFA imbalance; too many cortisone and antibiotic drugs; smoking; excess sugar and hard liquor consumption; heavy metal and environmental pollutants, (especially cadmium); anxiety and emotional stress.

See COOKING FOR HEALTHY HEALING by Linda Rector Page for a complete bone-building diet.

You Can Arrest or Avoid Post-Menopausal Bone Loss

Osteoporosis is far more complex than was thought even just 5 years ago. Bone and cartilage are an ever-changing infrastructure. Bone is living tissue, and like other body systems requires a wide variety of nutrients. Osteoporosis is partially a result of reduced nutrient (particularly mineral) absorption, which is highly bound to enzyme activity. High levels of phosphorous in meat, soft drinks and other common processed foods deprive the body of calcium. Lack of vitamin D from sunlight, and too little exercise also contribute to bone porosity.

What about calcium? It's a cornerstone of medical world treatment for osteoporosis. Calcium is the most abundant mineral in the body, and ninety-eight percent of all calcium is stored in the bones. But osteoporosis is the result of much more than a calcium deficiency. It involves both mineral and non-mineral components of bone. Calcium supplements, while playing a role in preventing bone loss, can't stand on their own as a viable treatment. In fact, bone strength is best enhanced when calcium is used with other nutrients, such as B vitamins, magnesium, silica, manganese and boron. **How do you know if you have a calcium deficiency?** Calcium deficiencies show up pre-menstrually as back pain, cramping, or tooth pain. Taking a natural calcium supplement before your period can let you know if this is your problem, because supplementation should help these symptoms disappear. However, women who think they are helping themselves by taking calcium-containing antacids may be doing just the opposite. Antacids are linked to bone pain and easy fracture, because they block stomach acids, causing, some specialists say, reduced bone growth.

There is a clear relationship between high protein consumption and osteoporosis, too. As amino acids from excess protein enter the kidneys they cause loss of water and excretion of large amounts of minerals, especially calcium, which is released from bone material in order to neutralize the acidity of the protein amino acids. Protein from animal sources is an even bigger danger for osteoporosis. Studies of vegetarians and nonvegetarians from age 60 through 90, reveal that the mineral content in meat eater's bones decreased 35% over time, while mineral content of a vegetarian's bones decreased only 18%. High levels of phosphorous in meat, soft drinks and other common processed foods also deprive the body of calcium.

Who is at high risk for osteoporosis? 1) post-menopausal small-boned white or Asian women, with a family history of osteoporosis, especially those who have not had children; 2) women over 75 years, especially those with a history of calcium and vitamin D deficiency; 3) women who have a consistently high consumption of tobacco, caffeine and animal proteins; 4) women who over use cortico-steroid drugs. If you are taking long courses of cortico-steroid drugs, consider reducing your dosage. Research indicates that over a long period of time these drugs tend to leach potassium from the system, weakening the bones; 5) women with long use of synthetic thyroid. The drug Synthroid can increase risk for both osteoporosis and high cholesterol, and may also aggravate weight problems; 6) hormone imbalances, especially for women who had their ovaries removed before menopause, or who had an early menopause, before 45 years old, or those with a history of irregular or no menstrual periods. Hormone and calcium deficiencies appear regularly in women with irregular menstrual cycles, notably when they result from excessive exercise, or eating disorders.

These risk factors really affect a lot of women, because over 50% of American women suffer from calcium deficiency alone. You can test yourself for probable osteoporosis. Use pH paper (sold in most health food stores), and test your urine. A habitual reading below pH 7 (acid) usually means calcium and bone loss. Above pH 7 (alkaline) indicates a low risk.

How do hormones fit into the bone building picture? Few men suffer osteoporosis because of their higher testosterone supply. For women, osteoporosis involves progesterone/estrogen balance, not just the amount of estrogen supply. Thyroid malfunction, and poor collagen protein development also contribute to osteoporosis. While it was first thought that estrogen was the only critical hormone that might defend against osteoporosis, we now know that progesterone is a key factor in laying down and strengthening bone. The medical world realizes this as well, and many doctors prescribe a combination of Premarin, (from pregnant mare's urine), conjugated man-made estrogens, and Provera, a synthetic progesterone, to address bone loss.

However, the newest research shows that neither Premarin nor Provera prevent osteoporosis. Both drugs are usually taken orally, passing through the liver where much of the substance is lost or altered. For this reason, and because hormones are readily absorbed through the skin, the estrogen patch has become popular. Our experience has been that neither work as well as natural, plant-derived progesterone therapy, delivered in herbal combinations. Early tests on women over 60 show that plant progesterone, such as that found in wild yam, along with an appropriate diet and supplements, may even reverse osteoporosis, something that no synthetic hormone in any combination has been able to demonstrate.

What about the new progesterone creams? Can rubbing a cream into the skin really stave off osteoporosis? Natural progesterone creams, usually derived from wild yam roots, are important news for osteoporosis. In a recent clinical study on women with osteoporosis, a bone scan showed that 5% new bone density occurred in an eighteen month period after the women used a natural wild yam progesterone cream, along with a specific nutritional program. Another 4 year study showed that plant-derived, progesterone creams increased new bone density anywhere from 10 to 40% for menopausal women who ranged from 45 to 60 years of age. Results were even better when a germanium supplement was added orally.

Can a weight loss diet really be harmful for bone density? While excessive fat intake has long been known to interfere with calcium absorption, a recent study of both pre-and post-menopausal women indicated that fat loss may also mean bone loss ....especially if the woman does not get an adequate range of nutrients for several months. Even taking calcium and multi-vitamin supplements is not enough to maintain bone mass during dieting. The test was particularly discouraging because although the diet was carried out slowly, as most nutritionists recommend, almost all the women gained all or a portion of the weight back. However, follow-up test results show promise for dieters when food and herb source minerals are added to a weight loss diet via green drinks and vegetable juices. Women who take in minerals from these sources don't seem to gain the lost weight back, either as quickly, or as much. Since a majority of American women readily admit to being on some sort of weight control diet most of the time, it seems that wisdom would indicate maintaining a broad spectrum of low fat foods in one's diet, and the addition of vegetable and herbal source mineral drinks for absorbable minerals to avoid bone loss while dieting.

Ovarian Cysts

Benign Ovarian Polyps & Small Tumors

Ovarian cysts, officially called polycystic ovary syndrome, are showing up in record numbers, especially in women with menstrual difficulties, in women who have irregular or no periods, and for women who have excessive bleeding during their periods. The cysts are small, non-malignant, chambered sacs filled with fluid. As with so many women's problems, they are thought to be hormone-driven, usually from too much estrogen, and aggravated by specific unhealthy body conditions. But they are not cancerous, nor are they cancer precursors. They normally cease to grow after menopause, but they are often painful, especially during intercourse, and can cause excessive menstrual bleeding and inter-period spotting.

Diet & Superfood Therapy

☙ Follow a low fat, vegetarian diet.

✾Reducing dietary fat intake is the first, best step to reducing cyst growth. High fats mean high circulating estrogen. Too much estrogen is the most common cause of cysts and their complications. Saturated fats from red meats and dairy foods are the worst offenders. Get your protein for healing from vegetable sources, whole grains, sprouts, soy products, and seafoods.

✾Increase intake of B vitamin foods-brown rice, wheat germ and brewer's yeast.

✾Add miso, sea vegetables, and leafy greens to alkalize the system.

✾Avoid fried and salty foods, especially during menses. Eliminate caffeine and refined sugars that cause iodine deficiency.

✾Avoid concentrated starches, full fat dairy products, and hard liquor.

✾Drink bottled water. Chlorinated water tends to leach vitamin E from the body.

✾Have some fresh apple or carrot juice every day. Vegetable green drinks (pages 168) alkalize the body.

☙ Effective superfoods:
✾Crystal Star SYSTEMS STRENGTH™
✾Transitions EASY GREENS.
✾Nature's Life GREENS PRO-96
✾Green Foods BETA CARROT drink.
✾Green Foods WHEAT GERM extract.
✾Solgar EARTH SOURCE GREENS and MORE protein plus greens.

Herbal Therapy

❧ Jump start herbal program:
Crystal Star WOMAN'S BEST FRIEND™ caps, 4 daily for 3 months, with ANTI-FLAM™ caps for inflammatory pain.
✾EVENING PRIMROSE OIL caps 4-6 daily for 3 months as an EFA.
✾Then FEMALE HARMONY™ capsules 2 daily as a hormone balancer.
✾Black cohosh extract to dissolve polyp adhesions.

❧ Iodine therapy is part of the key - often effective in 3-4 months. (Take with vit. E for best results.)
✾J.R.E. IOSOL.
✾Crystal Star IODINE/POTASSIUM™ caps or IODINE SOURCE™ extract.

❧ Make an infection-drawing vaginal pack with powders of echinacea, golden seal root, white oak, cranesbill, raspberry in water and glycerine to make a solution. Use 1 week on and 1 week off for 6 weeks. Take with a blood cleansing combination like Crystal Star DETOX!™ caps.

❧ Love your liver for proper estrogen metabolism:
✾MILK THISTLE SEED extract
✾Dandelion extract
✾Sun CHLORELLA 1 pkt. daily.

Supplements

✧ Anti-oxidants are important:
✾PCOs 100mg 3x daily
✾Nutricology germanium 150mg.
✾Vitamin E 400IU daily as an estrogen antagonist.
✾Vitamin C 5000mg daily with bioflavonoids. Bioflavonoids have estrogen-like effects to help balance the body's estrogen-progesterone ratio, and/or QUERCETIN w. BROMELAIN daily.

✾ B Complex 100mg daily to help the liver metabolize estrogen.

✾ Lane Labs BENE-FIN SHARK CARTILAGE as an anti-infective.

✾ Transitions PROGEST CREAM: rub on abdomen. Results in approx. 3 months.

✾ Pancreatin 1300mg for fat/protein metabolism.

✾ If you have a Type 2 PAP smear, begin the following program immediately:
✾Sun CHLORELLA daily, Crystal Star WOMAN'S BEST FRIEND™ caps 6 daily, or goldenseal/echinacea/myrrh caps, six SHARK CARTILAGE capsules daily, four PCO tablets daily, from grape seed oil or white pine, four 500mg EVENING PRIMROSE OIL capsules daily.

Lifestyle Support Therapy

☙ Pain in the heels, and swollen breasts at times other than menses, indicate ovarian cysts.

☙ Avoid IUDs, X-rays and radiation; they contribute to cyst occurrence.

☙ Reflexology has success in dissolving cysts.

☙ Reflexology point:

uterus
ovaries

Common Signs: pain in the fallopian tubes or ovaries, the inability to conceive, an erratic, painful menstrual cycle, unusual swelling and discomfort in the lower abdomen and breasts, often profuse uterine bleeding because of endometrial hyperplasia that results from unbalanced estrogen stimulation, painful intercourse, heel pain, fever and coated tongue, excess hair growth because of an imbalance between estrogen, progesterone and testosterone levels, unusual weight gain because of low thyroid activity.

Common Causes: Lifestyle habits: using an IUD, too much caffeine, a high fat diet, Frequent radiation treatments or X-rays, birth control pills, synthetic hormone replacement, obesity.

See ENDOMETRIOSIS page in this book for further information.

P.M.S.

Pre-Menstrual Syndrome ✳ Cramps ✳ Dysmenorrhea

PMS is by far the most common women's health complaint. It is estimated that a whopping 90% of all women between the ages of 20 and 50 experience some degree of PMS. For some women, it disrupts their whole lives. Over 150 symptoms have been documented, and new ones are being added all the time. The hormone shift in estrogen/progesterone ratios experienced during the menstrual cycle is the major factor in PMS symptoms. (Women have the widest variety of symptoms in the two week period before menstruation, when estrogen/progesterone ratios are the most elevated.) The modern women's lifestyle seems almost made to order for stress and imbalance. Both our foods and our environment are full of chemicals that clearly affect delicate hormone balance.

Diet & Superfood Therapy

Improve your diet first to control PMS. Women with severe PMS symptoms consume 60% more refined carbohydrates, 280% more refined sugars, 85% more dairy products, and 80% more sodium than women who don't get PMS.

❧ A low fat, vegetarian diet with some fish and seafood seems to produce the best results in terms of diminished symptoms.
☞Follow a mild Liver Cleansing or Hypoglycemia Diet for two months.

❧ Get plenty of low fat protein from vegetable sources, like whole grains, legumes, soy foods, sprouts, or sea foods. Or take a protein drink (see page 175) or see below.
☞Keep the diet low in fats, salt and sugar - high in greens and whole grains. Eat plenty of cultured foods, such as yogurt and kefir for friendly flora.
☞Avoid caffeine, red meat, sugars and saturated fat animal products. Eliminate dairy products during PMS days.
☞Drink 6 glasses of bottled water daily.
☞Have fresh apple or carrot juice every day during healing.

❧ Effective superfoods:
☞Crystal Star SYSTEMS STRENGTH™ drink for iodine-balancing sea vegetables.
☞Transitions EASY GREENS.
☞Solgar WHEY TO GO protein drink.
☞Lewis Labs BREWERS YEAST.

Herbal Therapy

❧ Jump start herbal programs:
Crystal Star FEMALE HARMONY™ capsules 2 daily each month, with EVENING PRIMROSE oil 4-6 daily the 1st month, 4 daily the 2nd month.
☞Before the period, use FEM SUPPORT™ for stress and to tonify; PRO-EST BALANCE™ roll-on to prevent cramping and pain.
☞During the period, use ANTI-SPZ™ caps, 4 at a time; FLOW EASE™ tea, or CRAMP BARK COMBO™ extract.
☞Apply LYSINE/LICORICE™ gel for mouth sores as needed.
☞Take an herbal diuretic like TINKLE TEA™ or caps for 5 days prior to your period to relieve pre-period edema.
☞Green tea, or Crystal Star GREEN TEA CLEANSER™ each morning as a mini detox.

❧ Relieving symptoms with herbs:
☞VITEX extract to normalize.
☞Bilberry for bioflavonoids.
☞Chamomile tea for cramping.
☞Bayberry capsules for heavy flow.
☞Ginger tea for cramping.
☞Burdock tea for hormone balance.
☞Yellow dock tea to build hemoglobin.
☞Cranesbill/red raspberry or FLOW EXCESS™ tea to normalize heavy flow.
☞Dandelion to relieve breast swelling.
☞Sarsaparilla for adrenal/fatigue help.
☞Wild Yam for DHEA-type activity.

Supplements

❧ Supplements for specific problems:
☞Transitions PRO-GEST CREAM - rub on abdomen for cramping.
☞Homeopathic Mag. Phos. to relieve cramping and congestion.
☞DLPA to alleviate mood swings.
☞Vitamin E 400IU to relieve breast swelling and soreness.
☞Apply liq. chlorophyll for face blemishes.
☞Omega-3 rich flax oil with quercetin and bromelain for lower back pain.
☞Vit. C 3000mg w. bioflavonoids, vitamin K 100mcg and Floradix IRON for excessive flow.
☞Calcium/magnesium to relax the uterus and help prevent cramping.

❧ Body normalizing multi-supplements:
☞Schiff PMS formula 1 & 2.
☞Biodynamics ATTUNE.
☞Country Life PRE-MENSES.
☞Biotanica EVERY WOMANS PHASE 1.
☞Enzymatic Therapy NUCLEOPRO F caps. (Chew for almost immediate results.)

❧ Iodine therapy for estrogen build-up:
☞J.R.E. IOSOL drops.
☞Crystal Star IODINE/POTASSIUM caps or IODINE SOURCE™ extract.

❧ Daily B vitamins for prevention:
☞B Complex 100mg, with extra B$_6$ 200mg, and Solaray 2000mcg B$_{12}$ daily.

Lifestyle Support Therapy

☙ Treat yourself to a good massage, sauna or shiatsu session before your period to loosen and release clogging mucous and fatty formations. Massage breasts and ovary areas to relax reproductive organs.
☞Stretching/relaxation exercises such as yoga with deep breathing and tai chi help.
☞End your morning shower with a cool rinse to stimulate circulation and relieve lymphatic congestion.
☞Switch from tampons to pads if you are very congested. Some research also shows that tampons may raise the risk of endometriosis.

☙ Be sparing with your schedule during premenstrual days. Give yourself some slack, and take some time out to read, listen to music and relax.
☞Light is linked to PMS. Get out in the sunshine at least 20 minutes a day.
☞Take a brisk walk every day possible.
☞Stop smoking and avoid second-hand smoke. Nicotine inhibits hormone function.

☙ Effective pelvic applications:
☞Ice packs to the pelvic area.
☞Fresh ginger rt. compresses over pelvic area, covered with a hot water bottle.
☞New Chapter ARNICA GINGER gel.
☞A compress of one drop each: aromatherapy oils of chamomile, marjoram, juniper and helichrysum in a quart of cool water.

Common Symptoms: Mood swings, tension, irritability, and depression; argumentative, aggressive behavior; water retention, bloating, and constipation; headaches; lower back pain; sore, swollen breasts; nausea; heavy cramping; low energy; food cravings for salt and sweets; acne and skin eruptions. Mouth sores with mood swings mean there is probably low progesterone or thyroid level.
Common Causes: Prostaglandin imbalance; estrogen excess or imbalance because of poor liver malfunction; thyroid insufficiency; lack of regular exercise; lack of B vitamins, mineral and protein deficiencies; endometriosis; too much salt, red meat, sugar and caffeine; stress and emotional tension.

See next page and the LIVER CLEANSING and HYPOGLYCEMIA DIETS for more information.

What's Really Going On With P.M.S.?

The intricacies of a woman's body are delicately tuned, and can become unbalanced or obstructed easily, causing pain, poor function, and lack of "oneness" that often results in physiological and emotional problems, especially during the menstrual cycle. One of the things women hate most about PMS is that they feel their whole body is out of control. Drugs, chemicals and synthetic medicines, standing as they do outside a woman's natural cycle, often do not bring positive results for women. Indeed the medical establishment, with its highly focused "one-treatment-for-one-symptom" protocols has not been successful in addressing PMS. Lifestyle therapy, including a highly nutritious diet, herbal tonifiers and balancers, and naturally-derived vitamin compounds, encourage the body to do its own work, providing balance and relief that is much more gratifying. PMS seems to be partially a consequence of the modern woman's emancipation. In times past, women were a silent, long-suffering lot, who felt that menstrual symptoms were just part of being a woman. Women were not out in the high profile workplace with men, and they could go to bed and suffer alone. In addition, our diets consisted of more whole and fresh foods than they do today. And our environment wasn't full of chemicals, nor our foods full of junk.

PMS symptoms tend to get worse for most women in their late thirties and beyond. They are often magnified after taking birth control pills, after pregnancy, and just before menopause because of hormone imbalances. But, with such a broad spectrum of symptoms affecting every system of the body, there is clearly no one cause and no one treatment. A holistic approach is far more beneficial, and self care allows a woman to tailor treatment to her own needs.

The Natural Keys To Controlling P.M.S.

MENSTRUATION IS A NATURAL PART OF OUR LIVES. PMS IS NOT. WOMEN CAN TAKE CONTROL OF PMS NATURALLY AND EFFECTIVELY.

A woman can expect a natural therapy program for PMS to take at least two months, as the body works through both ovary cycles with nutritional support. The first month, there is noticeable decrease in PMS symptoms; the second month finds them dramatically reduced. Don't be discouraged if you need 6 months or more to gently coax your system into balance. Even after many of the symptoms are gone, continuing with the diet recommendations, and smaller doses of the herb and vitamin choices, makes sense toward preventing the return of PMS.

•**Essential fatty acids balance prostaglandins.** Prostaglandins are vital hormone-type compounds that act as transient hormones, regulating body functions almost like an electrical current. Foods such as ocean fish, olive oil, and herbs such as EVENING PRIMROSE and flax oils, affect prostaglandin balance by supplementing and balancing the body's essential fatty acid supply. Too much saturated fat in the body, especially from meats and dairy products, inhibits both prostaglandin production and proper hormone flow. Essential fatty acids also promote the prostaglandins that decrease inflammation. Arachidonic acid, present in animal fats, tends to deplete progesterone levels and strain estrogen/ progesterone ratios. Three 1000mg capsules of EVENING PRIMROSE OIL daily, especially in conjunction with a broad spectrum herbal balancing compound, have shown excellent results for many women.

•**Love your liver to balance hormone (especially estrogen and progesterone) levels.** Lower your fat intake to help your liver do its job. A high-fat diet depletes liver function. A cup of green tea, or a green tea herbal cleanser, such as Crystal Star GREEN TEA CLEANSER™ each morning can go a long way toward relieving organ congestion and detoxifying the liver. Reduce your dairy product consumption to help your liver. Many dairy foods are also a source of synthetic estrogen from hormones injected into cows. At the very least, switch to non-fat dairy products. Estrogen is stored in fat; non-fat foods don't contribute to estrogen stores. Non-fat yogurt is a good choice because it also contains digestive lactobacillus. On PMS days, avoid dairy products altogether. Reduce caffeine to one cup of coffee or less a day. Caffeine also tends to deplete the liver, and lowers B vitamin levels, contributing to anxiety, mood swings, and irritability. Fifteen to 30% of women with breast tenderness find relief by stopping caffeine use. A little wine is fine, but hard liquor should be avoided to control PMS. Strong alcohol also lowers vitamin B levels and compromises liver function, reducing it's ability to break down excess estrogen.

•**The thyroid always seems to be involved in PMS.** Iodine is essential to the health of the thyroid gland, and estrogen levels are controlled by thyroid hormones. Herbs from the sea are an excellent choice for thyroid balance, because they provide iodine therapy. If the thyroid does not have enough iodine, insufficient thyroxine is produced and too much estrogen builds up. Enough iodine for therapeutic results from sea vegetables is about 2 tablespoons daily in a soup or salad. Other natural choices are IOSOL drops by J.R.E., Crystal Star POTASSIUM/IODINE SOURCE™ caps or IODINE SOURCE™ extract. Take your choice of iodine therapy with vitamin E for best results.

•**Phyto-hormone-rich herbal compounds to help balance body estrogen** levels. Phyto-estrogens are remarkably similar to human hormones. They can help raise body estrogen levels that are too low, by stimulating the body's own hormone production, or by attaching to estrogen receptor sites. Remarkably enough, plant estrogens can also lower estrogen levels that are too high. Plant estrogens are quite subtle. Even though they are only $1/400th$ or less of the strength of the body's own circulating estrogens, they are able to compete with human estrogens for receptor sites. When the weaker estrogens attach to receptors, the net overall effect is a lowering of the body's estrogen levels. Phyto-hormone-rich plants such as soybeans and wild yams, and hormone-rich herbs like black cohosh, panax ginseng, licorice root and dong quai, have a safety record of centuries. They offer a gentle, effective way to stimulate a woman's body to produce amounts of estrogen and progesterone in the right proportions for her needs. In fact, a broad-spectrum herbal combination like Crystal Star FEMALE HARMONY™ tea or capsules for women may be taken over a long period of time, as a stabilizing resource for keeping the female system female, naturally. Natural, whole, wild yam-based creams show success against PMS symptoms. As transdermal sources of plant progesterone, they offer women estrogen/ progesterone ratio balance.

•**Exercise is a must for female balance.** Exercise improves the way your body assimilates and metabolizes nutrients, especially hormones. It changes food habits, and decreases craving for alcohol or tobacco. It makes you feel better by increasing beta endorphin levels in the brain. It improves circulation to relieve congestion. It encourages regularity for more rapid elimination of toxins.

Pain Control

Using Pain's Information For Better Healing

Pain is a mechanism our bodies use to draw attention to a problem that the autonomic system cannot handle by itself. Pain signals us to consciously address its underlying cause. Pain is almost completely individual. It can stem from large pain centers that control certain areas of the body, and also from specific local areas that demand exact pinpointed action. Even mental trauma will eventually manifest itself as physical pain. There are different kinds of pain; physical, emotional, chronic, local, intermittent, throbbing, dull, spasmodic, sharp, shooting, etc. Every person feels and reacts differently to pain. Pain can be your body's best friend. It alerts you when something is wrong and needs your attention. It identifies the location, severity, and type of problem, so that you can treat the right area. Pain can be your body's worst enemy. Continuous, constant body trauma saps strength and spirit, causes irrational acts and decisions, and alters personality. Pain killers are obviously useful for these as well as other reasons. They allow you to think clearly, work and live, while addressing the cause of the problem. Chemical pain killing drugs, while strong, afford relief by masking pain, or deadening certain body mechanisms so that they cannot function. Herbal pain managers have much broader actions than analgesic drugs. They are more subtle and work at a deeper level, to relax, soothe, ease and calm the distressed area. You can use the pain for information about your body, yet not be overwhelmed by the trauma to body and spirit that unrelieved suffering can bring.

There are four basic pain centers in the body: 1) the cerebro-spinal area, controlling neural affliction, lower back pain and cramping; 2) the frontal lobe area, involved in earaches, toothaches, and headaches over the eyes; 3) the base of the brain, involved in migraines and tension headaches; 4) the abdominal area, affecting menstrual cramping, digestive and elimination pain. This page addresses chronic, lower back, joint and nerve pain. For many people natural therapies and herbs are superior to pharmaceutical drugs and their side effects.

Food Therapy

See "COOKING FOR HEALTHY HEALING" by Linda Rector-Page for an effective high mineral diet.

❧ Make sure your diet is rich in complex carbohydrates and vegetable proteins for strength: whole grains, broccoli, peas, brown rice, legumes, sea foods, etc.
⇒Add high mineral foods to the diet for solid body blocks. Emphasize magnesium and calcium foods for bone and muscle strength. Include bioflavonoid-rich foods, like fresh fruits and vegetables.
⇒Have a vegetable drink (pg. 168), and a green leafy salad every day.
⇒Avoid caffeine, salty and sugary foods that engender an overacid condition.

❧ Effective superfoods:
⇒Crystal Star SYSTEMS STRENGTH™.
⇒Crystal Star BIOFLAV., FIBER & C SUPPORT™ drink for bioflavonoids.
⇒Wakunaga KYO-GREEN.
⇒Sun CHLORELLA 1 pkt. daily.

Herbal Therapy

❧ Herbal pain management:
⇒Kava Kava extract for stress release.
⇒VALERIAN/WILD LETTUCE, a sedative and anti-spasmodic.
⇒White willow, anti-inflammatory/ analgesic.
⇒Cramp bark - cramping and spasms.
⇒Passionflower - gentle sedative.
⇒St. John's wort - nerve damage.
⇒Wild yam - anti-inflammatory.
⇒Capsaicin cream for nerve pain.
⇒Calendula for injury pain.

❧ An herbal combination works better than single herbs for pain:
Crystal Star ANTI-FLAM™ for inflammation; BACK TO RELIEF™ caps for lower back/ cerebro-spinal pain; ASPIR-SOURCE™ for headache, tooth and face pain; ANTI-SPZ™ caps, or CRAMP BARK extract for spasmodic/muscle pain; STRESSED-OUT™ tea or extract, and RELAX™ caps, for nerve pain and tension; AR EASE™ caps and tea for joint pain.

Supplements

⇝ Natural supplement analgesics:
⇒DLPA 500-750mg as needed daily, or
⇒PCOs from grapeseed or white pine 100mg 3x daily.
⇒CoQ₁₀ 60mg 3x daily.
⇒Twin Lab CSA for lower back pain.
⇒Enzymatic Therapy KAVA-TONE caps, and WILLOW/CIN with vitamin E.
⇒Country Life LIGATEND capsules as needed daily, and/or RELAXER caps. ♂
⇒Twin Lab GABA PLUS caps daily.

⇝ Fight pain with enzymes - especially proteolytic enzymes like bromelain and papain. Combine with Quercetin 1000mg and ascorbate vitamin C with bioflavonoids and rutin 5000mg daily for connective tissue formation.
⇒Biogenetics CELL-GUARD 6 daily.
⇒Solaray QBC 3 to 4x daily.

⇝ B Complex 100mg with extra B₁₂ internasal 2000mcg. ♀

⇝ B&T ARNI-FLORA homeopathic gel.

Lifestyle Support Therapy

⌘ Relaxation techniques like chiropractic adjustment, shiatsu massage, biofeedback, acupuncture, and massage therapy are effective in controlling pain.

⌘ Pain-relieving compresses:
⇒Plantain/marshmallow
⇒Wintergreen/cajeput
⇒Comfrey leaf
⇒Lobelia

⌘ Topical pain relief:
⇒Mullein oil
⇒Tea tree oil
⇒TIGER BALM
⇒CAPSAICIN creme

⌘ Acupressure: pinch and massage webs between the thumb and index finger.

⌘ Reflexology point:

spine
nerves

See also ARTHRITIS pages for more information.

Common Symptoms: Sharp shooting twinges or a dull ache; muscle wasting; poor reflexes; numbness; soreness in the sensory nerves, particularly the lower back.
Common Causes: Poor posture; poor nutrition with lack of green vegetables and calcium-rich foods; an overacid diet that eats away protective mucous membrane and nerve sheathing; poor muscle development; adrenal and pituitary gland exhaustion; recovery from disease, injury or surgery; flat feet; obesity; internal or external tumors or growths.

Parasite Infections

Intestinal Worms ✵ Amoebic Dysentery ✵ Giardia

Worm and parasite infestations can range from mild and hardly noticeable, to serious and even life-threatening in a child. Worms are parasites that live and feed in the intestinal tract. Amoebas cause dysentery, acute, unremitting diarrhea, usually contracted from parasite infested water or food in third world or tropical countries. Other parasites seem to be able to move all over the body, including the brain, weakening the entire system. Nutritional therapy is a good choice for thread and pin worms, but is very slow in cases of heavy infestation. Short term conventional medical treatment is often more beneficial for masses of hook and tape worms and blood flukes. A strong immune system is the best defense for all kinds of parasites.

Diet & Superfood Therapy

Amaranth grain is used successfully in South America to remove parasites.

♋ Go on an apple juice fast and mono diet for 4 days. (One day for a child). Take 8 garlic caps daily during the fast and chew fresh papaya seeds mixed with honey.
☞On the 3rd day, add papaya juice with 1 TB. wormwood tea, and 1 TB. molasses.
☞On the 4th day, add 2 cups senna/peppermint tea with 1 TB. castor oil, and eat raw pumpkin seeds every 4 hours.
☞A high resistance diet must be followed to prevent recurrence. Eat lots of onions and garlic. Avoid sweets, pasteurized milk and refined foods. Eat a green salad every day. No junk foods! ☺

♋ Herbal fast to expel tapeworms:
☞Mix 4 oz. cucumber juice with honey and water. Take only this mixture for 24 hours. Follow with 3 cups senna/pumpkin seed tea. Drink down all at once to use as a cathartic.

♋ For amoebic dysentery: Take carrot/beet/cucumber juice once a day for a week to clean the kidneys. Take a lemon juice/egg white drink each morning.
☞Take two TBS. epsom salts in a glass of water to purge the bowels.
☞After worms are gone, eat a high vegetable protein diet and lots of cultured foods, such as yogurt.

Herbal Therapy

♋ Jump start herbal program:
Crystal Star VERMEX™ capsules, 4 daily with 2 garlic capsules, after every meal for 2 weeks, and 4 cups fennel tea daily.
☞Then take Sonne bentonite in water 3x daily; 2 cups daily senna tea to purge.
☞BLACK WALNUT HULLS extract, or PAU D'ARCO/ECHINACEA extract 4x daily.
☞ANTI-BIO™ caps 4 daily as an anti-infective and lymph flush.
☞BITTERS & LEMON CLEANSE™ extract each morning.

or

♋ Take garlic oil capsules in the morning. Refrain from eating or drinking until bowels have moved. Repeat for 3 days.

♋ Effective vermifuge herbs:
☞Valerian caps
☞Barberry tea as an anti-infective
☞Solaray GARLIC/BLACK WALNUT caps
☞Una da gato capsules
☞UNI-KEY herbal parasite formulas.
☞Goldenseal caps esp. for giardia.
☞Myrrh extract
☞Witch hazel tea, 4 cups daily.
☞Cayenne/garlic capsules 6 to 8 daily.

♋ For giardia: BLACK WALNUT or MYRRH extract, 10 drops under the tongue every 4 hours, or tea tree oil, 4 drops in water 4x daily, and/or goldenseal extract in water over a 10 day period.

Supplements

New research shows that liver flukes may be a cause of cancer.

♋ American Biologics DIOXYCHLOR as directed for giardia infestation, or
☞Matrix Health H₂O₂ OXY CAPS.

♋ Nutribiotic GRAPEFRUIT SEED extract internally esp. for giardia.

♋ Support supplements:
☞Floradix HERBAL IRON liquid for strength during healing.
☞B Complex 50mg. daily.
☞Homeopathic Ipecac as directed.
☞Beta carotene 50,000IU daily as an anti-infective.
☞Enzymatic Therapy PHYTOBIOTIC.

♋ Pro-biotics are important: Prof. Nutrition Dr. DOPHILUS, Alta Health CANGEST, Natren TRINITY or other multi-culture powder, ¹/₂ teasp. 3x daily before meals to rebuild intestinal flora.

♋ Superfoods are important:
☞Sun CHLORELLA 2 pkts. daily.
☞AloeLife ALOE GOLD juice daily.
☞Chlorophyll liquid 1 teasp. 3x daily in water with meals.
☞ Crystal Star CHO-LO-FIBER TONE™ to clean the bowel.

Lifestyle Support Therapy

Parasites are often difficult to kill. The key is to stimulate the body's own immune response against them.

℞ Garlic enemas daily during healing.
☞Take a high colonic irrigation to clean the colon fast.

℞ Drink extra water. at least 8 to 10 glasses a day to flush out dead parasites.

℞ Apply zinc oxide to opening of anus. Then take a warm sitz bath using 1¹/₂ cups epsom salts per gallon of water. Repeat for 3 days. Worms will often expel into the sitz bath.

℞ For crabs and lice - apply: ☺
☞Thyme oil
☞Sassafras oil
☞Tea tree oil
☞Myrrh extract and tea tree oil mixed.

℞ Risk factors you can avoid:
☞Frequently eating raw or smoked fish.
☞Eating prosciutto or home-made sausages.
☞Kissing pets.
☞Not properly washing hands after using the restroom.
☞Drink only bottled water.

Common Symptoms: Round worms: fever and intestinal cramping. **Hookworms:** anemia, abdominal pain, diarrhea and lethargy; **Blood flukes:** cause lesions on the lungs and hemorrhages under the skin - typical in AIDS cases; **Protozoa, (amoebae)** cause arthritis-like pain, leukemia-like symptoms, frequent and often uncontrollable running of the bowels, pain, and dehydration. They can coat the inside lining of the small intestine and prevent absorption of nutrients, causing life-threatening malnutrition. **Tapeworms:** intestinal obstruction, gas and distress (even from a single worm). Tapeworm eggs in the liver have been mistaken for and treated with chemotherapy as if they were cancer. **Giardia:** causes diarrhea, weakness, weight loss, cramping, bloating and fever.

Common Causes: Low immune defenses; poor diet (low nutrition = low immunity); poor hygiene; fungal and yeast overgrowth conditions; infested, poorly cooked, or spoiled meat.

Parkinson's Disease

Central Nervous System Dysfunction

Parkinson's disease is a serious, degenerative central nervous system condition, characterized by a slowly spreading tremor, muscular weakness and body rigidity. Normal posture becomes stooped, walking becomes shambling, motion is trembling and life-span is shortened. The victim, whose thinking processes often remain normal, feels frozen in a position, and unable to make any voluntary movements. Parkinson's affects men and women equally, usually between the ages of 50 and 75; about 500,000 cases are found in the U.S. Although the direct cause of Parkinson's is unknown, it is thought that a neuro-toxin causes oxidative damage to the basal ganglia in the brain that controls muscle tension and movement.

Diet & Superfood Therapy

❧ Go on a completely fresh foods diet for 3 days to cleanse and alkalize the body. Use organically grown foods when possible.
☀Then, follow a modified macrobiotic diet (pg. 211) for 3-6 months until condition improves. Eat smaller meals more frequently. No large heavy meals.
☀Go on short 24 hour juice fasts (pg. 158) every two weeks during healing, with aloe vera juice each morning to accelerate toxin release.

❧ Live cell therapy from green drinks and chlorella has been notably successful in reducing symptoms. Take vegetable drinks (pg. 168) frequently, at least twice a week, and/ or Sun CHLORELLA once a day.
☀Drink only bottled water.
☀Make a mix of lecithin granules and brewer's yeast and take 2 TBS. daily. ♂

❧ Effective superfoods:
☀Crystal Star SYSTEMS STRENGTH™ drink to restore strength, return vitality.
☀AloeLife ALOE GOLD each morning.
☀**Y.S. or Beehive Botanicals ROYAL JELLY/GINSENG drink daily.**
☀Lewis Labs high potency LECITHIN and BREWER'S YEAST.
☀Sun CHLORELLA a.m./p.m. - 2 months.
☀Green Foods WHEAT GERM extract.
☀Wakunaga KYO-GREEN.

Herbal Therapy

❧ Jump start herbal program:
Crystal Star RELAX CAPS™ to help support rebuilding of the nerve sheath, and STRESSED OUT™ extract to ease shakiness.
☀**HAWTHORN extract for increased circulation and a feeling of well-being.**
☀**MENTAL CLARITY™ caps for brain and nerve nourishment.**
☀GINKGO BILOBA extract for leg cramps and tremor.
☀ADR-ACTIVE™ caps for deep energy.

❧ Critical EFAs for the nerves and brain:
☀EVENING PRIMROSE OIL 4-6 daily, ♀
☀Nature's Secret ULTIMATE OIL. ♀
☀Omega-3 flax oil 3x daily,

❧ Ginseng therapy is effective:
☀Ginseng/royal jelly vials daily. ♂
☀PAU d'ARCO/GINSENG extract.
☀Solaray GINSENG/DAMIANA and CAYENNE/GINSENG formulas.
☀Sun SIBERIAN GINSENG or Rainbow Light ADAPTO-GEM ginseng complex.

❧ **Health Aid America SIBERGIN with Enzymatic Therapy THYMU-PLEX caps.**

❧ Solaray EUROCALM to aid in serotonin formation.

Supplements

If taking L-Dopa, do not take vitamin B₆ which can block L-Dopa to the brain.

❧ **Anti-oxidants are critical in overcoming oxidative damage to the brain and slowing the progression of the disease:**
☀PCOs from grapeseed or white pine 100mg 3x daily. (also helps side effects from Sinemet).
☀Vitamin E 1000IU 2x daily.
☀Vitamin C 5000mg daily with bioflavonoids; (give as an ascorbic acid flush, pg. 445 for the initial 2 weeks for best results).
☀Twin Lab GABA plus, or Country Life RELAXER caps as needed.

❧ Brain neurotransmitters:
☀Solaray phosphatidyl choline (PC) 960mg 2 daily.
☀Phosphatidyl Serine (PS) 100mg 3 daily.
☀Tyrosine 500mg 2x for L-Dopa production. ♂
☀**DLPA 500-750mg for depression.**
☀**Lysine 500mg daily.** (Parkinson's victims are historically low.)

❧ Golden Pride FORMULA ONE oral chelation with EDTA as directed. ♂

❧ Niacin therapy: 500mg 2x daily, with B Complex 100mg, extra B₆ 500mg daily if not taking L-dopa, and Nature's Bounty B internasal gel every other day. ♂

❧ Magnesium 500mg daily. ♀

Lifestyle Support Therapy

L-dopa, a drug given for Parkinson's has serious hallucinatory side effects and leg cramps.

❧ Relaxation techniques like chiropractic treatment, massage therapy, acupuncture and acupressure have had notable success in reversing early Parkinson's.

❧ **Reflexology point:**

nerve points

❧ Regular aerobic exercise is critical for outlook and muscle health. A brisk walk every day is highly recommended.

❧ Use catnip enemas once a week to encourage liver/ kidney function.

❧ Avoid aluminum (cookware, deodorants with aluminum chloride, condiments with alum, etc.) and heavy metals that lodge in the brain and nerve centers.

Common Symptoms: Signs begin with a slight tremor in the hands or slight dragging of the foot, pronounced with stress or fatigue; then voluntary movement becomes increasingly difficult; walking becomes stiff and slow; lethargic movement and speech difficulty follow, often with vision problems; the face becomes expressionless and drooling develops because of muscle rigidity; there is numbness and tingling in the hands and feet; depression (which can show dramatic improvement with supplementation) often sets in.

Common Causes: Poor diet of chemicalized foods; hyperthyroidism; aluminum/heavy metal toxicity; pesticide residues; over-use of some psychotropic drugs; heroin abuse; allergy reaction; nerve malfunction; hereditary in multiplecase families.

See NERVE HEALTH page and M.S. diet suggestions in this book for extra help.

Phlebitis

Thrombo-Phlebitis ✤ Embolism ✤ Arterial Blood Clots

Phlebitis is vein inflammation, usually in the legs. It is a relatively common condition. An *embolism* is the obstruction of a blood vessel by a foreign substance or blood clot. *Thrombophlebitis* is the existence of a blood clot within the vascular system. Deep vein thrombosis is life-threatening because the clot can break free and occlude a vessel or lodge in the lung. Get medical help immediately!

Diet & Superfood Therapy

❧ **Take one glass of each every other day:**
➥Black cherry juice
➥Fresh carrot juice
➥A veggie drink (pg. 168), or see below.

❧ Have a leafy green salad every day.

❧ Eat plenty of onions, garlic and other high sulphur foods. Have an onion/garlic broth at least 2-3x week (pg. 171).

❧ Drink 6-8 glasses of bottled water daily.

❧ Make a mix of lecithin granules and brewer's yeast and take 2 TBS. daily.

❧ Avoid all starchy, fried and fatty foods. Avoid refined sugars, caffeine and hard liquor.
❧

❧ **Effective superfoods:**
➥Crystal Star BIOFLAV., FIBER & C SUPPORT™ drink for venous integrity.
➥Sun CHLORELLA packets or tabs daily.
➥**Wakunaga KYO-GREEN.** ♂
➥**Aloe Life ALOE GOLD drink.** ♂
➥Crystal Star ENERGY GREEN™ drink.
➥Green Foods WHEAT GERM extract.
➥Orange Peel GREENS PLUS.

Herbal Therapy

❧ **Jump start herbal program:**
Butcher's broom capsules or tea, or Crystal Star HEARTSEASE-CIRCU-CLEANSE™ tea with butcher's broom for 1 month.
➥**VARI-VEIN™ caps and roll-on** with grapeseed PCOs and horse chestnut to strengthen veins and capillaries.
➥USNEA extract to cleanse infection.
➥**HEARTSEASE/HAWTHORN caps or HAWTHORN extract 2-4x daily for 3 months to normalize circulation.**
➥GREEN TEA CLEANSER™ or kukicha tea with ANTI-FLAM™ caps as needed.
➥EVENING PRIMROSE oil 4-6 daily. ♀

❧ Reishi mushroom capsules or GINSENG/REISHI extract to rebuild immunity. ♂

❧ Herbal compresses are very successful applied right to the legs:
➥St. John's wort and St. John's wort oil.
➥Yarrow and Calendula flowers

❧ **Effective herbal bioflavonoids for vein health and integrity:**
➥GINKGO BILOBA extract
➥BILBERRY extract ♀
➥ECHINACEA extract also combats bacteria infection, always present in phlebitis
➥**Solaray CENTELLA-VEIN 3x daily.**

❧ Ayurvedic PADMA 28 for claudication.

Supplements

☙ **Vitamin E therapy, 800IU to keep body oxygen in good compound form. (also helpful for intermittent claudication.) Rapid improvement often noted.**

☙ **Bromelain 1500mg daily, or Solaray QBC, quercitin with bromelain as an anti-inflammatory and clot inhibitor for fragile veins.**

☙ **Twin Lab CSA capsules as directed for anti-thrombogenic and anti-coagulant activity.**

☙ **Free radical scavenging antioxidants:**
➥Biotec CELL GUARD 4 daily.
➥Nutricology germanium 150mg daily.
➥**PCOs from grapeseed or white pine 100mg 3x daily.**
➥Ascorbate vitamin C crystals with bioflavs and rutin, ¼ teasp. daily to bowel tolerance.

☙ High omega 3 flax oils 3 daily.

☙ **Niacin therapy: 500mg 3x daily.**

☙ Chromium picolinate 200mcg ♀ or Solaray CHROMIACIN daily. ♂

☙ Enzymatic Therapy LYMPH/SPLEEN COMPLEX as directed. ♂

☙ Apply Martin's PYCNOGENOL gel. ♀

Lifestyle Support Therapy

☙ Elevate legs whenever possible. No prolonged sitting. Consciously stretch and walk frequently during the day.

☙ Believe it or not, even too tight underwear or jeans can constrict circulation in the abdomen and groin where deep-vein phlebitis originates. Keep your weight down to relieve pressure on circulatory system instead of squeezing into tight clothes.

☙ Tale a brisk half hour walk daily.

☙ Avoid smoking and secondary smoke. It constricts blood vessels and restricts oxygen use.

☙ Avoid chemical anti-coagulants and oral contraceptives unless absolutely necessary.

☙ Take alternating hot and cold sitz baths, or apply alternating hot and cold ginger/cayenne compresses to stimulate leg blood circulation.

☙ **Effective applications:**
➥B&T ARNICA or CALIFLORA gel
➥Centipede, KITTY'S OXY-GEL.

☙ **Effective compresses:**
➥Plantain
➥Witch hazel
➥Fresh comfrey leaf
➥Alcohol compresses

Common Symptoms: Swelling, inflammation; redness and aching in the legs; fever with blood clots in the legs; pain and tenderness along course of a vein; swelling below obstruction.
Common Causes: Clogged and toxic bloodstream from excess saturated fats, especially from too much red meat and fried food; inactivity, lack of daily exercise, and sedentary life style; poor circulation from constipation, obesity or weak heart; oral contraceptive side effect; prolonged emotional stress.

See THE HEALTHY HEART DIET in this book for more information.

Pneumonia

Bacterial Pneumonia ✤ Viral Pneumonia ✤ Pleurisy

Pneumonias and pleurisy are inflammatory lung diseases caused by a wide array of viruses and other pathogenic organisms. *Bacterial pneumonia*, contracted most often by children, is caused by staph, strep or pneumo-bacilli; it responds to antibiotics, both medical and herbal. *Viral pneumonia* is an acute systemic disease, caused by a variety of virulent viruses, and does not respond to antibiotics. Herbal antivirals have shown some success. *Pleurisy* is an inflammation of the pleura membrane surrounding the lungs, and often accompanies pneumonia. Pneumonias drastically weaken the immune system. Typically, it can take 2 to 3 months to recover strength and up to 2 years to be able to resist a cold or flu without falling victim to another bout of pneumonia.

Diet & Superfood Therapy

♦ Go on a mucous-cleansing liquid diet for 1-3 days during the first and acute stages. (pg. 157). Drink plenty of fruit juices, herb teas and bottled water to thin mucous. Avoid alcohol.
  ☛Take a hot lemon and honey drink with water each morning.
  ☛Have a fresh carrot juice, a potassium broth (pg. 167) or see below.
  ☛Then follow a largely fresh foods, cleansing diet for 1-2 weeks.
  ☛Then eat a diet high in vegetable proteins, low in meat, dairy and animal fats, to allow lungs to heal easily.
  ☛Add cultured foods, such as yogurt and kefir.

♦ As an emergency measure, take fresh grated horseradish root in a spoon with lemon juice. Hang over a sink immediately to expel large quantities of mucous. ☞

♦ Effective superfoods:
  ☛Crystal Star SYSTEMS STRENGTH™.
  ☛Nature's Life PRO GREENS 96.
  ☛AloeLife ALOE GOLD drink.
  ☛Crystal Star BIOFLAV., FIBER & C SUPPORT™ drink daily for a month to 6 weeks of healing.
  ☛Sun Chlorella WAKASA GOLD extract.
  ☛Klamath BLUE GREEN SUPREME.
  ☛New Moon GINGER WONDER syrup.

Herbal Therapy

♦ Jump start herbal program:
Crystal Star ANTI-BIO™ caps or extract (or ANTI-VI™ extract or tea for viral pneumonia) 6x daily to flush toxins, with FIRST AID CAPS™ 3x daily to sweat out mucous.
  ☛After crisis has passed, take ANTI-OXIDANT™ caps, or RESPR™ caps and tea with ANTI-HST™ extract, to heal lungs and encourage oxygen uptake.
  ☛Add cayenne/ginger/goldenseal caps 6 daily, ♀ or garlic 8 caps daily, ♂ or mullein/lobelia extract in water. 🙂
  ☛HAWTHORN extract for circulation.

♦ For pneumonia with pleurisy (a burning sensation in the lungs, difficulty taking a deep breath, great fatigue even walking from one end of the house to the other):
  ☛Turmeric (curcumin) - anti-inflammatory.
  ☛GINSENG/LICORICE ELIXIR™ extract as a demulcent and adaptogen.
  ☛Thyme extract as a decongestant.
  ☛Pleurisy root or slippery elm tea for congestion.
  ☛Crystal Star ANTI-SPZ™ caps or lobelia extract - broncho-dilating anti-spasmodics.
  ☛Crystal Star X-PEC™ tea with extra ginger pinches as an expectorant.

♦ Herbal diuretics to reduce lung fluid:
Uva Ursi/cornsilk combination
Senna/dandelion combination

Supplements

✦ Vitamin C and antioxidant therapy:
  ☛Ascorbate vitamin C crystals with bioflavonoids and rutin, ¹/₄ teasp. every half hour to bowel tolerance, daily for 2 weeks; then every 2 hours for 2 weeks; then 3000mg daily for another month.
  ☛Twin Labs LYCOPENE 5-10mg.
  ☛Beta carotene 150,000IU
  ☛Vitamin E 400IU 2x daily.

✦ American Biologics INFLAZYME FORTE, an anti-infective with a full spectrum amino acid complex daily such as Country Life MAX AMINOS foe healing pro-proteins.

✦ Take several antioxidants during healing:
  ☛Matrix Health OXY-CAPS as directed or GENESIS 1000 OXY-SPRAY rubbed on the chest twice daily.
  ☛CoQ₁₀ 60mg 4x daily.
  ☛Quercetin with bromelain, 4 daily.
  ☛PCOs from grapeseed or white pine 100mg 3 daily.
  ☛Nutricology germanium 150mg 2 daily.
  ☛Carnitine 500mg 2x daily - lung protection.

✦ Rebuild immune strength w. probiotics:
  ☛Enzymatic Therapy THYMUPLEX caps.
  ☛Natren BIFIDO FACTORS, or Prof. Nut. Dr. DOPHILUS for both children and adults.
  ☛Enzyme therapy: Rainbow Light AD-VANCED ENZYME SYSTEM,

Lifestyle Support Therapy

Do not risk your health if you experience major difficulty in breathing. Short term heroic medicine may be necessary. Newer broad spectrum drugs, like CIPRO and amantidine are effective and less harmful to normal body functions than most primary antibiotics. Ask your physician.

❦ Get plenty of rest. Do conscious diaphragmatic breathing - esp. when recovering. Breathe in, pushing abdomen out, then from chest to completely fill upper and lower lungs.

❦ Apply a hot cayenne/ginger poultice: Mix powders - ¹/₂ teasp. cayenne, 1 TB. lobelia, 3 TBS. slippery elm, 2 TBS. ginger and enough water to make a paste. Leave on 1 hour.
  ✳Apply a mustard plaster to chest to stimulate lungs and draw out poisons: Mix 1 TB. mustard powder, 1 egg, 3 TBS. flour and water to make a paste. Leave on until skin turns pink.

❦ Take an oxygen bath. Use 1-2 cups 3% H₂O₂ to a tub of water. Soak 20 minutes.
  ✳Overheating therapy is effective, especially for viral pneumonia. See page 178 for home method.
  ✳Take hot and cold showers to stimulate lung circulation (pg. 177). Then use chest or back percussion with a cupped hand front and back to loosen matter.

See LUNG DISEASES page in this book for more suggestions.

Common Symptoms: *Inflamed lungs and chest pain; aggravated flu and cold symptoms, worsening after 5 days; swollen lymph glands; difficult breathing; heavy coughing and expectoration; back, muscle and body aches; chills and high fever; sore throat; inability to "get over it"; fluid in lymph and lungs; great fatigue which remains for six to eight weeks even after recovery.*

Common Causes: *Low immunity from poor nutrition; a preceding respiratory infection from a virus or bacteria; clogged lymph nodes; chemical sensitivity or allergy, especially to pesticides and herbicides; body stress and fatigue, especially from a long day outdoors in winter.*

Poisoning, Environmental

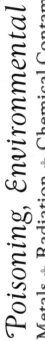

Heavy Metals ✵ Radiation ✵ Chemical Contaminants

Heavy metal poisoning is becoming a major problem of modern society. There seems to be no way to avoid toxic exposure. Chemical pollutants and toxic byproducts affect every facet of our lives, from our water and food supply to the workplace and our homes. The main effect of an unhealthy environment is on immune response, especially in the way that our filtering organs, the liver and kidneys, are impacted. Periodic detoxification needs to be a part of life so that the body can use its own cleansing mechanisms to maintain healthy immunity. A hair analysis is very helpful in determining nutrient deficiencies caused by environmental toxins.

Diet & Superfood Therapy

Do not go on an all-liquid diet when trying to release heavy metals or chemicals from the body. They enter the bloodstream too fast and heavily for the body to handle, and can poison you even more.

2) Go on a seven day brown rice and vegetable juice diet (pg. 158) to start releasing poisons from the body. Have a glass of fresh carrot juice, a potassium broth (pg. 167), and a cup of miso soup daily.

☛Green drinks are a key against all kinds of contaminants: Take veggie drinks (pg. 168) as detoxifiers and blood builders.

☛Then eat a diet full of leafy greens, and other mineral-rich foods, such as sea vegetables. Eat organically grown foods as much as possible. Avoid canned foods.

☛Make a mix of ¼ cup each: wheat germ, molasses, lecithin granules and brewer's yeast, and take 2 TBS. daily.

☛Avoid fried foods, red meats, pasteurized dairy products, fatty and sugary foods. Avoid caffeine - it inhibits liver filtering.

☛Drink only bottled or distilled water.

2) **Effective superfoods:**
☛Crystal Star ENERGY GREEN™.
☛**Crystal Star SYSTEMS STRENGTH™.**
☛**Salute ALOE VERA juice with herbs.**
☛Future Biotics VITAL K drink.
☛**Sun CHLORELLA drink daily, especially against radiation.**
☛Green Foods GREEN MAGMA.

Herbal Therapy

⚘ **Jump start herbal program:**
Crystal Star HEAVY METAL™ or DETOX™ caps for 2-3 months, with CLEANSING & PURIFYING™ tea. ☿
☛LIV-ALIVE™ caps with IODINE THERAPY™ extract or IODINE/POTASSIUM SOURCE™ caps 2-6 daily. ♂
☛EVENING PRIMROSE oil caps 4 daily with 2 cysteine caps each dose.
☛**FIRST AID™ caps - a source of white pine PCOs, for preventive measures when taken at 2 daily over several months.**

⚘ **Liver enhancers:**
☛MILK THISTLE SEED extract
☛GINSENG/LICORICE ELIXIR™.
☛Dandelion extract
☛Crystal Star LIV-ALIVE™ tea.
☛**Biostrath LIQUID YEAST w. herbs.** ☿

⚘ Herbal protectors/immune enhancers:
☛Astragalus extract ☿
☛**Propolis extract or lozenges** ☿
☛Kelp 8-10 tabs daily
☛Garlic 6-8 caps daily
☛**Siberian ginseng extract caps**
☛**Solaray ALFA-JUICE caps**
☛Crystal Star ANTI-OXIDANT™ caps
☛**Klamath POWER 3 (especially to overcome radiation/chemotherapy toxins); spirulina, Sun CHLORELLA tabs 20 daily for chemical toxins.**

Supplements

Avoid antacids - they interfere with enzyme production, and the ability of the body to carry off heavy metals.

✿ **Protective antioxidants are a key:**
☛PCOs 100mg from grapeseed 3x daily.
☛**CoQ10 60mg. 3x daily.**
☛Vit. E 400IU w/ selenium 200mcg.
☛Glutathione 50mg 2 daily. ♂
☛American Biologics OXY-5000 FORTE.

✿ Protection against contaminants:
☛Beta carotene 150,000IU
☛**Zinc 50-100mg daily** ♂
☛Solgar SOD 2000units
☛Source Naturals CHEM-DEFENSE

✿ **For radiation poisoning:** Ascorbate vitamin C powder with bioflavonoids and rutin, ½ teasp. every hour to bowel tolerance daily as a tissue flush.
☛Solaray CALCIUM CITRATE 6 daily, or Nature's Life CAL-MAG PHOS. FREE liquid.
☛J.R.E. IOSOL iodine caps. ♂
☛Enzymatic Therapy LIVA-TOX caps.

✿ **Golden Pride FORMULA ONE, oral chelation with EDTA daily.** ♂

✿ **Immune enhancers:**
☛Enzymatic Therapy THYMUPLEX.
☛Country Life LIFE SPAN 2000.
☛Nutricology GERMANIUM 150mg.

Lifestyle Support Therapy

☛ Protect against radiation syndromes: avoid foods labeled irradiated or electronically pasteurized.

☛ Use an inside air filter to remove toxins in the air. Use vinegar, baking soda and salt as cleansers if you are very sensitive.

☛ Protect yourself from EMF fields: avoid non-filtered computer screens, cellular phones, electric blankets; microwave ovens. (Don't use plastic wrap in the microwave. Its heat can drive the molecules into the food.) Look at EMF info on appliances.

★ Avoid smoking and secondary smoke, pesticides (sprinkle pepper on anthills instead), and herbicides, phosphorus fertilizers, fluorescent lights, aluminum cookware and deodorants.

★Get plenty of tissue oxygen. Take a walk every day, breathing deeply. Do deep breathing exercises on rising, and in the evening on retiring to clear the lungs and respiratory system.
★Centipede KITTY'S OXY-GEL on soles of feet every 2 days to keep tissue oxygen high.

☛ Take a hot seaweed bath, or a sweating bath, such as Crystal Star POUNDS OFF BATH™ to remove toxins. Use a dry skin brush before and after the bath to remove toxins coming out on the skin.

Common Symptoms: *Signs you may be chemically toxic: you smell things far better than most people. You can't take; even some vitamins make you feel worse. You feel worse in certain stores. Your reaction time when driving is noticeably poorer in city traffic. Other symptoms include seizures; schizophrenic-like, psychotic behavior; memory loss and senility; infertility and impotency; insomnia; small black spots along gum line; bad breath and body odor.*

Common Causes: *Body build-up of industrial pollutants and toxic chemicals; nicotine; insecticides; dental fillings; over-treated water; hair dyes; aluminum cookware and deodorants; smoke, smog; zinc depletion.*

See pages 38-40 on neutralizing the effects of chemotherapy and radiation.

Poisoning, Food
Salmonella ✴ Botulism ✴ Arsenic

Each year, more than 2 million Americans report cases of food poisoning; the actual number is thought to be far higher because food poisoning signs mimic flu and diarrhea symptoms. Even with all our government inspections, advanced packaging, refrigeration and chemical food preservatives, poisoning from food affects millions of people (mostly children and the elderly) and often leads to other diseases. **Botulism** is acute poisoning by a micro-organism similar to that causing tetanus. **Salmonella** is widespread, and comes from bacteria found in mainly hormone-injected beef and poultry.

Diet & Superfood Therapy

☘ Take $^1/_2$ cup olive oil very slowly through a straw to remove poison from the stomach or a glass of warm water with 1 teasp. baking soda.

➥Take no milk, juice, alcohol or vinegar until poison has moved from the stomach.

➥Eat high fiber foods, citrus fruits, wheat germ, whole grains, green and yellow vegetables. These foods act as protectors against pesticides and poisons in food.

➥Eat largely fresh foods for a week after poisoning to rebalance the system.

☘ **Effective toxin neutralizing foods:**
➥1-2 heads of iceberg lettuce
➥Bamboo shoots
➥Strong black tea
➥Burnt toast
➥2 raw eggs
➥Lemon water
➥Apple pectin caps.
➥Milk of magnesia
➥Onions and garlic ♂

☘ **Effective superfoods:**
➥George's high sulphur ALOE VERA JUICE morning and evening for a week after poisoning to cleanse the digestive tract.
➥Take a green drink every 4 hours to normalize body chemistry: Crystal Star ENERGY GREEN™ or Sun CHLORELLA 1 pkt.
➥Balance your intestinal structure with Solgar WHEY TO GO protein drink.

Herbal Therapy

☙ **Jump start herbal program:** Crystal Star CLEANSING & PURIFYING™ tea several times daily, with Sun CHLORELLA tabs, 10 every 4 hours to neutralize toxins and normalize body chemistry, with Bach Flower RESCUE REMEDY to rebalance the system.

or take

☙ Solaray CLAY & HERBS caps or bentonite clay powder as directed.

☙ Effective neutralizing teas:
➥Plantain ⊛
➥Scullcap
➥Elecampane
➥Wormwood

☙ **Yellow dock/nettles tea for arsenic poisoning.**

☙ Herbal protectors:
➥Garlic caps 2 with each meal.
➥Kelp tabs 8-12 daily. ♂

☙ MILK THISTLE SEED extract is used in Europe to fight liver disease caused by *Amanita*, death cap mushrooms.

also take

Enzymatic Therapy LIVA-TOX caps 3 daily.

☙ Water extract of guarana is toxic to salmonella.

Supplements

Protective food supplements can help you avoid many pathogenic organisms.

☞ **Take activated charcoal tabs to absorb poison; 3 to 5 every 15 minutes.** with **Ascorbate vitamin C powder, $^1/_2$ teasp. every $^1/_2$ hour to bowel tolerance to flush and alkalize the tissues.**

☞ Niacin therapy to sweat out poisons; 250-500mg every hour until improvement is felt (about 3-4 capsules). ♂

☞ Protective supplements against food poisons:
➥Vitamin E with selenium 400IU
➥Vitamin C with bioflavs and rutin
➥Beta carotene 25-50,000IU
➥Solgar SOD INDUCERS.
➥Glutathione 50mg.

☞ **Probiotics are a key:** bifidobacteria produce fatty acids and acidify the bowel to inhibit pathogenic micro-organisms, including *salmonella*.
➥Take acidophilus caps, or Alta Health CANGEST, or Natren BIFIDO FACTORS, or Dr. Dophilus powder before meals. (Take with Crystal Star ANTI-BIO™ extract if desired.)

☞ Nature's Life CAL-MAG LIQUID, phos. free. ♂

Lifestyle Support Therapy

Discard all bulging food cans.

☞ Use an emetic of *Ipecac*, or strong lobelia tea with $^1/_4 - ^1/_2$ teasp. cayenne, to throw up poisons and empty the stomach.
➥Follow with white oak tincture to neutralize and normalize the stomach.

☞ Use a coffee or catnip enema to flush the bowel and stimulate liver detox function.

☞ Sweat out pesticides and chemical poisons in a long, low heat sauna.

☞ Overheating therapy is effective. See page 178 in this book for correct technique.

☞ Use American Biologics DIOXY-CHLOR or NutriBiotic GRAPEFRUIT SEED extract in water as directed to decontaminate produce.

Common Symptoms: Diarrhea, nausea and vomiting; cold sweats after eating; severe abdominal pain and flatulence; severe headache; chills and fever; red, rashed skin. Botulism signs are weak, limp muscles 12 to 36 hours after eating, double vision, dry mouth, speech difficulty, vomiting, stomach cramps, even respiratory failure can results. (Do not give honey to infants for fear of botulism.)
Common Causes: Harmful bacteria in food; pesticides and fungicide residues in food; additives and preservatives in food; sulfites and MSG reactions; food allergy reaction; breathing noxious fumes; lack of proper cleaning of cutting boards and food preparation areas in both restaurants and homes.

Call the POISON CONTROL CENTER Hotline, 800-764-7661, if you need emergency information.

Poison Oak
Poison Ivy * Sumac

*Urushiol, the toxic oleoresin responsible for the poison oak/ivy reaction. is one of the most potent external toxins on earth! Its toxicity can survive for 100 years after the plant is dead. Even sap that has been diluted 50 million times can induce toxicity. **One quarter ounce of urushiol has the potential to affect everyone on earth.** Over 2 million people a year get a poison oak or ivy reaction; more than 60% of American are sensitive to it. Sensitivity during childhood is highest, but once you lose your sensitivity, an immunity sets in and remains for life.*

Diet & Superfood Therapy

❧ Apply cider vinegar, denatured alcohol, or a cornstarch paste to blisters to control itching and neutralize acid poisons.

❧ Follow a fresh foods diet during acute blistering to cleanse systemic poisons out of the bloodstream. No junk or fried foods.

❧ Take several veggie green drinks during acute phase (pg. 168 or see below).

❧ Apply oatmeal to rash areas to neutralize toxins.

❧ **Effective superfoods:**
 ❋**Alkalize your body with ALOE VERA juice and apply aloe vera gel.**
 ❋Green Foods GREEN ESSENCE.
 ❋Nature's Life SUPER GREEN PRO.

Herbal Therapy

❧ **Jump start herbal program:**
 Crystal Star P.O. #1 and P.O. # 2 capsules alternately as directed.
 ❋**Apply ANTI-BIO™ gel as needed**
 ❋Nature's Pharmacy GOLDEN MYRECAL lotion with golden seal; or apply a paste of honey and goldenseal powder and cover with a bandage.
 ❋**Crystal Star ANTI-HST™ capsules 4-6 daily until clear, to help curb the histamine allergy reaction.**
 ❋ADRN™ extract or ADR-ACTIVE™ caps 2x daily. to strengthen the adrenal glands against sensitivity.

❧ **Effective topical applications:**
 ❋Comfrey/aloe salve
 ❋Tea tree oil, which sloughs off old, affected tissue, and leaves healthy tissue intact.
  ❋B & T CALIFLORA gel
  ❋Calendula ointment
  ❋Witch hazel
  ❋Bioforce Echinacea cream
 ❋**Fresh plantain leaves**
 ❋**Goldenseal solution in water**
 ❋Sassafras tea

❧ Black walnut tincture. Apply locally. Take internally.

❧ Jewelweed tea. Apply locally. Take internally.

Supplements

❧ **Vitamin C therapy is a natural antihistamine:** ascorbate vitamin C crystals, $1/4$ teasp. every hour to bowel tolerance, until itching lessens, then reduce to $1/4$ teasp. 4x daily until clear.

❧ Nutribiotic GRAPEFRUIT SEED SKIN SPRAY. **Take internally. Apply locally.**

❧ Effective topicals:
 ❋Liquid chlorophyll
 ❋Centipede KITTY'S OXY GEL
 ❋Vitamin E oil to decrease healing time.
 ❋Nature's Life CAL-MAG liquid.

❧ **Homeopathic remedies:**
 ❋Homeopathic *Rhus Tox.*
 ❋Cell salts *Kali Sulph* and *Natrum Mur.*
 ❋Hylands homeopathic *Poison Oak* tabs to build resistance protection.

Lifestyle Support Therapy

❧ **Artemesia (mugwort) grows in the same vicinity as poison oak, and appears to be a naturally-occurring protective plant against it. Rub fresh mugwort leaves on any exposed skin before you go out in the woods or brush.**
 ❋Cover all exposed skin well before going out.
 ❋Wash within 30 minutes of contact in cold water with a non-oil soap. **(Oil soaps spread the urushiol.)**

❧ Effective bath additions:
 ❋Epsom salts
 ❋Apple cider vinegar
 ❋Baking soda
 ❋Oatmeal
 ❋Cornstarch
 ❋Green clay and salt water paste

❧ Swim in the ocean if possible - effective, neutralizing therapy.

❧ **Effective applications: wash off in cold water first.**
 ❋Aloe vera gel or aloe ice gel.
 ❋Chinese WHITE FLOWER OIL
 ❋Pau d'arco gel
 ❋Rubbing alcohol

See also Skin Itching page for more information.

Common Symptoms: Allergic reactions to the allergen in poison oak range from an annoying itch to a life-threatening condition. Itching blisters on the skin ooze, erupt and spread the systemic plant poisons. There may be throat swelling, cramps and diarrhea. People with sun-sensitive skin are most susceptible. Allergic reaction takes place within 72 hours after contact.

Common Causes: The resin responsible for the allergic skin reaction must touch the skin or clothing of the person to cause the reaction. Resins can even be carried in smoke of the burning plant, so don't burn it or try to uproot it. Kill poison oak and ivy with a systemic herbicide for best results. The blisters don't contain the oleoresin; you can't "pass it on."

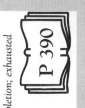

Prostate, Benign Hypertrophy (BPH)
Prostate Enlargement & Inflammation

A large number of men suffer from prostate enlargement problems. Disorders usually begin after age 35 and by age fifty, over 25 percent of all men have an enlarged prostate. By 70, it's over 50% and by age 80, over 80%. Lifestyle causes, (such as obesity), and hormonal changes, (such as increased estrogen levels and altered testosterone levels are at the root of the problem), but men can help themselves easily and naturally to manage prostate problems without the highly adverse side effects (often as bad as the prostate problem itself), and limited success of the drug approach. Watchwords should be: less fat, more fiber, stay fit.

Diet & Superfood Therapy

♦ Take lemon juice and water every morning for two weeks to cleanse sediment; then cider vinegar and honey in water daily for a month to prevent sediment recurrence.

➥Follow a fresh foods, high fiber diet for 1 week, with plenty of green salads, fresh fruits, juices and steamed vegetables.

➥Add simply cooked whole grains, soy foods, and sea foods for EFAs for 3 weeks. **Keep the diet very low in fats.**

➥Drink 6 to 8 glasses of water or cleansing fluids daily. Especially add 2 to 3 glasses of cranberry juice. Have a vegetable drink (pg. 168) every day for the first month of healing.

➥Avoid red meats, caffeine, hard liquor, carbonated drinks, and tomato juice, and especially beer during healing.

➥Avoid tobacco, and all fried, fatty and refined foods forever.

♦ Make a prostate health mix of lecithin granules, toasted wheat germ, pumpkin seeds, oat bran, brewer's yeast, sesame seeds, and crumbled dry sea vegetables; take 4 tbs. daily.

♦ **Effective superfoods:**
- Crystal Star SYSTEMS STRENGTH™ drink for iodine and potassium nutrients.
- **Nature's Life PRO GREENS 96.**
- ➥**Y.S. ROYAL JELLY/GINSENG drink.**
- ➥Green Foods GREEN MAGMA.
- ➥Sun CHLORELLA 1 pkts. daily.

Herbal Therapy

♦ **A highly successful herbal program:**
Crystal Star PROX™ caps or extract 4-6 daily for 1 month, then 2-4 daily for 1 month; RELAX™ caps to relax nerves/ease urination.

➥EVENING PRIMROSE oil 4-6 daily for 1 month, then 2-4 daily for 1 month with bee pollen caps 2 daily, and ANTI-BIO™ or ANTI-FLAM™ to reduce inflammation. ➥Then MALE PERFORMANCE™ for regeneration, IODINE/POTASSIUM™ caps, kelp tabs, or IODINE SOURCE™ extract for prevention, with vitamin E 400IU.

♦ **Other effective prevention herbals:**
- ➥Echinacea/goldenseal extract
- ➥GINSENG/LICORICE ELIXIR™ esp. to guard against prostate cancer.
- ➥White oak to shrink swollen prostate.
- ➥Una da Gato caps and/or nettles extract to relieve frequent urination.
- ➥Uva Ursi extract,anti-microbial/diuretic.
- ➥Marshmallow to soothe inflammation.
- ➥Pau d'arco for inflammation.
- ➥Omega-3 flax oil 3x daily to lower cholesterol.

- ➥Hydrangea to reduce sediment.
- ➥Garlic caps 8 daily - an anti-infective.

♦ **For prostatitis: A** saw palmetto/pygeum formula, with flax oil 3x daily, CHLORELLA-GINSENG extract, or GINSENG/ LICORICE ELIXIR™.

Supplements

♦ **Two month supplement program:**
➥**Zinc** 100mg daily for 1 month, then zinc 50mg daily for 1 month with B_6 200mg. ➥**Ascorbate vitamin C crystals,** $\frac{1}{2}$ teasp. every hour to bowel tolerance daily for 2 weeks, then $\frac{1}{2}$ teasp. 4x daily for 2 weeks, then 3000mg daily for 1 month.

➥Oceanic carotene 100,000IU to control infection.
➥Vitamin E 800IU daily.
➥**Melatonin 3mg at night for 1 month.**
➥Bromelain 1500mg daily for faster healing/anti-inflammatory enzyme therapy.
➥Biotec CELL GUARD 6 daily .

♦ **Effective brand products:**
➥Enzymatic Therapy NUCLEO-PRO M caps for prevention.
➥**Solaray PYGEUM or PROSTA-GEUM.**
➥Country Life PROSTA-MAX caps.
➥Flora PROSTA-KIT as directed.

♦ **Amino acid therapy:**
➥GABA for night time urination.
➥Glycine 500mg for sediment control.
➥Glutamine 500mg daily.

♦ **For prostatitis inflammation:**
➥**Bromelain** 750mg 2x daily, with zinc 50mg 2x daily, vitamin E 800IU 2x daily and vitamin C 5000mg with protective bioflavs. daily, or Alacer EMERGEN-C drink.

Lifestyle Support Therapy

Some studies show that a man should think twice before having a vasectomy, because of the increased risk of prostate cancer among vasectomized men. As sperm builds up in the sealed-off vas deferens, the body reabsorbs it and sometimes tries to mount an autoimmune response to its own tissue. In addition, the testes are a powerful focal point of the life force of a man. When something interferes with the movement of sperm, energy flow is blocked, eventually resulting in stagnation and degeneration.
A vasectomy can also result in liver blockage that leads to prostate inflammation, leg cramps, abdomen pain and irritability.

♦ Sexual intercourse during prostatitis irritates the prostate and delays recovery. After recovery sex life should be normal in frequency and desire with a natural climax.
➥Drugs like PROS-CAR and PROS-GUARD are reporting side effects of decreased potency and libido, and in some cases it is stifled entirely.

♦ **Avoid chemical antihistamines. Overuse impairs liver and prostate function.**

♦ Use chamomile tea enemas (pg. 177) once a week during healing to cleanse the body of harmful acids.
➥Or take warm chamomile sitz baths for 20 minutes at a time AM & PM.
➥Apply ice packs to reduce pain.
➥A brisk daily walk is important.

See also PROSTATE CANCER page for more information.

Common Symptoms: With BPH, the disease is basically the symptoms - see below. Inflamed, swollen, infected prostate gland, under the scrotum and testes; frequent, painful desire to urinate with reduced flow of urine; incontinence in severe cases; fever; lower back and leg pains; impotence and loss of libido, and/or painful ejaculation; reduced immune response; unusual insomnia and fatigue.
Common Causes: A high fat diet puts a man at greatest risk, as does a poor diet with too little fiber and too many over-acid, or spicy foods; too much alcohol and caffeine; EFA and prostaglandin depletion; exhausted lymph system from too many over-the-counter antihistamines; internal congestion and poor circulation; lack of exercise; zinc deficiency; venereal disease.

Rheumatic Fever
Severe Systemic Inflammation & Roseola

Rheumatic fever is a serious inflammatory condition following a strep infection. It normally affects small children between 3 and 12 years old. The severe inflammation of full blown rheumatic fever can affect the heart or brain; arthritis-like symptoms of pain and stiffness often settle in the joints. Rheumatic fever can be prevented if the strep virus is killed within ten to twelve days of infection, because it will not have become virulent enough in that time to overwhelm the body's immune defenses. However, once the disease has been contracted, recurrence is common, so natural treatment focuses on rebuilding a healthy immune system. **Roseola, often called scarlet fever,** is a similar young child's infectious disease accompanied by high fever, nausea and a similar skin rash.

Diet & Superfood Therapy

❧ Adhere to a fresh juice and liquid diet for the first bedridden stages of healing to reduce body work and strain.

➤Take potassium broth or essence, (page 167), and apple/alfalfa sprout juice daily during the acute period.

➤Take Organic Gourmet NUTRITIONAL YEAST or MISO broths, or miso soup with snipped sea vegetables daily for B vitamins and strength.

➤Then eat fresh and mildly cooked foods, including plenty of seafoods and vegetable protein from whole grains, tofu, sprouts, etc. Eat only small meals.

➤Drink only bottled water.

➤Avoid all sugars, salty, refined foods during healing. Keep fats low. No fried foods, caffeine or carbonated drinks during healing.

❧ Use superfoods to rebuild immunity: Crystal Star SYSTEM STRENGTH™ for iodine, potassium and broad spectrum nutrient support.

➤Sun CHLORELLA 1 pkt. daily.

➤Wakunaga KYO-GREEN drink.

➤Orange Peel GREENS PLUS drink (good tasting).

➤Amazake RICE DRINK for healing protein.

➤AloeLife ALOE GOLD drink.

Herbal Therapy

❧ Jump start herbal program: Crystal Star ANTI-BIO™ caps 4 daily for at least a month.

➤EVENING PRIMROSE OIL caps 4 daily.

➤Crystal Star AR-EASE™ tea or ANTI-FLAM™ extract drops as an anti-inflammatory for pain and stiffness symptoms.

➤Then Crystal Star HEARTSEASE/HAWTHORN™ caps, or HAWTHORN extract drops in water to normalize heart system.

➤Then GINSENG/CHLORELLA extract drops in water or GINSENG 6 SUPER TEA™ to strengthen against recurrence.

❧ Garlic tabs 6 daily to help overcome infection.

❧ Lobelia or dandelion extracts. ❀

❧ Apply wintergreen oil compresses to chest. Take wintergreen/white willow tea internally.

❧ High potency royal jelly 2 teasp. daily.

❧ Probiotics are important to replace friendly flora after lengthy antibiotic courses.

➤Prof. Nutrition DR. DOPHILUS 1/4 teasp. in water 4x daily. ❀

Supplements

Homeopathic treatment is very effective in the initial phase. See a homeopathic physician. It may be used even if chemical medications are already being taken. Remember to reduce doses for children.

❧ Ascorbate vitamin C crystals with bioflavonoids, 1/4 teasp. every hour in juice, or until stool turns soupy during acute periods, then reduce dosage to 3-5000mg daily. ❀

❧ Anti-infectives:
➤Beta carotene 50-100,000IU daily.
➤Colloidal silver as directed.
➤BENE-FIN SHARK CARTILAGE caps 2 daily as an antiviral.

❧ Effective anti-oxidants:
➤Vitamin E 4-800IU daily.
➤PCOs from grapeseed or white pine 50mg 3x daily.
➤Germanium 30mg 3x daily.
➤CoQ₁₀ 60mg. daily.
➤Solaray B₁₂ 2000mcg. daily during healing.

❧ Enzymatic Therapy THYMU-PLEX caps for immune stimulation. ❀

Lifestyle Support Therapy

❧ Plenty of bed rest is a key. Treatment may take months, or even years.

➤Yoga and mild muscle-toning exercises, and/or massage therapy during confinement (which can last for several weeks) will prevent loss and atrophy of body strength.

❧ Take a catnip enema once a week to reduce fever. ❀

❧ Do not use aspirin as an anti-inflammatory. ❀

➤Notify dentist of rheumatic heart disorder if having an extraction or anesthesia for any reason.

❧ Apply a tea tree oil rub on sore joints.

Common Symptoms: After an initial moderate fever, there is chronic extreme weakness; heart weakness may result; there is often a skin rash; poor circulation, shortness of breath and a continuing sore throat. The most common symptom of full-blown rheumatic fever is arthritis.

Common Causes: Inflammation of the main circulatory system causing holes in the heart ventricles; allergic reaction; low immunity, especially in children; often accompanied by acute viral disease; toxic exposure to harmful chemicals, environmental pollutants, or radiation.

See also INFECTIONS & INFLAMMATION page in this book for more information.

Schizophrenia

Psychosis ❧ Mental Illness ❧ Tardive Dyskinesia

Schizophrenia is a form of psychosis with severe perception disorder, characterized by hallucinations, delusions, extreme paranoia, and disturbed thought content. Personal relationships are abnormal, work is almost impossible, and the schizophrenic often withdraws emotionally and socially. Anti-psychotic (neuro-leptic) drugs may do more harm than good. Tardive dyskinesia is a side effect disorder, with slow, rhythmical, involuntary movements, caused exclusively by neuroleptic drugs used to treat schizophrenia and psychosis. It is bizarre in that the symptoms themselves are similar to a psychosis. Over 70% of the patients taking antipsychotic drugs develop this grim disorder which almost totally isolates them socially. Natural therapies have been successful in reversing TD.

Diet & Superfood Therapy

A diet for hypoglycemia has been very successful in controlling schizophrenia.

❧ **Improving body chemistry is a key:**
➤Start with a short juice and cleansing diet to normalize blood levels (pg. 157). Minimize fruit juices if hypoglycemia is involved.
➤Then, eat largely fresh foods for the remainder of the week. Eat niacin-rich foods like broccoli, carrots, potatoes and corn.
➤**Then, gradually add vegetable proteins, gluten-free grains (especially brown rice, millet and amaranth), fish (especially tuna and halibut), and sunflower seeds. Turkey is a good, calming tryptophan source.**
➤Eliminate all refined sugars, caffeine, red meats, food with additives and preserved foods. Especially eliminate arginine foods like peanut butter and nuts. They can be toxic to a schizophrenic's brain.

❧ **Effective superfoods:**
➤**Crystal Star CHO-LO-FIBER TONE™** with organic flax seed oil daily. ♂
➤**Nappi THE PERFECT MEAL protein.**
➤Solgar EARTH SOURCE GREENS & MORE.
➤**Nutricology PRO GREENS with flax.**
➤Beehive Botanicals or Y.S. GINSENG/ ROYAL JELLY.
➤Crystal Star SYSTEMS STRENGTH™.
➤Lewis Lab LECITHIN and BREWER'S YEAST.

Herbal Therapy

Avoid yohimbe in all herbal supplements - it may aggravate schizophrenia.

❧ **Herbal jump start program:**
Crystal Star **RELAX CAPS™ as needed for nerve rehabilitation; ANTI-HST™ to lower high histamine levels; WITHDRAWAL SUPPORT™ caps for tardive dyskinesia.**
➤**MENTAL CLARITY™ caps - 1 daily.**
➤ IODINE SOURCE™ drops, JRE IOSOL drops 2-3x daily, or kelp tabs 6-8 daily, and/or **DEPRESSEX™ extract caps 6-8 daily.**
and
➤**AMINO-ZYME™ or FEEL GREAT™ caps or tea for balance.** ♀✚

❧ **For cerebral circulation:**
➤GINKGO BILOBA extract
➤Siberian Ginseng extract.

❧ **EFAs are key nutrients:**
➤**EVENING PRIMROSE OIL 4-6 daily.**
➤Nature's Secret ULTIMATE OIL.
➤Rohe BALANCED EFAs 7 oils.
➤**Flax oil 1 TB. 3x daily.**

❧ Herbal balancing nervine herbs:
➤St. John's wort for depression.
➤Gotu kola to restore nerves
➤Valerian or VALERIAN-WILD LETTUCE.

❧ **For tardive dyskinesia:**
➤EVENING PRIMROSE oil 4 daily

Supplements

❧ **Balance body chemistry with amino acid therapy:**
➤Glutamine 1000mg daily.
➤Tyrosine 1000mg 2x daily.
➤Glycine 1000mg 2x daily.
with

❧ **Niacin & vitamin C therapy:**
➤1-3000mg daily or Solaray CHROMIACIN daily. (A baby aspirin before taking will remove niacin flush). ♂
➤Ascorbate vitamin C powder with bioflavonoids and rutin, ¼ teasp. every hour to bowel tolerance daily for the first month of healing. (Vitamin C will help in withdrawal from tranquilizers and drugs.)
or

❧ **B Complex 150mg with extra B₆ 500mg, and B₁₂ 2000mcg 3x daily.**
➤**Melatonin 3mg for 6 mos.** ♀
➤**Atrium LITHIUM 5mg as directed.**

❧ **For anxiety and depression:**
➤Phos. Chol. (PC55) 3x daily with zinc 50mg 2x daily, and GABA 500mg 2x daily.
➤Country Life MAX AMINO caps w. B₆
➤Country Life MOOD FACTORS. ♂

❧ **Effective for tardive dyskinesia:**
➤Am. Biologics MANGANESE FORTE.
➤**CoQ₁₀ 60mg 3x daily.**
➤Niacin 500mg 3x daily.
➤B₆ 200mg 2x and Vitamin E 800IU.

Lifestyle Support Therapy

New research shows that the herb rauwolfia serpentina (an Ayurvedic anti-psychotic remedy), works almost as well as reserpine, the drug for schizophrenia derived from it, with far fewer side effects like tardive dyskinesia.

❧ Get some exercise every day, especially running, walking or jogging. The oxygen will do wonders for your head.
➤Take ocean walks for sea minerals, or a visit to a mineral-rich spring and spa are effective.

❧ Regular massage therapy and spinal adjustment have had some success.

❧ Try to stick to an interesting daily schedule so you don't drift and lose the days to inertia.

❧ Avoid all pleasure drugs, and as many prescription drugs as possible. For many people, permanent brain change and psychosis can result.

Common Symptoms: *Severe mental depression; lethargy; emotional swings, often to violent actions; delusions and hallucinations; detachment from reality; the brain is without thought much of the time. What remains is scattered and chaotic like random shotgun fire. Tardive dyskinesia: social withdrawal, slow, shuffling gait, lethargy; grimaces and outbursts.*

Common Causes: *Hypoglycemia; diabetes; severe gluten and/or dairy allergies; heavy metal toxicity; too high copper levels; nutrient deficiency from too many junk foods, and refined sugars; prescription and/or pleasure drug abuse; vitamin B₁₂ deficiency; iodine deficiency; elevated histamine levels; hypothyroidism; glandular imbalance; when occurring in young children.*

See the HYPOGLYCEMIA DIET suggestions in this book for more information.

Sciatica

Neuritis of the Sciatic Nerve

Sciatica is neuritis of the sciatic nerve which runs from the low back across the buttocks, into the leg, calf and foot. Sciatic pain is caused by a compression of the sciatic nerve, characterized by sharp, radiating pain running down the buttocks and the back of the thighs. The inflammation is arthritic in nature - extremely sensitive to weather change and to the touch.

Diet & Superfood Therapy

A mineral rich diet is important:

- Take a potassium broth (pg. 167) every other day for a month to rebuild nerve health.
- Have a leafy green salad every day. Take a little white wine with dinner to relieve tension and nerve trauma.
- Eat calcium and magnesium rich foods, such as green vegetables, sea vegetables, shellfish, tofu, whole grains, molasses, nuts and seeds.
- Take a good natural protein drink, such as one from page 175, or see below.
- Drink bottled mineral water, 6-8 glasses daily.
- Avoid caffeine-containing foods, refined sugars and esp. chocolate.

Effective superfoods:

- Crystal Star ENERGY GREEN™ drink.
- **Wakunaga KYO-GREEN one packet daily for nerve rebuilding.**
- AloeLife ALOE GOLD juice.
- **Nappi THE PERFECT MEAL protein drink.**
- Green Foods GREEN ESSENCE.
- Beehive Botanicals or Y.S. GINSENG/ROYAL JELLY.
- **Crystal Star SYSTEMS STRENGTH™ drink for electrolyte minerals.**
- Future Biotics VITAL K, 3 teasp. daily.

Herbal Therapy

Herbal jump start program:
Crystal Star RELAX CAPS™ as needed for rebuilding the nerve sheath, with ANTI-FLAM™ as needed for inflammation.
and
Thyroid therapy is important:
- POTASSIUM/IODINE SOURCE™ caps or IODINE SOURCE extract on a regular basis. ♀

Aromatherapy:
- Mix wintergreen, cajeput, rosemary oils. Massage into area.
- Apply a cold compress of chamomile or lavender aromatherapy oils.

Liquid chlorophyll 3 teasp. daily with meals, or garlic/parsley caps 4-6 daily. ♂

Black cohosh extract drops in water.

Effective topical applications:
- St. John's wort oil
- Olive oil rubs
- TIGER BALM ♂
- Chinese WHITE FLOWER oil

Supplements

Country Life LIGATEND capsules as needed.
with
- Vitamin E 400IU daily.

Quercetin with bromelain 500mg, or Solaray QBC 3-4 daily as an anti-inflammatory.

Cal/mag/zinc 4 daily, with vitamin D 400IU, or Mezotrace sea mineral complex 4 daily with natural iodine and minerals.

Effective homeopathic remedies:
- *Lachesis*
- *Mag. Phos.* tabs.
- *Rhus Tox.*
- B & T *TRIFLORA* gel.

Ascorbate vitamin C or Ester C with bioflavonoids and rutin, 3-5000mg daily for connective tissue development.

DLPA 500-750mg 2x daily as needed for pain.

B Complex 100mg with extra B_1 100mg, B_6 250mg, niacin 250mg. ♀

Lifestyle Support Therapy

Treatment should focus on removing the pressure on the nerve - via chiropractic or massage therapy treatments.
- Apply alternating hot and cold, (finishing with cold), or hops/lobelia compresses to stimulate circulation.
- Apply ice packs or wet heat to relieve pain.

Gentle morning and evening stretches, and daily yoga exercises are effective.

Take hot epsom salts baths.

Reflexology point:

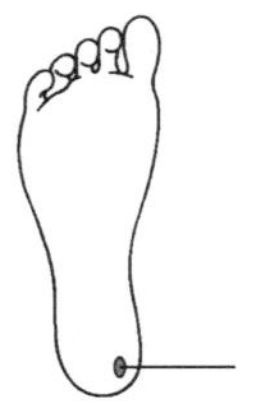

Common Symptoms: *Severe pain in the leg along the course of the sciatic nerve - felt at the back of the thigh, running down the inside of the leg; lower back pain; muscle weakness and wasting; reduced reflex activity.*
Common Causes: *Sciatic nerve compression resulting from a ruptured disc or arthritis, or an improper buttock injection; poor posture and muscle tone; poor bone/cartilage development; exhausted pituitary and adrenal glands; menopause symptoms; obesity; lack of exercise; high heels; protein and calcium depletion; not enough green vegetables; flat feet.*

See BACK PAIN AND NEURITIS/NEURALGIA *pages for more information.*

Seasonal Affective Disorder

S.A.D. ✻ Winter Blues ✻ Pineal Gland Imbalance

S.A.D. makes people sad. Wintertime for 25 million Americans (four times more women than men), means serious disruption of their lives. Work effectiveness is noticeably reduced, and relationships suffer. S.A.D. begins to manifest itself after the autumn equinox as sunlight hours lessen. The disorder is latitudinal - in Mexico, Florida and Texas, only 1.4% of the population suffers from S.A.D. In Canada, over 17% of the population suffer from acute S.A.D. In the Northeast U.S., up to 50% of the population is thought to have noticeable winter mood shifts. The unusual appetite and low energy aspects of S.A.D. show our ancient ties between seasonal rhythms, psychological well-being and nutritional factors as they affect our nervous system and behavior.

Diet & Superfood Therapy

Conscious diet improvement is the main key to reducing SAD symptoms. A diet for hypoglycemia has been effective.

☙ Make sure you are following a balanced diet with natural foods, rich in complex carbohydrates, (to shift the distribution of amino acids in the blood), and low in fats and sugars.

✻Include B-vitamin and mineral-rich foods, such as brown rice and fresh vegetables. Whole grains, legumes and soy products will help control sugar cravings.

✻Take a brewer's yeast supplement daily, such as Lewis Labs, as a source of B vitamins and chromium.

✻Add seafoods and especially sea vegetables to the diet for absorbable vitamin D and beta carotene. ℘

☙ **Effective superfoods:**
✻**Beehive Botanicals or Y.S. GINSENG/ROYAL JELLY.**
✻**Nutrex HAWAIIAN SPIRULINA, with B Complex 100mg to balance sugar use.**
✻**Crystal Star SYSTEMS STRENGTH™** drink for electrolyte minerals.
✻Biostrath original LIQUID YEAST.

Herbal Therapy

☙ **Herbal jump start program:**
Crystal Star DEPRESS-EX™ extract with St. John's wort throughout the winter.
✻**FEEL GREAT™ caps or tea for broad based rapid energy as needed.**

☙ **Pineal/pituitary stimulation is a key:**
✻Rosemary extract♀♂
✻Crystal Star MEDITATION™ tea.
✻Parsley/sage tea ♂♀
✻**GINKGO BILOBA extract 3 x daily.**

☙ **EFAs can help normalize the body's electrical connections:**
✻EVENING PRIMROSE oil 4 daily.
✻Nature's Secret ULTIMATE OIL♀♂
✻Omega-3 flax oil 3x daily.

☙ Herbal neurotransmitter stimulants:
✻Alfalfa
✻Cayenne

☙ **Ginsengs are key whole body nutrients, especially to control sugar cravings:**
✻Crystal Star GINSENG-LICORICE ELIXIR™.
✻Crystal Star ROYAL MU™ tea.♀♂
✻Ginseng/gotu kola capsules. ♂♀

☙ Effective herbal brain foods:
✻Royal jelly 2 teasp. daily
✻Kelp tabs 6 daily
✻Gotu kola

Supplements

☙ Take natural A & D supplements all during the winter.
✻**American Biologics EMULSIFIED A & D 2x daily.**
✻Twin Labs ALLERGY D, or A & D.
✻Solaray A & D 25,000/1,000IU.

☙ **B Complex 100mg daily with extra B₁ 100mg and B₆ 200mg daily,** with

✻Chromium picolinate 200mcg daily to control blood sugar levels and normalize brain chemistry.

☙ Well-balanced multi-vitamin and mineral complexes: Rainbow Light COMPLETE NUTRITONAL SYSTEM, Nature's Secret ULTIMATE MULTI PLUS, or Country Life MAXINE for women and MAX for men.

☙ Rainbow Light CALCIUM PLUS w. high magnesium 2x daily.

☙ Glutamine 500mg 2x daily. ♂

☙ Effective Homeopathic remedies:
✻Sepia 30x
✻Sulfur 30x

Lifestyle Support Therapy

☙ **Light therapy is the most widely accepted treatment for S.A.D.:** Indoor and fluorescent light is not effective. Full-spectrum light is necessary to shut off melatonin secretion through exposure to light and prevent or reduce SAD symptoms.

✻Light boxes have not been approved by the FDA but have shown definite effectiveness. Call the Winter Blues Information Network 1-800-FIX-BLUES. Depression typically begins lift about a week after "photo-therapy" begin. You will probably need to use light therapy from mid-fall until spring.

☙ **Going south for a winter vacation helps relieve symptoms temporarily, and also helps sufferers to function more normally for 3 to 4 weeks after they return. People who use this anti-depression therapy, say they can get through a whole winter with three or four southern trips.**

☙ Get outdoor exercise every day, especially running, walking or jogging. Those with an active lifestyle, especially in active winter sports like skiing, are disturbed less by winter.

✻Spend regular time in a greenhouse during the winter if possible. Light is a nutrient that does wonders for your pineal gland. The plant oxygen does wonders for your head.

See the HYPOGLYCEMIA DIET *in this book for more information.*

Common Symptoms: *Unexplained depression and mood swings; unusual sleepiness and inability to awake easily from sleep; reduced quality sleep and chronic fatigue; increased appetite, carbohydrate craving and weight gain; decreased sex drive; anxiety, irritability, low stress tolerance, low self-esteem; summertime high with very high energy and extended wakefulness for all daylight hours.*

Common Causes: *Not enough full spectrum light, especially during winter months; a result of the pineal gland not receiving enough light stimulation to stop secreting melatonin; hormone and body rhythm imbalance that results in unusual diet cravings (especially sweets) and weight gain.*

Sexuality
Lack Of Normal Libido

Reduced or inhibited sexual desire can stem from many reasons, both psychological and physical. For many of us these days, lack of time to turn our attention to our partners and body love seems to be the biggest problem. Both women and men today are overwhelmed with family and home care, career responsibilities, sports and activities that require all our energy, and leave us only able to collapse at the end of every day. This page offers some natural sexual energy tonics to turn your thoughts and mood to love.

Diet & Superfood Therapy

Lack of normal libido can often be overcome simply by improving a poor diet. Junk foods, chemical and processed foods are a key factor in the body's not feeling "up to it."

For women: increase consumption of soy foods; the phyto-estrogens in soy foods produce a mild, natural estrogenic effect.

➥Foods that enhance female sexual function include fennel, celery and parsley, flaxseed oil, nuts and seeds.

➥Add mineral-rich foods: shellfish, leafy greens, sea vegetables, whole grains, nuts, legumes and molasses.

➥Avoid red meats; keep fats, salt and sugar low. They all inhibit the free-flow of the system.

For men: Zinc is perhaps the most important nutrient for male sexual function. Zinc source foods include liver, oysters, nuts, seeds and legumes.

➥Dopamine (L-Dopa) is intimately associated with sex drive in men. Fava beans have high concentrations of L-dopa; one 16-oz. can offers almost a prescription dose!

Effective superfoods:
➥Nappi PERFECT MEAL protein drink.
➥Beehive Botanicals or Y.S. GINSENG/ROYAL JELLY drink and tabs.
➥Solgar WHEY TO GO protein.
➥Crystal Star SYSTEMS STRENGTH™ drink for electrolyte minerals.

Herbal Therapy

Herbs have a centuries-old reputation for effectiveness in working with the body toward sexual health and enhancement.

For men:
➥Yohimbe caps 750-1000mg to stimulate testosterone (Do not take yohimbe if you take diet products containing phenylpropanolamine, or have heart, kidney or liver disorders.)

➥**Crystal Star LOVE MALE™ caps, MALE GINSIAC™ or LOVING MOOD FOR MEN™ extracts, MALE PERFORMANCE™ caps; PRO-EST PROX™ roll-on for longer erections.**

➥Highest potency royal jelly 60,000-120,000mg daily.

➥Heart Foods KEEP IT UP tabs.
➥**GINKGO BILOBA for erectile dysf.**

For women:
➥Crystal Star LOVE FEMALE™ caps, or FEM-SUPPORT™ extract w. ashwagandha for several days before a special weekend.
➥Yohimbe 500mg capsules for a tingle. (See above for contra-indications.)
➥GINSENG/LICORICE ELIXIR™.

For both:
➥1 or 2 cayenne-ginger combination capsules for enhanced orgasm.
➥Ginseng/damiana caps, 4 as needed.
➥Crystal Star CUPID'S FLAME™ or GINSENG 6 SUPER tea or AMINO-ZYME™ caps.

Supplements

For men:
➥Unipro B₁₅, DMG liquid or SL tablets.
➥Premier GERMANIUM WITH DMG.
➥**Zinc 50mg 2x daily with lecithin caps for healthy seminal fluids.**

➥**Liquid niacin before sexual intercourse seems to be effective for men.**

➥Arginine 3000mg 45 minutes before sex for more blood flow to the penis; (not if you have herpes)

➥Carnitine 500mg 2x daily.
➥Life Enhancement PRO-SEXUAL PLUS.
➥Country Life ACTION MAX.
➥Solaray MALE caps with raw orchic.
➥Enzymatic Therapy NUCLEO-PRO M.

For women:
➥**Crystal Star WOMEN'S DRYNESS™, or lecithin caps for vaginal fluids.**

➥Transitions PROGEST cream, or Crystal Star PRO-EST BALANCE™ roll-on.
➥**Unipro B₁₅, DMG liquid or SL tablets.**
➥Enzymatic THYROID/TYROSINE.
➥Enzymatic Therapy KAVATONE.
➥**Highest potency YS royal jelly 60,000-120,000mg. daily, or Vitamin E 800IU daily.**

For both:
➥100mg niacin - 30 minutes before sexual activity to enhance sexual flush, mucous membrane tingling and the intensity of the orgasm.
➥Co. Life ADRENAL w. TYROSINE.

Lifestyle Support Therapy

❦ **Environmental estrogens in hormone-injected food animals, herbicides and pesticide affect male sperm counts and female hormone balance. Avoid hormone-injected meats and dairy products, and herbicide sprays to avoid the exogenous estrogens.**

❦ Exercise can increase sex drive, especially exercise with your mate. Regular exercise such as dancing, walking and swimming stimulates circulation and increases body oxygen.
➥Lose weight if you are obese.

❦ Hypnotherapy has been effective when the problem is psychologically based.

❦ **Lifestyle habits affect male sexual health:**
➥Look at your prescription drugs; some have the side effect of impaired sex drive.
➥**Prolonged recreational drug use inhibits sperm production.**

➥Heavy metal or radiation damages sperm and chromosome structure.
➥**Sexually transmitted diseases scar the vas deferens and testes, obstructing sperm delivery to the penis; infertility results.**
➥**Smoking, because the cadmium contained in cigarette papers interferes with the utilization and absorption of zinc.**

❦ Try aromatherapy oils on the sheets: ylang-ylang, jasmine, sandlewood.

Common Symptoms: Impotence; frigidity; lack of normal sexual interest.
Common Causes: Dissatisfaction with one's life, age, looks, etc.; emotional stress and tension from job, relationship unhappiness, or life style; poor diet resulting in physical malfunction; lack of exercise; childhood abuse and trauma; prescription and/or pleasure drug reaction.

See GLAND & HORMONE pages in this book for more information.

Sexually Transmitted Diseases
Venereal Infections

Sexually transmitted diseases have become a factor in every choice we make about our sexuality and our reproductive lives. No treatment for impotence, no questions about fertility or sterility, no decision about child conception can be made today without considering the STD quotient. We are in a STD health crisis. Sexually transmitted diseases are more prevalent and more varied than ever before. It has been estimated that one out of every five Americans has a sexually transmitted infection. Whether you believe our culture is paying for years of sexual freedom, (which is turning out not to be free, after all), or whether you believe that STDs are the result of irresponsible behavior and misinformation, they can't be ignored.

Diet & Superfood Therapy

Emphasis must be on optimal nutrient foods for body regeneration. See The Forever Diet in "COOKING FOR HEALTHY HEALING" by Linda Rector Page.

Follow a very cleansing liquid diet for 3-7 days (pg. 157) during acute stages. Take one each of the following juices daily: Potassium broth (pg. 167), fresh carrot juice, vegetable drink (pg. 168, or see below), apple/parsley juice to alkalize.

Then continue with a cleansing fresh foods diet to alkalize. Include several bunches of green grapes daily (an old remedy that still works).

Avoid refined, starchy, fried and saturated fat foods. Avoid red meats, pasteurized dairy products, and caffeine during healing.

Effective superfoods:
- Crystal Star ENERGY GREEN™.
- AloeLIfe ALOE GOLD concentrate, 14TBS. before meals. ♂
- Sun CHLORELLA 2 pkts. daily.
- Nutricology PRO-GREENS with flax.
- Wakunaga KYO-GREEN. ♀
- **Green Foods BETA CARROT.**

Herbal Therapy

For Gonorrhea:
Crystal Star ANTI-BIO™ or ANTI-VI™ formulas 4-6 x daily, with Crystal Star WHITES OUT #1 & #2 capsules alternately as needed.

For Chlamydia:
- Crystal Star DETOX™ caps with goldenseal. May also be opened and applied to sores.
- Enzymatic Therapy GARLINASE.
- **Mix powders of goldenseal, barberry and Oregon grape root with vitamin A oil and directly to the cervix via an all-cotton tampon.** ♀

For Trichomonas:
- Crystal Star WHITES OUT #1™ and WHITES OUT #2™ capsules for 2 months (alternate every 2 hours), with ZINC SOURCE™ extract.
- Bathe sores several times daily in a goldenseal/myrrh or gentian herb solution.
- Use a TEA TREE oil vaginal suppository nightly. ♀

For Syphilis: After antibiotics, use:
- Crystal Star DETOX™ with goldenseal.
- SARSAPARILLA extract for 4 months.
- PAU D'ARCO/ECHINACEA extract
- Calendula tea 3 cups daily.

Supplements

Many STDs benefit from GRAPEFRUIT SEED extract and/or SKIN SPRAY first.

For Gonorrhea:
- Beta carotene 150,000IU daily, with Vitamin C crystals ¹/₂ teasp. every hour to bowel tolerance during acute phase, reduced to 5000mg daily for a month.
- Vitamin E 400IU 2x daily.

For Chlamydia:
- Nutricology GERMANIUM 150mg.
- CoQ₁₀ 60mg 4x daily.
- Natren BIFIDO FACTORS.
- Zinc 50mg 2x daily, apply topically.
- Am. Biologics emulsified A & E.
- Lane Labs BENE-FIN SHARK CARTILAGE 4 caps daily as an anti-viral agent.
- Vitamin E 400IU 2x daily.

For Trichomonas:
- Zinc 50mg 2x daily, apply topically.
- Beta carotene 150,000IU daily, with Vitamin C crystals ¹/₂ teasp. every hour to bowel tolerance during acute phase, reduced to 5000mg. daily for a month.

For Syphilis:
- Calendula ointment
- CoQ₁₀ 60mg 4x daily.
- Nutricology GERMANIUM 150mg.
- Natren BIFIDO FACTORS.

Lifestyle Support Therapy

Strong doses of antibiotics are the usual medical treatment, but the most recent outbreaks (especially in teenagers) are showing resistance or non-response to these drugs.

Overheating therapy is very effective in controlling virus replication. Even slight body temperature increases can lead to considerable reduction of infection. See page 178 in this book for effective technique.

Smoking and a poor diet increase risk because they reduce immune defenses to create an environment for infection. Smokers are 3 times more at risk than non-smokers.

Oral contraceptives are known to potentiate the adverse effects of nicotine, and to decrease the levels of key nutrients like vitamins C, B₆, B₁₂, folic acid, and zinc. In addition, some oral contraceptives aggravate the formation of pre-cancerous lesions because of their imbalancing estrogen content.

Common Symptoms: *Symptoms usually appear two to three weeks after sexual contact. **Gonorrhea:** cloudy discharge for both sexes; frequent, painful urination, yeast infection symptoms; pelvic inflammation. **Syphilis:** First contagious stage; sores on the genitalia, rash and patchy, flaky tissue, fever, mouth sores and chronic sore throat. **Chlamydia:** thick discharge in both men and women, urethritis; pelvic pain, sterility. Can cause birth defects if present during pregnancy. **Trichomonas:** caused by a parasite, found in both men and women, usually contracted through intercourse, severe itchiness and thin, foamy, yellowish discharge with a foul odor.*

Call the National STD Hotline (800) 227-8922 for more information.

Sexually Transmitted Disease
Herpes Genitalis

Herpes Simplex 2 Virus is the most widespread of all STD's, affecting 60 to 100 million Americans. It is a lifelong infection that alternates between virulent and inactive stages. It may be transmitted even when there are no symptoms, by direct contact with infected fluids from saliva, skin: discharges or sexual fluids. Babies can pick up the virus in the birth canal, risking brain damage, blindness, even death. Recurrent outbreaks may be triggered by emotional stress, poor diet, food allergies, menstruation, drugs and alcohol, sunburn, fever, or a minor infection. Men are more susceptible to recurrence than women. Outbreaks are opportunistic in that it takes over when immunity is low and stress is high. Optimizing immune function is of primary importance.

Diet & Superfood Therapy

Good nutrition is critical against herpes - body chemistry balance is essential.

✿ Go on a short 3 day cleanse (pg. 157) to alkalize the body. Have plenty of fruit juices, and a carrot/beet/cucumber juice or potassium broth (pg. 167) each day. Take 2 teasp. sesame oil daily. Avoid citrus fruits during healing.

✱Then keep the diet consciously alkaline with miso soup, brown rice and vegetables frequently. Add cultured vegetable protein foods such as tofu and tempeh for healing and friendly G.I. bacteria. Increase consumption of fresh fish (rich in lysine).

✱Arginine-containing foods aggravate herpes. Avoid these foods until outbreak blisters have disappeared: chocolate, peanuts, almonds, cashews, and walnuts; sunflower and sesame seeds, and coconut. Eat wheat, soy, lentils, oats, corn, rice, barley, tomatoes, and squash with discretion.

Reduce dairy intake, especially hard cheeses, and red meat. Eliminate fried foods, nitrate-treated foods, and nightshade plants like tomatoes and eggplant.

✿ Effective superfoods:
✱Crystal Star ENERGY GREEN™ drink.
✱Nutricology PROGREENS w. flax oil.
✱George's ALOE juice every morning.
✱Green Foods GREEN MAGMA.
✱AloeLife FIBERMATE - internal cleansing.

Herbal Therapy

Herbal treatment has had remarkable success against herpes, both in remitting symptoms, and reducing outbreaks.

✿ Jump start herbal program:
Crystal Star HRPS™ capsules 4 daily, with ANTI-FLAM™ caps or extract, or turmeric (curcumin) caps as an anti-inflammatory, and extra ANTI-VI™ extract for 7 days if needed to overcome the virus.
✱Apply LYSINE/LICORICE GEL™.
✱In Life Energy Systems RED ALGAE. ♂
✱St. John's wort oil.♀
✱Lemon balm extract, cream or essential oil applied directly.♀
✱LIV-ALIVE™ caps cleanse the liver.

✿ Apply to sores and take orally:
✱Crystal Star THERADERM™ tea.†
✱Crystal Star ANTI-BIO™ caps (opened), or aloe vera gel/goldenseal solution.
✱Aloe vera juice and gel.
✱ECHINACEA-FAU D'ARCO extract - 1 dropper orally every 2 hrs.

✿ Effective body balancers:
✱BLACK WALNUT extract
✱Garlic 8 capsules daily.
✱GINSENG/REISHI extract

✿ Effective herpes tea: dandelion root, sarsaparilla root, astragalus, ligustrum, echinacea root.♀

Supplements

Lysine therapy fools the virus which needs the amino acid arginine to reproduce. Both amino acids, lysine and arginine look similar to the virus. So the virus takes lysine if it is available instead of arginine, thus blocking virus development, and keeping it from reactivating.

✍ Apply lysine cream frequently. Take lysine 500mg capsules 4-6 daily until outbreaks clear.
✱Apply AloeLife SKIN GEL frequently.

✍ Dr. Diamond HERPANACINE capsules as directed, with Enzymatic Therapy THYMU-PLEX caps as directed.♀
✱Quercetin Plus with bromelain for instant inflammation relief.

✍ Premier LITHIUM .5mg (also open a capsule, mix with water and apply.)♀

✍ Potentiate immune response:
✱B Complex 100mg 2x daily, tyrosine 500mg, and Nature's Bounty B₁₂.
✱Ascorbate vitamin C or Ester C powder ¼ teasp. every hour in water up to 10,000mg, or to bowel tolerance daily during an attack.
✱Beta carotene or emulsified Vitamin A 50,000IU daily, with Vit. E 400IU 3x daily. Also apply vitamin E oil directly.♀
✱Enzymatic Therapy ACID-A-CAL.
✱Nutricology ALIVE & WELL caps.

Lifestyle Support Therapy

✿ Apply ice packs to lesions for pain and inflammation relief. Ice may also be applied as a preventive measure when the sufferer feels a flare-up coming on.

✿ Get some early morning sunlight on the sores every day for healing Vitamin D.

✿ **Take hot baths frequently for overheating therapy (pg. 178).** ♂

✿ Wear cotton underwear.

✿ Practice stress reduction techniques like biofeedback, meditation and imagery to prevent outbreaks.
✱Acupuncture is effective for herpes.

✿ Cortico-steroid drugs taken over a long period of time for herpes greatly weakens both the immune system and bone density.
✱Immune-suppressing drugs, alcohol, and tobacco should be eliminated from your lifestyle.

✿ Effective applications:
✱Nutribiotic GRAPEFRUIT SEED SKIN SPRAY.
✱Body Essentials SILICA GEL.
✱Enzymatic Therapy HERPILYN ointment.
✱Crystal Star ANTI-BIO™ gel with una da gato.

Common Symptoms: *The first herpes outbreak is usually the most potent. It is accompanied by swollen glands and fever, as the body's immune system rallies to fight the infection. A cluster of painful blisters appears below the waist, over the groin, the thighs and buttocks, accompanied by a low grade fever, flu-like symptoms, and swelling of the groin lymph glands. There is headache, stiff neck, fever, pain, swelling, genital itching and blisters that swell and fester, and shooting pains through the thighs and legs. Blisters rupture after 1 to 3 days, then slowly heal in another 3 to 5 days.*

Common Causes: *Transmitted from kissing, oral sex, intercourse; excess arginine in the body; too many drugs; an acid-forming diet; hormone imbalance related to the menstrual cycle.*

Call the Herpes Hotline (919) 361-8488 for more information.

Sexually Transmitted Disease

Cervical Dysplasia ❦ Condyloma ❦ Venereal Warts (HPV)

Cervical dysplasia, a precancerous lesion in the cervix. is being called the newest sexually transmitted epidemic. It is silent, slow-growing and often unknown by the infected person. Researchers suspect that two sexually transmitted viruses, Human Papilloma Virus (Condyloma) and Herpes Simplex II are involved, because these viruses also play a role in cervical cancer. They are extremely contagious. Both conditions are the result of risky lifestyle habits and reduced immunity. Both can result in a pre-cancerous TYPE 4 PAP smear and are linked to cervical cancer. Natural treatments deal with the causes of genital warts and require strong commitment and significant lifestyle changes, with positive outlook and good mind/body connection for immune support.

Diet & Superfood Therapy

❧ A diet to encourage strong immune response against dysplasia:

❋Increase fresh fruits, vegetables (especially cruciferous veggies), and high fiber complex carbohydrates as protective factors. Add high folic acid foods like lima beans, whole wheat and brewer's yeast.

❋Add vegetable juices and/or green drinks (pg. 168) for immune support and supplementing vitamin deficiencies.

❋Add 2 TBS. chopped sea vegetables as a viable source of marine carotene. Add cold water fish like salmon for omega-3 oils.

❋Reduce dietary fat, especially from animal foods. Reduce caffeine, hard liquor and processed foods.

❋Avoid red meat and poultry foods. These may have been contaminated with estrogens or other hormone treatments.

❋Particularly avoid foods that aggravate herpes-type infections like sugary junk foods.

❧

Effective superfoods:

❋Sun CHLORELLA, 2 pkts. daily
❋Crystal Star SYSTEMS STRENGTH™ for detoxification ♂♀
❋Solgar EARTH SOURCE GREEN & MORE
❋Beehive Botanical ROYAL JELLY with Siberian ginseng 2 teasp. daily
❋George's ALOE VERA juice 2x daily
❋Lewis Labs BREWER'S YEAST

Herbal Therapy

❧ **Jump start herbal program:**
Crystal Star ANTI-VIT™ extract or tea to deal with the virus; ANTI-BIO™ extract or caps to help flush lymph glands.
❋**DETOX™ capsules for one month as a blood cleanser, followed by FIBER & HERBS COLON CLEANSE™ to rid the colon of re-infection.**

❋Use PAU d'ARCO/ECHINACEA extract, 2 cups daily of burdock tea, and a course of vaginal packs for both genital warts and dysplasia.

❋**CALCIUM SOURCE™ caps or extract to prevent pre-cancerous lesions from becoming cancerous.**

❋EVENING PRIMROSE oil, 6 daily.

For venereal warts:

❋Crystal Star ANTI-VI™ capsules 4 daily, with FIRST AID CAPS™ to raise body temperature during acute stages; one week off and one week on until improvement.

❋Golden seal/chaparral vaginal suppositories (powders mixed with vitamin A oil). This vag pack has been extremely helpful for women with venereal warts, rendering many disease-free. ♀
❋Aloe vera gel application along with 2 glasses of aloe vera juice daily; or steep several garlic cloves in a 4-oz. glass of high sulphur aloe vera juice and apply 2x daily.
❋Castor oil compresses.

Supplements

Women with high blood levels of folic acid have lower rates of cervical dysplasia.

☙ **Anti-oxidants are key factors:**
❋OPC's from grapeseed or pine bark 100mg 3x daily.
❋Nutricology germanium 150mg .
❋Marine or beta-carotene 200,000IU.
❋For 1 month, give your body an ascorbic acid flush with $\frac{1}{4}$ teasp. vitamin C powder with bioflav. every hour until the stool turns soupy. Then take ascorbate vitamin C 5000mg daily with bioflavonoids for a month.

❋Solaray QBC with bromelain 2 daily.
❋L-Cysteine or Nutricology NAC. ♂
❋Nature's Bounty internasal B$_{12}$. ♂

☙ **Increase immune support:**
❋Enzymatic Therapy THYMULUS.
❋Zinc picolinate 50mg daily.
❋B complex with extra folic acid 800mcg 2x during treatment, then once daily to help normalize abnormal cells.

❋Vitamin E 400IU with selenium 200mg 2x daily.

☙ Apply Transitions PRO-GEST CREAM or oil as directed. ♀

☙ **If there are mouth sores, treat as for thrush. (see page 262), or chew Enzymatic Therapy DGL tablets.**

Lifestyle Support Therapy

High-risk lifestyle factors must be eliminated for there to be permanent improvement and prevention of further invasive lesions. Recurrence often occurs after standard surgery alone.

☙ Eliminate smoking, oral contraceptives and multiple sexual partners.
❋Especially avoid hard alcohol.
❋Use a barrier contraceptive to prevent new contact with HPV or herpes II. ♂

☙ **Surgery may be avoided by using botanical vaginal packs, Nutribiotic GRAPE-FRUIT SEED extract, Body Essentials SILICA GEL, or chlorella powder paste, placed against the cervix to draw out toxic waste and slough abnormal cells. Abstain from sexual intercourse during vag pack treatment. (See page 446 for a pack you can make yourself.)**

❋Alternating hot and cold hydrotherapy or sitz baths will promote immune activity to the pelvic area.

☙ **For venereal warts:**
Matrix GENESIS H$_2$O$_2$ OXY-SPRAY daily for a month; then rest for a month, and resume if necessary. If noticeable improvement has occurred in this first month, returning to this treatment may not be necessary. The body's defense forces will have taken over and can better continue on their own.

See the previous pages for more information.

Common Symptoms: *Heavy painful periods; bleeding between periods; pain during intercourse; genital warts or herpes; chronic gonorrhea or any unusual vaginal discharge; fever and often, infertility.* **Symptoms of Venereal Warts (HPV):** *the most common STD, infects ovaries, fallopian tubes, cervix, and uterus. Chronic yeast infection with heavy, pus-filled discharge; painful intercourse; painful, infected sores in the genital area; high fever during infection.*
Common Risk Factors: *Early age of first intercourse, multiple sexual partners; lower socio-economic class with its traditionally nutrient-poor diet, smoking, and oral contraceptives.*

STDs and Birth Control

Contraceptive methods and sexually transmitted diseases must be considered together. Unless you are in a long-term relationship, in which you are *absolutely sure* that your partner is monogamous, you should take precautions against STDs. Even if you know your partner is monogamous you should be careful. Once a virus gets into your system, it never goes away. Sometimes people carry diseases from previous relationships and don't know it, or don't want to share the fact with a new partner. When considering your sexual lifestyle choices, remember that HIV and AIDS can kill you; herpes and HPV, (the virus that induces genital warts) are permanent. These STDs may become dormant, but they do not leave the body. Even others, that are not permanent, cause a great deal of pain and can leave you permanently infertile.

There are risks and benefits to every method of contraception, but the risks of contracting a sexually transmitted disease, abortion and unwanted pregnancy are obviously greater. Both partners, but especially women, need to earnestly evaluate their lifestyles, sexual discipline and partner's attitudes to make a responsible health choice.

1) **BARRIER METHODS** - condom, diaphragm, cervical cap and vaginal sponge - have become the most popular contraceptive devices since the advent of the AIDS epidemic. The latex (not lambskin) condom is the only method that offers almost complete protection from STDs. It encourages couples to share responsibility for birth and disease control. It should not, however, be used without a back-up, because the high failure rate from breakage, heat or wear is almost 15%. To further guard against unwanted pregnancy, a spermicide should be used in conjunction with a condom.

Because the pill shifted the responsibility for contraception from men to women, condom use has, unfortunately, become less common - especially among teenagers, where the greatest STD infection is being experienced. Young, unsophisticated lovers tend to think of the condom as a barrier to sexual enjoyment rather than as a part of a mature, responsible relationship. **The new female condoms,** polyurethane ringed sheaths that fit over the cervix, have been conceived as a solution to address this problem. They are comfortable, the effectiveness rate is high, and they can be inserted ahead of time, but they are clumsy, and unromantic, hanging slightly outside the vagina. However, they do give the woman a choice if the man refuses to wear a condom, and they do protect against STDs.

The diaphragm, fitted correctly, used with spermicide, without any tiny holes or cracks is an effective, unobtrusive method of birth control, and provides some protection against STDs. Unfortunately, many sensitive women get bladder infections from the rubbing of the diaphragm against the urethra, and yeast infections from the spermicide that must be used.

The cervical cap is used with spermicidal jelly to create a seal that prevents sperm penetration and inactivates sperm for contraception. It is effective for 48 hours at a time, and is effective for birth control if inserted properly, but is not effective against STDs.

The vaginal sponge is a simple device, impregnated with spermicide, that is inserted in the back of the vagina, and is effective for 24 hours. However, it is not a good choice for women who have had children, or for sensitive women who experience irritation from a large dose of spermicide. In addition, it may become a cause of toxic shock syndrome when the women is unable to remove the sponge or when fragments remain.

2) **SPERMICIDES** - such as creams, jellies, suppositories and foams, are put into the vagina to kill or immobilize sperm. They have some ability to kill sexually-transmitted viruses, but should always be used in conjunction with a barrier method of contraception.

3) **HORMONAL CONTRACEPTIVES** - although today's pills have much lower doses of hormones, overcoming many of the life-threatening side-effects, increased risk of breast cancer is still a controversy, and many women are still sensitive to the synthetic estrogen impact. High blood pressure, migraine headaches, depression, water retention, thrush, gum inflammation and changes in skin pigmentation are still frequent short-term effects - and of course the pill does not protect against STDs. Hormone implants are surgically inserted into the skin of a woman's upper arm, and release very small doses of hormone into the bloodstream. Even in these substantially smaller amounts of synthetic hormones, there are still some side effects of irregular menstruation, intra-period spotting, headaches, depression. They are effective birth control for five years, but do not protect against STDs.

4) **STERILIZATION** is the most rapidly increasing form of contraception in adult women in America, as the sexually active population ages past child-bearing years. A **tubal ligation** is a procedure where hormones, ovulation and menstruation continue as usual, but the egg disintegrates in the tubes and is absorbed by the bloodstream. Side effects are irregular bleeding, increased menstrual pain and excessively heavy periods, to the point, that in some cases, a hysterectomy becomes necessary to stop the bleeding. A **vasectomy** is a procedure where the tubes that carry the sperm to the penis are cut and tied. The man can continue to ejaculate semen without sperm, but many questions about side effects and long-term hormone imbalances are now being raised. (See page 390, Prostate Enlargement, for more information.) Neither sterilization form protects against STDs.

5) **IUDs** have fallen from favor because of their many complications, increased risk of infertility, and adverse health effects. The most recently discovered problem is that the string on an IUD acts as a wick for harmful organisms, thus spreading vaginal bacteria, including sexually transmitted diseases such as gonorrhea, into the uterus.

Shingles

Hives & Angioedema

Shingles are the eruption of acute, inflammatory, herpes-type blisters on the trunk of the body along a peripheral nerve. It is an acute central nervous system infection caused by the Herpes Zoster virus, and the blisters are infectious. Since the virus is the same as that causing chicken pox, there is proneness to shingles if one had chicken pox as a child. Hives are the same type of itching blisters, but are caused by an allergic reaction to a chemical, medication or food. The most common cause of shingles for adults is a reaction to certain medications. Both are very painful, inflammatory skin conditions.

Diet & Superfood Therapy

❧ Go on a short 3 day cleansing diet to eliminate acid wastes and alkalize the blood (pg. 157).
➛Take a carrot/beet/cucumber juice, and a natural cranberry juice each day. Take an apple juice or celery juice each night.
➛Then, eat only fresh foods for 1-2 weeks, with lots of salads and fruits.
➛Avoid arginine-forming foods
➛Keep the diet alkaline, with plenty of miso soup, whole grains, vegetables and leafy greens. Eat foods high in B vitamins, such as brown rice, green vegetables and brewer's yeast.
➛Include cultured foods, such as yogurt and kefir for friendly G.I. flora.
➛Avoid acid-forming foods, like red meats, cheese, salty foods, eggs, caffeine, fried foods, and carbonated drinks.
➛Avoid refined foods, sugars, aspirin, tetracyclines, and meats that may contain nitrates, nitrites and antibiotics.
➛**Eliminate allergy-causing foods, like those with preservatives, flavorings, additives and colorings.** ✿

❧ Effective superfoods:
➛Herbal Answers ALOE VERA juice w. herbs.
➛Crystal Star BIOFLAV. FIBER & C SUPPORT drink.
➛**Lewis Labs BREWER'S YEAST or Bio-Strath original LIQUID YEAST.**
➛**Crystal Star SYSTEMS STRENGTH™.**

Herbal Therapy

✤ Herbal jump start program:
➛Crystal Star ANTI-HST™ capsules as needed to help the body produce normalizing anti-histamines and open air passages.
➛THERADERM™ or HRPS™ capsules to help calm the itchy blistering.
➛**THERADERM™ tea, internally, and topically, patted on blisters to neutralize acids coming out through the skin.**
➛LYSINE/LICORICE™ skin gel.
➛RELAX CAPS™ to rebuild nerves.

✤ To help control the virus: Crystal Star ANTI-VI™ tea 2-4 cups daily, with ECHINACEA extract to flush and clear lymph glands, and high Omega-3 flax oil 3 teasp. daily.

✤ Herbal help for the nerves:
➛Scullcap extract
➛St. John's wort extract
➛Red clover/nettles tea
➛Reishi extract or GINSENG/REISHI extract to boost immunity.

✤ Effective topical applications:
➛**Lemon Balm cream or lemon balm essential aromatherapy oil directly.**
➛BioForce ECHINACEA cream.
➛AloeLife ALOE VERA SKIN gel, or aloe vera/golden seal solution.
➛Calendula extract gel

Supplements

✧ **Quercetin with bromelain as needed for instant action against inflammation. with**
➛**Lysine 1000mg internally, and apply LYSINE PLUS cream to blisters.**
➛Stress B complex 200mgx with extra B₆ 250mg and B₁₂ 2000mcg SL 2x daily.
➛Phosphatidyl choline (PC 55).

✧ **Vitamin C therapy is important in controlling eruptions:** Ascorbate vitamin C or Ester C powder with bioflavs., $\frac{1}{4}$ teasp. every hour in water up to 10,000mg or to bowel tolerance daily during an attack, then reduce to 5000mg daily until blisters heal.

✧ **Emulsified A & D 50,000/1,000IU 2x daily, with Vit. E 400IU 3x daily. Apply E oil directly.** ♂

✧ Effective homeopathics:
➛B & T CALIFLORA gel.
➛B&T SSSTING STOP gel.
➛Arsenicum.

✧ Lane Labs BENE-FIN shark cartilage, 6 daily. ♂

✧ **Cayenne caps, 2 daily to relieve pain, or DLPA 750mg for pain.** ♀

✧ Enzymatic Therapy HERPILYN caps. ♀

Lifestyle Support Therapy

☞ Effective topical applications for pain:
➛Petroleum jelly.
➛Ice compresses.
➛Flax seed compresses.
➛**CAPSAICIN cream or Biochemics PAIN RELEAF eucalyptus lotion.**
➛Epsom salt or oatmeal baths to neutralize acids.

☞ Get early morning sunlight on the body for healing vitamin D.

☞ Cortico-steroid drugs are frequently prescribed for shingles. Remember that corticosteroid drugs taken over a long period of time for shingles, weaken the immune system, allowing future attacks.

☞ Relaxation and tension control techniques are effective. Stress creates an acid body condition, and erodes protective nerve sheathing.

☞ Avoid acetaminophen pain killers such as Tylenol, that can aggravate the blisters.

Common Symptoms: Preliminary symptoms include chills, fever and an uncomfortable feeling before swollen, red skin blisters develop, usually around the upper part of the body; pain radiating along one or several nerves preceding outbreaks; attacks last from 2 days to 2 weeks, leaving irritated nerves even after blisters are gone; accompanied by fever, weakness, chills and nausea.
Common Causes: Food allergies, esp. to dairy products, shellfish, wheat, MSG, food additives and preservatives; reaction to antibiotic drugs like penicillin; over-chlorinated drinking water; stress; adrenal and/or liver exhaustion; histamine reaction; acidosis and HCl depletion; poor circulation and constipation; too many prescription drugs; too much caffeine or hard liquors.

See HERPES, page 397 in this book for more information.

Shock & Trauma Control

Shock is the condition that develops when blood flow is reduced below the levels needed to maintain vital body functions. Obviously, shock and trauma can happen during serious injuries or illnesses when a great deal of blood and other body fluids are lost. But it can also occur during severe infections, allergic reactions (such as anaphylactic shock), and malfunction of the nervous system (such as a severe reaction to a poisonous insect or snake bite).

Every significant injury is accompanied by some degree of shock, because the autonomic nervous system responds to the trauma of injury by altering blood flow. It is usually wise to treat any severely injured person for shock in addition to treating them for the injury. If there is lots of bleeding, major burns, or a head wound, treatment for shock should be very high priority.

✣   Have the person lie down with legs elevated slightly above the head. Don't bend the legs. Loosen clothing at neck, waist and chest. Protect the person from extremes of warmth and cold. If there is a chance of serious or life-threatening injury, do not move the person. Give small sips of fluids only if fully conscious - no solid food.

Get medical care immediately!

The following emergency measures are beneficial until medical help arrives:

• Deva Flowers FIRST AID remedy, or Bach Flowers RESCUE REMEDY; 2-4 drops on the tongue every 5 minutes until breathing normalizes.
• Dilute cayenne extract or powder in water (1-3 teasp. or 2-4 capsules); give with an eyedropper on the back of the tongue if necessary every 10 minutes to restore normal heart rate.
• Consciousness-reviving herbs such as strong incense, camphor, bay oil or musk can be used under the victim's nose as aromatherapy for revival.
• GINGKO BILOBA extract - a few drops in water, given on the tongue helps with stroke and allergic reactions such as dizziness, loss of balance, memory loss or ringing in the ears.
• *Arnica Montana* drops are usually the first homeopathic remedy to give for injury; every half hour to 1 hour on the tongue.
• Bromelain 500mg, or Quercetin with bromelain to control body trauma - open 1-2 capsules in water and give in small sips. Acts like aspirin, anti-inflammatory without stomach upset.
• Hops/valerian tincture, or VALERIAN/WILD LETTUCE; 5-6 drops in water. Give in small sips every 10-15 minutes for calmness.

Common Signs of Shock: Victim is weak, restless and unresponsive, with irregular deep breathing; the skin is cold and pale, and damp to the touch; the pupils are dilated; a rapid weak heartbeat; heart attack or stroke, sometimes with nausea; reduced alertness and consciousness; shallow breathing and confusion.

Common Causes: Major burns; heat prostration; major accident injury; loss of blood; head injury; poisonous insect or snake bite; bone breaks, sprains, and falls.

✣   **Cardiopulmonary resuscitation (CPR)** is an important medical emergency procedure, if a person's heart or breathing has stopped; CPR is essential in order to avoid brain damage, which usually begins in 4 to 6 minutes after cardiopulmonary arrest.

1. Be sure the person is truly unconscious. If tapping, shouting or shaking does not wake him or her, call immediately for help, giving precise directions and telephone number.
2. Lay the victim flat on the back on a straight, firm surface. If you have to roll the person over, roll him or her toward you with one of your hands supporting the neck as you turn.
3. Open the airway so the tongue is not blocking it. If you feel the person may have a neck injury, use your fingers to move the tongue out of the airway. If not, use the following procedure. Place one of your palms across the forehead, and using your other hand, lift the chin up and forward. At the same time, gently push down the forehead. This head and chin-tilt movement lifts the chin but does not fully close the mouth. As the jaw is tilted, the tongue will move out of the mouth. Remove any dentures if present.
4. Check to see if the person is breathing. Opening the airway may be all that is needed. If no signs of breathing are detected, move the tongue out of the airway again.
5. Begin mouth-to-mouth resuscitation. Remove your hand from the forehead and pinch the person's nostrils together. Take a deep breath and place your open mouth over the victim's mouth. Exhale completely into the person's mouth. Take your mouth away, inhale quickly, and repeat four times.
6. Check the pulse on the side of the neck. You should feel the pulse of the carotid artery here. Move your fingers around if you don't feel it at once, and keep trying for 10 to 15 seconds. If there is no pulse begin chest compression to maintain circulation until medical help arrives.
   • Kneel next to the victim's chest, midway between the shoulder and waist.
   • Find the tip of the breastbone, and place your hands one over the other, palms down on this point.
   • Shift your weight forward, and with your elbows locked, bear down on the victim's chest, compressing it 1¹/₂ to 2 inches.
   • Compress the chest for about a half second, then relax for a half second. Compress again, and relax again, etc. Count "1 and 2 and 3 and 4 and 5." Each time you reach 5 you should have done 5 compressions.
   • After you have done 15 compressions, take your hands off the chest and place them on the neck and forehead as before. Pinch the nostrils and administer 2 strong breaths into the victim's mouth.
   • Do 15 more chest compressions. After 4 cycles of chest compressions and mouth-to-mouth breathing, check again for pulse and breathing.
   • If neither pulse nor breathing have returned, resume until medical help arrives, or the victim revives, or you can no longer continue.

Don't give up too soon!

Thanks and credit to EVERYBODY'S GUIDE TO HOMEPATHIC MEDICINES for this section. It is needed for a family reference.

Sinus Problems

Sinus Infections & Sinusitis

The sinuses are thin, resonating air-filled chambers in the cartilage around the nose, on both sides of the forehead, between the nasal passages and the eye sockets and in the cheekbones. When sinus openings are obstructed, mucous and sometimes infected pus collect in these pockets causing pain and swelling. Acute sinusitis is an inflammation of the mucous membranes lining the sinuses. Sinus infections usually originate in the nose and chronic sinusitis often causes nasal polyps and scar tissue. Natural healing methods revolve around relieving the cause of the clogging and inflammation. Suppressive over-the-counter sinus medications can both trigger an infection by not allowing the draining of infective material, and aggravate it by driving the infection deeper into the sinus cavities.

Diet & Superfood Therapy

♋ Go on a short 3 day mucous cleansing liquid diet. (pg. 157).

➥Take a glass of lemon juice and water each morning to thin mucous secretions.

➥Take an onion/garlic, or mucous cleansing broth (pg. 171) each day.

➥Add fresh carrot juice the 1st day.

➥**Add a pineapple/papaya juice, or dilute pineapple juice the 2nd day.**

➥Add a glass of apple juice the 3rd day.

➥Mix fresh grated horseradish root with lemon juice in a spoon. Take and hang over a sink to expel lots of mucous all at once.

➥Then, eat only fresh foods for the rest of the week to cleanse encrusted mucous deposits. Drink 8 glasses of healthy liquids, including broths, herb teas and water.

➥Slowly add whole grains, vegetable protein, and cultured foods to your own tolerance.

➥Avoid heavy starches, red meats, pasteurized dairy products, caffeine and refined sugars for at least 3 months.
🌿

♋ **Effective superfoods:**

➥Beehive Botanicals ROYAL JELLY/ GINSENG drink and capsules.

➥**Crystal Star ZINC SOURCE™ drops in water as a nasal rinse or on back of the tongue.**

➥Sun CHLORELLA to regenerate immunity.

➥AloeLife ALOE JUICE CONCENTRATE 14 TBS. before meals.

Herbal Therapy

➷ **Herbal jump start program:**

➥**Crystal Star ANTI-BIO™ caps and FIRST AID CAPS™ 2-3x daily each for a week. Use Then ALRG™ caps, ALR-HST™ tea, or ALRG/HST™ extract for 1 week.**

➥USNEA extract for long term relief.

➥Apply Tiger Balm or Chinese WHITE FLOWER OIL to sinuses.

➷ **Propolis tincture drops ♂ or high potency royal jelly 2 teasp. daily. ♀**

➷ **Effective herbs to clear sinuses:**

➥Comfrey/fenugreek compresses

➥Fenugreek/thyme tea

➥Ephedra tea as a bronchodilator 🌀

➥Echinacea extract drops 🌀

➥Osha root as an anti-viral

➥Zand DECONGEST HERBAL

➥Lobelia extract

➥Calendula as a nasal wash

➷ Cleanse sinuses with sea salt water: make a solution of $1/4$ teasp. sea salt to 1 cup warm water. Close one nostril and inhale enough solution through other nostril to be able to spit it out your mouth. Repeat daily for 1 month.

➷ **For nasal polyps from sinus infection:**

➥Make a water solution of goldenseal, echinacea and myrrh powders - snuff enough up the nose to thoroughly rinse nasal sinus cavities.

Supplements

➷ **Quercetin with bromelain as a prime anti-inflammatory, at least twice daily. Use Source Naturals ACTIVATED QUERCETIN, or Solaray QBC caps.**

➷ **Vitamin C therapy:** Use ascorbate or Ester C powder with bioflavonoids, $1/4$ teasp. every hour to bowel tolerance daily during acute phase. Also, dissolve vitamin C crystals in water and drip into nose with an eye-dropper.

➥Add Beta carotene 50,000IU and NAC 500mg, each 2x daily.

➥Add zinc picolinate 50mg and zinc lozenges.

➷ **Enzyme therapy: use Prevail SINEASE.**

➷ Nutribiotic GRAPEFRUIT SEED extract diluted as directed - an antibiotic nasal rinse.

➷ Homeopathic remedies:

➥Boiron SINUSITIS tabs.

➥BioForce SINUS RELIEF drops or tabs.

➷ **Nutricology ALIVE & WELL CAPS.**

♌ **CoQ₁₀ 60mg 3x daily to rebuild immunity.**

➷ B complex 100mg with extra B₆ 250mg, pantothenic acid 500mg, and B₁₂ 2000mcg. sublingually 2x daily.

Lifestyle Support Therapy

☞ **Take a hot sauna for 20 minutes daily during acute phase.**

☞ Steam face and head with eucalyptus/ mullein, or a chamomile steam.

➥**Mix 1 teasp. 3% H₂O₂, or several drops of tea tree oil in a vaporizer. Use at night for clear morning sinuses.**

➥Apply a hot ginger compress to sinus areas; or use a hot mullein/lobelia compress. Alternate with cold compresses for best results.

☞ **Acupressure points:**

➥Massage under the big toes for 1 minute every day.

➥Squeeze ends of each finger and thumb hard for 20 seconds daily.

➥**Press your thumb and index finger gently on the top of your nose on either side for 5 seconds. Repeat 3 times.**

☞ Acupuncture is effective for chronic sinusitis.

☞ **Reflexology points:**

sinus points

See COOKING FOR HEALTHY HEALING by Linda Rector Page for a complete diet for respiratory health.

Common Symptoms: *Difficult breathing; pressure headaches and a mucous-clogged head; acute throbbing pain in the upper jaw and forehead; runny nose and inflamed nasal passages; post-nasal drip with yellowish discharge coughed up; sore throat; indigestion because of mucous overload; facial pain and pain behind the eyes; loss of smell and taste; bad breath from low grade infection.*

Common Causes: *A viral or bacterial infection, often triggered by an allergy condition; too many mucous-forming foods, such as pasteurized dairy products and refined sugar; too many salty, fatty foods; poor food combining; lack of green vegetables; constipation and poor circulation; lack of exercise and deep breathing.*

Skin
Health & Beauty

Beautiful skin is more than skin deep. The skin is the body's largest organ of both nourishment and elimination. The skin is the body's emotional state and our hormone balance, and is a sure sign of poor nutrition. (Allergies show up first on the skin.) Skin problems reflect a stressed lifestyle almost immediately. Our skin is the essence of renewable nature...it sloughs off old, dying cells every day, and gives a chance for a new start. Relaxation, nourishment and improved nutrition show quickly in skin health and beauty.

Diet & Superfood Therapy

Great skin starts with a good diet:
- Eat mineral-rich foods: leafy greens, bell peppers, broccoli, sesame and sunflower seeds, fish and sea vegetables.
- Eat cultured foods: yogurt, tofu and kefir.
- Eat cleansing foods: fresh fruit, vegetable and fruit juices, celery, cucumbers.
- Eat vitamin C, E and beta carotene-rich foods: sea foods and fresh vegetables.
- Drink 6 glasses of water every day.
- Drink watermelon juice whenever it is available - rich in natural silica to keep the system flushed and alkaline.
- Eliminate red meats, fried, fatty and fast foods. Reduce caffeine, dairy foods and salty, sugary foods. They show up on skin.

Kitchen cosmetic face lifts: apply, leave on 30 minutes and rinse off.
- Yogurt to balance pH
- Oatmeal to exfoliate
- Egg whites for wrinkles

Make your own AHA wrinkle treatment with a mix of honey and red wine. Smooth on; leave on 20 minutes. Rinse off.

Effective superfoods:
- Crystal Star BIOFLAV, FIBER & C SUPPORT™
- Salute ALOE VERA JUICE with herbs
- Crystal Star SYSTEMS STRENGTH™
- Premier 1 ROYAL JELLY/GINSENG

Herbal Therapy

Herbs are great for skin - packed with absorbable minerals, antioxidants, EFAs and bioflavonoids, to cleanse, hydrate, heal, alkalize, and balance.

Essential fatty acid sources:
- EVENING PRIMROSE OIL caps 4 daily.
- Nature's Secret ULTIMATE OIL 2 daily.
- Rohe 7 BLEND EFA oil, esp. nourishes while cleaning off eye make-up.

- Crystal Star BEAUTIFUL SKIN™ tea; internally and externally (pat on problem spots).
- GREEN TEA CLEANSER™- externally and internally to protect and heal the skin.

Blood cleansing skin health herbs:
- Crystal Star SKIN THERAPY #1™ caps, or PAU d'ARCO-ECHINACEA extract.
- Sage
- Burdock root.

Anti-oxidant herbs for skin:
- Rosemary or Dandelion capsules
- AloeLife ALOE SKIN GEL

Smoothing/hydrating herbs for skin:
- Lavender to reduce puffiness.
- Rose hips tea/lemon juice blend.
- Chamomile tea or CamoCare FACIAL THERAPY.
- Crystal Star SKIN THERAPY #2™ caps.
- Sandlewood or rose essential aromatherapy oils.

Supplements

Vitamins feed the skin, and improve nutrition deficiencies that show up in the skin.

Total skin support:
- Dr. Diamond HERPANACINE caps.
- Biotec AGELESS BEAUTY caps.
- Make a skin vitamin facial once a week: Prick open and squeeze a vit. A & D 25,000IU, and 1 vitamin E 400IU caps. Grind up 1 zinc 30mg tab and 1 PABA 100mg tab. Mix with 2 teasp. wheat germ oil or flax or jojoba oil and smear on face. Let dry and rinse off.

Effective collagen support:
- Flora VEGESIL 3 daily.
- PCOs 150mg. daily.
- Ascorbate vitamin C or Ester C with bioflavonoids, 3000mg daily.
- Jason ESTER C lotion.
- Alacer VITASTIC SPRAY.

Fatty acid liposomes for dry skin:
- High omega 3 flax oil caps 3 daily.
- Vitamin E 800IU daily.
- Vitamin A & D 25,000/1,000, or
- American Biol. emulsified A & E oil.
- American Health PEARL CREME.

Balancers for too oily, shiny skin:
- Matrix Health GENESIS OXY-SPRAY.
- Lavender essential aromatherapy oil
- Zia OIL CONTROL extract.
- Jojoba oil.

Lifestyle Support Therapy

- Use a gentle, balancing mask once a week, like Crystal Star NATURAL CLAY TONING™ mask, Reviva LIGHT SKIN PEEL, or Zia SUPER MOISTURIZING mask. Follow with a blend of aloe vera gel and vitamin E oil.

- **Get adequate rest and sleep.**
- Get 20 minutes of early morning sunlight on the skin for Vitamin D.
- Get regular aerobic exercise to increase circulation and tone.
- Cosmetic acupuncture and acupressure treatments are effective for skin problems..

- **Exfoliant/cleansers for glowing skin:**
- Loofa sponge, ayate cloth, dry skin brush
- Cucumber/papaya skins
- Honey/almond/oatmeal scrub
- Crystal Star LEMON BODY GLOW™

- **Skin detox cleansers and pH balancers:**
- Zia SEA TONIC with aloe
- Crystal Star HOT SEAWEED BATH™.
- Lemon juice to restore acid mantle.
- Olive oil soap.
- Zia FRESH PAPAYA PEEL.
- Jason SUMA moisturizer

- Nourishing make-up remover: Mix in a dark bottle, apricot, avocado, almond and sesame oils; good for all skin types - makes your skin feel wonderful.

See the following pages for more information about skin problems.

Common Symptoms: Unbalanced skin and acid mantle, with sores, spots, cracks, oiliness or dryness, scaling, itching, chapping, redness and rashes.
Common Causes: Emotional stress; poor diet of excess refined foods and sugars; too many saturated fats; caffeine overload; food allergies that cause redness; too high copper levels causing blotching; poor digestion and assimilation; PMS; too much sun; irritating cosmetics; essential fatty acid and bioflavonoid depletion; liver malfunction.

Skin, Aging

Dry & Wrinkling ✦ Age & Liver Spots

Age spots are an external sign of harmful waste accumulation (particularly in the liver, which shows up as sallow skin), and a result of free radical damage in skin cells. Lipofuscin is the age-related skin pigment that oxidizes to actually appear as the brown, age spots. The look of aging skin occurs when collagen becomes hard and crosslinked with neighboring collagen fibers, preventing it from holding water and maintaining elasticity. It collapses on itself, forming a kind of fish net below the surface of the skin, seen as wrinkles. The cause of the crosslinking is free radical formation. Free radicals attack skin cell membranes, collagen and elastin proteins, resulting in wrinkles, dry skin and sagging skin contours.

Diet & Superfood Therapy

♦ Age spots and a yellowish, old skin look are signs that the liver is throwing off metabolic wastes through the skin. Go on a short liver detox cleansing diet (pg. 163) to cleanse the liver of accumulated toxins.

➥Then drink carrot/beet/cucumber juice once a week for the next month to keep the liver clean.

➥The continuing diet should consciously include lots of vegetable proteins, from whole grains, seafoods, sprouts and soy foods; mineral-rich foods, like leafy greens, onions, root and cruciferous vegetables and molasses; and foods rich in beta carotene, vitamin E and C, such as carrots, greens, sea vegetables and broccoli.

➥Make a skin food mix of lecithin granules, wheat germ, brewer's yeast, molasses; take 2 TBS. daily in juice.

➥Drink 8 glasses of water or healthy liquids daily; include a glass of lemon juice and water; apply lemon juice to age spots.

➥Avoid refined sugars, red meats, and caffeine containing foods. They dry out your skin. Avoid rancid nuts and oils.

♦ Effective superfoods:
➥AloeLife aloe vera juice with herbs.
➥Crystal Star BIOFLAV. FIBER & C SUPPORT™.
➥**Lewis Labs Brewer's Yeast or Bio-Strath original LIQUID YEAST.**
➥Crystal Star SYSTEMS STRENGTH™.

Herbal Therapy

❧ **For age spots:**
➥Take high potency Premier One or YS ROYAL JELLY 2 teasp. daily, or Superior BEE SECRETION daily.
➥Zia Cosmetics EVEN SMOOTHER, CITRUS NIGHT TIME REVERSAL and other alpha hydroxy-acid products.
➥Apply chamomile tea or CamoCare CHAMOMILE CONCENTRATE♀.
➥Crystal Star ADR-ACTIVE™ caps for spots and freckling, GINKGO BILOBA extract 3x daily, IODINE POTASSIUM SOURCE™ caps and GINSENG SKIN REPAIR GEL™. ♂
➥Apply Dong Quai extract to spots.

❧ **For anti-wrinkle effects:** Estrogen is a key to tissue building, working with collagen to renew skin elasticity.
Effective phyto-estrogen herbs: Crystal Star EST-AID™ caps and FEM SUPPORT™ extract, sarsaparilla extract, Nature's Life ginseng cream, CamoCare FACIAL THERAPY.

➥ EVENING PRIMROSE OIL caps 4 daily with vit. E 400IU daily esp. for eye skin.

➥ Steam face with a mix of hydrating/aromatherapy herbs: chamomile flowers, eucalyptus leaves, rosemary and nettles.
➥Apply a facial mix: 1 teasp. each: vegetable glycerine, rosewater, witch hazel with 3 TBS. honey. Leave on 15-20 minutes.

Supplements

❧ **For age spots:** antioxidants help prevent the accumulation of lipofuscin.
➥Apply Matrix GENESIS OXY-SPRAY gel to wrinkles or age spots before bed. Results usually show in 1 to 3 months.
➥Vitamin E 400IU; prick oil caps and apply.
➥Reviva BROWN SPOT REMOVER.
➥Biotec AGELESS BEAUTY 4 daily to metabolize rancid fats and destroy free radicals.
➥High Omega-3 flax oil 3x daily.
➥PABA 100mg/pantothenic acid 1000mg.
➥Ascorbate vitamin C with bioflavonoids 3000mg daily.
➥Beta carotene A 100,000IU and vitamin D 400IU daily to clear the liver.
➥Nature's Secret ULTIMATE B with ULTIMATE OIL caps for EFAs, or EVENING PRIMROSE OIL 2-4 daily. ♂

❧ **Antioxidants for anti-wrinkle effects:**
Martin Pycnogenol Moisturizer.
➥Zia PAPAYA PEEL and aromatherapy treatment oils.
➥Apply Transitions PRO-GEST CREAM several times daily for 3 months. ♀
➥Apply 1 teasp. aloe vera gel mixed with 1 pricked vitamin E 400IU capsule.
➥**High potency royal jelly ampules.**
➥Revivia COLLAGEN AMPULES.
➥Jason PERFECT SOLUTIONS C cream.
➥Body Essentials SILICA gel.
➥**AloeLife ALOE SKIN GEL.** ♂

Lifestyle Support Therapy

Avoid all forms of tobacco. Tar and nicotine deprive skin of oxygen, causing shriveling and wrinkling.

☞ Use sunscreen regularly - SPF 15 or greater. Even minimal sun exposure is enough to sustain spots. **Sunscreens help prevent age spots from darkening.**

☞ **For facial rejuvenation:**
➥Get plenty of fresh air; exercise at least three times a week.
➥Cosmetic acupuncture treatments.
➥A gentle balancing mask once a week, such as Crystal Star CLAY TONING MASK.
➥Softening skin massages with jojoba oil, sesame oil, wheat germ oil, vitamin E oil, or AloeLife ALOE SKIN gel.
➥Anti-wrinkle food facials, like rubbing the insides of fresh papaya skins on the face, or patting on a mix of whipped egg white and cream. Let dry 20 minutes. Rinse off.
➥Facial exercises for elasticity and tone.
➥Massage therapy to release toxins from lymph glands and tone facial muscles.

☞ **Reflexology:** press point on stomach just above the navel. Stroke downward in the area of the liver under the right breast.

☞ **Reflexology point:**

liver

See the following pages for more information on other skin problems.

Common Symptoms: *Brown mottled spots on the hands, neck and face. Sallow, old-looking skin; dry skin with evident lines and wrinkles.*

Common Causes: *Free radical damage caused by smog and environmental pollutants, too much sun exposure, especially with a thinned ozone layer; stress, poor diet, liver malfunction and exhaustion; skin dehydration often caused by hormone (estrogen depletion); too much tobacco, fried foods, caffeine, and alcohol; broken capillaries; weak vein walls; long term use of hair colors and permanents; some birth control pills; lack of exercise; poor food assimilation and digestion, especially of saturated or rancid fats.*

Skin Infections

Dermatitis ❧ Inflamed Itches & Rashes ❧ Ulcerations

Dermatitis is an external skin condition caused by a systemic reaction to an allergen - usually in cosmetics, jewelry metals, drugs or topical medications. It can also be the body's reaction to emotional stress, or to a severe deficiency of essential fatty acids. Its systemic nature means that it can and does spread, and can become quite severe. Inflamed skin with itch and rash symptoms can come from a wide variety of causes, ranging from systemic to emotional stress, from food allergies to an infective reaction to cosmetics. Investigate the cause of your symptoms thoroughly before you attempt treatment to get best results.

Diet & Superfood Therapy

Rashes are often symptoms of food allergy, avoid common allergens, such as milk and wheat products, eggs, meats (that usually have nitrates), refined foods, sugar and fried foods.

❧ Go on a short 3 day juice cleanse (page 157) to clear acid waste from the system. Drink lemon water in the morning to neutralize acids if the condition is chronic body imbalance.

❧ Then eat a diet full of leafy greens, and other mineral-rich foods, such as sea vegetables to rebuild healthy tissue and good adrenal function.

❧ Use poly or mono-unsaturated oils. Reduce both dietary fats and total calories.

❧ Eat cultured foods frequently for healthy G.I. flora.

❧ Avoid fried foods, red meats, caffeine, chocolate, pasteurized dairy products, and acid-forming refined carbohydrates.

❧ Make a skin mix of ¼ cup each: wheat germ, molasses and brewers yeast; take 2 TBS. daily.

❧ Superfoods are very important:
➼Crystal Star BIOFLAV., FIBER & C SUPPORT™ drink.
➼Green Foods BETA CARROT and WHEAT GERM concentrates for liver support.
➼George's high sulphur ALOE juice.
➼Solgar WHEY TO GO protein drink.

Herbal Therapy

❧ Jump start herbal program:
Crystal Star ANTI-BIO™ gel, especially if skin is infected.
➼BEAUTIFUL SKIN TEA™ - apply as a wash to neutralize acids coming out through the skin; apply BEAUTIFUL SKIN™ gel to a minor rash.
➼ANTI-HST™ capsules, 4-6 daily to relieve a typical histamine weal-type rash. Very effective.
➼Solaray turmeric (curcumin) extract caps or THERADERM™ or BEAUTIFUL SKIN™ capsules as an anti-inflammatory.
➼SILICA SOURCE™-collagen formation.
➼GINKGO BILOBA extract 3-4x daily with Suma caps 3-4 daily. ♀

❧ Essential fatty acids for skin:
➼Evening primrose oil 4 daily
➼Omega-3 flax oil 2 teasp. daily
➼Nature's Secret ULTIMATE OIL ♀

❧ Apply and drink HERBAL ITCH TEA: dandelion root, burdock root, echinacea root, kelp, yellow dock root, chamomile.

❧ Effective herbal healing applications:
➼Aloe vera gel or AloeLife ALOE SKIN GEL and mix with goldenseal powder.
➼Beehive Botanicals DERMA CREAM.
➼St. John's wort oil esp. if infected.
➼Chamomile tea or CamoCare ointment or concentrate.

Supplements

➼ Stress B Complex 100mg 2x daily with extra B₆ 100mg and extra Biotin 600mcg.

➼ Vitamin C therapy: Ester C or ascorbate C powder; mix with water to a solution. Apply to area, and take 1 teasp. every hour for collagen/connective tissue growth.

➼ Flora VEGESIL for healthy new growth.

Effective natural applications:
➼Nutribiotic GRAPEFRUIT SEED extract. Mix 1 to 4 drops in 5 oz. water and apply directly, or use the spray.
➼Apply A, D & E oil, and take emulsified A & D or A & E oil caps. Apply wheat germ oil.
➼Enzyme Therapy DERMA-KLEAR skin treatment cream.

➼ Natural anti-inflammatories:
➼Solaray Quercetin w. bromelain 2 daily.
➼Nutricology GERMANIUM 150mg.

➼ Zinc 50mg. 2x daily. ♂

➼ Beta carotene 100,000IU daily.

➼ Country Life MAXIMUM SKIN CARE.

➼ Probiotics for system pH balance:
➼Prof. Nutrition Dr. DOPHILUS
➼Solaray PANCREATIN 1300mg. ♂

Lifestyle Support Therapy

❧ Get early morning sunlight on the skin every day possible for healing vitamin D.

❧ Avoid detergents on the skin. Use mild castile soap. Avoid perfumed cosmetics.

❧ Effective applications:
➼B & T CALIFLORA gel
➼Body Essentials SILICA GEL
➼Calendula gel, or NatureWorks MARIGOLD OINTMENT, esp. for ulcerations
➼Crystal Star LYSINE/LICORICE™ gel
➼Centipede KITTY'S OXY-GEL
➼Am. Biologics DIOXYCHLOR.
➼Mix lavender essential oil and aloe vera gel and apply
➼Fresh comfrey leaf compresses
➼Tea tree oil if fungus is the cause
➼Martin PYCNOGENOL GEL
➼Aubrey Org. COLLAGEN therapy cream

❧ Zia ALOE-CITRUS WASH, and PAPAYA PEEL to smooth skin after inflammation is gone.

❧ Skin cross-section:

Common Symptoms: Inflamed dry, thickened skin patches; oozing skin blisters; scaly, lumpy skin; itching skin. Tingling, unpleasant skin prickling; redness, rash; scaling and bumps on the skin.
Common Causes: EFA deficiency; allergic skin reaction to cosmetics, acid-forming foods like dairy products, pleasure or prescription drugs, or topical medications; emotional stress; poor liver activity resulting in poor metabolism. Liver malfunction or exhaustion; allergic reaction; stress and anxiety; detergents; over-acid system; drug after-effects and side-effects; poor diet with too many refined and chemical foods.

See also LIVER MALFUNCTION, ECZEMA, PSORIASIS and ACNE/BLEMISHES pages in this book for more information.

Skin, Damaged
Scars ❀ Sunburn ❀ Stretch Marks

For every sunburn you get that blisters, you double your risk of skin cancer. Even on a cloudy day, 80% of the sun's harmful UV rays come through. Sun damage is cumulative over a lifetime. Moderation is the key. Sunlight can help you avoid breast and prostate cancer (new research shows that a lack of protective vitamin D provided by sunlight may be involved). People who get almost no sun exposure are at higher risk for melanoma than those who get regular, moderate early morning sunshine. Practice good sun sense so that you don't fry now and pay later.

Diet & Superfood Therapy

☘ Have a veggie drink 3x a week during healing stage. (pg. 168 or see below). Eat a high vegetable protein diet for faster healing. Include plenty of whole grains, sprouts, tofu, and a protein drink every morning, (see below).

❈Make a healing skin mix of brewer's yeast, wheat germ, lecithin granules; take 2 TBS. daily. ♂

❈Drink 6-8 glasses of mineral water daily to rehydrate from within.

☘ **Take electrolytes for sunburn healing and skin fluid replacement:**
Alacer EMERGEN-C.
❈Potassium broth (pg. 167).
❈Crystal Star SYSTEMS STRENGTH™.
❈Knudsen's ELECTROLYTE drink. ♀

☘ Apply yogurt, honey, black tea, or vinegar to burned areas. Apply grated apple to burned eyelids for immediate relief. ♂

☘ **Effective superfoods:**
❈Crystal Star ENERGY GREEN™ drink. ♂
❈Nutricology PRO-GREENS with flax oil.
❈AloeLife ALOE GOLD juice.
❈Beehive Botanicals or Y.S. GINSENG/ROYAL JELLY. Take and also apply.

Herbal Therapy

☘ **Herbal jump start program:**
Crystal Star GINSENG SKIN REPAIR GEL with vitamin C™ for 2 to 3 months, especially for burned or scarred skin.
with
❈**AloeLife ALOE SKIN gel and EVENING PRIMROSE oil 4 daily for EFAs/healing.**
❈SILICA SOURCE™ drops for scarring.

☘ **Effective herbal topicals for scarring:**
❈Gotu kola extract capsules 4 daily.
❈Aloe vera or calendula gel
❈B&T *CALIFLORA* gel
❈Solaray CENTELLA ASIATICA.
❈BioForce *ECHINACEA* cream

☘ **Effective herbal topicals for sunburns:**
❈CamoCare CHAMOMILE OINTMENT
❈Beehive Botanicals PROPOLIS & HONEY
❈Tea tree oil
❈Green clay poultice
❈Calendula gel
❈A wheat germ oil, vitamin E oil, comfrey leaf and honey poultice (good for stretch marks, too).

☘ **Anti-oxidant herbs for free-radical damage:**
❈Rosemary
❈GINKGO BILOBA

☘ Phyto-estrogen herbs like dong quai, vitex, black cohosh help stimulate better estrogen supply for the skin healing.

Supplements

Prevention is the key. If your tissues are loaded with carotene A, vitamin C, E and B complex, whether from foods or supplements, your skin stands much less chance of being damaged by the sun.

☘ **Heal the skin with minerals:**
❈Mezotrace SEA MINERAL COMPLEX.
❈Flora VEGE-SIL 4 daily; apply Body Essentials SILICA GEL. Silicon healing treatments usually take from 3 to 4 months, depending on severity of the scar. ♀
❈Nutricology GERMANIUM 150mg for wound healing, for at least a month.
❈Zinc 50mg daily; apply zinc oxide cream. ♂

☘ **Anti-oxidants protect skin:**
❈Beta or marine carotene 100,000IU.
❈PCOs 50mg, 3x daily; and/or apply Martin PYCNOGENOL CREAM. ♀
❈Vitamin C therapy, for collagen production and connective tissue growth: ascorbate vitamin C with bioflavonoids 1/4 teasp. in water every hour during acute stage; pat a C solution on burned areas.
❈Tyrosine 500mg 2x daily - a tan activator and to improve the skin's resistance.
❈Vitamin E 400IU daily internally; prick a capsule and apply externally, too.
❈A & D oil capsules. Take 25-50,000IU internally daily. Prick a capsule and apply directly 2-3x daily.
❈B Complex 100mg daily with extra PABA caps 1000mg. and PABA cream. ♀

Lifestyle Support Therapy

☘ **Sun sense skin burn prevention:**
❈Minimize exposure to mid-day sun.
❈Wear sunglasses with 100% UV filters.
❈Use a sunscreen with SPF 15 or more. Make sure it contains Vitamin E.
❈Wear a lip balm with sunscreen.
❈Drink plenty of water before, after and during exposure to replenish and moisturize your skin from within.
❈Avoid photo-sensitive drugs: antibiotics, diuretics, hypoglycemia drugs, retinoic acid cosmetics, soaps w. hexa-chlorophene, and Phenergan in creams. Check labels.
❈**For sun damage** take a cool bath immediately (no soap or hot water); apply cold compresses.
❈Take an electrolyte drink, or a little salty water. No alcoholic beverages - they dehydrate. ♂

☘ **For scars:** Massage the scar thoroughly when rubbing in topical applications, to bring up healthy circulation and skin tone.
❈**Effective applications for scars:**
❈Home Health SCAR-GO.
❈Mtn. Ocean MOTHER'S BLEND oil.
❈Aubrey ROSA MOSQUETA creme.
❈**Centipede KITTY'S OXY-GEL.**
❈Sesame oil, wheat germ oil or avocado oil. Eat avocados for skin elasticity.

☘ **For stretch marks: Massage aloe vera gel mixed with vitamin E oil on stomach. Some women have had success with AHAs.**

See also BURNS page in this book for more information.

Common Symptoms: *Non-healing or slow healing skin wounds, often with continuing redness, roughness, and irregular weals. Sunburned, dehydrated skin; over-reaction to heat and sun exposure; loss of skin elasticity; headache; numbness; high blood pressure and/or rapid pulse; stretch marks from post-pregnancy stretching or serious weight-loss dieting.*

Common Causes and High Risk Factors: *Having had frequent sunburns as a child; living at high altitude; being on immuno-suppressive therapy; heavy use of sun lamps or a tanning bed; having light-colored eyes and hair, fair or freckled skin; moving from a northern climate to the south; working all day outdoors. Protein, vitamin A & D deficiency, zinc and other mineral deficiency.*

Therapy For Other Skin Problems

YOUR SKIN HEALS FROM THE INSIDE OUT. DON'T FORGET THE IMPORTANCE OF DIET AND NUTRITION TO SKIN REGENERATION.

❧ **WHITE HARD BUMPS ON THE UPPER ARMS & CHEST:** Emulsified vitamin A 25,000IU 2 daily, zinc picolinate 50mg daily, and Ester C 550mg with bioflavonoids and rutin 2-3 daily. Wash with diluted pineapple juice and take bromelain 750mg twice daily. Use a dry skin brush or an ayate cloth, and brush the areas morning and night until the skin is pink from increased circulation. This gives your skin oxygen, sloughs off dead cells and speeds up cell renewal. Apply AloeLife ALOE SKIN GEL to the areas.

❧ **VITILIGO (leukoderma)** - *a genetic immune system disorder causing depigmentation of the skin.* Some effectiveness has been shown when treated as for radiation poisoning (see that page in this book). The newest treatment is phenylalanine 1000mg one hour before exposure to UV light. Other good reports come from PABA 1000mg with 2 TBS. molasses daily as an iron source, pantothenic acid 1000mg; magnesium 1500mg daily; Solaray TURMERIC capsules 4 daily; vitamin C 3-5000mg daily with bioflavonoids; Flora VEGE-SIL tabs; Biotec AGELESS BEAUTY capsules 6 daily; Crystal Star IODINE SOURCE™ and ADRN™ extracts to address glandular deficiencies. EVENING PRIMROSE oil caps 6 daily, with egg yolk lecithin and GINKGO BILOBA extract. Calendula gel is an effective topical. Beware of long use of cortico-steroids given for vitiligo. There is some repigmentation, but higher risk of skin cancer.

❧ **ULCERATIONS** - Keep the diet simple and alkaline during healing. Add more fresh fruits and vegetables. Consciously add vegetable protein sources for faster healing - from whole grains, soy foods, sea foods and cultured foods. Include beta carotene-rich foods for both healing and prevention, from carrots, sweet potatoes, yellow-orange vegetables and sea vegetables. Include vitamin C-rich foods for collagen and interstitial tissue health. Include silicon-rich foods from vegetables, whole grains and seafoods to build healthy connective skin tissue. Take a skin healing mix of 1 teasp. each, wheat germ oil and brewer's yeast in a glass of aloe vera juice 2x daily. Drink 6-8 glasses of bottled water or other healthy liquids like juices and herbal teas daily to keep acid wastes flushed. Avoid saturated fats, sugars, caffeine and caffeine-containing foods.

Effective applications: hot comfrey compresses, dry mustard plaster. tea tree oil, propolis tincture, green clay poultice, B & T *CALIFLORA* gel. Apply Centipede Kitty's OXY-GEL to affected area, and on soles of feet; usually a noticeable change in 3 weeks. Make a paste of aloe vera gel and goldenseal powder and apply frequently. Take Bromelain 500mg with Omega-3 flax oil 3x daily. Take Crystal Star BEAUTIFUL SKIN™ caps and apply **Crystal Star GINSENG SKIN REPAIR GEL™, or ANTI-BIO™ gel** if there is infection. Make a lesion healing tea: Steep burdock and dandelion root and add 15 drops per cup of ECHINACEA EXTRACT; take 3 cups daily. For open ulcerations, use calendula gel, PABA 500-1000mg, Enzymatic Therapy DERMA-KLEAR cream, and Flora VEGE-SIL for connective tissue regrowth.

❧ **SCLERODERMA** - *a runaway healing process where the body inexplicably begins and continues to produce too much collagen and connective tissue, replacing normal cell structure, and causing scar tissue to build up on skin, lungs and circulatory organs. It begins with discolored skin, followed by lesions and swelling.* Take regular baths with aloe vera gel added to the water. Take **gotu kola (centella asiatica) extract** capsules for decreased skin hardening. Apply calendula gel to lesions and take bromelain 750mg 2x daily to reduce swelling. Get regular aerobic exercise to increase perspiration, stimulate metabolism, and rid the body of carbon dioxide build-up. Stop smoking and avoid secondary smoke. Add antioxidants like CoQ₁₀ 60mg 3x daily, beta carotene 25,000IU 4x daily, vitamin C with bioflavonoids, 5000mg daily, glutathione 50mg daily, PCOs from grapeseed or white pine 50mg 4x daily, B₆ 250mg daily, and zinc 30mg daily. Keep nutrition at the highest possible level with a protein drink like Nutricology PRO-GREENS with flax oil every day. Drink fresh carrot juice at least twice a week.

❧ **STRAWBERRIES & EXCESS PIGMENTATION:** Reduce too high copper levels by adding more zinc and iron-rich foods. Reduce clogging waste with a gentle herbal laxative. Apply B&T *CALIFLORA* ointment, take pantothenic acid 100mg and B₆ 500mg.

❧ **SKIN PROTECTION FROM ENVIRONMENTAL POLLUTANTS:** Nutricology GERMANIUM 150mg, suma root capsules 3-4 daily, **Biotec AGELESS BEAUTY capsules 6 daily,** Vitamin E with selenium 400IU, Twin Lab EGG YOLK LECITHIN capsules, ginkgo biloba extract, cosmetics and skin care products with azuline.

❧ **ROSACEA** - *chronic red skin spots on the face, neck and chest:* Generally caused by liver malfunction or a mineral deficiency. Keep your diet sugar-free. Reduce fats and concentrated proteins like red meats. Add Omega-3 rich flax oil in your salad dressings. Take EVENING PRIMROSE oil caps or Nature's Secret ULTIMATE OIL as a source of EFAs. Add B complex vitamins 100mg daily. Take anti-oxidants like beta carotene 100,000IU daily, vitamin E 400IU with selenium 200mcg, or American Biologics emulsified vitamin A & E. Take Crystal Star MINERAL SPECTRUM™ caps 2 daily, IODINE SOURCE™ caps for thyroid stimulation and minerals, or Mezotrace SEA MINERAL complex tabs. Apply GRAPEFRUIT SEED extract and also take GRAPEFRUIT SEED extract capsules internally as an effective antibiotic treatment for the skin. Add an herb combination such as Crystal Star THERADERM™ caps or BEAUTIFUL SKIN™ tea. Drink pau d'arco tea 3 to 4 cups daily as an anti-infective, or take as PAU d' ARCO/ECHINACEA extract to flush fats from the blood stream. Take **Dr. Diamond HERPANACINE** capsules as directed.

Smoking, How To Stop
Second-Hand Smoke * Smokeless Tobacco

Each cigarette takes 8 minutes off your life; a pack a day takes 1 month off your life each year; 2 packs a day, takes 12-15 years off your life. Cigarettes have over 4000 known poisons, any of which can kill in high enough doses. One drop of pure nicotinic acid can kill a man. Depending on the age that you quit, your life expectancy can increase from 2-5 years. Second-hand or passive smoke, and chewing tobacco are just as dangerous, especially for women. Passive smoke reduces fertility, successful pregnancies, and normal birth weight babies. It increases the instance of cervical, uterine and lung cancer, heart disease and osteoporosis in women and men. Don't be discouraged. Quitting is hard work, but it gets easier every day, as the body loses dependence on nicotine.

Diet & Superfood Therapy

There must be a lifestyle and diet change for permanent success against smoking.

❧ Start with a 3 day liquid cleansing diet (pg. 157), with fresh fruit and vegetable juices and miso soup to neutralize and clear the blood of nicotinic acid and to fortify blood sugar. Include lots of vegetable proteins. Add magnesium-rich foods like dark leafy veggies, whole grains, seafoods, sea vegetables and legumes.

⁎Then, follow with a fresh foods only diet for the rest of the week, with carrot juices, plenty of carrots and celery, leafy green salads, and lots of citrus fruits to promote body alkalinity. (pH 7 and above readings show decreased desire for tobacco.)

⁎Avoid junk foods and sugar that aggravate cravings. Avoid oxalic acid-forming foods like chocolate and cooked spinach or rutabaga that bind up magnesium in the body.

❧ Take a cup of green tea or Crystal Star **GREEN TEA CLEANSER™ daily to reduce body carcinogens.** ☙

❧ Effective superfoods:
⁎New Moon GINGER WONDER syrup.
⁎Crystal Star AMINO ZYME™ caps to control craving/weight gain after quitting.
⁎Nutricology PRO-GREENS with flax seed oil for EFAs.

Herbal Therapy

❧ **Jump start herbal program:**
Crystal Star NIC-STOP™ tea, with lobelia, 2 cups taken over the day in sips to keep tissues flooded with elements that discourage the taste for nicotine. (Add a pinch of ginger, or New Moon GINGER WONDER syrup for best results.)

⁎RELAX CAPS™ or GINSENG 6 SUPER™ caps to rebuild nervous system, WITHDRAWAL SUPPORT™ caps to calm tension. DEEP BREATHING™ tea to keep lungs clear.
⁎GINSENG/LICORICE ELIXIR™, an antioxidant that also helps blood sugar balance.

❧ Solaray TURMERIC caps to neutralize cancer-causing compounds.

❧ **Make a tobacco addiction-fighting tea to lessen desire, support nervous system, strengthen adrenals, and cleanse lungs and bronchi. One part each: Oat straw and seed, lobelia seed and tops, licorice, calamus root, sassafras.**

❧ Effective herbal aids:
⁎Echinacea to flush the lymph system.
⁎VALERIAN/WILD LETTUCE to calm.
⁎**Lobelia or oats/scullcap tea to reduce the craving.**

⁎Ephedra tea to help cleanse the lungs
⁎EVENING PRIMROSE for essential EFAs.
⁎Crystal Star ADRN-ACTIVE™ extract to support exhausted adrenals.

Supplements

❧ Enzymatic Therapy NICO-STOP for at least 2 months.

⁎Magnesium 400mg 2x daily. and B COMPLEX 100mg daily. ♀

❧ Homeopathic Natra-Bio *SMOKING WITHDRAWAL RELIEF.*

❧ **Anti-oxidants are a key lung protector:**
⁎Twin Labs LYCOPENE 10mg for lungs.
⁎Ascorbate vitamin C powder with bioflavonoids, $1/2$ teasp. in water every hour to bowel tolerance during acute stages of withdrawal, then reduce to 5000mg daily.
⁎Glutathione 50mg daily for secondary smoke.
⁎Nutricology GERMANIUM 150mg.
⁎CoQ 10 60mg 3x daily.

❧ **For nico-toxicity, take each 2x daily:**
1 Cysteine capsule
1 Glutamine capsule
2 Vitamin C 1000mg. tablets
2 EVENING PRIMROSE OIL capsules
10 Sun CHLORELLA tabs

❧ **Niacin therapy:** 500-1000mg daily, with beta-carotene 100,000IU daily. ♂

❧ Brain nourishers to overcome nicotine stimulation:
⁎Phosphatidyl choline
⁎Choline/inositol ♂

Lifestyle Support Therapy

☞ Do deep breathing exercises for more body oxygen whenever you feel the urge for tobacco until the desire decreases - about 4 minutes.

⁎To help curb craving for chewing tobacco, chew licorice root sticks, calamus root or cloves for oral gratification.

☞ **Information you may not know about smoking:**

⁎If your parents smoke, you may inherit a smoking addiction even before birth. Fetuses absorb nicotine, CO_2 and tar in the womb (some even pull away from the uterine wall), and second-hand smoke from **both** parents. The **family** of a heavy smoker experiences lung damage and lung cancer risk equal to smoking 1 to 10 cigarettes a day!

⁎Smokers are more prone to heartburn and ulcers. Smoking inhibits a natural, protective bicarbonate secretion in the small intestine that neutralizes acid.

⁎Smoking is a big contributor to high blood pressure because smoke narrows arteries. Nicotine revs up heartbeat; when the body calls for more oxygen-laden blood the arteries can't deliver it. Slow suicide.

Common Symptoms: *Chronic bronchitis; constant hacking cough; difficult and shortness of breath; lung and respiratory depletion and infection; emphysema and dry lungs; often eventual lung cancer and other degenerative diseases; adrenal exhaustion and fatigue; poor circulation affecting vision; high blood pressure; premature aging and wrinkled, dehydrated skin with poor color and elasticity (smoke decreases blood flow to the skin); stomach ulcers; osteoporosis; low immunity; etc., etc., etc. The cost of smoking-related illness is over 50 billion dollars today in medical bills alone.*

Common Causes: *System stress and disease from nicotine poisoning; emotional insecurity; hypoglycemia; dietary deficiencies; nicotine addiction.*

See POISONING, HEAVY METAL page in this book for more information.

Snake Bite
Poisonous Spider Bites ✦ Scorpions

Get emergency medical help immediately! Time is critical. The methods below are to be used only until this help arrives. There is anti-venin for snake bites, but it is often snake-specific and carries the risk of anaphylactic shock. There is anti-venin for black widow spiders, but none for brown recluse spiders. Shock and convulsions may occur.

Diet & Superfood Therapy

❧ **For snake bite:** wash bite with soap and water. No ice compresses for snake bite.
➻Give the victim only small sips of water. No alcoholic drinks. The poison will spread faster.
➻Make a tobacco and saliva poultice and apply to bite.
➻Plant onions and garlic around the house to keep snakes away.

❧ **Superfoods to rebuild after the bite:**
➻Sun CHLORELLA 2 packets daily.
➻Crystal Star SYSTEMS STRENGTH™ for iodine/potassium therapy.
➻Nutricology PRO-GREENS with flax seed oil.
➻Aloe vera juice to detoxify.

Herbal Therapy

In a life-threatening situation, where the victim may go into cardiac arrest, cayenne may save the person's life.

❧ Cayenne, 2 capsules or 8-10 drops of cayenne extract in warm water, as a shock preventive to strengthen the heart. Echinacea capsules or tea to flush poisons from the lymph glands.
➻Take Crystal Star ANTI-HST™ caps to help calm a histamine reaction.

❧ Take yellow dock tea with echinacea extract every hour until swelling goes down.

❧ **Effective applications:**
➻Black cohosh solution as an antidote to venom.
-Aloe/comfrey salve
-Aloe vera gel
-Comfrey tea
-Calendula gel or lotion
-Chinese WHITE FLOWER OIL

❧ **Effective compresses and poultices:**
➻Plantain
➻Rue
➻Fresh comfrey leaf
➻Slippery elm

Supplements

In a life-threatening situation, where the victim may go into shock or convulsions, massive doses of vitamin C may save the person's life.

❧ Calcium ascorbate vitamin C powder, ¼ teasp. in water every 15 minutes as a detoxifier during acute reaction phase.

❧ Vitamin E 400IU. Take internally; prick capsule and apply locally.

❧ Vitamin A & D 25,000IU - take internally; prick capsule and apply locally.

❧ **After the bite crisis has passed, and after poison is out of the body:**
➻Use Health Papers CETA CLEANSE oral chelation therapy with EDTA to detoxify the system.
➻Niacin therapy: up to 500mg daily, to dilate and tone blood vessels.

Lifestyle Support Therapy

☞ Take precautions if you are going on a camping trip, tropical hike, or working around snake havens like sheds and outhouses. Wear heavy boots and leggings that fangs can't penetrate.
➻Buy a snake bite kit before you go on any trip where you can'treach medical help in a reasonable time. Know what poisonous snakes are native to your area. If you can't identify a snake, treat it as if it is poisonous.
➻Only 2 spiders in the U.S. are poisonous - the black widow and the brown recluse.

☞ Keep victim still and calm. Immobilize the bite area and keep it lower than the heart.
➻Until medical help arrives, put a constricting band 2 to 4" above the bite. Do not cut off circulation. Move band up if swelling reaches it.
➻If you can't get to medical help within 15 minutes, and swelling is rapid and pain severe, make a small cut with a sharp knife up and down, not across, through each fang mark. Use suction by mouth or a suction cup for at least 30 minutes, repeatedly. Spit out blood. Rinse mouth immediately.

☞ Pouring alcohol on a bite is useless and may speed up the venom; ice packs are no good either because they may damage tissue.

See SHOCK & TRAUMA page in this book for more emergency information. (pg. 401)

Common Symptoms: Snake bite: slow upward spreading red lines as poison moves toward the heart, swelling, sometimes severe pain and nausea, sweating, increased heartbeat, dizziness, weakness and fainting, breathing difficulty. **Black widow bite:** severe chest and abdominal pain, labored breathing, headache, swollen face, fever, chills, profuse sweating and shock. **Brown recluse bite:** within a few days to a week after the bite, a small red, raised blister will form. then an ulcer that lasts for weeks or even months. There is general weakness, nausea, hive breakouts and kidney problems. California scorpions are not poisonous unless you are allergic. Texas/Southwest scorpions are poisonous. Get medical help.

Sore Throat • Strep Throat

Swollen Glands ✲ Laryngitis ✲ Hoarseness

Here are the differences between a strep throat and a sore throat irritation from a cold: Onset of a strep throat is rapid; a cold is slow. Throat is very sore with strep throat; not so sore with a cold. You have a fever and aches with strep throat; mild achiness with a cold. You have swollen, tender lymph nodes with strep throat; not with a cold. There are usually complications with strep throat, like streptococcal pneumonia or middle ear infections; sinusitis with a cold. Anti-biotics work for strep throat; not usually for a cold. Hoarseness, the result of inflammation of the vocal chords, is typically the result of a virus, or extensive yelling. Laryngitis, raspy, breathy voice, is often due to voice fatigue from a cold.

Diet & Superfood Therapy

☙ Go on a short 24 hr. liquid cleansing diet (pg. 158), or a 3 day mucous cleansing diet (pg. 162). Take citrus juices throughout the day.
❋Take lemon juice and honey in water, and a potassium broth (pg. 167) daily.
❋Then eat mainly fresh foods during healing. Have plenty of leafy greens.
❋Take Organic Gourmet NUTRITIONAL YEAST or miso broth at night before retiring.◯✢
❋Take garlic syrup. Soak a chopped garlic bulb in 1 pt. honey and water overnight; take a teasp. every hour.
❋Avoid all dairy foods, sugary, fried and fatty foods during healing.

☙ **Effective gargles:** Lemon juice and brandy, or black tea, or **pinches of cayenne, lemon juice and sea salt in water.**

☙ **For laryngitis and hoarseness:**
❋One teasp. **each:** cider vinegar and honey in water every hour until relief.
❋**Gargles:** Lemon juice and water, liquid chlorophyll in water.
☙

☙ **Effective superfoods:**
❋**New Moon GINGER WONDER syrup.**
❋**Crystal Star ZINC SOURCE™ drops (apply directly on throat).**
❋AloeLife ALOE GOLD juice.
❋Wakunaga KYO-GREEN drink.

Herbal Therapy

☙ **Jump start herbal program:**
Crystal Star ANTI-BIO™, ANTI-VI™ or FIRST AID CAPS™ depending on cause, 6 daily.
❋**GINSENG-LICORICE ELIXIR™ as needed.**
❋**COFEX™ tea** as needed. ⊛
❋**ECHINACEA extract as needed.**
❋**Garlic capsules 8 daily.**

☙ Lane Labs BENE-FIN SHARK CARTILAGE caps as an anti-strep factor.

☙ BioForce SANTASAPINA throat drops, or SANTASAPINA syrup. ⊛

☙ **Effective gargles (about every ¹/₂ hr.):**
❋**Goldenseal/myrrh solution.** ⊛
❋Fenugreek/honey in water.
❋Liquid chlorophyll ¹/₂ teasp. in water
❋Myrrh tincture, ¹/₂ teasp. in water. ◯+
❋Sage tea or white oak bark tea. ◯+

☙ **Effective herbal lozenges:**
❋Zand HERBAL INSURE lozenges
❋Olbas lozenges ◯+
❋Wild cherry lozenges

☙ **For laryngitis and hoarseness:**
❋Licorice root
❋**Beehive Bot. PROPOLIS THROAT SPRAY.** ◯+
❋Gargle tea tree oil, 3 drops in water.
❋**CamoCare CHAMOMILE MENTHOL throat spray and gargle.**

Supplements

☙ **For sore throat:**
❋**Zinc gluconate or propolis lozenges every few hours as needed.**
❋**Alacer EMERGEN-C every few hours. Hold in the mouth as long as possible for best absorption, and/or Vitamin C chewable 500mg every hour during acute stages.**
❋**Nutribiotic GRAPEFRUIT SEED extract in water, or capsules for infection.**

☙ Solaray MULTIDOPHILUS or Nature's Plus JUNIOR DOPHILUS chewables for strep infection. ⊛

☙ Hylands *Sore Throat* and *C Plus* tabs. ⊛

☙ **For strep throat:**
❋Enzymatic Therapy VIRAPLEX caps.
❋**Nutribiotic GRAPEFRUIT SEED extract in water, or capsules for infection.**
❋For chronic low-grade strep infection: take Enzymatic Therapy THYMU-PLEX caps w. vitamin C 5000mg daily, and Lysine 500mg with zinc lozenges as needed daily.

☙ **For laryngitis and hoarseness:**
❋Alacer EMERGEN-C.
❋Zinc gluconate lozenges.
❋Propolis lozenges. ◯+
❋Vit. E 400IU daily as a preventive.
❋**Nutribiotic GRAPEFRUIT SEED extract in water, or capsules for infection.**

Lifestyle Support Therapy

☙ **Effective throat applications:**
❋Hot ginger compresses
❋Massage throat with Centipede KITTY'S OXYGEL.
❋Eucalyptus steams.
❋Color therapy glasses: wear blue.
❋Hot parsley compresses on the throat.
•❋Drip black walnut extract in throat.

☙ Take hot 20 minute saunas daily.

☙ Stick tongue out as far as it will go. Hold for 30 seconds. Release and relax. Repeat 3 times to increase blood supply to the area.

☙ Take a catnip enema to cleanse infection from a strep throat. ⊛

☙ **For laryngitis and hoarseness:**
❋Apply ginger/cayenne compresses to throat.
❋Don't whisper. It's throat-abrasive.
❋A hot mineral or epsom salts bath.
❋Stop smoking; avoid secondary smoke.
❋Hum a little to reduce swelling.

☙ **Reflexology point:**

larynx
trachea
epiglottis

Common Symptoms: *Sore, aching, inflamed, throat and tonsils; swollen throat tissues; difficult talking; laryngitis (inability to speak above a whisper because of swollen throat tissues).*
Common Causes: *Viral or strep infection (if chronic, it may be mononucleosis); tonsillitis; beginnings of a cold or flu; consequence of smoking; lack of sleep; too many mucous-forming foods; adrenal exhaustion; stress.*

See COLDS & FLU, AND VIRAL, STAPH AND BACTERIAL INFECTION pages for more information

Sports Injuries

Torn Ligaments ❖ Sprains ❖ Muscle Pain ❖ Tendonitis

A strain or pulled muscle is any damage to the tendon that anchors the muscle. A sprain is caused by a twisting motion that tears ligaments that bind up the joints. It takes much longer to heal than a strain. Tendonitis is the painful inflammation of a tendon, usually resulting from a strain, and developing as a dull, dragging sensation after exercise. You can help yourself prevent sports injures. Start your workout slowly; warm your body up at least 2 degrees before you start pushing yourself; end your workout with a cool down period to prevent lactic acid build-up.

Diet & Superfood Therapy

❧ Concentrate on fresh foods (about 50% of the diet) during healing. Include vegetable proteins for faster healing. Muscles need complex carbs from green foods to heal.
  ❀Eat chromium-rich foods such as lobster, low fat cheeses, brewer's yeast.
  ❀Eat silicon-rich foods such as rice, oats, green grasses and leafy greens.
  ❀**Drink electrolyte replacements: Knudsens RECHARGE, Twin Labs CARBO FUEL powder, potassium broth (pg. 167).**
  ❀Eat magnesium-rich foods, like whole grains, nuts, beans, squashes for muscles.
  ❀Eat high vitamin C foods - a drink of lemon juice/honey/water at night; grapefruit or pineapple juice in the morning.
  ❀Avoid acid-forming foods, such as red meats, caffeine and carbonated drinks. Restrict intake of fats and sugars.

❧ **Foods to massage into injuries:**
  ❀Cider vinegar/sea salt paste
  ❀Hot flax oil
  ❀Cayenne/vinegar solution
  ❀Wheat germ oil

❧ **Healing superfoods:**
  ❀Nutrex HAWAIIAN SPIRULINA.
  ❀Crystal Star ENERGY GREEN™ drink.
  ❀Crystal Star SYSTEMS STRENGTH™.
  ❀Nutricology PRO-GREENS with flax.
  ❀Future Biotics VITAL K drink.

Herbal Therapy

🌿 **Jump start herbal program:**
  ❀**Crystal Star SILICA SOURCE™ or Flora VEGE-SIL caps 4 daily, for new collagen and interstitial tissue regrowth.**
  ❀**HIGH PERFORMANCE™ caps 24 daily to prevent lactic acid buildup,**
  ❀**ANTI-FLAM™ caps for inflammation.**
  ❀**BODY REBUILDER™ caps for new tissue.**
  ❀**RELAX CAPS™ to rebuild nerve sheath.**
  ❀**ANTI-SPZ™ or CRAMP BARK COMBO™** extract as needed for muscle pain.
  ❀**ADR-ACTIVE™** to rebuild adrenal cortex.

🌿 **Effective herbal healing topicals:**
  ❀Centipede KITTY'S OXY-GEL.
  ❀AloeLife ALOE VERA SKIN GEL.
  ❀A healing topical paste: mix one part *each*; goldenseal, comfrey root and slippery elm powders in 2 parts aloe vera gel.

🌿 **Ginseng and sports medicine:**
  ❀Siberian ginseng extract for lactic acid build-up, increased oxygen use.
  ❀Crystal Star GINSENG 6 SUPER ENERGY™, a non-overheating Am. ginseng source.
  ❀Ho-shou-wu for ligament, nerve healing.
  ❀Crystal Star GINSENG SKIN CARE™ gel with vit. C for abrasions, cuts and blisters.

🌿 **For cracked, sore feet: Miracle of Aloe MIRACLE FOOT REPAIR, or take a lavender or rosemary foot bath.**

Supplements

❧ **Effective anti-inflammatories:**
  ❀PCOs 100mg 2x daily.
  ❀**Country Life LIGATEND 4 daily.**
  ❀Enzymatic Therapy ACID-A-CAL, with MYOTONE caps.
  ❀DLPA 500-750mg as needed for pain.
  ❀**CoQ₁₀ 60mg 3x daily for pain.**
  ❀Vitamin E 800IU for torn cartilage.
  ❀Biotec CELL GUARD, 6 daily for arthritis-like symptoms.

❧ Enzyme combinations work well to heal soft tissue injuries and reduce inflammation.
  ❀Solaray QBC with bromelain 2-4 daily.
  ❀Mag./potassium/bromelain caps.
  ❀Rainbow Light ADVANCED ENZYME SYSTEM.

❧ Vitamin C crystals with bioflavs, ¹/₂ teasp. in water, or Alacer EMERGEN-C every hour during acute stress for collagen and connective tissue healing.

❧ Twin Lab CSA with zinc 75mg daily.

❧ **Homeopathic sports remedies:**
  ❀**Arnica for dislocations, sprains, bruises.**
  ❀*Ruta Graveolens* for pulled tendons.
  ❀*Hypericum* for damaged nerve tissue.
  ❀*Rhus Tox.* for swelling.
  ❀Boiron *Sportenine* for tendonitis.
  ❀Hylands *Arnicaid.*

Lifestyle Support Therapy

☞ **Elevate the injured area:**
  ❀Apply ice packs immediately. Leave on for 30 minutes. Remove for 15 minutes. Repeat process for 3 hours to decrease internal bleeding from injured vessels.
  ❀Wrap sprains with an ACE bandage (over the ice if necessary) to limit swelling. Rest injured area so injury is not extended.
  ❀Apply alternating hot and cold packs the next day for circulation, to take down swelling and relax cramps. Elevate legs and slap them hard with open palms to stimulate circulation.
  ❀Massage affected areas well and frequently. Massage therapy and shiatsu are both effective treatments.
  ❀Acupuncture and acupressure have been successful.

☞ **Healing applications for sports injuries:**
  ❀DMSO liquid roll-on with aloe
  ❀B&T *TRIFLORA* rub gel
  ❀TIGER BALM analgesic rub
  ❀Chinese WHITE FLOWER oil
  ❀St. John's wort salve
  ❀Calendula gel for blisters
  ❀ALOE ICE
  ❀CamoCare PAIN RELIEVING cream

☞ Effective compresses:
  ❀B&T *ARNIFLORA* GEL.
  ❀Tea tree oil.
  ❀Hot burdock/comfrey tea.

Common Symptoms: *Wrenched knees; twisted ankles; sprained wrists; shin splints; tennis elbows; torn ligaments; muscle pulls; arthritis-like symptoms; bruises; tendon inflammation; Achilles heel; shooting ankle, foot and knee pains. Cramping and soreness during and after muscle exertion; painful joints and nerve endings; limited range of motion; leg cramps at night.*
Common Causes: *Conditions that allow too many sports injuries - calcium, magnesium, and general mineral deficiency; poor diet, high in acid-forming foods, low in green vegetables and whole grains; too much saturated fat and sugar; HCL depletion; poor circulation.*

See also MAINTAINING HEALTH WITH EXERCISE, page 135 for more information.

Stress

Low Energy & Tension

Everyone is affected by varying degrees of stress. It is experienced by those who work in polluted atmospheres, by those who are immobilized at control desks with machines or instruments demanding continual attention, by those who travel coast to coast constantly, by those with mundane, boring jobs, etc. At best, stress causes useless fatigue; at worst, it is dangerous to health. Profound stress, such as that caused by job loss or the loss of a loved one can take a serious physical toll. But the human body is designed to handle stressful situations, if not indeed to thrive and be challenged by some of them. You can never avoid all stress, but you can maintain a high degree of health to handle and survive stress well. The failure to manage stress in your life can kill you.

Diet & Superfood Therapy
Good nutrition is a good answer to stress.

♨ As stress increases, protein needs increase. Protein and mineral-rich foods are the best choice - vegetable proteins from whole grains, sea vegetables, seafoods, soy foods, eggs and sprouts.
 ✳Have fresh carrot juice and fresh fish or seafood at least once a week.
 ✳Add magnesium-rich foods from green vegetables and whole grains.
 ✳Eat B-vitamin-rich foods like brown rice and other whole grains.
 ●Observe good food combining.
 ●Reduce caffeine intake.
 ✳Take a glass of wine before dinner. No liquids with meals. Drink bottled water.
 ✳Don't eat on the run, while working, between meals, or while watching TV.

♨ Make an anti-stress mix of brewer's yeast, toasted wheat germ, sunflower seeds, molasses, Omega-3 flax oil; take 2 TBS. daily in food.

♨ Nutritionally support your immune system and adrenals with foods like sea vegetables and green drinks (see below).

♨ **Effective superfoods:**
 ✳Y.S. or Beehive Botanicals ROYAL JELLY/GINSENG and honey tea,
 ✳Crystal Star SYSTEMS STRENGTH™
 ✳ProLogix GREEN SUPREME drink.
 ✳Nutricology PRO-GREENS.

Herbal Therapy

☙ **Feed your nerves:**
 Crystal Star RELAX CAPS™ 2-4 daily, or STRESSED OUT™ extract or tea as needed. ♂
 ✳Gotu kola or ginseng/gotu kola caps.
 ✳GINKGO BILOBA extract.

☙ **Feed your adrenals;**
 ✳Crystal Star ADR-ACTIVE™ caps/extract.
 ✳Licorice extract, or Crystal Star GINSENG/LICORICE ELIXIR™.

☙ **Add herbal minerals for stability:**
 ✳Crystal Star CALCIUM SOURCE™ caps or extract, or MINERAL SPECTRUM™ caps.
 ✳Kelp tabs 8 daily.

☙ **Balance your body with adaptogens:**
 –Siberian ginseng extract
 ✳Crystal Star MENTAL INNER ENERGY™ with kava kava, astragalus and suma
 ✳Una da gato for the immune system

☙ **Effective herbs for calm:**
 ✳VALERIAN/WILD LETTUCE extract. ☺
 ✳Bach Flower RESCUE REMEDY
 ✳Crystal Star RELAX™ tea ☺ or CALCIUM SOURCE™ caps with oatstraw. ♀
 ✳Rub St. John's wort oil on the temples.

☙ **Stress-balancing aromatherapy:**
 –Lavender oil, chamomile oil
 –Ylang-Ylang oil

Supplements

♒ **Fight stress with antioxidants:**
 ✳Ascorbate vitamin C with bioflav-onoids, 500mg every 4 hours during acute periods.
 ✳Premiere GERMANIUM with DMG. ♂
 ✳CoQ₁₀ 60mg daily.
 ✳Beta-carotene 25,000, 3x daily

♒ **Fight stress with B vitamins:**
 ✳Stress B Complex 100mg 2-3x daily, with extra B6 250mg and pantothenic acid 1500mg. ♀
 ✳Niacinamide for valium-like activity.

♒ **Support the adrenal glands:**
 ✳Enzymatic Therapy ADRENAL CORTEX COMPLEX caps.
 ✳Royal jelly ¹/₂ teasp. daily. ♀
 ✳Country Life RELAXER tabs under the tongue for fast relief. ♀

♒ **Stabilizing mineral supplements:**
 ✳Magnesium/potassium/bromelain ♂
 ✳Homeopathic *Mag. Phos.*
 ✳Mezotrace SEA MINERAL complex. ☺
 ✳Rainbow Light CALCIUM PLUS with high magnesium. ♀

♒ Effective supplements for nerves:
 ✳DLPA 500-750mg as needed daily
 ✳EVENING PRIMROSE oil 2-4 daily
 ✳Enzymatic Ther. THYROID/TYROSINE.
 ✳Hylands *Calms* and *Calms Forte.*
 ✳Twin Labs GABA PLUS w. taurine.

Lifestyle Support Therapy
You have to unwind before you can unleash.

☛ **Have a good laugh every day.**

☛ **Stress reduction and relaxation techniques are a key:**
 ✳**Massage therapy once a month.**
 ✳Quiet your mind with deep, rhythmic breathing exercises every day.
 ✳Regular aerobic exercise for tissue oxygen.
 ✳Consciously take a rest and relaxation period every day. Listen to soft music. Meditate. Do 3 minutes of neck rolls.
 ✳Walk your dog.
 ✳Go on a short vacation. Take a long weekend. It will do wonders for your head.

☛ **Work addiction is the health hazard of our time:**
 ✳Strengthen family and friendship ties.
 ✳Celebrate your life's rituals.
 ✳Build a good diet, adequate rest and exercise into your life.
 ✳Develop creative pastimes.
 ✳Delegate some responsibilities.
 ✳Live in the now.

☛ Hypnotherapy, aromatherapy, and shiatsu have all shown effective results against stress.

☛ Don't smoke. Nicotine constricts the blood vessels, causing increased stress.

Common Symptoms: *Four levels of stress symptoms: 1) losing interest in enjoyable activities, eye-corner sagging, forehead creasing, becoming short-tempered, bored, nervous; 2) tiredness, anger, insomnia, paranoia, sadness; 3) chronic head and neck aches, high blood pressure, upset stomach, looking older; 4) skin disorders, kidney malfunction, susceptibility to frequent infections, asthma, heart disease, mental and nervous breakdown. Symptoms of fight or flight reactions are elevated heart rate, breathing changes, muscle tension, mental focus and fear or anger.*

Common Causes: *Emotional and/or psychological problems; overuse of drugs or prescription medicines; work addiction; fatigue, lack of rest; too much tobacco, caffeine or alcohol; allergies; hypoglycemia; mineral depletion; noise, air, environmental pollutants; overcrowding; unemployment or job pressure; poverty; marital, social problems.*

Taste & Smell Loss
Deviated Septum

There is a broad variety of reasons for this dysfunction, including a deviated septum and response to several common drugs people take today for colds and flu. In addition, nerve endings may be damaged from arthritis or osteoporosis (one of the reasons this problem afflicts older people more than younger people). The natural healing emphasis on overcoming nutritional deficiencies is often able to successfully address many of the root causes. In most cases, if total atrophy has not developed, at least partial taste and smell can be restored.

Diet & Superfood Therapy

A mineral-rich, low fat, low salt diet is a key factor.

❧ Keep the diet free of mucous-clogging foods, such as heavy starches, red meats and pasteurized dairy foods.

→ Add in plenty of fresh, crunchy, high texture foods like celery and apples. Have a fresh green salad every day.

❧ Eat zinc rich foods like sea foods and fish and sea vegetables snipped over your salads or in soups.

→ Eat magnesium-rich foods like whole grains and green leafy vegetables.

→ Boost minerals and B-vitamins: Have some brown rice, miso soup, and sea vegetables every day for at least 3 months.

❧ Make sure the diet is low in salt and refined sugars.

→ Use herbal salt-free seasonings.

❧ **Effective superfoods:** Green drinks can sometimes do wonders. Use them for at least 3 months to see results.
→ Nutricology PRO-GREENS.
→ Orange Peel GREENS PLUS drink.
→ Crystal Star SYSTEMS STRENGTH™ drink daily, for at least 3 months.
→ Beehive Botanical ROYAL JELLY/ GINSENG drink.

Herbal Therapy

❧ **Jump start herbal program:** Crystal Star MINERAL SPECTRUM™ capsules 4 daily, to increase natural foundation minerals in the body.
→ **GINKGO BILOBA extract 3-4x daily, a primary sensory aid.**

❧ Kelp tabs 6 daily for several months. ♀

❧ Twin Lab propolis extract 3-4x daily. ♂

❧ **Herbal adaptogens like ginseng help normalize body systems:**
→ Siberian ginseng extract capsules 2 daily,
→ Superior ginseng/royal jelly vials 1 daily. ♀
→ Solaray ALFAJUICE caps.
→ Liquid chlorophyll, 1 teasp. before meals.

Supplements

❧ **Zinc, up to 100mg daily. Most people with sensory, especially taste, loss have a zinc deficiency.**
→ **Add beta-carotene 25,000IU 2x daily and flush-free niacin 100mg daily for best results.**

❧ **Magnesium improves the sense of smell. Take magnesium 800mg 2x daily.**

❧ Nature's Bounty B₁₂ internasal gel every other day. ♀

or

❧ B complex 100mg daily, with extra B₆ 100mg and B₁₂ 2000mcg. ♀
with
→ Ester C 550mg, with bioflavonoids 4-6 daily.

❧ Marine carotene up to 100,000IU daily.

❧ Solaray CAL/MAG CITRATE capsules 4-6 daily. ♀

❧ Glutamine 500mg 2 daily,
with
→ Mezotrace SEA MINERAL complex tabs 3 daily.

❧ Enzymatic Therapy LIQUID LIVER with Siberian ginseng capsules 3-4 daily.

Lifestyle Support Therapy

❧ Use a catnip or chlorophyll enema to cleanse clogging mucous.

❧ Regular exercise with deep breathing to keep passages clear.

❧ **Reflexology point:**

nose and tongue

See the LOW SALT DIET (pg. 209) for more information.

Common Symptoms: *Inability, or only partial ability to smell odors or taste foods.*
Common Causes: *Zinc and other mineral deficiencies; too many antibiotics, causing zinc excretion; side effect of chemotherapy; deviated septum; chronic low grade throat and sinus infection; poor circulation and mucous clogged system; atrophied nerve endings; high blood pressure medicine; over-the-counter cold medicines; chemical diuretics; gland imbalance and poor hormone secretions; hereditary proneness.*

Teething
Childhood Tooth & Mouth Pain

Although it may seem like an ailment to every parent who soothes a fussy child on numerous sleepless nights, teething is a natural process of the first baby teeth breaking through the gums. Normally beginning around the seventh or eighth month, a baby will add another tooth about every month, until the complete set of 20 teeth comes in - usually around thirty months. (Teething is also a natural reminder to Moms that it's time to wean the child from breast feeding.) Many of the same remedies apply for wisdom teeth breakthrough.

Diet & Superfood Therapy

☙ Effective food applications on gums:
 ☀Garlic oil rub if there is infection.
 ☀Sea salt and honey mix.
 ☀Wine or brandy if there is swelling.

☙ Include vitamin A-rich vegetables, vitamin D-rich eggs, fish and sea vegetables and high bioflavonoid foods in the child's diet.

☙ Feed plenty of chilled foods; fresh fruits, yogurt, etc. to relieve discomfort.
 ☀Give lots of cool water daily.

☙ Chilled food chews:
 ☀Give lots of cool water daily. Cold, hard cookies or bagels.
 ☀Let the child chew on cold raw carrot sticks.
 ☀Give a teething ring that has been kept in the fridge.

☙ Effective superfoods:
 ☀ New Moon GINGER WONDER syrup. Put a few drops in juice and rub on gums with a cotton swab.
 ☀Give a dilute solution of Crystal Star BIOFLAVONOID, FIBER & C SUPPORT™ drink several times a week.

Herbal Therapy

Gentle herbs have been used for centuries to help children over this rough growing patch in their lives.

☙ Effective rub-ons: use only a drop or two of the extract or oil; blend the oils with a few drops of flax oil to dilute; blend the extracts with a little water.
 ☀Lobelia extract.
 ☀Peppermint oil.
 ☀Myrrh extract.
 ☀Bilberry extract - anti-inflammatory.
 ☀Clove oil - especially good for cutting wisdom teeth, too.
 ☀Licorice root extract; or let the child chew on natural licorice sticks.

☙ Make a weak goldenseal solution in water. Give with an eye dropper on the back of the tongue. Rub on gums as an anti-infective.

☙ Effective weak teas: give internally and pat on with a soft-dipped cloth.
 ☀Slippery elm
 ☀Chamomile
 ☀Red raspberry
 ☀Catnip
 ☀Peppermint
 ☀Fennel

☙ Soak yarrow flowers in bran and water for 3 days. Strain and rub on gums.

Supplements

☙ Homeopathic remedies are an excellent, fast-working choice:
 ☀Natra-Bio *TEETHING* drops.
 ☀Hylands *TEETHING* tablets.
 ☀Hyland's *Calc.-Phos.* tabs (break in half, or dissolve in juice)
 ☀*Chamomilla.*
 ☀Rub *Plantago Majus* tincture directly on tender gums.

☙ Apply aloe vera gel to gums as needed.

☙ Ascorbate vitamin C powder with bioflavonoids - make a weak solution in water. Give internally and apply to gums every few hours.

☙ Chewable Mezotrace CHILDRENS SEA MINERAL complex. (Break in half or dissolve in juice.)

☙ Prevail CHILDREN'S VITASE formula for enzyme therapy against inflammation.

Lifestyle Support Therapy

☞ Make a weak tea tree oil solution with water, and rub on gums if there is swelling and infection.

☞ Let the child play in the sun for 15 to 20 minutes every morning for full-spectrum vitamins - especially sunlight vitamin D.

☞ Reflexology points:

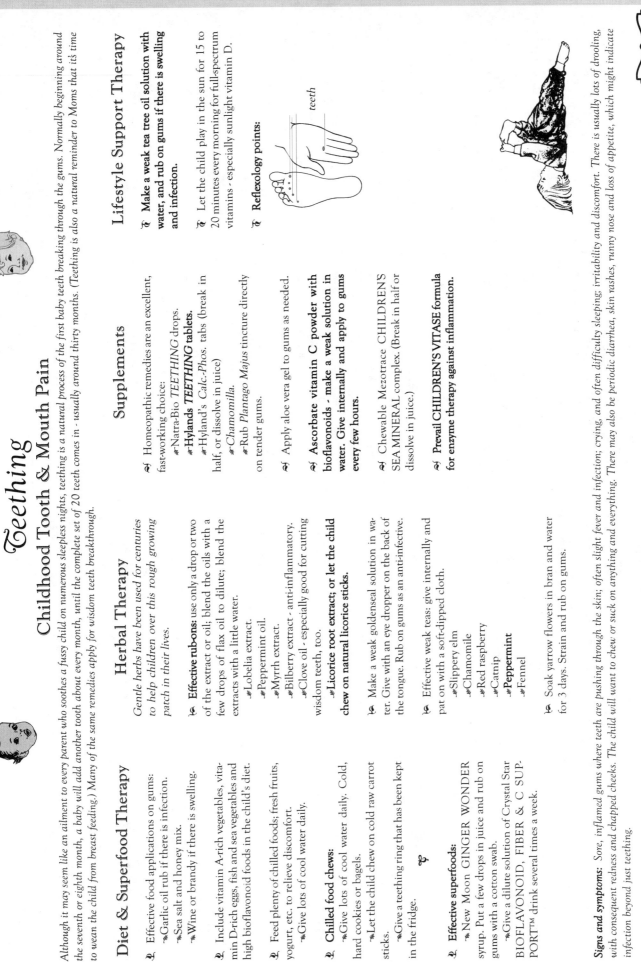

teeth

See CHILDREN'S REMEDIES in this book for more information, page 114.

Signs and symptoms: *Sore, inflamed gums where teeth are pushing through the skin; often slight fever and infection; crying, and often difficulty sleeping; irritability and discomfort. There is usually lots of drooling, with consequent redness and chapped cheeks. The child will want to chew or suck on anything and everything. There may also be periodic diarrhea, skin rashes, runny nose and loss of appetite, which might indicate infection beyond just teething.*

Tonsillitis
Tonsil Lymph Inflammation

The tonsils are part of the lymphatic gland tissue on either side of the entrance to the throat. Their normal activity is straining and processing poisons from the body. (Unnecessary removal of these glands reduces the body's ability to respond to harmful pathogens taken in by mouth.) Tonsillitis is tonsil inflammation, usually caused by streptococcal organisms. While the infection itself may not be serious, it always indicates a deeper immune response problem, and can lead to serious problems, such as rheumatic fever and nephritis. Scar tissue accumulates with every tonsillitis attack.

Diet & Superfood Therapy

❧ Go on a 24 hr. (pg. 158) or 3 day liquid cleansing diet (pg. 157) to clear out body toxins.
  ➛Then eat only fresh foods for the rest of the week during an attack. Get plenty of vegetable protein for healing.
  ➛Have lemon juice and water each morning with plenty of other high vitamin C juices throughout the day, such as orange, pineapple, and grapefruit juice.
  ➛Take a potassium broth or essence (pg. 167) once a day.
  ➛Have an onion/garlic broth each day (pg. 171).

❧ Avoid sugars, pasteurized dairy products, and all junk foods until condition clears.

❧ Drink 6-8 glasses of bottled water daily to keep the body flushed.

❧ Superfoods: *Glands need greens!*
  ➛Crystal Star BIOFLAV., FIBER & C SUPPORT™ drink.
  ➛Nutricology PRO GREENS w. flax
  ➛Solaray ALFAJUICE caps
  ➛Aloe Falls ALOE GINGER juice - sip as needed - very soothing.

Herbal Therapy

❧ **Jump start herbal program:** Herbal anti-inflammatories are a key to relief:
  ➛Crystal Star ANTI-FLAM™ caps or extract as needed.
  ➛ASPIR-SOURCE™ caps to relieve head and throat pain.
  ➛Licorice root or Crystal Star GINSENG/LICORICE ELIXIR™ extract.
  ➛Solaray TURMERIC (curcumin) caps.

❧ Crystal Star ANTI-BIO™ caps 4-6 daily, to flush lymph glands and clear infection, with FIRST AID CAPS™, 4-6 daily during the acute phase.
  ➛Crystal Star cold COFEX™ TEA as a soothing throat coat

❧ Mullein or lobelia tea as a throat compress.
  ➛**Thyme tea as a gargle.**

❧ **Effective herbs for symptoms of tonsillitis:**
  ➛ECHINACEA extract or cleavers tea as lymphatics to clear lymph tissue.
  ➛Garlic oil
  ➛Beehive Botanical PROPOLIS SPRAY.
  ➛Black walnut extract directly on throat.
  ➛Lobelia drops if there is high fever.

Supplements

Raw glandular extracts offer biochemical nutritional support for stress and fatigue affecting glands. They can improve gland health dramatically by delivering cell-specific and gland specific factors.

❧ **Zinc gluconate throat lozenges as needed.**
  ➛**Propolis lozenges or tincture as needed.**

❧ **Spray throat with Nutribiotic GRAPEFRUIT SEED extract as a gargle as directed, for anti-infective activity.**

❧ Solaray pantothenic acid 1500mg with B_6 250mg to take down swelling.
  ➛**Quercetin with bromelain to relieve inflammation.**

❧ Nature's Plus CHEWABLE ACEROLA C 500mg with bioflavonoids, 1-2 every hour during acute stages.
  ➛Beta carotene 100,000IU daily as an anti-infective.

❧ Enzymatic Therapy VIRAPLEX caps 4 daily.
  ➛THYMULUS extract for increased immune strength.

Lifestyle Support Therapy

If your tonsils do need conventional medical attention, ask about partial laser operation that just trim the tonsils with a carbon-dioxide laser. It's an inexpensive, out-patient procedure that leaves you with a minor sore throat instead of a major trauma, and leaves some tonsil-straining ability of the body intact.

🜨 Take a garlic or catnip enema during an attack to clear body poisons.
  ➛Chill the throat with a towel wrapped around crushed ice.

🜨 Get plenty of bed rest during acute stage.

🜨 **Effective gargles:**
  ➛Weak tea tree oil solution in water every 2-3 hours to counter inflammation.
  ➛Warm salt water gargles 3x daily.
  ➛Slippery elm tea to soothe.
  ➛Liquid chlorophyll 1 tsp. in water.
  ➛Goldenseal/myrrh solution in water.

🜨 Hot mineral salts baths frequently.

🜨 **Reflexology point:**

tonsils

Common Symptoms: Swollen tonsils and lymph glands; difficulty swallowing; fever, chills, and tender sore throat; aches and pains in the back and extremities; bad breath because of the infection; ear infection and hearing difficulty because of the swollen glands.
Common Causes: A strep infection; poor diet that aggravates a sporadic infection, with too many starches, sugars, and pasteurized dairy foods; not enough green vegetables and soluble fiber foods; constipation causing toxic build-up; food allergies, particularly to wheat and dairy; poor digestion, and non-assimilation of nutrients.

See Sore Throat page for more information.

Tooth Problems

Tooth Tartar ❀ Plaque ❀ Tooth Decay ❀ Salivary Stones

Plaque-causing bacteria can be formed and begin damaging teeth and gums within 12 hours after a meal. It is important to brush at least twice a day and to floss or water-pick just before going to bed. Relax more. Stress reduces salivary flow allowing bacteria to flourish in the mouth. About the safety of mercury amalgam fillings: although not all people with these fillings are sensitive to the mercury release, there seems to be no doubt that there are definite immuno-toxic effects for people who are. Mercury is a heavy metal that kills beneficial bacteria and allows antibiotic-resistant, to flourish. The best choice is still to have the fillings gradually removed and replaced. Go on a 2 to 3 month detox program to remove the mercury from the bloodstream.

Diet & Superfood Therapy

Various kinds of sweeteners, especially sucrose, and refined sugars are known to significantly increase plaque accumulation.

❧ Eat crunchy teeth-cleaning fresh vegetables; celery, carrots, broccoli, cauliflower, apples, etc. **Chew well.**

✱Eat high mineral foods for strong teeth - lots of green leafy vegetables and high fiber whole grains. Have a large fresh salad every day.

✱Eat cashews or chew cardamom seeds. The oil in either fights decay by interfering with production of plaque acid, and by washing away cavity-causing bacteria.

✱Reduce dietary fats. A high fat diet results in high lipid levels in the saliva and a higher risk of tooth decay.

✱Avoid soft, gooey foods, and dairy products such as ice cream or soft cheeses that leave a film on the teeth.

❧ Strawberries are a good tooth cleanser. Rub strawberry halves on the teeth.

✱Rinse the mouth with cider vinegar or lemon juice. Scrub teeth with lemon rind. ✍

❧ **Superfoods for teeth:**
✱Beehive Botanical ROYAL JELLY/ HONEY/PROPOLIS drink.
✱Crystal Star ENERGY GREEN™ and BIOFLAV, FIBER & C SUPPORT™ drinks.
✱Sun CHLORELLA 1 packet daily.

Herbal Therapy

Take care of your teeth. Studies show that the more natural teeth you are missing, the quicker you will age. If you're pregnant, breast-fed babies develop straighter teeth.

❧ **Jump start herbal program:**
Crystal Star GINSENG/LICORICE ELIXIR™ extract drops in water as a mouthwash daily to inhibit harmful bacteria that cause cavities and to better handle harmful sugars in the body.

✱SILICA SOURCE™ extract drops in **water as a mouthwash to build tooth enamel.** ☿
✱Beehive Botanical PROPOLIS & HERBS THROAT SPRAY.

❧ **Solaray ALFAJUICE capsules 4 daily or Klamath POWER 3 capsules.**

❧ Teeth teas:
✱Dandelion root and leaf tea
✱Parsley/Sage tea

❧ **For salivary duct stones:**
✱Rinse mouth with equal parts goldenseal root tea and white oak bark tea to reduce pain, swelling and bleeding. ☿
✱**Rinse mouth with ginger root solution, and apply ginger root compresses to affected area.**
✱Rinse mouth with J.R.E. IOSOL drops or Crystal Star IODINE SOURCE™ extract in water for potassium and iodine. ☿

Supplements

Floss daily, and brush well after every meal if you have a tendency to tartar build-up. Chew all food well for jaw growth and to prevent corrosion.

❧ **Beehive Botanicals PROPOLIS TINCTURE. Hold as long as possible.**

❧ Homeopathic remedies:
✱Mercurius (Merc. Sol.)
✱Chamomilla
✱Staphysagria

❧ Solaray CAL/MAG 500/500mg with vitamin D 1000IU for tooth strength. ☿
✱Enzymatic Therapy ACID-A-CAL. ☿

❧ **Ester C crystals with bioflavs. and rutin, 1/4 teasp. 3x daily in water. Swish and hold in mouth before swallowing for best results. Or use Ester C chewables as needed.**

❧ Enzyme therapy helps keep plaque and infections away.
✱CoQ 10, 30mg 3x daily, especially if there is gum disease present.
✱Papain chewables as anti-infectives.

❧ Massage gums with vitamin E oil; take internally 400IU daily.

❧ **For salivary duct stones:**
✱Potassium iodide drops.
✱Ester C, 3000mg equivalent daily.

Lifestyle Support Therapy

Fluoride build-up has been linked to health problems from skin eruptions to thyroid problems and immune weakening. If you are sensitive to fluoride, consider the options below.

❧ To remove tarter: Mix equal parts cream of tartar and sea salt, or baking soda and sea salt.

❧ **Beneficial oral care ingredients:**
✱**Xylitol** as a sweetener. It has been shown not to cause plaque formation.
✱**Papain powder or baking soda** as a tooth powder. Both help kill harmful bacteria, and are less abrasive than commercial toothpastes.
✱**Tea tree oil**, as an ingredient and by itself, is anti-bacterial and anti-fungal for almost every mouth problem.
✱**Peelu** contains a natural chlorine that whitens, removes tartar and controls plaque; it also has natural vitamin C.
✱**Myrrh** helps control mouth infections.
✱**Propolis**, a bee-collected product, is a natural immune booster and bacteriacide.

❧ **Effective natural mouthwashes:**
✱Dissolve 1 TB. food grade 3% H_2O_2 in 8-oz. of water, daily for a month.
✱**Nutribiotic GRAPEFRUIT SEED EXTRACT in water as a mouthwash.**
✱**Add 3 drops tea tree oil to water and use as a mouthwash.** ✍

Common Symptoms: *Bad breath; noticeable sticky film on the teeth; bad mouth taste. Salivary stones cause swelling and pain in the jaw just in front of the ear, and a stone-like growth that blocks saliva.*
Common Causes: *Too many refined carbohydrates and sugars; excess red meat, caffeine and soft drinks that cause constipation and acid in the system; vitamin and fresh food deficiency.; amalgamated fillings; stress.*

See next page and GUM DISEASE page in this book for more information.

Toothache

Wisdom Tooth Inflammation & TMJ (Temperomandibular Joint Syndrome)

Many dentists now realize that you need to see a nutritionist along with a dentist if you have chronic toothaches and infection. Diet, nutrition and lifestyle changes are indicated - not just more brushing and flossing. Natural healing wisdom about wisdom teeth - check to see that they're growing in straight; eat right so they don't decay; clean them well to keep them. They help the immune system of the mouth to work. TMJ is a painful syndrome that links various dental and other health problems to jaw misalignment. Approximately 10 million people suffer from TMJ, three times as many women as men.

Diet & Superfood Therapy

♄ Eat primarily fresh foods during acute stages to speed healing, with plenty of leafy greens and vegetable drinks (pg. 168).
　⌇Then, to prevent recurring tooth problems, eat lots of crunchy, crisp foods, such as celery, and other raw vegetables, nuts and seeds, and whole grain crackers.
　⌇Eat calcium-rich foods: greens and shellfish.
　⌇Go light on acid citrus juices if you have weak teeth. They are great for your insides, but not for your teeth. Avoid soft, gooey foods. No sweets, soft drinks or sodas, if your teeth are not strong.

♄ For pain:
　⌇Ice the jaw; take a little wine or brandy and hold on the aching area as long as possible.
　⌇Mix 20 drops of clove oil with 1-oz. brandy. Apply with a cotton swab to toothache area.
　⌇Chew food very well.

♄ Effective superfoods:
　⌇**Wakunaga KYO-GREEN - excellent for jaw arthritis.**
　⌇Nutricology PRO-GREENS with flax.
　⌇Crystal Star ENERGY GREEN™ drink.
　⌇Klamath BLUE GREEN SUPREME.

Herbal Therapy

☙ **Jump start herbal program:**
Take Crystal Star ANTI-BIO™ caps during infection period; apply ANTI-BIO™ extract with a cotton swab directly on infected area as an excellent disinfectant after a root canal.
　⌇Use Solaray TURMERIC caps, or Crystal Star ANTI-FLAM™ CAPS, 4 as needed for inflammation pain.
　⌇Or apply clove oil directly to painful tooth as needed.

☙ **Other effective herbal aids: take and apply directly:**
　⌇Black walnut extract, an anti-infective.
　⌇Twin Labs PROPOLIS extract
　⌇Lobelia tincture 🈲

☙ CALCIUM SOURCE™ and SILICA SOURCE™ extracts for building strong teeth.

☙ **Relaxing herbs help TMJ:**
　⌇Kava Kava caps
　⌇VALERIAN/WILD LETTUCE extract to calm from pain. 🈲
　⌇Crystal Star ASFIR-SOURCE™ capsules for nerve pain.
　⌇Cayenne/ginger

☙ Effective mouth rinses:
　⌇BILBERRY or HAWTHORN extract drops in water for on-the-spot bioflavonoids.
　⌇Echinacea/myrrh extract drops.

Supplements

Supplement your tooth health. Ignore your teeth and they'll go away.

❧ Take De Souza liquid chlorophyll in a small amount of water. Swish and hold in mouth as long as possible. ♂

❧ Nature's Plus CAL/MAG 500mg each, 4 daily, with boron 3mg for better tooth growth.
　⌇Nature's Life LIQUID CALCIUM PHOS. FREE with vitamin D.

❧ **For TMJ:**
　⌇B Complex 100mg with extra B₆ 100mg, niacin 100mg.
　⌇DLPA 500mg as needed for pain.
　⌇Take CoQ₁₀, 60mg daily on a regular basis as a preventive.

❧ Effective homeopathic remedies:
　⌇NatraBio *Teeth & Gums* tincture.
　⌇*Chamomilla* - neuralgic aches.
　⌇*Belladonna* - wisdom tooth pain and ache with pressure.
　⌇**For TMJ - *Cal. Phos.*, *Mag. Phos.*, and *Rhus Tox.***
　⌇*Hypericum* - pain after extraction.

❧ Flora VEGE-SIL silica caps 4 daily. ♀

❧ Bio culture the mouth with Bio Energy Systems BIO-CULTURE 2000, especially after wisdom tooth problems.

Lifestyle Support Therapy

🜊 Relaxation techniques are effective for TMJ, such as massage therapy, biofeedback and chiropractic adjustments.

🜊 Effective compresses:
　⌇Hot comfrey root
　⌇Ginger root

🜊 Apply directly to area with cotton swab:
　⌇Chinese WHITE FLOWER oil
　⌇Propolis tincture (Beehive Botanicals)
　⌇Eucalyptus oil

🜊 Rinse the mouth with a solution of equal parts goldenseal and white oak bark tea to take down pain and swelling.

🜊 Acupressure: Squeeze the sides of each index finger at the end. Hold hard for 30 seconds.

🜊 **Reflexology point:**

teeth & gums

See previous page in this book for more information

Common Symptoms: *Sore jaw and/or gums; dull or shooting pains; tooth or root nerve pain from a cavity; tooth and jaw crowding from wisdom teeth coming in too big, misaligned, etc.; pain from bruxism (tooth grinding at night); periodontal disease, and/or bleeding gums. TMJ symptoms, usually felt only on one side, include painful jaw movement; headaches, ringing in the ears, sinus pain, hearing loss, depression, dizziness and facial neuralgia.*

Common Causes: *TMJ - poor bite with frequent clenching of the teeth and grinding of the teeth at night (bruxism); stress.*

Toxic Shock Syndrome (TSS)
Virulent Staph Infection

Toxic shock is a virulent, often fatal staphylococcal infection that takes over the body incredibly quickly when immunity is depressed. Dangerously low blood pressure and circulatory collapse can take place within 48 hours. In fact, toxic shock syndrome has not disappeared, still victimizing one in 100,000 menstruating women every year. While absorbency ratings and safety procedures have improved, tampon absorbency is still the most important factor associated with toxic shock. Continuous high absorbency tampon use significantly alters vaginal flora, soaking up large amounts of protective magnesium, and allowing bacteria to respond by producing quantities of the deadly staph toxin. A strong immune system is the best and only defense. Get emergency care immediately!

Diet & Superfood Therapy

The following diet recommendations are to prevent recurrence, and to strengthen the immune system after emergency treatment and the hospital stay.

☙ The body will have suffered major deterioration. Optimum, concentrated nutrition must be followed for recovery. Make sure you are including several fresh vegetable juices and green drinks **every day** (pg. 168), or see one below.
 ✦Include high vegetable protein sources for faster recovery; plenty of whole grains, soy foods, sprouts and sea foods; complex carbohydrates for strength, and cultured foods for G.I. flora replacement.
 ✦Have nightly Organic Gourmet NUTRITIONAL YEAST or MISO broth. ❧

☙ **Green drinks and superfoods are key:**
 ✦**Crystal Star SYSTEMS STRENGTH™ drink, for rebuilding and strength.**
 ✦Sun CHLORELLA 2 pkts. daily.
 ✦Green Foods GREEN MAGMA.
 ✦Crystal Star ENERGY GREEN™.
 ✦Klamath BLUE GREEN SUPREME.
 ✦Wakunaga KYO-GREEN.
 ✦Solgar EARTH SOURCE GREENS & MORE.
 ✦Nature's Life SUPER-PRO 96 drink.
 ✦Y.S. GINSENG/ROYAL JELLY drink.
 ✦Future Biotic VITAL K drink.
 ✦Twin Lab PRE-DIGESTED LIQUID PROTEIN or YEAST AMINOS.
 ✦Lewis Labs BREWERS YEAST daily.
 ✦TRansitions EASY GREENS.

Herbal Therapy

☙ **Jump start herbal program:**
 Crystal Star rebuilding formulas:
 ADR-ACTIVE™ and BODY REBUILDER™ caps, 2 each daily.
 ✦GINSENG 6 SUPER TEA™.
 ✦IODINE/POTASSIUM SOURCE™ caps.

 ✦SILICA SOURCE™ extract.
 ✦HAWTHORN extract or HEARTSEASE/ HAWTHORN™ caps with vitamin E.
 ✦HEARTSEASE/ANEMIGIZE™ caps.
 ✦ GREEN TEA CLEANSER™ for cleansed blood and balanced body pH.

☙ Highest potency YS or Premier One ROYAL JELLY 100,000mg 3 teasp. daily. ♀

☙ **Ginseng is a body-normalizing key:**
 ✦**Crystal Star GINSENG 6 SUPER™ caps.**
 ✦GINSENG/CHLORELLA extract ♀
 ✦GINSENG/REISHI extract
 ✦GINSENG/LICORICE ELIXIR™
 ✦GINSENG/PAU d' ARCO extract

☙ Apply alternating hot and cold compresses to collapsed veins or numb extremities:
 ✦Cayenne/ginger compresses for the hot application; plain ice water for the cold.

☙ After tampon use, douche with a solution of GRAPEFRUIT SEED extract - 10 drops in 1 qt. water as a precautionary measure.

Supplements

✦ **Anti-oxidants are a key to healing:**
 ✦**Nutricology germanium 150mg daily.**
 ✦**Nutricology NAC (Acetyl-Cysteine).**
 ✦CoQ₁₀ 60mg 3x daily.
 ✦Grapeseed/white pine PCOs 100mg 3x daily.
 ✦Ester C pwdr. with bioflavs, ½ teasp. every 2 hrs. to bowel tolerance during healing period.
 ✦Biotec CELL GUARD enzymes 6 daily.
 ✦Centipede KITTY'S OXY-GEL; rub on feet at night.

✦ **Probiotics are important:**
 ✦Natren BIFIDO FACTORS
 ✦Jarrow JARRO-DOPHILUS

✦ **Enzyme therapy helps you heal faster:**
 ✦Bromelain 1500mg daily.
 ✦Enzymatic Therapy MEGA-ZYME.
 ✦Jarrow JARRO-ZYMES.

✦ **Minerals are body building blocks:**
 ✦Mezotrace SEA MINERALS 4 daily.
 ✦Zinc 50mg 2 daily.
 ✦Flora VEGE-SIL silica tabs for collagen.
 ✦Floradix HERBAL IRON liquid 3x daily.

✦ **B vitamins are a key for skin and hair regrowth:**
 ✦B Complex 150mg daily
 ✦Source Natural DIBENCOZIDE B₁₂ 10,000mcg. for 2 months.
 ✦Molasses 2 TBS. with PABA 1000mg and pantothenic acid 1000mg for hair regrowth.

Lifestyle Support Therapy

Emergency help can keep the victim alive if received in time. Natural therapies can help bring them back to health.

☞ **Seventy-five percent of all TSS occur in women who wear tampons. Take precautions:**
 ✦Use lower absorbency tampons - 100% cotton tampons if you can. The greater the absorbency of the tampon, the higher the risk of TSS. Use no super absorbent tampons at all.
 ✦Avoid all deodorant tampons. (They can cause irritation and even ulceration of the vaginal canal.)
 ✦Alternate tampon use with pads, especially if you are under a lot of emotional stress or have a poor diet. Or avoid them altogether.
 ✦Don't leave tampons in overnight. Never leave a tampon in for longer than 8 hours.

☞ Avoid all pleasure drugs as a preventive measure. The immune system is affected first.

☞ **Natural alternatives to tampons:**
 ✦Sea sponges - may be trimmed to fit, can be washed and re-used, and are inexpensive.
 ✦The Keeper - a menstrual cup.
 ✦Non-chlorine-bleached pads with no dioxins.
 ✦Re-usable, washable cotton pads.

Common Symptoms: High fever, (initially 102-105°), headache, sore throat, vomiting, diarrhea, dizziness, a painless sunburn-like rash; drifting in and out of consciousness with profound lethargy. The symptoms happen so fast and are so extreme, the victim has almost no time to examine or judge them. Only someone close to the victim can see the virulence and react.
Common Causes: Use of pleasure drugs, debilitating in their own right, with the chance of harmful poisons in the processing techniques; "New Age" eating on a long-term basis (low protein, primarily fruits and cleansing foods); tampon use; vitamin B depletion and deficiency; malnutrition, leaving the body with lowered immunity, wide open for a virulent virus to take over.

See SHOCK & TRAUMA procedures, page 401, and BUILDING & STRENGTHENING IMMUNITY on page 340 for more information.

Tumors
Malignant

Malignant tumors should be addressed as soon as possible to control spreading to other tissues. Tumors may be internal, as brain, gland or organ tumors, or external. Brain tumors especially should be acted upon immediately, because both malignant and benign tumors can cause irreversible neurological damage. Brain tumors are likely to return if not completely excised. Immune enhancement is the key in natural treatment. A whole foods diet and natural supplementation program has been successful in both reducing and in some cases, completely eliminating tumors.

Diet & Superfood Therapy

❧ Begin with a short liquid cleansing diet (pg. 157). For 1 month, have one each of the following juices daily:
  -Potassium broth (pg. 167)
  -A veggie drink (pg. 168), or see below.
  -Cranberry/pineapple juice
  ⚘Add whole grains, high fiber foods and steamed vegetables during the 4th week. **Eat primarily fresh foods, especially sprouts, for the next month.**
  ⚘Keep the system clean and clear and the liver functioning well with a diet high in greens, and low in dairy products and saturated fats.
  ⚘Avoid heavy starches, refined sugars, and all fried foods.
  ⚘Drink only distilled bottled water - 6-8 glasses daily to quickly clear toxic wastes.

❧ **Add high sulphur foods:**
  ⚘AloeLife ALOE VERA juice with herbs.
  ⚘Schiff GARLIC/ONION capsules.
  ⚘Garlic, onion and cruciferous vegetables.
  ❦

❧ **Superfoods are very important:**
  ⚘Crystal Star ENERGY GREEN™ for both iodine and green therapy.
  ⚘Sun CHLORELLA drink.
  ⚘Transitions EASY GREENS, especially for hormone driven tumors.
  ⚘Green Foods GREEN MAGMA, 2 pkts daily.
  ⚘AloeLife ALOE GOLD drink.

Herbal Therapy

❧ **Iodine therapy is important:**
  ⚘Crystal Star IODINE SOURCE™ extract, or IODINE/POTASSIUM caps. ♀
  ⚘J.R.E. IOSOL drops 3-4x daily, or kelp tabs 8-10 daily, with vitamin E 800IU. ♂

❧ **EFAs are important balancing nutrients:**
  ⚘EVENING PRIMROSE OIL 6 daily
  ⚘Nature's Secret ULTIMATE OIL especially for tumors caused by radiation/chemical carcinogens. ♀

❧ **Effective tumor-reducing herbs:**
  ⚘Comfrey tea 4-5 cups daily. ♂
  ⚘Pau darco/butternut for natural quercetin.
  ⚘Calendula gel, esp. if too late for an operation.
  ⚘Reishi mushroom capsules.
  ⚘Crystal Star PAU d'ARCO/ECHINACEA extract and/or pau d'arco gel. ♂
  ⚘Apply Aloe Life ALOE SKIN GEL.
  ⚘Garlic capsules 8 daily.

❧ **Ginseng is a key to normalize cells:**
  ⚘Crystal Star GINSENG SKIN REPAIR GEL™ with germanium and vitamin C for several months.
  ⚘Siberian ginseng extract 3-4x daily, or Health Aid SIBERGIN to retard growth.
  ⚘GINSENG/REISHI extract.
  ⚘GINSENG 6 SUPER™ CAPS or TEA with panax ginseng and suma (both proven tumor inhibitors). ♂

Supplements

❧ **Tumor-specific nutrients:**
  ⚘Quercetin Plus with bromelain 2 daily.
  ⚘Vitamin K 100mcg to inhibit growth.
  ⚘CoQ₁₀ 60mg 6x daily.
  ⚘Nutricology CAR-T-CELL emulsified shark cartilage as directed.

❧ **Anti-oxidants are a key:**
  ⚘Nutricology GERMANIUM 150mg.
  ⚘Matrix Health OXY-CAPS 2 daily, and apply GENESIS OXY-SPRAY directly.
  ⚘Ascorbate vitamin C with bioflavonoids, ½ teasp. every 2-3 hours to bowel tolerance during healing.
  ⚘Marine carotene 100,000IU daily.
  ⚘Nutricology MODIFIED CITRUS PECTIN as directed to reduce tumor spread. ♂
  ⚘Solaray TRI-O2, 2 daily. ♂
  ⚘Matrix Health OXY-CAPS; and apply directly GENESIS OXY-SPRAY for 3 months.

❧ **For brain tumors:** Phosphatidyl choline (PC 55) 4 daily, and carnitine 500mg 2 daily.
  ⚘Vitamin C therapy: see above, with folic acid 400mcg for neuroblastoma. ®
  ⚘Natren BIFIDO FACTORS, ½ teasp. with meals, and Vita Carte BOVINE TRACHEAL CARTILAGE as directed.

❧ B Complex 150mg daily, with extra B₆ 250mg, pantothenic acid 500mg, and folic acid 400mcg to help deter spread of cancerous cells. ♀

Lifestyle Support Therapy

❧ **Tumor-reducing poultices:**
  ⚘Blue violet
  ⚘Mullein/lobelia
  ⚘Fresh comfrey leaf
  ⚘Green clay
  ⚘Chaparral - good results from both poultices and 4 capsules daily.

❧ Una da gato poultices, or Crystal Star ANTI-BIO™ gel with una da gato.

Common Symptoms: Growing and mutating lumps and nodules; often inflamed, weeping, and painful; many times with adhesions to other tissue. Brain tumor signs include chronic headaches, unexplained vomiting, weakness and lethargy, personality changes, double vision, recent incoordination and intellectual deterioration; sometimes seizures and stupor.
Common Causes: Poor diet with years of excess acid and mucous-forming foods; environmental, heavy metal or radiation poisoning; X-rays and low grade radiation tests, such as mammograms, causing iodine deficiency and thyroid malfunction; viral infection such as Epstein-Barr, herpes simplex and Kaposi's sarcoma.

See BREAST AND UTERINE CANCER and SKIN CANCER pages for more information.

Ulcers

Stomach ❀ Peptic ❀ Duodenal

Approximately 14 million Americans now have, or have recently had, an ulcer. Ten thousand people die of peptic ulcer complications every year. A peptic ulcer is an open sore, an erosion of the lining in either the stomach (a gastric ulcer), or the duodenum (the first part of the small intestine). Most ulcers are caused by H. pylori, a common stomach bacterium which liberate copious amounts of damaging ammonia and carbon dioxide when the body's intestinal protective devices fail. Natural therapy focuses on gastric mucosal support and re-establishing intestinal balance.

Diet & Superfood Therapy

☙ Go on a short 3 day liquid diet (pg. 157) to cleanse and alkalize the G.I. tract. Take 3 glasses of your choice of juices daily:
➥Potassium broth (pg. 167)
➥Veggie drinks (pg. 168) or see below
➥Cabbage/celery/parsley juice
➥Apple/alfalfa sprout juice with 1 teasp. spirulina powder added.

☙ Add easily digestible, fresh alkalizing foods, like leafy greens, steamed vegetables, whole grains and non-acidic fruits.
➥**A raw cabbage salad daily during healing.**
➥Include cultured foods, such as yogurt, kefir and buttermilk for friendly G.I. flora.
➥**Avoid sugars, fatty foods (interfere with buffer activity of protein and calcium), pasteurized dairy foods, red meat, heavy, spicy, refined foods. Reduce alcohol (a little wine is ok).**
➥Drink 2-3 glasses mineral water daily. Avoid cola drinks–provoke *acid production.*
➥Diet watchwords: Chew all food slowly and well. Eat small meals. No large, heavy meals. Avoid late night snacks.
❦

☙ **Superfoods are very important:**
➥New Moon GINGER WONDER syrup.
➥Sun CHLORELLA tabs 15 daily, or liquid chlorophyll 3 teasp. daily with meals.
➥**Aloe Falls ALOE/GINGER juice, or AloeLife ALOE GOLD drink.**
➥Wakunaga KYO-GREEN.

Herbal Therapy

☙ **Jump start herbal program:**
➥**Crystal Star ULCR COMPLEX™ caps with meals, and ginger capsules before meals.**
➥**GINSENG/LICORICE ELIXIR™ to inhibit H. pylori and balance G.I. tract.**
➥**RELAX™ caps or ANTI-SPZ™ caps** to calm and help rebuild nerve structure.
➥**CHLORELLA/GINSENG extract to normalize immune response/rebuild mucosa.**
➥ANTI-BIO™ caps 6 daily against H. pylori.
➥Tea tree oil mouth rinse as needed.

☙ Una da gato tea, 3 cups daily.

☙ Herbal flavonoids have anti-ulcer properties and inhibit H. pylori bacteria:
➥Goldenseal/myrrh extract
➥GINKGO BILOBA EXTRACT
➥Garlic or garlic/parsley capsules 8 daily
➥**Duodenal ulcers: BILBERRY extract drops in calendula flower tea.**

☙ Effective soothing/healing teas:
➥**Slippery elm to heal mucous membranes and inflamed tissue.**
➥Marshmallow root, a demulcent.
➥Comfrey/fenugreek tea
➥Chamomile 3 cups daily.

☙ **Anti-inflammatory herbs:**
➥**Solaray TURMERIC capsules**
➥Goldenseal/cayenne caps

Supplements

✔ Supplements fight H pylori:
➥**Quercetin 1000mg w. bromelain 1500mg daily.**
➥**NAC (acetyl-cysteine) as directed.**
➥**Acidophilus complex like Natren TRINITY, $\frac{1}{2}$ teasp. before meals.**
➥**Enzymatic Therapy DGL chewables as needed before meals.**

✔ Antioxidants help to improve the integrity of the gastrointestinal mucosa:
➥Ascorbate vitamin C or Ester C, 3000mg daily, for 3 months.
➥High potency YS or Premier One ROYAL JELLY 2 teasp. daily. ♀
➥Propolis tincture as needed. ♂
➥**Vitamin E 400IU 2x daily.**
➥Emulsified A 100,000IU daily.
➥Zinc 30mg daily.
➥Glutamine 500mg daily.
➥Chromium picolinate 200mcg daily. ♂

✔ Stress B Complex 100mg with extra pantothenic acid 500mg and B₆ 50mg. ♀

✔ **EVENING PRIMROSE oil or Omega-3 flax oil for prostaglandin synthesis.**

✔ **For duodenal ulcers:** a mild olive oil flush - 2 TBS. oil through a straw before retiring for a week, and Gamma Oryzanol (GO) as directed, - a rice bran oil extract.

Lifestyle Support Therapy

☜ Avoid hard liquor, smoking, caffeine, NSAIDS drugs and aspirin - key culprits in aggravating ulcers. Smoking particularly inhibits a natural bicarbonate secretion that neutralizes harmful acids.

☜ Take a catnip or garlic enema once a week during healing to detoxify the G.I. tract.

☜ Calcium carbonate antacids, such as TUMS and ALKA-2 actually produce increased gastric acid secretions when medication is stopped, and may cause kidney stones. Sodium bi-carbonate antacids, such as Alka-Seltzer and Rolaids elevate blood pH levels interfering with metabolism and they can increase blood pressure. Aluminum-magnesium antacids, such as Maalox and Mylanta can cause calcium depletion and contribute to aluminum toxicity.
★Tagamet and Zantac drugs (over 1 billion dollars in sales yearly) suppress HCL formation in the stomach, inhibit bone formation, and cause eventual liver damage. Both drugs also interfere with the liver's ability to metabolize and excrete toxic chemicals, making a person vulnerable to poisons from pesticides, herbicides, etc. Take DGL (deglycyrrhizinated licorice) to normalize after these drugs.

Common Symptoms: *Open sores or lesions in the stomach/duodenum walls, causing burning, nausea and diarrhea; pain right after eating for a stomach ulcer - two or three hours later for a duodenal ulcer. If the vomit is bright red, and the feces are very dark, it is a duodenal ulcer.*
Common Causes: *Mental and emotional stress creating an acid system; gastrointestinal irritants like smoking, aspirin, NSAIDS drugs, coffee, alcohol; poor food combining and food irritants; eating too fast; excessive use of commercial antacids; food allergies; too many sugary foods; anemia; Candida albicans; hypoglycemia.*

See also the HYPOGLYCEMIA DIET in this book, or COOKING FOR HEALTHY HEALING by Linda Rector-Page.

Vaginal Yeast Infections
Leukorrhea ❖ Gardnerella ❖ Vulvitis

Trichomonas - caused by a parasite, found in both men and women, usually contracted through intercourse. *Leukorrhea* - a yeast type infection occurring during low resistance times and when normal vaginal acidity is disrupted. *Gardnerella* - a bacterial infection that thrives when vaginal pH is disturbed. *Vulvitis* - an inflammation of the vulva, caused by allergic reaction, irritation, bacterial or fungal infection. Natural therapies are very successful for most vaginal yeast infections, but a long-term cure is not likely unless dietary/lifestyle changes are made. Be kind to your mate: many of these infections bounce back and forth between sexual partners. Avoid sex during an infection, or at the very least, use barrier protection.

Diet & Superfood Therapy

♌ The diet should be primarily fresh foods during healing. Have a large green salad with alfalfa sprouts every day. Keep meals very light, without heavy starches, fatty foods, sugars, or dairy products.
　✸**Eat plenty of fermented foods, such as yogurt and kefir, for friendly G.I. flora, especially if you have been taking antibiotics.**

♌ Acidify the system: drink 3-4 glasses of cranberry juice from concentrate daily.
　✸Avoid red meats, hard liquor, sugar and caffeine while clearing.

♌ Schiff GARLIC/ONION caps 6 daily with watermelon seed tea if there is also a bladder infection.

♌ Effective food douches:
　✸Cider vinegar - 2 TBS. to 1 qt. water.
Add ¼ teasp. cayenne or 2 TBS. green clay if desired.
　✸Diluted mineral water.
　✸Baking soda 2 teasp., honey 1 teasp. in 1 qt. water.
　✸Chlorophyll liquid 1 tsp. to 1 qt. water.

♌ **Green drinks may be used both orally and as douches:**
　✸**Crystal Star ENERGY GREEN™ drink.**
　✸Sun CHLORELLA 1 packet daily.
　✸Wakunaga KYO-GREEN drink.

Herbal Therapy

♒ **Jump start herbal program:**
　✸Crystal Star WOMAN'S BEST FRIEND™ caps 6 daily, **with Crystal Star WHITES OUT DOUCHE™ for 4 days for a mild infection.**
　✸**WHITES OUT™ #1 and #2 capsules for more severe problems.**
　✸Use extra **ANTI-BIO™ caps to boost effectiveness.**

♒ **Herbals to use orally and as douches:**
　✸Black walnut hulls extract
　✸Pau d'Arco tea 3 cups daily.
　✸Garlic 8 capsules daily.
　✸Berberine-containing herbs like Goldenseal or Oregon grape

♒ Phyto-estrogen herbs show long range body-balancing effects against yeast infections: Crystal Star EST-AID™ caps and tea as a douche, or other formula containing licorice, dong quai, squaw vine, alfalfa, etc.

♒ **Vaginal herbal suppositories:**
　✸Mix powders of cranesbill, goldenseal, echinacea root, white oak bark, and raspberry with cocoa butter to bind. Insert at night. Seal with a napkin or tampon. **Especially for chronic vaginitis - more than a yeast infection.**
　✸Garlic powder or capsules.

Supplements

✍ **Nutribiotic GRAPEFRUIT SEED concentrate 20 drops in 1 gal. water. May also use orally according to instructions.**

✍ **Acidophilus therapy:**
　DR. DOPHILUS ½ teasp. or contents of 5 capsules in 1 TB. yogurt. Smear on a tampon and insert upon retiring. Douche in the morning with ¼ teasp. or contents of 3 caps in water. Take ¼ teasp. in water orally, or 6 capsules daily.

✍ For recurrent infections, take American Biologics DI-OXYCHLOR.

✍ Vitamin therapy effective for most vaginal yeast infections:
　✸Beta carotene 100,000IU daily.
　✸Vitamin E 400IU 2x daily.
　✸Vitamin C (ascorbic acid) crystals, ½ teasp. every 2 hours during healing, up to 5000mg daily. A weak water solution may also be used as a douche.
　✸B Complex 100mg daily, with extra B₆ 100mg.
　✸Vitamin K 100mcg 3x daily.

Lifestyle Support Therapy

ॐ **Effective vaginal douches: Add 1-oz.** herbs to 1-qt. water. Steep 30 min., strain.
　✸Calendula - esp. for candida infections
　✸Tea tree oil
　✸Witch hazel bark and leaf
　✸Sage or white oak bk./white vinegar
　✸Dilute 3% H₂O₂, 1 TB. in 1 qt. water.

ॐ Vaginal packs and suppositories to rebalance vaginal pH: Apply on a tampon, or mix with cocoa butter or simply insert.
　✸**Dilute tea tree oil or Calendula oil.**
　✸**Natren GY-NA-TREN.**
　✸Plain yogurt or cottage cheese
　✸Acidophilus powder or capsules
　✸Boric acid/alternate with acidophilus.
　✸Dolisos *homeopathic Yeast Clear.*

ॐ **For vulvitis:**
　✸Crystal Star FUNGEX™ gel. Don't use fluorinated cortisone creams. They cause thinning and atrophy of the skin.

ॐ **For gardnerella and trichomonas:**
　✸Drink cranberry juice, insert tea tree oil suppositories for 14 days, alternate salt water and vinegar douches for a week, and take vitamins B complex and C daily each.

ॐ **For trichomonas and candida infections - be sure to treat your sexual partner with a penis soak as well.**

Common symptoms: Leukorrhea: itching, irritation, inflammation of the vaginal tissues; foul odor, "cottage cheese" discharge; painful sex. **Trichomonas:** severe itchiness and thin, foamy, yellowish discharge with a foul odor. **Gardnerella:** especially foul, fishy odor, white discharge, moderate itchiness. **Vulvitis:** itching, redness, swelling, often with fluid-filled blisters resembling genital herpes.
Common Causes: Often a condition, not a disease, in which vaginal pH is imbalanced. Causes range from long exposure to antibiotics, to a weakened immune system, and hormone imbalances. The active chemical in many spermicidal creams, nonoxynol-9, aggravates recurrent cystitis and Candida yeast infections, and also kills friendly lactobacilli that protect the vagina against disease-causing micro-organisms.

See SEXUALLY TRANSMITTED DISEASES *and* CANDIDA ALBICANS *healing suggestions for more information.*

Varicose Veins

Spider Veins ✧ Peripheral Vascular Problems

Peripheral vascular problems like varicose veins are more than a cosmetic nuisance. They can be painful, cause unusual fatigue and heaviness, and leg and ankle swelling and cramping. Varicose veins develop when a defect in the vein wall causes dilation in the vein and damage to the valves. When the valves are not functioning well, the increased pressure results in bulging. Spider veins are thin, red, unsightly lines on the face, upper arms and thighs. Vasculitis is an inflammation of the peripheral blood vessels. Women are affected four times as frequently as men. Vein fragility increases with age due to loss of tissue tone, muscle mass and weakening of vein walls.

Diet & Superfood Therapy

Varicose veins are rarely seen in parts of the world where unrefined, high fiber diets are consumed.

♙ Go on a short 24 hour (pg. 158) liquid diet to clear circulation.

❋Then, eat only fresh foods for the rest of the week - plenty of green salads and juices. Add a glass of cider vinegar and honey each morning. **Then follow a vegetarian, high fiber diet for the rest of the month.** Include sea foods, beans, whole grain cereals, brown rice, and steamed vegetables.

❋Reduce dairy products, fried foods, prepared meats, red meats, and saturated fats of all kinds.

❋Avoid salty, sugary and caffeine-containing foods.

♙ **Have a high vitamin C juice every day, such as pineapple, carrot, citrus, fruit, or a veggie drink (pg. 168), or see below. ❋Eat foods with high PCOs, like cherries, berries, currants and grapes.**

♙ **Effective superfoods:**
❋Crystal Star ENERGY GREEN™ drink.
❋Crystal Star BIOFLAV., FIBER & C SUPPORT™ drink for venous integrity.
❋Sun CHLORELLA 1 packet daily.
❋Aloe Falls ALOE JUICE with ginger, or George's ALOE VERA juice..
❋Nutricology PRO GREENS w. flax oil.

Herbal Therapy

Herbal formulas are good choices for vascular fragility because they can stimulate circulation and restore venous tone.

❧ **Jump start herbal program: Crystal Star VARI-VAIN™ Kit, roll-on gel and capsules for 3 months (with horse chestnut and grape seed PCOs).**
❋HEMR-EASE™ caps 4 daily.
❋HEARTSEASE/HAWTHORN™ caps 3 daily.
❋**CHO-LO FIBER TONE™ drink or capsules morning and evening.**
❋CRAMP BARK COMBO™ - pain/heaviness.
❋**Butcher's broom tea and compresses for circulation increase.** ♂
❋Apply aloe vera gel 2x daily.

❧ **Herbal flavonoids help vein tone:**
❋GINKGO BILOBA extract
❋Gotu kola (centella asiatica)
❋HAWTHORN extract
❋BILBERRY extract
❋Enzymatic Therapy HERBAL FLAVONOIDS extract caps 4 daily. ♀

❧ **For spider veins:**
❋Solaray CENTELLA VEIN capsules to help maintain connective tissue.

❧ **Effective fibrinolytic spices:**
❋**Capsicum 4 daily.**
❋Ginger root caps, 6 daily.
❋Schiff GARLIC/ONION capsules

Supplements

✿ **Bioflavonoids are a key:**
❋**Quercetin with bromelain 500mg 4 daily, or Solaray QBC caps.**
❋**PCOs from grapeseed or white pine caps 50mg. 6 daily.**
❋Vitamin C crystals with bioflavonoids and rutin, ¹/₂ teasp. every 2 hours to bowel tolerance daily for 1 month, for connective tissue and collagen formtion.
with
❋Vitamin E 400IU with zinc 30mg daily, and apply a mix of ¹/₄ teasp. vitamin E oil and 2 TBS. liquid lecithin. (The feet and legs will tingle and feel hot as if thawing out).

✿ **Enzyme therapy: Bromelain 1500mg daily to help break down fibrin.**

✿ **Enzymatic Therapy CELLU-VAR cream and capsules to improve venous tone.**

✿ B₁₅ DMG sublingual daily, or Premier GERMANIUM with DMG. ♂

✿ Homeopathic remedies:
❋BioForce *Varicose Veins Relief* tincture.
❋B&T *CALIFLORA* gel.

Lifestyle Support Therapy

✿ Walk every day; swim as much as possible, for the best leg exercises. Elevate the legs when possible. Avoid standing for long periods.
❋Massage feet and legs every morning and night with diluted myrrh oil.
❋Go barefoot, or wear flat sandals.
❋Walk in the ocean whenever possible for strengthening sea minerals.
❋Walk in the early morning dewy grass.

✿ Apply calendula lotion or gel, or Crystal Star CEL-LEAN™ gel. Elevate legs while application soaks in.
❋A mineral salt or epsom salts bath once a week.
❋Use alternating hot and cold hydrotherapy (pg. 177) daily.

✿ Apply Centipede KITTY'S OXYGEL to the legs and feet, 2x daily for 2 months.

✿ **Effective compresses:**
❋White oak bark. (Also take 8 white oak capsules daily.)
❋Witch hazel
❋Plantain
❋Bayberry bark
❋Marshmallow root
❋Cider vinegar
❋Fresh comfrey leaf

✿ Do not use knee high hosiery. The elastic band at the top impedes circulation.

See Circulation page in this book for more information.

Common Symptoms: *Distended, swollen, painful, bulging leg veins; legs feel heavy, tight and tired, sometimes with numbness and tingling; thin red, unsightly spider veins; muscle cramps.*
Common Causes: *Low-fiber, meat and dairy based diet with too many refined foods; vitamin E, C, and A deficiency; EFA (essential fatty acid) deficiency; constipation and straining at the stool; pressure on the veins from excess weight or pregnancy; weakness of vascular walls due to weak connective tissue; poor posture and circulation; liver malfunction; long periods of standing or heavy lifting; damage to veins from inflammation and blood clots in the vein.*

Vertigo

Dizziness ❀ Inner Ear Malfunction ❀ Meniere's Syndrome

Vertigo is a result of equilibrium (inner ear) disturbance with the sensation of moving around in space, or of having objects move around you. It occurs when the brain and central nervous system get conflicting messages from the body sensors that affect and maintain balance - the ear, eyes, and skin pressure receptors. Meniere's syndrome is a recurrent and usually progressive group of symptoms that include ringing and pressure in the ears (also usually with some hearing loss), and dizziness. Rest, relaxation techniques and proper nutrition are the key to preventing attacks.

Diet & Superfood Therapy

❧ The diet should be low in saturated fats and cholesterol, high in vegetable proteins and B vitamin foods, such as brown rice, broccoli, tofu, sea foods, and sprouts.
  ✹Have a potassium broth (pg. 167) or a green drink like those below once a week.
  ✹Make a mix of brewer's yeast and wheat germ (or 2 teasp. wheat germ oil), take 2 TBS. daily on a fresh salad.
  ✹Eliminate common allergy foods: wheat, corn, dairy products, sprayed foods like oranges and lettuce.
  ✹Avoid salty, fried foods, chemical-containing foods and preserved foods.
  ✹Avoid caffeine, especially full-strength coffee.

❧ Effective superfoods:
  ✹Crystal Star ENERGY GREEN™ drink.
  ✹New Moon GINGER WONDER syrup daily.
  ✹Wakunaga KYO-GREEN.
  ✹Beehive Botanicals or Y.S. ROYAL JELLY/GINSENG drink.
  ✹Future Biotics VITAL K drink daily.
  ✹Aloe Falls ALOE juice with ginger.
  ✹Lewis Labs NUTRITIONAL YEAST.
  ✹Nature's Life GREENS PRO 96.

Herbal Therapy

❧ Jump start herbal program:
  ✹GINKGO BILOBA extract drops as needed to promote circulation to the brain, for at least 1 month.
  ✹Ginger capsules 4 daily for 3 months.
  ✹Crystal Star RELAX CAPS™ for nerve rebuilding, and MEDITATION TEA™ to restore mental stability.
  ✹GINSENG/REISHI mushroom extract™.

❧ Make a tea for excess fluid elimination: 1 part each - uva ursi, parsley leaf, red clover, fennel seed, flax seed.

❧ Effective circulation balancing herbs:
  ✹Butcher's broom capsules or tea.
  ✹Crystal Star HEARTSEASE/CIRCU-CLEANSE™ tea with butcher's broom.
  ✹Catnip ☺
  ✹St. John's wort
  ✹Cayenne/ginger capsules
  ✹Peppermint if there is nausea.

❧ Bee products are a specific:
  ✹Superior royal jelly/ginseng vials♂
  ✹High potency YS or Premier One royal jelly 2 teasp. daily.
  ✹Ginseng/honey in water as a daily drink. ♀

Supplements

✍ B Complex 100mg with extra B6 100mg, B₁₂ 2000mcg SL and pantothenic acid 500mg.

✍ Antioxidant therapy:
  ✹Premier GERMANIUM with DMG B₁₅ daily.
  ✹Vitamin E 800IU daily.
  ✹CoQ10 30mg. 3x daily.
  ✹Rosehips vitamin C or Ester C with bioflavonoids and rutin, up to 5000mg daily.

✍ Glutamine 500mg daily. ♂

✍ Niacin Therapy: to clear circulation blocks, 250mg 3x daily. ♂

w Rainbow Light ADVANCED ENZYME SYSTEM with meals, and CALCIUM PLUS capsules with high magnesium 4 daily.

✍ Twin Lab CHOLINE 600mg 3x daily. ♂

✍ Enzymatic Therapy RAW ADRENAL complex caps.

Lifestyle Support Therapy

❧ Take preventive measures: Remove stress from your life as much as possible.
  ✹Practice stress management or relaxation techniques, such as meditation, soft music, yoga and body stretches.
  ✹Chiropractic adjustment and shiatsu massage have also shown effective improvement.

❧ Acupressure point:
  ✹Pinch between the eyebrows 3x for 10 seconds each time during an attack.
  ✹Press top of the arm, just above the wrist line for 15 seconds at a time.

❧ Get plenty of good quality sleep.

❧ Attain ideal body weight for better body balance.

❧ Avoid alcohol, marijuana, methamphetamines, cocaine, hallucinogens, and balance-changing drugs.

❧ Reflexology points:

ear points

Common symptoms: *Starting with ear pain, ringing and pressure, and a feeling of faintness and lightheadedness, the victim has a feeling of falling and lack of steadiness; lightheadedness upon standing quickly; off-balance feeling. Vertigo victims also frequently have hearing loss and nausea.*

Common Causes: *Poor circulation and blood pressure imbalance (which shows up if you stand or move too quickly); lack of brain oxygen or brain tumors; food and chemical allergies; neurological disease; chronic stress and anxiety; hypoglycemia; excess ear wax; B vitamin deficiency.*

See MOTION SICKNESS AND NAUSEA page for more information.

Warts
Moles

Moles are congenital, discolored growths elevated above the surface of the skin, and may appear because of a liver or lung condition. They are harmless unless continually irritated. **Warts** are single or clustered soft, irregular skin growths found on the hands, feet, arms and face, ranging in size from a pinhead to a small bean. They can also occur on the throat or voice box and affect the speaking voice tone. Usually caused by a virus, they are contagious and will spread if picked, bitten, or nicked through shaving.

Diet & Superfood Therapy

❧ Add vitamin A rich foods to the diet, such as yellow and green fruits and vegetables, eggs, and cold water fish.

➼Add sulphur-containing foods, such as asparagus, garlic and onion family foods, fresh figs, citrus fruits and eggs.

➼Include high vitamin C foods with bioflavonoids, and a concentrated source, such as Crystal Star BIOFLAV, FIBER & C SUPPORT™ drink.

➼Take a vegetable drink (pg.168) or see below.

❧ **Effective applications:**
➼**Use very soft brown-black bananas. Place a small section of peel (inside down) on the wart. Cover with a bandage and leave on 24 hours. Repeat until wart is gone.**
➼Mixture of lemon juice, sea salt, onion juice and vitamin E oil.
➼Papaya skins
➼Raw potato ✿

❧ **Superfoods are very important:**
➼Crystal Star ENERGY GREEN™ drink with sea vegetables, every day for a month.
➼AloeLife ALOE GOLD drink.

Herbal Therapy

☙ **Jump start herbal program:** **Crystal Star ANTI-BIO™ caps or extract if there is inflammation or bacterial infection. Use ANTI-VI™ extract and apply ANTI-VI™ tea directly for warts.**
➼Crystal Star GINSENG SKIN REPAIR™ GEL with germanium, vitamin C and bioflavonoids.
➼**ANTI-BIO™ gel with una da gato**
➼**BIO-VI™ extract with usnea.**
➼**AloeLife ALOE SKIN GEL**

☙ **Apply tea tree oil religiously for 1-2 months, 3-4 times daily. Wonderful results.** 🜨

☙ Enzymatic Therapy LIQUID LIVER w. Siberian ginseng caps.

☙ Applications for warts and moles:
➼B&T CALIFLORA ointment
➼Jojoba oil
➼Cinnamon oil drops 🜨
➼Nutribiotic Grapefruit seed extract
➼Crystal Star PAU d'ARCO/ECHINACEA extract ♂
➼Nettles extract ♀
➼Martin PYCNOGENOL GEL.

☙ Garlic oil 2x daily or garlic/parsley caps 6 daily. Apply a paste of garlic cloves directly and cover with a plastic strip. ♀

Supplements

The high dosages recommended here should be used for no longer than 2-3 months at a time.

✑ **Beta carotene or emulsified A 100,000-150,000IU as an anti-infective. (Nothing seems to happen for 1 to 2 months, then growths seem to disappear in a week or so, all at once).**

✑ **Vitamin C crystals with bioflavonoids; take internally, $\frac{1}{2}$ teasp. in water every 4 hours daily. Apply locally to affected area. Also important for immunity against warts.**

✑ Vitamin E 800IU daily. (Also prick a capsule and apply.)
➼Take with zinc 75mg daily.

✑ Cysteine 500mg 2x daily.

✑ For wart and moles caused by a virus: (not HPV-caused warts)
➼Enzymatic Therapy VIRAPLEX.
➼**Rough up a viral wart with the smooth side of an emery board and apply a drop of 3% H_2O_2 to kill the virus.** ♂

✑ Flora VEGE-SIL 4 daily.

✑ B Complex up to 200mg daily, with extra B_6 250mg daily. ♀

Lifestyle Support Therapy

☜ For plantar warts: soak foot in the hottest water you can stand about 30 minutes daily for a month.
Then apply Centipeded KITTY'S OXYGEL or H_2O_2 3% solution. Rough up the wart with the smooth side of an emery board, and apply 1 drop 2-3x daily. Wart or mole will slowly shrink and slough off. Do not squeeze or pick.

☜ Hypnosis therapy has been successful in controlling warts and moles.
➼Some skin therapists now use a electric current passed through a wart to make it shrink.

☜ Effective applications: soak warts in hot water first.
➼**NutriBiotic GRAPEFRUIT SEED extract full strength, or SKIN SPRAY 2 to 3x daily.**
➼A paste of charcoal and water.
➼**Home Health CASTOR OIL PACKS.**
➼Lysine cream applications, and take lysine capsules 500mg 3-4x daily.
➼Wheat germ oil.

☜ Avoid smoking. It cuts off oxygen to the tissues.

Common Symptoms: Warts are flat or raised nodules on the skin surface, with a rough, pitted discolored surface, sometimes causing pain and discomfort when rubbed or chafed; if virally caused, warts are often contagious. Moles are generally smooth and rounded.

Common Causes: Vitamin A and mineral deficiencies; viral infection; widespread use of anti-biotics and vaccinations that depress normal immunity.

See GENITAL WARTS AND CYSTS, WENS & LIPOMAS for more information.

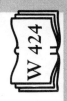
W 424

Water Retention
Bloating ✢ Edema

Water retention, the excessive accumulation of fluid in body tissues and cavities, is often a problem of not enough water - a condition of body imbalance. If we don't get sufficient water, fluid levels go out of balance, and the body begins to retain more water in an effort to compensate. Kidney, liver, blood pressure, circulation, pre-menstrual and pregnancy problems are all associated with water retention. Dieting can take away foods that previously provided water. Medical diuretics, alcoholic drinks and other drugs can dehydrate. Or you may just not be drinking enough healthy fluids. A natural healing program should concentrate on balancing body chemistry rather than simply releasing water.

Diet & Superfood Therapy

❀ Reduce salt and salty foods intake.

✹Eat largely fresh foods for 3-5 days to increase the body's food water content without density.

✹Have a leafy green salad every day with plenty of cucumbers, parsley, alfalfa sprouts and celery.

✹Avoid starchy, sugary, foods. Reduce meats, dried foods and dairy foods that demand more water to dissolve.

✹ Take electrolyte drinks daily like Alacer MIRACLE WATER or Knudsen's RECHARGE.

❀ Drink at least 6-8 glasses of bottled water daily for free flowing functions, waste removal, and appetite suppression. Caffeine drinks are diuretic, but should be avoided by women with pre-period edema.
♣

❀ Green drinks can provide both needed minerals and body acid/alkaline balance:
✹**Orange Peel GREENS PLUS.**
✹**Green Foods Green Magma.**
✹Future Biotics VITAL K 2-4 teasp. daily in water.
✹**Crystal Star SYSTEMS STRENGTH™ drink with sea vegetables for potassium.**
✹**Be Well VEGETABLE JUICE.**

Herbal Therapy

❀ **Jump start herbal program:**
✹**Crystal Star BLDR-K™ caps (with anti-infective activity) or TINKLE CAPS™, 4-6 daily, and/or BLDR-K™ flushing tea.**
✹**Dandelion leaf tea, 3 cups daily.**
✹**CEL-LEAN™ caps 3-4 daily for 1-3 months for enhanced liver function.**
✹HAWTHORN extract as needed to increase circulation. ♂
✹**ADR-ACTIVE™ caps 2-4 daily for salt and water balance.**
✹BILBERRY extract for tissue tone.

❀ Hormones balance affects fluid balance for women.
✹Crystal Star FEMALE HARMONY™ caps and tea have proven effective. ♀

❀ **ECHINACEA extract with 2 cups daily of burdock tea to flush lymph glands and balance hormones.**
✹Solaray ALFA-JUICE caps for hormone balance and as a detoxifier. ♀

❀ **Effective diuretic herbal teas: take 2 cups daily for a week.**
✹Cornsilk/dandelion ♀
✹Juniper/Parsley/uva ursi tea or uva ursi extract drops in water
✹**Crystal Star TINKLE TEA™ 2x daily as needed for pre-period edema.**

Supplements

If taking prescription diuretics, be sure to include a potassium supplement in your daily diet.

❀ Ascorbic acid therapy: Vitamin C crystals with bioflavonoids and rutin, $1/2$ teasp. in water or juice every 2-3 hours until relief. Then 3-5000mg daily for prevention.
✹B Complex 100mg daily with extra B_6 250mg 2x daily. ♀

❀ Proteolytic enzymes for correct nutrient assimilation leading to body balance:
✹Bromelain 750mg 2x daily.
✹Betaine HCL 3x daily.

❀ Enzymatic Therapy ACID-A-CAL caps 3 daily for acid/alkaline balance, with KIDNEY/LIVER COMPLEX.

❀ Natural diuretics:
✹Richardson Labs CHROMA SLIM.
✹Flora VEGE-SIL as a natural diuretic.

❀ MEZOTRACE sea minerals for mineral balance ⊛ very important if you have low adrenal function with water retention.

Lifestyle Support Therapy

Be careful of overusing chemical/medical diuretics. They can cause potassium and mineral loss, and eventually muscle weakness and fatigue.

☙ Take hot 20 minute saunas, often.

☙ **Crystal Star POUNDS OFF™ bath as a strong diaphoretic for sweating, once a week.**

☙ Exercise every day to keep circulation and body metabolism free-flowing.

☙ Elevate head and shoulders for sleeping.

See PMS pages for more information about pre-period edema.

Common Symptoms: Swelling of hands, feet, ankles and stomach; PMS symptoms; headache and bloating.

Common Causes: Too much salt, red meat or MSG; kidney or bladder infection; oral contraceptives reaction; hypothyroidism; PMS symptoms; adrenal exhaustion; protein and B Complex deficiency; hormonal changes, especially estrogen output; climate changes; allergies; poor circulation; potassium depletion; allergies; corticosteroid drug reaction; obesity; constipation; lack of exercise. Persistent edema is linked to kidney, liver, bladder and circulatory problems.

Weight Loss
Excess Fat Retention

Weight loss is a national obsession in America. Yet 34 million American adults are obese. Another 45 million are overweight. (And this doesn't count kids, who are rapidly becoming an overweight generation.) At any given time, 25 million Americans are seriously dieting. As fried, fatty foods have increased in our diets, and physical labor has decreased, there has been a 500-800% increase in obesity in the 20th century. Wow!

The answers to weight control aren't simple. Most serious dieters are able to lose about 10% of their body weight on a strict diet, yet, typically, two-thirds of that weight is gained back within a year, and 90% is regained within five years. Even drastic diets don't make much of a difference in the long run. Most people who repeatedly diet and fail, follow a "crash and burn" philosophy... crash dieting to burn calories fast, without any real change in lifestyle or eating habits. Crash diets, especially those that are almost totally fat-free, are impossible to stick with, intolerable for a normal lifestyle, and even dangerous to health because they are so imbalanced. In the end, crash dieters get burned by gaining the weight back.

Weight control today is a strategy of prevention lifestyle - an attitude of keeping weight down. Even though Americans are always looking for the "miracle magic bullet" for slimness and body tone, everyone is slowly realizing that a good nutritional diet has to be front and center for permanent results. Weight loss is a component of a sound nutritious eating plan, rather than a try at the latest fad. People are becoming more motivated for health reasons to lose weight and want to change their way of eating to insure both looks and health.

Healthy Healing Publications conducts a continuing review of weight loss products, at both a manufacturer and a consumer level. The following products have proven viable aids to weight loss problems.

Diet & Superfood Therapy

The four keys to an effective weight control diet: low fat, high fiber, regular exercise, lots of water.

✿ Changing diet composition is the passport to weight control. The importance of cutting back on fat cannot be overstated. You can eat two to three times more volume of low-fat foods than high fat foods, and still lose weight.

✦**Fat is not all bad.** It is your body's chief source of energy, and essential for good body function in small amounts. The average overweight person often has **too high blood sugar** and **too low** fat levels. This causes constant hunger - the delicate balance between fat storage and fat utilization is upset, and the body's ability to use fat for energy decreases. Eating fast, fatty, fried, or junk foods particularly aggravates this imbalance. The person winds up with "empty calories" and more cravings. Fat becomes non-moving energy, and fat cells become fat storage depots.

✦Saturated fats are the hardest for the liver to metabolize. Stay away from them to control fat storage.

✦**Water** can get you over weight loss plateaus. Drink it, and all liquids before eating to suppress appetite.

✦Small amounts of caffeine after a meal can raise thermogenesis (calorie burning) increasing metabolic rate.

Herbal Therapy

Herbs have a double-whammy for weight control: enzyme therapy and metabolic stimulants for thermogenesis.

❧ Recommended herbal weight loss supplements:

✸Enzyme therapy: Bromelain 500mg 3x daily for maximum metabolism; Pancreatin to help suppress appetite. ♂

✸Country Life DIET POWER, FAT DEFENSE and DIET EASE.

✸Rainbow Light SPIRULINA HERBAL DIET COMPLEX for appetite control. ♂

✸Chae CONTOUR CREAM for cellulite with aminophylline. ♀

✸Crystal Star TIGHTENING & TONING HERBAL WRAP™ for cellulite loss.

✸Gymnema sylvestre caps to reduce sugar cravings.

✸Source Naturals CITRI-MAX.

✸Natrol CITRI-MAX PLUS, and Now CITRI-MAX with kelp and ginseng.

✸Silver Sage Thermogenics.

✸Spirulina and bee pollen for high proteins, energy and blood sugar balance.

✸High Omega-3 flax oil to overcome binging and an addictive need for food.

✸Wild yam caps for highest natural DHEA, an appetite suppressor. ♀

Supplements

Take all regular supplements after meals to avoid appetite stimulation.

✍ **For carbohydrate metabolism**, take B Complex vitamins and pantothenic acid.

✍ **For compulsive eating**, take tyrosine 500mg 2-3x, with zinc 30mg 1 daily.

✍ **For better thermogenesis of fat calories**, carnitine 500mg 2x daily; arginine/ornithine 1000mg at bedtime.

✍ **For effective appetite suppression**, phenylalanine 500mg before meals. (Do not take if sensitive to phenylalanine.)

✍ **For breaking down fat into energy:** take CoQ_{10} 60mg 2x daily.

✍ **Recommended dieting supplements:**

✸Enzymatic Therapy THYROID/TYROSINE caps for metabolic increase. ♂

✸Enzymatic Therapy RAW PITUITARY, MAMMARY, THYROID/TYROSINE for sluggish gland and pear-shaped problems. ♂

✸Prevail FAT DIGEST enzyme formula.

✸Action Labs FAT BURNERS.

✸Lewis Labs WEIGH DOWN w. chromium for retaining muscle while losing fat. ♂

✸ Strength Systems LIQUID FAT BURNERS or Richardson Labs CHROMA-SLIM - a lipotropic/carnitine formula. ♂

✸Kal DIET MAX plan.

Lifestyle Support Therapy

No diet will work without exercise; with it, almost every diet will.

☞ Daily exercise is the key to permanent, painless weight control. Even if eating habits are just slightly changed, you can still lose weight with a brisk hour's walk, or 15 minutes of aerobic exercise.

One pound of fat represents 3500 calories. A 3 mile walk burns up 250 calories. In about 2 weeks you will have lost a pound of real extra fat. That amounts to 3 pounds a month and 30 pounds a year without changing your diet. It's easy to see how cutting down even moderately on fatty, sugary foods in combination with exercise can still provide the look and body tone we all want.

✸Exercise promotes an "afterburn" effect, raising metabolic rate from 1.00 to 1.05-1.15 per minute for up to 24 hours afterwards. So calories are used up at an even faster rate after exercise.

✸Weight training exercise increases lean muscle mass, replacing fat-marbled muscle tissue with lean muscle. Muscle tissue uses up calories; the greater the amount of muscle tissue you have, the more calories you can burn. This is very important as aging decreases muscle mass. Exercise before a meal raises blood sugar levels and thus decreases appetite, often for several hours afterward.

See next page for products for specific weight control problems.

The Six Most Common Weight Control Problems

There are almost as many different weight loss problems as there are people who have them. The following categories represent the most common weight loss obstacles. I have developed comprehensive, natural product programs to address them. Each of the six plans has years of empirical study and success behind it. Once you make the big decision to be a thin person, analyze what your weight loss block really is. Identify the most prominent weight control problem, especially if there seems to be more than one. Best results will be achieved by working on the worst problem first. As improvement is realized in the primary area, secondary problems are often overcome in the process. If lingering problems still exist, they may be addressed with additional supplementation after the first program is well underway and producing noticeable results.

After identifying your personal difficulty, choose the weight loss products within that area that most appeal to you. Follow directions carefully. Since natural products work with the body to rebalance gland and hormone functions, product activity may be subtle and long-range for more permanent results.

Overdosing is not productive, nor will it increase activity. Go slow, stick to it, improve your diet and your daily habits if necessary. *Don't Weight!*

✦LAZY METABOLISM & THYROID IMBALANCE

A poorly functioning thyroid results in sluggish metabolism. Most people with underactive thyroids (hypothyroidism), have a weight problem. Factors that decrease thyroid activity and the rate at which the body burns calories, include certain nutrient deficiencies, thyroid exhaustion from overstimulation by caffeine, sugar and other stimulants, and substances that inhibit thyroid function, like alcohol.

•**Therapy choices:** Herbal supplements, like sea plants, rich in iodine and potassium, help metabolism. Crystal Star META-TABS™, and RAINFOREST ENERGY™ tea and capsules, and HOT SEAWEED BATH™; Enzymatic Therapy THYROID/TYROSINE caps, EVENING PRIMROSE OIL for EFAs, and BEE POLLEN as an adrenal booster. Other natural aids for normalizing metabolism include: vitamin C - especially in the Ester C™ form; Carnitine, 500mg daily; CoQ₁₀ 60mg 3x daily; Vitamin B complex 100mg daily to help the liver; Chromium, 200mcg daily to help activate metabolism by mediated thermogenesis; Tyrosine 500mg as a thyroid precursor.

✦CELLULITE DEPOSITS & LIVER MALFUNCTION

Cellulite is a combination of fat, water, and wastes. When circulation and elimination become impaired, connective tissue weakens, and unmetabolized fats and wastes become trapped just beneath the skin instead of being eliminated by the body. Cellulite forms in areas of sluggish circulation, building up where normal cell exchange slows down.

•**Therapy choices:** Crystal Star CEL-LEAN™ diet caps, CEL-LEAN RELEASE™ tea, CEL-LEAN™ gel, and CEL-LEAN™ HERBAL BODY WRAP PROGRAM or HOT SEAWEED BATH™ as needed. Crystal Star BITTERS & LEMON CLEANSE™ extract, morning and before bed. Other aids for eliminating cellulite include: Thigh creams with ephedra extracts of aminophylline appear to work. Vitamin C with bioflavonoids helps.

✦OVEREATING & EATING TOO MUCH FAT

Overeating on empty calories, like junk food is the downfall of most dieters. Overeaters usually diet by eating one large meal a day and then try to eat nothing the rest of the time. Gnawing hunger for long periods makes the dieter irritable and miserable. This type of so-called diet taxes willpower to the max and makes the dieter want a food binge.

•**Therapy choices:** Crystal Star APPE-TIGHT™ caps, SCALE DOWN DIET™ extract, and RAINFOREST ENERGY TEA™. Super green supplement foods help control appetite for the overeater. Crystal Star ENERGY GREEN™ may be used between meals to almost instantly decrease the craving for high-calorie foods; take with AMINO-ZYME™ for energy lift. Herbal appetite control is a good choice for overeating; Crystal Star APPE-TIGHT™ with META-TABS™. Other aids for reducing a fatty diet: 5-Hydroxy Tryptophan 50-100mg ½ hour before meals; the amino acids Phenylalanine and Carnitine 500mg, and bromelain 1500mg.

✦POOR CIRCULATION & LOW BODY ENERGY

For some dieters, initial weight loss is quite rapid, but then a plateau is reached and further weight loss becomes difficult, because restricted food intake slows down metabolism. Herbal stimulants, along with exercise, can help reactivate thyroid activity and the rate at which the body burns calories, help convert stored fat to energy, and energize circulation to help a dieter get over this plateau.

•**Therapy choices:** Ginseng-containing formulas can be a key: Crystal Star GINSENG 6 SUPER™ caps or tea, or MENTAL INNER ENERGY™, or ACTIVE PHYSICAL ENERGY™, or RAINFOREST ENERGY™ tea and capsules boost energy and circulation, AMINO-ZYME™ capsules with glutamine and carnitine 500mg, ADRN™ extract to boost adrenal activity, and HAWTHORN extract to activate circulation as needed. Other natural aids for normalizing elimination include: CoQ10, 60mg, daily for anti-oxidant enzyme activity; bee pollen and royal jelly for B complex vitamins.

✦POOR ELIMINATION - DETOXING THE COLON, BOWEL, KIDNEY & BLADDER

Today, people make rich foods like red meats, rich cheeses, cream, butter, sugars and sweets, once reserved for festive occasions, a part of every meal. These foods are poor nutrition providers and difficult to eliminate. The environmental pollutants, pesticides, and chemical by-products in these foods also obstruct body processes. Clogged elimination systems especially impede the weight loss process.

•**Therapy choices:** Herbal cleansing supplements can help reactivate normal elimination and body functions. Crystal Star LEAN & CLEAN DIET™ capsules and tea, or SUPER LEAN DIET™ capsules and tea, CHO-LO FIBER TONE™ morning and evening, GREEN TEA CLEANSER™ every morning, and POUNDS OFF™ bath once a week. To flush elimination systems, alternate use of the bladder/kidney program (pg. 161) for a week, with the colon/bowel program (pg. 159) for a week: Crystal Star BLDR-K™ caps and TINKLE TEA™, FIBER & HERBS COLON CLEANSE™ caps and LAXA-TEA™. Other natural aids for normalizing elimination include: Flax seed oil, for EFAs; acidophilus for efficient digestion, and green superfoods like Klamath POWER 3 caps.

✦SUGAR CRAVING & BODY SUGAR IMBALANCE

Sugar provides a temporary "insulin rush," but is then followed by a craving for more food caused by low blood sugar levels. After a sugar binge, raised insulin levels mean more calories are transformed into fat. A low glycemic diet is a good answer for fewer calories turned into fat and more are burned for energy.

•**Therapy choices:** Avoid sugary foods. Eat a plant-based, low-glycemic diet with plenty of fresh vegetables. Crystal Star CHO-LO FIBER TONE™ a.m. and p.m. GINSENG/LICORICE ELIXIR™ to balance sugar levels, and Beehive Botanicals GINSENG/ROYAL jelly drink. Other aids for sugar cravers include: Chromium picolinate 200mcg daily, stevia as a sugar substitute and gymnema sylvestre caps before meals, and a dry sauna twice a week.

See COOKING FOR HEALTHY HEALING by Linda Rector Page for complete weight loss diets for both kids and adults.

Weight Control After 40

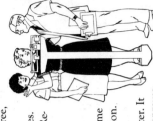

There's no doubt about it. Weight loss gets more difficult after 40. Everybody goes through a change of life. The hormone changes of our middle years affect our body shapes, too......for both men and women. One of the problems people face as they reach their late 40's and 50's is a disconcerting body thickening and a slow upward rise in body weight. This seems to happen with everybody, even for people who have always been slender, who have a good diet, and who exercise moderately. Changes in estrogen levels for women and testosterone levels for men mean that our body chemistry is in transition. Clearly, metabolic rates slow as we age, so it takes food longer to digest, and more of it goes into storage. People who could always lose weight when they were younger just by going on a crash diet for a weekend or a week whenever they gained a few pounds, find that strategy doesn't work anymore. Most of us also become less physically active as we age, which leads to muscle loss, an important factor for a youthful body.

Weight control solutions have to be approached differently when your metabolism slows down. Just eating all the low fat or even no-fat foods available today doesn't seem to make a difference. We tend to think we're getting a free ride, and eat too many of them, or we eat too much of something else to fill up the hunger hole left by not eating any fat. Even the free ride isn't free, because most of the low fat foods have plenty of calories.

I have been working for several years to develop natural weight control techniques for people trying to maintain healthy body weight and tone after their metabolism changes. The program is showing promise and results. For success after 40, begin with two basic weight loss starting points: 1) Improve body chemistry at the gland and hormone level. 2) Re-establish better, long-lasting metabolic rates.

We can do something about our weight, our body tone and our looks. Here are some of the natural techniques to boost metabolism after 40.

#1)   **LOVE YOUR LIVER.** The liver is the basic organ responsible for fat metabolism. It is also intricately involved with the hormone functions of the body, so it is the prime target to optimize for weight loss after 40. Weight gain and energy loss are often the result of a liver which has become enlarged through overwork, alcohol exhaustion and congestion. Typically, a man whose body is slim everywhere but his stomach is one who has a very enlarged, often inflamed, liver.

***Ginseng compounds are a key for body chemistry change and improvement. Ginseng supports every area of metabolism. Ginseng helps the liver to metabolize fats better. It helps the body to metabolize and regulate sugars better. It has phyto-hormone qualities to balance estrogen levels in women and helps normalize testosterone levels in men. It improves digestion for better nutrient use, and less food storage. It energizes the body so you don't eat as much. It enhances thermogenic activity in the body, by helping re-activate brown fat activity, and extending the effects of other thermogenic herbs. Formulas like Crystal Star THERMO-GINSENG™ extract and capsules work extremely well.

#2)   **CONSCIOUSLY EAT LESS.** As metabolism slows, you don't need to fuel it up as much, because your body doesn't use up the nutrients like it once did. If you eat like you did in your 20's and 30's, your body will store too much, mostly as fat.

***Make sure you are eating a low fat diet. Even with all the fat-conscious foods on the market today, Americans still consume almost 40% of their calories as fat. Your fat intake should be about 20% for **weight control,** 15% or less for **weight loss.** No-fat is not good for weight loss, though. The body goes into a survival mode if you eliminate **all** fat, shedding its highly active lean muscle tissue to reduce the body's need for food. If lean muscle tissue decreases, fat burning slows or stops.

***Consciously control your food portions. Portion control is a cornerstone for weight control. Even though your diet may be healthy and the foods reasonably low in fat, there's no way you can eat all you want of anything. This is hard if you like to eat a lot of your favorite foods. One way to do this effectively is to eat smaller meals every two to three hours to keep your appetite hole from gnawing, and to keep metabolic rates high. Small meals virtually prevent carbohydrates and proteins from being converted into fat.

***Control your appetite with safe, gentle herbal appetite suppressants. Superfood herbs like barley grass, spirulina, sea vegetables and alfalfa help control appetite, and may be used between meals to almost instantly decrease the craving for high-calorie foods. They offer an energy lift that carries throughout the day. Herbal compounds like Crystal Star ENERGY GREEN™ or Green Foods GREEN MAGMA can raise both metabolic rate and activity levels.

#3)   **RAISE YOUR METABOLISM.** A higher metabolic rate means you burn more fat, lose weight easier, and maintain your ideal body weight more comfortably.

***Don't skip meals.....especially breakfast. Many people skip breakfast because it's so easy to rush out the door to work and not miss it. But breakfast is the worst meal to skip if you want to raise metabolism. It sends a **temporary fasting signal** to the brain that food is scarce. So stress hormones increase, and the body begins shedding lean muscle tissue in order to decrease it's need for food. By the time you eat again, your pancreas is so sensitized to a lack of food, that it sharply increases blood insulin levels, the body's signal to make fat.

***Avoid **both sugars and fats** because they slow metabolism. Fats not only have twice the calories, gram for gram, as protein and complex carbohydrates; they also use only 2% of their calories before the fat storage process begins. Protein and carbohydrates burn almost 25% of their calories before storing them as fat. Limit alcohol consumption, even wine, to two glasses or less a day. With seven calories per gram, sugars from alcohol shift metabolism in favor of fat depositing; alcohol can also burden the liver and stimulate the appetite.

***Eat fat-burning foods. Foods that raise metabolism are vegetables, whole grains, legumes and fruits. Eat fruits for breakfast or between meals. If you eat them with or after meals, the fructose is likely to be converted to fat by the liver. Eat early in the day to lose weight, when your metabolism is at its best, and when you have hours of activity ahead of you to burn fats.

***Re-activate your fat-burning systems. Use herbs to stoke the metabolic fire. A formula like Crystal Star FEEL GREAT™ with herbal adaptogens such as ginseng, suma, gotu kola, and licorice root, balances the body's homeostasis, especially after 40. Herbal spices, such as cinnamon, ginger, cayenne and cardamom, are thermogenic. Sea vegetables, such as kelp and dulse possess oceanic iodine to aid the thyroid gland, which governs metabolism.

*** *Add three amino acids to boost metabolism.* L-PHENYLALANINE (LPA), suppresses appetite and reduces food craving. When LPA crosses the blood-brain barrier, the body converts it into two neurotransmitters, dopamine and norepinephrine, to suppress appetite. But, remember that phenylalanine is strong, and should be avoided by those taking anti-depressant medication, those who have high blood pressure, pregnant women, children, and people with phenylketonuria. L-TYROSINE also helps produce norepinephrine and dopamine and reduces appetite. L-CARNITINE accelerates fat metabolism and helps control sugar levels. It is also an appetite suppressant important in the thermogenesis process because it carries fatty acids into the cells' mitochondria furnace. Crystal Star AMINO-ZYME™ caps have these amino acids and others to help you keep metabolism high while dieting.

*** *Drink plenty of water.* Water naturally suppresses appetite, and helps maintain a high metabolic rate. In fact, water may be the most important catalyst for increased fat burning. It increases the liver's main functions of detoxification and metabolism, and allows it to metabolize more fats. For those concerned with fluid retention, high water intake actually **decreases bloating,** because it flushes out sodium and toxins. Expert dieters drink eight glasses of water a day. They know each pound of fat burned releases 22 ounces of water which is flushed away along with the by-products of fat breakdown.

*** *Get moderate doses of sunlight.* The sun receives a lot of criticism today, but sunlight in moderation increases metabolism and food digestion. One of the best choices is to eat outdoors. Sunlight produces metabolic effects in the body similar to that of physical training.

#4) **EXERCISE FOR SURE.** Exercise especially before you eat, because exercise suppresses appetite and increases metabolism. Walking is considered to be superior to running as a fat-burning exercise. Walking burns fat and increases your metabolic rate for hours afterwards. An exercise heart rate around 60% of the maximum burns mostly fat. Intense exercise that causes the heart rate to rise over 80% of the maximum actually decreases metabolism, because it burns muscle tissue instead of fat. Studies on walking and weight loss showed that in test groups who walked at different rates for six months or more, the slowest walking group lost the most weight. Kinda blows a hole in the old excuse that exercise is too hard, right?

*** *Exercise to build and maintain lean muscle.* Loss of calorie-gobbling lean muscle tissue almost guarantees that you'll gain any weight you've lost, back. Lean muscle is highly metabolic tissue. Pound for pound, it burns five times as many calories as other body tissue. Adding just 10 pounds of muscle tissue can burn one pound of fat per week, or 52 pounds of fat per year. The best way to increase lean muscle mass is through resistance training, or weight lifting. All it takes to add 10 pounds of muscle is a weight training program for 30 minutes, 3 times a week, for about six months.

Thermogenesis May Be The Key

We hear so much about thermogenesis today. What does it do? What is brown fat? Why is it good for weight control after 40?

Thermogenesis is all about fat burning. About 75% of all the calories you eat goes to keeping you alive and supporting your resting metabolic rate. The rest can be stored as white fat, or can be burned up by special body cells known as brown adipose tissue, or BAT. Brown fat tissue is really a fat-burning factory, burning up calories your body doesn't need, a process called thermogenesis. The more active your brown fat is, the easier it is to maintain a desirable weight. People who eat light but still can't lose weight may have a genetic basis for their obesity. They may not have been born with enough brown fat. If their weight problems started around middle age, the little brown fat they did have may not be working well.

Too much fat-making means too little thermogenesis. Everybody produces heat and increases metabolism after eating, a process known as diet-induced thermogenesis. But the amounts of heat vary widely. Lean people experience a 40% increase in heat production after a meal. Overweight people may have only an increase of 10%. Obesity occurs primarily when brown fat isn't working properly, because thermogenesis doesn't take place, and the body deals with excess calories by storing them as fat. This is especially true in the phenomenon known as middle-aged spread. During middle years, beginning in our late 30's and early 40's, a genetic timer shuts down the thermogenic mechanism. Turning this timer back on is the secret to re-activating thermogenesis and a more youthful metabolism.

Thermogenic herbal stimulants can re-activate brown fat in middle age. Brown fat is present in the body in smaller quantities than white or storage fat, and is located between the shoulder blades, in the armpits, on the back of the neck and surrounding the large blood vessels in the chest and abdomen. Under the right circumstances the body can convert white fat back into calories that can then be disposed of through thermal combustion. This is how, for instance, the famous herbal spa body wraps work.

Here's how thermogenesis works. A special protein, called uncoupling protein, has been identified in brown fat cells. This substance breaks down, or uncouples, the train of biochemical events that the cells use to turn calories into energy. Research shows that sometimes, even though the uncoupling protein produces heat, the resulting energy may not go anywhere, so thermogenesis doesn't happen. Brown fat cells, however, will continue to convert calories into heat as long as they are stimulated, and as long as there is white fat for them to work on. Brown fat activity is also self-perpetuating, because it energizes more uncoupling proteins, produces more brown fat cells, and results in substantially more excess calories being burned off as heat through thermogenesis.

Thermogenic herbal compounds are a good choice for activating the process of thermogenesis. Thermogenic herb formulas have the following effects:
• Herbs can increase thermogenesis without additional support of diet or exercise, although these things offer additional benefits.
• Thermogenic herbs increase blood flow and oxygen to muscle tissue.
• Thermogenic herbs suppress appetite. You eat less with less effort.

•The longer you take thermogenic herbs, the more effective they tend to become, because your body steps up its thermogenic activity.

What about ephedra and thermogenesis? It's effective. Is it safe? Ephedra, an herb used safely for centuries as a broncho-dilator for chest congestion, also has thermogenic properties. Many thermogenic products are formulated with ephedra, because tests show that one of its constituents, ephedrine, stimulates thermogenesis. The advantage of ephedra-based products over calorie-restricted crash dieting is that the body actually loses fat tissue.

Ephedrine acts as an analog to adrenaline, helping to turn on brown fat tissue that has become dormant. Yet ephedrine is tricky to use because the body sets up natural barriers to prevent what it perceives as wasted energy, and requires high dosages of ephedra to overcome them. Unfortunately, high doses of ephedrine, especially if in an isolated concentrate, also act as a central nervous system stimulant, similar to coffee, which sometimes precipitates side effects such as increased blood pressure, heart rate, insomnia and anxiety. Most experts acknowledge that an ephedra-based product should not be used continuously because of potential long-term strain to the adrenal glands. But since the body adapts to the increased stimulation by growing more active brown fat, the thermogenic need for the product **naturally decreases** over time.

In order to use less ephedrine, some thermogenic weight loss products now combine ephedrine with caffeine and aspirin, about 75mg of ephedrine, 150mg of caffeine, and 300mg of aspirin, claiming that this ratio is still effective for weight loss with much less ephedrine. To me, this is a highly stimulative compound with even more dangerous side effects than the original ephedrine. It's the kind of chemical mix that's easy to over-dose on.

There are better answers from herbs. There are brown fat stimulating herbs that can be used in place of ephedra without heart-speeding effects. SIDA CORDIFOLIA, an Ayurvedic herb from India, contains a form of ephedrine that also raises metabolic rate and increases energy, but is gentler in its action than ephedra. Undesirable effects like nervousness, insomnia and heart palpitations rarely, if ever, occur with sida cordifolia. Sida cordifolia is especially effective in activating brown fat that has gone dormant due to genetic signals and the process of aging. It gently raises the levels of thermogenesis after 40. Crystal Star THERMO-GINSENG™ extract is an effective herbal compound that includes sida cordifolia and ginseng as well as other thermogenic benefits.

We've all heard a lot about HCA. Does it really boost thermogenesis? HCA, hydroxy-citric acid, known commercially as CITRIN™ or CITRI-MAX™, comes from the fruit garcinia cambogia. It is an effective appetite suppressant, especially when used with biologically active chromium. Twenty-five years of study indicate that HCA is both safe and effective in weight control, especially after metabolism slows down in middle age years.

HCA influences three important weight control processes: 1) it inhibits the body's fat storage; 2) it controls appetite; and 3) it increases calorie burning. HCA also works through enzyme function. Our bodies convert the calories we eat into energy. Excess calories are stored in the liver and muscles as glycogen, the major form of energy stored in the body. When blood sugar levels drop and we need more energy, hormones send a message to the liver or muscles to release glycogen. Enzymes then split the glycogen molecules into glucose, which travel to the brain and other organs to provide energy.

But, this process breaks down when we take in more calories than we need to meet our energy demands. The liver holds the glycogen for a few hours, but when it reaches its capacity, the leftover amount is converted to acetyl-coenzyme A, and then into fatty acids, which are stored throughout the body. The body accomplishes this conversion with an enzyme called ATP-citrate lyase. HCA inhibits ATP-citrate lyase action by a process called competitive inhibition. It allows the liver to synthesize more glycogen, and increase the fullness signal to the brain, suppressing appetite.

The appetite-suppressing action of HCA is different than over-the-counter appetite suppressants, such as phenyl-propanolamine, and prescription medications like amphet-amines, methamphetamines, fenfluramine, phenmetrazine and di-ethyl-propion. They act on the brain and central nervous system, and may lead to depression, nervousness, insomnia, hypertension and rapid heart rate, especially with long term use. HCA's appetite-suppressing activity works peripherally. It doesn't enter the central nervous system directly, but instead stimulates an increase in the amount of glycogen that the liver produces to curb appetite. HCA is thus able to inhibit lipogenesis, the process by which the body produces and stores fat. A New York study found that HCA inhibited lipogenesis quickly, within 150 minutes of administration.

The most valuable research on HCA shows that it efficiently activates thermogenesis, preserving lean muscle tissue during fat loss on a reduced-calorie diet. Reducing calories below what it takes to maintain your current weight always causes some lean muscle loss along with the fat, but preserving as much of lean muscle tissue as possible is vital to long-lasting weight control, because it is the body's most metabolically active tissue. It can burn calories even at rest while fat tissue is dead weight.

Loss of calorie-gobbling lean muscle contributes to the yo-yo syndrome. Your body regains fat tissue on less calories after your diet is over. An extremely low-calorie diet, below 1200 calories for women and 1500 for men, usually results in loss of more lean muscle tissue. HCA along with exercise helps maintain and build muscle, making it possible to control your weight even with more calories. A balanced, effective herbal formula like Crystal Star THERMO-CITRIN GINSENG™ caps includes HCA as well as other thermogenic herbs. Taking thermogenic herbs with 500mg of Carnitine, and 200mcg of Chromium Picolinate offers even better results.

Weight loss is not easy in today's lifestyle. Reaching your ideal weight is a victory. Keeping it requires vigilance, especially in light of today's processed foods and fast lifestyle. But it can be successful on a long-term basis, and without side effects.

Here are some watchwords:

•Try to lose 1% of your body weight per week. More than that and the body doesn't adjust properly. You will probably end up regaining the weight.

•Don't worry about the pounds and the calories. Worry about the inches and the fat. Muscle is heavy. Adding exercise to your life and correcting your diet composition will take inches off a lot faster than pounds. Watch your clothing size go down! It is a real achievement!

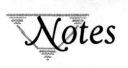

Notes

Notes

Section 8

Diagnostics:
A How-To Section

One of the most valuable assets of conventional medicine is its diagnostic arsenal of medical tests and laboratory analyses. Yet, without taking any of the authority away from these important medical tools, there are many personal information techniques that we can use to determine a nutrient deficiency or measure our body's status during a healing program.

Most of these methods have been part of traditional natural healing for centuries, but seem to have been forgotten, or underestimated in our society's current enchantment with high tech science.

This section includes personal body element deficiency tests you can do yourself, and home healing protocols and techniques you can use to maximize your healing program. Many tests allow you to chart your progressive improvement if you perform them over the course of the healing process....a very interesting part of watching your body and immune system at work.

A correct food combining chart is also included as a guide if you wish to maximize your nutrient assimilation.

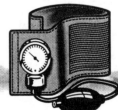

Self Diagnosis Nutrient Tests

Ailment diagnosis has historically been the unchallenged prerogative of conventional protocol. The medical world has maintained that only its complex, expensive and sometimes painful testing proce dures can correctly diagnose health problems. **But is this actually the case?**

Many people feel that much diagnostic testing has little to do with necessary diagnosis, being instead a lawsuit preventive measure, or the result of the enormous, profit-driven establishment between health care providers and health care insurers. These people question the seemingly endless round of annoying, often invasive tests, as they try to take more responsibility for their health.

CAN YOU REALISTICALLY DIAGNOSE YOUR OWN HEALTH PROBLEMS? I believe in many cases, you **can** appraise your health status, especially in uncovering nutrient and gland deficiencies that are based in life-style choices. Key questions in this section can point you in the right direction to determine your health needs.

Note: If you have more than half of the "signs and symptoms" listed after each nutrient you are probably deficient in that nutrient. If you have one-quarter of the symptoms, you are probably slightly deficient. By referencing the Alpha-Index ALTERNATIVE HEALTH CARE ARSENAL *in this book you can learn more about each nutrient and how to get more from your diet or supplements.*

Signs and symptoms of a folic acid deficiency:
- frequent hangnails or slow growing nails and hair
- chronic diarrhea or constipation
- constantly chapped or cracked lips, and chronic gum infections or receding/ bleeding gums
- a history of intestinal parasitic and/or fungal infection
- a history of abnormal pap smears, cervical dysplasia and/or cervical cancer
- a history of chronic anemia unresponsive to iron or B_{12} therapy
- one or more children with birth defects, such as spina bifida
- celiac disease and/or wheat allergy
- chronic mental illness, such as psychosis, anxiety, depression or schizophrenia
- breathing difficulties or a chronic cough
- diminished resistance to infection; slow wound healing, frequent muscle cramps

Factors that contribute to folic acid deficiency:
- eating mostly microwave cooked, canned, boiled or fried foods that kill food enzymes
- smoking cigarettes, cigars or pipes, or using chewing tobacco
- taking long courses of birth control pills, antibiotics, Dilantin, Tagamet, Zantac or Methotrexate
- taking antacids or aspirin on a daily basis
- chemotherapy or radiation therapy

✣

Signs and symptoms of a Vitamin B_{12} deficiency:
- dark circles under the eyes, usually from chronic constipation
- chronic fatigue, usually because of anemia; frequent bursitis attacks
- lack of appetite and taste, or unexplained weight loss
- premature graying of the hair
- frequent depression, anxiety, or psychotic behavior
- a history of Crohn's disease, ulcerative colitis or IBS, and swollen and/or inflamed tongue

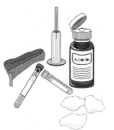

Other factors contributing to B_{12} deficiency:
- taking antacids, Tagamet or Zantac on a daily basis, regularly using cortisone or cortisone creams
- having your stomach stapled or a portion removed, or your lower small intestine removed
- a completely vegetarian diet with no meat or dairy protein sources
- long courses of birth control pills

✣

Signs and symptoms of a biotin deficiency:
- alopecia or hair loss from the scalp, usually with dandruff/ seborrhea, or cowlicks
- mood swings or long lasting, unexplained depression
- nausea, lack of appetite, or intolerance to sweets, or a history of diabetes or high blood sugar
- muscle pains and aches, dermatitis skin inflammation, pallor of the skin and loss of skin pigment
- delayed body development or growth, a current and/or family history of male pattern baldness
- a history of candida albicans infections, or high cholesterol and/or triglyceride levels

Other factors contributing to biotin deficiency:
- taking long courses of antibiotics, eating large amounts of refined sugar, or drinking hard alcohol beverages daily.

Note: The preceding problems are B vitamin deficiencies. B vitamins work best when taken together. I recommend taking a complete B vitamin supplement rather than any of the B vitamins separately.

Signs and symptoms of a Vitamin C deficiency:
- easy bruising, easy muscle and tendon injury, frequent nosebleeds, delayed wound healing
- bleeding, purplish gums, loose or sore teeth, tendency to form plaque or tartar
- heightened susceptibility to infections and colds, and sensitive to extremes in temperature
- arthritis, a history of degenerative joint disease, or lower back pain
- liver spots, spots or floaters in the eyes, frequent hemorrhoids
- thinning and/or premature aging of the skin
- insomnia, depression or listlessness, loss of appetite
- a history of learning or reading impairment

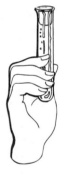

Other factors contributing to Vitamin C deficiency:
- low dietary intake of fresh fruits and vegetables
- high stress life-style
- regularly taking aspirin, or anti-inflammatory drugs like Motrin; or birth control pills
- taking cortisone or applying cortisone cream on a daily or weekly basis
- prolonged use of cocaine, crack, heroin or marijuana; or prolonged periods in the past
- smoking cigarettes or exposure to second-hand smoke on a regular basis
- exposure to excessive quantities of chemical or exhaust fumes, or exposure on a regular basis to X-rays

Those at highest risk for Vitamin C deficiency:
- patients taking anticoagulants, or long courses of cortisone, antibiotics or aspirin
- cigarette smokers, their children and spouses; chewing tobacco users, alcoholics and recreational drug users
- nursing home occupants
- workers exposed to Vitamin C- destroying chemicals, such as gas station attendants, beauticians chemical and nuclear plant employees, or anyone who works with toxic chemicals, truck drivers and heavy equipment operators, employees of synthetic fiber plants, dry cleaners, airline mechanics and ground crews, oil and gas refinery employees, and sewage treatment plant employees.

Signs and symptoms of a Vitamin D deficiency:
- insomnia, irritability or sadness, especially in winter or long rainy seasons
- rapid and/or irregular heartbeat, frequent muscle cramps or spasms
- nearsightedness or cataracts, easy bruising and/or nosebleeds
- chronic diarrhea, chronic back or leg pain, or arthritis joint pain
- chronic psoriasis or eczema, adult acne or rosacea
- very fair skin
- low dietary intake of Omega-3 oils from fish like salmon, halibut, mackerel, sardines or herring
- a strict vegetarian diet with no meat or dairy protein sources
- dietary lactose intolerance, a history of duodenal ulcer
- a history of high blood pressure, liver, kidney or pancreatic disease, celiac disease or gluten intolerance

Other factors contributing to Vitamin D deficiency:
- not getting enough sunlight.
- taking long courses of Dilantin, phenobarbital, Tagamet or Zantac.
- living in an area with heavy air pollution.

✤

Signs and symptoms of a Vitamin K deficiency:
- easy bruising with peripheral blood vessels bursting easily
- a history of hemorrhoids or bursting blood vessels in the eyes
- spider or varicose veins
- spontaneous hemorrhaging from the ears, nose or rectum.
- intermittent and/or chronic diarrhea
- a history of repeated miscarriages
- low intake of dark green leafy vegetables
- a portion of the small intestines or colon removed
- intestinal parasitic infection, or chronic candidiasis yeast infections
- a history of Crohn's disease, irritable bowel syndrome, dumping syndrome or ulcerative colitis
- a history of pancreatic or liver disease
- a history of gallbladder attacks or gallstones, or gallbladder removal
- a very low cholesterol diet and/or long courses of cholesterol-lowering medication
- a history of celiac disease or gluten intolerance
- suffering a stroke or a significant family history of stroke
- having osteoporosis
- taking mineral oil or castor oil on a regular basis

Other factors contributing to Vitamin K deficiency:
- taking antibiotics and/or birth control pills on a regular basis, or over long periods of time in the past
- taking Coumadin or Heparin, blood thinners
- consuming chlorinated water
- low dietary intake of sprouts and other rich greens

✤

Signs and symptoms of a calcium deficiency:
- joint pain
- slow pulse rate
- nervousness and irritability
- muscle tics and twitches, and/or leg cramps
- chronic back and/or hip pain
- loose teeth, and tendency to form cavities
- brittle or vertically ridged nails
- a history of high blood pressure
- chronic headaches
- numbness and/or tingling of the extremities
- spastic stomach, or irritable bowel syndrome
- chronic muscle and neck tension
- little or no exposure to sunshine
- a dislike of fresh fish and/or milk products
- taking long courses of calcium channel blockers
- having undergone or undergoing chemotherapy
- bedridden and/or wheelchair-bound
- little or no exercise

Other factors contributing to a calcium deficiency:
- consuming large amounts of coffee and/or sugar; smoking cigarettes, pipes or cigars
- long courses of cortisone or using cortisone creams, or regularly taking antacids or tetracycline

Signs and symptoms of a chromium deficiency:

- blood sugar disturbances; intolerance to sugar or starch, elevated blood sugar and/or diabetes
- difficulty losing weight, a tendency to gain weight after eating sugars and/or starches; chronic obesity
- chronic fatigue, chronic depression and/or anxiety
- cravings for sugars and/or starches, feeling sleepy after eating starchy or sugary foods
- poor muscle tone and/or muscular weakness; nearsighted or frequent blurry vision
- unexplained, sudden loss of weight, episodes of shakiness
- a history of infertility and/or reduced sperm count
- a history of cataracts or macular degeneration
- a history of arterial blockage, hardening of the arteries, or coronary artery disease
- high blood cholesterol and/or triglyceride levels
- eating lots of white flour products, like white bread, buns, muffins, pasta, crackers or doughnuts

Other factors contributing to chromium deficiency:
- consuming refined sugar (as hidden sugar in foods or beverages) on a daily basis.
- consuming alcoholic beverages - 4 or more drinks per week.

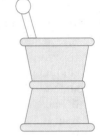

Signs and symptoms of a copper deficiency:

- heart rhythm disturbances, suffering from hardening of the arteries
- alopecia (patchy hair loss); chronic skin rashes, or rosacea
- chronic diarrhea; a long history of high cholesterol
- chronic fatigue, usually because of anemia; infertility
- fragile or brittle bones, or osteoporosis; slow healing of fractures or sprains
- frequent numbness in the extremities; difficulty breathing
- heavy perspiration and bitter taste in the mouth
- a personal history of diabetes, or a significant family history of diabetes
- heavy and regular intake of sugar, particularly fructose; eating primarily processed foods

Certain people are at exceptionally high risk for copper deficiency. These groups include:
- those undergoing high-dose zinc therapy; gastrectomy patients; people with wheat intolerance
- people taking multiple medications; cancer patients undergoing chemotherapy or radiation
- people who eat a high sugar diet; patients with chronic liver disease, including cirrhosis and hepatitis
- individuals who have had a portion of their intestines or stomach removed

Signs and symptoms of an iodine deficiency:

- cystic and/or sore ovaries or fibrocystic breast disease
- severe menstrual cramps or heavy menstrual bleeding
- heightened susceptibility to infections like bronchitis, pneumonia, ear infections or strep throat
- chronic fatigue or lethargy, especially morning fatigue that improves as the day goes on
- chronic skin infections, such as boils, acne, fungal infections
- excess mucous and/or thick mucous in the throat; stuffy sinuses
- cold extremities or reduced body temperature
- having an overactive or underactive thyroid; a history of goiter
- if you are on a low sodium diet
- low dietary intake of fish or sea food; eating a total vegetarian diet with no seafood or sea vegetables
- a history of infertility and/or low sperm count, a history of low libido
- heavy cellulite patches
- having high cholesterol, above 220

Thyroid-nourishing, iodine-rich nutrients include:
potassium, tyrosine, magnesium, vitamin C, thiamine, riboflavin, pantothenic acid, niacin, folic acid, coenzyme Q-10, zinc and copper. Sea foods and sea vegetables are primary thyroid health foods.

Signs and symptoms of an iron deficiency:
- chronic fatigue; lack of appetite; constipation
- spoon shaped nails, or vertical ridges on the fingernails, brittle hair and/or nails
- confusion or memory loss; irritability or depression, usually with chronic headaches
- rapid heartbeat after minimal exercise
- inflamed and/or sore tongue, difficulty swallowing
- fragile, brittle bones; hair loss, especially in females
- tingling of the fingers or toes and sensitivity to cold; a history of rheumatoid arthritis
- heavy menstrual flow for a prolonged time; paleness of the facial skin, usually from anemia

Other factors contributing to Iron deficiency:
- taking antacids on a regular basis
- drinking three or more cups of black or green tea every day
- taking aspirin or anti-inflammatory drugs, like Naprosyn, Indocin, Clinoril, etc., on a daily basis

✣

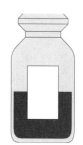

Signs and symptoms of an potassium deficiency:
- adult acne; arthritis and/or swollen joints
- chronic constipation, or chronic or intermittent diarrhea
- chronic depression and headaches; blood sugar disturbances
- abdominal bloating and edema, yet frequent urination with large volumes
- irregular or rapid heartbeat; light-headedness and/or episodes of fainting
- frequent muscle weakness or cramps, constant fatigue
- facial tics and twitching of the muscles, or tremors; vomiting frequently (once a week or more)
- easy injuries during exercise
- ow intake of fresh fruits, vegetables, nuts and seeds
- a history of high blood pressure, a recent stroke, or other heart/circulatory disease

Other factors contributing to potassium deficiency:
- using diuretics on a daily or weekly basis. Taking antacids or Zantac or Tagamet on a daily basis
- consuming aspirin, Motrin or similar anti-inflammatory drugs on a daily or weekly basis
- taking commercial laxatives daily; taking drugs containing cortisone
- consuming hard liquor on a daily basis

Potassium deficiency is a proven contributing cause of a number of illnesses, including:

arthritis, kidney stones, atrial fibrillation, adrenal insufficiency, celiac disease, high blood pressure, coronary artery disease, ulcerative colitis, hypothyroidism, irritable bowel syndrome, Alzheimer's disease, multiple sclerosis, myasthenia gravis, Crohn's disease, lupus, atherosclerosis, diabetes and stroke.

✣

Signs and symptoms of a bioflavonoid deficiency:
- easy bruising; retinal hemorrhages
- inflammation and/or swelling of the joints; arthritis or swollen extremities
- fragile blood vessels, varicose and/or spider veins; a tendency to form blood clots
- heavy menstrual bleeding, and repeated miscarriages; blood in the urine or stool or hemorrhoids
- fever blisters; shingles or genital herpes outbreaks
- a history of coronary artery disease or hardening of the arteries
- a history of stomach and/or duodenal ulcers
- having had a stroke or have a significant family history of stroke
- low dietary intake of fresh fruits and/or vegetables
- suffer from failing vision; glaucoma

Other factors contributing to bioflavonoid deficiency:
- consuming aspirin, Motrin or other anti-inflammatory drugs on a daily or weekly basis
- a low dietary inertia of fresh fruits and vegetables

Signs and symptoms of enzyme deficiency:

- excessive gas, fullness and/or bloating after meals
- constipation or poorly formed stools, or chronic diarrhea
- greasy, pale or gray stools with undigested food particles in stool; ropy mucous in the stool
- chronic heartburn and rectal burning; low stomach acid and/or a history of pancreatitis
- eczema and/or psoriasis;
- hives and/or other severe allergic reactions
- slow growing nails and/or hair, white spots on the fingernails
- a history of diabetes; a significant family history of diabetes
- low dietary intake of fresh fruit and vegetables, and eating mostly cooked or microwaved foods
- eating ravenously or excessively fast

Other factors contributing to enzyme deficiency:
- consuming foods/beverages containing artificial sweeteners on a daily basis
- a diet high in refined sugar; consuming hard alcoholic beverages on a daily basis
- eating processed foods or fast foods on a daily basis; drinking five or more cups of coffee per day
- smoking or using chewing tobacco

❖

Signs and symptoms of Co-Q10 deficiency:

- high blood pressure; a history of congestive heart failure
- muscular weakness; severe muscle pain, particularly after exercising
- heart rhythm disturbances, enlarged heart
- increasing susceptibility to colds, flu and infections; delayed wound healing
- receding gums; chronic gum infections and foul breath
- chronic kidney disease;
- chronic lung infection and/or asthma
- accelerated aging of the skin
- great difficulty losing weight even while dieting
- an immune deficiency disorder, such as HIV or lupus
- a history of angina and/or coronary artery disease
- eating a completely vegetarian diet with no meat, fish or poultry protein sources

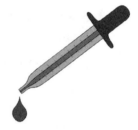

❖

Signs and symptoms of essential fatty acid (EFA) deficiency:

- dry, flaky skin, brittle hair and/or fingernails; adult acne and/or enlarged facial pores
- chronic eczema, psoriasis or dermatitis
- chronic diarrhea; Crohn's disease or irritable bowel syndrome
- easy bruising and slow wound healing; tingling in the arms and legs
- have attention deficit disorder
- irritability and/or nervousness, or PMS
- dryness of the mouth and throat, especially when speaking, dryness or cracks behind the ears
- have Sjogren's syndrome and/or lupus
- have emphysema, asthma, or other chronic lung disease
- suffer from chronic joint pain or arthritis
- a history of sluggish kidneys, chronic kidney disease, and/or bladder infections
- a history of prostate problems
- a history of infertility or impotence, or a history of repeated miscarriages

Other factors contributing to EFA deficiency:
- taking aspirin or other anti-inflammatory drugs, cortisone or prednisone on a daily or weekly basis
- consuming margarine or refined sugars on a daily or weekly basis
- drinking hard liquor on a daily or weekly basis
- smoking or chewing tobacco

❖

Signs and symptoms of low hydration and water deficiency:

- chronic constipation and headaches; hemorrhoids or varicose veins
- adult acne
- dry mouth and/or eyes; dry, leathery skin, dry nasal membranes, dry or chapped lips
- easily shocked by static electricity
- large, daily coffee or beer intake; large amounts of black tea on a daily basis
- low water intake - consuming less that 2 glasses of water per day
- dark colored and/or foul smelling urine, recurrent urinary tract infections
- taking diuretics on a daily or regular basis; a history of kidney stones

Signs and symptoms of a lactobacillus deficiency:

- intestinal gas; constipation and alternating diarrhea; a history of diverticulitis or diverticulosis
- hard pebble-like stools and hemorrhoids; mucous in the stool, foul-smelling stools
- easy bruising; recurrent nosebleeds
- psoriasis and/or eczema
- indigestion and/or heartburn
- long courses of antibiotics; a history of chronic candidiasis
- regularly eat commercial meat and poultry
- rarely or never eat fermented milk products; bottle fed instead of breast fed as a baby
- frequent intestinal flus or bouts of food poisoning
- frequent bouts of ulcerative colitis, irritable bowel syndrome, or Crohn's disease
- drinking lots of chlorinated water

Diseases associated with a deficiency of lactobacillus include:

chronic candidiasis, psoriasis, eczema, lymphoma, high cholesterol, hepatitis, irritable bowel syndrome, colitis, diverticulitis, dermatitis, acne, heart disease, stomach acidity, intestinal parasites, lupus and colon cancer.

THE FOLLOWING QUESTIONNAIRE CAN HELP YOU DETERMINE THE HEALTH STATUS OF YOUR GLANDS AND HORMONES, CRITICALLY IMPORTANT PARTS OF YOUR BODY - INVOLVED IN ALMOST EVERY AILMENT AND SIGNIFICANT TO YOUR WELL-BEING.

Sluggish Thyroid Syndrome is perhaps the most commonly occurring hormonal disturbance in America today. It afflicts millions of people of all ages and sexes, although adult women are its usual victims. Experts estimate as many as one in four Americans suffer from sluggish thyroid function.

As the master of metabolism, the thyroid gland exerts control over body temperature (reduced body temperature is the most common consequence of low thyroid function), digestive enzyme synthesis, stomach acid production, calorie burning (thermogenesis), fat and protein synthesis, and white blood cell activity. The thyroid is also a crucial player in the synthesis and activity of sex hormones.

Signs and symptoms of a sluggish thyroid:

- lethargy, especially tired in the morning and energetic at night; chronically low body temperature
- slow or slurred speech; inability to translate thoughts into action; hoarseness or coarse voice
- swelling of the face and/or eyelids; swelling of hands and/or ankles
- chronically cold hands and feet; require long periods to get "warmed up" after exposure to cold
- bloating and indigestion after eating; easily constipated
- hair loss from the outer third of the eyebrows; brittle; slow growing nails or dry or coarse hair and/or skin
- depression which is worse in the winter or on overcast days
- chronic weight problems; chronic headaches
- PMS and/or menstrual difficulties; generally nervous or emotionally unstable; frequent heart palpitations
- infertility; a history of repeated miscarriages; lack of sexual desire
- inability to sweat, or sometimes to tear

- severe muscle cramps, especially at night; tendency to bruise easily
- poor hand-to-eye coordination; a history of carpal tunnel syndrome
- a history of ovarian cysts
- chronic breast inflammation and/or infections, or fibrocystic breast disease (lumpy breasts)
- low stomach acid and generally poor digestion
- don't feel rested even after sleeping long hours
- skin has developed a yellowish tint with enlarged facial pores
- a history of high cholesterol and/or triglyceride levels
- chronic cracks in the bottom of the heels

Some diet choices impair thyroid function. Avoid refined sugar, fluoride toothpaste, hard liquor, hydrogenated fats and excessive caffeine. A number of foods contain substances called goitrogens, which interfere with thyroid activity. They should be eaten cooked to inactivate the thyroid-blocking components. This mainly includes cruciferous vegetables, and legumes - cabbage, kale, cauliflower, broccoli, brussels sprouts, peanuts, beans, and spinach.

Adrenal Failure Syndrome is a condition of adrenal insufficiency suffered by tens of millions of Americans. Its incidence is rising every year largely due to extreme nutritional deficiency from an over-processed food diet and chronic emotional strain. The adrenal glands are the primary body system for fighting stress. Keep them healthy to ward off mental or physical stresses. Emotional strain and anger are the most significant adrenal disrupters, with profound negative effects. Stress-reducing techniques along with improved nutrition usually result in regenerating exhausted adrenals, and a return to normal function.

Virtually all people with adrenal insufficiency suffer from severe allergic tendencies, because the adrenals are the primary means for preventing or reversing allergic reactions. Adrenal failure is also associated with hypoglycemia, because the adrenals exert potent control over blood sugar status in order to prevent sugar levels from dropping during stress. Weakened adrenal glands allow Blood Sugar Collapse Syndrome. (See next page.)

Adrenal glands, located atop the kidneys, are normally golf-ball size. If nutrition is poor, or high stress are prolonged, they become significantly enlarged (known as cellular hypertrophy), a state where adrenal gland cells multiply excessively in an attempt to supply the body with enough steroid hormones to handle the stress. Poor nutrition aggravates the problem, because proper nutrients are required for steroid synthesis to normalize. If high stress continues and nutritional deficits are neglected, the adrenal glands become so weak that even insignificant stresses can precipitate a noticeable decline in health.

In fact, the adrenals can ultimately self-destruct and shrink, a condition known as adrenal atrophy, which may result in a potentially life-threatening disorder called Addison's Disease, where the adrenals are totally incapable of producing steroid hormones. People with Addison's disease are unable to cope with stress at all.

ADRENAL HEALTH SELF-TEST: A common diagnostic performed by many chiropractors, massage therapists and naturopaths. Home blood pressure testing kits make this test an easy way to monitor your own adrenal health.

1. Lie down and rest for 5 minutes. Take a blood pressure reading.
2. Stand up and immediately take another blood pressure reading. If your blood pressure is lower after you stand up, your adrenals are probably functioning poorly. The amount of drop in blood pressure is usually in ratio to the amount of adrenal dysfunction.

Signs and symptoms of exhausted adrenals or adrenal failure:
- constant fatigue and muscular weakness; sweating or wetness of hands and feet caused by nervousness
- mood swings, sometimes paranoia; depression often relieved by eating
- frequent heart palpitations; light-headed sensation and/or fainting spells
- chronic heartburn; vague indigestion or abdominal pain; low blood pressure
- alternating constipation and diarrhea; infrequent urination
- blood sugar disturbances; cravings for salt or sweets; lack of thirst; food sensitivities/allergies
- headaches, particularly migraines, along with insomnia
- extreme sensitivity to odors and/or noises; intolerance to alcohol, tobacco or exhaust smoke
- clenching and/or grinding of teeth, especially at night; chronic pain in the lower neck and upper back
- inability to concentrate and/or confusion, usually along with clumsiness
- easily frustrated with a tendency to cry; tendency to have guilt feelings
- compulsive behavior; panic attacks

- an unusually small jawbone or chin; lower teeth crowded, unequal in length, or misaligned
- a chronic breathing disorder, particularly asthma
- a tendency to develop yeast or fungal infections
- an excessively low cholesterol level (below 150mg/dl)
- bouts of severe infections, like TB, blood poisoning, sepsis or hepatitis?

Other factors that affect adrenal health:
- taking cortisone pills, creams or ointment (or prednisone) for more than a month at a time
- drinking caffeinated beverages on a daily basis; consuming alcoholic beverages on a daily basis
- consuming large amounts of refined sugar throughout your life
- smoking cigarettes

❖

Blood Sugar Imbalance Syndrome is a result of exceedingly common blood sugar disorders in the U.S., primarily a result of the high sugar consumption most Americans practice. Some experts believe as many as one in two Americans are affected.

As with all body needs, balance is the key. Both too little and too much blood sugar is dangerous. Blood glucose is the primary fuel for the cells. Too much blood sugar and too little balancing insulin, invites diabetes to develop. Too little available blood sugar, and too much blood-sugar-depressing insulin invites hypoglycemia or low blood sugar to develop. (See DIABETES & HYPOGLYCEMIA)

Yet the Blood Sugar Imbalance Syndrome is the most under-diagnosed, as well as misdiagnosed, of all medical conditions in America today. Physicians are generally unaware of how prevalent blood sugar disorders are. Yet, the most accurate method for diagnosing blood sugar disorders, the 6-hour glucose tolerance test, is only rarely performed by physicians even if a blood sugar disorder is suspected. To complicate matters, the symptoms of blood sugar disorders occur in a wide variety of other illnesses. For example, depression, fatigue, and anxiety are among its most common symptoms.

In fact, most visible symptoms are mental and personality related, because the brain consumes a greater amount of glucose for its weight than any other organ. It relies almost exclusively on glucose as its energy source. As a result, a sudden drop in the blood sugar causes disorientation, anxiety, anger, agitation, depression, and frustration. Some people simply fall asleep or faint when their blood sugar level collapses.

Signs and symptoms of blood sugar imbalance
- mood swings; crying spells
- fatigue after eating, worse if dessert is included; sleepiness after eating sugar, fruit, or starch
- insomnia (especially waking up after falling asleep)
- episodes of agitation or temper tantrums
- dizziness and/or fainting spells; legs feel rubbery or weak; episodes of blurry vision
- episodes of shakiness and/or tremors; clumsiness; heart rhythm disturbances
- headaches (worse after skipping a meal)
- episodes of cold sweats and/or nausea; frequent indigestion
- attention deficit (or childhood behavioral problems); paranoia and/or anxiety; panic attacks
- sudden drop in energy level during mid-morning or mid-day
- indecisiveness, constant worrying; poor concentration
- episodes of uncontrollable eating (binging)
- constantly craving sweets and/or starches; an intense craving for salty foods
- a history of liver and/or pancreatic disease; a significant family history of diabetes

Other factors that affect sugar balance:
- heavy alcohol consumption; consuming sweets on a daily basis
- eating fast food on a weekly basis (pizza, hot dogs, hamburgers, subs, doughnuts, etc.)
- taking birth control pills on a regular basis or having done so in the past for two years or more
- taking large doses of cortisone, orally or injectable

❖

Yeast Fungus Syndrome and fungal infections have become prominent plagues of Western civilization. As many as one in four Americans suffer from chronic fungal infections. Many feel this is another consequence of our sugary, starchy Western diet, because fungi use sugars and starches as their primary food. Fungal growth is only moderately influenced by natural sugars in fruits; it is excessively stimulated by refined or heated sugar.

Western medicine's overuse of antibiotics is an another factor for the increase in yeast infections. Most physicians regard antibiotics as non-toxic, and prescribe them repeatedly without concern or warning about side effects. Tens of millions of Americans consume antibiotic drugs every year. Yet with each dose, the risk for chronic fungal infections rises. Add to this the consumption of cortico-steroid drugs like prednisone, Tagamet, Zantac, antacids, and asthma medications, and the number of Americans regularly using drugs which enhance fungal growth exceeds 500 million!

Antibiotics are particularly aggressive in destroying the body's protective intestinal bacteria, leaving the entire digestive tract vulnerable to yeast and fungus colonization. Fungus invasions cause severe inflammation, and produce highly toxic biochemicals which disrupt immune function; chemicals so powerful that immune response against the yeast or fungus is neutralized. The mucous membranes are the primary site of damage; the liver, spleen, kidneys, ovaries, thyroid gland, and adrenals are all susceptible. Fungi also commonly infect the skin and nails. Sites which retain moisture between the toes, the scalp, the groin, and the umbilicus are especially vulnerable.

Signs and symptoms of a chronic yeast infection:
* low body temperature; reduced white blood count
* indigestion or abdominal discomfort after eating fruits or other sweet foods
* itching of the vagina, penis, groin and/or rectum; itching of the ear canals or belly button
* rectal or vaginal burning, especially during or after urination; recurrent urinary tract infections.
* chronic vaginal discharge (a white, off-white, or cottage-cheese consistency, with a foul odor)
* bloating after meals; persistent indigestion and/or heartburn
* intolerance to alcoholic drinks of any kind; sensitivity to chemicals, their odors, and/or cigarette smoke
* seborrhea or heavy dandruff on the scalp, face, or hands; skin or scalp itching after eating sugar or fruit
* a history of eczema and/or psoriasis;
* chronic athlete's foot, toenail or finger nail fungus, ringworm infection, or oral, rectal or vaginal thrush
* chronic constipation or diarrhea; a history of ulcerative colitis or Crohn's disease
* attention deficit disorder and spaciness
* severe intolerance to cold weather, usually with a hanging-on sore or scratchy throat
* a history of fungal infection of the internal organs, e.g. lungs, brain, kidneys, bladder, etc.
* sensitivity to airborne molds, or moldy or fermented foods like aged cheeses, soy sauce, or baker's yeast
* craving sweets; consuming large amounts of fruit sugars daily, from fruits and fruit juices
* a history of endometriosis and overly painful menstrual cramps

Other factors that aggravate yeast or fungus overgrowth:
* consuming refined sugar on a daily basis; eating commercially raised meats on a daily basis.
* taking antibiotics daily, weekly or monthly; using steroids (cortisone) on a regular basis
* regular use of Tagamet, Zantac or other antacids.

⁑

Intestinal Parasite Infections are the activity of microbes which infect and live off of human tissue. Parasitic illnesses are a major plague of modern society. They both cause and accompany many of today's most virulent diseases, account for many otherwise unexplained conditions, and can be exceedingly difficult to kill. One estimate contends that 25% of New Yorkers currently have a parasitic infection: by the year 2025, experts say 50% of the world's 8.3 billion people will be infested.

Most doctors don't recognize the risk factors or clinical symptoms of parasite infections, and don't test for them. This is probably because parasite symptoms mimic so many other problems: joint and muscle aches, anemia, allergies, skin conditions, nervousness, diarrhea, bloating, constipation, chronic fatigue, or immune dysfunction. Members of the same family can have the same species of parasites yet have completely different clinical symptoms.

Parasites include protozoans like amoebas, giardia and Trichomonas, and various worms, like roundworms, pinworms, hookworms and tapeworms. The major distinction between parasites and bacteria or viruses is that intestinal parasites are larger, in some cases visible to the naked eye. Bacteria and viruses can be seen only through a microscope. Parasites are particularly dangerous because they can infect people three ways - by the live organism itself, its eggs or its cysts.

Both acute and chronic diseases may result from parasitic infections. Acute diseases include flu syndromes, hepatitis, food poisoning, diarrhea, appendicitis, and gallbladder attacks. Chronic diseases include anemia, colitis, intestinal ulcers, liver disease (including cirrhosis), arthritis, immune deficiency, and lung disease. The key to getting rid of a parasite infection is to stimulate immune response against them.

Signs and symptoms of a parasite infection

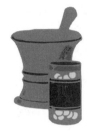

- rectal itching and/or pressure; diarrhea; mucous in stools and poorly formed stools
- muscular wasting and/or weakness
- chronic vague abdominal pain with constant belching
- ravenous appetite; constant or frequent heartburn after eating
- bloating after eating; especially digestive distress after eating fatty foods
- unexplained weight loss or inability to gain weight
- night sweats and insomnia; itchy skin, worse at night; chronic dark circles under the eyes
- severe fatigue usually with a history of chronic anemia
- unexplained nausea and/or vomiting; unexplained fever and/or chills
- illness after a trip overseas or to Mexico that just doesn't go away
- developing diarrheal disease or severe fever while traveling abroad
- living overseas for an extended period of time, especially in Africa or other tropical countries
- drinking untreated or unfiltered water in the wilderness or when traveling overseas

Other factors that put you at risk for a parasite infection:
- frequently eating raw or smoked fish; eating prosciutto and/or home-made sausage
- kissing or sleeping with pets; not properly washing hands after using the restroom

❖

Estrogen Imbalance - until recently, regarded as a scourge of menopause, but becoming a health problem for rising numbers of women as environmental and dietary estrogens enter our lives in greater amounts. (Environmental estrogens are also affecting men, in terms of reduced sperm counts and sperm vitality.)

Estrogen is essential to womanhood itself, but imbalanced estrogen causes undeniable health problems. Estrogen deficiency is only one aspect of the dilemma, because many women have enough estrogen but cannot utilize it properly. Others produce excess estrogen, which becomes toxic. Abnormally high estrogen levels are associated with breast, uterine, and ovarian cancer, and less serious conditions such as cystic ovaries and fibrocystic breast disease. The symptoms of too little, too much, or poorly utilized estrogen are similar. The estrogen is simply imbalanced, as shown through the following test.

Signs and symptoms of estrogen imbalance
- hot flashes or night sweats; insomnia or interrupted sleep
- chronic PMS; breast engorgement, worse during or before periods
- mood swings, worse during or before periods; headaches occurring prior to or during menses
- heavy menstrual bleeding; excessive or painful menstrual cramps; a history of endometriosis
- poor vaginal lubrication; general loss of libido; a history of infertility and/or repeated miscarriages
- a family history or current history of breast cancer or ovarian cancer
- a family history or current history of uterine fibroids; a family history or current history of ovarian cysts
- a family history or current history of fibrocystic breast disease
- becoming weak or tired prior to or during menses; an abnormal pap smear, or cervical dysplasia
- excessive hair growth, especially on the face; excessive amounts of weight on your hips and/or breasts

Other factors that create estrogen imbalance:
- taking birth control pills over a long period of time, or having taken them for 5 or more years in the past
- a partial or complete hysterectomy
- consuming refined sugar, alcohol and/or caffeine on a daily or weekly basis
- consuming margarine, refined vegetable oils and/or deep-fried foods on a daily or weekly basis

❖

Liver Dysfunction is at the heart of a wide variety of diseases and toxic conditions. The liver is the primary organ responsible for the detoxification and decomposition of all molecular compounds in the body. It is the only organ which can efficiently rid the body of wastes from products we commonly consume, like alcohol, drugs, fat-soluble vitamins, preservatives, artificial additives and/or hormones.

Diseases of the liver, like liver cancer, hepatitis, parasite infestation, diabetes, and cirrhosis, are occurring with alarmingly high frequency. Alcoholism is rising today; it is the number one cause of liver disease. As many as 30 million Americans suffer liver damage and hepatitis because of alcohol abuse.

All obese individuals suffer from impaired liver function, because the liver is the first internal organ to become infiltrated with fat. Fat is deposited within the liver cells, known as hepatocytes, greatly impairing their ability to function. In the extreme, fat infiltration causes balloon degeneration of the liver cells or, put simply, cellular death. Usually, when the weight is lost, the liver cells regenerate and function returns to normal. Certain nutrients, notably biotin, lipoic acid, thiamine, inositol, choline, and methionine, aid in liver cell regeneration by reversing fatty liver.

Signs and symptoms of liver dysfunction
- intolerance to alcohol and to sugar with blood sugar disturbances
- tendency to gain weight easily
- chronic constipation; pale, greasy stools that float; foul-smelling bowel gas
- chronic indigestion unrelieved by antacids; intolerance to fatty foods and/or cooking oils
- high cholesterol and/or triglycerides (or excessively low cholesterol - below 140 mg/dl)
- persistent sleepiness and/or fatigue; sudden hair loss; dark circles and/or bags under the eyes
- chronic itching (pruritus); thick ridges on the fingernails
- a history of hepatitis an/or cirrhosis; a history of intestinal or hepatic parasites
- gallbladder removal, or a history of gallstones
- recent chemotherapy treatments
- a history of impaired immunity and/or immune deficiency
- a history of diabetic, or a significant family history of diabetes
- poor blood clotting
- giardia infection, intestinal worms, or amoebic dysentery

Other factors that harm good liver function:
- over-consumption of hard alcohol (5 or more drinks per week)
- being 20 or more pounds overweight
- taking Tylenol on a daily or weekly basis; taking two or more prescription medications on a daily basis
- taking cholesterol-lowering drugs; taking birth control pills for one year or longer at a time
- working with or near toxic chemicals or having worked with them in the past

❖

Malabsorption syndrome occurs when the body can't absorb nutrients from the food into the blood. Millions of Americans suffer from this condition, many unknowingly.

Nutrients are absorbed primarily in the small intestine by billions of microscopic organ systems called intestinal villi that control the absorption of nutrients from the intestine into the bloodstream. Deficiency of certain nutrients, notably zinc and folic acid, leads to the destruction of intestinal villi.

Food allergy is perhaps the most common cause of malabsorption. A dramatic example is allergy to grains (gluten intolerance), which may lead to wholesale destruction of the intestinal villi. Other primary causes include intestinal parasitic infection, enzyme deficiency, intestinal flora imbalance, alcoholism, and reduced stomach acid.

Malabsorption can lead to widespread nutritional deficiencies. Deficiency-induced illnesses, like osteoporosis, lung disease, chronic fatigue syndrome, immune deficiency, emaciation, Crohn's disease, arthritis, anemia, and liver disease, are associated with chronic malabsorption. Some people develop deficits of virtually every major nutrient.

Signs and symptoms of malabsorption
- excessive weight loss or gain
- greasy foul-smelling stools; constipation, particularly after eating certain foods, like aged cheeses
- chronic diarrhea; undigested food in the stool
- bloating and indigestion after meals unrelieved by antacids; foul-smelling intestinal gas
- belch after meals or have chronic heartburn
- premature graying of the hair; hair loss and/or balding; seborrhea and/or severe dandruff

- hangnails, ridges on the nails and/or brittle nails; dry flaky and/or chapped skin
- chronic fatigue with blood sugar disturbances
- spots on the tongue and/or red or inflamed tongue
- a history of diabetes, or hypoglycemia
- a lactose or milk intolerance; a history of celiac disease or gluten intolerance
- an active intestinal or stomach ulcer; liver or pancreatic disease, or cystic fibrosis, or chronic anemia
- a history of Crohn's disease, ulcerative colitis, or irritable bowel syndrome
- a history of intestinal parasitic infection
- systemic skin diseases such as psoriasis, eczema or dermatitis

Other factors that aggravate malabsorption:
- taking antacids, or Zantac or Tagamet on a daily basis; taking antibiotics on a daily or weekly basis
- consuming alcohol on a daily basis
- taking laxatives, including mineral and castor oil, on a daily or weekly basis
- chemotherapy treatments

❖

Do you have an eating disorder?

Not everyone who is on a strict weight loss diet, or who is a strict vegetarian is walking a fine line between health and self-destruction. But if you are concerned about yourself or someone else, the following questions can help you determine whether there might be a problem.

- Do you constantly feel fat?
- Have you repeatedly tried and failed to lose weight?
- Do you ever fast or put yourself on incredibly strict diets?
- Are you preoccupied with food?
- Is there any relationship between your eating and your self-esteem? Do you feel you have lost control?
- Do you sometimes binge, or eat large amounts of food in a short period of time?
- Have you ever tried to "undo" the damage of eating by vomiting, taking laxatives or fasting?
- Do you exercise compulsively? Do you feel guilty or fat if you miss your regular exercise schedule?
- Do you eat when you are under stress or depressed?
- Do you try to hide your eating habits from others?
- Are you a vegetarian solely to be thin, or is it for other reasons?
- Do you feel guilty when you eat meat and dairy, or caloric and high-fat vegetarian foods?
- Do you prepare food for others but refuse to eat it yourself? Do you stick to a rigid routine of eating?
- Do you still think you're fat even after losing a substantial amount of weight?
- How do your weight loss goals compare with what weight charts suggest for someone of your height?

❖

Be careful how you live.

You may be the only Bible some people ever read.

Home Tests & Healing Protocols
A HANDS-ON REFERENCE FOR HEALING TECHNIQUES AND SELF DIAGNOSIS METHODS

Taking Your Basal Body Temperature:

Body temperature reflects metabolic rate, largely determined by hormones secreted by the thyroid gland. Thyroid health can be measured by basal body temperature. You will need a thermometer.

1. Shake down thermometer to below 95°F and place it by your bed before going to sleep at night.
2. On waking, place the thermometer in your armpit for a full 10 minutes. Lie quietly with your eyes closed, making as little movement as possible for the best results.
3. After 10 minutes, read and record the temperature and date.
4. Record temperature for at least 3 mornings. Menstruating women must perform the test on the 2nd, 3rd, and 4th days of menstruation. Men and post-menopausal women can perform the test any time. Normal basal body temperature is between 97.6° and 98.2°.

Giving Your Body An Ascorbic Acid Flush:

This procedure accelerates detoxification programs, changing body chemistry to neutralize allergens and fight infections, promoting more rapid healing, and protecting against illness.

1. Use ascorbate vitamin C or Ester C powder with bioflavonoids for best results.
2. Take $1/2$ teasp. every 20 minutes until a soupy stool results. *Note:* Use $1/4$ teasp. every hour for a very young child; $1/2$ teasp. every hour for a child six to ten years old.
3. Then reduce amount taken slightly so that the bowel produces a mealy, loose stool, but not diarrhea. The body continues to cleanse at this point. You will be taking approximately 8-10,000mg. daily depending on body weight and make-up. Continue for one to two days for a thorough flush.

Bentonite Clay Colonic Cleanse:

Bentonite clay is a mineral substance with powerful absorption qualities; it can pull out suspended impurities in the body. It helps prevent proliferation of pathogenic organisms and parasites, and sets up an environment for rebuilding healthy tissue. It is effective for lymph congestion, cellulite in fatty tissues, blood cleansing and reducing toxicity from environmental pollutants. It may be used orally, anally, or vaginally. It works like an internal poultice, drawing out toxic materials, then draining and eliminating them through evacuation. For best results, avoid refined foods, especially sugars and flour, and pasteurized dairy products during this cleanse.

1. To take as an enema, mix $1/2$ cup clay to an enema bag of water. Use 5 to 6 bags for each enema set to replace a colonic. Follow the normal enema procedure on page 177, or the directions with your enema apparatus.
2. Massage across the abdomen while expelling toxic waste into the toilet.
Note: Bentonite clay packs are also effective applied to varicose veins and arthritic areas.

Coca's Pulse Test:

Dr. Arthur Coca, an immunologist, discovered that when people eat foods to which they are allergic, there is a dramatic increase in the heartbeat - 20 or more beats a minute above normal. Pulse rate is normally remarkably stable, and unaffected by digestion or ordinary physical activities or normal emotions. Unless a person is ill or under great stress, pulse rate deviation is probably due to an allergy. By performing Coca's PULSE TEST one can find and eliminate foods that harm.

1. Take your pulse when you wake in the morning. Using a watch with a second hand, count the number of beats in a 60-second period. A normal pulse reading is 50 to 70 beats per minute.

2. Take your pulse again after eating a suspected allergy food. Wait 15 to 20 minutes and take your pulse again. If the pulse rate has increased more than 10 beats per minute, omit the food from your diet.

Muscle Kinesiology Testing:

Muscle kinesiology attributes can often be used to determine an individual's response to a food or substance. Muscle testing is a good personal technique to use before buying a healing product, because it lets you estimate the product's effectiveness for your individual body needs and make-up. You will need a partner for the procedure.

1. Hold your arm out straight from your side, parallel to the ground. Have a partner take hold of the arm with one hand just below the shoulder, and one hand on the forearm. Your partner should then try to force down towards your side, while you exert all your strength to hold it level. Unless you are in ill health, you should easily be able to withstand this pressure and keep your arm level.

2. Then, simply hold the item that you desire to test against your diaphragm (under the breastbone) or thyroid (the point where the collarbone comes together below the neck). The item may be in or out of normal packaging, or in its raw state, like a fresh food.

3. While holding the item as above, put your arm out straight from your side as before and have your partner try to press it down again. If the substance or product is beneficial for you, your arm will retain its strength, and your partner will be unable to force it down. If the substance or product is not beneficial, or would worsen your condition, your arm can be easily pushed down by your partner.

Herbal Vaginal Packs

A cleansing herbal combination may be used as a vaginal pack by placing it against the cervix, or as a bolus inserted in the vagina. The herbs act as an internal poultice to draw out toxic wastes from the vagina, rectum or urethral areas. An herbal pack is effective for cysts, benign tumors, polyps and uterine tumors, and against cervical dysplasia. It takes 6 weeks to 6 months for complete healing, depending on the problem and severity. Here is a choice of two formula combinations:

1. Mix either combination with warmed cocoa butter to form finger-sized suppositories. Place in waxed paper in the refrigerator to chill and harden slightly.

2. A suppository may then be smeared on the end of a cotton tampon and inserted; or inserted as is, along with the use of a sanitary napkin to catch drainage. Use suppositories at night and rinse out in the morning with white oak bark tea, or yellow dock root tea to rebalance vaginal pH.

3. Repeat for 6 days. Rest for one week. Resume and repeat.

Formula #1: Mix 1 part each with cocoa butter to form a suppository: squaw vine, marshmallow root, slippery elm, goldenseal root, pau d'arco, comfrey root, mullein, yellow dock root, chickweed, acidophilus powder.

Formula #2: Mix 1 part each with cocoa butter to form a suppository: cranesbill powder, goldenseal root, red raspberry leaf, white oak bark, echinacea root, myrrh gum powder.

Therapeutic Sitz Bath:

A sitz bath is a mild form of alternating hot and cold hydrotherapy (see page 177). It may be used as a healing technique for a patient who cannot take a full shower. It is especially beneficial for increasing circulation in the pelvic and urethral area.

1. Fill a bathtub with water to cover the hips when seated. Start with water about 100° and increase the temperature by letting hot water drip continuously into the tub, until the temperature reaches approximately 112°. Place your feet at the faucet end of the tub so that they are soaking in slightly hotter water as the water drips in.

2. Soak in the bath for 20 to 30 minutes. Cover the upper body with a towel, and place a cool, wet washcloth on the forehead.

3. Then take a quick, cool rinse in the shower, or splash the body with cool water before drying off to further stimulate circulation.

4. Epsom salts, Crystal Star HOT SEAWEED BATH, Breh or Batherapy bath salts, ginger powder, comfrey or chamomile may be added to the bath water for therapeutic results.

Enemas:

Enemas are an important therapeutic aid for a congestion cleansing program. They accelerate the release of old, encrusted colon waste, encourage discharge of parasites, freshen the G.I. tract, and cleanse your body more thoroughly. Use enemas during both mucous and colon cleansing diets for optimum results. They are helpful during a healing crisis, or after a serious illness or drug-treated hospital stay to speed healing. Some headaches and inflammatory skin conditions can be relieved with enemas. Herbal enemas can immediately alkalize the bowel area, help control irritation and inflammation, and provide local healing action for ulcerated tissue. There are several herbs particularly helpful for enemas. USE 2 CUPS OF VERY STRONG BREWED TEA OR SOLUTION TO 1 QT. OF WATER PER ENEMA.

✤ Garlic, helps kill parasites and cleanse harmful bacteria, viruses and mucous. BLEND SIX GARLIC CLOVES IN 2 CUPS COLD WATER AND STRAIN. FOR SMALL CHILDREN, USE 1 CLOVE GARLIC TO 1 PINT WATER.

✤ Catnip helps stomach, digestive problems and cramping; also for childhood disease.

✤ Pau d' arco helps when system chemistry is imbalanced, as in chronic yeast and fungal infections.

✤ Spirulina is effective when both blood and bowel are toxic.

✤ Lobelia helps in cases of food poisoning, especially when vomiting prevents antidotal herbs from being taken by mouth.

✤ Aloe vera helps heal tissues in cases of hemorrhoids, irritable bowel and diverticulitis.

✤ Lemon Juice is an internal wash to rapidly neutralize an acid system, cleanse the colon and bowel.

✤ Acidophilus helps gas, yeast, and candidiasis infections. Mix 4-oz. powder to 1-qt. water.

✤ Coffee enemas have become a standard in natural healing for liver and blood related cancers. Caffeine used in this way stimulates the liver and gallbladder to remove toxins, open bile ducts, encourage increased peristaltic action, and produce necessary enzyme activity for healthy red blood cell formation and oxygen uptake. Use 1 cup of regular strong brewed coffee to 1 qt. water.

Herbal implants:

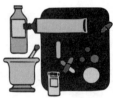

Implants are concentrated enema solutions which can be used for serious health problems, such as colitis, arthritis or prostate inflammation. Prepare for the implant by taking a small enema with warm water to clear out the lower bowel, allowing you to hold the implant longer. Then mix 2 TBS. of your chosen powder, such as spirulina, or wheat grass, in $1/2$ cup water. Lubricate the tip of a syringe with vaseline or vitamin E oil, get down on your hands and knees and insert the nozzle into the rectum. Squeeze the bulb to insert the mixture, but do not release pressure on the bulb before it is withdrawn, so the mixture will stay in the lower bowel. Hold as long as you can before expelling.

HOW TO TAKE A DETOXIFYING, COLONIC ENEMA:

Place the enema solution in a water bag, and hang or hold about 18 inches higher than your body. Attach the colon tube, and lubricate with vaseline or vitamin E oil. Expel a little water from the tube to let out air bubbles. Lying on your left side, slowly insert the tube about 18 inches into the colon. Never use force. Rotate tube gently to ease insertion, removing kinks, so liquid will flow freely. Massage your abdomen, or flex and contract stomach muscles to relieve any cramping. When all solution has entered the colon, slowly remove the tube and remain on your left side for 5 minutes.

Then move to a knee-chest position with the weight of your body on your knees and one hand. Use the other hand to massage the lower left side of the abdomen for several minutes. Massage releases encrusted fecal matter. Roll onto your back for another 5 minutes, massaging up the descending colon, over the transverse colon to the right side, and down the ascending colon. Then move onto your right side for 5 minutes, and repeat. Get up and quickly expel fluid into the toilet. Sticky grey or brown mucous, small dark, chunks, or long, tough ribbon-like pieces are frequently loosened and expelled during a colonic enema. These poisonous looking things are usually the obstacles and toxins interfering with normal body functions. The good news is that they are no longer in you. You may have to take several enemas before there is no more evidence of these substances.

Arthritis Elimination Sweat:

A surprising amount of toxic material that can aggravate arthritis can be eliminated by the body via the skin in an arthritis sweat bath with Epsom salts or Dead Sea salts. Herbs with a diaphoretic action, can play a part in the success of the bath. Elderflowers, peppermint, yarrow can be taken as a tea, and should be drunk as hot as possible before the bath.

Here's how:

Use about 3 pounds of Epsom salts or as directed for Dead Sea salts. Add to very hot bath water. Rub the affected joints with a stiff brush in the water for 5 - 10 minutes; try to stay in the bath for 10-25 minutes. On emerging, do not dry yourself. Wrap up immediately in a clean sheet and go straight to bed, covering yourself with several blankets. The osmotic pressure of the Epsom salt solution absorbed by the sheet will draw off heavy perspiration, and for this reason the mattress should be protected with a sheet of plastic. The following morning the sheet will be stained with products excreted through the skin - sometimes the color of egg yolk. (Take care if you have a weak heart or hypertension.)

Improvement after the Epsom salt bath experience is notable. Continue treatment once every two weeks until the sheet is no longer stained, a sign that the body is well cleansed by then. Drink plenty of water throughout the procedure to prevent dehydration and loss of body salts.

You can purchase the following home tests at most pharmacies. Ask if you don't see it on the shelf.

Home Ovulation Predictors:

An ovulation test can help women to get pregnant. Pregnancy can only occur during part of the monthly menstrual cycle, for a week or so after ovulation. Ovulation occurs about the midpoint between periods, but many women have irregular cycles, making it difficult for them to know when they are fertile. Ovulation predictors enable women to pinpoint their fertile days by measuring the concentration of luteinizing hormone (LH) in urine. The level of LH increases significantly 12 to 24 hours before ovulation.

These tests instruct women to test their urine daily with activating strips, for several days early in the menstrual cycle. The strips turn a color, which establishes an LH baseline. When LH concentration rises, shortly before ovulation, the test strip turns a different color. A woman can then better plan sexual intercourse for procreation.

Home Bladder Infection Tests:

Bladder infections develop when bacteria ascend the urine tube (urethra) and enter the bladder where they reproduce and infect. Bladder infections most commonly appear in women, and cause painful, overly frequent urination, and sometimes, back and groin pain, and fever. A bladder infection increases the concentration of nitrites in urine. A home test can detect the nitrites with dip strips that change color when urine comes in contact with the impregnated chemicals.

Note: Some women develop symptoms of a bladder infection, but don't show the expected amounts of bacteria or nitrites in their urine. When test results conflict with symptoms of infection, practitioners give more weight to the person's symptoms than to the test. You should too. If you experience symptoms of bladder infection, but your home test turns out negative or marginally positive, call your practitioner. Treatment is usually recommended regardless of test results, because of the risk of kidney infection.

Home Blood Pressure Monitor:

Chronic high blood pressure, or hypertension, is a major risk factor for heart disease and stroke, which together account for almost half of U.S. deaths. If you are considerably overweight, have a history of hypertension, heart disease, or stroke, or have a family history of cardiovascular disease, you might give serious thought to investing in a home blood pressure monitor for peace of mind.

Simply slip your arm into the provided cuff and fill it with air using a bulb-shaped hand pump. When you release the air, the monitor determines your pressure electronically and displays it digitally. (Although available and more convenient, finger cuffs are not as accurate as the arm cuffs.)

For some people, home blood pressure testing is more accurate than professional testing, because the anxiousness of being in a doctor's office raises their blood pressure. Home testing eliminates this "white coat hypertension," and the medications that might be unnecessarily prescribed to treat it.

Home Blood Glucose Monitor:

Blood glucose monitors have become indispensable for people with diabetes. Glucose is the simple sugar that fuels the body, but diabetics can't process it properly because they lack the hormone insulin, or can't use the insulin they produce. Glucose monitoring at home allows diabetics to adjust their insulin and/or diet to control their blood glucose level. (Urine glucose testing, also available for home use, is easier, but gives a less accurate blood glucose reading.)

A drop of blood is placed on a test strip and inserted into the monitor, which electronically measures the glucose level. Calibrations differ; you may need to match your monitor's calibration to that of a test lab. Check.

Home Colorectal Cancer Screening Tests:

All colorectal cancers can not be detected by this test. False positives are not uncommon. A variety of factors besides cancer can introduce small amounts of blood into the stool. Aspirin, hemorrhoids, gastrointestinal problems, as well as some foods, like popcorn, may cause blood in the stool. To reduce the risk of false results, follow package directions scrupulously.

The test is based on the fact that early-stage colorectal tumors release a tiny amount of blood, which becomes incorporated into the stool. Some tests rely on chemically impregnated toilet paper to detect the blood. If the toilet paper changes color after use, it indicates a positive result. Others require the user to place a sheet of test paper in the toilet bowl following a bowel movement. If a color change appears on the paper, blood is present in the stool.

Home Thyroid Test:

The thyroid gland produces hormones which increase protein synthesis in all body tissues, as well as certain important enzymes that influence the rate at which fat is burned for energy. If the thyroid is not functioning properly, a slow metabolism results. Many people with underactive thyroids also have weight problems. Thyroid dysfunction is almost always involved with women's problems.

A common method for testing thyroid function is to place a basal thermometer under the arm for ten minutes before getting out of bed in the morning. The thermometer must read to tenths of a degree. Normal body temperature ranges for this test are between 97.8 and 98.2 degrees Fahrenheit. A reading below 97.8 may indicate hypothyroid activity (low thyroid); a reading above may indicate hyperthyroid activity (excess thyroid). Some of the factors which can cause thyroid problems, and decrease the rate at which the body burns calories, include malnourishment because of nutrient deficiencies, thyroid and/or pituitary exhaustion because of overstimulation from caffeine, sugar, or other stimulants, and the presence of substances which inhibit thyroid function, such as hard liquor.

Home pH Testing:

pH testing measures acidity or alkalinity. The degrees of acidity or alkalinity of a substance are expressed in pH values. The neutral point, where a solution is neither acid or alkaline, is pH 7. Water has a pH of 7.0. Anything with a pH below 7.0 is acid while anything with a pH above 7.0 is alkaline. The ideal pH range for saliva and urine is 6.0 to 6.8. Our bodies are naturally mildly acidic. Therefore, values below pH 6.3 are considered too acidic; values above pH 6.8 are too alkaline. Maximum acidity is pH 0 and maximum alkalinity is pH 14.

Saliva and urine pH can be measured on litmus paper. Normal saliva pH is 6.4. If saliva pH is above 6.8, it could indicate digestive problems, while a saliva reading below 6.0 might mean liver and blood toxicity. Urine pH cycles from a low of 5.5 to 5.8 in the morning, to a high of 7.0 during the day, averaging 6.4 in a 24hr. period. If it is too acid, below 6.0, it can indicate dehydration as well as over-acidity. Colon pH is a critically important area. It should be in a narrow range of 6.8 to 7.0. If it is too alkaline (above 7.0), yeasts and pathogenic bacteria grow. To lower the pH of the colon, implant a good L. bifidus colon culture. Most of the bacteria in the colon is bifidus.

You can determine whether your body fluids are either too acidic or too alkaline, causing acidosis or alkalosis. Purchase nitrazine paper, available at any drugstore, and test saliva and/or urine. Perform the test either before eating or at least one hour after eating. The paper will change color to indicate if your system is overly acidic or alkaline. If your test indicated one extreme or another, omit the acid-or alkaline-forming foods from your diet until another pH test shows that you have returned to normal.

Home Therapeutic Use For Food Grade Hydrogen Peroxide: See also ALTERNATIVE ARSENAL page 72
How to use H_2O_2 orally:

Purchase 35% food grade H_2O_2, or magnesium peroxide from your local health food store. Do not use household, beauty supply or any other form of peroxide for internal use - many of these products have added chemicals to stabilize the H_2O_2. You will also need an eye dropper.

- Do not use with carrot juice, carbonated drinks or alcohol. Take on an empty stomach 1 hour before or 3 hours after meals.
- If you get the 35% H_2O_2 on your skin, rinse it under running water a few minutes.
- Do not ever take 35% H_2O_2 internally without first diluting.
- If your stomach is upset at any level, go back one level. Then proceed to increase your daily dosage again.

You may experience slight nausea. In addition, as dead bacteria or various forms of poisons are released you will experience a cleansing effect as they are eliminated through the skin, lungs, kidneys and bowels. Some reactions to the cleansing effect could include skin eruptions, nausea, headaches, sleepiness, unusual fatigue, diarrhea, head or chest cold, ear infections, boils or any other ways the body uses to loosen toxins. This is natural cleansing of the body and should be of short duration.

In most applications, especially those where anti-infective and antifungal properties are needed, we have found it more beneficial to use H_2O_2 in an alternating series - usually 10 days of use, and then 10 days of rest, or 3 weeks of use, and 3 weeks of rest, in more serious cases.

Matrix Health GENESIS OXY-SPRAY GEL, combined with aloe vera juice, vegetable glycerine and red seaweed extract, is useful for general application as an antiseptic and antifungal. It may be applied topically to affected areas on the skin, or massaged into the soles of the feet where the pores are large.

Here's an easy chart to determine number of days, drops and times per day to take H_2O_2:

Count Day	Number of drops	Times per day
1	3	3
2	4	3
3	5	3
4	6	3
5	7	3
6	8	3
7	9	3
8	10	3
9	11	3
10	12	3
11	13	3

Topical therapeutic use: at a 3% solution, H_2O_2 can effectively be used externally. Make a 3% solution by mixing 1 part 35% H_2O_2 with 11 parts of water. Place in a spray bottle or dip a cotton ball in the solution and use as a facial freshener after bathing, being careful to avoid the eyes, eyebrows and hair.

Douche: mix 6 TBS. of 3% solution to a quart of warm distilled water. Do not exceed this amount.

Colonic enema: add 1 cup 3% solution to 5 gallons warm water. Do not exceed this amount.

Regular enema: add 1 tablespoon of 3% solution to a quart of warm distilled water.

Detox bath: add about 2 quarts 3% H_2O_2 to a tub of warm water.

Foot soak: add 3% H_2O_2 to a gallon of warm water as needed.

For animals: 1-oz. of 3% H_2O_2 can be added to 1 qt. of your pets drinking water if they are ill.

Humidifiers and steamers: mix 1 pint 3% solution to 1 gallon of water.

Vegetable soak: add $1/4$ cup 3% H_2O_2 to a full sink of cold water. Soak light skinned vegetables (like lettuce) 20 minutes, thicker skinned (like cucumbers) for 30 minutes. Drain, dry and chill to prolong freshness. If time is a problem, spray produce with a solution of 3%. Let stand for a few minutes, rinse and dry.

To freshen kitchen: use a spray bottle of 3% to wipe off counter tops and appliances. It will disinfect and give the kitchen a fresh smell. Works great to clean refrigerator and kids' school lunch boxes.

Laundry: add 8 oz. of 3% to your wash in place of bleaches.

Sprouting seeds: add 1 oz. 3% to 1 pint of water and soak the seeds overnight. Add the same amount of H_2O_2 each time you rinse the seeds.

House and garden plants: put 1 oz. 3% in 1 quart water. Water of mist plants with this solution.

Insecticide spray: Mix 8-oz. black strap molasses or sugar and 8-oz. 3% H_2O_2 to 1 gallon of water.

Home Urinary Tract Infection Test:

You can purchase a product called DIPSTICK from your pharmacy. It contains a chemical re-agent to indicate the presence of a bacterial infection when dipped in urine. If you are at frequent risk for bladder infections, check yourself weekly.

Home Low Blood Sugar Self Test:

The importance of correct diagnosis and treatment of sugar instabilities is essential. The human body possesses a complex set of checks and balances to maintain blood glucose concentrations within a narrow range. Blood sugar control is influenced by the pituitary, thyroid and adrenal glands, as well as the pancreas, liver, kidneys and even the skeletal muscles. Hypoglycemia symptoms are often mistaken for other problems. Low blood sugar is the biological equivalent of a race car running on empty. It is not so much a disease as a symptom of other disorders. The symptoms can be improved right away by eating something, but this does not address the cause.

Children are also subject to hypoglycemia widely indicated as a cause of both hyperactivity and learning disorders. Chronic negativism, hyperkinesis, and obstinate resentment to all discipline are reasons for at least the self-test below and probably a Glucose Tolerance Test. (With children, the condition can only be managed by a diet from which all forms of concentrated sugars have been removed, including fruit juices, until the body achieves glucose homeostasis.)

The following questionnaire is for self-determination, reprinted from the Enzymatic Therapy Notebook. It can help you decide, in cooperation with a health care professional, whether you need low blood sugar support, and whether professional help is necessary.

Mark the following symptoms as they pertain to you: (1) for mild symptoms, occurring once or twice a year; (2) for moderate symptoms, occurring several times a year; (3) severe symptoms, occurring almost constantly.

( ) Irritability
( ) Anti-social behavior
( ) Craving for sweets
( ) Blurred vision
( ) Heart palpitations
( ) Rapid pulse
( ) Mental confusion, spaciness
( ) Forgetfulness
( ) Constant phobias, fears
( ) Constant worry and anxiety
( ) Nightmares
( ) Cold sweats and shaking
( ) Frequent headaches
( ) Faintness and dizziness
( ) Nervousness
( ) Convulsions, trembling
( ) Poor concentration
( ) Crying spells
( ) Weak spells
( ) Extreme fatigue, exhaustion
( ) Lots of sighing and yawning
( ) Insomnia; inability to return to sleep after awakening
( ) Twitching, involuntary muscle jerks
( ) Digestive problems
( ) Indecisiveness
( ) Unexplained depression
( ) Nervous breakdown
( ) Suicidal intent

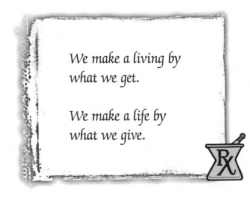

We make a living by
what we get.

We make a life by
what we give.

Correct Food Combining Chart

USE AS A REFERENCE TOOL FOR A GOOD HEALING DIET

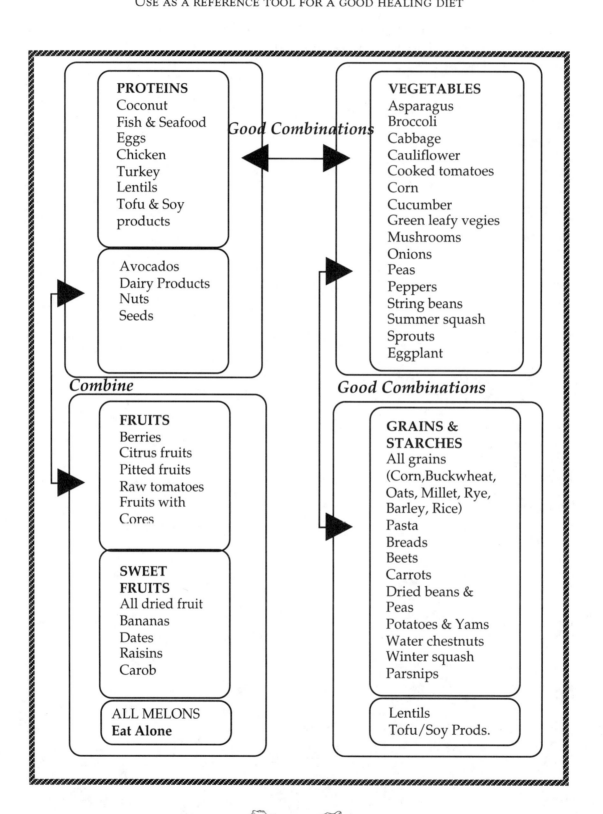

PROTEINS
Coconut
Fish & Seafood
Eggs
Chicken
Turkey
Lentils
Tofu & Soy
products

Avocados
Dairy Products
Nuts
Seeds

Good Combinations

VEGETABLES
Asparagus
Broccoli
Cabbage
Cauliflower
Cooked tomatoes
Corn
Cucumber
Green leafy vegies
Mushrooms
Onions
Peas
Peppers
String beans
Summer squash
Sprouts
Eggplant

Combine

Good Combinations

FRUITS
Berries
Citrus fruits
Pitted fruits
Raw tomatoes
Fruits with
Cores

**SWEET
FRUITS**
All dried fruit
Bananas
Dates
Raisins
Carob

ALL MELONS
Eat Alone

**GRAINS &
STARCHES**
All grains
(Corn,Buckwheat,
Oats, Millet, Rye,
Barley, Rice)
Pasta
Breads
Beets
Carrots
Dried beans &
Peas
Potatoes & Yams
Water chestnuts
Winter squash
Parsnips

Lentils
Tofu/Soy Prods.

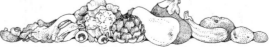

Product Resources

here you can get what we recommend.....

The following listing is included for your convenience and assistance in obtaining further information about the products recommended in this book. The list is unsolicited by the companies named. Each company has a solid, successful history of testing and corroborative data that has been invaluable to me and my staff, as well as confirmation by empirical observation from the stores that carry these products who have shared their experiences with us. In addition, we hear from thousands of readers about the products they have used. All of this information is considered with every edition of HEALTHY HEALING. I realize there are many other fine companies and products who are not listed here, but I feel you can rely on the companies who are, for the highest quality products and the best results.

Aloe Life International, 4822 Santa Monica Ave. #231, San Diego, CA 92107, 800-414-2563, 619-258-0145
Ageless Products, Inc., 24101 N.C. 138 Highway, Albemarle, NC 28001, 704-982-7551
Alta Health Products Inc., 1979 E. Locust St., Pasadena, CA 91107, 626-796-1047
American Biologics, 1180 Walnut Ave., Chula Vista, CA 91911, 800-227-4473
AmeriFit Inc., 166 Highland Park Dr., Bloomfield, CT 06002, 800-990-3476
Atkins Ginseng Farm Ltd., R.R. #1, P.O. Box 1125, Waterford, Ontario CAN NOE1Y0
Be Well, 12420 Evergreen Dr., Mukilteo, WA 98275, 206-348-4900
Beehive Botanicals, Route 8, Box 8257, Hayward, WI 54843, 800-233-4483
Bio-Botanica, Inc., 75 Commerce Dr., Hauppauge, NY 11788, 800-645-5720
Bioforce of America Ltd., 2 Broad St., 2nd Floor, Kinderhook, NY 12106, 800-645-9135
Bio-Research Ltd., 2389 N.W. Military Dr., Ste. 588, San Antonio, TX 78231, 210-492-4966
Bio-Tech Foods Ltd., 250 S. Hotel St., Ste. 200, Honolulu, HI 96813-2869, 800-468-7578
(B & T) Boericke & Tafel Inc., 2381 Circadian Way, Santa Rosa, CA 95407, 800-876-9505
Boiron, #6 Campus Blvd. Building A, Newtown Square, PA 19073, 800-258-8823
Bricker Labs, 18722 Santee Ln., Valley Center, CA 92082, 800-274-2537
Canine Care Inc. (Terminator), P.O. Box 11436, Costa Mesa, CA 92627, 800-242-9966
Cartilage USA Inc., 200 Clearbrook Rd., Elmsford, NY 10523, 800-700-7325
Centipede Industries Inc., 6511 Manchester Ln., Eden Prarie, MN 55346, 612-937-2354
Champion Nutrition, 2615 Stanwell Dr., Concord, CA 94520, 800-225-4831
Country Life, 28300 B Industrial Blvd., Hayward, CA 94545, 510-785-1196
Crystal Star Herbal Nutrition, 16050 Via Este, Sonora, CA 95370, 800-736-6015
Desert Essence, 9510 Vassar Ave., Unit A, Chatsworth, CA 91311, 800-848-7331
De Souza Food Corp., P.O. Box 395, Beaumont, CA 92223, 909-849-5172
Diamond/Herpanacine Associates,138 Stout Rd., P.O. Box 544, Ambler, PA 19002, 215-542-2981
(Dr. Dophilus) Professional Nutrition, 811 Cliff Dr. , Suite C-1, Santa Barbara, CA 93109, 800-336-9301
Dr. Goodpet Labs, Inc., P.O. Box 4489, Inglewood, CA 90309, 800-222-9932
Earthrise Co., 424 Payran St., Petaluma, CA 94952, 800-949-7473
EAS, 400 Corporate Circle Dr., Ste. J, Golden, CO 80401, 800-923-4300
Educated Beauty, Hollywood Florida, 1-888-323-8423
Enzymatic Therapy, Dept. L, P.O. Box 22310, Green Bay, WI 54305, 800-783-2286
Ethical Nutrients, 971 Calle Negocio, San Clemente, CA 92673, 714-366-0818
Flora, Inc., P.O. Box 950, Lynden, WA 98264, 800-446-2110
Flora Labs Inc., 50 Warner Rd., Trout Lake, WA 98650, 800-395-6093
Food Science Labs, 20 New England Dr., Essex Junction, VT 05453, 800-874-9444
Futurebiotics, 72 Cotton Mill Hill, Unit A24, Brattleboro, VT 05301-8614, 800-367-5433
Ginseng Co., Inc., 2279 Agate Ct., Simi Valley, CA 93065, 800-423-5176
Green Foods Corp., 320 N. Graves Ave., Oxnard, CA 93030 800-777-4430
Halo, Purely For Pets, 3438 East Lake Rd., #14, Palm Harbor, FL 34685, 800-426-4256
Health Plus Inc., 13325 Benson Ave., Chino, CA 91710, 800-822-6225
Heart Foods Co., 2235 E. 38th St., Minneapolis, MN 55407, 800-229-3663
Herbal Products & Development, P.O. Box 1084, Aptos, CA 95001, 408-688-8706
Herbs For Kids, Inc., 151 Evergreen Dr., Suite D, Bozeman, MT 59715, 406-587-0180
Home Health Products, P.O. Box 8425, Virginia Beach, VA 23450-8425, 800-468-7313

Hyland's-Standard Homeopathic Co., P. O. Box 61067, Los Angeles, CA 90061, 800-624-9659
Jarrow Formulas Inc., 1824 S. Robertson Blvd., Los Angeles, CA 90035, 800-726-0886
Klamath, P.O. Box 626, Mt. Shasta, CA 96067, 800-327-1956
Knudsen & Sons Inc., Speedway Ave., Chico, CA 95928, 916-899-5000
Lane Labs, 172 Broadway, Woodcliff Lake, NJ 07675, 800-526-3005
Lewis Laboratories Int'l. Ltd., 49 Richmondville Ave. Westport, CT 06880-2052, 800-243-6020
Long Life Herb Classics, 111 Canfield Ave., Randolph, NJ 07867-1114, 908-580-9252
Lotus Brands, P.O. Box 325, Twin Lakes, WI 53181, 414-889-8561
Maitake Products, Inc., 222 Bergan Tpk., Ridgefield Park, NJ 07660, 800-747-418
Makers of KAL, Inc., Park City, UT 84060, 800-755-4525
Matrix Health Products, 8400 Magnolia Ave., Ste. N, Santee, CA 92071, 800-736-5609
Motherlove Herbal Co., P. O. Box 101, Laporte, CO 80535, 970-493-2892
Natra Bio, 1441 West Smith Road, Ferndale, WA 98248, 800-232-4005
Natren Inc., 3105 Willow Ln., Westlake Village, CA 91361, 800-992-3323
Natrol Inc., 20731 Marilla St., Chatsworth, CA 91311, 800-326-1520
Nature's Life, 7180 Lampson Ave., Garden Grove, CA 92641, 800-854-6837
Nature's Path, P.O. Box 7862, Venice, FL 34287, 800-326-5772
Nature's Plus, Farmingdale, NY 11735, 800-645-9500
Nature's Secret, 5485 Conestoga Court, Boulder, CO 80301, 800-525-9696
Nature's Way Products, 10 Mountain Springs Pkwy., Springville, UT 84663, 800-962-8873
New Moon Extracts Inc., 99 Main St., Brattleboro, VT 05301, 800-543-7279
Next Nutrition, Inc., P. O. Box 2469, Carlsbad, CA 92018, 800-468-6398
NuAge Laboratories Ltd., 4200 Laclede Ave., St. Louis, MO 63108, 800-325-8080
Nutrapathic, 10934 Lin-Valle Dr., St. Louis, MO 63123, 800-747-1601
Nutrex Inc., 73-4460 Queen Kaahumanu, Kailua-Kona, HI 96740, 800-395-1353
Nutribiotic, 865 Parallel Dr., Lakeport, CA 95453, 800-225-4345
NutriCology, 400 Preda St., San Leandro, CA 94577, 800-545-9960
Nutritech Inc./All One People, 719 E. Haley St., Santa Barbara, CA 93103, 800-235-5727
Olbas Products From Switzerland, 603 N Second St., Philadelphia, PA 19123-3098, 800-523-9971
Orange Peel Enterprises, 2183 Ponce de Leon Circle, Vero Beach, FL 32960, 800-643-1210
Pharm-Aloe, 10743 Main St., Woodford, WI 53599, 800-972-2981
Premier Labs, 27475 Ynez Rd. Suite 305, Temecula, CA 92591, 800-887-5227
Prevail Corp., 2204-8 NW Birdsdale, Gresham, OR 97030, 800-248-0885
Prologix / Ultra Life, P.O. Box 2094, Fullerton, CA 92633-2094, 714-738-1269
Radiant Life Formulas, HCR 73 Box 553, San Jose, NM 87565, 888-348-7587
Rainbow Light, P.O. Box 600, Santa Cruz, CA 95061, 800-635-1233
Richardson Labs 3475 Commerical Court, Meridian, ID 83642, 888-564-7239
Rockland Corp., The, 6846 S. Canton, Ste. 100, Tulsa, OK 74136, 800-421-7310
Root To Health, / Hsu's Ginseng Enterprises, T6819 Cty. Hwy. W, Wausau, WI 54403, 800-388-3818
Solaray, Inc., 1104 Country Hills Dr., Suite 300, Ogden, UT 84403, 800-669-8877
Solgar, 500 Willow Tree Rd., Leonia, NJ 07605, 800-645-2246
Sonne P.O. Box 2160, Cottonwood, CA 96022, 916-347-5868
Spectrum Naturals, Inc., 133 Copeland St., Petaluma, CA 94952, 707-778-8900
Sun Chlorella, 4025 Spencer #104, Torrance, CA 90503, 800-829-2828
Threshold Enterprises & Source Naturals Inc. & Planetary Formulas 23 Janis Way, Scotts Valley, CA 95066, 800-777-5677
Thursday Plantation Inc., P.O. Box 5613, Montecito, CA 93150, 800-848-8966
Tom's of Maine, 302 Lafayette Ctr., Kennebunk, ME 04043, 207-985-2944
Trace Minerals Research, P.O. Box 429, Roy, UT 84067, 800-624-7145
Transitions For Health, 621 SW Alder, Suite 900, Portland, OR 97205, 800-888-6814
Tushies, 675 Industrial Blvd., Delta, CO 81416, 303-874-7536
Twin Laboratories, Inc., 2120 Smithtown Ave., Ronkonkoma, NY 11779, 516-467-3140
USA Laboratories, 5610 Rowland Rd., Ste #110, Minnetonka, MN 55343, 800-422-3371
Viobin Corp., 226 W. Livingston, Monticello, IL 61856, 217-762-2561
Wakunaga of America Co., Ltd., 23501 Madero, Mission Viejo, CA 92691-2764, 800-825-7888
World Organics Corp., 5242 Bolsa Ave., #3, Huntington Beach, CA 92649, 800-926-7455
Yerba Prima, Inc., 740 Jefferson Avenue, Ashland, OR 97520-3743, 800-488-4339
Y.S. Royal Jelly & Organic Bee Farms, RR 1 Box 91A, Sheridan, IL 60551-9629, 800-654-4593
Zand Herbal Formulas, P.O. Box 5312, Santa Monica, CA 90409, 310-822-0500
Zia Cosmetics, 410 Townsend St., 2nd Floor, San Francisco, CA 94107, 800-334-7546

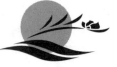

About Crystal Star Herbal Nutrition

Crystal Star Herbal Nutrition is an exceptional herb supplier that you can be confident in using for therapeutic strength medicinal herbs. As the formulator for Crystal Star, I rely on a firm commitment to excellence, knowing that consistent quality is never an accident, and always the result of sincere effort, intelligent direction and skillful ability.

My formulating philosophy is based on personal experience and on many years of working with herbs and the health conditions they can address. As a professional herbalist, I have been creating herbal formulas since 1978. I use combination formulas because in most cases they work more efficiently with complex body functions and multiple body needs. The synergistic activity of herbs in combination provides balanced healing properties to normalize body chemistry and performance. I find that combinations stimulate the body much more readily to rally its own self-healing processes.

I am including the Crystal Star products and their ingredients in HEALTHY HEALING to give you an opportunity to see what is in each herbal compound I recommend. Also, I feel it may be helpful for those who might have a sensitivity to a particular herb.

Detailed information about other companies' products recommended in this book is proprietary and unavailable. However, a complete listing of these companies, and their addresses is on page 453 if you wish to obtain further information.

A Guide To Herbal Selections.....

All Crystal Star Herbal Nutrition capsules are in **vegetarian capsules,** Vegicaps® with the exception of Evening Primrose Pearls. Vegicaps® are a superior vegetarian capsule free of animal products, sugar, starches, and preservatives. Vegicaps® offer greater stability, faster dissolution and non-interference in digestion.

Following each product name in parentheses is the herbal selection category code reflecting specific areas of interest.

Herbal Selection Category Codes

A - Animal Formulas
B - Breath of Life Formulas
BB - Beautiful Body Formulas
CD - Cleansing & Detox Formulas

CO - Comfort Formulas
D - Dieting Formulas
E - Energy Formulas
H - Heartsease Formulas

M - Men's Formulas
PD - Prevention/Defense Formulas
Rx - Relaxing Formulas
SA - Superfood Advantage Formulas
W - Women's Formulas

Combination Capsule Formulas

ACTIVE PHYSICAL ENERGY™ Caps (E)
Ingredients: American Panax Ginseng, Chinese Kirin Ginseng, Siberian Ginseng, Suma Rt., Fo Ti Rt., Gotu Kola Herb, Prince Ginseng Rt., Dong Quai Rt., Sarsaparilla Rt., Ginkgo Biloba Lf.

ADR-ACTIVE™ Caps (E)
Ingredients: Licorice Rt., Sarsaparilla Rt., Bladderwrack, Uva Ursi Lf., Irish Moss, Ginger Rt., Astragalus Rt., Capsicum Fruit, Rose Hips Ext., Ascorbate Vit. C, Pantothenic Acid 25 mg, Vit B_6 20 mg, Betaine HCL.

AGELESS VITALITY™ Caps (SA)
Ingredients: Ginkgo Biloba, White Pine Am. Panax Ginseng, Wild Yam, Bilberry, Siberian Ginseng Rt., Suma, Alfalfa, Gotu Kola, Spirulina, Damiana, Sarsaparilla Rt., Hawthorn, Ashwaghandha, Reishi and Maitake Mushroom, Dong Quai Rt., Licorice Rt., Echinacea Rt., Ginger, Royal Jelly, Capsicum Fruit.

ALRG™ Caps (B)
Ingredients: Marshmallow Rt., Burdock, Mullein, Goldenseal Rt., Parsley, Acerola Cherry, Ma Huang, Capsicum, Rosemary Lf., White Pine, Pantothenic Acid 25 mg.

AMINO ZYME™ Caps (D)
Ingredients: Ginger, Chickweed, Gotu Kola, L-Lysine 85mg, Gymnema Sylvestre, L-Ornithine 60mg, L-Glycine 60mg, DL-Phenylalanine 40mg, Lecithin 40mg, L-Tyrosine 30mg, Carnitine 25mg, Bromelain, GTF-Chromium 200mcg.

ANTI-BIO™ Caps (PD)
Ingredients: Echinacea Angustifolia Rt., Goldenseal Rt., Capsicum Fruit, Myrrh gum, Yarrow, Marshmallow Rt., Echinacea Purpurea Rt. & Lf., Black Walnut Hulls, Elecampane Rt., Turmeric Rt., Potassium Chloride 15mg.

ANTI-FLAM™ Caps (CO)
Ingredients: White Willow Bk., St. John's Wort, Echinacea Angustifolia Rt., Echinacea Purpurea Rt., White Pine Bk., Gotu Kola, Red Clover., Devil's Claw Rt., Alfalfa, Burdock, Dandelion Rt., Chamomile, Uva Ursi Lf., Ginger Rt., Bromelain 22mg.

ANTI-HST™ Caps (B)
Ingredients: Marshmallow Rt., Ma Huang, Bee Pollen, White Pine Bk., Goldenseal Rt., Burdock Rt., Juniper Bry., Parsley Rt., Acerola Cherry, Rosemary, Mullein Lf., Capsicum Fruit, Lobelia Herb, Pantothenic Acid 20mg, Vit B_6 20mg.

ANTI-OXIDANT CAPS™ (PD)
Ingredients: White Pine Bk., Rosemary, Siberian Ginseng Rt., Ginkgo Biloba, Ascorbate Vit. C, Echinacea Purp. Rt., Echinacea Angustifolia Rt., Pau d'Arco Bk., Red Clover Blm., Licorice Rt., Astragalus, Lemon Peel, Lemon Balm, Garlic, Hawthorn Lf., Flr. & Bry., Bilberry Bry., Spirulina, Capsicum, Ginger Rt.

ANTI-SPZ™ Caps (CO)
Ingredients: Cramp Bark, Black Haw Bk., Rosemary Lf., Kava Kava Rt., Passionflowers, Red Raspberry Lf., Wild Yam Rt., St. John's Wort Herb, Kelp, Lobelia Herb, Valerian Rt.

APPE-TIGHT™ Caps (D)
Ingredients: Chickweed Lf., Gotu Kola Lf., Kelp, Fennel Sd., Hawthorn Bry., Lf. & Flr., Safflowers, Black Walnut Lf., Licorice Rt., Guar Gum, Kola Nut, Echinacea Purpurea Rt., Lecithin, Ginger Rt., Sida Cordifolia extract, Ornithine 20mg, Vit. B_6 20mg, Niacin 10mg.

AR-EASE™ Caps (CO)
Ingredients: Yucca Rt., Alfalfa Sd., Devil's Claw Rt., Guggul Resin, Buckthorn Bk., Dandelion Lf. & Rt., Bilberry Bry., Parsley Rt., Burdock Rt., Black Cohosh Rt., Rose Hips Ext./ Ascorbate Vit. C, Slippery Elm Bk., St. John's Wort Herb, Yarrow Flr., Hydrangea Rt., Licorice Rt., Hawthorn Lf., Flr. & Bry., Turmeric Rt., Ligusticum, Poria Mushroom, Pantothenic Acid 15mg, DL-Phenylalanine 10mg, Vitamin B_6 10mg.

ASPIR-SOURCE™ Caps (CO)
Ingredients: White Willow Bk., Rosemary Lf., Wood Betony Lf., Heartsease Lf., Scullcap Lf., Valerian Rt., Red Raspberry Lf., Ginger Rt., Blue Vervain Herb, European Mistletoe.

ASTH-AID™ Caps (B)
Ingredients: Bee Pollen, Bupleurum, White Pine Bk., Elecampane, Scullcap, Royal Jelly, Ma Huang, Acerola Cherry, Ginger.

BACK TO RELIEF™ Caps (CO)
Ingredients: Wild Lettuce Lf., Valerian Rt., White Willow Bk., St. John's Wort Herb, Capsicum Fruit, DL-Phenylalanine 20mg, Magnesium (Gluconate) 20mg.

BEAUTIFUL SKIN™ CAPS (SA)
Ingredients: Barley Grass, Horsetail Herb, Sage Lf., Dulse, Rosemary Lf., Echinacea Angustifollia, Goldenseal Rt., Cranberry Jce. Ext. Pwdr., Dandelion Rt. & Lf., Nettles Herb.

BLD-K COMFORT™ Caps (CD)
Ingredients: Juniper Bry., Uva Ursi Lf., Mullein Lf., Goldenseal Rt., Parsley Rt., Marshmallow Rt., Ginger Rt., Stone Rt., Lobelia Herb, Dandelion Lf., Hydrangea Rt., Vit. B_6 25mg.

BODY RE-BUILDER™ Caps (SA)
Ingredients: Spirulina, Bee Pollen, Alfalfa, Rose Hips, Ascorbate Vit. C, Hawthorn Lf., Flr. & Bry., Free Form Amino Acid Complex 30mg, Barley Grass, Carrot Crystals, Siberian Ginseng Rt., Sarsaparilla Rt., Red Raspberry Lf., Kelp, Wild Cherry Bk., Chlorella, Goldenseal Rt., Mullein Lf., Zinc Gluconate 4mg.

BWL-TONE I.B.S.™ Caps (CD)
Ingredients: Peppermint Herb & Oil, Aloe Vera, Slippery Elm Bk., Marshmallow, Pau d' Arco, Wild Yam, Lobelia, Ginger.

CALCIUM SOURCE CAPS™ (SA)
Ingredients: Watercress, Oatstraw, Rosemary Lf., Dandelion Rt., Alfalfa Lf., Pau d'Arco Bk., Borage Sd., Carrot Crystals.

CAN-SSIAC™ Caps (PD)
Ingredients: Sheep Sorrel, Burdock Rt., Red Clover, American Panax Ginseng Rt., Pau d'Arco, Turkey Rhubarb Rt.

CAND-EX™ Caps (CD)
Ingredients: Pau d'Arco, DDS-1® Stabilized Veg. Acidophilus, Black Walnut Hulls, Garlic, Barberry, Sodium Caprylate, Spirulina, Cranberry Juice, Licorice, Burdock, Echinacea Angustifolia, Echinacea Purpurea, Peppermint, Thyme, Rosemary, Dong Quai, Damiana, Rose Hips, Ascorbate Vit. C, DL-Phenylalanine 10mg, Zinc (Gluc.)3mg, Cal Citrate 3mg.

CEL-LEAN™ Caps (D)
Ingredients: Fenugreek Sd., Gotu Kola, Black Cohosh Rt., Quassia wood chips, Red Sage, Goldenseal Rt., Lecithin, Garlic, Bilberry Bry., Guggul Resin, Choline, Vit B_6 20 mg, Betaine HCL. mg, Poria Mushroom, Fennel Sd., Turmeric Rt., Milk Thistle Sd., Kola Nut, Kelp, Vit. B_6 10mg.

CHOL-EX™ Caps (H)
Ingredients: Hawthorn, Lecithin, Rose Hips, Guar gum, Apple Pectin, Plantain, Fenugreek, Stabilized Veg. Acidophilus, Siberian Ginseng Rt., Capsicum, Barley Grass, Psyllium Husks, Heartsease, Niacin 10mg, Vit. B_6 10mg.

CHO-LO FIBER-TONE™ Caps (H)
Ingredients: Organic Oat Bran, Organic Flax Seed, Psyllium Husks, Guar Gum, DDS-1® Stabilized Vegetable Acidophilus, Apple Pectin, Acerola Cherry Fruit, Fennel Sd., Heartsease Lf., Grapefruit Seed Extract.

CLUSTER™ Caps (CO)
Ingredients: Feverfew, Ashwagandha, Valerian, Wild Lettuce, Ginkgo Biloba, Goldenseal Rt., Capsicum, Niacin.

COLD SEASON DEFENSE™ Caps (PD)
Ingredients: Garlic, Acerola Cherry, Bayberry Bk., Ascorbate Vit. C, DDS-1® Stabilized Veg. Acidophilus, Bee Pollen, Parsley Rt., Ginger Rt., Rosemary, Boneset Herb, St. John's Wort, Echinacea Angustifolia Rt., Capsicum.

DEPRESSEX™ Caps (CO)
Ingredients: ST. John's Wort, Kava Kava, American Ginseng Rt., Ashwagandha, Gtu Kola, Scullcap, Siberian Ginseng Rt., Rosemary, Wood Betony, FoTi Root, Ginger Root.

DETOX™ Caps (CD)
Ingredients: Red Clover Blsm., Licorice Rt., Ascorbate Vit. C, Burdock Rt., Pau d' Arco Bk., Sarsaparilla Rt., Kelp, Alfalfa Lf., Echinacea Purpurea Rt., Butternut Bk., Garlic, Goldenseal Rt., Astragalus Rt., Yellow Dock Rt., Buckthorn Bk., Prickly Ash Bk., Poria Mushroom, American Panax Ginseng Rt., Dandelion Rt., Milk Thistle Sd.

EASY CHANGE™ Caps (W)
Ingredients: Black Cohosh Rt., Scullcap Lf., Damiana Lf., Triphala Fruit, False Unicorn Rt., Sarsaparilla Rt., Dong Quai Rt., Squaw Vine Lf., Uva Ursi Lf., Red Raspberry Lf., Bayberry Bk., Cramp Bk., Ginger Rt., Rosemary Lf., Pennyroyal Herb, Blessed Thistle Herb.

EST-AID™ Caps (W)
Ingredients: Black Cohosh Rt., Sarsaparilla Rt., Licorice Rt., Dong Quai Rt., Damiana Lf., False Unicorn Rt., Squaw Vine Lf., Wild Yam Rt., Blessed Thistle.

ENERGY GREEN™ Caps (SA)
Ingredients: Barley Grass & Sprouts, Alfalfa Leaf & Sprouts, Rice Protein, Bee Pollen, Spirulina, Siberian Ginseng Root, Sarsaparilla Root, Acerola Cherry, Dandelion Root, Quinoa Sprouts, Oat Sprouts, Licorice Root, Hawthorn Bry., Lf., Flower, Gotu Kola, Dulse, Kelp.

EVENING PRIMROSE OIL PEARLS 1000mg (W)

EVENING PRIMROSE OIL PEARLS 500mg (W)

EYEBRIGHT COMPLEX™ Caps (CO)
Ingredients: Eyebright Herb, Parsley Rt., Bilberry Bry., Ginkgo Biloba Lf., Goldenseal Lf., Bayberry Bk., Hawthorn Lf., Flr & Bry., Red Raspberry Lf., Angelica Rt., Capsicum Fruit, Passionflowers.

FEEL GREAT™ Caps (E)
Ingredients: Bee Pollen, Siberian Ginseng Rt., Gotu Kola, Sarsaparilla, Licorice, Suma, Schizandra, Rice Protein Pwd., Alfalfa, Wild Cherry, Black Cohosh, Kelp, Goldenseal Rt., Hawthorn, American Panax Ginseng, Spirulina, Barley Grass, Ginkgo Biloba Lf., Capsicum Fruit, Nutritional Yeast Choline 10mg, Zinc (Gluconate) 3mg.

FEMALE HARMONY CAPS™ (W)
Ingredients: Dong Quai Rt., Damiana Lf., Burdock Rt., Sarsaparilla Rt., Licorice Rt., Red Raspberry Lf., Oat Straw, Nettles Herb, Dandelion Rt., Yellow Dock Rt., Rosemary Lf., Hawthorn Bry., Lf. & Flr., Peony Rt., Angelica Rt., Fennel Sd., Rose Hips, Ashwagandha Rt., & Lf., Ginger Rt., Rehmannia Rt., Cinnamon Bk., Chamomile Flr.

FIBER & HERB CLEANSE™ Caps (CD)
Ingredients: Butternut Bk., Cascara Sagrada, Turkey Rhubarb Rt., Psyllium Husks, Barberry Bk., Fennel Sd., Licorice Rt., Ginger Rt., Irish Moss, Capsicum Fruit.

FIRST- AID CAPS™ (PD)
Ingredients: Ascorbate Vit. C, Bayberry, Ginger Rt., White Pine Bk., Rose Hips, White Willow, Cloves, Capsicum.

GINSENG SIX™ Super Energy Caps (E)
Ingredients: Bee Pollen, Siberian Ginseng, Gotu Kola, Fo Ti Root, Kirin Ginseng root, Aralia Root, Prince Ginseng Root, Suma Root, Alfalfa Leaf Extract, Dong Quai Root, L-Glutamine 10mg.

HEARTSEASE/HAWTHORN Caps (H)
Ingredients: Hawthorn Lf., Flr. & Bry., Siberian Ginseng Rt., Motherwort Lf., Bilberry Bry., Capsicum Fruit, Astragalus Rt., Lecithin, D-Alpha Vit. E Pwd. 20IU, Ginkgo Biloba Lf., Heartsease Lf., Choline 15mg, Niacin 15mg.

HEARTSEASE H.B.P.™ Caps (H)
Ingredients: Garlic, Hawthorn Lf., Flr. & Bry., Siberian Ginseng Rt., Dandelion Rt., Parsley Rt., Ginger Rt., Capsicum Fruit, Heartsease Lf., Goldenseal Rt., Bilberry Bry., Vit. B$_6$ 15mg.

HEAVY METAL CLEANSE™ Caps (CD)
Ingredients: Ascorbate Vit. C, Bladderwrack, Kelp, Bugleweed Herb, Astragalus Rt., Barley Grass, Prickly Ash Bk., Licorice Rt., Parsley Rt.

HEMR-EASE™ Caps (CO)
Ingredients: Stone Rt., Slippery Elm Bk., Cranesbill, Goldenseal Rt., Butcher's Broom Rt., Witch Hazel Lf., Mullein Lf., Bilberry Bry., Rose Hips Ext., Ascorbate Vit. C.

HERBAL DEFENSE TEAM™ Caps (PD)
Ingredients: Siberian Ginseng Rt., Bee Pollen, Pau d'Arco Bk., Garlic, Bayberry Bk., Ascorbate Vit. C, Hawthorn Lf., Flr. & Bry., Burdock Rt., Echinacea Angustifolia Rt., Barley Grass, Suma Rt., Alfalfa Lf., Astragalus Rt., Schizandra Bry., Goldenseal Rt., Red Sage Lf., Elecampane Rt., Kelp, Yarrow Flr., Acerola Cherry Fruit, Capsicum Fruit, Dandelion Rt., Zinc Gluconate 3mg.

HI-PERFORMANCE™ Caps (E)
Ingredients: Siberian Ginseng Root, Bee Pollen granules, Sarsaparilla Rt., Licorice Rt., Gotu Kola Lf., Yeast Flakes, Spirulina, Suma Rt., Dandelion Rt., Yarrow Flws., Wild Yam Rt., Alfalfa Lf., Ginger Rt., Capsicum, Barley Grass Pwd., Ornithine, Arginine.

HRPS™ Caps (CO)
Ingredients: Astragalus Rt., Yellow Dock Rt., L-Lysine 75 mg, Echinacea Angustifolia Rt., Bupleurum Rt., Gentian Rt., Red Sage Lf., Oregon Grape Rt., Myrrh Gum, Marshmallow Rt., Wild Yam Rt., Sarsaparilla Rt., Natural Vit.E 15mg, Poria Mushroom.

IODINE/POTASSIUM SOURCE CAPS™ (SA)
Ingredients: Kelp, Alfalfa Lf., Dandelion Rt., & Lf., Dulse, Spirulina, Barley Grass, Nettles Herb, Borage Sd., Watercress Lf., L-Glutamine.

IRON SOURCE CAPS™ (SA)
Ingredients: Beet Rt., Yellow Dock Rt., Dulse, Dandelion Rt., & Lf., Borage Sd., Parsley, Rosemary Lf., Alfalfa Lf.

LEAN & CLEAN DIET™ Caps (D)
Ingredients: Spirulina, Kelp, Senna Lf. & Pods, Bancha Lf., Bee Pollen, Cascara Sagrada Bk., Alfalfa Sd., Fennel, Ginger Rt., Guar gum, Uva Ursi, Vit. B$_6$ 20mg.

LIV-ALIVE™ Caps (CD)
Ingredients: Beet Rt., Oregon Grape Rt., Dandelion Rt., Wild Yam Rt., Milk Thistle Sd., Yellow Dock Rt., Ginkgo Biloba Lf., Wild Cherry Bk., Licorice Rt., Gotu Kola Herb, Ginger Rt., Barberry Bk., Choline 10mg, Inositol 10mg.

LOVE FEMALE™ Caps (W)
Ingredients: Damiana., Dong Quai Rt., Burdock Rt., Licorice Rt., Guaraña Sd., Ashwagandha Rt. & Lf., Kola Nut, Sarsaparilla Rt.,Gotu Kola Lf., Parsley Lf., Ginger Rt.

LOVE MALE™ Caps (M)
Ingredients: Damiana, Guaraña, Saw Palmetto, Siberian Ginseng Rt., Kava Kava Rt., Yohimbe Bk., Sarsaparilla Rt., Muira Pauma wood chips, Suma Rt., Wild Yam Rt., Gotu Kola, Ginger, Niacin 15mg., Zinc (Gluconate) 3mg.

MALE PERFORMANCE CAPS™ (M)
Ingredients: Saw Palmetto Bry., Damiana Lf., Siberian Ginseng Rt., Sarsaparilla Rt., Royal Jelly, Muira Puama Wood Chips, Gotu Kola Herb, Wild Yam Rt., Licorice Rt., Dandelion Rt., American Panax Ginseng Rt., Fo Ti Rt., Yellow Dock Rt., Capsicum Fruit.

MENTAL CLARITY™ Caps (E)
Ingredients: American Panax Ginseng Rt., Gotu Kola Herb, Fo Ti Rt., Kelp, Ginkgo Biloba Lf., L-Glutamine 40mg, Siberian Ginseng Rt., Rosemary Lf., Schizandra Bry., Choline 20mg, Prickly Ash Bk., Capsicum, L-Phenylalanine 10mg, Zinc Gluconate 3mg.

MENTAL INNER ENERGY™ Caps (E)
Ingredients: Kava Kava Rt., Chinese Kirin Ginseng Rt., Siberian Ginseng Rt., American Panax Ginseng Rt., Dong Quai Rt., Suma Rt., Fo Ti Rt., Gotu Kola Herb, Prince Ginseng Rt., Ginkgo Biloba, Ashwagandha Root & Leaf.

META-TABS™ Active Caps (D)
Ingredients: Irish Moss, Kelp, Parsley Rt. & Lf., Watercress Lf., Sarsaparilla Rt., Mullein Lf., Lobelia Herb, Carrot Crystals, L-Glutamine 15mg.

MIGR-EASE™ Caps (CO)
Ingredients: Feverfew Herb, Valerian Rt., Wild Lettuce Lf., Rosemary Lf., Catnip Herb, European Mistletoe, Gentian Rt., Licorice Rt., DL-Phenylalanine.

MINERAL SPECTRUM CAPS™ (SA)
Ingredients: Nettles Herb, Irish Moss, Watercress Lf., Alfalfa Lf., Yellow Dock Rt., Dandelion, Barley Grass, Kelp, Parsley, Borage Sd., Dulse, L-Glutamine 10mg.

NIGHT CAPS™ (Rx)
Ingredients: Valerian, Scullcap, Passionflowers, Kava Kava, Hops, Carrots, GABA. 20mg, Taurine 20mg, Niacin 10mg.

PROX FOR MEN™ Caps (M)
Ingredients: Saw Palmetto, Licorice, Gravel Rt., Juniper Bry., Parsley Rt., Potency Wood, Goldenseal Rt., Uva Ursi Lf., Marshmallow, Ginger, Pygeum Africanum, Hydrangea, Capsicum, Vit. E Pwd. 20IU, Zinc Gluconate 7mg.

RAINFOREST ENERGY™ Caps (E)
Ingredients: Guaraña Sd., Kola Nut, Suma Rt., Bee Pollen, Ginger Rt., Capsicum, Astragalus, L-Glutamine 30mg.

RELAX CAPS™ (Rx)
Ingredients: Ashwaghndha Rt., & Lf., Black Cohosh Rt., Scullcap, Kava Kava Rt., Black Haw Bk., Hops Flr., Valerian Rt., Eur. Mistletoe, Wood Betony, Lobelia, Oatstraw.

RESPR™ Caps (B)
Ingredients: Mullein Lf., Wild Cherry Bk. & Oil, Ginkgo Biloba Lf., Slippery Elm Bk., Marshmallow Rt., Chickweed Herb, Licorice Rt., Kelp, Acerola Cherry Fruit, Cinnamon Bk., Ma Huang Herb, Capsicum.

SKIN #1™ Caps (BB)
Ingredients: Dandelion Rt., Burdock Rt., Echinacea Purpurea Rt., Blackthorn Bk., Sarsaparilla Rt., Red Clover Blsm., Licorice Rt., Yellow Dock Rt., Chamomile Flr., Vit. B$_6$ 25mg, L-Glutamine 12mg.

SKIN #2™ Caps (BB)
Ingredients: Licorice Rt., Dandelion, Burdock, Chickweed, Yellow Dock Rt., Alfalfa Lf., Sarsaparilla Rt., Rosemary, White Oak Bk., Bilberry Bry., Wild Yam Rt., Rose Hips, Ginger, L-Glutamine 10mg., Zinc (Gluconate) 3mg.

STN-EX™ Caps (CO)
Ingredients: Dandelion Rt., Parsley Rt., Wild Yam Rt., Marshmallow Rt., Hydrangea Rt., Licorice Rt., Gravel Rt., Lecithin, Lemon Balm Herb, Ginger Rt., Milk Thistle Sd.

SUGAR STRATEGY HIGH™ Caps (D)
Ingredients: Cedar Bry., Licorice Rt., Dandelion Rt., Elecampane Rt., Mullein Lf., Guar Gum, Wild Yam Rt., Uva Ursi Lf., Kelp, Horseradish, Bilberry Bry., Spirulina, Capsicum Pantothenic Acid 20mg, Glycine, Manganese 5mg.

SUGAR STRATEGY LOW™ Caps (D)
Ingredients: Licorice Rt., Dandelion, Cedar Bry., Alfalfa Lf., Wild Yam Rt., Gotu Kola Herb, Spirulina, Barley Grass, Guar Gum, Amino Acid Comp., Horseradish, Suma Rt.

SUPER LEAN DIET CAPS™ (D)
Ingredients: Gotu Kola, Chickweed, Gymnema Sylvestre, Guaraña, Ornithine 25mg, Carnitine 25mg, Lysine 25mg, Glycine 25mg, Bromelain, Rose Hips, Asc. Vit C 25mg, Phenylalanine 10mg, Vit.B$_6$ 10mg, GTF Chromium 10mg.

SUPERMAX™ Caps (SA)
Ingredients: Bee Pollen, American Panax Ginseng Rt., Siberian Ginseng Rt., Spirulina, Barley Grass, Suma Rt., Gotu Kola Lf., Kelp, Alfalfa Lf., Full Spectrum Amino Acid Compound, Pantothenic Acid 10mg.

SYSTEMS STRENGTH™ (SA)
Ingredients: The Food Blend: Yellow Miso, Soy Protein, Bee Pollen, Cranberry juice, Nutritional Yeast, DDS-1® Stabilized Vegetable Acidophilus. *The Herbal Blend:* Alfalfa, Oatstraw, Dandelion, Yellow Dock Rt., Borage Sd., Licorice Rt., Barley Grass, Watercress, Pau d'Arco, Raspberry, Horsetail, Nettles, Fennel, Parsley, Sib. Ginseng Rt., Schizandra, Bilberry, Rosemary. *Sea Vegetable Blend:* Spirulina, Dulse, Wakame, Kombu, Chlorella, Sea Palm.

THERA-DERM™ Caps (BB)
Ingredients: Burdock Rt., Dandelion Rt., Cleavers Herb, Yellow Dock Rt., Echinacea Purpurea Rt., Nettles Herb, Kelp, St. John's Wort Herb, Turmeric Rt., L-Lysine.

THERMO-CITRIN™ GINSENG™ caps (D)
Ingredients: Spirulina, Citrin™, Sida Cordifolia Rt., Lf., Seed extract, American Panax Ginseng Rt., Bancha Leaf, Kukicha Twig, Guarana Seed, Capsicum, Chromium Picolinate 200mcg.

TINKLE™ Caps (CD)
Ingredients: Uva Ursi , Corn Silk, Parsley, Dandelion, Juniper, Cleavers, Marshmallo, Ginger, Kelp, Vit.B$_6$ 25mg.

U.L.C.R.™ Complex Caps (CO)
Ingredients: Goldenseal Rt., Slippery Elm Bk., Licorice Rt., Myrrh Gum, Capsicum Fruit, Calendula Flr., Bilberry Bry.

VARI-VAIN™ Caps (BB)
Ingredients: Bilberry Bry., Hawthorn Lf., Flr. & Bry., Lemon Peel, Rose Hips, Hibiscus Flr., Grape Sd.Pwd.Ext.

VERMEX™ Caps (CD)
Ingredients: Black Walnut Hulls, Garlic, Pumpkin Sd., Gentian Rt., Butternut, Fennel Sd., Cascara Sagrada Bk., Mugwort, Slippery Elm Bk., False Unicorn, Wormwood.

WHITES OUT #1™ Caps (W)
Ingredients: Goldenseal Rt., Myrrh Gum, Pau d' Arco Bk., Echinacea Angustifolia Rt., DDS-1® Stabilized Vegetable Acidophilus, Ginkgo Biloba Lf., Dandelion Rt.

WHITES OUT #2™ Caps (W)
Ingredients: Burdock Rt., Juniper Bry., Squaw Vine Lf., Bayberry Bk., Parsley Rt., Dandelion Rt., Gentian Rt., Black Walnut Hulls, Uva Ursi Lf.

WITHDRAWAL SUPPORT™ Caps (CD)
Ingredients: Scullcap, Siberian Ginseng Rt., Ascorbate Vit. C, Kava Kava, Valerian, Alfalfa., Wood Betony, DL-Phenylalanine 35mg, Niacin 35mg, Licorice, Capsicum.

WOMAN'S BALANCE FIBRO™ Caps (W)
Ingredients: Pau d'Arco Bk., Burdock Rt., Goldenseal Rt., Black Cohosh Rt., Dandelion Rt. & Lf., Yellow Dock Rt., Ashwagandha Rt. & Lf., Dong Quai Rt., Ginger Rt., Astragalus Rt., Licorice Rt., Red Raspberry Lf.

WOMEN'S BEST FRIEND™ Caps (W)
Ingredients: Goldenseal Rt., Cramp Bark, Squaw Vine Lf., Red Raspberry Lf., Rose Hips, Dong Quai Rt., False Unicorn Rt., Sarsaparilla Rt., Peony Rt., Uva Ursi Leaf, Blessed Thistle Herb, Ginger Root, Rehmannia Root, Lobelia Herb.

ZINC SOURCE™ Caps (SA)
Ingredients: Echinacea Angustifolia Rt., Spirulina, Gotu Kola Herb, Barley Grass, Peppermint Herb, Alfalfa Lf., Bilberry Bry., Yellow Dock Rt.

Combination Extract Formulas

ACTIVE PHYSICAL ENERGY™ Ext. (E)
Ingredients: Fresh American Panax Ginseng, Kirin Ginseng, Prince Ginseng Rt., Siberian Ginseng Rt., Fo-Ti Rt., Suma Rt., Dong Quai Rt., Gotu Kola Lf., Wild Oats, Sarsaparilla Rt., Alcohol content 30%.

ADRN™ Extract (E)
Ingredients: Licorice Rt., Sarsaparilla Rt., Bladderwrack, Irish Moss, Alcohol content 45%.

AFTER MEAL ENZ.™ Extract (CO)
Ingredients: Mint Mix (Peppermint Lf., Spearmint Lf., Orange Peel, Lemon Peel), Papaya Sd., Licorice Rt., Hibiscus Flr., Glycerin. Alcohol content 40%.

ALRG/HST™ Extract (B)
Ingredients: Ma Huang Herb, Mullein Lf., Marshmallow Rt., Goldenseal Rt., Burdock Rt., Wild Cherry Bk., Licorice Rt., Cinnamon Bk., Essential Oils of Wintergreen & Lime. Alcohol content 50%.

ANTI-BIO™ Extract (PD)
Ingredients: Echinacea Angustifolia and Purpurea Rt., Lf. & Flr., Goldenseal Rt., Pau d'Arco, Myrrh Gum, Vegetable Glycerine, Wintergreen Oil. Alcohol content 55%.

ANTI-FLAM™ Extract (CO)
Ingredients: Curcumin (an isolated extract of Tumeric), St. John's Wort Lf., Butcher's Broom Herb, White Willow Bk., Bromelain. Alcohol content 50%.

ANTI-OXIDANT™ Extract (PD)
Ingredients: White Pine Bk., Siberian Ginseng Rt., Ginkgo Biloba, White Willow Bk., Sarsaparilla Rt., Spearmint, Lemon Peel & Oil. Alcohol content 50%.

ANTI-VI™ Extract (PD)
Ingredients: Lomatium Rt. 50%, St. John's Wort Lf. 50%, Honey, Tangerine Oil. Alcohol content 50%.

BILBERRY Extract (H)
Ingredients: Bilberry Berries (Vaccinium myrtillus). Alcohol content 45%.

BIO-VI™ Extract (PD)
Ingredients: Usnea Barbata, Wintergreen Oil, Alcohol 40%.

BITTERS AND LEMON™ Extract (CD)
Ingredients: Oregon Grape Rt., Gentian Rt., Cardamom Pods, Lemon Peel, Senna Lf., Dandelion Rt., Peppermint Lf., Honey. Alcohol content 40%.

BLACK WALNUT HULLS Extract (CD)
Ingredients: Black Walnut Hulls. Alcohol content 45%.

BLDR-K™ Extract (CD)
Ingredients: Cornsilk, Juniper Berry, Uva Ursi, Dandelion Root, Marshmallow Root, Goldenseal Root, Ginger Root, Parsley Root & Leaf, Honey. Alcohol content 55%.

BRNX™ Extract (B)
Ingredients: Mullein Leaf, Grindelia Squar Herb, Usnea Barbata Moss, Osha Root, Coltsfoot, Licorice Root, Goldenseal Root, Lobelia Leaf, Tangerine essential oil, Alcohol content 50%.

CALCIUM SOURCE™ Extract (SA)
Ingredients: Watercress Lf., Oatstraw, Rosemary Lf., Dandelion Lf., Borage Sd., Alfalfa Lf., Horsetail Herb. Alcohol content 55%.

CAN-SSIAC™ Extract (PD)

Ingredients: Sheep Sorrel, Burdock Rt., Red Clover Blm., Fresh American Ginseng Rt., Slippery Elm Bk., Turkey Rhubarb, Pau d'Arco Bk. Alcohol content 40%.

CHLORELLA/GINSENG Herbal Revitalizer Extract (SA)

Ingredients: Fresh American Panax Ginseng Rt., Chlorella. Alcohol content 30%.

CRAMP BARK COMBO™ Extract (CO)

Ingredients: Black Haw Bk., Cramp Bark, Kava Kava Rt., Rosemary Lf., Lobelia Lf., Honey, Vegetable Glycerine, Orange Essential Oil. Alcohol content 50%.

DEPRS-EX™ Extract (CO)

Ingredients: Scullcap Lf., Ashwagandha, St. John's wort, Rosemary Lf., Hops, Catnip, Wood Betony, Peppermint, Celery Sd., Cinnamon, Lime Essential Oil. Alcohol 45%.

DONG QUAI/DAMIANA Extract (W)

Ingredients: Dong Quai Rt., Damiana, Alcohol 55%.

ECHINACEA 100% Extract (PD)

Ingredients: Organically grown Echinacea Angustifolia Rt., Lf., Flr. & Sd. 50%, Echinacea Angustifolia., Lf., Flr. & Sd. 50%. Alcohol content 50%.

EASY CHANGE™ Extract (W)

Ingredients: Wild Yam Rt., Dong Quai Rt., Chaste Tree Bry., Damiana Lf., Licorice Rt. Alcohol content 40%.

EST-AID™ Extract (W)

Ingredients: Black Cohosh Rt., Dong Quai Rt., Damiana, Licorice Rt., Sarsaparilla Rt., Burdock Rt., Peony Rt., Oatstraw, Raspberry, Rosemary, Honey. Alcohol 55%.

FEM SUPPORT™ C.F.S. with Ashwaghandha (W)

Ingredients: Ashwaghandha Rt. & Lf., Dong Quai Rt., Damiana Lf. Alcohol content 38%.

GINKGO BILOBA Extract (H)

Ingredients: Ginkgo Biloba Lf. Alcohol content 55%.

GINSENG/LICORICE ELIXIR™ (D)

Ingredients: Fresh American Panax Ginseng Rt., Licorice Rt. Alcohol content 40%.

HAWTHORN 100% Extract (H)

Ingredients: Hawthorn Lf. Berry & Flower. Alcohol 45%.

HERBAL DEFENSE TEAM™ Extract (PD)

Ingredients: Garlic, Echinacea Angustifolia Rt., Siberian Ginseng Rt., Rose Hips, Hawthorn Lf. & Bry., Goldenseal Rt., Guggul, Pau d'Arco Bk., Astragalus Rt., Elecampane Rt., Honey, Peppermint Oil. Alcohol content 45%.

IODINE SOURCE™ Extract (SA)

Ingredients: Kelp, Kombu, Dulse, Wakame, Horsetail Herb, Alfalfa Lf., Irish Moss, Watercress Lf., Lemon & Orange Essential Oil. Alcohol content 40%.

IRON SOURCE™ Extract (SA)

Ingredients: Yellow Dock, Dulse, Watercress, Dandelion Lf., Nettles, Borage, Wintergreen Oil. Alcohol cont. 45%.

LIV-ALIVE™ Extract (CD)

Ingredients: Oregon Grape, Milk Thistle Sd., Yellow Dock Rt., Dandelion Rt., Licorice Rt., Red Sage Lf., Ginkgo Biloba Lf., Wild Yam, Fennel Sd., Alcohol content 60%.

LOVING MOOD EXTRACT FOR MEN™ (M)

Ingredients: Damiana Lf., Siberian Ginseng Rt., Licorice Rt., Wild Oats, Dandelion Rt., Capsicum Fruit , Yohimbe Bk. Alcohol content 50%.

MALE GINSIAC™ Extract (M)

Ingredients: Fresh Panax Ginseng, Damiana, Ginkgo Biloba, Muira Puama chips, Gotu Kola, Saw Palmetto Bry., Fresh Ginger Rt., Capsicum Fruit. Alcohol content 30%.

MENTAL INNER ENERGY™ Ext. (E)

Ingredients: Kava Kava Rt., Kirin Ginseng Rt., American Ginseng, Siberian Ginseng, Prince Ginseng, Dong Quai, Fo-Ti, Suma, Kola Nut, Gotu Kola. Alcohol content 45%.

MILK THISTLE SEED EXTRACT (CD)

Ingredients: Milk Thistle Sd. Alcohol content 60%.

MIGR™ Extract (CO)

Ingredients: Feverfew Flr., Ginkgo Biloba Lf., Siberian Ginseng Rt., Capsicum Fruit. Alcohol content 50%.

NIGHT ZZZ'S™ Extract (Rx)

Ingredients: Valerian Rt., Scullcap Lf., Hops, Passionflowers, Wild Lettuce Lf., Lime Oil. Alcohol content 50%.

PAU D' ARCO/ECHINACEA Ext. (PD)

Ingredients: Pau d'Arco Bk., Echinacea Angustifolia Rt. Alcohol content 45%.

PAU D' ARCO/GINSENG Ext. (PD)

Ingredients: Pau d'Arco Bk., Fresh American Panax Ginseng. Alcohol content 40%.

PRE-MEAL ENZ™ Extract (CO)

Ingredients: Ginger, Peppermint, Fennel, Catnip, Cramp Bark, Spearmint, Turmeric, Papaya. Alcohol content 45%.

PRO X™ for Men, with Pygeum Africanum (M)

Ingredients: Saw Palmetto, White Oak, Potency Wood, Echinacea Angust., Pau d' Arco, Goldenseal Rt., Marshmallow, Pygeum Afric., Uva Ursi. Alcohol cont. 45%.

REISHI/GINSENG Extract (PD)

Ingredients: Fresh American Panax Ginseng Rt., Reishi Mushrooms. Alcohol content 30%.

SCALE DOWN DIET™ Extract (D)

Ingredients: Chickweed Lf., Gotu Kola Lf., Licorice Rt., Dulse, Spirulina, Lemon Peel, Fennel Seed, Ma Huang, Senna Lf., Honey. Alcohol content 45%.

SIBERIAN GINSENG Extract (E)

Ingredients: Eleutherococcus. Alcohol content 35%.

STRESSED OUT™ Extract (Rx)

Ingredients: Black Cohosh Rt., Scullcap Lf., Black Haw Bk., Wood Betony Lf., Kava Kava Rt., Carrot Crystals, Honey, Lime Oil. Alcohol 50%.

SUPER MAN'S ENERGY™ Ext. (M)
Ingredients: Sarsaparilla rt., Saw Palmetto Bry., Suma Bk., Siberian Ginseng Rt., Gotu Kola Lf., Capsicum, Tangerine Essential Oil. Alcohol content 45%.

SUPER SARSAPARILLA Extract (W)
Ingredients: Organically grown Sarsaparilla. alcohol content 45%.

THERMO-GINSENG™ Extract (D)
Ingredients: Extract of Sida Cordifolia, Kukicha, Guaraña Sd., Fresh American Ginseng Rt., Spirulina, Bee Pollen, Hibiscus Flr., Fresh Ginger Rt., Capsicum Fruit, Chromium Picolinate 50mcg per dosage. Alcohol content 30%.

TRAVELER'S COMFORT™ Extract (CO)
Ingredients: Fresh Ginger Root, Ginkgo Biloba Leaf, Passionflowers, Wild Yam Root, Peppermint Leaf, & Oil, St. John's Wort Herb, Lavender Flowers, Capsicum Fruit, Alcohol content 50%.

VALERIAN/WILD LETTUCE EXT. (Rx)
Ingredients: Valerian Rt., Wild Lettuce Lf., Lemon and Lime Oil. Alcohol content 45%.

VITEX Extract (W)
Ingredients: Chaste Tree Berries (Vitex agnus castus). Alcohol content 45%.

WOMEN'S DRYNESS EXTRACT™ (W)
Ingredients: Licorice Rt., Dendrobium Rt., Alcohol content 45%.

ZINC SOURCE EXTRACT™ (PD)
Ingredients: Echinacea Angustifolia Rt., Spirulina, Gotu Kola Lf., Peppermint Herb, Bilberry Bry., Yellow Dock Rt., Alfalfa Lf., Barley Grass, Propolis, Peppermint Oil. Alcohol content 45%.

Combination Tea Formulas

ALLR/HST™ Tea (B)
Ingredients: Horehound Herb, Peppermint Leaf, Rose Hips, Ma Huang Herb, Rosebuds, Bee Pollen, Anise Seed & Oil, Ginger Root & Oil, Orange Peel, Cloves Fruit & Oil, Burdock Rt.

ANTI-VI™ Super Tea (PD)
Ingredients: Osha Rt., St. John's Wort Herb, Prince Ginseng Rt., Astragalus Root, Echinacea Purpurea Root, Peppermint Leaf & Oil.

ASTH-AID™ Tea (B)
Ingredients: Marshmallow Rt., Fenugreek Sd., Mullein, Ma Huang Herb, Wild Cherry Bk., Ginkgo Biloba, Rosemary Lf., Angelica, Passionflowers, Cinnamon, Lobelia.

BEAUTIFUL SKIN™ Tea (BB)
Ingredients: Licorice Rt., Burdock Rt., Rosemary Lf. & Oil, Rose Hips, Sarsaparilla Rt., Fennel Sd., White Sage Lf. & Oil, Thyme Lf., Parsley Leaf, Chamomile Flr., Dandelion Lf., Stevia Herb.

BLDR-K™ Tea (CD)
Ingredients: Uva Ursi Lf., Juniper Bry. & Oil, Corn Silk, Parsley Lf., Dandelion Lf., Plantain Lf., Ginger Rt. & Oil, Cleavers Herb, Marshmallow Rt.

CEL-LEAN RELEASE™ Tea (D)
Ingredients: Lemon Juice Pwd., Lemon Peel, Hawthorn Bry., Rose Hips, Hibiscus Flr., Bilberry Bry.

CHINESE ROYAL MU™ Tea (E)
Ingredients: Prince Ginseng Rt., Sarsaparilla Rt., Licorice Rt., Dandelion Rt., Burdock Rt., Ginger Rt. & Oil, Star Anise Sd. & Oil, Cloves Fruit & Oil, Orange Peel, Cinnamon Bk. & Oil, Aralia Rt., Cardamom Pods.

CLEANSING & PURIFYING™ Tea (CD)
Ingredients: Red Clover, Hawthorn, Horsetail, Echinacea Purpurea Lf., Milk Thistle Sd., Pau d' Arco Bk., Gotu Kola Herb, Lemongrass & Oil, Blue Malva Flr., Yerba Santa Lf.

COFEX™ Tea (B)
Ingredients: Slippery Elm Bk., Wild Cherry Bk., Licorice Rt., Fennel Sd., Orange Peel, Cinnamon Bk. & Oil, Cardamom Pods, Ginger Rt., Anise Oil.

CONCEPTIONS TEA™ (W)
Ingredients: Dong Quai, Black Cohosh, Royal Jelly, Licorice Rt., Sarsaparilla, Damiana, Wild Yam Rt., Fo-Ti, Burdock, Yellow Dock Rt., Scullcap, Ginger Rt., Bladderwrack.

CRAN-PLUS™ Tea (CD)
Ingredients: Pau d' Arco Bk., Cranberry Juice, Rose Hips, Damiana, Burdock Rt., Echinacea Purpurea, Myrrh Gum, Lemon Balm, Cinnamon Bk. & Oil, Hibiscus Flowers.

CREATIVI-TEA™ (E)
Ingredients: Gotu Kola, Kava Kava Rt., Prince Ginseng Rt., Damiana Lf., Cloves & Oil, Licorice Rt. & Oil, Spearmint Lf. & Oil, Juniper Bry., Muira Pauma wood chips.

CUPID'S FLAME™ Tea (E)
Ingredients: Damiana, Prince Ginseng Rt., Sarsaparilla Rt., Gotu Kola, Licorice Rt., Saw Palmetto., Muira Puama Chips, Kava Kava, Angelica Rt., Angelica Rt., Fo-Ti Rt., Ginger Rt. & Oil, Allspice Fruit & Oil, Anise Seed Oil.

DEEP BREATHING™ Tea (B)
Ingredients: Wild Cherry Bk. & Oil, Safflowers, Mullein Lf., Ma Huang Herb, Sage Lf., Ginger Rt., Pleurisy Rt., Thyme Lf., Blackberry Lf., Parsley Lf., Lobelia Lf.

EASY CHANGE™ Tea (W)
Ingredients: Burdock Rt., Licorice Rt., Black Cohosh, Dong Quai, Damiana Lf., Scullcap Lf., Red Raspberry Lf., Sarsaparilla Ginkgo Biloba, Ginger Rt., Bayberry Bk.

EST-AID™ Tea (W)
Ingredients: Motherwort Lf., White Sage Lf. & Oil, Licorice Rt., Blessed Thistle Herb, Dong Quai Rt., Damiana Lf., Rosemary Lf., Wild Yam Rt., Anise Oil.

EYEBRIGHT™ Tea (CO)
Ingredients: Eyebright, Bilberry, Passionflower, Plantain, Elder Flr., Rosemary, Goldenseal, Red Raspberry Lf.

FEEL GREAT TEA™ (E)
Ingredients: Red Clover, Alfalfa, Hawthorn Lf., Flr. & Bry., Prince Ginseng Rt., Spearmint, Dandelion Rt., White Sage Lf., Lemongrass, Dulse, Licorice Rt., Stevia Herb.

FEMALE HARMONY™ Tea (W)
Ingredients: Raspberry, Licorice Rt., Nettles Herb, Spearmint Herb & Oil, Rose Hips, Lemongrass & Oil, Strawberry Lf. & Oil, Sarsaparilla Rt., Burdock Rt., Rosebuds.

FIRST-AID TEA FOR KIDS™ (PD)
Ingredients: Chamomile Flr., Catnip Herb, Lemon Balm Herb, Fennel Sd., Acerola Cherry Fruit, Cinnamon Bk. & Oil, Cherry Oil, Stevia Herb.

FLOW EASE™ Tea (W)
Ingredients: Cramp Bark, Spearmint, Sarsaparilla Rt., Ginger Rt., Angelica Rt., Chamomile, Squaw Vine Lf.

GINSENG SIX SUPER TEA™ (PD)
Ingredients: Prince Ginseng Rt., Kirin Ginseng Rt., Echinacea Angustifolia, Pau d' Arco Bk., Suma Rt., Astragalus Rt., Echinacea Purpurea Rt., St. John's Wort Lf., Aralia Rt., Ashwagandha Rt. & Lf., Chinese White Ginseng Rt., Siberian Ginseng Rt., Reishi Mushroom, Fennel Sd., Tienchi Ginseng Rt., Ginger Oil.

GOOD NIGHT TEA™ (Rx)
Ingredients: Chamomile Flr., Spearmint Herb & Oil, Scullcap Lf., Passionflowers, Hops Flr., Lemongrass & Oil, Blackberry Lf., Orange Blm. & Oil, Rosebuds, Catnip Herb, Rose Hips, Stevia Herb.

GREEN TEA CLEANSER™ (CD)
Ingredients: Bancha Lf., Kukicha Twig, Burdock Rt., Gotu Kola Herb, Fo-Ti Rt., Hawthorn Bry., Orange Peel, Cinnamon Bk. & Oil, Orange Blossom Oil.

HEALTHY HAIR & NAILS™ Tea (BB)
Ingredients: Horsetail Herb, Nettles Herb, Rosemary Lf. & Oil, Alfalfa Lf., Lemongrass & Oil, Fenugreek Sd., Dandelion Rt., Coltsfoot Herb, White Sage Lf., Parsley Lf., Peppermint Lf. & Oil, Stevia Herb.

HEARTSEASE CIRCU-CLEANSE™ Tea (H)
Ingredients: Hawthorn Lf., Flr. & Bry., Bilberry Bry., Kukicha Twig, Ginger Rt. & Oil, Heartsease Lf., Ginkgo Biloba Lf., Pau d' Arco Bk., Red Sage Lf., Licorice Rt., White Sage & Oil, Astragalus Rt.

HEARTSEASE H.B.P.™ Tea (H)
Ingredients: Hawthorn Lf., Flr. & Bry., Scullcap Lf., Dandelion Rt. & Lf., Prince Ginseng Rt., Ginger Rt. & Oil, Heartsease Lf., Valerian Rt.

HERBAL DEFENSE TEAM TEA™ (PD)
Ingredients: Red Clover, Hawthorn Lf., Flr. & Bry., Burdock Rt., Licorice Rt., Suma Rt., Schizandra Bry., Astragalus Rt., White Sage, Aralia Rt., Lemongrass & Oil, Marshmallow Rt., Boneset Lf., St. John's Wort, Anise Oil.

HI-ENERGY™ Tea (E)
Ingredients: Gotu Kola Lf., Peppermint Lf. & Oil, Damiana Lf., Red Clover, Cloves Fruit & Oil, Prince Ginseng Rt., Kava Kava Rt., Aralia, Raspberry Lf.

INCREDIBLE DREAMS™ Tea (Rx)
Ingredients: Kava Kava Rt., Mugwort Lf., Rosemary Lf. & Oil, Lemongrass, Red Raspberry Lf., Alfalfa Lf., Stevia.

LAXA™ Tea (CD)
Ingredients: Senna Lf., Fennel Sd. & Oil, Papaya Lf., Peppermint Lf. & Oil, Ginger Rt. & Oil, Lemon Balm Herb, Parsley Lf., Hibiscus Flr., Calendula Flr.

LEAN & CLEAN DIET™ Tea (D)
Ingredients: Flax Sd., Fennel Sd. & Oil, Uva Ursi Lf., Parsley Lf., Senna Lf., Chickweed Lf., Senna Pods, Red Clover Blm., Hibiscus Flr., Lemon Peel, Burdock Rt., Cleavers.

LEAN & CLEAN SUPER DIET™ Tea (D)
Ingredients: Flax Sd., Fennel Sd. & Oil, Gotu Kola Lf., Uva Ursi Lf., Senna Lf. & Pods, Fenugreek Sd., Parsley Lf., Bancha Lf., Gymnema Sylvestre Lf., Burdock Rt., Red Clover Blm., Lemon Peel, Hibiscus Flr., Bladderwrack.

LIV-ALIVE™ Tea (CD)
Ingredients: Dandelion Rt., Watercress Lf., Yellow Dock Rt., Pau d'Arco Bk., Hyssop Herb, Parsley Lf., Oregon Grape Rt., Red Sage, Licorice Rt., Milk Thistle Sd., Hibiscus Flr., White Sage Oil.

MEDITATION TEA™ (Rx)
Ingredients: Cardamom, Cinnamon Bk. & Oil, Cloves Fruit & Oil, Black Peppercorns, Fennel Sd., Ginger Rt. & Oil.

MIGR.™ TEA (CO)
Ingredients: Feverfew Herb, Ashwagandha Rt. & Lf., Valerian Rt., Wild Lettuce Lf., Ginkgo Biloba Lf., Cardamom Sd. Pods, Niacinamide 60mg.

MOTHERING TEA™ (W)
Ingredients: Red Raspberry Lf. & Oil, Spearmint Herb & Oil, Alfalfa Lf., Nettles Herb, Lemongrass & Oil, Fennel Sd., Strawberry Lf., Ginger Rt., Stevia Herb.

NIC-STOP TEA™ (PD)
Ingredients: Lobelia Lf., Licorice Rt., Oats, Peppermint Lf. & Oil, Sarsaparilla Rt., Egyptian Chamomile Flr., Stevia.

RAINFOREST ENERGY™ Super Tea (E)
Ingredients: Guaraña Sd., Kola Nut, Suma Rt., Yerba Mate, Cinnamon Bk. & Oil, Stevia Herb.

RELAX TEA™ (Rx)
Ingredients: Lemon Balm Herb, Lemongrass & Oil, Spearmint Herb & Oil, Licorice Rt., Orange Peel, Yerba Santa Lf., Cinnamon Bk., Rosemary Lf., Passion flowers, Rosebuds, Anise Oil.

RESPR™ Tea (B)
Ingredients: Fenugreek Sd., Hyssop Herb, Horehound Herb, Ginkgo Biloba Lf., Rose Hips, Ma Huang Herb, Marshmallow Rt., Boneset Herb, Anise Sd. & Oil, Peppermint Lf. & Oil, Wild Cherry Bk., Lobelia Herb, Stevia Herb.

STRESSED OUT" TEA™ (Rx)
Ingredients: Rosemary Lf. & Oil, Chamomile Flr., Catnip Herb, Peppermint Herb & Oil, Heartsease Lf., Wood Betony Lf., Blessed Thistle Herb, Gotu Kola Herb, White Willow Bk., Feverfew Flr.

SUGAR STRATEGY LOW™ Tea (D)
Ingredients: Licorice Rt., Dandelion Rt., Alfalfa Lf., Gotu Kola Lf., Prince Ginseng Rt., Peppermint Lf. & Oil, Nettles Herb, Bee Pollen, Anise Oil.

TINKLE™ TEA (CD)
Ingredients: Uva Ursi, Senna Lf., Parsley Lf., Fennel Sd. & Oil, Lemon Peel & Oil, Dandelion Lf., Ginger Rt., Dulse.

WOMAN'S STRENGTH ENDO™ Tea (W)
Ingredients: Dandelion Rt., Wild Yam Rt., Sarsaparilla Rt., Burdock Rt., Pau d' Arco Bk., Chaste Tree Bry., Milk Thistle Sd., Echinacea Purpurea Rt., Dong Quai Rt., Cinnamon Bk. & Oil, Ginger Rt., Orange Peel, Orange Blossom Oil, Stevia Herb.

X-PECT-TEA™ (B)
Ingredients: Ma Huang Herb, Licorice Rt., Pleurisy Rt., Mullein Lf., Rose Hips, Marshmallow Rt., Peppermint Lf. & Oil, Fennel Sd. & Oil, Boneset Herb, Ginger Rt. & Oil, Calendula Flr., Stevia Herb.

Drink Mixes

BIOFLAVONOID FIBER & VIT.C SUPPORT™ CITRUS & Herb Drink Mix (PD)
Ingredients: Pear Flakes, Cranberry Pwd., Apple Pectin, Acerola Cherry, Honey Crystals, Rose Hips, Lemon Peel, Orange Peel, Hawthorn Bry., Hibiscus Flr., Ginkgo Biloba Lf., Rutin, Bilberry Lf.

CHO-LO FIBER-TONE™ (H)
Ingredients: Organic Oat Bran, Organic Flax Seed (high in Omega 3 Oils), Psyllium Husks, Guar Gum, Vegetable Acidophilus, Apple Pectin, Fennel Sd., Acerola Cherry, Wild Cherry Oil or Orange Oil, Grapefruit Sd. Ext.

ENERGY GREEN™ Drink Mix (SA)
Ingredients: Rice Protein, Barley Grass & Sprouts, Alfalfa Leaf & Sprouts, Bee Pollen, Acerola Cherry, Oat & Quinoa Sprouts, Apple Pectin, Siberian Ginseng Root, Sarsaparilla, Spirulina, Chlorella, Dandelion, Dulse, Licorice Root, Gotu Kola, and Apple Juice.

LIGHT WEIGHT™ Vanilla Spice, Nutritional Meal Replacement (D)
Ingredients: Brown Rice Protein, Honey Crystals, Guar Gum, Oat Bran, Acerola Cherry, Beet Root, Soy Protein, Cherry concentrate, Bee Pollen, Senna Lf. & Pods, Fennel Sd., Maple Sugar Granules, Apple Pectin Powder., Papaya Leaf, Pineapple Juice Powder, Gymnema Sylvestre, Vanilla Powder, Red Raspberry, Cinnamon Bk., Rutin, Wild Yam Root, Nutritional Yeast, Spirulina.

LIGHT WEIGHT™ Pineapple/Orange, Nutritional Meal Replacement (D)
Ingredients: Brown Rice Protein, Honey Crystals, Guar Gum, Oat Bran, Acerola Cherry, Soy Protein, Safflowers, Pineapple Juice Pwd., Bee Pollen, Senna Lf., Fennel Sd., Maple Sugar Granules, Apple Pectin Pwd., Papaya Lf., Gymnema Sylvestre, Barley Grass, Orange concentrate, Red Raspberry Lf., Cinnamon Bk., Wild Yam Rt., Rutin, Spirulina, Orange Oil, Nutritional Yeast.

SYSTEMS STRENGTH™ Drink Mix (SA)
Ingredients: Herbal Blend: Alfalfa, Borage Sd., Yellow Dock Rt., Oatstraw, Dandelion, Barley Grass, Licorice Rt., Watercress Lf., Pau d'Arco, Nettles, Horsetail Herb, Red Raspberry, Fennel Sd., Parsley, Bilberry Bry., Siberian Ginseng Rt., Schizandra, Rosemary Lf. *Sea Vegetable Blend:* Dulse, Wakame, Kombu, Sea Palm. *Food Blend:* Miso, Soy, Tamari, Cranberry Juice, Nutritional Yeast.

Phyto-Therapy Gels

ANTI-BIO™ Gel (BB)
Ingredients: Extracts of Una de Gato Bk., Pau d' Arco Bk., and Calendula Flr. in a natural gel base (Distilled Water, Aloe Vera Gel, Vegetable Glycerine, Lecithin, Grapefruit Sd. Ext., Cellulose thickener and Agar.)

BEAUTIFUL SKIN™ Gel (BB)
Ingredients: Extract of Licorice Rt., Burdock Rt., Rosemary Lf., Rose Hips, Sarsaparilla Rt., White Sage Lf., Chamomile Flr., Parsley Lf., Fennel Sd., Thyme Lf., Dandelion Lf: Royal Jelly 175mg, Propolis 100mg, Bee Pollen 100mg, Korean Ginseng; in a natural gel base (Distilled Water, Aloe Vera, Vegetable Glycerine, Lecithin, Honey, Grapefruit Sd. Ext., Cellulose Thickener and Agar.)

FUNGEX SKIN™ Gel (BB)
Ingredients: Extracts of Pau d'Arco Bk., Dandelion Rt., Gentian Rt., Myrrh Gum, Goldenseal Rt., Witch Hazel Lf., Lomatium Dissectum Rt. and Grapefruit Sd: Vit. D; in a natural gel base (Distilled Water, Aloe Vera Gel, Vegetable Glycerine, Lecithin, Cellulose Thickener and Agar.)

GINSENG SKIN REPAIR™ Gel (BB)
Ingredients: Ext. of Ginseng (American Ginseng, Chinese Ginseng), Suma, White Pine and Calendula, Vit. C, Germanium, in a natural base (dist. Water, Aloe Vera, Veg. Glycerine, Lecithin, Grapefruit Sd. Ext., Cellulose, Agar).

HEMR-EASE™ Gel (CO)
Ingredients: Extracts of Slippery Elm Bk., Stone Rt., Rose Hips/ Vit.C, Goldenseal Rt., Bilberry, Mullein, Cranesbill Rt., Butcher's Broom, Witch Hazel Lf. in a natural base (Distilled Water, Aloe Vera Gel, Vegetable Glycerine, Lecithin, Grapefruit Sd. Ext., Cellulose thickener and Agar).

LYSINE/LICORICE HEALING™ Gel (BB)
Ingredients: Extracts of Licorice and Myrrh; 800mg Lysine in a natural base (Distilled Water, Aloe Vera, Veg. Glycerine, Lecithin, Grapefruit Sd. Ext., Cellulose and Agar).

Pro-Est Roll-On Gels

PRO-EST BALANCE™ (W)
Ingredients: Aloe Vera Juice, Dist. Water, Grapeseed Oil, Extracts (Wild Yam, American Ginseng Rt.,Dong Quai., Damiana, Licorice Rt., Black Cohosh, Burdock Rt., Sarsaparilla, Raspberry, Dandelion, Echinacea Angustifolia Rt., Red Clover, Peony Rt., Oatstraw), Vegetable Glycerine, Lecithin, Cellulose, Ginseng Rt., Phytosomes, Licorice Rt. Phytosomes.

PRO-EST EASY CHANGE™ (W)
Ingredients: Aloe Vera Juice Conc., Dist. Water, Grape Seed Oil, Herbal Extract (Extract of: Wild Yam Rt., Fresh Am. Ginseng Rt., Licorice Rt., Dong Quai Rt., Damiana Lf., Black Cohosh Rt., Scullcap, Sarsaparilla Rt., Burdock Rt., Alfalfa Lf., Peony Rt., Ginkgo Biloba, Dandelion Lf., Uva Ursi, Bayberry Bk., Red Raspberry), Vegetable Glycerine, Lecithin S-10, Cellulose thickener, Methyl &Propyl Paraben, Ginseng Rt. Phytosomes, Licorice Rt Phytosomes.

PRO-EST OSTEO-PLUS™ Roll-on (PD)
Ingredients: Aloe Vera Juice Conc., Distilled Water, Grape Seed Oil, Herbal Extract (Extracts of: Wild Yam Rt., Fresh American Ginseng Rt., Dong Quai Rt., Horsetail Herb, Black Cohosh Rt., Dandelion Lf., Alfalfa Lf., Borage Seed, Sarsaparilla Rt., Burdock Rt., Red Raspberry Lf., Dulse, Oatstraw), Vegetable Glycerine, Lecithin S-10, Cellulose thickener, Methyl Paraben, Propyl Paraben, Ginseng Root Phytosomes, Licorice Root Phytosomes.

PRO-EST PROX™ Roll-on (M)
Ingredients: Aloe Vera Juice Conc., Distilled Water, Grape Seed Oil, Herbal Extract (Extracts of: Wild Yam Rt., Fresh American Ginseng Rt., Saw Palmetto Bry., White Oak Bk., Potency Wood, Echinacea Angustifolia Rt., Goldenseal Rt., Pau d'Arco Bk., Licorice Rt., Burdock Rt., Oregon Grape Rt., European Mistletoe, Marshmallow Rt., Uva Ursi Lf., Pygeum Africanum Bk.), Vegetable Glycerine, Lecithin S-10, Cellulose thickener, Methylparaben, Propylparaben, Ginseng Rt. Phytosomes, Licorice Rt. Phytosomes.

PRO-EST WOMAN'S DEFENSE™ (W)
Ingredients: Aloe Vera Juice Distilled Water, Grape Seed Oil, Herbal Extract (Extracts of Wild Yam Rt., Fresh American Ginseng Rt., Dong Quai Rt., Damiana, Licorice Rt., Black Cohosh Rt., Burdock, Sarsaparilla Rt., Raspberry Lf., Dandelion, Echinacea Angustifolia Rt., Red Clover Blm., Peony Rt., Oatstraw), Veg. Glycerine, Lecithin, Cellulose, Ginseng Rt. Phytosomes, Licorice Rt. Phytosomes.

Euro Spa

ALKALIZING ENZYME HERBAL BODY WRAP (CD)
Ingredients: The Wrap: Bladderwrack, Alfalfa Lf., Ginger Rt., Dandelion Rt., Spearmint Herb, Capsicum, Cinnamon Bk. in a base of Aloe Vera Gel, Olive Oil, Grapeseed Oil, Lecithin, Veg. Glycerine and Beeswax. *The Drink:* Miso Granules, Dulse, Barley Grass, Turmeric Rt., Ginger Rt. *The Capsules:* Spirulina, Alfalfa, Vegetable Acidophilus.

CEL-LEAN GEL™ & WAFER KIT (D)
Ingredients: The Gel: Extract of Bladderwrack, Gotu Kola Lf., Rosemary Lf., Uva Ursi Lf., Lemon Peel, Butcher's Broom Rt., Plantain Lf., Eucalyptus Lf., Capsicum, Vanilla in a base of Aloe Vera Gel, Vegetable Cellulose, Distilled Water, Vegetable Glycerine, Grapefruit Sd. Ext., Ascorbate Vit.C and Vit.E, Cinnamon Oil for Fragrance. *The Wafers:* Lemon Juice Pwd., Lemon Peel, Bilberry Bry., Hibiscus Flr., Rose Hips, Hawthorn Bry., Fruitsource Sweetener.

HOT SEAWEED BATH (CD)
Ingredients: Kelp, Kombu, Bladderwrack, Dulse, Sea Grasses.

LEMON BODY GLOW™ (BB)
Ingredients: Sundried Sea Salt, Aloe Vera Powder, Lemon Peel Granules, Almond Oil, Lemon Oil.

THERMO-CEL-LEAN™ Gel (D)
Ingredients: Aloe Vera Juice Conc., Distilled Water, Grape Seed Oil, Herbal Extract (Extracts of: Bladderwrack, Gotu Kola Lf., Kola Nut, Bancha Lf., Guarana, Rosemary Lf., Uva Ursi Lf., Lemon Peel, Butcher's Broom Rt., Eucalyptus Lf., Horsetail Herb, Dulse, Wakame, Kombu, Capsicum), Escin, Lecinol S-10, Vegetable Glycerine, Cellulose Thickener, Methyl Paraben, Propyl Paraben.

TONING MASQUE (BB)
Ingredients: French White Clay, Chamomile Flr., Calendula Flr., Lemon Peel, Eucalyptus Lf., Rosemary Lf., Spearmint Lf., Fennel Sd., Goldenseal Rt.

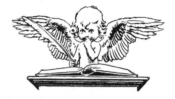

Miscellaneous Combinations

POUNDS OFF™ BATH (D)
Ingredients: Jaborandi Lf., Thyme Herb, Angelica R., Elder Flower, Orange Peel, Pennyroyal Herb, Kesu Flower, Orange Blossom Oil.

WHITES OUT DOUCHE™ (W)
Ingredients: Witch Hazel Lf. & Bk., Comfrey Root, Juniper Bry., Myrrh Gum, Goldenseal Rt., Pau d'Arco Bk., Buchu Lf., Squaw Vine Lf., Oatstraw, White Oak Bk.

Animal Formulas

AR-EASE FOR ANIMALS™ (A)
Ingredients: Nutritional Yeast, Alfalfa Lf., Sodium Ascorbate Vit.C, Garlic, Alfalfa Sd., Yucca, Kelp, Turmeric Rt., Devil's Claw Rt., Bilberry Bry., Black Cohosh Rt., Buckthorne Bk., Yarrow Flr., Licorice Rt., Parsley Rt., Slippery Elm Bk., Dandelion Rt. & Lf., Acidophilus, Papaya Lf., Comfrey Rt., Bromelain.

HEALTHY LIFE ANIMAL MIX™ (A)
Ingredients: Nutritional Yeast, Alfalfa Lf., Lecithin, Kelp, Wheat Bran & Germ, Comfrey Lf., Barley Grass, Garlic, Soy Protein, Dandelion Lf., Spirulina, Sodium Ascorbate Vit. C, Rosemary Lf.

MOTH-FREE™ (A)
Ingredients: Cedarwood Chips, Rosemary Lf., Lemongrass, Lavender Flr., Bay Lf., Basil-Egypt, Cellulose, Rosemary Oil, Eucalyptus Oil, Cedar Oil.

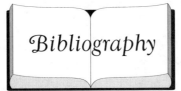

Bibliography

Thanks to four dedicated, hard-working research assistants: Barbara Howard, Kim Tunella, Sarah Abernathy.

Your Health Care Choices Today

Mowrey, Daniel B., Ph. D. *The Scientific Validation of Herbal Medicine.* 1986

Krizmanic, Judy. "The Best of Both Worlds." *Vegetarian Times.* 1995

Mowrey, Daniel B., Ph.D. *Next Generation Herbal Medicine.* 1990

Ruch, M. Gould, "Feeling Down?" *Natural Health.* 1993

Grimm, Ellen. "Increase Your Energy with Self-Massage." *Natural Health.* 1994

Blate, Michael. "Headaches & Backaches." *Healthy and Natural Journal.* 1994

Weiss, Rick. "Medicine's Latest Miracle Acupuncture." *The Natural Way.* 1995

Steefel, Lorraine R.N, M.A. "Use of Acupuncture for Detoxification." *Alternative & Complementary Therapies.* 1995

Bowles, Willa Vae, "Enzymes for Energy," *Total Health.* 1993

Cichoke, Anthony J., D.C. *Enzymes & Enzyme Therapy.* 1994

Cichoke, Anthony J., D.C. "Enzyme Therapy." *Let's Live.* 1993

Gregory, Scott J., *A Holistic Protocol for The Immune System,* 1995

Valnet, Jean, M.D. *The Practice of Aromatherapy.* 1990

Tisserand, Robert. *Aromatherapy to Heal and Tend the Body.* 1988

Price, Shirley. *Practical Aromatherapy, How to Use Essential Oils to Restore Vitality.* 1987

Robbins, John. *Diet For A New America.* 1987

Gates, Donna. *The Body Ecology Diet.* 1993

Liberman, Jacob, O.D., Ph. D. *Light - Medicine Of The Future.* 1991

Myss, Caroline, Ph.D & C. Norman Shealy, M.D., Ph.D. *The Creation of Health.* 1993

Herbal Healing

Chen, Ze-lin M.D. & Mei-fang Chen, M.D. *Comprehensive Guide to Chinese Herbal Medicine.* 1992

Reid, Daniel. *Chinese Herbal Medicine.* 1993

Yen-Hsu, Hong. *How to Treat Yourself with Chinese Herbs.* 1993

Frawley, David O., M.D. "Ayurveda, the Science of Life." *Let's Live.* 1993

Treadway, Scott Ph.D. & Linda Treadway Ph.D. *Ayurveda & Immortality.* 1986

Weil, Andrew, M.D. *Spontaneous Healing.* 1995

Zucker, Martin. "Women's Health - Ayurveda Offers Ancient Solutions for Modern Times." *Let's Live.* 1995

Werbach, Melvyn R., M.D. *Nutritional Influences On Illness - A Sourcebook Of Clinical Research.* 1988

Baar, Karen. *The Real Options in Healthcare.* 1995

Marshall, Lisa Anne. "The Roots of Western And Herbal Medicine." *Natural Foods Merchandiser.* 1994

Wolfson, Evelyn. *From the Earth To Beyond the Sky - Native American Medicine.* 1993

Hultkrantz, Ake. *Shamanic Healing & Ritual Drama.* 1992

Fillius, Thomas J., et al. "Chief Two Moons Meridas: Indian Miracle Man?" *HerbClip-American Botanical Council.* 1995

Colbin, Annemarie. *Food and Healing.* 1986

Laux, Marcus. *Cures from the Rainforest Pharmacy.* 1995

Arnold, Kathryn. "Rain Forest Medicine." *Delicious Magazine.* 1994

Schwontkowski, Donna. *Herbal Treasures from the Amazon.* 1995

Mendelsohn, Robert & Michael J. Balick. "More Drugs Await Discovery in Rainforests." *ABC.* 1995

Rodger, Katie. "Back To Our Roots." *Pharmacists Explore the Potential of Phytomedicinals." Drug Topics.* 1995

Hevelingen, Andy Van. "Growing Seeds." *The Herb Companion.* 1993

Baar, Karen. "Grow Your Own Pharmacy." *Natural Health.* 1995

Healing Programs For People With Special Needs

Zand, Janet , LAc, OMD, et al. *Smart Medicine For a Healthier Child.* 1994

Denda, Margare E. & Phyllis S. Williams. *The Natural Baby Food Cookbook.* 1982

Wigmore, Ann. *Recipes for Longer Life.* 1978

Bauman, Edward, Ph.D. "Eating For Health - A Regenerative Five Food Group System." 1994

Tunella, Kim, C.D.C. "Enzymes...The Spark of Life." 1994

Howell, Dr. Edward. *Enzyme Nutrition - The Food Enzyme Concept.* 1985

Peiper, Howard & Nina Anderson. *Over 50 Looking 30!* 1996.

Jones, Susan Smith. *The Main Ingredients of Health & Happiness.* 1995

Peiper, Howard & Nina Anderson. *All Natural Anti-Aging Skin Care.* 1996

Martlew, Gillian, N. D. *Electrolytes the Spark of Life.* 1994

Murray, Michael T., N.D. *The Healing Power of Foods.* 1993

Murray, Michael T., N.D. *Healing Power of Herbs.* 1992

Fontaine, Darryl & David Minard. *Forever Young - How To Energize Your Body Naturally.* 1993

Murray, Michael T., N.D. *The Complete Book of Juicing.* 1992

Passwater, Richard A., Ph.D. *The New Super Nutrition.* 1991

Hoffman, Dr. Jay M. *Hunza - 15 Secrets of the World's Healthiest & Oldest Living People.* 1979

Hobbs, Christopher. *Ginkgo - Elixir of Youth.* 1995

Batmanghelidj, F. , M.D. *Your Body's Many Cries for Water.* 1996

Kugler, Hans, Ph. D. "Interview." *Nutrition & Healing.* 1995

Samuels, Mike, M.D. & Nancy Samuels. *The Well Adult.* 1988

Brown, Donald J., N.D. *Herbal Prescriptions for Better Health.* 1995

Tierra, Lesley, L. AC. *The Herbs of Life.* 1992

Loehr, Dr. James E. & Dr. Jeffrey A. Migdow. *Take A Deep Breath.* 1986

Siegal, Bernie, M.D. *How To Live Between Office Visits.* 1993

Dossey, Larry, M.D. *Healing Words.* 1993

Borysenko, Joan & Miroslav. *The Power of the Mind to Heal - Renewing Body, Mind & Spirit.* 1994

Colgan, Dr. Michael. *Optimum Sports Nutrition.* 1993

Phillips, Bill. *Supplement Review 1996* (Athletes & Bodybuilders)

Burgstiner, Carson B., M.D. "You Are What You Eat." *Health Counselor.* 1991

Hobbs, Christopher. "Herbs For Fitness." *Let's Live.* 1991

Peiper, Howard & Nina Anderson. *Are You Poisoning Your Pets?* 1995

Pitcairn, Richard H., D.V.M., Ph.D. & Susan H. Pitcairn *Natural Health for Dogs & Cats.* 1995

Stein, Diane. *Natural Healing for Dogs & Cats.* 1993

A Guide to Detoxification, Fasting & Body Cleansing

Larson, Joan Mathews, Ph.D. *Seven Weeks To Sobriety.* 1992

Jensen, Bernard, D.C., Nutritionist. *Tissue Cleansing Through Bowel Management.* 1981

Schechter, Steven R., N.D. *Fighting Radiation & Chemical Pollutants With Foods, Herbs & Vitamins* - Documented Natural Remedies That Boost Your Immunity & Detoxify. 1994

Cassata, Carla. "How To Balance Body Chemistry." *Let's Live.* March 1995

Baker, Elizabeth & Dr. Elton. *The Uncook Book - Raw Food Adventures To A New Health High.* 1983

Benninger, Jon. 'Detox." *The Energy Times.* July 1994

Thomson, Bill. "Rejuvenate Yourself in Three Weeks." *Natural Health.* January 1993

Langer, Stephen, M.D. "Keeping Environmental Toxins At Bay," *Better Nutrition For Today's Living.* July 1993

Hobbs, Christopher. "Tonics, Bitters, Digestion, and Elimination." *Let's Live.* August 1990

Easterling, John. "Rainforest Bio-Energetics." *Healthy & Natural Journal.* October 1994

Rogers, Sherry A., M.D. "Doctors' Dialogue - Toxic Encephalopathy." *Let's Live.* March 1995

Hobbs, Christopher. "Herbs For Health - Losing Addictions Naturally." *Let's Live.* April 1993

Zand, Janet, L.Ac., O.M.D. "Nutrients and Herbs for the Recovering Addict." *Health World.* July 1992

Duncan, Lindsey, C.N. "Internal Detoxification." *Healthy & Natural Journal.* October 1994

Blauer, Stephen. *Rejuvenation.* 1980

Airola, Paavo, Ph.D. *How To Get Well.* 1974

Walker, Norman, D.SC., Ph. D. *Colon Health.* 1979

Goldberg, Burton. "Detoxification Therapy." *Alternative Medicine - The Definitive Guide.* 1993

Diagnostics

Igram, Dr. Cass. with Judy K. Gray, M.S. *Self Test Nutrition Guide.* 1994

Chilnick, Lawerance D., et al. *Pill Book.* 1994

Castleman, Michael. "Diagnose Yourself." *Natural Health.* July 1993

LeBeau, James, DN. *Balance Your PH*

Murray, Michael T., N.D. *Natural Alternatives to Over-the-Counter and Prescription Drugs.* 1994

Ody, Penelope. *The Complete Medicinal Herbal,* 1993

Duke, James Alan & Rodolfo Vasquez. *Amazonian Ethnobotanical Dictionary.* 1994

Thomas, Clayton L., M.D., M.P.H. *Taber's Cyclopedic Medical Dictionary.* 1989

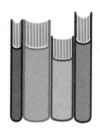

Jackson, Mildred, N.D. & Terri Teague, N.D., D.C. *The Handbook of Alternatives to Chemical Medicine,* 1991

Gaia Herbal Research Institute, *Gaia Symposium Proceedings-Naturopatic Herbal Wisdom,* 1994

Golin, Mark. "Morning Forecast - A 14 Point Health Checklist." *Men's Health.* July 1995

Stein, Diane. *The Natural Remedy Book For Women,* 1995

Chaitow, Leon, N.D., D.O. & James Strohecker with The Burton Goldberg Group. *You Don't Have To Die - Aids Can Be Controlled.* 1994

Gottlieb, Bill (Editor-in-Chief Prevention Magazine Health Books). *New Choices in Natural Healing* - Over 1,800 of the Best Self-Help Remedies from the World of Alternative Medicine. 1995

Medline (The Physician's National Medical Research Database). *Physical Conditions Affected By A Deficiency Of The Metabolic Catalysts.* Hawaii Medical Library, Inc.

Herbal Research Publications. *The Protocol Journal Of Botanical Medicine,* 1995

Werbach, Melvyn R., M.D. *Nutritional Influences On Illness - A Sourcebook Of Clinical Research.* 1988

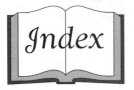

Index

A

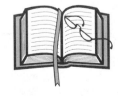

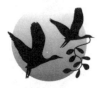

HEALTHY HEALING PUBLICATIONS
Books

HEALTHY HEALING - *Tenth Edition, A Guide to Self Healing for Everyone* - by Dr. Linda Rector Page, N.D., Ph.D. - A 500 page alternative healing reference used by professors, students, health care professionals and private individuals. $28.95 ISBN# 1-884334-85-7

HOW TO BE YOUR OWN HERBAL PHARMACIST - *Herbal Traditions, Expert Formulations* - by Dr. Linda Rector Page, N.D., Ph.D. A complete reference guide for herbal formulations and preparations. $18.95-ISBN# 1-884334-77-6

COOKING FOR HEALTHY HEALING - *Diets and Recipes for Alternative Healing* - by Dr. Linda Rector Page, N.D., Ph.D. - Over 900 recipes and 33 separate diet and healing programs. $29.95-ISBN# 1-884334-56-3

PARTY LIGHTS - *Healthy Party Foods & Earthwise Entertaining* - by Dr. Linda Rector Page. N.D., Ph.D., and Doug Vanderberg - A party reference book with over 70 parties and more than 500 original recipes you can prepare at home. $19.95 ISBN# 1-884334-53-9

THE BODY SMART SYSTEM - *The Complete Guide to Cleansing & Rejuvenation* - by Helene Silver - A complete 21 day regimen and guide that includes diet, relaxation techniques, massage and bath, exercise programs and recipes. $19.95 ISBN# 1-884334-60-1

THE HEALTHY HEALING LIBRARY SERIES - by Dr. Linda Rector Page, N.D., Ph.D. - $3.50 each. ISBN#'s - 1884334 -

30-X **RENEWING MALE HEALTH & ENERGY**

49-0 **DETOXIFICATION & BODY CLEANSING**

32-6 **THE ENERGY CRUNCH & YOU**

34-2 **BOOSTING IMMUNITY WITH POWER PLANTS**

35-0 **ALLERGY CONTROL & MANAGEMENT**

47-4 **COLDS, FLU & YOU** - Building Optimum Immunity

13-X **REVEALING THE SECRETS OF ANTI-AGING**

29-6 **FIGHTING INFECTIONS WITH HERBS**

33-4 **STRESS MANAGEMENT, DEPRESSION & OVERCOMING ADDICTIONS**

37-7 **A FIGHTING CHANCE FOR WEIGHT LOSS & CELLULITE CONTROL**

27-X **DO YOU WANT TO HAVE A BABY?**

14-8 **FATIGUE SYDROMES & IMMUNE DISORDERS** - New - 46 Page Book - $3.95

New Expanded 48 Page Format:

64-4 **RENEWING FEMALE BALANCE** - $4.50

65-2 **MENOPAUSE & OSTEOPOROSIS** - $4.50 36-9 **CANCER** - $4.50

11-97

Continental U.S. shipping info: $4.50 each for books, .75 each for booklets. FREE SHIPPING FOR ORDERS OVER $75.00!

NAME_____ ADDRESS_____

CITY_____ STATE_____ ZIP_____ PHONE_____

☐ Check(Make payable to Healthy Healing) ☐ Visa   ☐ Mastercard   ☐ American Express   ☐ Discover

CARD #_____ EXP. DATE_____ SIGNATURE_____

QTY.	BOOK	PRICE	SHIPPING	TOTAL
	CA Residents add 7.25% tax			

Mail to: Healthy Healing Publications, P.O. Box 436, Carmel Valley, CA 93924.
Or, fax your order to: 408-659-4044. Or, Call 1-800-289-9222.
Or order online @ healthyhealing.com.

TOTAL _____

Natural Health Questions? Get help. Have a private consultation with a professional. Call 1-900-903-5885 M-F, 9 to 5 Pacific Time

$2.29 per minute - ave. call 5 min. - must be 18

Take Control and Stay Informed
With Monthly Updates From Dr. Page!

Dear Reader:

This book, *Healthy Healing, A Guide to Self Healing For Everyone*, is truly a valuable resource. I know you will refer to it for years to come. You are joining the hundreds of thousands, including top experts both in the natural health industry and the field of conventional medicine, who regard this book as their "health bible."

New information floods into my research department each and every day. And, more and more people are asking me to address controversial issues that occur on a daily basis. I hear a lot of success stories from my readers, and I get a lot of questions. Like DHEA: Are there any drawbacks to taking DHEA? Is DHEA natural?

That is why I've started my own newsletter, **THE NATURAL HEALING REPORT.** This newsletter will be packed full of the latest and most exciting health care topics for men, women, teens, seniors, children and even pets! Plus, I'll include a series of natural product reviews (a mini-consumer report), special healing diets with recipes, health secrets and tips, the latest studies on natural therapies and treatments, a personal question and answer section, and much, much more every month!

I've gathered a very special group of expert professionals, medical doctors, naturopathic doctors, chiropractors, licensed acupuncturists, homeopaths, doctors of Oriental medicine, and Ph.Ds, whose opinions I value and trust to serve on my board of advisors. I want you to have the best possible health choices for yourself and your loved ones.

THE NATURAL HEALING REPORT is **one of the only national newsletters from an alternative medicine healer**. I believe this is the newsletter you have been waiting for. Remember, in order for us to take more responsibility for our health choices, we all need to be better informed. Take control and stay informed!

Stay Well!

Linda Page

Special Offer!

As part of the Healthy Healing "family," you can get **THE NATURAL HEALING REPORT** at the special discount rate of $48.95 for a one year subscription (it's regularly $79.95). Simply complete the reply card and send it in!

Yes! I want to receive monthly updates from Dr. Page.
Please sign me up for:

____2 years $89.95 (regularly $159.90). As part of the Healthy Healing "family," I receive a $69.95 discount.

____1 year $48.95 - a 39% discount off the regular rate

Risk Free! If you are not fully satisfied with your first issue of **THE NATURAL HEALING REPORT**, simply write cancel on your invoice and return it to us - no questions asked.

Name_____

Address_____

City, State, Zip_____

For faster service, call Howard at **800-289-9222.** Or, fax him at 561-625-6685. (Our fax never sleeps.)

THE NATURAL HEALING REPORT, PO Box 109665, Palm Beach Gardens, FL 33410

THE NATURAL HEALING REPORT
PO BOX 109665
PALM BEACH GARDENS, FL   33410-9835